Postgraduate
Gynecology

Postgraduate Gynecology

Joydeb Roychowdhury

MBBS, MD, FICOG, FICMCH

Professor and Head
Department of Obstetrics and Gynecology
ESI–Postgraduate Institute of Medical Sciences and Research
and ESIC Medical College
Joka, Kolkata, WB

Ex-Associate Professor
NRS Medical College
Kolkata

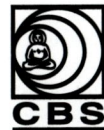

CBS Publishers & Distributors Pvt Ltd

New Delhi • Bengaluru • Chennai • Kochi • Kolkata • Mumbai
Hyderabad • Jharkhand • Nagpur • Patna • Pune • Uttarakhand

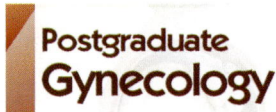

Postgraduate
Gynecology

ISBN: 978-93-86310-71-2

First Edition 2017

Published by Satish Kumar Jain and Produced by Varun Jain for
CBS Publishers & Distributors Pvt Ltd
4819/XI Prahlad Street, 24 Ansari Road, Daryaganj, New Delhi 110 002, India.
Ph: 23289259, 23266861, 23266867   Fax: 011-23243014   Website: www.cbspd.com
e-mail: delhi@cbspd.com; cbspubs@airtelmail.in.
Corporate Office: 204 FIE, Industrial Area, Patparganj, Delhi 110 092, India
Ph: 4934 4934   Fax: 4934 4935   e-mail: publishing@cbspd.com; publicity@cbspd.com

Branches

- **Bengaluru:** Seema House 2975, 17th Cross, K.R. Road,
  Banasankari 2nd Stage, Bengaluru 560 070, Karnataka, India
  Ph: +91-80-26771678/79   Fax: +91-80-26771680   e-mail: bangalore@cbspd.com
- **Chennai:** 7, Subbaraya Street, Shenoy Nagar, Chennai 600 030, Tamil Nadu, India
  Ph: +91-44-26260666, 26208620   Fax: +91-44-42032115   e-mail: chennai@cbspd.com
- **Kochi:** Ashana House, No. 39/1904, AM Thomas Road, Valanjambalam, Ernakulam 682 016, Kochi, Kerala, India
  Ph: +91-484-4059061-65   Fax: +91-484-4059065   e-mail: kochi@cbspd.com
- **Kolkata:** No. 6/B, Ground Floor, Rameswar Shaw Road, Kolkata-700014 (West Bengal), India
  Ph: +91-33-2289-1126, 2289-1127, 2289-1128   e-mail: kolkata@cbspd.com
- **Mumbai:** 83-C, Dr E Moses Road, Worli, Mumbai-400018, Maharashtra, India
  Ph: +91-22-24902340/41   Fax: +91-22-24902342   e-mail: mumbai@cbspd.com

Representatives

- **Hyderabad** 0-9885175004
- **Jharkhand** 0-9811541605
- **Nagpur** 0-9021734563
- **Patna** 0-9334159340
- **Pune** 0-9623451994
- **Uttrakhand** 0-9716462459

Printed at International Print-o-Pac Limited, Noida, U.P., India

to
My Medical Students
and
My Family

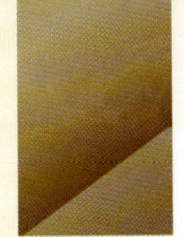
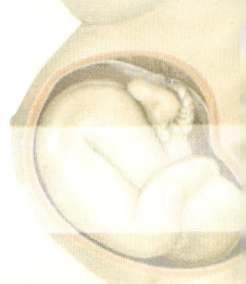

Preface

This is my first endeavour to write a textbook on gynecology for students of obstetrics and gynecology. I have always desired to publish a book in which all possible information of recent updates can be compiled to serve maximum benefits to my postgraduate and aspiring undergraduate students who want to build their careers in obstetrics and gynecology.

I have authored this book on the basis of recent knowledge, updates and national and international guidelines along with my teaching experience for the last twenty years, to make the information as updated as possible.

I am aware of the fact that due to fast and rapid advancement in medical sciences, the information laid down in the book at 2017 will become old as the year advances. I can assure my readers that any new and relevant advancement will be added in the next edition.

I have tried to put down the important information in a format which will be best suited for the students to make them prepared for their examinations. RCOG, FOGSI guidelines are added in many chapters for their ready reference. Its elegant printing, pictures and overall getup will, I believe, make the book exciting for them to read and understand.

I sincerely pay tribute to my teachers through this small endeavour, who constantly encouraged me to adopt this initiative to help students. I also cannot forget my students who have been my constant source of encouragement in publishing this book which they insisted on for long.

Finally, the publisher deserves my heartfelt thanks and congratulations for taking this bold initiative, and for guiding me to perform this unique and difficult task quite easily and efficiently.

Joydeb Roychowdhury

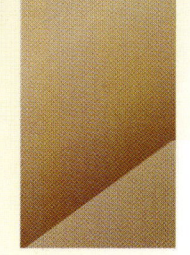

Acknowledgments

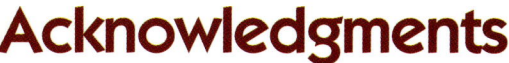

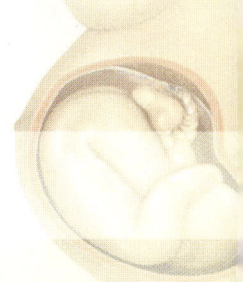

I express my sincere gratitude to all my colleagues and friends for their constant moral support in this academic endeavour. I am also indebted to all my senior residents at NRS Medical College and ESI-PGIMSR, Joka who have shared with me lot of scientific knowledge and information. I like to congratulate my PG students in ESIC Medical College, Kolkata who contributed many of the photographs in this book.

I am also grateful to all my patients and students who are always the best form of aspiration for my academic endeavour. I am equally grateful to my wife and daughters who have helped me day and night and shared with me all the hardship required to give the book a final shape.

Finally I acknowledge the best efforts by my typist Mr. Subrata Roy and composer and designer–CBS Publishers for the herculean task they have rendered for publication of this book in such an exciting design.

Finally, I seek blessings from the almighty God and all my well-wishers to make this book successful and worthwhile for my students.

Joydeb Roychowdhury

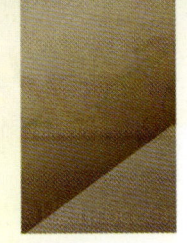

Contents

Anatomy of Female Reproductive System

1

The female reproductive organs can be subdivided into the internal and external genitalia. The internal genitalia are those organs that are within the true pelvis. These include the vagina, uterus, cervix, uterine tubes or fallopian tubes, and ovaries. The external genitalia lie outside the true pelvis. These include the perineum, mons pubis, clitoris, urethral (urinary) meatus, labia majora and minora, vestibule, greater vestibular (Bartholin) glands, Skene's glands, and periurethral area.

External Genitalia

The vulva, also known as the pudendum, is a term used to describe those external organs that may be visible in the perineal area. The boundaries include the mons pubis anteriorly, the rectum posteriorly, and the genitocrural folds laterally (Fig. 1.1).

Mons Pubis

The mons pubis is the rounded portion of the vulva where sexual hair development occurs at the time of puberty. This area may be described as directly anterosuperior to the pubic symphysis.

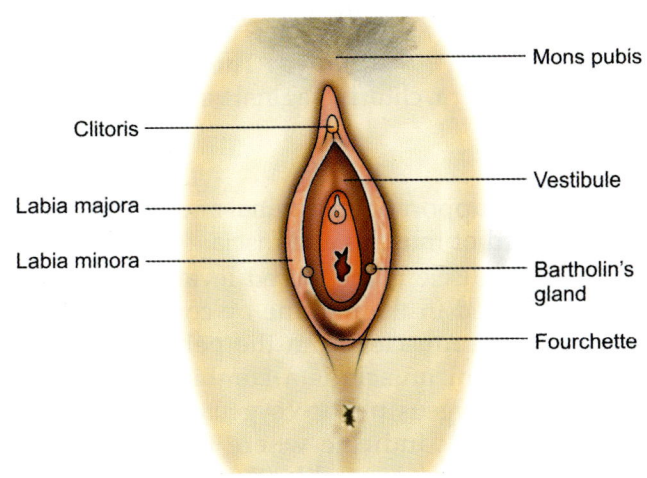

Fig. 1.1: External genitalia

Labels: Mons pubis, Clitoris, Vestibule, Labia majora, Labia minora, Bartholin's gland, Fourchette

Labia

The **labia majora** are two large, longitudinal folds of adipose and fibrous tissues. They vary in size and distribution from female to female, and the size is dependent upon adipose content. They extend from the mons anteriorly to the perineal body posteriorly. Posteriorly the majora do not join, they are separated by a depression known as the posterior commissure. The labia majora have hair follicles.

The **labia minora**, also known as nymphae, are two small cutaneous folds that are found between the labia majora and the introitus or vaginal vestibule. The medial part joins anteriorly in the midline behind the clitoris which is known as the frenulum of the clitoris. The lateral part joins anteriorly in the midline in front of the clitoris which is known as the clitoral hood or prepuce. Posteriorly, both folds join at the midline to form the fourchette (Fig. 1.2).

Hymen

The hymen is a thin membrane found at the entrance to the vaginal orifice. Often, this membrane is perforated before the onset of menstruation, allowing flow of menses. The hymen varies greatly in shape (Fig. 1.3).

Clitoris

The clitoris is an erectile structure found beneath the anterior joining of the labia minora. Its width in an adult female is approximately 1 cm, with an average length of 1.5–2.0 cm. The clitoris is made up of 2 crura, which attach to the periosteum of the ischiopubic rami. It is a very sensitive erectile structure, analogous to the male penis. It is innervated by the dorsal nerve of the clitoris, a terminal branch of the pudendal nerve.

Vestibule and Urethra

Between the clitoris and the vaginal opening is a triangular area known as the vestibule, which extends

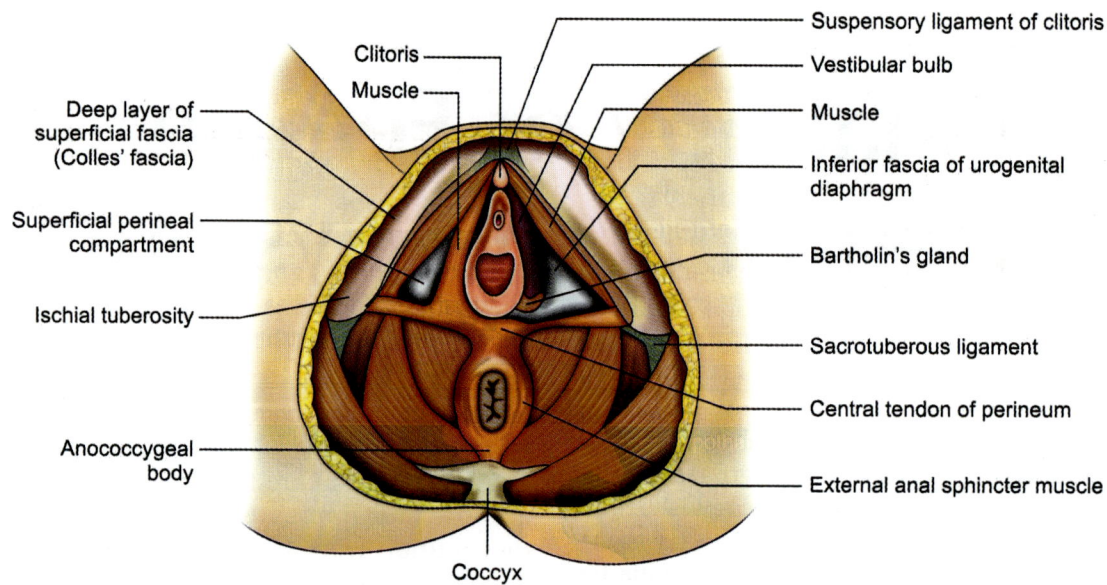

Fig. 1.2: Deeper view of external structures

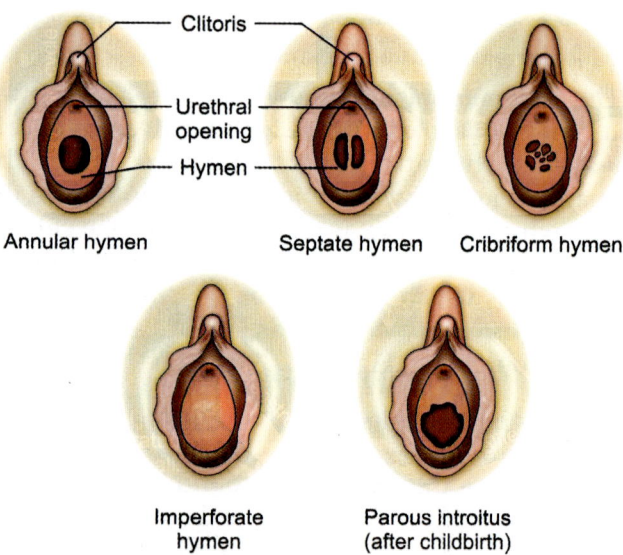

Fig. 1.3: Various types of hymens

to the posterior fourchette. The vestibule is where the urethral meatus is found, approximately 1 cm anterior to the vaginal orifice and it also gives rise to the opening of the Skene's glands bilaterally. The urethra is composed of membranous connective tissue and links the urinary bladder to the vestibule externally. A female urethra ranges in length from 3.5 to 4.0 cm.

Skene and Bartholin Glands

The Skene's glands secrete lubrication at the opening of the urethra. The greater vestibular (Bartholin) glands are also responsible for secreting lubrication to the vagina, with openings just outside the hymen, bilaterally, at the posterior aspect of the vagina. Each gland is small, similar

to a kidney bean in shape. **The G-spot** (Gräfenberg spot) is considered to be an area around the urethra in the anterior wall of the vagina. Stimulation of the G-spot acts directly on the Skene's glands to lubricate vagina.

Greater Vestibule Gland

This is homologous to the Cowper's gland of the male. It produces mucus as a lubricant.

Vestibular Bulbs

The vestibular bulbs are to masses of erectile tissue that lie deep to the bulbocavernosus muscles bilaterally.

Urogenital triangle: Its base is the line between ischial tuberosities and apex is the pubic symphysis.

Anal triangle: Its base is the line between ischial tuberosities and apex is the coccyx.

Contents of urogenital triangle: The vulva, with labia majora and minora, clitoris, vaginal vault and vestibule.

Pelvic Floor

This helps in support of abdominal and pelvic viscera. It is composed of muscles and fascia.

The main muscle is the paired levator ani muscles which are joined in the midline by connective tissue. The levator ani muscles form the pelvic diaphragm. Each levator ani muscle is a combination of three muscles: Iliococcygeus, pubococcygeus and puborectalis. These names just indicate where the fibres attach, otherwise they work in combination. The other muscle of the pelvic diaphragm is the coccygeus muscle.

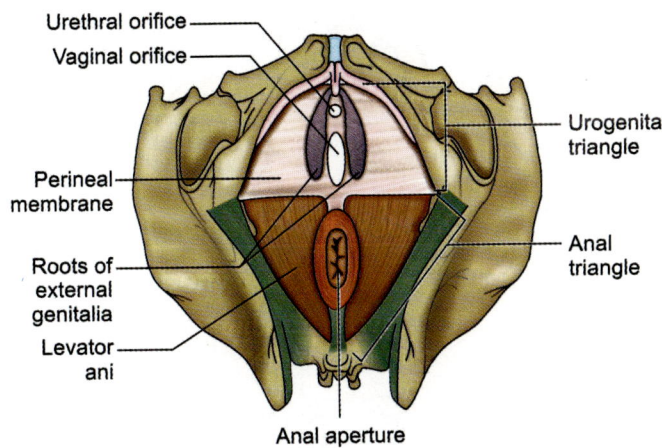

Urethral orifice

Vaginal orifice

Perineal membrane

Roots of external genitalia

Levator ani

Urogenital triangle

Anal triangle

Anal aperture

Fig. 1.4: Perineum

There are three apertures in the pelvic floor (two in males). From front to back, there is the urethra, vagina and then the rectum. All three apertures are enclosed by the puborectalis part of the levator ani muscle.

The shape of the diaphragm is U-shape anteriorly due to the urogenital system. The anterior portion is supported by the perineal membrane and muscles of the deep perineal pouch. Vagina and urethra pass through the perineal membrane. The anal canal passes posteriorly through the pelvic diaphragm.

There are two triangles in the perineum—urogenital and anal. The urogenital triangle is covered by the perineal membrane, whereas the anal triangle is not (Fig. 1.4).

Internal Genital Organs

Vagina

The vagina is a muscular, hollow tube that extends from the vaginal opening to the cervix of the uterus. It is situated between the urinary bladder and the rectum. It is about three to five inches long in an adult woman. The muscular wall allows the vagina to expand and contract. The muscular walls are lined with mucous membranes of stratified squamous epithelium which keep it protected and moist. A thin sheet of tissue with one or more holes in it, called the hymen, partially covers the opening of the vagina.

The vagina is composed of three layers. The first layer is made up of a stratified squamous non-keratinized epithelium and is an underlying lamina propria of connective tissue (a layer of connective tissue that is highly vascular under the base area lining the epithelium). This layer forms the folds or rugae and facilitates the vagina's ability to expand large enough for child birth. The rugae are a series of ridges produced by folding of the wall of the outer third of the vagina;

they are transverse epithelial ridges and their function is to provide the vagina with increased surface area for extension and stretching. The second layer is the muscular layer, which is composed of smooth muscle fibers and situated longitudinally and circularly. The third layer is the adventitia, which is a dense connective tissue that blends with the fascia surrounding the area.

Cervix

The cervix (from Latin "neck") is the lower, narrow portion of the uterus where it joins with the top end of the vagina. The location where they meet forms an almost 90° angle (angle of version). It is cylindrical or conical in shape and protrudes through the upper anterior vaginal wall.

During menstruation, the cervix stretches open slightly to allow the endometrium to be shed. This stretching is believed to be part of the cramping pain that many women experience. The portion projecting into the vagina is referred to as the portio vaginalis or exocervix. On an average, the exocervix is 3 cm long and two and a half cm wide. It has a convex, elliptical surface and is divided into anterior and posterior lips. In women who have not had a vaginal birth, the external os appears as a small, circular opening. In women who have had a vaginal birth, the exocervix appears bulkier and the external os appears wider, more slit-like and gaping. The endocervical canal varies widely in length and width and is flattened anterior to posterior, the endocervical canal measures 7 to 8 mm at its widest in reproductive-aged women. The endocervical canal terminates at the internal os which opens into the uterine cavity. During childbirth, contractions of the uterus will dilate the cervix up to 10 cm in diameter to allow the child to pass through. During orgasm, the cervix convulses and the external os dilates.

Uterus

The uterus is shaped like an upside-down pear, with a thick lining and muscular walls. Located near the floor of the pelvic cavity, it is hollow to allow a blastocyte, or fertilized egg, to implant and grow. It also allows for the inner lining of the uterus to build up until a fertilized egg is implanted, or it is sloughed off during menses (Fig. 1.5).

The uterus contains some of the strongest muscles in the female body. These muscles are able to expand and contract to accommodate a growing fetus and then help push the baby out during labor. These muscles also contract rhythmically during an orgasm in a wave-like action. It is presumed to help push or guide the

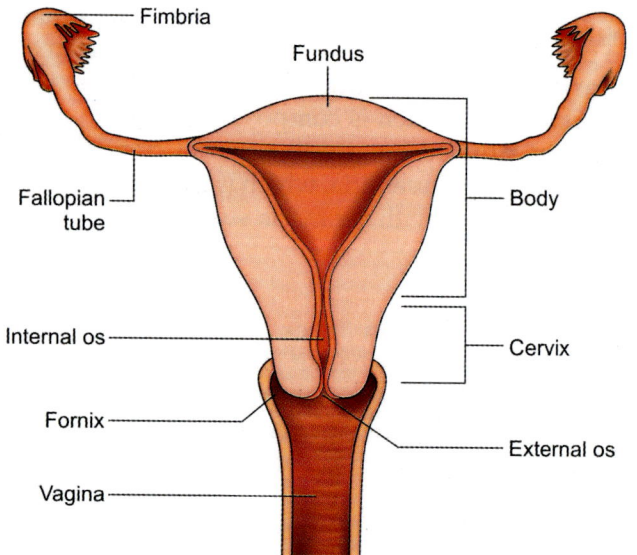

Fig. 1.5: Uterus

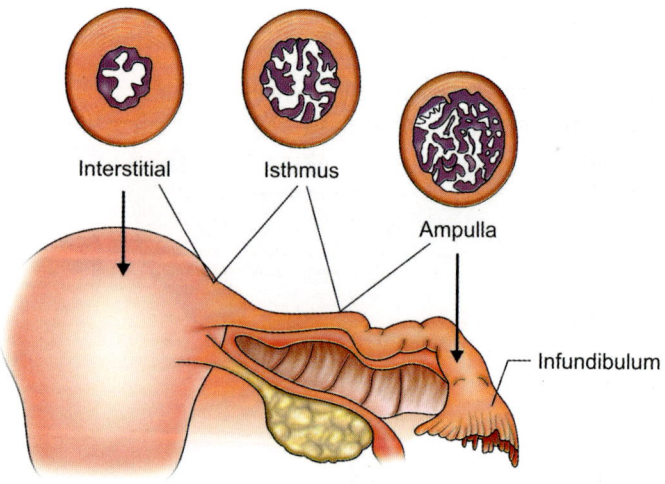

Fig. 1.6: Fallopian tubes

sperm up the uterus to the fallopian tubes where fertilization may be possible.

The uterus is only about 3 inches long and two inches wide, but during pregnancy it changes rapidly and dramatically.

Uterus has a rounded superior end—fundus. The uterine cavity is a narrow slit in the lateral view and triangular in the anterior view. At the inferior end is the cervix. The uterus is usually anteflexed (125°) on the cervix and is anteverted (90°) on the vagina. The cervix projects into the vagina and as a result a gutter is formed known as the fornix. The canal in the cervix has two openings—the external os into the vagina and an internal os into the uterine cavity.

Fallopian Tubes

At the upper corners of the uterus are the fallopian tubes. They are placed one on each side of the uterus attached to cornu of the uterus and connects to the ovary on the same side. They are positioned between the ligament of the ovary posteriorly and round ligament anteriorly (Fig. 1.6).

The fallopian tubes are about 4 inches (10 cm) long. At the other end of each uterine tube is a fringed area that looks like a funnel. This fringed area, called the infundibulum, lies close to the ovary, but is not attached. Starting from the uterus and proceeding outward, these are the:

- Interstitial segment—extends from the uterine cavity through the uterine muscle (1.25 cm)
- Isthmic segment—narrow muscular portion adjacent to the uterus (3 cm)

- Ampullary segment—wider and longer middle part of the tube (5 cm)
- Infundibular segment—funnel-shaped segment next to the fimbrial end (1.25 cm)
- Fimbrial segment—wide opening at the end of the tube facing the ovary.

The ovaries generally alternately release an egg every month. When an ovary ovulate, or release an egg, it is swept into the lumen of the uterine tube by the fimbriae. Once the egg is in the uterine tube, ciliated epithelium in the tube helps push it down the narrow passageway toward the uterus. The oocyte, or developing egg cell, takes four to five days to travel down the length of the uterine tube. Fertilization most often occurs in the ampullary segment of the fallopian tube. After fertilization occurs, the zygote, or fertilized egg, continues down to the uterus and implants itself in the uterine wall where it will grow and develop until birth. If a zygote does not move down to the uterus and implants itself in the uterine tube, it is called a ectopic or tubal pregnancy.

Ovaries

The ovaries are paired, oval organs located within the pelvic cavity lateral to the uterus. In an adult, ovaries are slightly larger than an almond about 2 to 3 cm long, 2 cm wide, and 1 to 1.5 cm thick. Their size usually varies during each menstrual cycle as well as during pregnancy.

The ovaries are anchored within the pelvic cavity by special "cords" and sheets of tissue. A double fold of peritonuem called the mesovarium, attaches to each ovary at its hilum. The hilum is the anterior surface of the ovary where blood vessels and nerves enter the ovary.

The mesovarium secures each ovary to a broad ligament, which is a drape of peritoneum that hangs over the uterus. Each ovary is anchored to the posterior aspect of the broad ligament by an ovarian ligament.

A suspensory ligament attaches to the lateral edge of each ovary and projects superolaterally to the pelvic wall. The ovarian blood vessels and nerves are housed within each suspensory ligament, and they join the ovary at its hilum.

Smooth muscle fibers within both the mesovarium and the suspensory ligaments contract at the time of ovulation to bring the ovaries into close proximity with the uterine tube openings. Each ovary is supplied by an ovarian vein and artery. The ovarian arteries are branches that come directly off the aorta immediately inferior to the renal vessel. The ovarian veins exit the ovary and drain into either the inferior cava (right) or one of the renal veins (left).

Traveling with the ovarian artery and vein are autonomic nerves. Sympathetic axons come from the T10 segments of the spinal cord whereas para-sympathetic axons come from 10th cranial nerve.

Arterial Supply to Pelvis (Table 1.1 and Fig. 1.7)

Internal iliac artery is the major artery feeding the pelvis. It arises from and the common iliac at L5–S1 level and passes anteromedial to the sacroiliac joint into the pelvic inlet where it bifurcates into an anterior and posterior trunk.

Posterior Trunk

It supplies the lower posterior abdominal wall, posterior pelvic wall and the gluteal region. Branches are:

- *Iliolumbar artery:* This turns back up and out of the pelvic cavity to supply the posterior abdominal wall (lumbar) and iliac fossa (iliac).

- *Lateral sacral arteries:* Two from each side to supply areas of the sacrum and posterior pelvic wall.

- *Superior gluteal artery:* Terminal continuation of the posterior trunk and is the largest branch. It leaves the pelvic cavity through the greater sciatic foramen to supply the gluteal region.

Anterior Trunk

Supplies the pelvic viscera, perineum, gluteal region and adductor region of the thigh as well as placenta and fetus in pregnancy. Branches in order are:

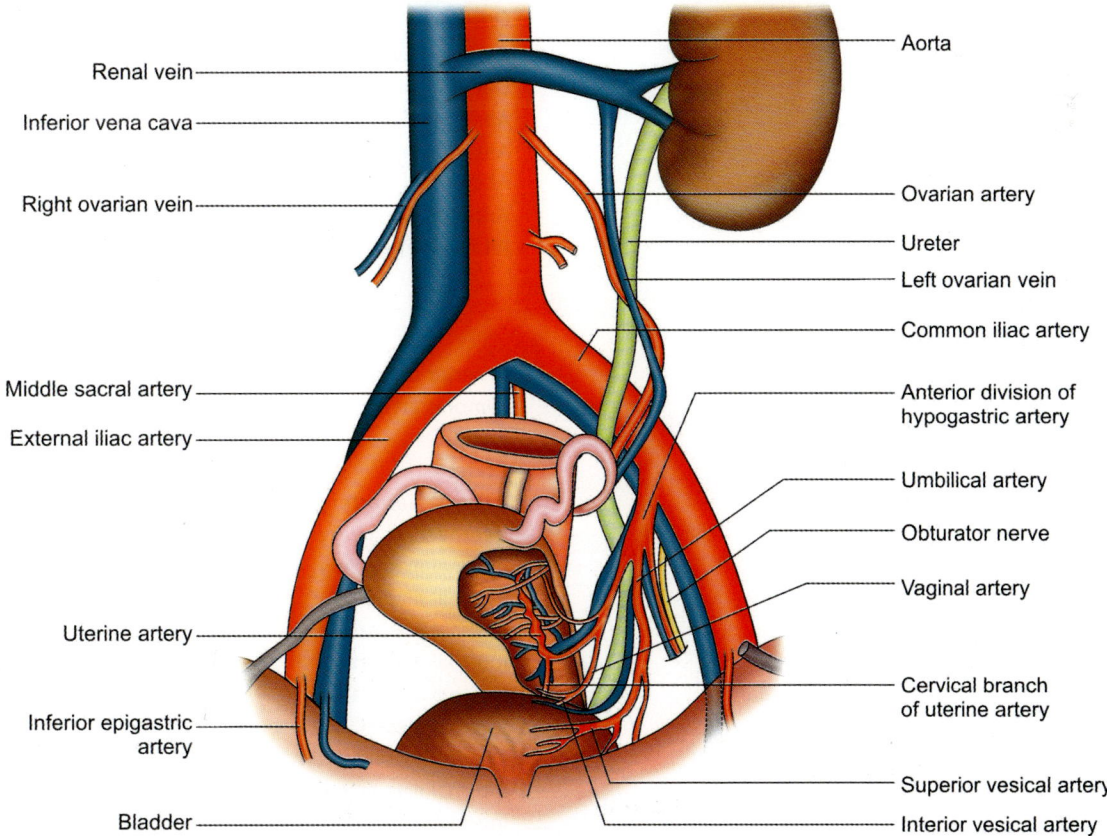

Fig. 1.7: Arterial supply to pelvis

Umbilical artery: This gives rise to the **superior vesical artery** which supplies the superior region of the bladder and distal parts of the ureter. The umbilical artery carries blood from fetus to placenta and is large (there are two arteries, one on each side). After birth, the umbilical arteries fibrose and become the medial umbilical ligaments. It also leaves a fold in the peritoneum—medial umbilical fold.

Inferior vesical artery: This occurs in men only, in females it is the **vaginal artery**. In men, it supplies inferior region of bladder, ureter, seminal vesicle and prostate. In females, the vaginal artery supplies the vagina and surrounding parts of the bladder and rectum.

Middle rectal artery: Supplies the rectum and anastomoses with superior rectal (from inferior mesenteric) and inferior rectal (which is the branch of internal pudendal) arteries.

Obturator artery: Leaves pelvic cavity through obturator canal supplying adductor region of thigh.

Internal pudendal artery: Leaves pelvic cavity through greater sciatic foramen but re-enters through the lesser sciatic foramen with the pudendal nerve. It supplies the perineum region as well as erectile tissues of penis and clitoris. It also gives rise to **inferior rectal** artery.

Inferior gluteal artery: Large terminal branch of anterior trunk. Supplies lower gluteal and hip region.

Uterine artery: It travels along the root of the broad ligament and crosses above and in front of the ureter approximately 2 cm anteromedially from the cervix. It reaches the lateral fornices and then supplies the cervix. From here, it travels tortuously along the lateral margin of the uterus and then the fallopian tubes. Here it anastomoses with the ovarian artery. Uterine artery supplies most of the uterus and cervix. One of its branches anastomoses with the vaginal artery to produce azygos artery of vagina. It enlarges during pregnancy.

Ovarian artery: This originates from the abdominal aorta and enters the pelvic inlet to supply the ovaries. It anastomoses with the uterine arteries. It is found traveling in the suspensory ligament of the ovary. The reason for a different supply is due to the descent of ovaries from the abdomen during development.

Table 1.1: Artery supply of pelvic organs		
Organ	*Artery*	*Origin*
Uterus	Uterine	Anterior division of internal iliac artery
	Ovarian	Direct branch from abdominal aorta
Ovary	Ovarian	Abdominal aorta
	Uterine	Anterior division of internal iliac artery
Fallopian tube	Ovarian	Abdominal aorta
	Uterine	Anterior division of internal iliac artery
Vagina	Vaginal	All from anterior division of internal iliac artery
	Uterine	
	Internal pudendal	
	Middle rectal	
Vulva	Internal pudendal	Anterior division of internal iliac artery
	External pudendal	Femoral artery
Ureter	Renal	Aorta
	Ovarian	Aorta
	Uterine	Internal iliac artery
	Superior vesical	Internal iliac artery
	Inferior vesical	Internal iliac artery
Bladder	Superior vesical	Internal iliac artery
	Inferior vesical	Internal iliac artery
Urethra	Interior vesical	Internal iliac artery
	Internal pudendal	Internal iliac artery
Sigmoid colon	Left colic	Interior mesenteric artery
Rectum	Superior rectal	Inferior mesenteric artery
	Middle rectal	Internal iliac artery
	Inferior rectal	Internal pudendal (branch of anterior division of internal iliac) artery

Median sacral artery: Descends from the bifurcation of the aorta in the midline from L4 to the coccyx. It gives rise to last pair of lumbar arteries and anastomoses with lateral sacral and iliolumbar artery.

Veins

Veins follow arteries except for umbilical and iliolumbar. The other veins drain into the internal iliac veins. Drainage from the pelvic cavity is through plexuses of veins and the name given depends on the region. Internal and external rectal plexuses can give rise to hemorrhoids if enlarged. Other veins are:

Deep dorsal vein: It is a single vein that drains the penis and clitoris. It does not follow the internal pudendal artery. Instead it drains into the prostatic plexus in males and vesical plexus in females.

Umbilical vein is present only in the fetus. It travels from the umbilicus to the liver. It travels alongside the falciform ligament to the liver and then splits into two branches. A larger branch joins the portal vein. The smaller branch ductus venosus joins the IVC. After birth, the umbilical vein obliterates to become the round ligament of the liver (or the ligamentum teres). This is continuous with the ligamentum venosum which splits the liver into left and right lobes.

Lymphatics

Main drainage is either through nodes associated with internal iliac artery or external iliac artery.

Lymph drainage from the ovaries and parts of the uterus and fallopian tubes leave the pelvic cavity with the ovarian artery and drain in lateral aortic and pre-aortic nodes.

Important Nerves of Pelvis and Perineum (Fig. 1.8)

Pudendal nerve: Comes from the sacral plexus (S2–S4)

Motor nerve
- Skeletal muscles in the perineum
- External urethral sphincter and external anal sphincter
- Levator ani

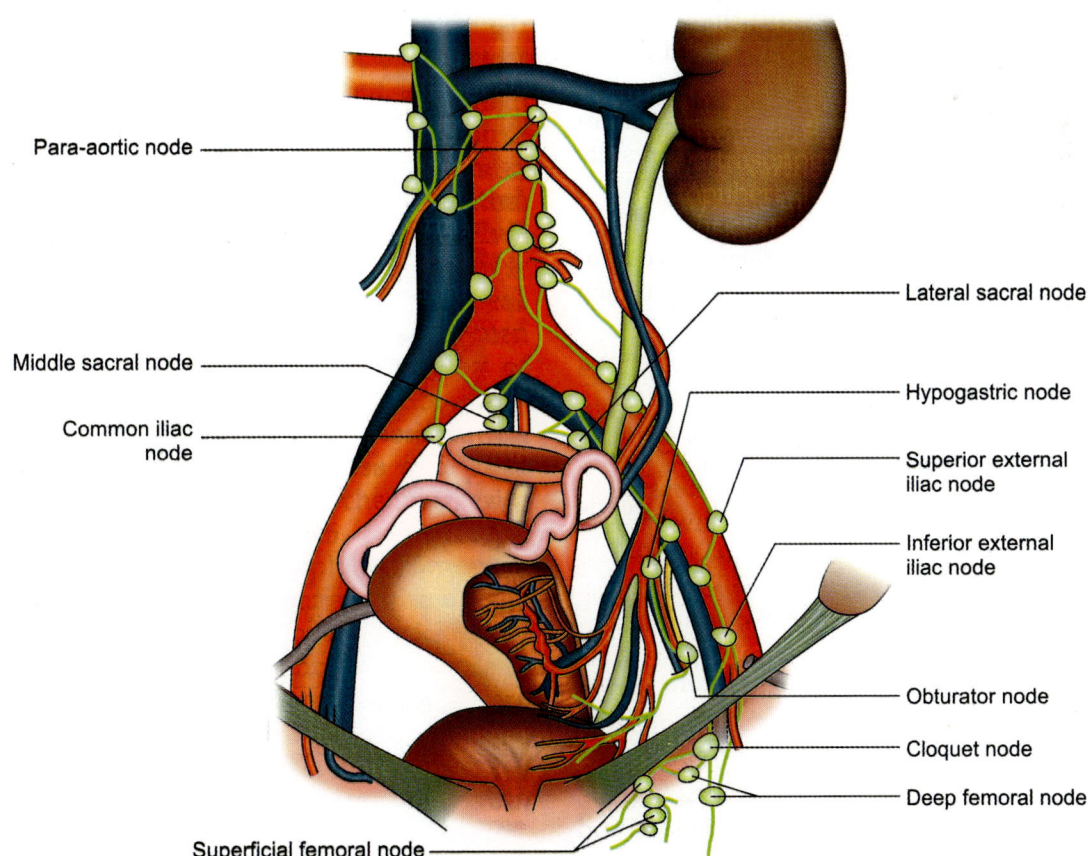

Fig. 1.8: Lymph nodes distribution from pelvis

Sensory nerve

- To supply skin of the perineum, penis and clitoris.

  A pudendal block helps relieve pain during childbirth.

Apart from the pudendal nerve, there are fibers that go straight from the S4 spinal nerve to the levator ani, coccygeus and external anal sphincter as well as sensory function to the patch of skin between the anus and coccyx.

There is also the anococcygeal nerve from the coccygeal plexus (S4 to coccyx) which has sensory function to the perianal area.

The organs receive parasympathetic and sympathetic stimulation from the inferior hypogastric plexus. This is formed by fibres from the hypogastric nerve (which comes from the superior hypogastric plexus). The hypogastric nerve carries sympathetic fibers from the lumbar splanchnic nerves. The hypogastric nerve forms the inferior hypogastric plexus by joining the sacral splanchnic nerves (sympathetic) and the pelvic splanchnic nerves (parasympathetic).

The inferior hypogastric plexus is located on either side of the rectum and vagina in females (rectum in males). The inferior hypogastric plexus gives rise to smaller plexuses—rectal, uterovaginal, prostatic, vesical. The terminal branches of the inferior hypogastric plexus penetrate the deep perineal pouch and innervate erectile tissues in the penis or clitoris.

Sympathetic stimulation of the organs (from hypogastric nerve and sacral splanchnic nerves) results in:

- Vasoconstriction
- Smooth muscle contraction of internal urethral sphincter in men and internal anal sphincter in men and women.
- Smooth muscle contraction of the reproductive tract and accessory glands of reproductive system.
- Secretion from epididymis and other glands to urethra to form semen during ejaculation.

Parasympathetic stimulation of organs (from pelvic splanchnic nerves) causes:

- Vasodilatation
- Bladder contraction (detrusor muscle)
- Stimulate erection
- Communicate with enteric nervous system in the inferior mesenteric plexus.

Breast

Mammary glands are composed of glandular tissue and a variable amount of fat. They have a complex secretory product called breast milk. Breast milk travels through a passageway called the lactiferous duct, which travels from the alveoli to the nipple. The nipple is a centrally located projection on the breast comprised partly of erectile tissue. The areola is the darkened region of the breast that surrounds the nipple. An areola may vary in color depending on whether or not a woman has given birth.

The breast overlies the pectoralis major muscle between the second and sixth ribs as well as the uppermost portion of the rectus abdominis muscle inferomedially. The gland is anchored to the pectoralis major fascia by the suspensory ligaments first described by Astley Cooper in 1840. These ligaments run throughout the breast tissue parenchyma from the deep fascia beneath the breast and attach to the dermis of the skin. Since they are not taut, they allow for the natural motion of the breast. These ligaments relax with age and time, eventually resulting in breast ptosis. The lower pole of the breast is fuller than the upper pole. The tail of Spence extends obliquely up into the medial wall of the axilla (Fig. 1.9).

The nipple should lie above the inframammary crease and is usually level with the fourth rib and just lateral to the midclavicular line. The average nipple-to-sternal notch measurement in a young well-developed breast is 21–22 cm; an equilateral triangle formed between the nipples and sternal notch measures an average of 21 cm per side.

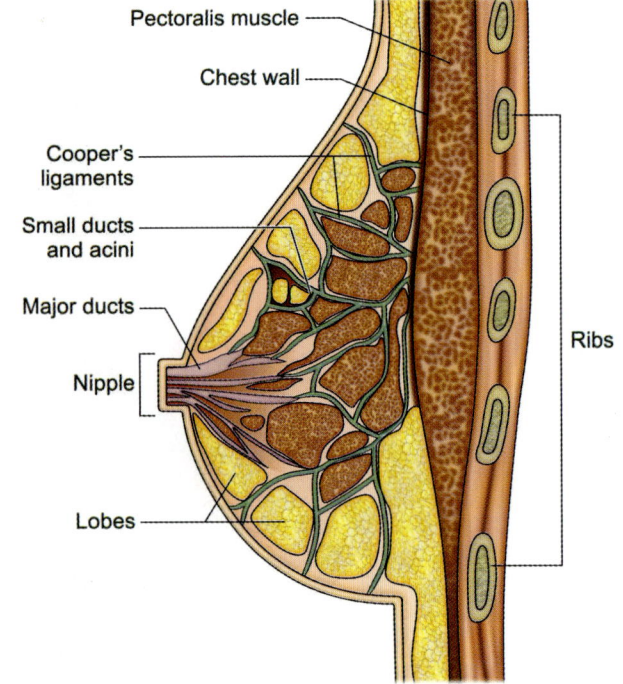

Fig. 1.9: Breast

The blood supply to the breast skin depends on the subdermal plexus, which is in communication with deeper underlying vessels supplying the breast parenchyma. The blood supply is derived from the following:

- The internal mammary perforators (most notably the second to fifth perforators)
- The thoracoacromial artery
- The vessels to serratus anterior
- The lateral thoracic artery
- The terminal branches of the third to eighth intercostal perforators

The superomedial perforator supply from the internal mammary vessels is particularly robust and accounts for some 60% of the total breast blood supply.

Sensory innervation of the breast is dermatomal in nature. It is mainly derived from the anterolateral and anteromedial branches of thoracic intercostal nerves T3–T5. Supraclavicular nerves from the lower fibers of the cervical plexus also provide innervation to the upper and lateral portions of the breast to the nipple derives largely from the lateral cutaneous branch of T4.

Anatomy of Hypothalamus and Pituitary Glands

2

The hypothalamus is a region of the brain composed of many small nuclei with diverse functions. Located above the midbrain and below the thalamus, the hypothalamus makes up the ventral diencephalon. The diencephalon is an embryologic region of the vertebrate neural tube that gives rise to posterior forebrain structures. By synthesizing and secreting neuro-hormones, the nuclei of the hypothalamus act as a conduit between the nervous and endocrine systems via the pituitary gland (hypophysis), regulating homeostatic functions such as hunger, thirst, body temperature, and circadian rhythms.

Gross Anatomy

The hypothalamus occupies the ventral diencephalon and is composed of numerous fiber tracts and nuclei situated symmetrically around the third ventricle. In sagittal section, the hypothalamus is diamond shaped. Cranially, the hypothalamus extends from the anterior commissure, lamina terminalis, and optic chiasma. Caudally, the hypothalamus extends to the periaqueductal gray matter of the midbrain, approximated by (from ventral to dorsal) the mammillary bodies, interpeduncular fossa, and cerebral peduncles (Fig. 2.1).

In the coronal plane, the boundaries of the hypothalamus are more distinct. Superiorly, the hypothalamus is divided from the thalamus by a groove in the lateral wall of the third ventricle, the hypothalamic sulcus. The lateral surface is contiguous with the thalamus and subthalamus and is bordered by the internal capsule and optic tracts. Medially, the hypothalamus is bounded by the ependyma of the third ventricle. Finally, the inferior surface is continuous with the floor of the third ventricle.

The external surface of the hypothalamic floor projects into the interpeduncular cistern. A median protuberance, the tuber cinereum, lies between the optic chiasma cranially and mammillary bodies caudally and

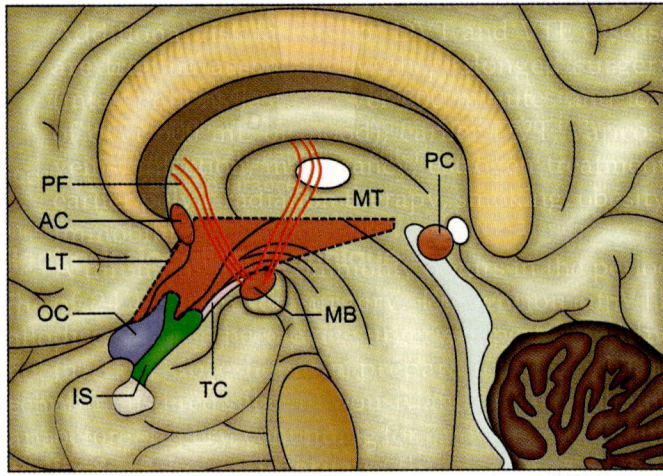

Fig. 2.1: Sagittal section of the hypothalamus, with schematic boundary landmarks. AC: anterior commissure. PC: posterior commissure. LT: lamina terminalis. OC: optic chiasm. MB: mammillary bodies. IS: infundibular stalk. TC: tuber cinereum. MT: mammillothalamic tract. PF: postcommissural fornix

is continuous anteriorly with the lamina terminalis. This projection continues as the infundibulum, terminating inferiorly on the pituitary gland.

Microscopic Anatomy

The nuclei of the hypothalamus are organized into the following three subdivisions:

1. Anterior (or chiasmatic) region, which extends between the lamina terminalis and the anterior infundibular recess.
2. Median (or tuberal) region, which proceeds to the anterior column of the fornix.
3. Posterior (or mammillary) region, which stretches to the caudal mammillary bodies.

These subdivisions are derived primarily from the hypothalamic blood supply. The anterior hypothalamus is supplied by branches of the anterior cerebral and anterior communicating arteries; the tuberal hypothalamus is supplied by the posterior communicating artery and the mammillary region is supplied by the posterior communicating, posterior cerebral, and basilar arteries.

Anatomic subdivisions can be further segregated into three morphological and functional areas: Lateral, medial, and periventricular. The medial and lateral regions are anatomically divided by the anterior column of the fornix and the mammillothalamic tract; the periventricular region is a further subdivision of the medial hypothalamus that lacks a gross anatomic boundary. Although the lateral region is the most voluminous, the medial and periventricular regions contain the majority of hypothalamic nuclei.

The lateral region is largely composed of a massive bidirectional fiber pathway, the medial forebrain bundle (MFB), which connects the hypothalamus to the limbic system and brainstem autonomic centres. Through the MFB, signals from the brainstem, amygdala, hippocampus, retina, and olfactory system are conveyed to hypothalamic nuclei, underlying the crucial role of the hypothalamus in systemic homeostasis as shown in Fig. 2.2.

Anterior Hypothalamic Nuclei

Nuclei within the anterior subdivision of the hypothalamus include the medial/lateral preoptic, periventricular, supraoptic, suprachiasmatic, and anterior/lateral hypothalamic nuclei.

The medial preoptic nucleus abuts the third ventricle and periventricular nucleus medially and is bounded laterally by the lateral preoptic nucleus, superiorly by the anterior commissure, and inferiorly by the supraoptic and suprachiasmatic nuclei. The medial preoptic nucleus generates gonadotropin-releasing hormone (GnRH).

The supraoptic nucleus lies dorsal to the optic tract and ventral to the medial preoptic nucleus, adjoining the intrapeduncular cistern. It is composed of neurosecretory cells, which produce vasopressin (or antidiuretic hormone) and oxytocin; the axons of these neurons are conveyed ventrally through the median eminence and infundibulum (in the supraoptico-hypophyseal tract), and vesicle contents are released from the posterior pituitary gland.

The paraventricular nucleus (PVN) adjoins the third ventricle ventral to the fornix and dorsal to the anterior hypothalamic nucleus and extends across the rostrocaudal axis of the hypothalamus. Like the supraoptic nucleus, it maintains systemic osmotic balance through secretion of vasopressin and oxytocin from the posterior pituitary gland. Additionally, it houses parvocellular neurosecretory neurons projecting to the median eminence, where axon terminals release corticotropin-releasing hormone (CRH), thyrotropin-releasing hormone (TRH), GnRH, growth hormone-releasing hormone (GHRH), and somatostatin into the

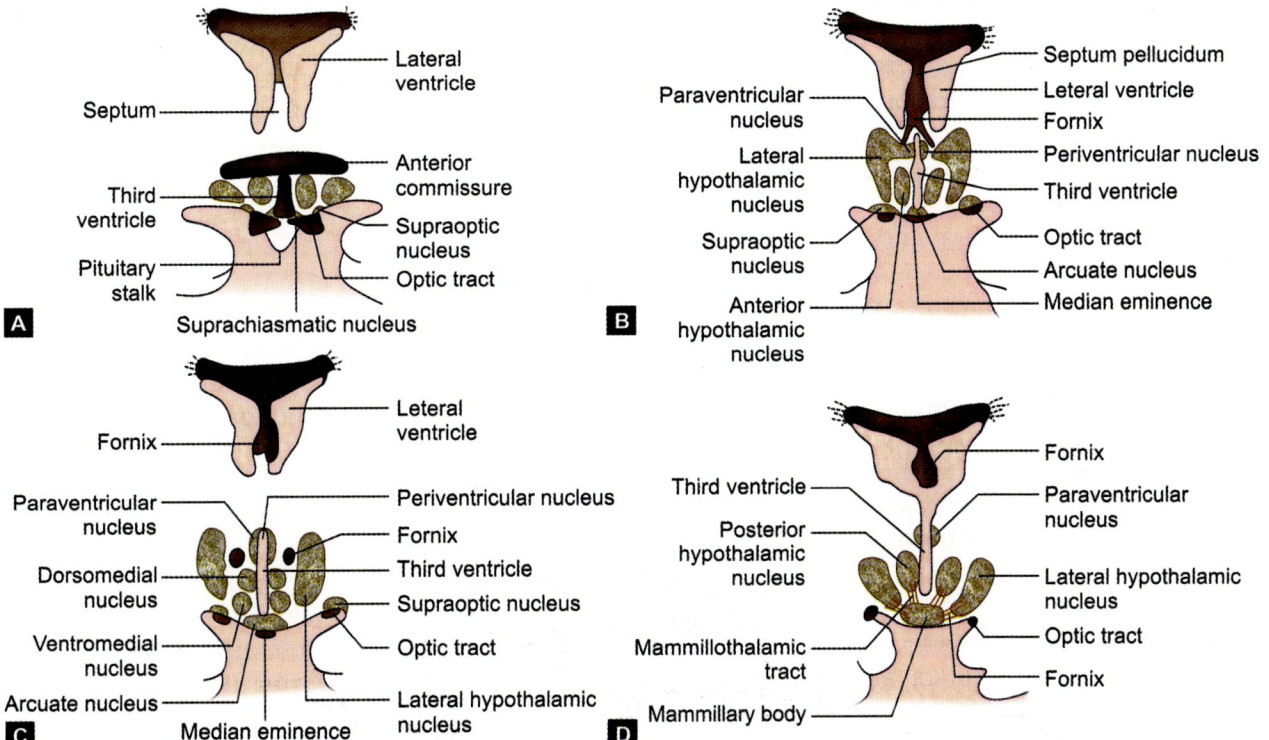

Fig. 2.2: Rostral to caudal (A–D) coronal sections of the hypothalamus, reflecting relative positions of hypothalamic nuclei

perivascular spaces of the hypothalamic–pituitary portal system.

The anterior hypothalamic nucleus plays a critical role in thermoregulation and circadian rhythms. It is situated at the inferior border of the PVN and is bounded dorsolaterally by the lateral hypothalamic nucleus (LHN), ventromedially by the arcuate nucleus, and ventrolaterally by the supraoptic nucleus.

The suprachiasmatic nucleus (SCN) lies dorsal to the optic chiasma and optic tracts at the floor of the third ventricle. This position allows the SCN to receive afferent input directly from the retina, as well as projections from the lateral geniculate nucleus and superior colliculus. With these afferents, the SCN acts as a dominant regulator of circadian rhythms.

The lateral preoptic nucleus mediates non-rapid-eye movement sleep onset. It is contiguous caudally with the LHN, which extends through the tuberal and posterior divisions of the hypothalamus. The LHN responds to blood glucose concentrations to regulate hunger.

Tuberal Hypothalamic Nuclei

The tuberal region is the largest of the hypothalamus with the most pronounced anatomic distinction between medial and lateral hypothalamic areas. The dorsomedial and ventromedial nuclei abut the third ventricle, ventrolateral to the PVN and ventromedial to the fornix. Both nuclei regulate hunger and satiety, although the more voluminous ventromedial nucleus appears to be the dominant regulator. The ventromedial nucleus additionally appears to play a role in fear and aggression.

The arcuate nucleus overlies the median eminence at the floor of the third ventricle. Apparently horseshoe-shaped, it surrounds the lateral and caudal exit of the infundibulum. The arcuate nucleus contains the bodies of neuroendocrine neurons, which produce GHRH and dopamine for release into the hypophyseal portal circulation. Consequently, it plays a critical role in the function of the hypothalamic–pituitary–gonadal (HPG) axis. Arcuate neurons also have diverse projections to other hypothalamic nuclei, particularly the lateral hypothalamus, PVN (a pathway critical in regulating hunger), and medial preoptic nucleus (regulating sexual drive).

Posterior Hypothalamic Nuclei

The posterior nucleus lies dorsal to the mammillary bodies and medial to the caudal end of the LHN, adjoining the third ventricle. It is primarily involved in thermoregulation.

The mammillary nuclei, situated at the caudal hypothalamic floor, lie within the mammillary bodies. Although functionally a component of the limbic system, neuroanatomists frequently categorize them as hypothalamic constituents. Mammillary neurons act as a conduit for signals originating in the ipsilateral amygdala and hippocampus, and they convey these signals to the thalamus via the mammillothalamic tract (a limb of the circuit of Papez, which regulates cortical control of emotion). Mammillary nuclei are additionally critical in recognition memory.

The tuber cinereum lies dorsal to the median eminence, interposed between the mammillary bodies and infundibulum. It houses the tuberoinfundibular nucleus, which globally governs alertness through histamine secretion.

Median Eminence, Tuberoinfundibular Portal System, and Hypophyseal Portal System

The median eminence of the hypothalamus projects from the hypothalamic floor ventral to the arcuate nucleus. It is an integral component of the hypophyseal portal system, which allows the hypothalamus to regulate anterior pituitary gland function. The median eminence is organized into three zones across a dorsoventral axis: The ependymal zone, the zona interna, and zona externa. The ependymal zone forms the floor of the third ventricle and is primarily characterized by the bodies of specialized ependymal cells called tanycytes. Tanycytes extend along the dorsoventral axis of the median eminence, with protrusions both into the cerebrospinal fluid (CSF) of the third ventricle and ventral projections deep into the median eminence.

The zona interna (internal zone) lies directly ventral to the ependymal zone and is primarily composed of unmyelinated axons passing from hypothalamic nuclei (principally the paraventricular nucleus and supraoptic nucleus) to the posterior pituitary. These axons transport vasopressin and oxytocin in neurosecretory granules that are secreted directly from terminals in the posterior pituitary gland. The zona interna additionally contains axons passing from the tuberoinfundibular system into the zona externa. These unmyelinated axons originate at hypothalamic nuclei, principally the arcuate, paraventricular, and medial preoptic nuclei, and terminate in the portal capillary plexus within the zona externa. At the portal capillary plexus, vesicles containing hypophysiotropic ("releasing") hormones (i.e. CRH, GnRH, TRH, GHRH, dopamine, somatostatin) are secreted. These hormones percolate through the fenestrated capillary endothelium to reach the anterior pituitary gland.

Vascular supply to the pituitary gland comes primarily from two branches of the internal carotid artery—the superior and inferior hypophyseal arteries. The superior hypophyseal artery forms a ring around the dorsal infundibulum, while the inferior hypophyseal artery similarly encircles the ventral infundibulum and anterior pituitary. These arteries disseminate into connected capillary plexuses within the median eminence and anterior pituitary. Hormones deposited into the zona externa of the median eminence make a brief ventral transit to the capillary plexus of the anterior pituitary, where they diffuse into the parenchyma of the gland to modulate its endocrine activity (Fig. 2.3).

Pathophysiological Variants

The best-known variant of hypothalamic dysfunction leads to Kallmann syndrome, a condition characterized by delayed or absent puberty and anosmia. Under normal circumstances, gonadotropin-releasing hormone—secreting neurons migrates to the hypothalamus (primarily the arcuate and paraventricular nuclei) from the olfactory placode during embryogenesis. Failure of this migration results in absence of these hypothalamic neurons, with downstream effects on the hypothalamic–pituitary–gonadal axis, mediated by the anterior pituitary gland. Although this deficiency is not evident grossly, a diminution in paraventricular nucleus volume is microscopically evident.

Numerous disease processes may impinge on the hypothalamus, causing secondary detriment of normal function. Tumors of the hypothalamus, pituitary gland, or suprasellar region may impinge on nuclei and fiber tracts, disrupting the endocrine conduit between the hypothalamus and pituitary gland and globally modifying normal hormone concentrations. Systemic infiltrative disease may also affect the hypothalamus or pituitary, disrupting function and distorting anatomy.

Certain developmental disorders (particularly Prader-Willi and Bardet-Biedl syndromes) are known to arise in part from disrupted hypothalamic function, but are not associated with aberrations in hypothalamic anatomy. The lateral hypothalamic nucleus is severely affected by Huntington disease, and neuronal loss in the area has even been used as a marker for disease progression. Histologic changes of the mammillary

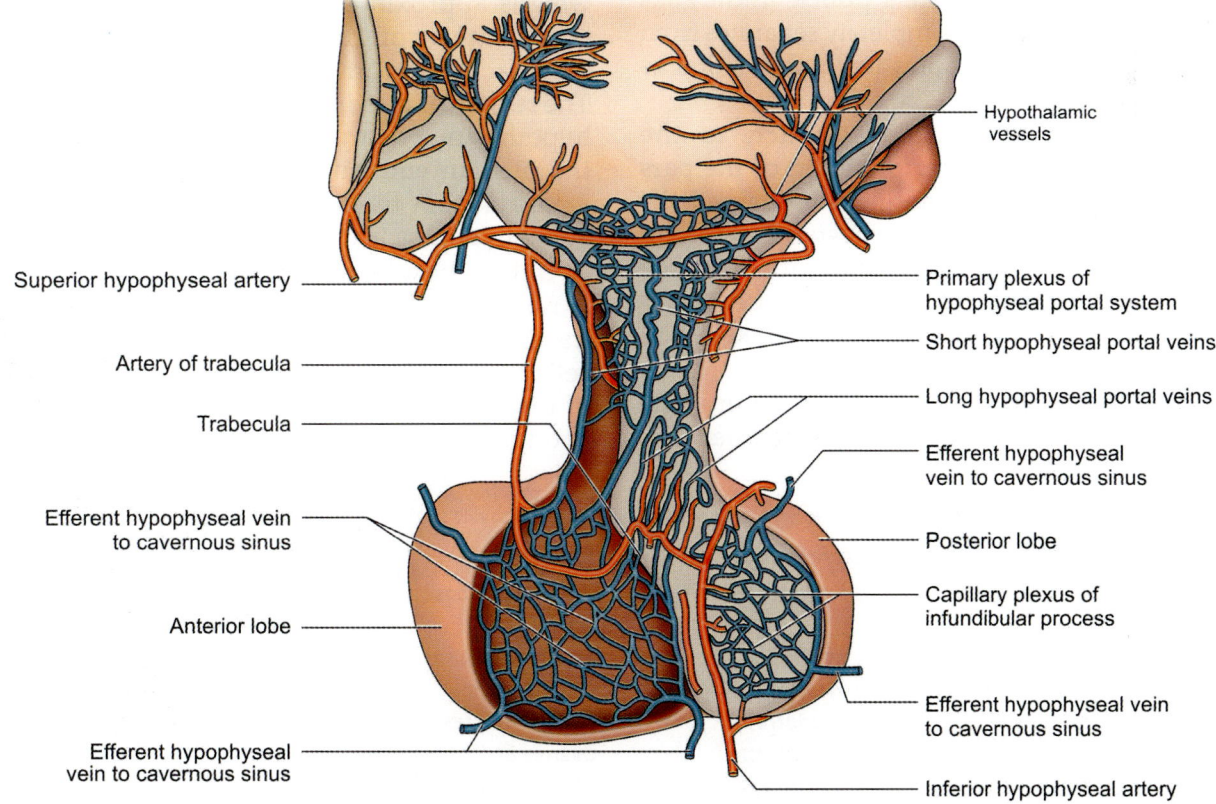

Fig. 2.3: Illustration of the hypophyseal portal system

nucleus occur with Alzheimer and Parkinson diseases, but no gross changes or microscopic cell loss have been observed.

Anatomy of Pituitary Gland

The pituitary gland is a pea-sized endocrine gland that sits at the base of the brain. Often referred to as the "master gland", the pituitary gland synthesizes and releases various hormones that affect several organs throughout the body. These are mentioned below.

Embryologic Development

The pituitary gland is entirely ectodermal in origin but is composed of two functionally distinct structures that differ in embryologic development and anatomy: The adenohypophysis (anterior pituitary) and the neurohypophysis (posterior pituitary) (Fig. 2.4).

The adenohypophysis develops from Rathke's pouch, which is an upward invagination of oral ectoderm from the roof of the stomodeum; in contrast, the neurohypophysis develops from the infundibulum, which is a downward extension of neural ectoderm from the floor of the diencephalon. The oral ectoderm and neural ectoderm that form the pituitary anlagen are in close contact during early embryogenesis, and this connection is critical for pituitary development.

Over several weeks, Rathke's pouch undergoes constriction at its base until it completely separates from the oral epithelium and occupies its final position as the adenohypophysis.

The transition from Rathke's pouch to the adenohypophysis involves the formation of the pars distalis from the rapidly proliferating anterior wall, the pars intermedia from the less active posterior wall, and the pars tuberalis from an upward outgrowth of the anterior wall. The incomplete obliteration of Rathke's pouch can lead to remnants that form Rathke's cleft cysts.

The neurohypophysis develops from the differentiation of neural ectoderm into the pars nervosa,

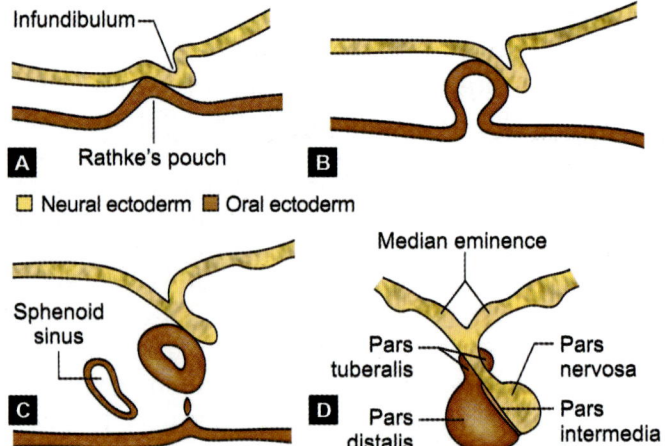

Fig. 2.4: Illustration of the hypophyseal portal system. Anatomy of pituitary gland. (A) Infundibulum and Rathke's pouch develop from neural ectoderm and oral ectoderm, respectively. (B) Rathke's pouch constricts at base. (C) Rathke's pouch completely separates from oral epithelium. (D) Adenohypophysis is formed by development of pars distalis, pars tuberalis, and pars intermedia; neurohypophysis is formed by development of pars nervosa, infundibular stem, and median eminence

the infundibular stem, and the median eminence. The infundibular stem is surrounded by the pars tuberalis.

Gross Anatomy

The fully developed pituitary gland is pea-sized and weighs approximately 0.5 g. The adenohypophysis constitutes roughly 80% of the pituitary and manufactures an array of peptide hormones (Table 2.1). The release of these pituitary hormones is mediated by hypothalamic neurohormones that are secreted from the median eminence (a site where axon terminals emanate from the hypothalamus) and that reach the adenohypophysis via a portal venous system (Fig. 2.5).

Unlike the adenohypophysis, the neurohypophysis is not glandular and does not synthesize hormones. Instead, it is a site where axons project from neuronal cell bodies in the supraoptic and paraventricular nuclei of the hypothalamus. These hypothalamic cell bodies produce hormones that undergo axonal transport

Table 2.1: Hormones secreted by adenohypophysis (anterior pituitary)			
Hormone	*Secretory cell type*	*Target*	*Effects*
Growth hormone (GH)	Somatotroph	Liver and adipose tissue	Stimulation of growth and metabolism of carbohydrates and lipids
Prolactin (PRL)	Lactotroph	Mammary glands	Production of milk
Thyroid-stimulating hormone (TSH)	Thyrotroph	Thyroid gland	Secretion of thyroid hormones
Follicle-stimulating hormone (FSH)	Gonadotroph	Ovaries and testes	Regulates reproductive functioning
Luteinizing hormone (LH)	Gonadotroph	Ovaries and testes	Production of sex hormones
Adrenocorticotropic hormone (ACTH)	Corticotroph	Adrenal gland (cortex)	Secretion of glucocorticoids
β-Endorphin	Corticotroph	Opioid receptors	Opioid receptors

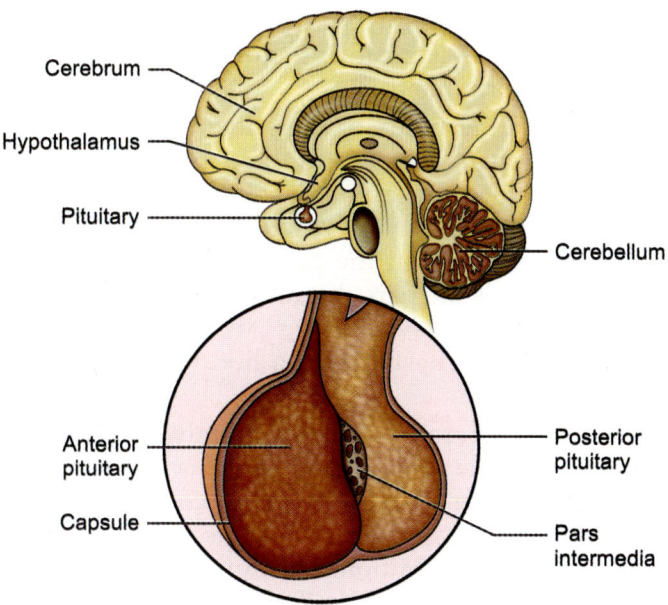

Fig. 2.5: Illustration of pituitary gland, sagittal section

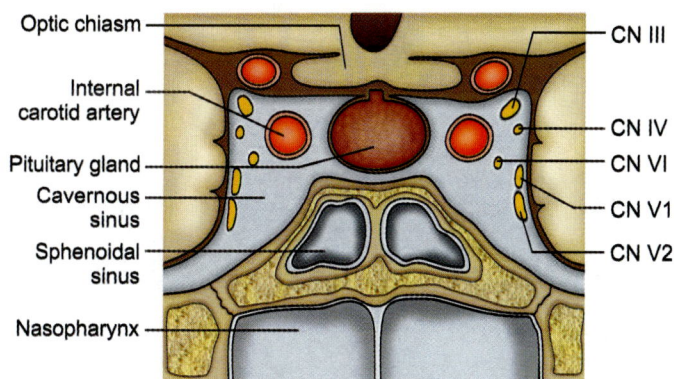

Fig. 2.6: Coronal depiction of pituitary gland and surrounding structures. Lateral aspects of pituitary gland are in close proximity to internal carotid artery and several cranial nerves

through the pituitary stalk and into terminal axons within the neurohypophysis. The hormones are then stored and released directly into the systemic vasculature (Table 2.2).

The pituitary gland is enveloped by dura and sits within the sella turcica of the sphenoid bone. The sella turcica is a saddle-shaped depression that surrounds the inferior, anterior, and posterior aspects of the pituitary. The superior aspect of the pituitary is covered by the diaphragma sellae, which is a fold of dura mater that separates the cerebrospinal fluid-filled subarachnoid space from the pituitary. The infundibulum pierces the diaphragma sellae in order to connect the pituitary to the hypothalamus.

The lateral aspects of the pituitary are adjacent to the cavernous sinuses. From superior to inferior, the cavernous sinus contains cranial nerves III (oculomotor), IV (trochlear), VI (abducens), V1 (ophthalmic branch of trigeminal nerve), and V2 (maxillary branch of trigeminal nerve). The internal carotid artery also courses through the cavernous sinus, medial to these nerves (Fig. 2.6).

Different pneumatization patterns of the sphenoid sinus (conchal, presellar, sellar, and postsellar) describe the location of the sphenoid sinus relative to the sella turcica and thus dictate the extent of exposure of the sellar floor. In the conchal type, pneumatization is absent, and thus the sphenoid sinus does not contain an air cavity. In the presellar type, there is minimal posterior extension of an air cavity, whereas in the postsellar type, there is posterior extension of an air cavity past the level of the sella turcica.

Vasculature

The adenohypophysis receives the majority of its blood supply from the paired superior hypophyseal arteries, which arise from the medial aspect of the internal carotid artery, within the ophthalmic segment. The superior hypophyseal artery commonly emerges within 5 mm distal to the origin of the ophthalmic artery and eventually forms the primary capillary network found in the median eminence.

The neurohypophysis is supplied by the inferior hypophyseal arteries (Fig. 2.7). These vessels are terminal branches of the meningohypophyseal trunk, which arises from the cavernous portion of the internal carotid artery.

The hypophyseal portal veins drain the primary capillary plexus formed by the superior hypophyseal arteries, which deliver blood to the pars distalis. The pars distalis in turn houses the secondary capillary plexus. Thus, a portal venous system allows delivery of hypothalamic prohormones to the adenohypophysis, and the neurohypophysis secretes hormones directly into the venous draining system of the pituitary.

Table 2.2: Hormones secreted by neurohypophysis (posterior pituitary)		
Hormone	*Acts on*	*Effects*
Oxytocin	Uterus and mammary gland	Uterine contractions and lactation
Antidiuretic hormone (ADH)	Kidneys and arterioles	Water retention and increased blood pressure

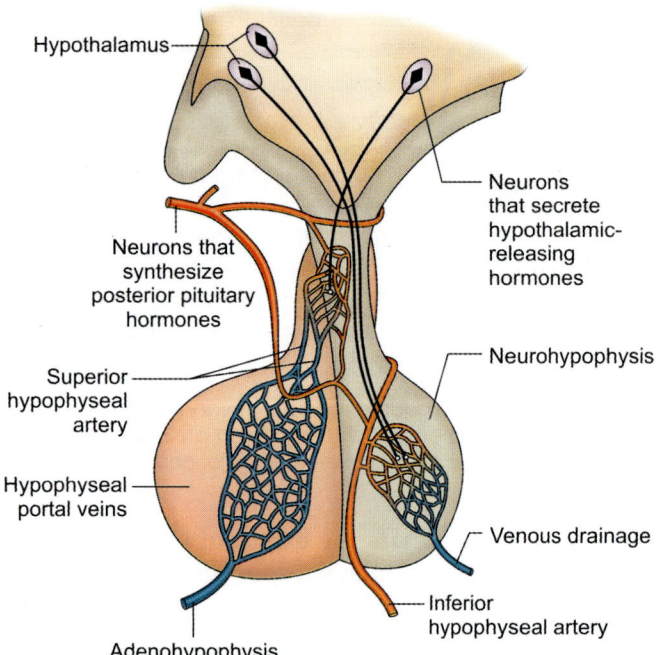

Fig. 2.7: Vasculature of pituitary gland. Adenohypophysis and neurohypophysis receive majority of their blood supply from superior hypophyseal arteries and inferior hypophyseal arteries, respectively

Microscopic Anatomy

The pars distalis forms the majority of the adenohypophysis and resembles a typical endocrine gland. Cords and clusters of cuboidal secretory cells within the pars distalis contain hormones stored in cytoplasmic granules that are released via exocytosis and taken up by nearby sinusoidal capillaries. Histochemical staining of these granules with pH-dependent dyes allows categorization of the cells into acidophils, basophils, or chromophobes.

In general, acidophilic cells contain polypeptide hormones, basophilic cells contain glycoprotein hormones, and chromophobes have minimal to no hormone content. The most common cell type is the acidophilic somatotrope, which is concentrated in the lateral regions of the adenohypophysis and secretes growth hormone (GH). Lactotropes are also acidophilic but are more scattered throughout the adenohypophysis and secrete prolactin (PRL).

The basophilic cells include corticotropes, thyrotropes, and gonadotropes. Although corticotropes secrete nonglycosylated polypeptides such as adrenocorticotropic hormone (ACTH), these cells are basophilic as a result of the glycoprotein composition of the precursor hormone pro-opiomelanocortin (POMC). Thyrotropes are among the least prevalent secretory cells of the pars distalis; they release thyroid-stimulating hormone (TSH), whereas gonadotropes secrete follicle-stimulating hormone (FSH) and luteinizing hormone (LH).

The pars intermedia of the adenohypophysis lies between the pars distalis and the pars nervosa of the neurohypophysis. In humans, this region is not well developed and has poor vascularization. Although secretory cells within the pars intermedia, like the corticotropes of the pars distalis, produce POMC, the principal hormones synthesized by the pars intermedia include melanocyte-stimulating hormone (MSH) and β-endorphin.

The pars tuberalis is a thin, highly vascularized component of the adenohypophysis that surrounds the infundibular stem. The principal secretory cell type within this tissue is the gonadotrope, which contains FSH and LH. In addition, melatonin receptors exist within the pars tuberalis that may play a role in rhythmic gene expression.

The pars nervosa of the neurohypophysis contains unmyelinated axons that project from neuronal cell bodies in the hypothalamus. Oxytocin and antidiuretic hormone (ADH) synthesized in the cell bodies are transported via the axons and accumulate at the terminal ends within swellings called Herring bodies. A network of capillaries surrounds the axon terminals and facilitates the uptake of released hormones into the vasculature.

Specialized glial cells known as pituicytes are also interspersed within the pars nervosa and have been hypothesized to actively participate in the modulation of hormone release.

Pathophysiologic Variants

Pituitary tumors are relatively common, accounting for about 15% of all primary brain tumors. The vast majority originate in the adenohypophysis and are typically nonsecretory benign adenomas. These adenomas frequently go undiagnosed, and there is an 11–14% overall prevalence of silent pituitary adenomas in the general population. Tumors of the neurohypophysis are rare and include metastasis, and granular cell tumors.

Pituitary adenomas are arbitrarily classified as **microadenomas** (<1 cm) or **macroadenomas** (>1 cm). Macroadenomas, when large, have a mass effect on adjacent structures, with clinical consequences. Compression of the pituitary gland itself may cause hypopituitarism, and compression of the optic chiasm results in bitemporal hemianopsia. Headache is also a common symptom of pituitary tumors.

Secretory adenomas are typically monoclonal, i.e. they secrete a single hormone. Approximately 1 to 2% of adenomas secrete 2 or more hormones, with growth hormone (GH) and prolactin (PRL) being the hormones most commonly elevated concomitantly.

Prolactinomas are the most common secretory adenomas. Even small microadenomas can involve secretion sufficient to produce symptoms, but there is also a direct correlation between the tumor mass of prolactinomas and hormone production. Although prolactinomas classically present with galactorrhea, this symptom is not always present.

GH-secreting adenomas are next most common adenomas, followed by adrenocorticotropic hormone (ACTH)-secreting tumors and gonadotroph adenomas (tumors that secrete luteinizing hormone [LH] and follicle-stimulating hormone [FSH]); thyrotroph tumors account for fewer than 1% of pituitary adenomas. Pituitary carcinomas are quite rare.

Macroadenomas, particularly those with suprasellar extension, and head trauma may cause hyper-prolactinemia unrelated to prolactinoma. Normally, dopamine is secreted by the hypothalamus and is transported via the pituitary stalk to the adenohypophysis, where it inhibits the high basal secretory rate of the pituitary lactotrophs. When tumors grow large enough, a "stalk effect" occurs, and this transport is disrupted. As a result, prolactin secretion is no longer inhibited appropriately, and pituitary lactotroph hyperplasia develops.

Remnants of Rathke's pouch have the potential to produce signs and symptoms associated with mass effect. Although commonly asymptomatic, **Rathke's cleft cysts** can accumulate proteinaceous fluid and subsequently expand, compressing nearby structures. Vestigial remnants of Rathke's pouch can also form craniopharyngiomas, slow-growing benign tumors that most often present in either the very young or the very old women.

Although **craniopharyngiomas** can be encapsulated and solid, they are often cystic and multiloculated. The adenomatous form frequently contains calcifications and projects into adjacent brain tissue, eliciting an intense inflammatory reaction. It is often filled with a rich, cholesterol-containing cystic fluid. The papillary form lacks calcification, keratin, and cysts and therefore, is much more amenable to surgical resection.

Inflammatory conditions can affect the pituitary but are rare. Lymphocytic hypophysitis is a primary inflammatory disorder that typically presents during or shortly after pregnancy. Although of unknown etiology, lymphocytic hypophysitis is believed to be caused by autoimmune process.

Empty sella syndrome describes a sella turcica that appears to be empty on radiologic imaging as a consequence of a shrunken or flattened pituitary gland. Primary empty sella syndrome is thought to result from chronic intracranial hypertension with a defect in the diaphragma sella that allows intradural contents to herniate into the sella, compressing the pituitary and resulting in endocrine abnormalities and even visual symptoms from mass effect.

Secondary empty sella syndrome results from either iatrogenic treatment of a sellar mass or spontaneous (typically ischemic) necrosis of such a mass. Hypopituitarism can be seen in both primary and secondary empty sella syndrome.

Sheehan syndrome, also referred to as postpartum hypopituitarism, is attributed to infarction of the pituitary gland caused by hypovolemia from obstetric hemorrhage. The first clinical manifestation of the syndrome is typically the absence of milk production during the postpartum period. Multiple hormone deficiencies are common, and pituitary function can decline further over time.

Pituitary apoplexy is a potentially life-threatening syndrome that occurs as a result of hemorrhage, infarction, or hemorrhagic infarction within a pituitary tumor. The pressure resulting from edema and the accumulation of blood compresses adjacent structures and leads to symptoms that include sudden onset of visual dysfunction, severe headache, and pituitary insufficiency. This syndrome is a neurosurgical emergency that calls for immediate treatment.

Diagnostic Imaging

Magnetic resonance imaging (MRI) is the study of choice for evaluating the pituitary gland. This multiplanar imaging modality has the advantages of providing superior contrast differentiation of soft tissues and not exposing the subject to potentially harmful ionizing radiation. Coronal and sagittal T1-weighted sequences with 3 mm thick sections are typically recommended for detecting pituitary lesions. As a supplement, T2-weighted images are often useful.

Hyperintense signals on T1-weighted images can be due to numerous disease processes, such as hemorrhage, Rathke's cleft cyst, and craniopharyngioma. Microadenomas commonly appear hypointense on noncontrast T1-weighted images but can occasionally appear isointense.

The sensitivity of lesion detection with MRI can be improved by repeating T1-weighted sequences after administration of a single dose (0.1 mmol/kg) gadolinium-containing contrast agent.

Computed tomography (CT) is useful as an adjunct to MRI when increased detail of bone structure is required. CT is superior in demonstrating erosions of bone and calcifications and can also be used in evaluating bone anatomy before transsphenoidal surgery. Furthermore, CT can detect many pituitary lesions and provides a reasonable screening method when MRI is not available.

Surgical Approaches

Transsphenoidal surgery is currently the principal technique employed for resecting pituitary lesions within the sellar and parasellar regions. This operative procedure commonly involves using an endonasal incision to create a route to the anterior wall of the sphenoid sinus. If greater exposure is required, a sublabial incision can be employed instead. Once the sphenoid bone is reached, it is fractured to provide entry into the sphenoid sinus. The sellar floor is then penetrated, and a durotomy is performed to provide an unobstructed view into the sellar region.

For more than half a century, the transsphenoidal approach has been coupled with the operative microscope to enhance visualization of the surgical field. However, the relatively recent development of endoscopic transnasal transsphenoidal techniques offers a significant advance from microscopic methods which include increased patient comfort, decreased use of nasal packing and decreased hospital stay.

Hypothalamic–Pituitary–Gonadal Axis

The hypothalamic–pituitary–gonadal axis is a critical part in the development and regulation of a number of the body's systems, such as the reproductive and immune systems. Fluctuations in the hormones cause changes in the hormones produced by each gland and have various widespread and local effects on the body.

The hypothalamus produces gonadotropin-releasing hormone (GnRH). The anterior portion of the pituitary gland produces luteinizing hormone (LH) and follicle-stimulating hormone (FSH), and the gonads produce estrogen and testosterone.

Endocrine Control of HPO Axis

GnRH is a decapeptide synthesized in the hypo-thalamus. GnRH neurons can be detected in the fetal hypothalamus as early as 9–10 weeks of gestation. These neurons originate from the olfactory area and later migrating to olfactory placode to rest in the arcuate nucleus of hypothalamus. Three types of GnRH (GnRH-I, GnRH-II, GnRH-III) have been detected in humans. GnRH-I is the classic hypothalamic hormone responsible for the regulation, synthesis, and secretion of the pituitary gonadoptropins FSH and LH. GnRH-II is detected in the brain tissue and in many other peripheral tissues like endometrium, breast and ovaries. GnRH-III is also found in neurons from hypothalamus but its role is not clear.

GnRH-I is synthesized from a 92 amino acid precursor; it then travels to the median eminence of the hypothalamus and is released in the portal circulation in a pulsatile fashion. The half life of GnRH-I is very short (2–4 min) as it is cleaved rapidly. It acts on the anterior pituitary leading to synthesis, storage and secretion of gonadotropins. For this action to take place, pulsatile GnRH release is necessary. Continuous GnRH secretion leads to suppression of FSH and LH release and this property is utilized for creating pharmacological hypogonadotropic hypogonadism.

GnRH-II differs from GnRH-I by three amino acids at positions 5, 7 and 8. It is released from the placenta in a pulsatile fashion. Estrogen suppresses GnRH-I secretion in negative feedback fashion but increase GnRH-II mRNA levels.

Structure of GnRH-I (Table 2.3)

Pyro-Glu^1-His^2-Trp^3-Ser^4-Tyr^5-Gly^6-Leu^7-Arg^8-Pro^9-Gly^{10}-NH$_2$

GnRH analogues have been developed by changing the amino acid sequence of the GnRH molecule. There are two major groups of GnRH analogues: GnRH agonists and GnRH antagonists. In case of GnRH agonist use, the continuous activation of GnRH receptor results in desensitization due to a conformational change of the receptor, internalization and reduced

GnRH analogue	Structural changes	Half life	Route of admins
Nafarelin	Decapeptide at pos 6-Nal flr Gly	3–4 hr	IV, SC, intranasal
Triptorelin	Decapeptide; at pos 6-Trp for Gly	3–4 hr	SC, IM depot
Leuprolide	Nonapeptide; Pos 6-Leu for Gly; Pos 10-NHE for Gly	1.5 hr	SC, IM depot
Buserelin	Nonapeptide; Pos 6-Set for Gly and pos 10-NHE for Gly	1.5 hr	SC, intranasal

Table 2.3: Structure of GnRH-I

synthesis of the receptor. Prior to the desensitization by GnRH agonist there is an initial flare with increased gonadotropin secretion. Desensitization then takes place 7–14 days later. Unlike GnRH agonists, GnRH antagonists do not cause flare effect upon initial administration; but it causes an immediate suppression of gonadotropin secretion that is rapid and reversible. GnRH analogues are available in injectable form in the treatment of precocious puberty, endometriosis, uterine fibroid and in IVF cycle. Oral form of GnRH analogues are under investigation. Elagolix is an orally active GnRH antagonist under investigation.

GnRH acts on the anterior pituitary to secrete gonadotropins—FSH and LH. FSH is a glycoprotein dimer consisting of two subunits—α and β. The α-subunit consists of 92 amino acids and is common in FSH, LH as well as in TSH, hCG. The β subunit of FSH consists of 118 amino acids and five sialistic acid residues which determine the half-life of the hormone. FSH has half-life of several hours and addition of sialic acid to recombinant FSH leads to their longer half life. However, FSH β-subunit synthesis is dependent on the presence of activin. FSH is responsible for follicular growth and starts rising from day 25 of the previous cycle and continues to rise till day 7 of the current cycle when it starts declining in response to negative feedback from follicular rise of estrogen. It induces granulosa cell growth and activates aromatase activity which converts follicular androgens to estrogens. But the dominant follicle continues to grow due to recruitment of highest concentration of FSH receptors and produce positive feedback rise of LH before ovulation. The small rise of progesterone also produce positive feedback rise of FSH also just at the time of ovulation to help in dissolution of ovarian cumulus by increased plasminogen activity to help in rupture of the dominant follicle during ovulation.

LH is also a glycoprotein dimer consisting of two subunits—α and β. The β subunit consists of 121 amino acids and one to two sialic acid residues with a shorter half-life of approximately 20 mins. Because of this shorter half-life, LH needs to be rapidly synthesized and typically has pulses higher in amplitude than FSH. The surge of LH secretion is mainly preovulatory and is in response to positive feedback of estrogen rise from the dominant follicle. FSH receptors exist predominantly on granulosa cells while LH receptors are present on theca cells. In the presence of estradiol, FSH induces LH receptors on granulosa cells which are essential for LH surge to act.

Endogenous opiates (opioids) are naturally occurring narcotics produced by the brain. There are three classes of opiates—encephalin, endorphin, and dynorphin. Endorphin levels increase throughout the menstrual cycle; they are at their lowest at the time of menses and highest in luteal phase. An increase in endorphin release decreases LH secretion by suppressing hypothalamic GnRH release. Therefore, treatment with opioid receptor antagonist, like naltrexone, appears to correct the problem of hypothalamic amenorrhea particularly which is stress related (Table 2.4).

Ovarian peptide hormones, such as inhibin, activin and AMH, play a role by modulating central nervous system hormone release. They all belong to transforming growth factor (TGF-β) of ligands.

Inhibin is a polypeptide mainly secreted by granulosa cells. It consists of two subunits—α and β and two forms of Inhibin—A and B are produced. Both forms of inhibin consist of same α subunit but they vary in β subunits. Inhibin B is found predominantly in follicular cells and inhibin A is found mainly in luteal cells. Inhibin is released by granulosa cells in response to FSH and selectively inhibits FSH release from anterior pituitary by negative feedback.

Activin in contrast secreted by granulosa cells augments secretion of FSH by enhancing GnRH receptor in hypothalamus and hence its action is blocked by inhibin and follistatin.

AMH (anti-müllerian hormone) is a polypeptide produced from granulosa cells in preantral and antral follicles and reflects the ovarian reserve. Its role in females after birth is not very clear. It is believed that AMH through paracrine effect in the ovary inhibits FSH-stimulated follicular growth and contribute to the emergence of dominant follicle. AMH (normal 2–4 ng/ml) determines follicular response to gonadotropin stimulation in ART cycles. If it is < 2 ng/mL, it indicates poor ovarian reserve. In PCOS, it is elevated (>5 ng/mL).

Leptin is a protein cytokine secreted by adipocytes. It consists of 167 amino acids and is secreted by adipose tissue. Its secretion is regulated by insulin, glucose and obesity which enhance its secretion and its release is inhibited by fasting, androgens and thyroid hormones.

Table 2.4: Effect of neurotransmitter on GnRH	
Neurotransmitter	*Effects*
Dopamine	Inhibits GnRH release
Endorphin	Inhibits GnRH release
Serotonin	Inhibits GnRH release
Norepinephrine, epinephrine	Stimulates GnRH release

The reduction in leptin release stimulates CRH release from the brain explaining stress and weight loss-related amenorrhea. Its role in reproductive system is not clear. Leptin indirectly affects release of LH, and FSH in ART cycles.

Estrogens are 18 carbon steroid hormones and include estrone, estradiol, and estriol. The most potent estrogen is estradiol which is produced from the ovary. Albumin carries approximately 60% of estradiol, while sex-hormone binding globulin binds 38% of estradiol with 2% remaining free in the bloodstream. At the early follicular growth, estradiol level does not increase beyond 50 ng/mL but in peak follicular growth it increases to 200–250 pg/mL. Estradiol level drops after ovulation but a secondary rise occurs in luteal phase reflecting its secretion from corpus luteum. Circulating estrogens are conjugated in the liver to form sulfates and glucuronides; 80% excreted in the urine and 20% in the bile. There are two known estrogen receptors—estrogen receptor-alfa (ER-α) and estrogen receptor-beta (ER-β). The receptor is nuclear in location; once estrogen is bound to its receptor, activation of gene transcription takes place.

Progesterone is a steroid hormone with a 21-carbon molecule and is the main steroid of the corpus luteum. In the follicular phase, progesterone level is <2 ng/mL and it reaches its peak in the midluteal phase with levels exceeding 5 ng/mL. The majority of progesterone in the bloodstream is bound to albumin (80%) and corticosteroid-binding globulin 18%) and to SHBG (0.5%). The remaining progesterone is free in the circulation. The liver is responsible for clearing progesterone from the circulation by converting progesterone to pregnanediol which is conjugated to glucuronic acid and excreted in the urine. There are three progesterone receptors—progesterone receptor-A (PR-A), progesterone receptor-B (PR-B) and progesterone receptor-C (PR-C). PR-B is the positive regulator of progesterone effects while PR-A and PR-C antagonize PR-B. At high concentration, progesterone inhibits FSH and LH secretion through effects on both the hypothalamus and pituitary. The presence of progesterone in the luteal phase also causes decline in GnRH pulse frequency in the hypothalamus. At low concentration, progesterone can stimulate LH release only after exposure to estrogen and progesterone.

Androgens are 19-carbon steroids and include androstenedione, testosterone and dehydroepiandrostenedione (DHEA). The principal secreted androgen by theca cells is androstenedione. The most of the testosterone is the product of peripheral conversion of androstenedione through the action of 17β-hydroxy-steroid dehydrogenase. Under the effect of FSH, androstenedione and testosterone are further aromatized to granulosa cells and converted to estrogens. The androgen receptor exists in full length B and shorter A form. Androgens and progesterone cross-react to their receptor only when present in high concentration.

In the preovulatory follicles, the preferred steroid pathway for androgen and estrogen synthesis is the "delta pathway", which involves the conversion of pregnenolone to 17-OH pregnenolone. In the theca cells, 17-OH pregnenolone is converted to androgens and later diffuse to the granulose cells for aromatization to estrogens.

In contrast, in the corpus luteum the preferred pathway is the delta4 pathway of steroidogenesis which deals with the conversion of pregnenolone to progesterone. The rate-limiting step in steroidogenesis is the side-chain cleavage of cholesterol to pregnenolone. In the ovary, this step is regulated by LH which stimulates increased cAMP production and increased LDL, the major form of cholesterol used for steroidogenesis in ovary.

Function of HPG Axis (Fig. 2.8)

I. Reproduction

One of the most important functions of the HPG axis is to regulate reproduction by controlling the uterine and ovarian cycles. In females, the positive feedback loop between estrogen and luteinizing hormone helps to prepare the follicle in the ovary and the uterus for ovulation and implantation. When the egg is released, the ovary begins to produce progesterone to inhibit the hypothalamus and the anterior pituitary, thus stopping the estrogen-LH positive feedback loop. If conception occurs, the fetus will take over the secretion of progesterone; therefore, the mother cannot ovulate again. If conception does not occur, decreasing excretion of progesterone will allow the hypothalamus to restart secretion of GnRH. These hormone levels also control the uterine cycle causing the proliferation phase in preparation for ovulation, the secretory phase after ovulation, and menstruation when conception does not occur. The activation of the HPG axis in both males and females during puberty also causes individuals to acquire secondary sex characteristics.

In males, the production of GnRH, LH, and FSH is similar, but the effects of these hormones are different. FSH stimulates sustentacular cells to release androgen-binding protein, which promotes testosterone binding. LH binds to the interstitial cells, causing them to secrete testosterone. Testosterone is required for normal spermatogenesis and inhibits the hypothalamus. Inhibin is produced by the spermatogenic cells, which, also through inactivating activin, inhibits the hypothalamus. After puberty, these hormone levels remain relatively constant.

II. Life Cycle

The activation and deactivation of the HPG axis also helps to regulate life cycles. At birth, FSH and LH levels are elevated, and females also have a lifetime supply of primary oocytes. These levels decrease and remain low through childhood. During puberty, the HPG axis is activated by the secretions of estrogen from the ovaries or testosterone from the testes. This activation of estrogen and testosterone causes physiological and psychological changes. Once activated, the HPG axis continues to function in men for the rest of their life but becomes deregulated in women, leading to menopause. This deregulation is caused mainly by the lack of oocytes that normally produce estrogen to create the positive feedback loop. Over several years, the activity of the HPG axis decreases and women are no longer fertile.

Although males remain fertile until death, the activity of the HPG axis decreases. As males age, the testes begin to produce less testosterone, leading to a condition known as post-pubertal hypogonadism. The cause of the decreased testosterone is unclear. Post-pubertal hypogonadism results in progressive muscle mass decrease, increase in visceral fat mass, loss of libido, impotence, decreased attention, increased risk of fractures, and abnormal sperm production.

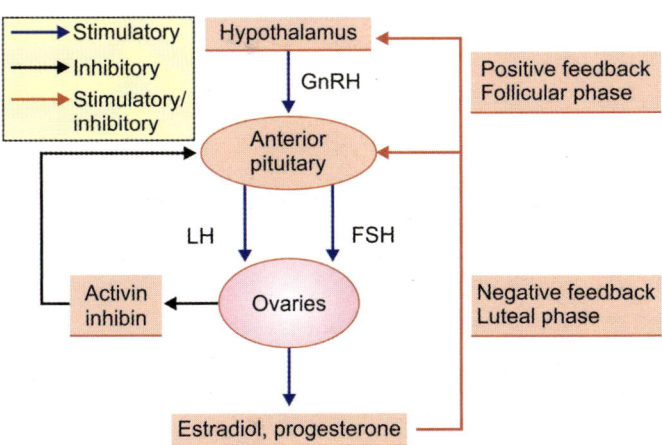

Fig. 2.8: Hypothalamus, pituitary and ovaries form a functional endocrine axis, known as HPG axis with hormonal regulations and feedback loops

III. Sexual Dimorphism and Behavior

Sex steroids also affect behavior, because sex steroids affect brain structure and functioning. During development, hormones help determine how neurons synapse and migrate to result in sexual dimorphisms. These physical differences lead to differences in behavior. While GnRH does not have any direct influence on regulating brain structure and function, gonadotropins like FSH, sex steroids, and activin may have important role in brain development and differentiation. Testosterone levels have been shown to relate to aggression and sex drive.

Clinical Relevance
Disorders

Disorders of the hypothalamic–pituitary–gonadal axis are classified by the World Health Organization (WHO) as:
- *WHO group I of ovulation disorders:* Hypothalamic–pituitary failure.
- *WHO group II of ovulation disorders:* Hypothalamic–pituitary dysfunction. WHO group II is the most common cause of ovulation disorders, and the most common causative member is polycystic ovary syndrome (PCOS).
- *WHO group III of ovulation disorders:* Premature ovarian failure with hypergonadotropic hypogonadism.

Gene Mutations

Genetic mutations and chromosomal abnormalities are two sources of HPG axis alteration. Single mutations usually lead to changes in binding ability of the hormone and receptor leading to inactivation or over-activation. These mutations can occur in the genes coding for GnRH, LH, and FSH or their receptors. For example, the male mutation of the GnRH coding gene can result in hypogonadotropic hypogonadism. A mutation that causes a gain of function for LH receptor can result in a condition known as testotoxicosis, which causes puberty to occur between ages 2 and 3 years. Loss of function of LH receptors can cause male pseudohermaphroditism.

Medications

Hormone levels can be altered in the case of hormonal birth control and hormone replacement therapy. Although often described as preventing pregnancy by mimicking the pregnancy state, hormonal birth control is effective because it works on the HPG axis to mimic the luteal phase of a woman's cycle. The primary active ingredients are synthetic progesterones, which mimic biologically derived progesterone. The synthetic progesterone prevents the hypothalamus from releasing GnRH and the pituitary from releasing LH and FSH; therefore, it prevents the ovarian cycle from entering the menstrual phase and prevents follicle development and ovulation.

Environment Factors

Environment can have a large impact on the HPG axis. One example is women with eating disorders suffer from oligomenorrhea and secondary amenorrhea. Starvation from anorexia nervosa or bulimia causes the HPG axis to deactivate causing women's ovarian and uterine cycles to stop. Stress, physical exercise, and weight loss have been correlated with oligomenorrhea and secondary amenorrhea. Similarly environmental factors can also affect men such as stress causing impotence.

3

Gynecology: Case History and Examination

Gynecological history taking involves a series of methodical questioning of a gynecological patient with the aim of developing a diagnosis or a differential diagnosis on which further management of the patient can be arranged. This further treatment may involve examination of the patient, further investigative testing or treatment of a diagnosed condition.

There is a basic structure for all gynecological histories but this can differ slightly depending on the presenting complaint.

When taking any history in medicine, it is essential to understand what the presenting complaint means and what the possible causes (differential diagnosis) of the presenting complaint may be.

Basic Structure of a Gynecological History

Introduction

- Name of patient
- Age of patient
- Parity of the patient
- Consent for questioning

Presenting Complaint

It is important to ask a question as open as possible in this part of the history and to ensure the complaint is understood as everything else follows on from here.

History of Presenting Complaint

This will elaborate in details all the presenting complaints in the following structure:
- If pain is involved ascertain site, radiation (if any) and character
- Onset
- Periodicity
- Duration
- Recurrence

Marital Status

Age and health of children: Social supports, employment.

Menstrual History

- Age at menarche or menopause
- Last menstrual period (LMP)—date of the first day of bleeding.
- Cycle length and frequency, e.g. 5/28, 5 days of bleeding every 28 days.
- How heavy is the bleeding? Number of tampons per day/clots/flooding/double protection.
- Any intermenstrual bleeding (IMB).
- Any postcoital bleeding (PCB).
- Age of menarche/menopause.
- Any postmenopausal bleeding (PMB).

Discharge

- Color
- Amount
- Smell
- Itchiness
- Duration
- Rash
- Any symptoms in a partner.

Pain or Discomfort

- Duration, type, alleviating or aggravating factors, radiation.
- Any relation to cycle (mid-cycle or period-related).
- Any possibility of pregnancy (ectopic).
- Bowel problems.
- A feeling of "something coming down below" may be a prolapse.
- Dyspareunia—superficial or deep.

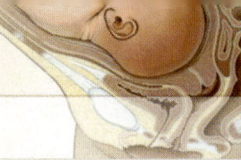

Urinary Symptoms

- Leakage
- Cloudiness
- Hematuria
- Hesitancy
- Dysuria
- Frequency
- Strangury
- Stress or urge incontinence.

Obstetric History

- Number of children, details of pregnancy, labor and delivery, birth weights.
- Any problems with the babies.
- Miscarriages/terminations.
- Any postnatal problems, e.g. depression.
- Conception difficulties/subfertility.

Past Gynecological History

- Gynecological symptoms
- Gynecological diagnoses
- Gynecological surgery
- Abnormal smear

Contraception

- Contraceptive history.
- Any recent unprotected intercourse.
- Reliability of method and user.
- Potential contraindications to different methods, e.g. combined pill.
- Permanent or temporary method required.

Infection

- Any past history of pelvic inflammatory disease.
- Was it adequately treated, including contact tracing?
- Any known contact with sexually transmitted diseases.
- Assess the risk of HIV and hepatitis
- Date of last cervical smear.

Family History

- *Medical conditions:* Tuberculosis, hypertension, thyroid disease, diabetes.
- Gynecological conditions
- Malignancies

Past Medical/Surgical History

- Current or past illnesses
- Hospital admissions
- Past surgeries

Drug History

- *Prescribed medications:* Thyroid drugs, antihypertensives, antidiabetic, anticoagulants, anti-Loch's, OC pills.
- Non-prescribed medications/herbal remedies
- Recreational drugs

Social History

- Occupation
- Support network
- Smoking
- Alcohol

Physical Examination

General Health

- Smoking/alcohol/drugs (especially intravenous usage).
- Note any other health symptoms or concerns, e.g. arthritis, physical mobility problems, any breast symptoms (such as breast tenderness, discharges, lumps), history of breast cancer, etc; acne, hirsutism, abnormal weight gain or loss, etc.
- Scar of past gynecological operations.

Examination: It is always done in the presence of female attendant with her full consent. Examination is done in covered place, initially with full bladder and then empty bladder. Any exposure of private parts is done by the patient herself. She has to be adequately explained about the reason of the examination and the family member accompanying her has to be informed. The patient may be provided a blanket or other clean cover to cover herself.

General Appearance

- Paleness
- Jaundice
- Smoke-stained fingers
- Obesity
- Extreme thinness
- Swollen abdomen
- Ankle swelling
- Look for pyrexia, shock, swelling
- Blood pressure, breast examination (if indicated)
- Abdomen palpation for:
  - Peritonitis.

– Abnormal lumps including enlarged kidney, liver, spleen, nodes in the groin and umbilicus, enlarged uterus, ovaries, bladder.
– Ascites, distended veins, peritoneal secondaries.
– To percuss the bladder, if palpably enlarged, or indicated from history.

Vaginal Examination

- Ask the patient to empty the bladder. All gynecologic examination is done with empty bladder except in a few situations like demonstration of GSI, cystocele, etc.
- Usually done with the patient on her back.
- Look at the vulva for any abnormalities of skin texture, lumps, excoriation, lichenification and whitening.

Speculum Examination

- Choose an appropriately sized speculum—usually Sims' or Cusco's bivalve speculum—for the patient. Sims is used to see the anterior vaginal wall lesion like VVF; Cusco is used for looking to cervix for its lesions (Fig. 3.1).
- Warm the speculum before use.
- Part the labia with your hand from above and introduce the speculum at a slight tilt to the vertical and twist it gently to the horizontal.
- Point the speculum downwards, at about 45°; open, making sure that the handle is not impinging on the clitoris.
- Look at the vaginal mucosa and locate the cervix.
- Take a vaginal swab, if there is discharge.
- Check for any retained tampon.
- Look for warts/herpes, polyp, erosion, growth.

If no Cervix is Visualized

- Try partially withdrawing and try again with speculum.
- Perform a bimanual examination to establish the position of the cervix.

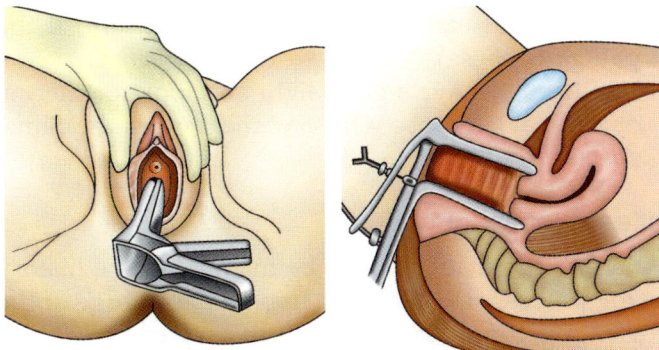

Fig. 3.1: How to insert Cusco speculum

- Ask the patient to hold on to her knees or put hands under the sacrum to tilt the pelvis. A pillow can also be used.
- The left lateral position may be more successful.

Examination in Sims' Position (Fig. 3.2)

- Position patient in the left lateral position
- Left leg extended
- Right knee drawn up to chest
- Hold back anterior vaginal wall with lubricated speculum—helpful to see VVF.

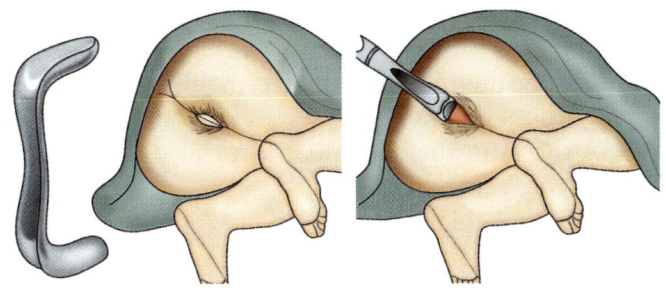

Fig. 3.2: Examination in Sims' position

Taking a Smear (Fig. 3.3)

- Ideally, this should take place mid-cycle.
- Visualize the cervix, clear excess mucus/discharge, unless using liquid-based cytology (LBC).
- If using a spatula, make two full 360° sweeps of the cervix to sample the transformation zone. Fix the slide immediately, as drying before fixing spoils the smear.
- If there is an obviously abnormal area on the cervix, note the position on the form/notes and include the area in your smear sweep.

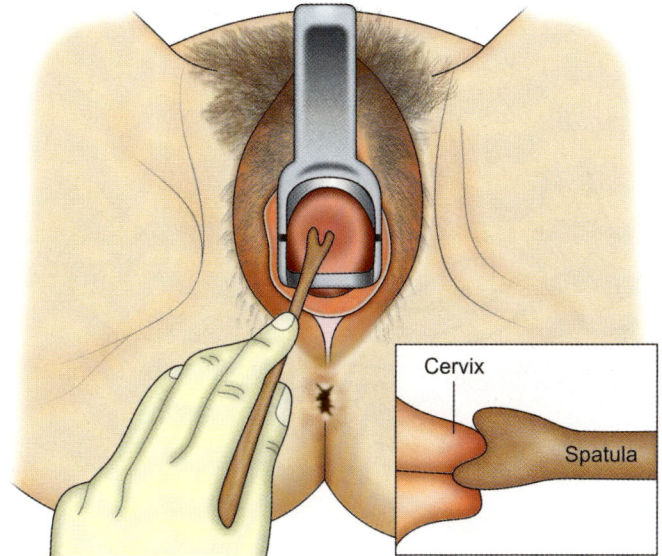

Fig. 3.3: To take smear

- If using a brush and LBC, take 5 anticlockwise sweeps of the transformation zone. Then (depending on the brush type) either push the end of the brush into the liquid, or agitate the brush in the liquid for 15–20 seconds to ensure there are adequate cells in the specimen. LBC has reduced the rate of inadequate smears. Training is provided locally.

Bimanual Examination

- Use your left hand to palpate abdomen and your right for internal (if examining from the right).
- Feel for any abnormalities of the vagina.
- Feel the cervix for areas of roughness, hardness, lumps.
- Assess the uterine position, size, mobility, lumpiness, tenderness (Fig. 3.4).
- Feel the adnexae bimanually for any swelling or tenderness (Fig. 3.5).
- Uterosacral thickening.
- *Pouch of Douglas:* Any tender nodule (endometriosis, metastatic ovarian cancer, pelvic Koch)

Uterine Size

- Within the pelvis (size of an orange) = 8 weeks.
- Suprapubic = 12 weeks.
- Mid-suprapubic umbilicus = 16 weeks.
- To umbilicus = 20 weeks.
- To xiphisternum = 36 weeks.
- To assess its position, mobility.

PR Examination

- To assess anal sphincter tone

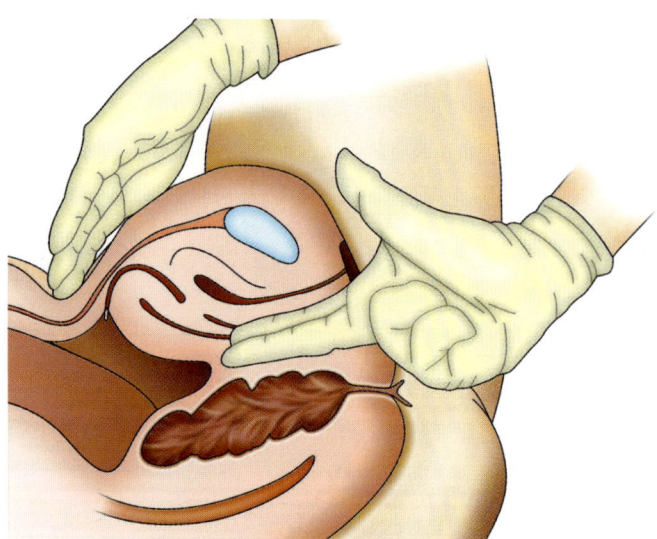

Fig. 3.4: Bimanual uterine examination

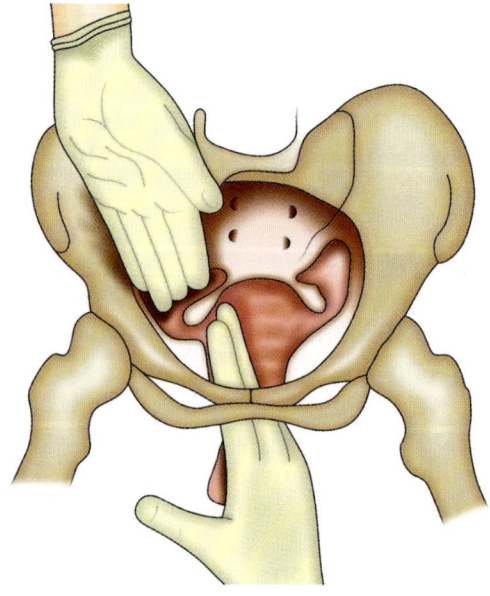

Fig. 3.5: Bimanual adnexal palpation

- To assess any CPT or anal injury or anal mucosal prolapse
- To assess pelvic tumor spread into parametrium or rectal involvement or any pelvic abscess

Rectovaginal Examination

- For diagnosis of rectovaginal nodule in endometriosis
- For staging of cancer cervix
- For diagnosis of enterocele

Urinary Incontinence

Confirmation of leakage can be done by asking the patient to cough whilst holding a tissue over the urethral opening, either lying or standing with the feet slightly apart. However, if there is a history of urinary incontinence, then refer for urodynamics.

Prolapse

- Vaginal examination needs to be performed with a Sims' speculum in the left lateral position looking for a cystocele or rectocele.
- An assistant can hold the leg at 30° (useful if the patient is obese).
- You need to have a good light and look for uterine or vaginal prolapse whilst withdrawing the Sims' speculum.

Differential Diagnosis

A differential diagnosis can be made after the history taking process. This is based upon a knowledge of the presenting complaints and the history of presenting complaints in relation to certain disease states.

Although there is a general structure for history taking in gynecology, there are small differences in the approach depending on what the presenting complaint is. It is essential for a physician to know the causes of each symptom and the other manifestations of those causes before taking a history.

Postcoital Bleeding

This is bleeding after intercourse. Causes include:
- Cervicitis
- Cervical erosion
- Cervical carcinoma
- Cervical polyps
- Vaginitis
- Vaginal cancer

Intermenstrual Bleeding

This is vaginal bleeding between menstrual periods. Causes include the following:

Cervical causes
- Carcinoma
- Ectropion
- Cervicitis
- Polyps

Endometrial causes
- Carcinoma
- Polyps
- Endometritis
- Intrauterine contraceptive device.
- Oral contraceptive pill or contraceptive injection

Vaginal causes
- Atrophic vaginitis
- Infective vaginitis
- Carcinoma

Ovarian causes
- Estrogen-secreting tumor
- Irregular ovulation

Fallopian tube causes
- Carcinoma

Post-menopausal Bleeding

This is vaginal bleeding more than 6 months after the menopause. Causes include:

Vaginal causes
- Atrophic vaginitis

Cervical causes
- Carcinoma
- Polyps

Endometrial causes
- Atrophic endometritis
- Carcinoma
- Polyps
- Hyperplasia

Ovarian causes
- Estrogen-secreting tumor

Other causes
- Ring pessary
- Exogenous estrogens (HRT)

Menorrhagia

This is history of heavy cyclical blood loss over several consecutive menstrual cycles in the absence of any intermenstrual or postcoital bleeding. Causes include the following:

Pelvic Pathology
- Uterine fibroids
- Endometriosis and adenomyosis
- Pelvic inflammatory disease
- Endometrial polyps

Endocrine causes
- Dysfunctional uterine bleeding
- Hypothyroidism

Hematological causes
- Disorders of coagulation
- Thrombocytopenia
- Leukemia

Oligomenorrhea and Amenorrhea

Oligomenorrhea is infrequent menstruation defined by a cycle length between 6 weeks and 6 months. Amenorrhea is absent menstruation for at least 6 months. They both have the same list for causes with one exception—primary failure of elements of the hypothalamic–pituitary–ovarian axis cause complete amenorrhea, not oligomenorrhea. Causes include:

Endocrine Causes
Hypothalamic disorders
- Kallman's syndrome—hypogonadotropic hypo-gonadism
- Psychogenic—stress/shift work

- Exercise
- Excessive weight gain/loss
- Tumors, e.g. craniopharyngioma
- Post-oral contraceptive use

Pituitary lesions
- Pituitary adenomas
- Sheehan's syndrome—infarction necrosis
- Granulomatous infiltration, e.g. sarcoidosis

Ovarian lesions
- Turner's syndrome—ovarian dysgenesis
- Polycystic ovarian syndrome
- Resistant ovary syndrome
- Premature ovarian failure
- Androgen-secreting ovarian tumors

Other
- Primary hypothyroidism/hyperthyroidism
- Poorly controlled diabetes mellitus
- Cushing's syndrome
- Addison's disease

Dysmenorrhea

This is painful menstruation which can be primary (absence of pelvic pathology) or secondary (attributed to pelvic pathology). Causes include the following:
- Endometriosis
- Pelvic inflammatory disease
- Submucosal fibroids
- Endometrial polyps
- Pelvic congestion syndrome
- Intrauterine contraceptive device
- Ovarian cysts
- Adenomyosis

Dyspareunia

This is pain during intercourse. Causes include:

Superficial
- Infection
- Vaginal atrophy
- Inadequate episiotomy repair
- Vaginal/rectal tumor

Deep
- Pelvic inflammatory disease
- Endometriosis

- Adenomyosis
- Cervicitis

Cervical Carcinoma

Age: This condition usually affects women between the ages of 35 and 55.

Clinical features
- Postcoital bleeding
- Intermenstrual bleeding
- Postmenopausal bleeding

Risk factors
- Early age of first experience of intercourse
- High number of sexual partners of patient or patient's current or past sexual partners
- HPV infection
- Smoking
- Low socioeconomic status

Endometrial Carcinoma

Age: >40 years

Clinical features
Post-menopausal bleeding

Risk factors
- Obesity
- Nulliparity
- Late menopause
- Unopposed estrogen stimulation
- Diabetes mellitus

Fibroids

Age: Women of child-bearing age

Clinical features
- Menorrhagia
- Abdominal swelling
- Frequency of micturition
- Pain

Risk factors
- Pregnancy

Endometriosis

Age: Women of child-bearing age

Clinical features
- Cyclical pelvic pain
- Dysmenorrhea
- Dyspareunia

Pelvic Inflammatory Disease

Clinical features

- Bilateral lower abdominal pain
- Fever
- Vaginal discharge
- Deep dyspareunia

Risk factors

- Multiple sexual partners

Polycystic Ovary Syndrome

Clinical features

- Oligomenorrhea
- Amenorrhea
- Hirsutism
- Infertility
- Acne
- Obesity

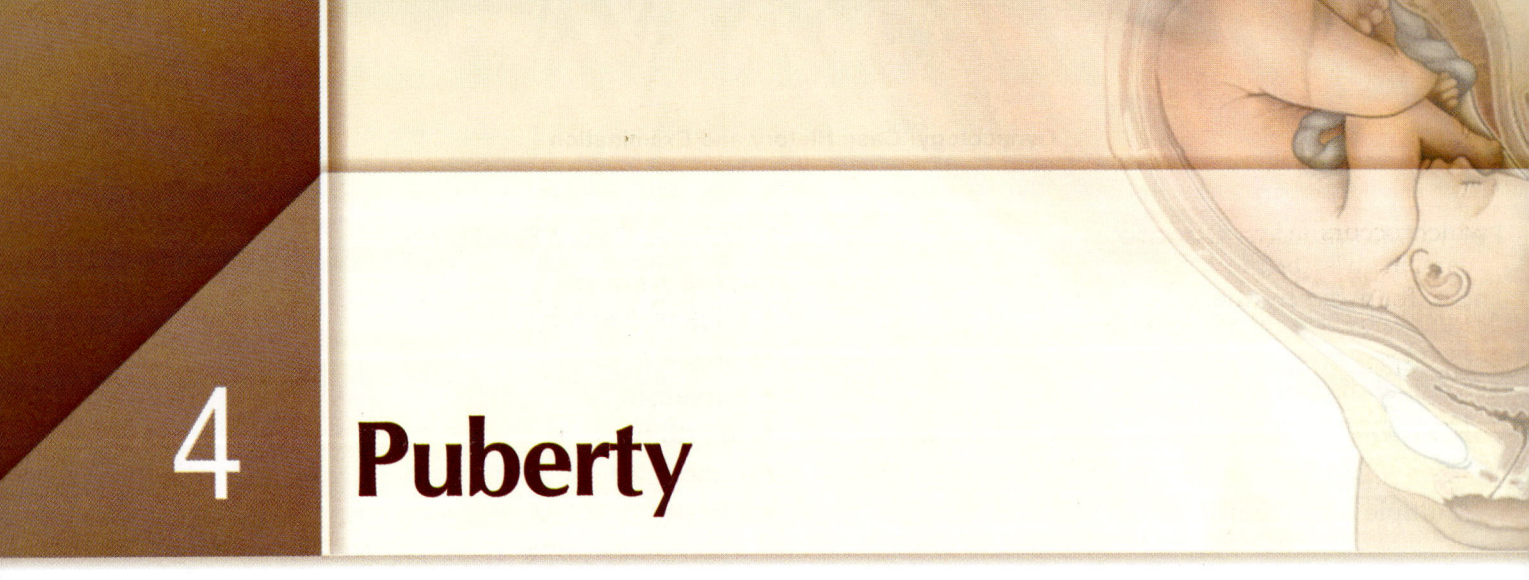

4 Puberty

Definition

Puberty is the stage of physical maturation in which an individual becomes physiologically capable of sexual reproduction. Puberty is originated from Latin word *"pubscere"*.

Physical changes that occur during puberty include:

1. *Adrenarche:* Activation of the adrenal glands whose hormonal stimulation is partially responsible for onset of body odor, increase in sweat rate, increase in skin oil production, acne and facial hair growth in both genders.
2. *Pubarche:* The appearance of pubic hair
3. *Thelarche:* The appearance of breast tissue
4. *Menarche:* The first menstrual bleeding

Factors Influencing on Puberty

Hypothalamus is responsible for puberty onset. The onset of puberty varies among individuals. Puberty usually occurs in girls between the ages of 10 and 14, while in boys it generally occurs later, between the ages of 12 and 16. The timing of the onset of puberty is not completely understood and is likely determined by a number of factors.

One theory proposes that reaching a critical weight or body composition may play a role in the onset of puberty. Therefore, increase in childhood obesity may be related to the overall earlier onset of puberty in the general population in recent years.

The primary stimulus of adrenarche is unknown. There is shift towards secretion of $\Delta 5$-3β-hydroxy-steroid intermediates (17α-hydroxypregnenolone, DHEA) and decreased production of $\Delta 4$-ketosteroids (17α- hydroxyprogesterone, androstenedione) and thus the serum DHEA concentration increases to 40 μg/dL. Adrenarche generally precedes activation of the hypothalamic–pituitary–gonadal axis by 2–3 years.

Leptin, a hormone produced by fat cells (adipocytes) in the body, has been suggested as a possible mediator of the timing of puberty. Further, girls with higher concentrations of the hormone leptin are known to have an increased percentage of body fat and an earlier onset of puberty than girls with lower levels of leptin. The concentration of leptin in the blood is known to increase just before puberty in both boys and girls.

Leptin is likely to one of multiple influences on the hypothalamus, an area of the brain that releases a hormone known as gonadotropin-releasing hormone (GnRH), which in turn signals the pituitary gland to release luteinizing hormone (LH) and follicle-stimulating hormone (FSH). LH and FSH secretion by the pituitary is responsible for sexual development.

Growth hormone is secreted from anterior pituitary in pulsatile fashion and at the onset of puberty GH pulse amplitude increases especially during sleep. GH gene is family of five distinct genes are located at chromosome17(17q22). GH secretion is controlled primarily by hypothalamus GH releasing hormone (GHRH) and peripherally by **ghrelin** which stimulates and **somatostatin** which inhibits GH release. The rate of increase in circulating GH levels is the most important determinant of the pubertal growth rate. Its peripheral action is mainly mediated through insulin-like growth factor-1 (IGF-1). IGF-1 is synthesized and secreted by the liver in response to GH stimulation. IGF-1 augments the effects of FSH and LH in the ovary, ACTH on steroidogenesis and thyroid response to TSH. IGF-1 level rises 7-fold from very low concentration at birth to peak values at puberty, falls rapidly by 50% by age of 20 and then declines slowly.

A gene has been identified that appears to be critical for the normal development of puberty. The gene, known as GPR54, encodes a protein that appears to have an effect on the secretion of GnRH by the hypothalamus. Individuals who do not have a functioning copy of this gene are not able to enter puberty normally.

The changes that happen during the process of puberty have a typical pattern with a generally predictable sequence of events. In most girls, the first sign of puberty is the beginning of breast development, which occurs at an average age of approximately 11 years. In girls, the growth of pubic hair typically begins next, followed by the growth of hair in the armpits. The onset of menstruation usually occurs around 2½ years after the onset of puberty.

A regular pattern of ovulation, usually develops rapidly once a girl begins menstrual periods. However, studies have shown that one-half of adolescent girls who begin to menstruate after age 13 will not ovulate regularly over the next 4½ years.

In boys, an increase in the size of the testicles is the first change observed at the onset of puberty. Enlargement of the testicles begins at an approximate average age of 11½ years in boys and lasts for about six months. After enlargement of the testicles, the penis also increases in size. Enlargement of the testicles and penis almost always occurs before the development of pubic hair. The next stage is the growth of pubic hair and hair in the armpits. Next, the voice becomes deeper and muscles increase in size. The last step is usually the development of facial hair. Fertility is achieved in males near the onset of puberty, when a surge in testosterone triggers the production of sperm.

The sequence of changes in puberty has been characterized as sexual maturity rating (SMR) or Tanner stages, named after a physician who described sequence of physical changes in puberty in 1969. Tanner stages are determined by the development of the secondary sex characteristics and encompass changes in the size and appearance of the external genitalia, the development of pubic hair, and breast development in girls. Tanner stages classify the extent of development of sex characteristics into five distinct steps ranging from stage 1 (prepubertal) to stage 5 (mature adult type).

Physical Changes during Puberty

Secondary Sex Changes

For any child experiencing puberty, the profound hormonal changes that are occurring center around the reproductive organs. This evolution commonly requires approximately five years from onset to completion.

In 1970, Dr WA Marshall and Dr JM Tanner published a landmark paper standardizing this sequence, and the series of changes have subsequently been known as the Tanner stages. These sequential stages of sexual maturity are listed below.

Males

- *Tanner I:* Preadolescent.
- *Tanner II:* Testicular enlargement and thinning of scrotal skin.

- *Tanner III:* Penile enlargement and continued increase in testicular size.
- *Tanner IV:* Further testicular/penile enlargement and appearance of pubic hair.
- *Tanner V:* Adult testicular/penile size and pubic hair distribution.

Females

- *Tanner I:* Preadolescent breast.
- *Tanner II:* Breast tissue development with onset of areolar enlargement sparse longitudinal labial pubic hair.
- *Tanner III:* Increase in breast tissue volume and areolar enlargement coarser and curlier pubic hair.
- *Tanner IV:* Adult breast shape and elevation of the nipple thickening and broader distribution of pubic hair.
- *Tanner V:* Mature adult breast shape and contour; adult pubic hair character and distribution.

The onset of puberty in males should take place between 9 and 14 years of age; females should experience the initial pubertal changes between 8 and 13 years of age. Precocious puberty is defined as the onset of the complete changes of puberty prior to these ages. Delayed onset of puberty implies lack of pubertal onset by the above time table. There are several medical conditions (both physiologically normal and abnormal) that may give rise to problems with only adrenarche, pubarche, or thelarche.

Table 4.1 describes the physical changes and their age of onset as described by Marshall and Tanner. There exists a standard deviation of approximately one year. It is important to note that while some adolescents have a methodical step-by-step march through this period of their life, others seem to follow a much more erratic timetable of maturation.

Several observations are notable when reviewing Table 4.1.

Table 4.1: Physical changes and their age of onset (Marshall and Tanner)		
Pubertal event	*Mean age of onset for boys*	*Mean age of onset for girls*
Breast development	N/A	11.2 years
Testicular enlargement	11.6 years	N/A
Pubic hair development	13.4	11.7
Peak height velocity	14.1	12.1
Menarche	N/A	13.5
Adult pubic hair configuration	15.2	14.4
Adult type breast	N/A	15.3

1. The duration of puberty for both genders is approximately five years.
2. Girls generally start puberty approximately one year ahead of boys.
3. Peak height velocity indicates that time of maximal acquisition of height ("growth spurt")
4. The onset of menstrual periods coincides with the slowing of rapid growth and is generally about 2½ years after the onset of puberty (Tanner II). This growth spurt occurs in females during the earlier stages of pubertal events while this occurs during the later stages of puberty in males. It is during this rapid height attainment in boys that a more muscular physique is established.

As children, both genders have a growth velocity of 3–4 cm/year. At the maximum pubertal growth rate, boys have a greater velocity (10.3 cm/yr) than their female counterparts (9 cm/yr).

- Adolescent growth spurt later in males than girls and not until genitalia stages 3–4.

Pubertal Stages (Tanner) Female (Figs 4.1 and 4.2)

- **P1:** Prepubertal.
- **P2:** Early development of subareolar breast bud +/- small amounts of pubic hair and axillary hair.
- **P3:** Increase in size of palpable breast tissue and areolae, increased amount of dark pubic hair and of axillary hair.
- **P4:** Further increase in breast size and areolae that protrude above breast level with adult pubic hair.
- **P5:** Adult stage, pubic hair with extension to upper thigh.

Pubertal Stages (Tanner) Male (Fig. 4.2)

- **P1:** Prepubertal, testicular length less than 2.5 cm
- **P2:** Early increase in testicular size, scrotum slightly pigmented, few long and dark pubic hair.
- **P3:** Testicular length 3.3–4 cm, lengthening of the penis, increase in pubic hair.
- **P4:** Testicular length 4.1–4.5 cm, increase in length and thickening of the penis, adult amount of pubic hair.
- **P5:** Testicular length greater than 4.5 cm, full spermatogenesis.

The "Growth Spurt"

A rapid increase in height, referred to as a growth spurt, usually accompanies puberty. This rapid increase in height typically lasts for two to three years. About 17–18% of adult height is attained during puberty. Although the increase in height affects both the trunk and the limbs, growth in the limbs usually happens first. The growth spurt characteristically occurs 2 years earlier in girls than in boys. In girls, the growth spurt peak height velocity typically precedes the onset of menstruation by about six months.

Bone Growth and Mineralization

Puberty is accompanied by growth of bones and increases in bone density in both boys and girls. In girls, bone mineralization peaks around the time of the onset of menstrual periods, at about 9–12 months after the time of peak height velocity (growth spurt). In females, approximately 50% of lifetime total body calcium is

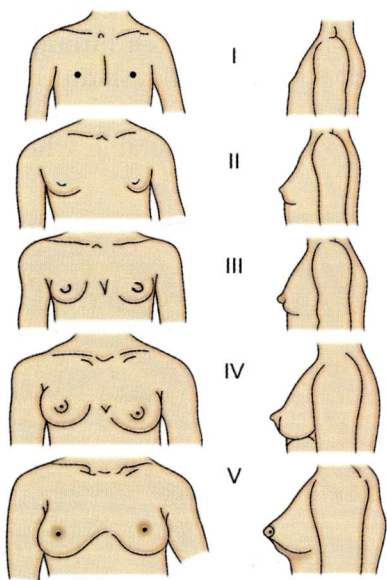

Fig. 4.1: Stages of breast development

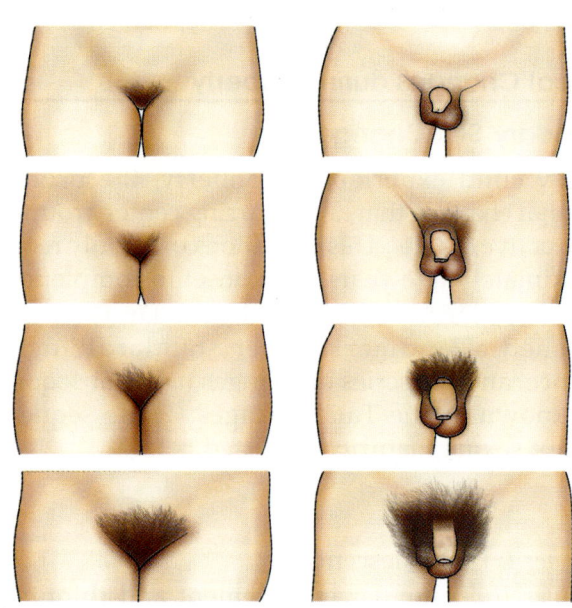

Fig. 4.2: Puberty in boys and girls

deposited into bones during puberty. In males, 50–65% of lifetime total body calcium is laid down, with males having approximately 50% more total body calcium than females. A woman's maximal calcium deposition in bones occurs during the first half of puberty. Studies have shown that bone width increases first, followed by bone mineral content, and lastly by bone density. Because of the lag between bone growth and achievement of full bone density, adolescents may be at increased risk for fractures during this time.

Weight Changes

Changes in weight and body composition occur in both boys and girls. Adolescent girls develop a greater proportion of body fat than boys, with redistribution of the fat toward the upper and lower portions of the body, leading to a curvier appearance. While boys also have an increase in the growth of body fat, their muscle growth is faster. By the end of puberty, boys have a muscle mass about one and a half times greater than that of comparably sized girls.

What Initiates Puberty?

GPR54 and its cognate ligand, kisspeptin-1mRNA, are found localized in the hypothalamus GnRH neurons. Kissepeptin activates LH and FSH release at the time of puberty. The mechanisms by which kisspeptin activates GnRH release, at the onset of puberty, are yet to be elucidated (Fig. 4.3).

Activation of the Hypothalamic–Pituitary-Gonadal Axis

- Induces and enhances the progressive ovarian and testicular sex hormone secretion.

- Is responsible for the profound biological, morphological, and psychological changes to attain adolescence.
- Enables sex steroid production for appearance and maintenance of sexual characters and attain capacity for reproduction.

During early infancy, GnRH activity starts from age 2 weeks to 6 months in boys and 12 months in girls. Testes secrete small amounts of testrosterone and ovaries estradiol. But there is always immature feedback to pituitary.

During childhood, feedback matures after 6 months with decline in FSH and LH. Lowest levels of FSH and LH are observed at about 4 years and in ovaries activity increases after 6 years.

During late prepuberty, increasing amplitude and frequency of GnRH are observed leading to increase in diurnal rhythms of LH, FSH and steroids release from about 6 years in girls. Estrogen then sensitises pituitary to release more GnRH.

During puberty, transition from childhood to adult occurs with growth acceleration, development of secondary sexual character and fertility (Fig. 4.4).

Uterine Development

- The prepubertal uterus is teardrop-shaped, with the neck as isthmus accounting for up to two-thirds of the uterine volume.
- With the production of estrogens, it becomes pear-shaped, with the uterine body increasing in length and thickness proportionately more than cervix.

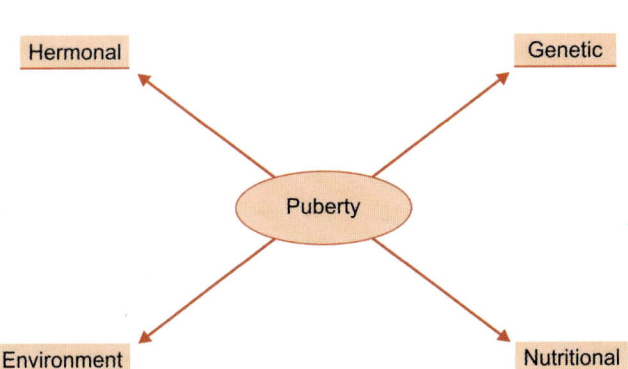

Fig. 4.3: Factors influencing on puberty

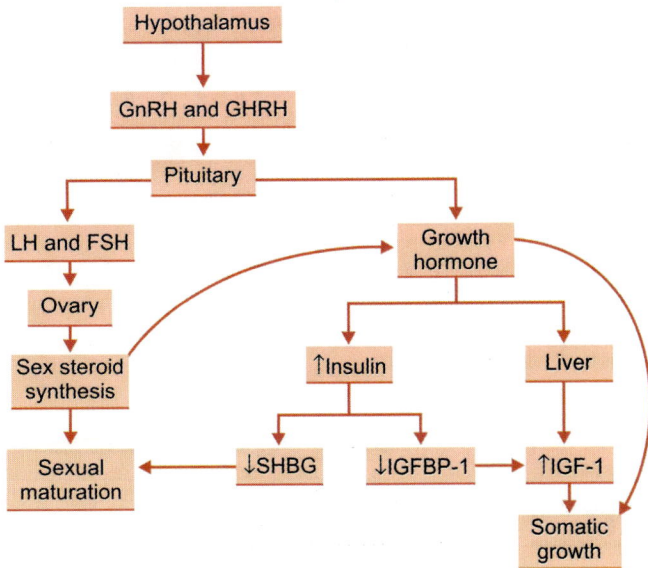

Fig. 4.4: Physiological effects of puberty

Ovarian Development

- The rising levels of plasma gonadotropins stimulate the ovary to produce increasing amounts of estradiol.
- Estradiol is responsible for the development of secondary sexual characters, i.e. growth and development of the breasts and reproductive organs, fat redistribution (hips, breasts), and bone maturation.
- The maturation of the ovary at adolescence correlates well with estradiol secretion and the stages of puberty.

- In prepuberty, the ovarian volume extends from 0.3 to 0.9 cm³. More than 1.0 cm³ indicates that puberty has begun.
- During puberty, the ovarian increases rapidly to a mean postpubertal volume of 4.0 cm³ (1.8 to 5.3 cm³).

Ovulation (Fig. 4.5)

- Plasma testosterone levels also increase at puberty although not as markedly as in males.
- Plasma progesterone remains at low levels, even if secondary sexual characters have appeared.

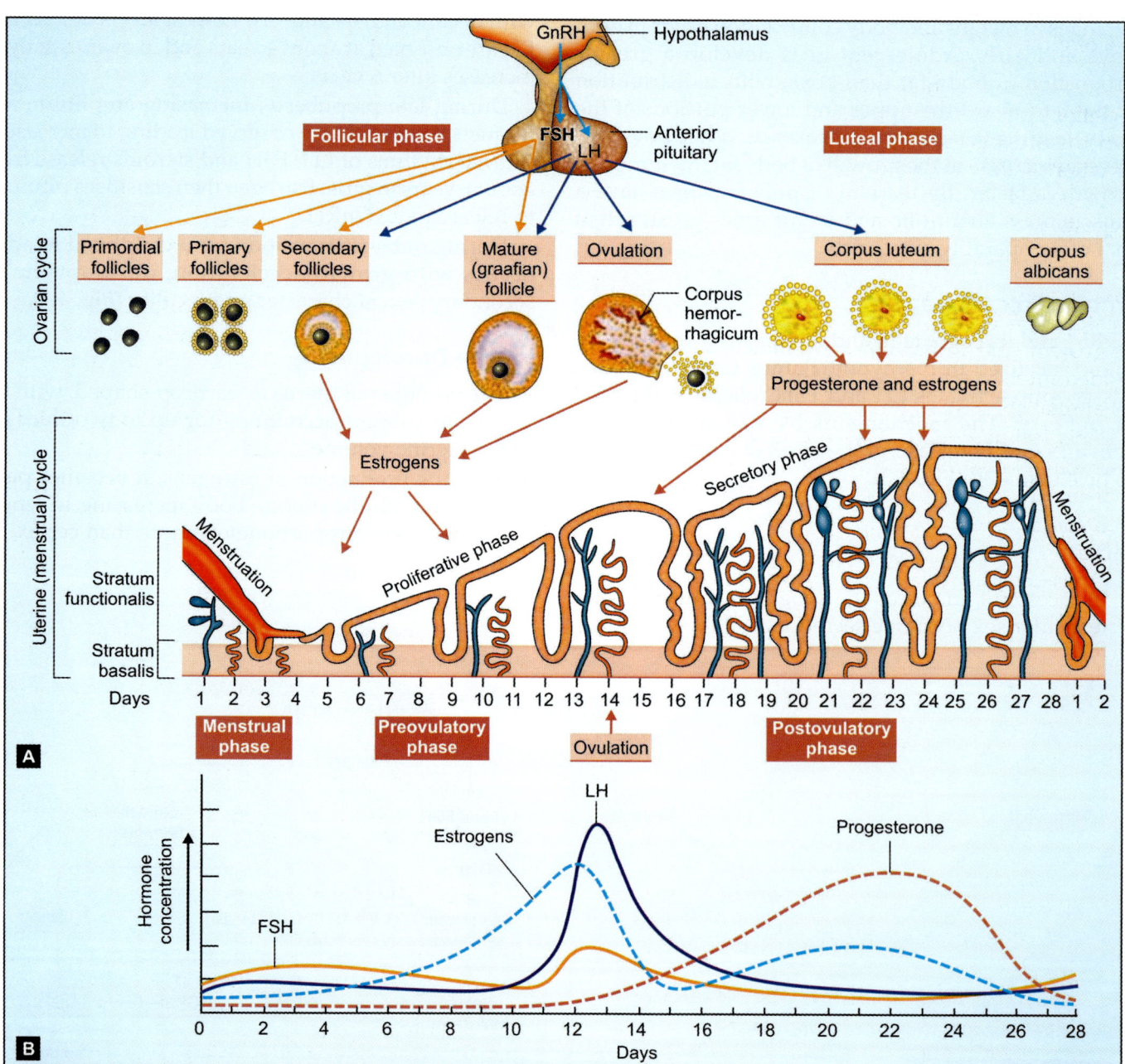

Fig. 4.5: (A) Hormonal regulation of changes in the ovary and uterus; (B) Changes in concentration of anterior pituitary and ovarian hormones

- A rise in progesterone after menarche indicates ovulation.

The first ovulation does not take place until 6–9 months after menarche because the positive feedback mechanism of estrogen is not developed.

Problems associated with Puberty

Delayed Puberty

Delayed onset of puberty is defined as occurring older than 2 SD of the average age of girls >13.4 years old and boys >14 years old. Breast development, usually the first sign, begins by the age of 12 years in more than 95% of girls.

Short stature is defined as height that is two standard deviations below the mean height for age and sex (less than the 3rd percentile) or more than two standard deviations below the mid-parental height. The child's rate of growth is important. A downward growth trend suggests a slowdown in growth.

A growth velocity disorder is defined as an abnormally slow growth rate, which may manifest as height deceleration across two major percentile lines on the growth chart. The causes of short stature can be divided into three broad categories:

- Familial short stature.
- Constitutional delay of growth and development.
- Chronic disease, including malnutrition and genetic disorders.

In some cases, short stature or slow growth is the initial sign of a serious underlying disease in an otherwise healthy child.

Epidemiology

- Delayed puberty occurs in approximately 3% of children.
- Constitutional delay in growth and puberty (CDGP) is more common in boys than in girls.

Causes of Delayed Puberty

I. *General*
- Constitutional delay of growth and puberty
- Malabsorption
  - Coeliac/imflammatory bowel disease
- Underweight
  - Dieting, anorexia nervosa, over-exercise
- Chronic illness
  - Asthma, malignancy, beta thalssemia major gonadal failure (hypergonadotropic hypo-gonadism)

II. *Constitutional delay*
- Positive family history, short stature, delayed epiphyseal maturation, relatively short upper body.
- Bone age is less than chronological age.
- Treatment for psychological reasons, with low dose ethinylestradiol: onset of breast development with a growth spurt and problem usually resolves

III. *Hypergonadotropic hypogonadism (43%)*
- a. Turner's syndrome
- b. Post-malignancy chemotherapy/radiotherapy/surgery
- c. Polyglandular autoimmune syndromes
- d. Gonadal deficiency
- e. Rare gene mutations inactivating FSH/LH or their receptors

IV. *Hypogonadotropic hypogonadism (31%)*
- Idiopathic
- *Kallmann's syndrome (X-linked):* Impaired migration of GnRH neurons; anosmia, disturbance in color vision, dyskinesis.
- *Prader-Willi syndrome (autosomal, dominant chromosome 15):* Obesity, muscle hypotonia, mental retardation, short stature, small hands/feet, cryptorchidism.
- Mutations in pathway for GnRH secretion and action (KAL, DAX1, GnRH receptor, etc.)

History

- *Growth pattern:* Adolescents with constitutional delay in growth and puberty (CDGP) have a long-standing history of short stature.
- *General health:* Any symptoms of chronic ill health.
- *Gonadal impairment:* History of cryptorchidism, orchidopexy, and gonadal irradiation, smell (for Kallmann's syndrome).
- *Family patterns:* Age at menarche in female members of family, delayed growth spurt.
- *Social and educational aspects:* Any indication of psychosocial problems.

Examination

- Height, weight; any suspicion of malnutrition.
- Measured parental and sibling heights (reported heights are much less reliable). Pubertal staging.
- Dysmorphic features.
- General examination, including fundoscopy and visual fields (pituitary tumor) and any indication of chronic disease, e.g. finger clubbing.

Investigations

Most boys and girls with delayed puberty have constitutional delay and do not need detailed investigation. In selected cases:

- *Investigations for chronic disease:* FBC, ferritin, renal function tests and electrolytes, coeliac screening, urinalysis for blood and protein, etc.
- Investigations related to disorders of gonadal axis.
- Chromosomes (e.g. for Turner's syndrome and Klinefelter's syndrome).
- Basal FSH and LH, thyroid function and serum estradiol/testosterone.
- Pelvic ultrasound in girls.
- *Bone age:* A delayed bone age may occur in constitutional delay, growth hormone deficiency and hypothyroidism.
- GnRH test and tests for prolactin and growth hormone; some cases of central delay are difficult to assess and the GnRH test cannot distinguish between physiological delay and gonadotropin deficiency.
- MRI or CT scan of the pituitary and surrounding structures may be indicated.
- A karyotype is obtained in girls with primary ovarian failure to detect chromosomal defects.

Calculate Expected Final Height

- The mid-parental height provides an estimation of the expected final height. If a child's height lies within the target centile range, then their height is normal with regard to their genetic potential.
- A calibrated stadiometer should be used for measuring standing height and the heights of the parents should be accurately measured rather than rely on reported heights. The mid-parental height is unreliable, if the parents' heights are very different.
- Mid-parental height (cm) = (Father's height – 14) + (Mother's height) divided by 2.

Bone Age

- Bone age can predict the final adult height by estimating skeletal maturation from an assessment of the ossification of the epiphyseal centers.
- The most widely used method is based on comparing frontal radiograph of the left hand and wrist with standards from the Greulich-Pyle atlas.
- Overemphasis of bone age evaluation can be misleading, if not used in the proper settings. The predictions do not apply to children with endocrine or bone pathologies affecting growth.

- Bone age is considered delayed, if it is two standard deviations below the chronological age.
- Bone age is usually normal for age in children with familial short stature. In children with constitutional delay of growth and puberty (CDGP), the bone age corresponds with height age and is delayed (up to two standard deviations). In children with pathological short stature, the bone age is severely delayed (more than two standard deviations).

Dental Age

This can provide an indirect assessment of skeletal age. The eruption of primary and secondary teeth may be delayed for up to 1.3 years in children with growth hormone deficiency, up to 1.5 years in children with constitutional delay of growth and puberty, and more than two years in children with severe hypothyroidism.

Management

1. *Constitutional delay in growth and puberty (CDGP):*
   - Medical treatment is usually not necessary and reassurance and monitoring are sufficient. However, short courses of sex hormones are an option, if delayed growth and puberty are causing psychological distress.
   - *CDGP in girls:* Gradually increasing doses of estrogen treatment, with cyclical progesterone therapy once adequate estrogen levels have been achieved.

   Dose: Oral or transdermal estrogen in doses below that used in adults (0.25–0.5 mg) micronized estradiol increasing gradually every 3–6 months to complete sexual maturation over a period of 2–3 years. Once breast development and menses are established, hormone therapy may be discontinued to assess the spontaneous response.

2. *Chronic disease*
   - Treat the underlying cause if possible; induction of puberty and hormone treatment may be required.

3. *Primary ovarian failure*
   - Estrogen replacement should be gradual to avoid premature fusion of the epiphyses and prevent overdevelopment of the areolae of the breast.
   - Gradually increased doses of ethinyl estradiol with cyclical progesterone therapy, once adequate estrogen levels have been achieved or if breakthrough bleeding occurs.
   - A low-dose combined oral contraceptive pill can then be used.

4. *Central delay*

- Treatment of any underlying cause like craniopharyngioma.
- Pubertal induction and hormone replacement.
- Pulsatile GnRH or gonadotropin therapy in documented GH deficiency or pituitary failure.

Precocious Puberty

Precocious onset of puberty is defined as puberty occurring younger than 2 SD before the average age in girls <8 years old and in boys <9 years old. They are of two types:

1. Gonadotropin-dependent (true/central)
2. Gonadotropin-independent

Premature menarche is one variant of central precocious puberty with isolated bleeds without any signs of sexual maturation. It is due to sporadic activation of H–P–G axis with estrogen too low for breast changes to occur. But one must exclude:

- Local lesions genital tract
- Estrogen intake
- Child abuse

Gonadotropin Dependent Causes ("true" or "central" precocious puberty)

- Idiopathic cause
- Family history may be present
- Overweight/obese
- Accounts for 74% girls (60% boys)
- TGF-α may stimulate GnRH secretion

Gonadotropin-independent Causes (FSH and LH Suppressed)

- CAH
- Sex steroid-secreting tumors
  - Adrenal or ovarian, Peutz-Jeghers syndrome
- McCune-Albright syndrome
  - Irregular areas of skin pigmentation, polyostotic fibrous dysplasia, ovarian functional cysts due to autonomous ovarian activation.
- Gonadotropin-secreting ovarian/adrenal tumors.
- Estrogen intake

Precocious puberty refers to the appearance of physical and hormonal signs of pubertal development at an earlier age than is considered normal. For many years, puberty was considered precocious in girls younger than 8 years; however, recent studies indicate that signs of early puberty (breasts and pubic hair) are often present in girls (particularly black girls) aged 6–8 years.

For boys, onset of puberty before age 9 years is considered precocious.

Early onset of puberty can cause several problems. The early growth spurt initially can cause tall stature, but rapid bone maturation can cause linear growth to cease too early and can result in short adult stature. The early appearance of breasts or menses in girls and increased libido in boys can cause emotional distress for some children.

Premature pubarche and premature thelarche are two common, benign, normal variant conditions that can resemble precocious puberty but are nonprogressive or very slowly progressive. **Premature thelarche** refers to the isolated appearance of breast development, usually in girls younger than 3 years; **Premature pubarche** refers to appearance of pubic hair without other signs of puberty in girls or boys younger than 7–8 years. A thorough history, physical examination, and growth curve review can help distinguish these normal variants from true sexual precocity.

If the history, physical examination, and laboratory data suggest that a child exhibits early and sustained evidence of pubertal maturation, the clinician must differentiate central precocious puberty (CPP) from precocious pseudopuberty. **Central precocious puberty**, which is gonadotropin-dependent, is the early maturation of the entire hypothalamic–pituitary–gonadal (HPG) axis, with the full spectrum of physical and hormonal changes of puberty. **Precocious pseudopuberty** is much less common and refers to conditions in which increased production of sex steroids is gonadotropin-independent. Correct diagnosis of the etiology of sexual precocity is critical, because evaluation and treatment of patients with precocious pseudopuberty is quite different than that for patients with central precocious puberty.

Pathophysiology

Most patients, particularly girls suspected of having central precocious puberty, are otherwise healthy children whose pubertal maturation begins at the early end of the normal distribution curve. CNS imaging studies of these otherwise healthy 6–8 years old girls usually reveal no structural abnormalities. The onset of puberty is caused by the secretion of high-amplitude pulses of gonadotropin-releasing hormone (GnRH) by the hypothalamus. Normally the hypothesized mechanisms that suppress onset of puberty include: (1) the HPG axis, which is highly sensitive to feedback inhibition by small amounts of sex steroids, and (2) central neural pathways that suppress the release of GnRH pulses.

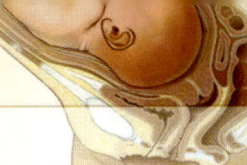

CNS abnormalities associated with precocious puberty include the following:

- Tumors (e.g. astrocytomas, gliomas, germ cell tumors secreting hCG.
- Hypothalamic hamartomas.
- Acquired CNS injury caused by inflammation, surgery, trauma, radiation therapy, or abscess.
- Congenital anomalies (e.g. hydrocephalus, arachnoid cysts, suprasellar cysts).

High-amplitude pulses of GnRH cause pulsatile increases in the release of pituitary LH and FSH. Increased LH levels stimulate production of sex steroids by ovarian granulosa cells. Pubertal levels of estrogens cause the physical changes of puberty, including breast development and pubic hair in girls. These levels also mediate the pubertal growth spurt. Increased FSH levels promote follicular maturation in girls.

Mortality/Morbidity

Isolated sexual precocity of unknown etiology carries no increased risk of mortality; however, distinguishing between children with idiopathic central precocious puberty and the rare patient with a CNS, adrenal, or ovarian tumor is important because the latter group may be at risk for tumor-related complications. Some studies have found an association between early puberty in girls and a higher risk of breast cancer.

Children with precocious puberty may be stressed because of physical and hormonal changes they are too young to understand. Girls with a history of early puberty have a slightly earlier age of initiation of sexual activity.

Children with precocious puberty more frequently exhibit behavioral problems and are less socially competent than age-matched peers. The distress associated with early menses can be decreased if parents are encouraged to prepare their daughters for this event when they reach stage III–IV of breast development.

Early puberty accelerates growth. These children may initially be considerably taller than their peers. Because bone maturation is also accelerated, growth may be completed at an unusually early age, resulting in short stature. Short stature is more likely if puberty starts very early (i.e. before age 6 years) than if it begins moderately early (i.e. ages 6–8 years).

History

Precocious puberty in girls:

- The first and most obvious sign of early puberty is usually breast enlargement, which may initially be unilateral.

- Pubic and axillary hair may appear before, at about the same time, or well after the appearance of breast tissue. Axillary odor usually starts about the same time as the appearance of pubic hair.
- Menarche is a late event and does not usually occur until 2–3 years after onset of breast enlargement.
- The pubertal growth spurt occurs early in female puberty and usually is evident by the time of initial evaluation.

Physical Examination

- The most reliable sign of increased estrogen production is breast enlargement. Initially, breast budding may be unilateral or asymmetric. Gradually, the breast diameter increases, the areola darkens and thickens, and the nipple becomes more prominent. Distinguishing glandular breast tissue from fat, which can mimic true breast tissue, is essential. Examining the patient while she is in the supine position usually minimizes the chance of misinterpreting fat as true breast enlargement.
- Genital examination may or may not reveal pubic hair, but enlargement of the clitoris indicates significant androgen excess that must be promptly evaluated. The vaginal mucosa, which is a deep-red color in prepubertal girls, takes on a moist pastel-pink appearance as estrogen exposure increases.
- Mild acne may be normal in early puberty, but rapid onset of severe acne, like clitoral enlargement, should increase suspicion of an androgen-excess disorder.

Causes

The timing of puberty has a genetic component. A history of early puberty in a parent or sibling is relevant and early puberty may not have any organic cause. Precocious puberty is familial in one-fourth of cases and that the predominant mode of inheritance is autosomal dominant. An increased body mass index (BMI) has been associated with early puberty.

Laboratory Studies

Sex steroid levels

- For girls, estradiol measurements are less reliable indicators of the stage of puberty. Levels that exceed 20 pg/mL usually indicate puberty. Girls who have ovarian tumors or cysts often have estradiol levels that exceed 100 pg/mL.
- Levels of adrenal androgens (e.g. dehydroepiandrosterone [DHEA], dehydroepiandrosterone sulfate [DHEA-S]) are usually elevated in girls with premature pubarche. DHEA-S, the storage form of

DHEA, is the preferred steroid to measure. In most children with premature pubarche, DHEA-S levels are 20–100 µg/dL, whereas in patients with virilizing adrenal tumors, levels may exceed 500 µg/dL.

- Serum level of 17-OH progesterone is needed when mild or nonclassic congenital adrenal hyperplasia is suspected. If basal level is below 200 ng/dL, the diagnosis of nonclassic congenital adrenal hyperplasia can be excluded; however, if the random 17-OH progesterone level is elevated, a corticotropin stimulation test provides the greatest diagnostic accuracy, with a post corticotropin 17-hydroxy-progesterone of greater than 1000 ng/dL being diagnostic.

Gonadotropins

- Because of the development of more sensitive third-generation assays for LH, which can detect levels as low as 0.1 IU/L or lower, LH is now the best screening test for central precocious puberty (CPP).
- Random follicle-stimulating hormone (FSH) levels do not discriminate between prepubertal and pubertal children. Suppressed levels of LH and FSH accompanied by highly elevated testosterone or estradiol levels point suggest precocious pseudopuberty rather than central precocious puberty.
- A definitive diagnosis of central precocious puberty may be confirmed by measuring LH and FSH levels 30–60 minutes after stimulation with gonadotropin-releasing hormone (GnRH) at 100 µg or with a GnRH analog.
- The GnRH analog leuprolide (aqueous form) at a dose of 20 µg/kg, up to a maximum of 500 µg is used. An increase in FSH levels much greater than the increase in LH levels suggests that the child is prepubertal.
- Some studies suggest that an increase in LH levels to more than 8 IU/L is diagnostic of central precocious puberty, but this depends on the specific LH assay used.

Thyroid

Thyroid tests are not a routine requirement in the evaluation of precocious puberty. Severe hypothyroidism rarely leads to precocious puberty. Major clues of severe hypothyroidism include growth arrest instead of growth acceleration, goiter, and symptoms of thyroid hormone deficiency (fatigue, cold intolerance).

Radiography

Radiography of the hand and wrist used to determine bone age is a quick and helpful means to estimate the likelihood of precocious puberty and its speed of progression. If bone age is within one year of chronological age, puberty has not started or the duration of the pubertal process has been relatively brief. If bone age is advanced by 2 years or more, puberty likely has been present for a year or more or is progressing more rapidly.

Imaging Studies

MRI of brain

- MRI may be indicated to look for a tumor or a hamartoma after hormonal studies indicate a diagnosis of central precocious puberty.
- For healthy girls aged 6–8 years with no signs or symptoms of CNS disease, the likelihood of finding a tumor or hamartoma is only about 2%; therefore, this test may be unnecessary depending on the clinical situation.
- The younger the child with central precocious puberty, the greater the chance of finding CNS pathology (among children younger than 6 years).

Pelvic ultrasonography

- Ultrasonography is unnecessary for girls with a definite diagnosis of central precocious puberty. If performed, however, ultrasonography usually reveals bilaterally enlarged ovaries, often with multiple small follicular cysts, and an enlarged uterus with an endometrial stripe.
- Pelvic ultrasonography is essential when precocious pseudopuberty is suspected in girls where an ovarian tumor or cyst may be detected.

Histological Findings

If central precocious puberty is caused by a tumor in the hypothalamic–pituitary area, the histology of the tumor can be important to the patient's prognosis.

Gliomas tend to grow more rapidly than astrocytomas, whereas hamartomas are benign.

Treatment of precocious puberty associated with a hamartoma suppresses gonadotropin production by the pituitary without effect on the hamartoma itself.

Surgical Care

When central precocious puberty (CPP) is caused by a CNS tumor other than a hamartoma, a resection should be attempted to the extent possible without impinging on vital structures such as the optic nerves. Radiation therapy is often indicated, if surgical resection is incomplete. Unfortunately, removal of the tumor rarely causes regression of precocious puberty.

Gonadotropin-releasing Hormone Analog

Continuous administration of LHRH and GnRH agonists provides negative feedback and results in decreased levels of LH and FSH 2–4 weeks after initiating treatment.

GnRH agonist: Suppresses ovarian and testicular steroidogenesis by decreasing LH and FSH levels. It is available in a monthly depot formulation in 7.5-, 11.25-, and 15-mg dose. Duration of therapy is individualized according to age and maturity of child and predicted adult height; in most cases, continuing treatment after age of 10–11 years is unnecessary.

LHRH agonist: LHRH agonist is a potent inhibitor of gonadotropin secretion when administered long term. It desensitizes responsiveness of pituitary gonadotropin. Circulating LH and FSH levels initially increase following administration, leading to transient increase in concentration of gonadal steroids. However, long-term administration decreases LH and FSH levels. Implant can provide continuous SC release of LHRH at nominal rate of 50–65 μg/day over 12 months. It is indicated for treatment of central precocious puberty (neurogenic or idiopathic).

Progestin: Before availability of GnRH agonists, these agents were the mainstay of therapy. Progestins work by providing feedback suppression of pituitary gonadotropin secretion. They lack significant androgenic or estrogenic activity.

Medroxyprogesterone acetate: It inhibits secretion of pituitary gonadotropin and effect of LH. It is effective by slowing breast growth and preventing or stopping menstruation although breakthrough bleeding may occur. It is used less now due to relative ineffectiveness in reversing rapid advancement of skeletal maturation seen in CPP.

Oral contraceptive: Low dose oral contraceptive tablets containing 15–30 μg ethinyl estradiol daily is used till epiphyses are closed. It should be started from 10–12 years. The efficacy is monitored by serial measurement of bony age every 6–12 months. The mean reduction in height ranges from 1–6 cm.

Follow-up

a. For patients with precocious puberty on treatment with gonadotropin-releasing hormone (GnRH) agonists:
   - Follow up every 4–6 months to ensure that progression of puberty has been arrested.
   - Favorable signs include normalization of accelerated growth, reduction (or at least no increase) in size of breasts, and suppression of gonadotropin levels after a challenge of GnRH.
   - Monitor bone age yearly to confirm that the rapid advancement seen in the untreated state has slowed, typically to a half year of bone age per year or less.

b. For patients not treated with GnRH agonists: In many cases, the physician may elect to observe the child with central precocious puberty (CPP), either because the age is borderline (i.e. 7–8 yrs) and the progression of puberty is not rapid and the bone age is only mildly advanced so that predicted adult height falls well within the reference range. In these cases, follow-up at 6-month intervals is appropriate. Testing and treatment may be initiated, if the growth of puberty begins to accelerate and predicted adult height deteriorates.

Prognosis

Without treatment

- Most girls with early puberty who are aged 6–8 years at the onset of puberty achieve an adult height within the reference range. Treatment with GnRH analogues is usually associated with only a modest gain in final height in this age group.
- Consider therapy following initial evaluation for girls who have predicted heights less than 4 ft 11 inch or who are well below their target height (i.e. average of parents' heights, less 2.5 inch) or when the patient has very advanced bone age but a height below the 25th percentile, or both.

With treatment

- Most studies show significant improvement in adult height compared with height predicted at the start of therapy, but the extent of this improvement depends to some extent on the age of onset of central precocious puberty.
- Height gained in girls after discontinuation of GnRH analogue therapy at age 11–12 years (and bone age 12–12.5 yers) is greater for girls with onset of central precocious puberty before age 6 years than at age 6–8 years or after age 8 years. The benefit of treatment in terms of increased adult height is the greatest in patients who are diagnosed with central precocious puberty and started on GnRH analogues at younger ages.
- Normal adult height can be achieved in most cases, if treatment is started before bone maturation is too advanced (>12 yr in girls, >13 yr in boys) and if good gonadal suppression is maintained for several years. Treatment allows growth to continue while dramatically slowing the rate of bone maturation.

Preoperative Care in Gynecologic Surgery

Introduction

Surgical treatment of the patients with gynecologic diseases is warranted only when all the conservative treatment has failed to deliver. Surgical treatment is associated with risks and complications which may be life-threatening. Surgery may be performed after the patient has been informed and her written consent is obtained regarding the risks associated with surgery. In order to avoid the risks and complications of surgery, preoperative patient preparation constitutes an important step and is done according to a precise sequence of procedures and measures.

During preoperative care, the gynecologic surgeon is fully acquainted with the patient's physical condition, and all the relevant data obtained during the interview with the patient must be inserted into the history of disease. The patient must be fully acquainted with procedures and risks of the surgery planned and must not be persuaded to undergo surgery against her own will. The patient must submit an informed written consent to confirm that she takes the risk of the planned surgical treatment. There are two groups of indications for gynecological surgery:

1. Absolute—when surgery must be undertaken, and its cancellation is life-threatening,
2. Relative—when surgery can be postponed till the most appropriate occasion for its performing. Before making a decision on surgery, one of the three requirements must be fulfilled: (a) relief of pain and suffering, (b) preservation of life, and (c) correction of an existing deformity.

Preoperative Examination

Preoperative examination should help a gynecologic surgeon to prepare patients for operation. In most cases, it involves a physical examination, various tests, risk stratification and modification of risk factors. The surgeon can thus reduce any delays in the preparation phase, to improve patient's safety, to recognize and treat complex medical problems, and to reduce costs and surgery cancellations.

A systemic assessment is done by the following steps:

1. *Detailed history*
2. *General medical history:* A gynecologic surgeon must know about the patient's cardiovascular diseases (congenital anomalies, blood pressure, arrhythmias), respiratory system (chronic obstructive pulmonary disease), endocrine and gastrointestinal diseases, neurologic status, hematologic condition (anemias, bleeding and coagulation disorders), health habits (smoking, intake of alcohol, drugs, diets, physical exercise) and socioeconomic status (marital status, occupation, education).
3. *Gynecologic and obstetric history*
4. *Clinical examination:* An adequate examination consists of the parameters such as vital signs, physical appearance, airways and lung auscultation, heart auscultation with rhythm determination; neurologic condition with mental status observation, sensorimotor abilities and detailed examination of the abdomen and pelvis. The physical examination should serve the surgeon to assess the severity and urgency in treatment of the disease process without which life carries a substantial risk.
5. *Complete gynecologic examination:* A proper clinical diagnosis is always mandatory for achieving success in treatment. This can be always corroborated by necessary investigations. A differentiation between benign and malignant nature of the disease process makes a huge difference in patient counseling before surgery. The route of surgical approach—abdominal, vaginal or laparoscopy must be determined judiciously on the basis of nature of underlying disease pathology, surgical expertise and maximum safety to the life of the patient.

6. *Preoperative indications for laboratory tests:* Laboratory analyses of the blood involve blood group determination, complete blood count, ESR, bleeding and coagulation time, thrombocytes, and fibrinogen. Renal and liver functions are checked. General analysis of the urine and urine-culture, chest X-ray, ECG is routine investigating procedure.

7. *Anesthesiologic preoperative examination:* Anesthesiologic surgical risk is assessed based on the assessment of physical status created by the American Society of Anesthesiology (ASA), classifying them into six categories defining the risk of death:
    i. Group—original disease, if it is without a systemic impact;
    ii. Group—moderate systemic disease without functional impediments;
    iii. Group—severe systemic disease with serious functional impediments;
    iv. Group—severe systemic life-threatening disease;
    v. Group—moribund patient, with life expectancy below 24 hours;
    vi. Group—confirmed brain death

8. *Preoperative use of antibiotics:* A recommended regimen for patients undergoing vaginal hysterectomy, abdominal or radical hysterectomy consists of a dose of IV cefazolin (1 g) or cefotetan (1 g) at the induction of anesthesia, or aminoglycosides with metronidazole. The regimes are as follows:
    a. Cephalosporins first generation: up to 2.0 g
    b. Metronidazole 0.5–1.0 g + gentamicin 1.5 mg/kg IV.
    c. Clindamycin 600–900 mg IV + gentamicin 1.5 mg/kg
    d. Ciprofloxacin 400 mg IV

9. *Risk factors of developing postoperative infection in gynecologic surgery:*
    a. Age of patient
    b. Body mass
    c. Presence of regional infection
    d. Chronic disease (malignant disease, diabetes, hypertension, liver, lung disease, etc.)
    e. Duration of operation (risk of infection doubles after 60 min following the first hour)
    f. Patient's weak immune system
    g. Problems with intestinal tract (ileus, previous operations, radiations, etc.)
    h. Bad surgical technique (stitching bigger tissue parts than necessary, tissue maceration, etc.)
    i. Imperfect hemostasis
    j. Noise and conversation in the operating theatre, air-borne contamination

10. *Prevention of thromboembolic disease:* Deep venous thrombosis (DVT) and venous thromboembolic (VTE) disease are significant and statistically confirmed complications of surgical treatment. The rate of postoperative VTE ranges from 15 to 40% in women undergoing major gynecologic surgery without thromboprophylaxis. Important factors in the occurrence of postoperative venous thrombosis in gynecologic surgery are age (years) and extent of the surgery. Additional risk factors for DVT and VTE disease are trauma associated with prolonged surgery (interventions lasting over 300 minutes and loss of over 600 mL of blood), earlier DVT, varicose veins, infection, malignancy, estrogen treatment, earlier pelvic radiation therapy, smoking, obesity, immobility.
    A thrombus most commonly occurs in the period of 24 hours after surgery. Prevention of VTE disease in gynecologic surgery is performed by: (a) Low-dose heparin preparations which are administered subcutaneously and initiated 2 hours before surgery, continuing for 7 postoperative days in 8–12 hours intervals; (b) by use of elastic stockings for prevention of thromboembolic disease in the medium- and high-risk patient group (Table 5.1).

11. *Immediate preparation of patients for gynecologic surgery:* A patient list should contain all the agents and procedures performed during preoperative patient preparation.
    a. It is necessary to use laxative like bisacodyl for bowel emptying 24 hours before surgery, and if required, a deep enema in the evening before or morning on the day of operation.
    b. In the evening before surgery, a nurse should remove all pubic hair from the patient's external genitals, performs vaginal toilette and applies an antiseptic vaginal tablet, and the patient may take a shower and clean her anterior abdominal wall, if abdominal surgery is planned.
    c. A dose of sedative is given after dinner on the night before surgery.
    d. In developed country, particularly for obese patients, on the day of operation, two hours before surgery, a planned low-dose heparin is administered, and prophylactic administration of antibiotics and bandaging of the lower extremities with an elastic bandage or

Table 5.1: Risk groups according to thromboembolic disease prevention

Low risk	Moderate risk	High risk	Highest risk
1. Do not have risk factors	1. Surgery lasting less than 30 minutes in patient with additional risk factors	1. Major surgery in patients older than 40 years or with additional risk factors	1. Major surgery in patient older than 60 years plus deep vein thrombosis, cancer or hypercoagulable state
2. Younger than 40 years of age	2. Surgery lasting less than 30 minutes in patients aged 40–60 years with no additional risk factors	2. Surgery lasting less than 30 minutes in patients older than 60 years or with additional risk factors	2. Pelvic exenteration
	3. Major surgery in patients younger than 40 years with no additional risk factors		3. Radical vulvectomy with inguinofemoral lymphadenectomy
			4. Major surgery + deep vein thrombosis history and lung thrombosis

compressive stockings is done 30 minutes before surgery.
  e. Before the induction of anesthesia, disinfection of the vagina and anterior abdominal wall is performed, and a Foley catheter is placed into the bladder. The operation field is delineated with sterile surgical clothes before the operation is commenced.

Consent for Surgery

The medical professional liability issues of the 1970s and 1980s were nothing in comparison to the circumstances affecting physicians today. Information about medicine and health has become a staple of consumer interest, yet the consumer is often inadequately prepared to appreciate the limitations of science despite its advances. In reality, whatever the intended effect of a medical or surgical intervention, an unsatisfactory outcome has often resulted in the full use of one's legal rights and remedies.

The informed consent process epitomizes this sharing of information and represents a partnership between physician and patient. It is a process because it takes some time to share information, exchange queries and answers, to reflect and consider the alternatives, and to make a decision. Informed consent is a deliberative and interactive session.

Traditionally, physicians have considered themselves most capable of making medical decisions for their patients. This logical but paternalistic attitude was not only accepted but also not expected by our patients. The doctrine of informed consent has, in a pragmatic way, significantly altered this approach. It has taken medical decision-making away from the sole proprietorship of the physician and given an important role to the patient.

The foundational elements of informed consent are, therefore:
1. The knowledge between the doctor and the patient is not in parity.
2. A competent adult has the right to decide whether to submit to lawful medical treatment.
3. Consent to treatment must be informed.
4. The patient is dependent on the doctor for information to make an informed choice.

What Information is to be Disclosed in Consent?

1. Patient's diagnosis of disease
2. Alternative treatments or options
3. Material risks and complications
4. Consequences of non-treatment
5. Any personal interests

Exceptions to Informed Consent

In balancing the decision-making equation, the courts have allowed certain exceptions to the informed consent doctrine. Under either the majority or minority rules, there are specific situations that make disclosure unnecessary.

Disclosure is reasonably believed to be unnecessary in the following circumstances:
1. If the risk is not reasonably foreseeable and not inherent in the procedure.
2. If full disclosure would be detrimental to the patient's best interest.
3. If the danger is commonly known and it can be assumed that the patient knows the danger.
4. If the patient has requested that she not to be told of the risk.

5. If the patient is already aware of the risk.
6. If the doctor can establish that the patient would have proceeded with the treatment whether or not she knew of the risks.
7. If the risks have no apparent materiality or relation to the patient's decision.
8. If the risk concerns improper performance of an appropriate procedure.
9. If an emergency situation exists requiring prompt treatment in the face of immediate possibility of permanent injury or death and the patient is in no condition to make a decision.

6 Principles of Surgical Techniques in Gynecology

Introduction

The success of a gynecologic procedure performed through an abdominal incision depends on careful selection of the incision site and proper closure of the wound. The surgeon needs to consider multiple factors before making an abdominal incision. These factors include the disease process, body habitus, operative exposure, simplicity, previous scars, cosmesis, and the need for quick entry into the abdominal cavity. The most important factor is adequate exposure to the operative field.

Complications during surgery can occur because of inadequate exposure, which is often due to the unwillingness of the surgeon to extend the incision. Incision location is particularly important when the patient has a gynecologic malignancy. These patients may need a colostomy, urinary diversion, or extraperitoneal lymph node dissection to satisfactorily manage the clinical situation.

A thorough understanding of abdominal wall anatomy is essential for choosing and making the proper surgical incision. The musculature of the abdominal wall is composed of 2 muscle groups.
1. The flat muscles consist of the external oblique, internal oblique, and the transversus abdominis.
2. The second group is composed of 2 muscles that run vertically, the rectus abdominis and the pyramidalis.

Group 1

The **external oblique muscle** is the largest and most superficial of the flat muscles of the abdominal wall. Arising from the lower 8 ribs, the external oblique courses transversely to insert upon the iliac crests. The aponeurosis is a strong tendinous sheath that ends medially in the linea alba.

The **internal oblique muscle** arises from the upper surface of the inguinal ligament, the iliac crest, and the thoracolumbar fascia. This muscle courses at a right angle to the fibers of the external oblique muscle. The aponeurosis of the internal oblique splits at the edge of the rectus muscle to envelope the rectus. The anterior layer blends with the aponeurosis of the external oblique. Posterior to the rectus muscle, this aponeurosis blends with the aponeurosis of the transversus abdominis to form a portion of the posterior rectus sheath.

The innermost of the flat muscles is the **transversus abdominis**. This muscle arises from the inguinal ligament, the iliac crest, the thoracolumbar fascia, and the lower costal cartilages. Coursing transversely to the midline, the upper three-fourths of the transversus aponeurosis lies behind the rectus muscle. The lower one-fourth of the aponeurosis passes in front of the rectus muscle. The aponeurosis of each flat muscle joins medial to the rectus muscle to form the linea alba.

Group 2

The **rectus abdominis** muscle originates from the pubic crest, runs vertically to insert into the xiphoid process and the fifth, sixth, and seventh costal cartilages. The rectus is surrounded by the rectus sheath, which consists of the aponeuroses of the oblique muscles and the transversus abdominis.

A small, vestigial, triangular-shaped muscle, the **pyramidalis,** arises from the symphysis and inserts upon the linea alba. This muscle marks the midline and assists in the identification of the medial borders of the rectus muscle.

Blood Supply

The primary blood supply to the abdominal wall is from the superficial and deep vasculature. The superficial vasculature originates from branches of the femoral artery and includes the superficial epigastric, the superficial circumflex, and the superficial external pudendal arteries. These vessels course through the tissues anterior to the rectus sheath.

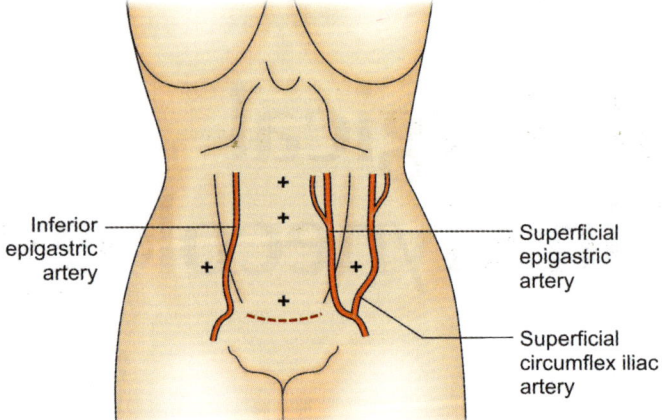

Fig. 6.1: Deep and superficial vessels of the anterior abdominal wall

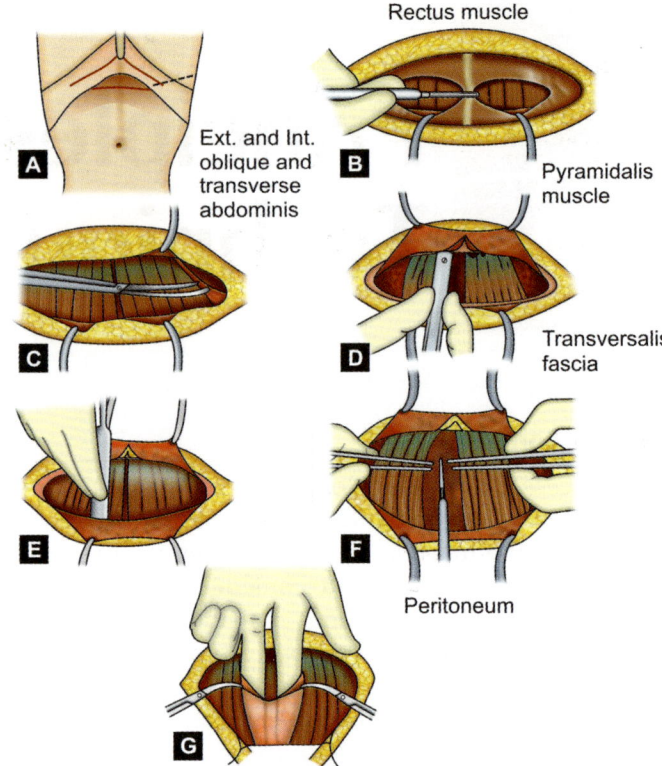

Fig. 6.2: Layers of abdominal wall

The deep vasculature is composed of vessels from the external iliac artery and the internal thoracic artery. The inferior epigastric artery originates from the external iliac artery and courses posterior to the lateral one-third of the rectus muscle. Another branch of the external iliac is the deep circumflex artery, which courses cephalad lateral to the inferior epigastric artery. The superior epigastric artery is the terminal branch of the internal thoracic artery. This artery has multiple branches leading to the rectus muscle and has an anastomosis with the inferior epigastric artery. The internal thoracic artery is the source of the musculophrenic artery, which has an anastomosis with the deep circumflex artery. This large network of vascular anastomoses in the abdominal wall provides an excellent blood supply to all areas of the abdominal wall (Fig. 6.1).

Abdominal Incisions

Abdominal incisions used for most gynecologic procedures are divided into transverse and vertical incisions (Table 6.1).

Pfannenstiel Incision

The incision is usually made 1–2 fingerbreadths above the pubic crest. An incision length of 10–14 cm is sufficient. Increasing the length of the skin incision usually does not improve exposure due to the rectus muscles. The incision is made through the subcutaneous fat to the fascia. The superficial epigastric vessels are often near the lateral edges of the incision (Fig. 6.2).

The anterior fascia is incised in the midline with a scalpel or electrocautery. Using curved scissors or electrocautery, the fascia is incised in a curvilinear fashion 1–2 cm lateral to the rectus muscle. The upper edge of the fascia is grasped with 2 Allis forceps on either side of the midline. Using electrocautery, the rectus muscle is dissected free from the fascia. Electrocautery allows coagulation of multiple small vessels that perforate the rectus muscle to the fascia. The rectus muscles are mobilized off the fascia to the level of the umbilicus. Next, the lower fascial edge is grasped with 2 Allis forceps. Electrocautery is used again to dissect the rectus and the pyramidalis muscles from the fascia. The rectus muscles are separated. The peritoneum is opened and incised vertically to complete a Pfannenstiel incision.

Closure of the Pfannenstiel incision is straightforward. The peritoneum does not need to be closed separately as re-epithelialization occurs within 48 hours. Closure of the peritoneum does not add to the strength of the incision. The rectus muscles should be thoroughly irrigated with water or saline, and any bleeding areas should be cauterized or ligated. Bleeding from small perforating vessels through the rectus muscle is the most common source of rectus sheath hematoma. The fascia is approximated with a delayed absorbable suture. Usually, a separate suture is started at each end of the fascial incision with 2 cm gap and thickness and all layers of the anterior rectus sheath are incorporated. Unless a large area of dead space exists between the fascia and the skin, closure of the Scarpa fascia is not needed. Placement of a closed

Table 6.1: Advantages and disadvantages of transverse and vertical incisions

	Transverse incisions	Vertical incisions
1. Cosmesis	Best consmetic results	Less cosmesis
2. Strength	30 times stronger	Vertical incisions are weak
3. Pain	Less painful	More painful
4. Relation with postoperative	Least respiratory discomfort	More respiratory discomfort
5. Risk of wound dehiscence	Least with transverse incision	More with paramedian incision
6. Exposure	Exposure to central pelvis is more	More with further extension upwards
7. Entry to abdomen	Slow in transverse incision	Fast in vertical incision
8. Bleeding	Bleeding risk more	Bleeding is less
9. Nerve injury	More frequent	Rare

drainage system, like a Jackson-Pratt drain, may be needed, if a large amount of fluid collection is anticipated (Fig. 6.3).

Maylard Incision

In an effort to improve surgical exposure to the lateral pelvic sidewall with a transverse incision, Maylard

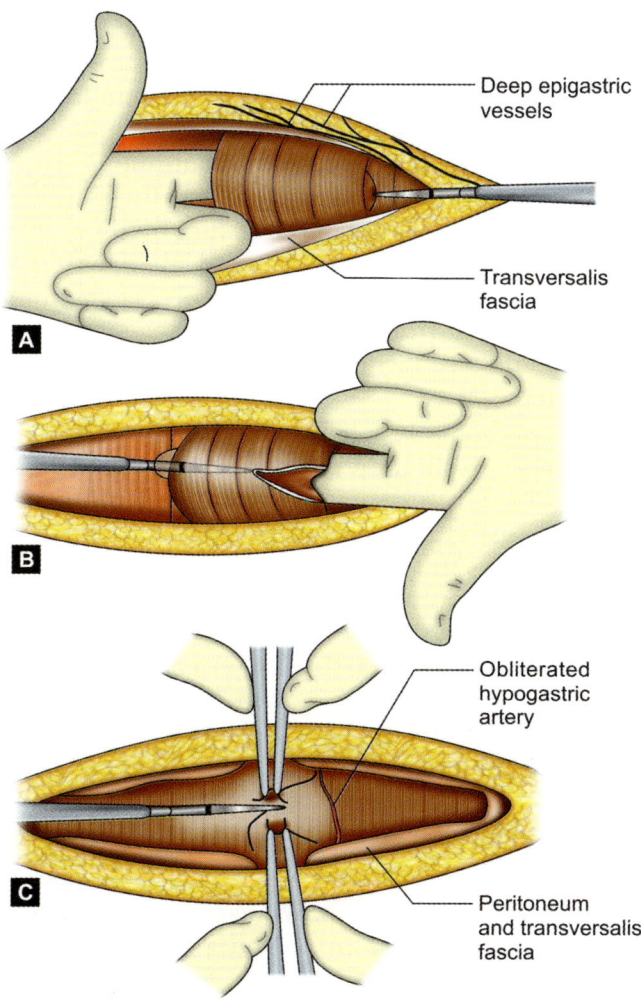

A

B

C

Fig. 6.3: Steps of entry into abdominal cavity

Deep epigastric vessels

Transversalis fascia

Obliterated hypogastric artery

Peritoneum and transversalis fascia

proposed a transverse muscle-cutting incision. For gynecologic surgery, the incision is made 3–8 cm superior to the pubis symphysis. The anterior rectus sheath is cut transversely. The inferior epigastric vessels are identified under the lateral edge of each rectus muscle and then are ligated. Patients with significant peripheral arterial disease may experience ischemia from ligation of the inferior epigastric vessels. These patients may have collateral flow from the epigastric vessels to the lower extremities. After ligation of the inferior epigastric vessels, **electrocautery is used to transversely cut the rectus muscle**. The peritoneum is opened and cut laterally.

During closure, the peritoneum is first closed with an absorbable suture. The cut edges of the rectus muscles are examined for any bleeding areas. The fascia and underlying rectus muscle can be closed with a monofilament absorbable suture.

Cherney Incision

Cherney described a transverse incision that allows excellent surgical exposure to the space of Retzius and the pelvic sidewall. The skin and fascia are cut in a manner similar to a Maylard incision. The rectus muscles are separated to the pubis symphysis and separated from the pyramidalis muscles. A plane is developed between the fibrous tendons of the rectus muscle and the underlying transversalis fascia. Using electrocautery, the rectus tendons are cut from the pubic bone. The rectus muscles are retracted and the peritoneum to be opened.

Closing a Cherney incision begins with closure of the peritoneum. The cut ends of the rectus muscle are attached to the distal end of the anterior rectus sheath with interrupted nonabsorbable sutures. Fixing the rectus muscle to the pubis symphysis can result in osteomyelitis. The fascia is then closed with 2 continuous, delayed-absorbable sutures (Table 6.2).

Table 6.2: Comparative study of characters of different skin incisions

Incisions	Pfannenstiel	Cherney	Maylard	Vertical
Pelvic exposure	++	+++	++++	+++
Upper abdomen exposure	—	+	++	++++
Potential blood loss	++	+	++	+++
Potential hernia	+	+	++	+++
Evisceration risk	—	+	++	+++
Speed	++	+++	+	++++

Modified Gibson Incision

Gynecologic oncologists perform an extraperitoneal lymph node dissection using a modification of the Gibson incision. This incision can be made on each side of the midline, but often, the skin is cut only on the left. The incision is started 3 cm superior and parallel to the inguinal ligament. Extension is made vertically 3 cm medial to the anterior superior iliac spine to the level of the umbilicus. The fascia is cut and the peritoneum bluntly dissected. The round ligament and the inferior epigastric vessels are ligated to facilitate surgical exposure. This incision is needed for extraperitoneal approach to pelvic space particularly for lymph node dissections.

Vertical Incision

Several types of vertical abdominal incisions have been used in gynecologic surgery, including midline, paramedian, and wide paramedian incisions.

a. A midline incision is almost exclusively the type of vertical incision used in gynecologic oncology surgery. The midline incision is the easiest and most versatile vertical incision for performing gynecologic cancer surgery. This incision allows quick entry into the abdominal cavity with a little blood loss, and it is easily extended in length to accommodate the operative findings. The presumed increased risk of wound dehiscence and hernia formation have been now challenged and it is advocated that a little difference exists in dehiscence rates between properly closed midline incisions and transverse incisions.

b. For a midline abdominal incision, the skin and subcutaneous fat are incised to the level of the fascia. The scalpel or electrocautery can be used to incise this tissue. Some surgeons believe the infection rate is higher with the use of electrocautery. However, more recent prospective studies indicate no increased wound complications with electrocautery compared with a scalpel in midline abdominal incisions.

Using either instrument, the principle is to make long smooth strokes through the subcutaneous fat to the fascia. The subcutaneous fat should not be dissected from the fascia because this creates unnecessary dead space. Next, the fascia is incised, and the rectus muscles are separated vertically in the midline. The midline may not be evident in patients with previous abdominal surgery. It can be identified where the rectus muscles diverge around the umbilicus or locating the pyramidalis muscles assists in identifying the midline. Once the rectus muscles are divided, the peritoneum is grasped between 2 hemostats, opened with a scalpel, and extended afterward the length of the incision.

If the operative findings necessitate extending the incision above the umbilicus, cutting through the umbilicus is avoided. Postoperative wound infections may be increased due to bacterial colonization of the umbilicus. Extension of the incision should pass to the left of the umbilicus to avoid cutting through the ligamentum teres.

Closure of the midline incision by layered closure using interrupted sutures is still the choice of many surgeons. Today, many surgeons prefer to close the abdominal wall with a continuous running suture using delayed absorbable sutures. Two basic techniques are used to close the abdomen with continuous suture: (a) Single-layer mass closure, and (b) Internal mass closure. The **single-layer mass closure** involves using a heavy monofilament delayed-absorbable or permanent suture. Fascial closure involves penetrating the fascia 1.5 cm from the edge with the suture. The suture should also include the underlying muscle and peritoneum.

Some surgeons close the wound using **the internal mass closure** technique advocated by Smead-Jones. This is a far-far, near-near suturing technique. The anterior fascia is included in the near-near bite. The initial stitch is similar to the single-layer mass closure. The second bite only includes the anterior rectus fascia, approximately 0.5 cm from the fascial edge. Either technique requires starting from each end of the incision. Securing the suture with 5 knots at each end is sufficient. In patients who are slender, burying the knot is helpful (Fig. 6.4).

Incisions in Obese Patients

Surgery in patients who are obese represents a challenge for every surgeon. Wound complication rates are uniformly higher in patients who are obese, regardless of the type of incision. Obtaining adequate surgical exposure requires patience, understanding of

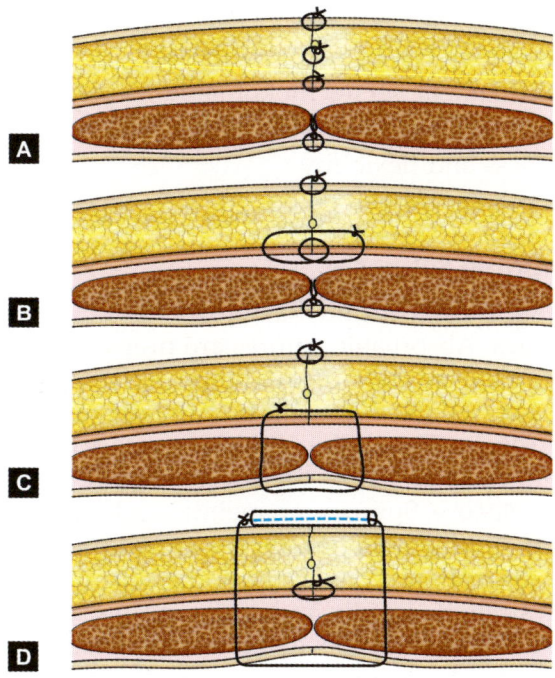

Fig. 6.4: Techniques of abdominal wall closure

changes in anatomical landmarks, and proper surgical equipment. Problems in obese patients are:

a. The abdominal wall landmarks are distorted in patients who are obese, particularly in the presence of a large panniculus. The umbilicus is located caudal to its normal position. If a vertical incision is needed, first the panniculus is pulled downward. A periumbilical incision is made and the fascia is incised to the symphysis. Care is needed not to buttonhole the skin under the panniculus. Use of a ring retractor, such as the Bookwalter, optimizes surgical exposure.

b. The site of a transverse incision in patients who are obese should never be made under the fold of the panniculus. Wound complications are invariably higher compared with an incision made away from the panniculus.

c. Ideally, a paraumbilical midline incision should be made. In some patients, this will not allow for adequate exposure to the pelvic organs. The surgeon may find the distance to the pelvic structures exceeds the length of the surgical instruments and the retractors. In this scenario, a panniculectomy should be performed. A panniculectomy allows the fascial incision to be within several centimeters of the pubis symphysis, allowing easier access to the pelvic organs. Large suction drains should be placed above the fascial closure with a panniculectomy, and kept in place until the drainage is less than 25 mL in 24 hours.

Wound Healing and Inflammatory Responses

The physiology of wound healing has traditionally been segmented into three phases—inflammation, proliferation, maturation and remodeling.

Phase I: Inflammation (Onset of Injury to Days 4–6)

The initial stage of wound healing is marked by a hypoxic, ischemic environment populated by macrophages, neutrophils, and platelets. Within moments after tissue injury, the body responds to limit further injury and repair damage that has already been done. Cell membrane damage results in the immediate release of thromboxane A_2 and prostaglandin $F_{2\alpha}$ both of which are potent vasoconstrictors. Damage to blood vessels exposes the vascular endothelium, to initiate both the intrinsic and extrinsic coagulation cascade. Collagen, platelets, thrombin, fibrin, and complement: (a) expresses cellular mediators (cytokines, prostaglandins, serotonin, etc.) into the area of inflammation, and (b) provides a support matrix for the arriving inflammatory cells. Finally, it excites monocytes to become macrophages that ignite angiogenesis, and fibroblast development while neutrophils consume bacteria and necrotic tissue in the wound.

Phase II: Proliferation (Days 4–14)

The second stage of wound healing is characterized by the rapid formation of new tissue. Macrophages from the previous stage emit nitrous oxide and previously constricted vessels dilate to accommodate influx of new cells. Under the influence of various growth factors, epithelial cells on the skin edge proliferate to form an eschar and then migrate across the wound to re-create an intact protective layer. Simultaneously, endothelial cells begin to build new capillaries. Angiogenesis at this stage is critical because continued proliferation requires large amounts of adenosine triphosphate and this cannot occur without adequate oxygen and nutrient delivery. Granulation tissue begins to form. Fibroblasts are recruited from surrounding intact tissue and begin to synthesize and deposit collagen and a temporary matrix of (weaker) type III collagen, fibronectin, and glycosaminoglycans is laid down in the wound.

Phase III: Maturation and Remodeling (Week 1–Year 1)

The third and final stage of wound healing is marked by the evolution of the matrix into a highly refined and ordered collagen complex. Inability to mature results in a weak and ineffective scar; overzealous refining results in keloid formation. Myofibroblasts begin to shrink and contract the wound to minimize the amount of collagen deposition that is required; the wound further contracts as collagen fibers crosslink to increase their strength. Collagen deposition continues to occur over 4 to 6 weeks. Initially, the collagen is laid down in thin fibrils that run parallel to the wound's surface. As the wound matures, the thin collagen fibers become progressively thicker and reorient themselves in such a fashion as to minimize stress. This is reflected as increasing tensile strength of the wound over the postoperative period. At 1 week, the wound has 3% of its final strength, at 3 weeks it has 30% of its final strength, and at 3 months and beyond, it has approximately 80% of its final strength. Wounds will never regain the strength of uninjured tissues.

Effects of Sutures on Wound Healing

The presence of suture material in wounds induces excessive inflammatory tissue responses that lower the body's defense mechanism against infection, interfere with the proliferative phase of wound healing and ultimately lead to inferior wound strength due to excessive scar tissue formation. Although normal wound healing from surgical trauma involves an inflammatory process, these reactions typically subside within a week as phase I transitions into phase II. However, inflammatory tissue reactions due to the presence of suture material will persist as long as the foreign body remains within the tissue. The degree of tissue reaction in turn depends largely on the chemical nature and physical characteristics of the various suture materials.

Sutures

A suture is any strand of material used to approximate tissue or ligate vessels. Materials incorporated into sutures include horsehair, linen, silk, animal intestines, and wire.

A perfect suture would have the following properties:
- Adequate strength for the time and forces needed for the wounded tissue to heal
- Minimal tissue reactivity
- Comfortable handling characteristics
- Unfavorable for bacterial growth and easily sterilized
- *Non-electrolytic, non-capillary, non-allergenic, and noncarcinogenic.*

Classification and Characteristics of Suture Materials

There are numerous ways to classify suture material depending on natural versus synthetic fibers, coated versus uncoated, dyed versus undyed, etc.

These are:
- Absorbable versus non-absorbable
- Multifilament versus monofilament
- Suture size and tensile strength
- Stiffness and flexibility
- Smooth versus barbed

Absorbable Sutures

Sutures are classified based on their absorptive properties. Absorbable sutures are prepared from the collagen of animals or synthetic polymers. These sutures are removed from the body by enzymatic action or hydrolysis. The ability of the suture to retain tensile strength dictates where the suture should be used in wound closure. Sutures can maintain adequate tensile strength until wound healing is complete, followed by rapid absorption. Conversely, some sutures may lose tensile strength rapidly and undergo slow absorption. All absorbable sutures eventually completely dissolve.

Absorbable sutures have some limitations. For patients with fever, infection, or poor nutritional status, absorption of absorbable suture may accelerate and lead to premature diminution of tensile strength. If these sutures are exposed to significant moisture, such as ascites, absorption rates are accelerated. The common absorbable sutures used in gynecologic surgery are as follows:
- Surgical gut
  - Plain
  - Chromic
  - Fast absorbing
- Polyglactin 910
  - Uncoated
  - Coated
- Polyglycolic acid
- Poliglecaprone
- Polydioxanone (PDS)
- Polyglyconate

Surgical gut sutures can be used to reapproximate mucosal surfaces or peritoneal edges, but they lack the tensile strength for use in fascial closure. Poliglecaprone (Monocryl) is an absorbable suture that retains 50% of its tensile strength after 2 weeks. This suture should not be used to reapproximate the abdominal wall fascia.

Synthetic absorbable sutures are used extensively in many gynecologic surgeries. Polyglactin and polyglycolic acid are frequently used to ligate pedicles during hysterectomy. These sutures can be used to close a transverse incision in a healthy patient, although monofilament sutures are preferred by many surgeons for fascial closure of a transverse incision.

Two monofilament delayed absorbable sutures useful in fascial closure are polyglyconate and polydioxanone (PDS). Both of these sutures invoke a little tissue reaction and maintain 50% of their tensile strength at 4 weeks. These sutures are often used with midline incision closures in gynecologic surgeries. Studies indicate that using a delayed absorbable suture in a mass closure of all layers of the abdominal wall is efficient and safe.

The long-lasting absorbable polydioxanone suture is typically used for deeper tissue closures and subcuticular closure. This suture has a helical barbed design that does not require tying knots to secure the suture.

Nonabsorbable Sutures

Enzymatic activity or hydrolysis does not digest nonabsorbable sutures. These sutures are composed of multiple filaments of metal, synthetic fibers, and organic fibers fashioned into a strand by twisting, braiding, or spinning. The commonly used non-absorbable sutures are as follows:

- Natural
  - Silk
  - Cotton
  - Stainless steel wire
  - Nylon
  - Polypropylene (Prolene)
  - Braided synthetics

Use of nonabsorbable sutures, polypropylene or polybutester is recommended to close the fascia in a midline abdominal incision. There is a 32% decreased risk of incisional hernia when the fascia is approximated with nonabsorbable sutures compared with absorbable sutures. But there may be no difference in incisional hernia rates between delayed absorbable sutures and nonabsorbable sutures.

Absorbable versus Nonabsorbable

All foreign bodies induce some degree of tissue reaction that impedes wound healing. The longer a suture material stays in the body, the more likely it is to serve as a nidus for undesirable tissue reactions that can delay or interfere with normal wound healing. Thus, the perfect suture material should retain adequate strength throughout the healing process and disappear afterward with minimal associated inflammatory reaction.

In terms of lasting performance, suture materials are classified into absorbable and nonabsorbable based on whether they lose their entire tensile strength within 2 to 3 months or retain their entire strength for longer than 2 to 3 months.

Surgical catgut is available in 2 preparations—plain and chromic. Both varieties involve the same basic initial processing. The submucosa of sheep intestines or serosa of cow intestines are split into longitudinal ribbons and treated with formaldehyde. Several ribbons are then twisted into strands, dried, ground down, and polished into the correct suture size. The resulting untreated product is called *plain catgut*. If the plain gut is further tanned in a bath of chromium trioxide, it is called *chromic catgut*. The chromium treatment delays the absorption of the chromic gut and thereby extends its tensile strength for longer periods than plain gut.

Although plain and chromic gut have served the surgical world admirably for many years and millions of procedures, the inherent nature of the material's processing and composition makes this suture material less ideal today. First, the grinding and polishing process of the twisted multifilament suture produces unpredictable amounts of weak points and fibril tears that lead to the sutures' characteristic fraying with use. Besides, as because surgical gut is a foreign protein, it is degraded and absorbed mainly via proteolytic enzymes from phagocytes and other cells and tends to have a less predictable absorption rate and elicit a much more intense tissue reaction than the newer, synthetic absorbable sutures.

The first commercial synthetic absorbable polyfila-ment sutures are based on polyglycolic acid-polyglycolide and glycolide-l-lactide copolymer or polyglactin 910. The fibers are stretched to several hundred percent of their original length and heat-set to improve their dimensional stability and inhibit shrinkage. These individual smaller fibers are braided into final multifilament strands of various sizes.

Despite these advances, there becomes a need for an absorbable, synthetic monofilament suture. Both polydioxanone and polyglycolide-trimethylene carbonate copolymer or polyglyconate are absorbable monofilament sutures that have the predictable strength and absorption requirements for a monofilament configuration.

Multifilament versus Monofilament

Multifilament refers to the use of more than 1 fiber in the manufacturing of a single finished strand of suture.

From the perspective of wound healing alone, there are no advantages of a multifilament suture over a monofilament suture.

a. Multifilament sutures inflict more microtrauma as they pass through tissues.

b. Multifilament sutures also induce more intense inflammatory response and contribute to larger knot volumes than monofilaments of equal sizes.

c. Finally, multifilament sutures demonstrate enhanced capillarity with a resultant increase in the transport and spread of microorganisms.

Suture Size and Tensile Strength

Sutures of all compositions are available in a variety of sizes. The higher the first number, the smaller is the suture diameter. Sutures with increasing size increases its tensile strength. For example, 0 chromic gut suture has a minimum diameter of 0.40 mm with an average minimum knot-pull tensile strength of 2.77 kilogram-force (kgf), whereas 0 polydioxanone suture has a minimum diameter of 0.35 mm with an average minimum knot-pull tensile strength of 3.90 kgf.

Stiffness and Flexibility

Suture stiffness and flexibility is equally important as strength and its absorption. The stiffness makes the suture soft or hard, gives it memory or recoil, and determines the ease with which knots can be tied. As a general rule, monofilament suture materials tend to have higher bending stiffness than multifilament, braided configuration irrespective of its sizes.

Smooth versus Barbed Suture

Smooth Suture

Knot tying of suture is almost integral to surgery as the suture itself. Given the smooth nature of most suture materials, there is a need for a knot as an anchor to the tissue to avoid suture slippage. First, knot-secured smooth suture creates an uneven distribution of tension across the wound. This tension gradient across the wound may subtly interfere with uniform healing and remodeling.

Irrespective of the knot configuration and material, the weakest spot in a surgical suture is the knot and the second weakest point is the portion immediately adjacent to the knot. However, surgical knots, when tied too tightly, can cause localized tissue necrosis, reduced fibroblast proliferation, and excessive tissue overlap, leading to reduced strength in the healed wound. A surgical knot represents the highest amount and density of foreign body material in any given suture line and the volume of a knot is directly related to the total amount of surrounding inflammatory reaction. If minimizing the inflammatory reaction in a wound is integral to improved wound healing, then minimizing knot sizes or the number of knots should be beneficial

as long as the tensile strength of the suture line is not compromised.

Barbed Suture

Currently available bidirectional barbed suture materials include polydioxanone (PDO), poligleca-prone, nylon, and polypropylene. Bidirectional barbed sutures are manufactured from monofilament fibers via a micromachining technique that cuts barbs into the suture around the circumference in a helical pattern. The barbs are separated by a distance of 0.88 to 0.98 mm, and are divided into 2 groups that face each other in opposing directions from the suture midpoint (Fig. 6.5).

Needles are swaged on to both ends of the suture length. Owing to its decreased effective diameter as a result of the process of creating barbs, a barbed suture is typically rated equivalent to 1 suture size greater than its conventional equivalent. For example, a 2-0 barbed suture equals a 3-0 smooth suture. The advantages of use of barbed suture are:

a. Elimination of need for a knot because barbed sutures self-anchor and are balanced by the countervailing barbs securing tissue in the opposing direction, no knots are needed on the ends.

b. Knotless barbed suture does not display weak spots and demonstrates equal to better *in vitro* and *in vivo* wound breaking strengths.

c. The elimination of a knot effectively reduces the overall foreign body load and thereby reduces the total wound tissue reactions.

d. In minimally invasive laparoscopic procedures where knot-tying is difficult, the use of knotless bidirectional barbed suture can securely re-approximate tissues with less time, cost, and aggravation.

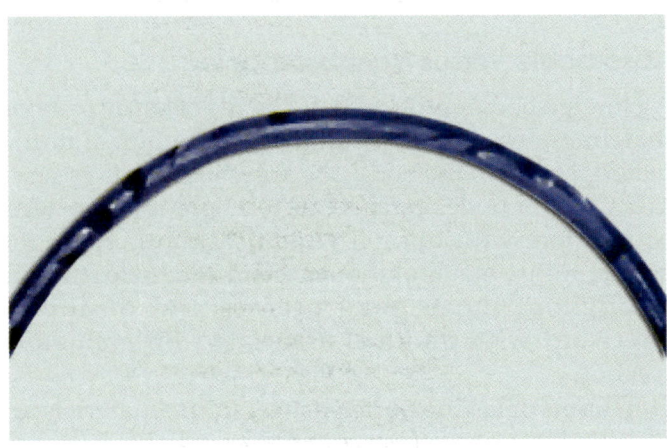

Fig. 6.5: Barbed suture

e. Because barbed suture self-anchors at approximately every 1 mm of tissue, there is a more uniform distribution of wound tension across the suture line.

f. The anchoring of barbed suture resists migration and can be conceptualized as a "continuous interrupted" suture without any knots.

g. This process of more evenly distributed tension may yield stronger wounds by eliminating the high tension spots that are more prone to disrupted healing.

h. For a procedure in which cavity leakage may be an issue, the secure anchoring of barbed suture at 1 mm intervals may provide a reduction in gaps and thereby create a more "watertight" seal than conventional suturing techniques.

Reapproximation of Tissues

A. Rectus Fascia Reapproximation

Techniques and materials for reapproximating abdominal wall fascia have been extensively researched, with most of the studies focusing on incisional hernia formation as the primary endpoint. The majority of incisional hernias appear to develop following the mechanical disruption of fascial wounds occurring during the initial "lag phase" of the wound healing process. Laparotomy wound disruptions progressing to incisional hernias begin to form within 30 days of laparotomy wound closure. There is essentially no real gain in wound strength for the first 4 to 5 days after injury, followed by a rapid increase in strength with the maximal slope at around postoperative day 15 and a subsequent leveling off, with wound strength approximating 70 to 90% of original tissue strength around 120 days. The fascia rarely regains the strength of normal unwounded tissue, and in any case never before 4 months.

Because of the high natural disruptive forces on rectus fascia, sutures used in repair of these wounds need relatively longer tensile strength retention than materials used in other areas of obstetric and gynecologic surgery. The suture selection for closing rectus fascia in obstetric and gynecologic operations seem to be one of the delayed absorption monofilament materials such as polydioxanone or polyglyconate and polyglycolic acid-based sutures as well. Whether this suture should be smooth or barbed remains to be determined.

B. Uterine Reapproximation

The excellent historical record of chromic gut in obstetrics imply 2 important principles: (1) the knotted tensile strength of 0 chromic gut (average minimum of knot-pull tensile strength of 2.77 kgf) is adequate to withstand the disruptive forces on the repaired hysterotomy, and (2) the complete loss of tensile strength (14–21 days) and reabsorption profile of chromic gut is adequate for cesarean delivery repair. Building off these 2 principles, a more reasoned suture choice might focus on a monofilament suture that causes less tissue trauma and induces less intense inflammatory response than the twisted multifilament surgical gut. Thus the most logical suture materials of choice for closing the well-vascularized uterus during a cesarean delivery seem to be either poliglecaprone 25 or polyglactin 910. For closing the uterus in the less vascular nonpregnant state, either the same sutures or longer lasting polydioxanone or polyglyconate seem to be the best options.

C. Vaginal Cuff Closure

Closing the vaginal cuff after hysterectomy is a common complex procedure. Bacterial contamination from the vaginal vault is a major cause of febrile morbidity and infectious complications, such as vaginal cuff cellulitis and pelvic abscess after hysterectomy. Even in the absence of infection, the vaginal cuff is prone to persistent granulation tissue with postoperative vaginal discharge and bleeding. Finally, the introduction of newer minimally invasive techniques has increased the use of thermal energy rather than a knife to enter the vagina. This change leads to less viable tissue at cuff edges, with subsequent potential delays in wound healing.

The ideal suture for vaginal cuff closure should inhibit bacterial growth, elicit minimal tissue reactivity, be pliable, and maintain a reasonable amount of tensile strength for at least 2 to 4 weeks even though absorbable. The chromic catgut leads to more postoperative granulation tissue. Reasonable choices include one of the multifilament polyglycolic acid-based sutures, if stiffness is a greater concern than capillarity, or one of the delayed absorption monofilament materials such as polydioxanone or polyglyconate, if minimizing inflammation is the goal. The knots or suture edges of the delayed absorption monofilaments should face intra-abdominally rather than intravaginally to mitigate the potentially irritating effects of the stiffer suture.

7 | Postoperative Care and Its Complications

The postoperative period is a time when the patient recovers from complex surgical procedures and need very close monitoring of vitals. The preoperative assessment and preparation and the eventual surgical procedure determines its outcome to a large extent. The successful anesthetic recovery also influences the outcome of surgery in the immediate postoperative period. Therefore, the postoperative care is divided in the following areas of care:

1. Anesthetic Recovery

Day care surgeries and laparoscopy in gynecology have rapidly become popular in modern day surgical practice. Evolution has occurred in anesthetic practice to provide stable hemodynamic, adequate analgesia with minimal complications, rapid recovery and early ambulation. Though general anesthesia (GA) has been the choice for long surgery but selective spinal anesthesia (SSA) has been developed and modified for selective short duration analgesia, which facilitates ambulation at the end of the surgical procedure. Spinal anesthesia is usually simple and quick, provides good postoperative pain relief and minimizes postoperative nausea. It is modified to reduce duration of motor block without compromising analgesia for day care surgeries, involving the use of short-acting local anesthetics and combinations of a low dose of local anesthetic with an analgesic adjuvant, usually an opioid.

Postoperative nausea and vomiting (PONV) is inconvenient, and uncomfortable. Dromperidol and ondansetron are the most consistently reliable agents for PONV prophylaxis.

2. Fluid Infusion

Intraoperative fluid administration in patients undergoing intra-abdominal procedures should range from 10 to 15 mL/kg/hr. The fluid regimen should consist of 12–15 mL/kg for the first hour and 6–10 mL/kg for the next 2 hr. It is observed that cardiovascular stability during major operations is much better preserved when intraoperative crystalloids are given at the rate of 10–15 mL/kg/hr.

The physiological alteration in the postoperative period is mainly because of release of profuse water in response to tissue breakdown following any major intra-abdominal surgery. This free water is often retained in the body particularly in the 3rd space of surgical field due to increased level of ADH and Aldosterone in response to surgical stress. The development of ileus occurs when 1–3 L of fluid is sequestered in the bowel lumen, bowel wall and peritoneal cavity. Since the kidney continues to excrete a minimum of 30–60 mEq/L of potassium daily, hypokalemia may develop, if potassium is not replaced. In the first postoperative day, release of intracellular potassium in response to tissue damage is adequate to replenish the loss but potassium replacement is essential to replace the loss from the 2nd postoperative day. After the first few postoperative days, third space fluid returns to intravascular space and ADH, aldosterone levels return to normal. The excess fluid retained is now excreted through kidneys. Patients with decreased cardiac and renal reserve are at risk of fluid overload during this time, if intravenous fluids are not appropriately reduced. Therefore, close monitoring of daily weight, urine output, serum hematocrit, hemodynamic parameters determines the need of crystalloid replacement. Ideally isotonic crystalloid Ringer lactate solution is the best replacement fluid in the postoperative period.

3. Specific Electrolyte Disorders

a. *Hyponatremia:* Inappropriate replacement of body salt losses with water alone can result in hyponatremia. This typically occurs when patients lose large amount of electrolytes due to vomiting, diarrhea, nasogastric suction and gastrointestinal fistula and only receive hypotonic solutions. Simple replacement with isotonic fluids and potassium usually corrects the abnormality. Rarely, hypertonic saline (3%) infusion can be administered with caution.

b. *Hypernatremia:* This is defined when serum sodium is greater than 160 mEq/L and occurs in extracellular fluid deficit and mainly in central nervous system causing disorientation, seizures and death. The treatment includes correction of fever, replacement with 5% dextrose intravenous infusion.

c. *Hypokalemia:* This is characterized by symptoms like muscle weakness, flaccid paralysis, CV abnormalities like hypotension, bradycardia, and arrhythmias. This mainly occurs when serum potassium level is less than 3 mEq/L. This arises when potassium free parenteral fluid is administered for prolonged period in patients who are restricted from oral feeding. This may be compounded by the events of prolonged emesis, diarrhea, NG suction or intestinal fistulas. The treatment is potassium replacement which can be given oral or parenteral in doses that should not exceed 10 mEq/hr.

d. *Hyperkalemia:* This happens occasionally in association with renal impairment, massive GI bleeding or hemolysis when serum potassium goes high above 7 mEq/L. This can result in bradycardia, ventricular fibrillation and cardiac arrest. 10 mL of 10% calcium gluconate given IV with 5% dextrose and insulin cause a rapid shift of potassium into cells.

4. Pain Relief

Almost one-fourth to half of postoperative patients suffer moderate to severe pain unnecessarily. The 'patient-controlled analgesia' devices provide electronically controlled infusion pumps that deliver a preset dose of narcotic into IV catheter on patient's request. But use of PCA is associated with increase in respiratory depression.

Epidural analgesia with bupivacaine provides excellent analgesia for 1st 72 hours in the postoperative period. Epidural opioids have a longer duration of action. The respiratory depression is less with epidural fentanyl which is quickly absorbed into the spinal cord. Pruritus, hypotension, nausea, vomiting and respiratory depression are drawback of epidural analgesia.

Anti-inflammatory analgesic drugs are useful and used in postoperative period for sustained pain free periods for next 7–10 days. It is started with parenteral formulations for 1st 72 hours followed by oral route when patient starts her motion regularly. These drugs along with sedatives like diazepam is a good adjunct

for purpose of pain relief. These drugs also sometimes prove toxic and is usually backed up by H_2 inhibitor drugs to decrease its acidic effect on gastric mucosa.

5. Antibiotic Prophylaxis in Surgery

The purpose of this is to increase immunity in host tissues to resist infections in surgical site. **Cephalosporines, like cefazolin, cefotetan, cefotaxime, cefoxitin,** are the commonly prescribed drugs in prophylaxis. 1 gm is the standard dose for average weight women and in patients with BMI >35, 2 gm is administered. But it is also not without risks. Anaphylactic reactions, pseudomembranous colitis by *Clostridium difficile* are not uncommon. Therefore, all gynecological surgeries do not need antimicrobial prophylaxis. The diagnostic or operative hysteroscopy or laparoscopy, endometrial aspiration, and endometrial biopsy do not need routine antibiotic prophylaxis. The timing of administration is ideally within 30 minutes of start of surgery. A delay of 3 hours or more between time of skin incision and antibiotic administration may result in ineffective prophylaxis. Usually, one single dose is sufficient, but if surgery is prolonged beyond 3 hours or longer, then one-half dose of the drug is used or in addition blood loss is greater than 1.5 liters, 2nd dose is administered to maintain adequate levels in tissues after 6 hrs (Table 7.1).

Table 7.1: Antibiotics used in gynecologic surgical prophylaxis

Procedure	Antibiotics	Dose recommended
1. MTP	Doxycycline	100 mg oral 1 hr before surgery and 200 mg after the procedure
	Metronidazole	1–1.2 gm daily for 5 days
2. HSG	Doxycycline	100 mg oral twice daily × 5 days
3. Hysterectomy	Cefazolin	2 gm IV strugle dose
4. Urogynecology procedures	Quinolone+ Clindamycin	400 mg IV 900 mg IV hrly

6. Postoperative Infections

Surgical site infections (SSI) are a serious form of postoperative morbidity. The risk factors include:

a. Poor nutrition

b. Chronic illness

c. Pre-existing systemic infections

d. Poor surgical technique

e. Immune compromised state

f. Contamination of wound by spillage of infected tissues or intestinal contents.

The postoperative infection may include surgical site, vaginal cuff, abdominal wound, urinary tract and pelvis which result in cellulitis, pelvic collection or fever, intestinal distension, secondary hemorrhage and wound dehiscence.

The postoperative febrile morbidity is defined when there is a rise in temperature of 100.4°F and above on two occasions at least 4 hours apart during the postoperative period after the first 24 hours. When fever appears anytime with two consecutive elevations greater than 101°F, this may be due to cause not related to surgical sepsis.

The assessment of febrile surgical patient is a great challenge to help fast recovery. This include:

a. Review of patients' history in regard to risk factors

b. Any history of blood transfusion

c. Inspection of pharynx, respiratory tract

d. Any lymphadenopathy, epigastric and loin tenderness

e. Symptoms of dysuria, urgency, diarrhea, vomiting, urinary or fecal incontinence

f. Evidence of thrombophlebitis in area of drip sites or deep or superficial thromboembolism in the legs

g. Abdominal tenderness, distension, hepato-splenomegaly, ascites

h. Any evidence of wound sepsis, vault sepsis

i. Pelvic and per-rectal examination for parametritis, broad ligament hematoma and pelvic abscess.

The important investigations required are:

a. Blood for hemoglobin, leukocytosis, malaria

b. Urine RE/ME and C/S

c. LFT, KFT, electrolytes

d. USG whole abdomen and pelvis

e. Blood culture

f. Chest X-ray and straight X-ray abdomen.

The presence of foreign body inside is a serious life-threatening and medicolegal condition. The treatment basically includes the prompt diagnosis of the cause and treat them accordingly. The common steps are:

a. Change to higher antibiotics according to sepsis culture report

b. Restore adequate hydration

c. Blood transfusion

d. Drainage of pelvic abscess

e. Correction of electrolyte deficit

f. Aggressive pulmonary support with spirometry

g. Wound dressing and secondary suture

h. Repair of burst abdomen.

7. Postoperative Ileus

For most gynecological surgeries, the postoperative ileus is less common and GI function returns rapidly. The patients who have persistently diminished bowel sounds, abdominal distension, need evaluation and more aggressive treatment. An ileus following endoscopic surgery most likely represent GI injury including thermal burns from diathermy. Abdominal X-ray to evaluate the abdomen in the supine and the upright positions helps in its diagnosis by the presence of dilated loops of small and large intestines and air-fluid levels in between. The management includes:

1. Patients remain in NPO status with IV fluids and electrolytes.

2. A nasogastric tube is given to decompress the gastric contents.

3. Fluid and electrolyte replacement must be adequate.

4. Titration with I/O and electrolytes to measure the amount and type of fluids are to be determined daily.

5. Most cases begin to improve by 72–96 hours with passage of flatus and stool and reduction of intestinal distension.

6. Timely removal of NG tube, start of liquid diet and enema for bowel motion are given when IPS returns.

7. If there is no sign of improvement after 72 hours, other causes are to be ascertained like gut injury, ongoing sepsis, pyoperitoneum, ureteral injury and left out foreign body. CT scan with oral contrast assists in diagnosis of gut injury. For that often relaparotomy is done to save the patient. In most of the cases, release of band obstruction will be enough to release the small gut obstruction though rarely resection and anastomosis may be needed in some of the cases. Postoperative large gut obstruction is rare following gynecological surgery except in case of genital malignancy when dilatation of cecum of >12 cm in diameter need immediate colostomy and repair of large gut wall because conservative treatment for large gut obstruction is not effective and any large gut injury may carry a high mortality.

8. Thromboembolism

Though not very common in women of our country, deep venous thrombosis and pulmonary embolism are responsible for sudden postoperative deaths following prolonged gynecological surgery. Therefore, **low-dose heparin** is given SC at 2 hours preoperative and every 8–12 hours postoperative in patients of high-risk factors like obesity, >60 yr of age, of heart disease, cancer and previous history of DVT/PE. If low dose heparin is continued for more than 4 days, platelet count should be checked since thrombocytopenia is seen in 6% of patients after gynecologic surgery.

The low molecular weight heparin (LMWH) which has more anti-Xa and less antithrombin activity has more convenient once a day dosing advantage because of its long half-life and less bleeding complications.

Besides, mechanical methods like compression stockings and intermittent pneumatic compression particularly calf suppression during and after gynecologic surgery reduces the incidence of DVT.

9. Urinary Tract-related Morbidity

a. *Urinary tract infection:* It occurs more commonly following prolonged catheterization, ureteric stenting or bladder injury. It is one of the commonest reasons for postoperative fever mainly caused by the microbials through vaginal route or catheterization. Appropriate antibiotics on the basis of culture-sensitivity report is adequate to control infection.

b. *Fistulae:* Both vesicovaginal and ureterovaginal fistulae are serious though relatively uncommon complications. They mainly result from anatomical distortion of pathology, ischemia, kinking or direct surgical injury. Repair is the only key to solve this problem.

10. Wound Sepsis

a. *Superficial dehiscence:* This occurs mainly in obese patients. Thorough daily cleansing with high order antibiotics on the result of swab culture reports work very well.

b. *Complete dehiscence:* This mainly is evident from 3rd postoperative day with local site edema, foul smelling discharge, fever, redness, and total wound breakdown after removal of stitch. Often dehiscence involves deep up to rectus sheath. It is often essential to rule out **burst abdomen** when peritoneum gives way to expose the intestines. Immediate repair is mandatory in case of suspected burst abdomen. Otherwise, wound will be made healthy by control of infection and to wait till the healthy red granulation tissue generates. Secondary suture is done with interrupted monofilament nylon with an indwelling drain in the dead space below the rectus or in the subcutaneous space. Stitches are usually removed on 8–10th postoperative day. During this time, anemia, and hypoproteinemias are corrected and euglycemia is strictly maintained.

8 Pelvic Infections

8A. PELVIC INFLAMMATORY DISEASE

Pelvic inflammatory disease (PID) is infection of a woman's reproductive organs. Infection spreads upward from the cervix to the uterus, fallopian tubes, ovaries, and surrounding structures resulting in:

- Cervicitis
- Endometritis
- Salpingitis
- Peritonitis

Causes

The two most commonly involved bacteria that cause PID are *Chlamydia trachomatis* and *Neisseria gonorrhoae*.

However, microorganisms that comprise the vaginal flora (e.g. anaerobes, *G. vaginalis*, *Haemophilus influenzae*, and *Streptococcus agalactiae*) also have been associated with PID. In addition, cytomegalovirus (CMV), *M. hominis*, *U. urealyticum*, and *M. genitalium* might be associated with some cases of PID. All women who have acute PID should be tested for *N. gonorrhoeae* and *C. trachomatis* and should be screened for HIV infection.

- PID can cause a wide variety of symptoms. Pain in the lower abdomen, acute or subacute, and fever are the most common symptoms. Others may remain asymptomatic. Thus, PID is not always easy to diagnose.
- Sexually active adolescent females and women younger than 25 years are at greatest risk, although PID can occur at any age.

Diagnosis

Woman with PID may have any of these symptoms:
- Lower abdominal pain or tenderness
- Back pain
- Abnormal uterine bleeding
- Unusual or heavy or foul-smelling vaginal discharge
- Painful urination
- Painful sexual intercourse

Symptoms not related to the female reproductive organs include fever, nausea, and vomiting.

PID symptoms may be worse at the end of a menstrual period and during the first several days following a period.

RCOG Recommendation for Diagnosis

A low threshold for empiric treatment of PID is recommended because of lack of definitive clinical diagnostic criteria and risk of potential harm, if not treated in early stage of the disease. The following clinical features are suggestive of diagnosis of PID:
- Bilateral lower abdominal tenderness sometimes radiating to legs.
- Abnormal vaginal or cervical discharge.
- Fever >38°C.
- *Abnormal vaginal bleeding:* Intermenstrual, postcoital or breakthrough bleeding.
- Deep dysparunia.
- Cervical motion tenderness on bimanual pelvic examination.
- Adnexal tenderness on bimanual vaginal examination with or without a palpable mass.

Following women are at risk for pelvic inflammatory disease:
- Women with sexually transmitted diseases—especially gonorrhea and chlamydia—are at greater risk for developing PID.
- Women who have had a prior episode of PID are at higher risk for another episode.
- Sexually active teenagers are more likely to develop PID than older women.
- Women with many sexual partners are at greater risk for sexually transmitted infections (STIs) and PID.

Laboratory tests may include the following:

- Urine or serum pregnancy test, if the female is of child-bearing age.
- Urinalysis to check for bladder and kidney infection.
- Hb, complete blood count, ESR.
- Cervical cultures for gonorrhea and chlamydia.
- Tests for other sexually transmitted diseases, including syphilis and HIV.

Special tests, if more severe symptoms are present:

1. Testing for gonorrhea and chlamydia should be done with endocervical culture or using a nucleic acid amplification test (NAAT) and if found positive, antibiotic sensitivity is also examined.
2. Taking an additional sample from urethra also increase diagnostic yield for gonorrhea and chlamydia. A clean catch urine or self-collected vulvovaginal swab can be an alternative source of collection for examination.
3. The absence of pus cells from endocervical and vaginal swab on a wet mount smear has a 95% negative predictive value for diagnosis of PID but its presence has poor 17% positive predictive value.

The most specific criteria for diagnosing PID include:

- Endometrial biopsy with histopathologic evidence of endometritis.
- TVS or MRI show thickened, fluid-filled tubes with or without free pelvic fluid or tubo-ovarian complex, or tubal hyperemia on Doppler.
- Laparoscopic abnormalities consistent with PID include (Fig. 8.1):
  1. Hyperemias in pelvic organs.
  2. Flimsy adhesions in periadnexal region, pouch of Douglas (POD).
  3. Draining of pus from fimbrial orifice.
  4. Hydrosalpinx.
  5. Fimbrial stenosis and tubal phimosis
  6. Tubo-ovarian abscess.
  7. Fluid collection in pouch of Douglas

Treatment

PID treatment regimens must provide broad-spectrum coverage of likely pathogens. Treatment should be initiated as soon as the presumptive diagnosis has been made because prevention of long-term sequele is dependent on early administration of appropriate antibiotics.

In women with PID of mild or moderate clinical severity, outpatient therapy yields short- and long-term clinical outcomes similar to inpatient therapy. **The decision of whether hospitalization is necessary should be based on the judgment of the provider and whether the patient meets any of the following suggested criteria (RCOG).**

- Surgical emergencies (e.g. appendicitis) cannot be excluded.
- The patient is pregnant.
- The patient does not respond clinically to oral antimicrobial therapy.
- The patient is unable to follow or tolerate an outpatient oral regimen.
- The patient has severe illness, nausea and vomiting, or high fever.
- The patient has tubo-ovarian abscess.

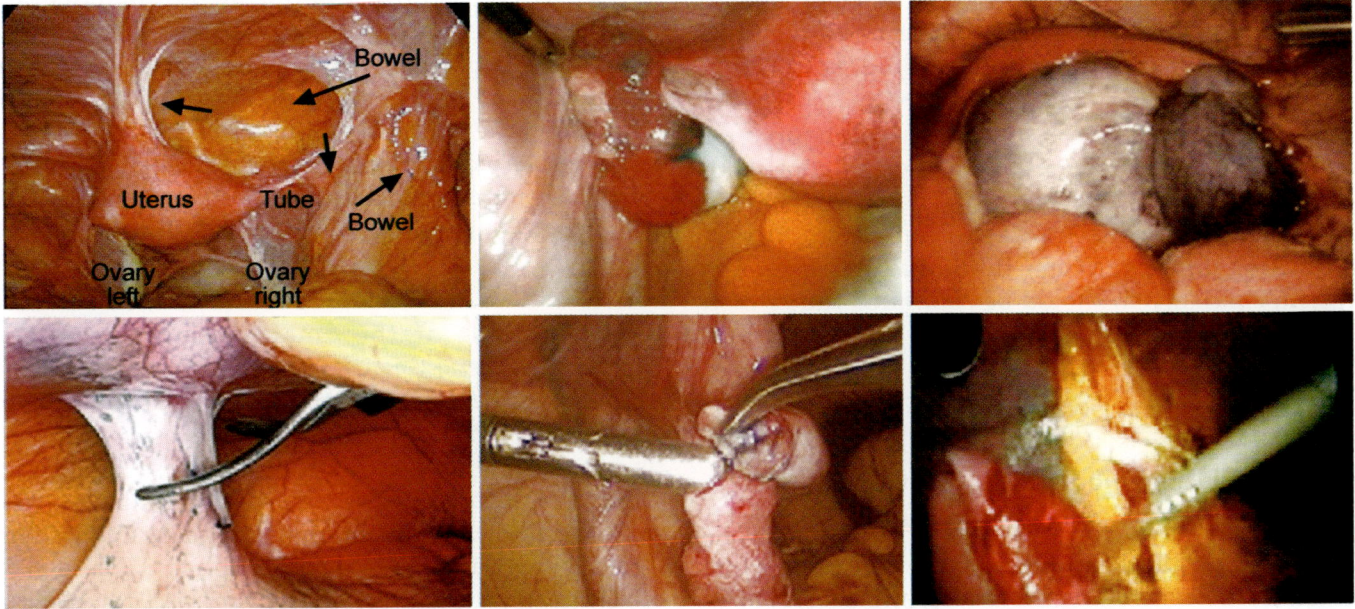

Fig. 8.1: Findings of diagnostic laparoscopy—adhesions, tubal phimosis, ovarian abscess

Parenteral Treatment

For women with PID of mild or moderate severity, parenteral and oral therapies appear to have similar clinical efficacy. Clinical experience should guide decisions regarding transition to oral therapy, which usually can be initiated within 24–48 hours of clinical improvement.

Recommended Parenteral Regimen A

- **Inj. Cefotetan** 2 g IV every 12 hours or
- **Inj. Cefoxitin** 2 g IV every 6 hours +
- **Doxycycline** 100 mg orally or IV every 12 hours

Because of the pain associated with intravenous infusion, doxycycline should be administered orally when possible.

Parenteral therapy can be discontinued 24 hours after clinical improvement, but oral therapy with doxycycline (100 mg twice a day) should continue to complete 14 days of therapy. When tubo-ovarian abscess is present, clindamycin or metronidazole with doxycycline can be used for continued therapy rather than doxycycline alone because this regimen provides more effective anaerobic coverage.

There are other second- or third-generation cephalosporins (e.g. ceftizoxime, cefotaxime, and ceftriaxone), which are also effective therapy for PID and can potentially replace cefotetan or cefoxitin. However, these cephalosporins are less active than cefotetan or cefoxitin against anaerobic bacteria.

Recommended Parenteral Regimen B

Inj. Clindamycin 900 mg IV every 8 hours + **gentamicin** loading dose IV or IM (2 mg/kg of body weight), followed by a maintenance dose (1.5 mg/kg) every 8 hours.

Parenteral therapy can be discontinued 24 hours after clinical improvement; ongoing oral therapy consists of doxycycline 100 mg orally twice a day, or clindamycin 450 mg orally four times a day to complete a total of 14 days of therapy. When tubo-ovarian abscess is present, clindamycin should be continued rather than doxycycline, because clindamycin provides more effective anaerobic coverage.

Alternative Parenteral Regimens

- **Inj. Ampicillin/sulbactam** 3 g IV every 6 hours +
- **Doxycycline** 100 mg orally or IV every 12 hours.

Ampicillin/sulbactam plus doxycycline is effective against *C. trachomatis, N. gonorrhoeae*, and anaerobes in women with tubo-ovarian abscess.

High short-term clinical cure rates are also observed with azithromycin, either as monotherapy for 1 week (500 mg IV for 1 or 2 doses followed by 250 mg orally for 5–6 days) or combined with a 12-day course of metronidazole.

Primary Oral Treatment

Outpatient, oral therapy can be considered for women with mild-to-moderately severe acute PID, because **the clinical outcomes among women treated with oral therapy are similar to those treated with parenteral therapy**. Patients who do not respond to oral therapy within 72 hours should be re-evaluated to confirm the diagnosis and should be administered parenteral therapy on either an outpatient or inpatient basis.

Recommended Regimen

i. **Inj. Ceftriaxone** 250 mg IM in a single dose +
   Doxycycline 100 mg orally twice a day for 14 days
   with or without
   Metronidazole 500 mg orally twice a day for 14 days or
ii. **Inj. Cefoxitin** 2 g IM in a single dose and Probenecid 1 g orally administered concurrently in a single dose
   +
   Doxycycline 100 mg orally twice a day for 14 days
   with or without
   Metronidazole 500 mg orally twice a day for 14 days.

The optimal choice of a cephalosporin is unclear; although cefoxitin has better anaerobic coverage, ceftriaxone has better coverage against *N. gonorrhoeae*. A single dose of cefoxitin is effective in obtaining short-term clinical response in women who have PID. However, the theoretical limitations in coverage of anaerobes by recommended cephalosporin antimicrobials may require the addition of metronidazole to the treatment regimen. Adding metronidazole also will effectively treat BV, which is frequently associated with PID.

As a result of the emergence of quinolone-resistant *Neisseria gonorrhoeae*, regimens that include a quinolone agent are no longer recommended for the treatment of PID. If parenteral cephalosporin therapy is not feasible, use of fluoroquinolones (levofloxacin 500 mg orally once daily or ofloxacin 400 mg twice daily for 14 days) with or without metronidazole (500 mg orally twice daily for 14 days) can be considered, if the community prevalence and individual risk for gonorrhea are low.

Diagnostic tests for gonorrhea must be performed before instituting therapy and the patient managed as follows, if the test is positive:

- If the culture for gonorrhea is positive, treatment should be based on results of antimicrobial susceptibility.
- If the isolate is determined to be quinolone-resistant *N. gonorrhoeae* (QRNG) or if antimicrobial susceptibility cannot be assessed, parenteral cephalosporin is recommended. However, if cephalosporin therapy is not feasible, the addition of azithromycin 2 g orally as a single dose to a quinolone-based PID regimen is recommended.

Treatment in Pregnancy and in Young Women

- A pregnancy test should be performed in all women suspected of having PID to help exclude an ectopic pregnancy. When the risk of ectopic pregnancy is judged clinically to be high, pregnancy test should be repeated 21 days after the date of last intercourse.
- PID is rare in women with an intrauterine pregnancy except in case of septic abortion. Cervicitis may, however, occur in pregnancy and is associated with increased maternal and fetal morbidity. Treatment regimen will be dependent upon the organisms isolated. Drugs like tetracyclines are avoided in pregnancy.
- A combination of cefotaxime, azithromycin and metronidazole for 14 days may be used. The risks associated with metronidazole are uncertain—better to avoid in 1st trimester of pregnancy.

For Younger Women

- Ofloxacin should be avoided in young women when bone development is occurring though no problems are found in humans. Doxycycline can be safely used in children over the age of 12 years.
- IUD should be removed in women presenting with PID, if symptoms are not resolved in 72 hours.

Surgery

- When PID causes an abscess, antibiotics therapy will not be very effective. Surgery is often needed to drain the abscess to prevent them from rupturing and

causing widespread infection throughout the pelvis and abdomen. Depending on the conditions, this may be done with a laparoscope or by laparotomy.

- If abscess is formed on the uterus or ovaries, drainage of abscess is often required either by colpotomy or by laparotomy.
- Abdominal hysterectomy and/or oophorectomy is otherwise recommended in widespread peritonitis.
- Excision of TO mass or pyosalpinx is a life-saving procedure.
- Sometimes nerve ablation surgeries can be effective in eliminating pain.

Follow-up

Patients should demonstrate substantial clinical improvement of reduced rebound abdominal tenderness; and uterine, adnexal, and cervical motion tenderness within 3 days after initiation of therapy.

Women with documented chlamydial or gonococcal infections have a high rate of reinfection within 6 months of treatment. Repeat testing of all women who have been diagnosed with chlamydia or gonorrhea is recommended 3–6 months after treatment, regardless of whether their sex partners were treated. All women diagnosed with acute PID should be offered HIV testing.

Management of Sex Partners

Male sex partners of women with PID should be examined and treated, if they had sexual contact with the patient during the 60 days preceding the patient's onset of symptoms.

Patients should be instructed to abstain from sexual intercourse until therapy is completed or both of them are free of symptoms. Evaluation and treatment are necessary because of the risk for reinfection of the patient and the strong likelihood of urethral gonococcal or chlamydial infection in the sex partner. Male partners of women who have PID caused by *C. trachomatis* and/or *N. gonorrhoeae* frequently are asymptomatic. Sex partners should be treated empirically with regimens effective against both of these infections, regardless of the etiology of PID or pathogens isolated from the infected woman.

Introduction

A spontaneous complaint of abnormal vaginal discharge in terms of quantity, color or odor is most commonly a result of vaginal infection. It may in rare cases be caused by mucopurulent STI-related cervicitis. *T. vaginalis, C. albicans* and bacterial vaginosis (BV) are the commonest causes of vaginal infection. *N. gonorrhea,* and *C. trachomatis* cause cervical infection. The clinical detection of cervical infection is difficult because many of them with gonococcal and chlamydial infections are asymptomatic. The symptom of abnormal vaginal discharge is highly indicative of vaginal infection but poorly predictive of cervical infection.

Diseases Characterized by Vaginal Discharge

Most women will have a vaginal infection, characterized by discharge, itching, or odor, during their lifetime.

A careful history, examination, and laboratory testing to determine the etiology of vaginal complaints are warranted. Information on sexual behaviors, gender of sex partners, menses, vaginal hygiene practices (such as douching), and other medications should be elicited. The three diseases most frequently associated with vaginal discharge are **bacterial vaginosis** (caused by the replacement of the vaginal flora by an overgrowth of anaerobic bacteria including *Prevotella* sp., *Mobiluncus* sp., *G. vaginalis, Ureaplasma, Mycoplasma,* etc.), **trichomoniasis** (caused by *T. vaginalis*), and **candidiasis** (usually caused by *Candida albicans*). Cervicitis can also sometimes cause a vaginal discharge.

Various diagnostic methods are available to identify the etiology of an abnormal vaginal discharge. The cause of vaginal symptoms might be determined by pH, a potassium hydroxide (KOH) test, and microscopic examination of fresh samples of the discharge.

a. The pH of the vaginal secretions can be determined by narrow-range pH paper; an elevated pH (i.e. >4.5) is common with BV or trichomoniasis.

b. Because pH testing is not highly specific, discharge should be further examined microscopically by first diluting one sample in one to two drops of 0.9% normal saline solution on one slide and a second sample in 10% KOH solution (samples that emit an amine odor immediately upon application of KOH suggest BV or trichomoniasis infection).

c. On examination under a microscope at low and high power fields, the saline-solution specimen may yield motile *T. vaginalis*, or clue cells (i.e. epithelial cells with borders obscured by small bacteria), which are

characteristic of BV, whereas the presence of WBCs without evidence of trichomonads or yeast in this solution is suggestive of cervicitis. The KOH specimen typically is used to identify the yeast or pseudohyphae of Candida species.

However, the absence of trichomonads or pseudohyphae in KOH samples does not rule out these infections. The sensitivity of microscropy is approximately 50% compared with P58 Nucleic acid amplification test (NAAT for trichomoniasis) or culture (for yeast).

Bacterial Vaginosis (BV)

BV is the most prevalent cause of vaginal discharge or malodor; but most women with BV may remain asymptomatic. Bacterial vaginosis is a polymicrobial clinical syndrome resulting from replacement of the normal hydrogen peroxide producing Lactobacillus sp. in the vagina with high concentrations of anaerobic bacteria. BV is associated with:

a. Multiple male or female partners or a new sex partner

b. Douching

c. Lack of condom use

d. Lack of vaginal lactobacilli; women who have never been sexually active can also be affected.

The cause of the microbial alteration that characterizes BV is not fully understood. Nonetheless, women with BV are at increased risk for the acquisition of some STDs (e.g. HIV, *N. gonorrhoeae, C. trachomatis,* and HSV-2), complications after gynecologic surgery, complications in pregnancy, and recurrence of BV. Treatment of male sex partners has not been beneficial in preventing the recurrence of BV.

Diagnostic Considerations

BV can be diagnosed by the use of clinical criteria (i.e. Amsel' Diagnostic Criteria) or Gram stain. A Gram stain (considered the gold standard laboratory method for diagnosing BV) is used to determine the relative concentration of lactobacilli (i.e. long Gram-positive rods), Gram-negative and Gram-variable rods and cocci (i.e. *G. vaginalis, Prevotella, Porphyromonas, and peptostreptococci*), and curved Gram-negative rods (i.e. *Mobiluncus*) characteristic of BV. If a Gram stain is not available, clinical criteria can be used and require three of the following symptoms or signs:

• Homogeneous, thin, white discharge that smoothly coats the vaginal walls;

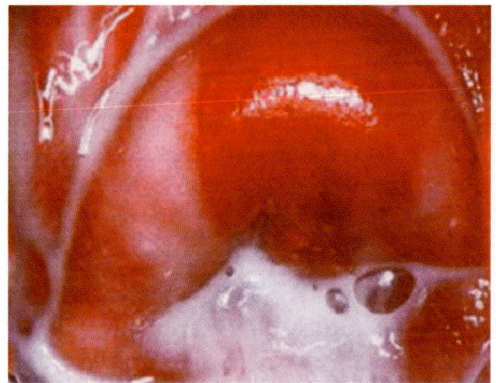
Creamy vaginal discharge

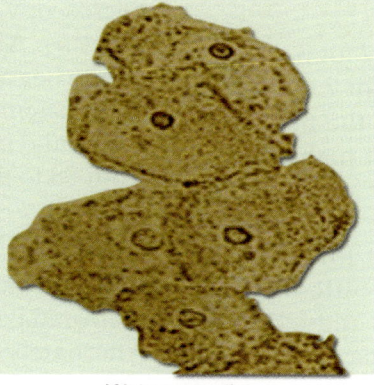
Wet preparation

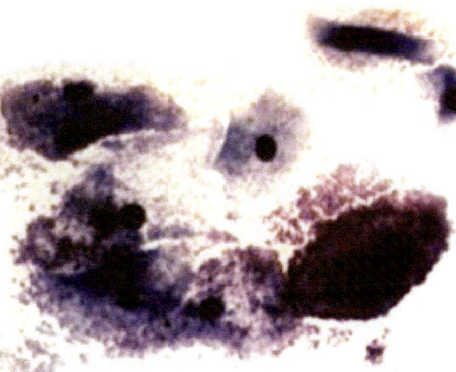
Pap smears showing clue cells

Fig. 8.2: Bacterial vaginosis

- Presence of clue cells on microscopic examination;
- pH of vaginal fluid >4.5; or
- A fishy odor of vaginal discharge before or after addition of 10% KOH (i.e. the whiff test).

Detection of three of these criteria has been correlated with results by Gram stain. Culture of *G. vaginalis* is not recommended as a diagnostic tool because it is not specific. Cervical Pap tests have no clinical utility for the diagnosis of BV because of their low sensitivity (Fig. 8.2).

1. *The characteristic* milky or creamy vaginal discharge of bacterial vaginosis is associated with a high vaginal pH and a fishy odor.
2. Wet preparation of vaginal fluid, absence of WBCs and stippling of epithelial cells support a diagnosis of bacterial vaginosis.
3. Pap smear showing clue cells consistent with bacterial vaginosis.

Treatment

Treatment is recommended for women with symptoms. The established benefits of therapy in non-pregnant women are to relieve vaginal symptoms and signs of infection. Other potential benefits to treatment include reduction in the risk for acquiring *C. trachomatis* or *N. gonorrhoeae*, HIV, and other viral STDs.

Recommended Regime

- Metronidazole, 500 mg orally twice daily for 7 days (in India, 400 mg tablets are available), Or
- Metronidazole gel 0.75%—one full applicator of 5 gm intravaginally once a day for 5 days, Or
- Clindamycin cream 2%—one full applicator of 5 gm intravaginally once a day for 7 days.

Consuming alcohol during treatment with metronidazole is avoided for 24 hours. Clindamycin cream is oil based and, therefore, can weaken the latex condom or diaphragm for 7 days after its use.

Women should be advised to refrain from intercourse or to use condoms consistently and correctly during the treatment regimen.

Alternative regimens: Tinidazole 1 gm orally once daily for 5 days or clindamycin 300 mg orally twice daily for 7 days.

Follow-up

- Follow-up visits are unnecessary, if symptoms resolve. Because recurrence of BV is common, women should be advised to return for evaluation, if symptoms recur.
- For women with multiple recurrences after completion of a recommended regimen, metronidazole gel twice weekly for 4–6 months can reduce recurrences.
- Monthly oral metronidazole administered with fluconazole is another option as suppressive therapy.

Management of Sex Partners

The results of clinical trials indicate that a woman's response to therapy and the likelihood of relapse or recurrence are not affected by treatment of her sex partner(s). Therefore, routine treatment of sex partners is not recommended.

Pregnancy

Treatment is recommended for all pregnant women with symptoms. Although BV is associated with adverse pregnancy outcomes, including premature rupture of membranes, preterm labor, preterm birth, intra-amniotic infection, and postpartum endometritis, the only established benefit of therapy for BV in pregnant women is the reduction of symptoms and signs of vaginal infection.

Recommended Regime for Pregnant Women

Metronidazole 500 mg orally twice a day for 7 days or clindamycin 300 mg orally twice a day for 7 days.

But evidence is insufficient to assess the impact of screening for BV in pregnant women at high risk for preterm delivery. Similarly, data are inconsistent regarding whether the treatment of asymptomatic pregnant women with BV who are at low risk for preterm delivery reduces adverse outcomes of pregnancy. But there may occur 40% reduction in spontaneous preterm birth among women using oral clindamycin during weeks 13–22 of gestation.

HIV Infection

BV appears to recur with higher frequency in HIV-positive women. Patients who have BV and also are infected with HIV should receive the same treatment regimen as those who are HIV negative.

Trichomoniasis

Trichomoniasis (Fig. 8.3) is caused by the protozoan *Trichomona vaginalis*. Some women have symptoms characterized by diffuse, malodorous, yellow-green vaginal discharge with vulvar irritation. However, many women have minimal or no symptoms. Screening for *T. vaginalis* in women can be considered in those at high risk for infection (i.e. women who have new or multiple partners, have a history of STDs, multiple sex partners). Diagnosis of vaginal trichomoniasis is usually performed by microscopy of vaginal secretions, but this method has a sensitivity of only approximately 60–70% and requires immediate evaluation of wet preparation slide for optimal results.

Culture is another sensitive and highly specific method of diagnosis. Among women in whom trichomoniasis is suspected but not confirmed by microscopy, vaginal secretions should be cultured for *T. vaginalis*. An FDA-cleared PCR assay for detection of gonorrhea and chlamydial infection has been modified for *T. vaginalis* detection in vaginal or endocervical swabs and in urine from women; with sensitivity ranges from 88 to 97% and specificity from 98 to 99%.

Recommended Regimes

Metronidazole 2 gm orally in a single dose or metronidazole 500 mg orally twice a day for 7 days. Alternately, tinidazole 2 gm orally in a single dose is also effective.

Recommended metronidazole and tinidazole regimens have resulted in cure rates of approximately 90–95%, and 86–100%, respectively.

Follow-up

- Because of the high rate of reinfection, rescreening for *T. vaginalis* at 3 months following initial infection is recommended for sexually active women.
- Most recurrent *T. vaginalis* infections result from having sex with an untreated partner though some recurrent cases are attributed to diminished susceptibility to metronidazole. Low-level metronidazole resistance is identified in 2–5% of cases of vaginal trichomoniasis.
- Fortunately, infections caused by most of these organisms respond to tinidazole or higher doses of metronidazole. Tinidazole has a longer serum half-life and reaches higher levels in genitourinary tissues than metronidazole.

Management of Sex Partners

Sex partners of patients with *T. vaginalis* should be treated. Patients should be instructed to abstain from sex until they and their sex partners are cured. Male

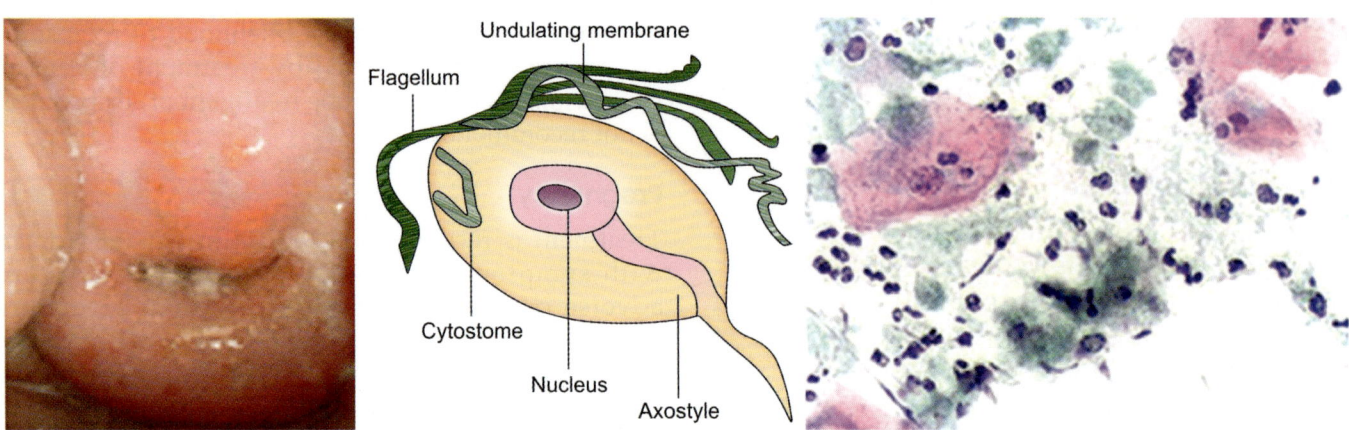

Fig. 8.3: Trichomoniasis

partners should be evaluated and treated with either tinidazole in a single dose of 2 g orally or metronidazole twice a day at 500 mg orally for 7 days.

Pregnancy

Vaginal trichomoniasis is associated with adverse pregnancy outcomes, particularly premature rupture of membranes, preterm delivery and low birth weight. However, metronidazole treatment has not been shown to reduce perinatal morbidity. Treatment of *T. vaginalis* relieve symptoms of vaginal discharge in pregnant women and thus prevent respiratory or genital infection of the newborn.

Clinicians should counsel patients regarding the potential risks and benefits of treatment and communicate the option of therapy deferral in asymptomatic pregnant women until after 37 weeks' gestation.

All symptomatic pregnant women should be considered for treatment regardless of pregnancy stage and counsel for condom use and the continued risk of sexual transmission.

Women can be treated with 2 g metronidazole in a single dose at 2nd and 3rd trimesters of pregnancy. The safety of tinidazole in pregnant women, however, has not been well evaluated.

In lactating women who are administered metronidazole, withholding breastfeeding during treatment and for 12–24 hours after the last dose will reduce the exposure of the infant to metronidazole. For women treated with tinidazole, interruption of breastfeeding is recommended during treatment and for 3 days after the last dose.

HIV Infection

- There is increasing evidence for epidemiologic and biologic interaction between HIV and *T. vaginalis*.

T. vaginalis infection in HIV-infected women enhances HIV transmission by increasing genital shedding of the virus and treatment for *T. vaginalis* has been shown to reduce HIV shedding.

- Rescreening 3 months after completion of therapy is recommended among HIV-positive women with trichomoniasis.
- In women coinfected with trichomoniasis and HIV, metronidazole 500 mg twice daily for 7 days is more effective than a single dose.

Vulvovaginal Candidiasis (VVC)

VVC usually is caused by *C. albicans*, but occasionally is caused by other *Candida* sp. or yeasts. Typical symptoms of VVC include pruritus, vaginal soreness, dyspareunia, external dysuria, and abnormal vaginal discharge. None of these symptoms is specific for VVC. An estimated 75% of women will have at least one episode of VVC, and 40–45% will have two or more episodes within their lifetime (Fig. 8.4).

On the basis of clinical presentation, microbiology, host factors, and response to therapy, VVC can be classified as either uncomplicated or complicated. Approximately 10–20% of women will have complicated VVC that necessitates diagnostic and therapeutic considerations.

Classification of Vulvovaginal Candidiasis

1. Uncomplicated VVC
- Sporadic or infrequent vulvovaginal candidiasis or mild-to-moderate vulvovaginal candidiasis
- Likely to be *caused by C. albicans*
- Non-immunocompromised women are affected

2. Complicated VVC
- Present as recurrent vulvovaginal candidiasis
- It can be severe vulvovaginal candidiasis

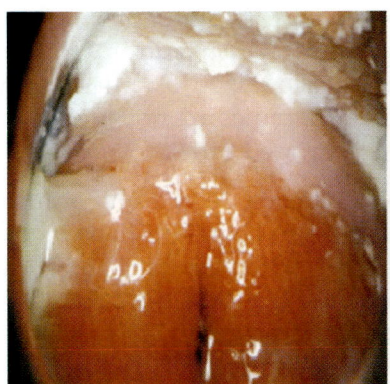

Candidiasis in cervix

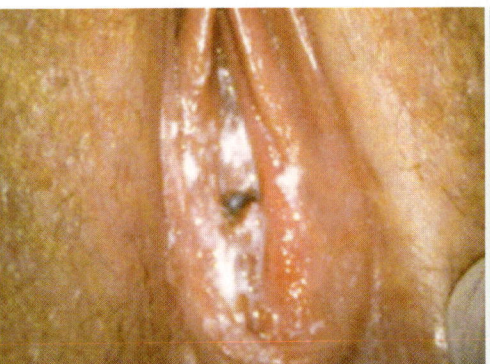

Vulvovaginal candidiasis

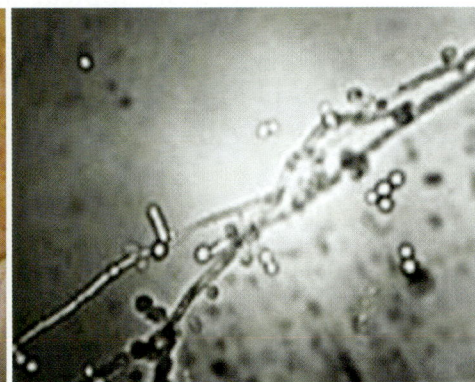

Blastospores, hyphae, pseudohyphae of vulvovaginal candidiasis

Fig. 8.4: Candidiasis

- It may be non-albicans candidiasis
- Women with uncontrolled diabetes, debilitation, or immunosuppression are affected.

Uncomplicated VVC

Diagnostic considerations: A diagnosis of *Candida* vaginitis is suggested clinically by the presence of external dysuria and vulvar pruritus, pain, swelling, and redness.

Signs include vulvar edema, fissures, excoriations, or thick, curdy vaginal discharge.

The diagnosis can be made in a woman who has signs and symptoms of vaginitis when either:

1. A wet preparation (saline, 10% KOH) or Gram stain of vaginal discharge demonstrates yeasts, hyphae, or pseudohyphae, or
2. A culture or other test yields a yeast species. *Candida* vaginitis is associated with a normal vaginal pH (<4.5), and therefore, pH testing is not a useful diagnostic tool. Use of 10% KOH in wet preparations improves the visualization of yeast and mycelia by disrupting cellular material that may obscure the yeast or pseudohyphae. Examination of a wet mount with KOH preparation should be performed for all women with symptoms or signs of VVC, and women with a positive result should receive treatment.

For women with negative wet mounts who are symptomatic, vaginal cultures for *Candida* should be considered. If the wet mount is negative and *Candida* cultures cannot be done, empiric treatment can be considered for symptomatic women with any sign of VVC on examination. Identifying *Candida* by culture in the absence of symptoms or signs is not an indication for treatment, because approximately 10–20% of women harbor *Candida* sp. and other yeasts in the vagina.

Treatment: Short-course topical formulations effectively treat uncomplicated VVC. The topically applied azole drugs are more effective than nystatin. Treatment with azoles results in relief of symptoms and negative cultures in 80–90% of patients who complete therapy.

Recommended regimens

1. Butoconazole 2% cream 5 g intravaginally for 5 days, Or
2. Clotrimazole (1% cream): 5 g or 100 mg vaginal suppository intravaginally for 7–14 days, Or
3. Miconazole (2% cream): 5 g intravaginal for 7 days, or
4. Tioconazole (6.5% ointment): 5 g intravaginal as a single dose.

Follow-up: Patients should be instructed to return for follow-up visits, only if symptoms persist or recur within 2 months of onset of the initial symptoms.

Management of sex partners: VVC is not usually acquired through sexual intercourse; no data support the treatment of sex partners. A minority of male sex partners might have balanitis, which is characterized by erythematous areas on the glans of the penis in conjunction with pruritus or irritation. These men benefit from treatment with topical antifungal agents to relieve symptoms.

Adverse reactions

- Topical agents usually cause no systemic side effects, although local burning or irritation might occur. Oral agents occasionally cause nausea, abdominal pain, and headache.
- Therapy with the oral azoles has been associated rarely with abnormal elevations of liver enzymes.
- Clinically important interactions can occur when these oral agents are administered with other drugs, including astemizole, calcium channel antagonists, cisapride, cyclosporin A, oral hypoglycemic agents, phenytoin, protease inhibitors, rifampin, and warfarin.

Complicated VVC

Recurrent vulvovaginal candidiasis (RVVC): RVVC, usually defined as four or more episodes of symptomatic VVC in 1 year, affects a small percentage of women (<5%).

The pathogenesis of RVVC is poorly understood, and most women with RVVC have no apparent predisposing or underlying conditions.

Vaginal cultures should be obtained from patients with RVVC to confirm the clinical diagnosis and to identify non-albicans species particularly *Candida glabrata*. Although *C. glabrata* and other non-albicans *Candidia* species are observed in 10–20% of patients with RVVC. *C. glabrata* does not form pseudohyphae or hyphae and is not easily recognized on microscopy. Conventional antimycotic therapies are not as effective against these species as they are against *C. albicans*.

Treatment: Each individual episode of RVVC caused by *C. albicans* responds well to short-duration oral or topical azole therapy. However, to maintain clinical and mycologic control, a longer duration of initial therapy (e.g. 7–14 days of topical therapy or a 150 mg, oral dose of fluconazole every third day for a total of 3 doses (day 1, 4, and 7) is recommended to attempt mycologic remission before initiating a maintenance antifungal regimen.

Maintenance regimens: Oral fluconazole (100 mg, 150 mg, or 200 mg dose) weekly for 6 months is the first line of treatment. If this regimen is not feasible, topical treatments used intermittently as a maintenance regimen can be considered.

However, 30–50% of women will have recurrent disease after maintenance therapy is discontinued. Routine treatment of sex partners is controversial.

Severe VVC: Severe vulvovaginitis (i.e. extensive vulvar erythema, edema, excoriation, and fissure formation) is associated with lower clinical response rates in patients treated with short courses of topical or oral therapy. Either 7–14 days of topical azole or 150 mg of fluconazole in two sequential doses (second dose 72 hours after initial dose) is recommended.

Non-albicans VVC: The optimal treatment of non-albicans VVC remains unknown. Options include longer duration of therapy (7–14 days) with a nonfluconazole azole drug (oral or topical) as first-line therapy. If recurrence occurs, 600 mg of boric acid in a gelatin capsule is recommended, administered vaginally once daily for 2 weeks. This regimen has clinical and mycologic eradication rates of approximately 70%.

Pregnancy: VVC frequently occurs during pregnancy. Only topical azole therapies, applied for 7 days, are recommended for use among pregnant women.

HIV infection: The incidence of VVC in HIV-infected women is unknown. Vaginal *Candida* colonization rates among HIV-infected women are higher than among those for seronegative women with similar demographic characteristics and high-risk behaviors, and the colonization rates correlate with increasing severity of immunosuppression.

Symptomatic VVC is more frequent in seropositive women and similarly correlates with severity of immunodeficiency.

Therapy for VVC in HIV-infected women should not differ from that for seronegative women. Although long-term prophylactic therapy with fluconazole at a dose of 200 mg weekly has been effective in reducing *C. albicans* colonization and symptomatic VVC, this regimen is not recommended for routine primary prophylaxis in HIV-infected women in the absence of recurrent VVC.

Despite the frequency at which RVVC occurs in the immmunocompetent healthy population, the occurrence of RVVC should not be considered an indication for HIV testing among women previously testing HIV negative.

8C. TUBERCULOSIS OF FEMALE GENITAL TRACT

Introduction

Genital tuberculosis (TB) in females is by no means uncommon, particularly in communities where pulmonary or other forms of extragenital TB are common. TB can affect any organ in the body, can exist without any clinical manifestation, and can recur.

TB is considered the most important communicable disease in the world. Since the beginning of the 20th century, the incidence of TB in general and genital TB more particularly has been steadily declining in developed countries. However, TB remains a major health problem in many developing countries, and in these areas, genital TB is responsible for a significant proportion of females presenting with infertility. An estimated 30 million persons have active TB, and 7–10 million people die each year of TB. It has been estimated that approximately 5% of females presenting to subfertility clinics worldwide have genital TB. However, estimates of incidence vary from less than 1% in the United States to 19% in India. Genital TB is mostly a secondary manifestation of primary TB, the most common primary site being the lungs and the genital tract is vulnerable to this disease after puberty, and during the childbearing period.

Pathogenesis

Genital TB is almost always secondary to TB elsewhere in the body—usually pulmonary and sometimes renal, gastrointestinal, bone, or joint; occasionally it is part of a generalized miliary disease process. If the bacilli are not eradicated, there is a lifelong risk of reactivation, especially in conjunction with diseases or drugs that cause attenuation of T cell response (e.g. Hodgkin's lymphoma, AIDS, steroids, stress, or malnutrition). The mode of spread is usually hematogenous or lymphatic and occasionally occurs by way of direct contiguity with an intra-abdominal or peritoneal focus. The focus in the lung often heals, and the lesion may lie dormant in the genital tract for years, only to reactivate at a later time.

Hematogenous Spread

After tubercle bacilli invade the lung, in most cases, the bacilli are disseminated by way of the bloodstream within a matter of hours and deposited in various organs of the body. This bacillemia may persist for 6 weeks or longer, if the disease is not recognized and treated promptly with antituberculous drugs. No organ or tissue of the human body is immune from the attack of the tubercle bacillus, although there are marked differences in the frequency with which different organs are infected.

Tubercle bacilli may also reach the bloodstream and thus the genital tract from extrapulmonary and chronic pulmonary lesions. The fallopian tube forms a most favorable nidus for tubercle bacilli, with the earliest lesion found in the mucosa. The tendency of the tubercle bacillus to affect bilateral organs results in both tubes being involved in the tuberculous process. There is almost uniform initial pelvic involvement of the tubes, with subsequent dissemination to other genital organs and the peritoneum. Tuberculous peritonitis is commonly seen with genital tract involvement and may also be associated with rupture of a caseous abdominal lymph node or, less frequently, with spread from an intestinal focus.

Lymphatic Spread

A less common mode of infection, lymphatic spread, occurs when the primary lesion is in the abdominal cavity.

Direct Spread from a Neighboring Viscus

Direct extension to the genital tract organs from tuberculous abdominal viscera, such as the bladder, rectum, appendix, and intestines, has been observed along the peritoneal surface. However, peritoneal involvement can also be the result of spillage of infected material from the fallopian tubes; thus, the primary process is not always clear. It also may occur when adhesions bind the bladder or intestine to the fallopian tubes and perforation of a tuberculous ulcer results in direct spread to the genital organs.

Most pathologists state that primary infection of the female genital organs does not occur. It is known that tuberculous foci may exist in the body and remain undetected for a long time. These lesions may precede the genital lesions and heal without leaving traces demonstrable on clinical examination. The criteria necessary for a diagnosis of primary genital TB are that (1) the genital lesions should be the first tuberculous infection in the body and (2) regional lymph nodes should demonstrate the same stage of tuberculous development as do the genital organs.

There are reports of primary cervical and vulvar disease in which sexual partners have been thought to be the source of infection. This type of disease may also occur in a woman who has TB of another organ and who excretes tubercle bacilli in her stool, urine, or sputum. When these excretions come into contact with the external genitalia, TB of the vulva or vagina may result, particularly if the skin is abraded or broken. The lesions in the cervix and vagina are rare and usually present as isolated, chronic, ulcerative lesions. The infectious agent in TB is usually *M. tuberculosis;* occasionally *Mycobacterium bovis* may cause human disease, including genital tract infection, especially in underdeveloped countries lacking facilities for pasteurization of milk and an effective TB control program for cattle.

Pathology

When the tubercle bacilli infect a susceptible host, the initial reaction is a polymorphonuclear inflammatory exudate. Within 48 hours, this is replaced by mononuclear cells, which become the prime sites for intracellular tubercle replication. As cellular immunity develops, destruction of tubercle bacilli takes place and caseation necrosis occurs. Later reactivation of a focus of infection results in proliferative granulomatous lesion, classically with central caseation necrosis surrounded by concentric layers of epithelial and giant cells, with peripheral lymphocytes, monocytes, and fibroblasts.

Tuberculosis of the Pelvis

Pelvic TB may exist as tuberculous adenitis, of either the mesenteric or the pelvic lymph nodes, without involvement of the genital tract. Generalized miliary peritoneal TB, in which grayish white tubercles stud the abdomen, may involve the serosal surface of both abdominal and pelvic organs without penetrating to the mucosa. Such superficial lesions do not usually impair the reproductive function of the pelvic organs. It should be emphasized that pelvic TB is not the same disease as genital TB.

Tuberculosis of the Fallopian Tubes

Various sources on the topic of genital TB appear to agree that the fallopian tubes are likely the initial source of infection, because both tubes are involved in nearly 100% of cases. The fallopian tubes constitute the initial focus of genital TB in the overwhelming majority of cases (Table 8.1), and TB has accounted for approximately 5% of all cases of salpingitis in many areas of the world.

In more than 90% of patients with genital TB, the tubes are involved bilaterally. In the early stages, the

Table 8.1: Frequency of tuberculosis in genital organs

Organ	Frequency (%)
Fallopian tubes	90–100
Endometrium	50–60
Ovaries	20–30
Cervix	5–15
Vulva and vagina	1

tubes show a little change, but as progression occurs, the diameter of the tube becomes larger. Usually, the ampullary region shows the earliest and most extensive changes, the fimbrial processes become greatly swollen, and the ostia remain open or closed. The isthmus and the adjacent interstitial portion of the tube may remain free of TB. As the process continues, the tubes become softer, and caseation develops in the inner wall. At times, the peritoneal surfaces of the tubes will be studded with tubercles, and the cross-sections may show them to be filled with caseous material. In 25–50% of cases of genital TB, the tubes remain patent with recognizable everted fimbriae, even if the remaining tube is enlarged and distended, the so-called tobacco-pouch appearance.

Microscopic Appearance

Microscopically, granulomata and a chronic inflammatory infiltrate may involve the full thickness of the tubal wall, and caseation necrosis is common in advanced states. Some tubercles have a caseous center, which, as they progress, involves the overlying mucous membrane or causes pressure atrophy. After liquefaction, the caseous foci pour their bacilli into the lumen and form an ulcer at the site. Caseation or a pyogenic membrane lines the ulcer; beyond the inner zone is an area of vascular granulation tissue containing epithelioid and giant cells. Adhesion of the individual foci may occur, resulting in large cystic spaces—*pseudofollicular salpingitis.* Tuberculous salpingitis may contain **Schaumann bodies,** which are conchoidal, laminated, calcified structures surrounded by foreign body giant cells (Fig. 8.5).

Types of Tuberculous Salpingitis

Exudative: In the exudative type, the tube may be significantly enlarged. Although a large pyosalpinx may form, these tubes show a few adhesions and usually are reasonably mobile, if surgery is needed. Frequently, the organs contain a large amount of caseous material plus purulent exudate from secondary infection. This is a relatively acute phase of the process.

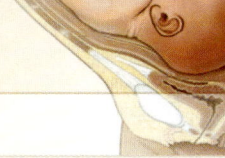

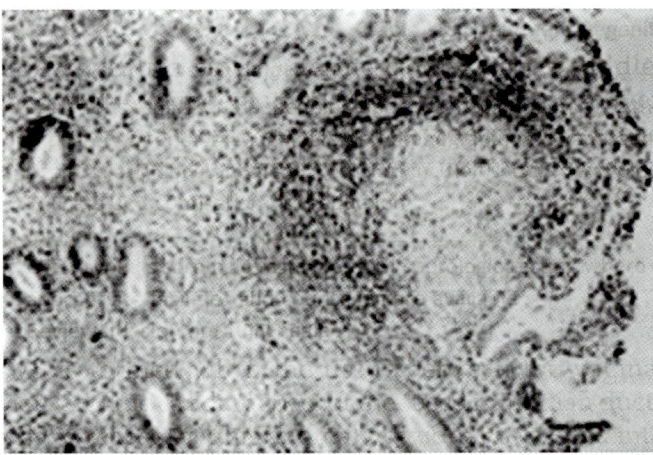

Fig. 8.5: *Schaumann bodies*

Productive–adhesive: In the productive–adhesive form, which is found most frequently at laparoscopy or laparotomy, the tubes are studded with tubercles and are densely adherent to the surrounding organs. The tubercles are seen mostly near the attachment of the tube to the mesosalpinx. The tube wall is thickened and nodular, and the fimbriae and tube are slightly swollen. Eventually, when the process starts healing, it results in calcification and fibrosis.

Mode of Spread from Tubes

After the initial involvement of the tubes, the tuberculous infection spreads to the uterus and ovaries by direct extension. Extension to the uterus is along the endometrium and rarely into the myometrium. Direct hematogenous spread to the uterus as part of a generalized hematogenous TB has rarely been reported.

The ovaries may be involved by direct spread from adjacent organs. In most cases, infection spreads from the tube, and the lesion is seen on the surface of the ovaries. Rarely, the infection extends from the peritoneum to the ovary. Hematogenous spread usually affects the center of the ovary, and the periphery appears normal.

The cervix is involved by spread from the endometrium or as part of the hematogenous infection. Tuberculous infection of the vagina and vulva may follow injury or abrasions to these structure in the presence of tubercle bacilli from the upper genital tract, intestinal tract, or lungs.

Tuberculosis of the Endometrium

Grossly, the size and shape of the uterus may appear normal. The tuberculous process generally is localized to the endometrium, is most extensive in the fundus, and decreases toward the cervix. The myometrium is not usually involved. In premenopausal patients, much of the infected tissue is shed during the menstruation, only to have the endometrium reinfected from the tubes with each cycle. In genital TB, the incidence of involvement of the endometrium is 50–60%.

Microscopic Appearance

TB of the endometrium resembles TB in other tissues, but the advanced stages—caseation, fibrosis, and calcification—are rarely seen during the reproductive period of the regular cyclical shedding of the endometrium. The classic lesion in tuberculous endometritis is the noncaseating granuloma, composed of epithelial cells, Langhans giant cells, and lymphocytes. These granulomata are located throughout the endometrium but occur in greater density in the more superficial layers.

Tuberculosis of the Ovary

Usually, the involvement is bilateral, although this cannot always be recognized with certainty at laparotomy. Two forms of ovarian TB are described: perioophoritis, in which the ovary may be surrounded by or encased in adhesions and studded with tubercles caused by direct extension from the tube; and oophoritis, in which infection starts in the stroma of the ovary, presumably from a hematogenous source that produces a caseating granuloma within the parenchyma.

Tuberculosis of the Cervix

The usual incidence of cervical involvement in genital TB is 5–15%. The diagnosis can be made with certainty only by histologic or bacteriologic examination. Bacteriologic examination of endocervical mucus performed for tuberculous infection, can detect cases of tuberculous cervicitis accurately. The cytopathologic examination of the cervix may reveal multinucleated giant cells, histiocytes, and epithelioid cells arranged in clusters, simulating the appearance of the granulomata that are characteristic of the Papanicolaou smear in cervical TB.

Tuberculosis of the Vulva and Vagina

TB of the vulva and vagina is the rarest form of genital TB, occurring in less than 2% of cases. In most cases, the lesions appear to be secondary to disease higher up in the genital tract but, rarely, the disease may be acquired from the male partner with an infected epididymis or seminal vesicles. In the vulva, it begins as a nodule on the labia or in the vestibular region, which breaks down and forms an irregular ragged ulcer, sometimes with sinuses discharging caseous material and pus. TB of Bartholin's gland is rare. Rarely, a vulvar lesion presents as a hypertrophic, irregular warty growth sometimes resembling elephantiasis.

Tuberculous Peritonitis

Tuberculous peritonitis is seen in combination with female genital tract TB approximately 45% of the time and is thought to be responsible for the often extensive adhesions seen in patients with pelvic TB. Two types of tuberculous peritonitis have been described: The plastic variety and the serous variety.

The *plastic variety* is less common and is characterized by tender abdominal masses and an abdomen "doughy" to palpation. The *serous variety* is seen more commonly and is characterized by ascites, signs of peritoneal inflammation, fever, abdominal pain, weight loss, and anorexia. Most cases of the serous variety are insidious. Patients may be asymptomatic or may present acutely with chills, fever, ascites, and sometimes, rebound tenderness. In the plastic variety, one may observe symptoms suggestive of partial intestinal obstruction.

With advanced diseases, all pelvic organs are densely matted together, often with tubercles studding peritoneal surface, foci of caseation, and calcified plaques, which represent attempts at healing. The peritoneal fluid is exudative in character and generally contains 500–2000 cells, with a predominance of lymphocytes.

Clinical Features

The clinical diagnosis of genital TB requires a high index of suspicion. About 20% of patients with genital TB give a history of TB in their immediate family. Approximately 50% of patients might have had tuberculous pleurisy, peritonitis, erythema nodosum, or renal, osseous, or pulmonary TB. A history of primary infertility in a woman in whom examination reveals no apparent cause and who gives a family history or personal history of TB should raise suspicion of genital TB.

A history of poor general health persisting over months or years and associated with weight loss, undue fatigue, low-grade fever, or vague lower abdominal discomfort is often elicited in patients with genital TB.

Age: Female genital TB is typically understood as a disease of young women, with 80 to 90% of cases diagnosed in patients 20–40 years old, often during work up for subfertility.

Symptoms

Systemic symptoms (Table 8.2) tend to be relatively mild, if present, and may include weight loss, fatigue, and a tendency toward a persistent mild evening elevation of temperature. Approximately 11% of patients are asymptomatic.

In women with genital TB, four major presenting complaints are described with varying frequencies—infertility, abnormal bleeding, pelvic pain, and amenorrhea.

The most common initial symptom is infertility. Infertility is the presenting complaint in 40–50% of patients affected with TB.

Lower Abdominal Pain

The second most frequent complaint is lower abdominal pain or pelvic pain, present in approximately 25 to 50% of patients. The pain is not usually severe and may be accompanied by swelling of the abdomen, although episodes of acute lower abdominal pain owing to secondary infection by pyogenic organisms may occur.

Menstrual Disorders

The third most common symptom is abnormal uterine bleeding in genital TB found in 10 to 40% of patients. The commonly observed menstrual disorders are oligohypomenorrhea (54%), menorrhagia (19.9%), amenorrhea (14.3%) and postmenopausal bleeding in 1.6% of cases.

Other symptoms seen less frequently with pelvic TB include vaginal discharge, abdominal swelling, pelvic relaxation, and symptoms associated with fistula formation. Uterovesical, tubointestinal, and

Table 8.2: Symptoms related to genital tuberculosis
Systemic
Weight loss
Fatigue
Low-grade fever
Infertility
Primary
Secondary
Menstrual disturbances
Amenorrhea
Menorrhagia
Metrorrhagia
Oligomenorrhea
Abdominal swelling
Postcoital bleeding
Vaginal discharge
Dyspareunia

tuboperitoneal fistulas have all been described. Genital TB can mimic ovarian cancer. These patients commonly present with adnexal masses and ascites. To further confuse the picture, serum CA-125 levels can be elevated as well in genital TB, and diagnosis is often made only after laparotomy.

Physical Signs

The physical examination can be normal in up to 35–50% of cases of female genital TB. When abnormal findings are present, they usually consist of adnexal masses, signs of ascites or fixation of pelvic organs. Tuberculous tuboovarian masses are less tender than those due to pyogenic infection, although secondary infection and acute exacerbation may produce sharp pain and tenderness (Table 8.3).

Abdominal examination may reveal a "doughy" sensation, which has been ascribed to tubercle formation on the intestines and peritoneum. Ascites, either general or sacculated, may produce distention of the abdomen. Irregular masses caused by the matting together of intestines, omentum, and pelvic organs may be palpated. In an adolescent female presenting with ascites, pain, and low-grade fever, the cause is frequently TB.

In menopausal women, genital TB may cause an enlarged uterus that is tense and tender on examination, the result of pyometra formation. A fistulous tract between the genital tract and the bowel, bladder, or cutaneous area may suggest ovarian malignancy. These are usually caused by rupture of a tuberculous pyosalpinx into adjacent organs. Less common findings include lesions of the cervix and external genitalia.

Diagnosis

- The possibility of TB infection of the genital tract should always be considered, especially in a patient from an area where TB is endemic, a patient with a family history of exposure to TB, or a patient with

Table 8.3: Physical signs in genital tuberculosis

Normal
- Abdominal mass
- Pelvic mass
- Adnexal mass
- Abdominal tenderness
- Pelvic/adnexal tenderness
- Ascites
- Excessive vaginal discharge
- Ulcer in the vulva, vagina, and cervix
- Enlarged uterus with pyometra
- Fistula

some proven extragenital manifestations of the disease.
- Infertility for which no obvious cause can be found, chronic pelvic inflammatory disease refractory to standard antibiotic therapy, or adnexal disease with ascites in virgin females should alert the clinician to look for TB of the genital tract.

Laboratory Investigations (Table 8.4)

Chest Radiograph

Though genital TB is believed to be secondary to primary pulmonary infection in most cases, chest radiograph abnormalities are identified in only 10–50% of cases. Most of the abnormalities found were suggestive of prior pulmonary TB, whereas active pulmonary TB in association with genital TB is rare.

Tuberculin Test

The tuberculin skin test has been the traditional method of demonstrating infection with *M. tuberculosis*. The reaction to intracutaneously injected tuberculin is the classic example of a delayed (cellular) hypersensitivity reaction. Characteristically, this reaction begins at 5–6 hours, and is maximal at 48–72 hours. The typical method of performing the tuberculin test is the intracutaneous, or Mantoux method. Here 0.1 mL of PPD is injected intracutaneously into the dorsal or volar surface of the forearm. A discrete wheal should be produced. The test is read between 48 and 72 hours after the injection. A reaction of greater than or equal to 15 mm is classified as positive in all other groups of patients. It only indicates past infection.

Menstrual Blood Analysis

Definitive diagnosis of TB requires isolation of tubercle bacilli via culture, although histological presence of

Table 8.4: Investigations to confirm the diagnosis of genital TB

Complete blood count
　　Chest radiographs
　　Tuberculin test
Menstrual blood, peritoneal fluid for culture for *Mycobacterium tuberculosis*
Endometrial curettage for histologic examination
Peritoneal biopsy for culture and histology
Hysterosalpingography
Ultrasonography
Cervical cytology
Endoscopy
　　Laparoscopy
　　Hysteroscopy
　　Cystoscopy

characteristic granulomata is confirmatory to make the diagnosis of genital TB. Because the endometrium is involved in the majority of cases and is readily accessible to sampling, menstrual blood is considered the easily available sample for diagnosis. Bacteriologic examination of menstrual blood with acid-fast bacilli (AFB) smear and culture is recommended by some; however, sensitivity of these tests is quite low.

Endometrial Curettage

In investigating the possibility of genital tract TB, the most accessible tissue for study with a high frequency of involvement is the endometrium. The histologic examination of endometrial tissues removed by biopsy or curettage, especially from the cornual area, affords a rapid method of diagnosing genital TB in at least 50% of cases. AFB stain and culture and, occasionally, guinea pig inoculation, yield better microbiologic assessment. The optimal time for sampling is at the end of the menstrual cycle or within 12 hours after the onset of menstrual flow to allow the endometrial granulomata maximal time to develop.

Polymerase Chain Reaction

Faster and more accurate in diagnosis. But it has also high false positive rate of diagnosis and, therefore, is not recommended for start of ATT for FGTB unless other evidence of TB is present.

Radiography

No characteristic radiographic features are pathognomonic for genital tract TB, although certain findings should raise suspicion of its possibility.

Hysterosalpingography may reveal certain abnormalities that suggest the possibility of pelvic TB.

1. The uterine cavity is classically shriveled and deformed, with associated intrauterine adhesions and lymphatic extravasation (Fig. 8.6).
2. The fallopian tubes often show ragged outlines with multiple strictures, giving a beaded appearance (Fig. 8.6).
3. The entire tube appears rigid and may exhibit small terminal sacculations of the ampullary end (Fig. 8.7).
4. Occlusion of the digital end of the fallopian tubes is common, and marked hydrosalpinx is not uncommon (Figs 8.8 and 8.9).
5. Calcification of the organs, lymph nodes may be visualized.

Hysterosalpingography is contraindicated in the presence of recent acute pelvic infection, and there is

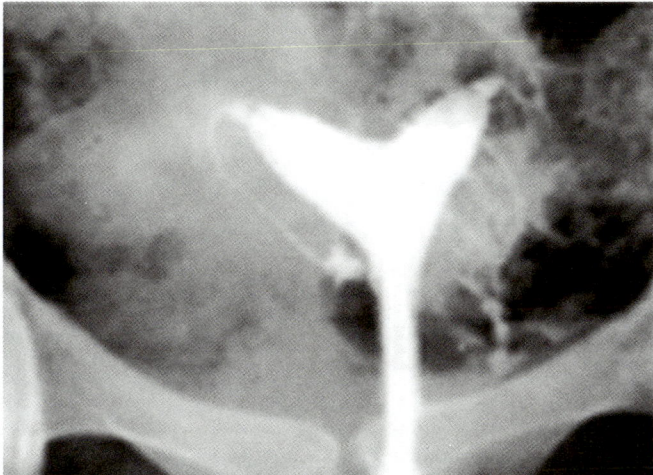

Fig. 8.6: Radiograph demonstrates lymphatic extravasation, a deformed uterine cavity, and a narrow-rigid fallopian tube with a dilated and closed fimbrial end on the right side

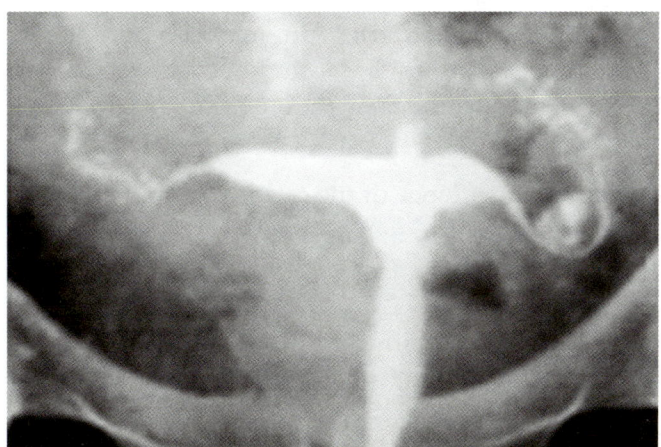

Fig. 8.7: The fallopian tubes show a rigid, ragged outline with a beaded appearance

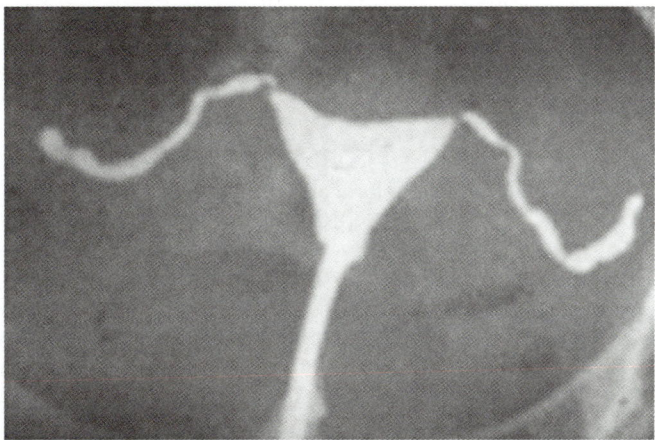

Fig. 8.8: The entire fallopian tube appears rigid and exhibits small terminal sacculations

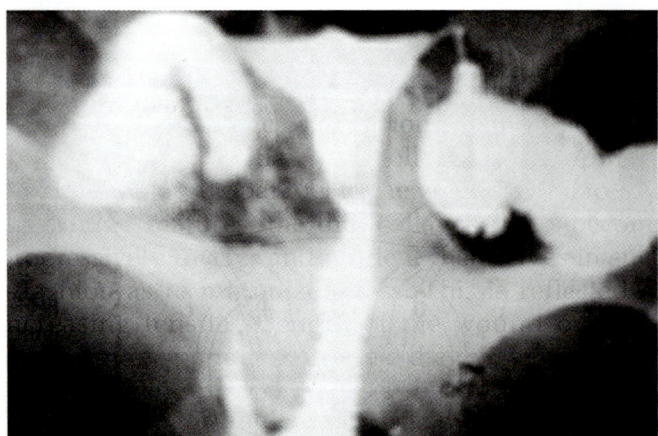

Fig. 8.9: Gross dilatation and occlusion of both f allopian tubes is visible on this radiograph

possibility of exacerbation of pelvic TB following the procedure.

Uterus

1. Small contracted uterus with irregular outline.
2. Endometrial adhesions with deformity.
3. Serrated appearance of endometrium.

Cervix

1. Sunray appearance of the cervical canals
2. Cervical stenosis

Ultrasonography

High-resolution abdominal and transvaginal ultrasonography may demonstrate loculated ascites;

bilateral, predominantly solid, adnexal masses containing scattered small calcification; thickened omentum; thickened peritoneum; and endometrial involvement, which might alert the clinician to suspect genital tract TB.

CT scan: May be useful to differentiate from ovarian cancer by low-density ascites and caseating lymphadenopathy.

MRI can differentiate from ovarian cancer and avoid laparotomy. The presence of hypodense masses with rim enhancement abutting the pelvic sidewalls is diagnostic of TB.

Tumor Markers

CA-125 never exceeds 200 U/mL whereas it is much high in ovarian cancer.

Endoscopy

Hysteroscopy: Abnormal contour of uterine cavity, flimsy adhesions, dense adhesions, blocked cornual ostia, poor distensibility, pale endometrium, cervical constrictions are suspicious.

Laparoscopy: Different findings are:
a. Yellow, small nodules on tubes
b. Short swollen tubes with agglutinated fimbria
c. Unilateral or bilateral hydrosalpinx with retort shape tubes
d. Pyosalpix or caseosalpinx
e. Presence of bowel adhesions

	Type of patients	Initial phase of TB regime	Continuation phase of TB regime
Category I	New smear +ve PTB, new smear −ve PTB with extensive pulmonary involvement Severe forms of FGTB and other EPTB	2 HRZE; INH (600 mg), Rifampicin (450 mg/600 mg if BW >50 kg), Ethambutol (800 mg), PZN (1500 mg) for 2 months:	4 HR (INH 600 mg); Rifampicin (450 mg/600 mg, if body wt. >50 kg) for 4 months
Category II	Previously treated sputum +ve PTB, relapse in FGTB, treatment failure in FGTB	2 months of KRZES: INH, Rifampicin, Ethambutol same as category 1 + Inj. Streptomycin 0.75 mg/day or thrice a week for 2 months followed by 1 month of HRZE	5 HRE: INH, ethambutol, rifampicin for 5 months
Category III	New smear −ve PTB (other than category I) Less severe form of EPTB	2 HRZ	4HR
Category IV	Chronic/multidrug-resistant TB (MDR-TB) cases/culture +ve or histopatho- logically proven FGTB	Kanamycin IM: dose—500–750 mg daily; Ofloxacin oral: dose—600–800 mg daily; Ethionamide oral: dose— 500–750 mg daily; Pyrazinamide oral: dose—1250–1500 mg/day; Ethambutol oral: dose—800–100 mg/ day; Cycloserine oral; 500–750 mg/day Ofloxacin : 600–800 mg/day Ethambutol: 800–1000 mg/day Cycloserine: 500–750 mg/day	For 6–9 months intensive phase For 18 months continuation phase

Table 8.5: Anti-Koch's regime

f. Tubercles on gut and tubal serosa

g. Peritoneal/enlarged lymph node biopsy

Treatment

All PTB are treated in DOTS category 1 with thrice weekly 4-drug regime which includes INH, pyrazinamide, ethambutol, and rifampicin for 2 months. This is followed by INH, rifampicin for 4 months. Those showing relapse or irregular treatment may be put in DOTS category 2 where inj. streptomycin along with 4 drugs were given for 2 months, followed by 4 drugs for another 1 month. This is followed by 3 drugs INH, rifampicin, ethambutol for another 5 months. All these drugs are given thrice a week (Table 8.5).

Treatment of Infertility in FGTB

Pregnancy rate is higher in IVF procedures in patients without endometrial damage. Tuboplasty results in poor pregnancy outcome as the tubes are mostly badly damaged. Ectopic pregnancy is another sequela of tuboplasty in TB salpingitis. There are reports of 17.3% conception rate in IVF-ET procedures. Silent latent TB is considered as one of the important causes of idiopathic infertility and outcome of results improve with good implantation rate in IVF procedures following ATT with ciprofloxacin. Adoption is better, if endometrium is badly damaged like in TB synechia.

8D. SYNDROMIC MANAGEMENT

In many developing country, health facilities lack laboratory equipment or skills required for etiological diagnosis of STI. To overcome this, a syndrome-based approach to the management of STI patients was developed and promoted in a large number of countries in the developing world. Syndromic management is based on the identification of consistent groups of symptoms and easily recognized signs (syndromes), and the provision of treatment that will deal with the majority or most serious organisms responsible for producing this syndrome. WHO developed a simplified tool (a flowchart or algorithm) to guide health workers in the implementation of syndromic management.

WHO have developed syndromic case management algorithms for women with symptoms of vaginal discharge and/or lower abdominal pain. However, it is important to recognize the limitations of the vaginal discharge algorithms, particularly in the management of cervical (gonococcal and chlamydial) infections.

Risk Factors for STI-related Cervicitis

Clinical observations that have been consistently found to be associated with cervical infection are the presence of cervical mucus, cervical erosions, cervical friability and bleeding between menses or during sexual intercourse. A number of demographic and behavioral risk factors have also been frequently associated with cervical infection. These include: these whose age are below 21 years, being unmarried, more than one sexual partner in the last 3 months, new partner in the previous 3 months, current partner who has a sexually transmitted infection and recent use of condoms by the partner.

Selection of Drugs

Antimicrobial resistance of several sexually transmitted pathogens has been increasing in many parts of the world and this has rendered some low-cost regimens ineffective. Recommendations to use more effective drugs frequently raise concerns about cost and possible misuse.

The drugs used for STI in all healthcare facilities should be at least 95% effective. Criteria for the selection of drugs are listed in Box 8.1.

Treatment of STI-associated Syndromes

Urethral Discharge

Male patients complaining of urethral discharge and/ or dysuria should be examined for evidence of

Box 8.1: Criteria for the selection of STI drugs

Drugs selected for treating STI should meet the following criteria:
- High efficacy (at least 95%)
- Low cost
- Acceptable toxicity and tolerance
- Organism resistance unlikely to develop or likely to be delayed
- Single dose
- Oral administration
- Not contraindicated for pregnant or lactating women.

discharge. If none is seen, the urethra should be gently massaged from the ventral part of the penis towards the meatus.

If microscopy is available, examination of the urethral smear may show an increased number of polymorphonuclear leukocytes and a Gram stain may demonstrate the presence of gonococci. In the male, more than 5 polymorphonuclear leukocytes per high power field ($\times$ 1000) are indicative of urethritis.

The major pathogens causing urethral discharge are *N. gonorrhoeae* and *Chlamydia trachomatis*. In the syndromic management, treatment of a patient with urethral discharge should adequately cover these two organisms (Table 8.6).

Genital Ulcer (Table 8.7)

The relative prevalence of causative organisms for genital ulcer disease varies considerably in different parts of the world and may change dramatically over time. Clinical differential diagnosis of genital ulcers is inaccurate, particularly in settings where several etiologies are common. Clinical manifestations and patterns of genital ulcer disease may be further altered in the presence of HIV infection.

After examination to confirm the presence of genital ulceration, treatment appropriate to local etiologies and antibiotic sensitivity patterns should be given. For example, in areas where both syphilis and chancroid are prevalent, patients with genital ulcers should be treated for both conditions at the time of their initial presentation to ensure adequate therapy in case of loss to follow-up. In areas where granuloma inguinale or lymphogranuloma venereum (LGV) is prevalent, treatment for these conditions should be included. In many parts of the world, genital herpes is the most frequent cause of genital ulcer disease. Where HIV infection is prevalent, an increasing portion of cases of

Table 8.6: Recommended syndromic treatment—urethral discharge

Treatment options for gonorrhea	Treatment options for chlamydia
Ciprofloxacin	Doxycycline
Azithromycin	Azithromycin
Ceftriaxone	
Cefixime	
Spectinomycin	
Alternatives:	*Alternatives*
Kanamycin	Amoxycillin
Trimethoprim/sulfamethoxazole	Erythromycin (if tetracycline contraindicated)
	Ofloxacin
	Tetracycline

WHO recommends that, where possible, single dose therapy be utilized.

Table 8.7: Recommended syndromic treatment—genital ulcer

Drug options for syphilis	Drug options for chancroid	Drug options for granuloma inguinale	Drug options for LGV
Benzathine	Ciprofloxacin	Azithromycin	Doxycycline
Benzylpenicillin	Erythromycin	Doxycycline	Erythromycin
	Azithromycin		
Alternatives	*Alternatives*	*Alternatives*	*Alternatives*
Procaine	Ceftriaxone	Erythromycin	Tetracycline
Benzylpenicillin		Tetracycline	
		Trimethoprim/sulfamethoxazole	
Penicillin allergy and non-pregnancy			
Doxycycline			
Tetracycline			

Depending upon local availability, management for herpes could include specific antiviral therapy (acyclovir 500–800 mg 3–5 times daily), but in all settings, appropriate counseling is essential.

genital ulcer disease is likely to harbour herpes simplex virus. Herpetic ulcers may be atypical and persist for long periods in HIV-infected patients.

Laboratory-assisted differential diagnosis is rarely helpful at the initial visit, as mixed infections are common. In addition, in areas of high syphilis prevalence, a reactive serological test may reflect a previous infection and give a misleading picture of the patient's present condition.

Genital Ulcer and HIV Infection (Table 8.8)

There have been a number of anecdotal reports in the literature suggesting that the natural history of syphilis may be altered as a result of concomitant HIV infection.

There is evidence to suggest that HIV infection may increase rates of treatment failure in chancroid, especially when single-dose therapies are given.

Herpes simplex lesions may present as persistent multiple ulcers that require medical attention, as opposed to self-limiting vesicles and ulcers which occur in immunocompetent individuals. Thus, antiviral treatment may have to be considered therapeutically or prophylactically to offer comfort to the patient. Adequate education needs to be given to the patient to explain the nature and purpose of treatment in order to avoid false expectations of cure.

Vaginal Discharge (Fig. 8.10)

A spontaneous complaint of abnormal vaginal discharge is most commonly due to a vaginal infection. Rarely, it may be the result of mucopurulent STI-related cervicitis. *T. vaginalis, C. albicans* and bacterial vaginosis are the commonest causes of vaginal infection and *N. gonorrhoeae* and *C. trachomatis* cause cervical infection. The clinical detection of cervical infection is difficult because a large proportion of women with gonococcal or chlamydia cervical infection is asymptomatic. The symptom of abnormal vaginal discharge is highly indicative of vaginal infection, but poorly predictive for cervical infection. Thus, all women presenting with vaginal discharge should receive treatment for trichomoniasis and bacterial vaginosis (Tables 8.9 and 8.10).

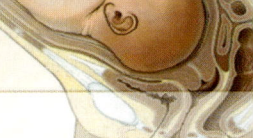

Table 8.8: Treatment of genital ulcer and hopes simplex infection

Genital ulcer disease management	*Herpes simplex management*
• Treat for syphilis, and depending upon local epidemiology, either chancroid, granuloma inguinale or lymphogranuloma venereum	• Advise on basic care of the lesion (keep clean and dry)
• Aspirate any fluctuant glands (surgical incision should be avoided)	• Educate and counsel on compliance and risk reduction
• Educate and counsel on risk reduction	• Offer syphilis and HIV serologic testing where appropariate facilities and counseling are available
• Offer syphilis serologic testing and HIV serologic testing where appropriate facilities and counseling are available	• Promote and provide condoms
• Review if lesion not fully healed	• Advise to return in 7 days, if lesion is not fully healed, and if there is clinical deterioration

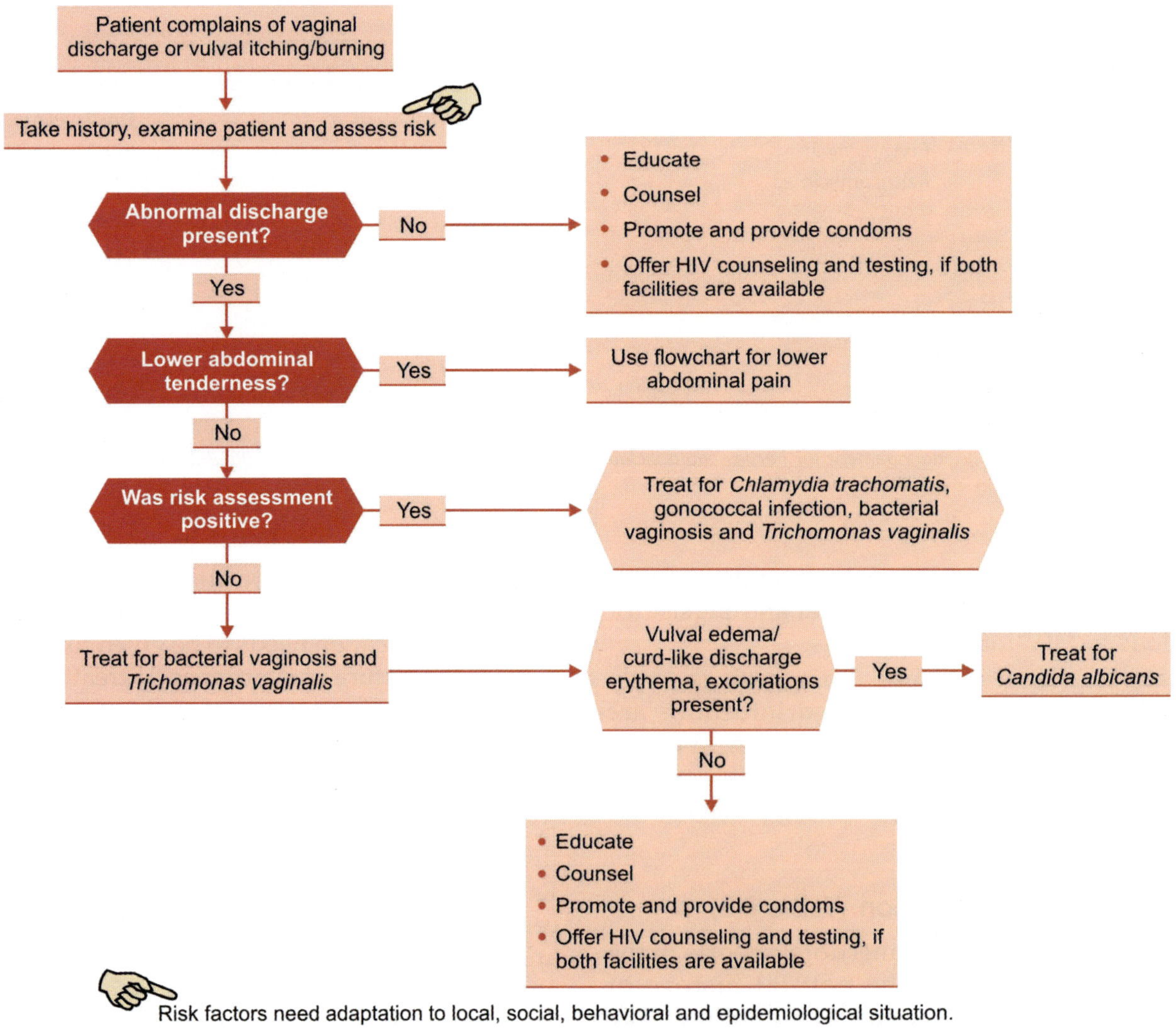

Patient complains of vaginal discharge or vulval itching/burning

Take history, examine patient and assess risk

Abnormal discharge present? — No →
- Educate
- Counsel
- Promote and provide condoms
- Offer HIV counseling and testing, if both facilities are available

Yes ↓

Lower abdominal tenderness? — Yes → Use flowchart for lower abdominal pain

No ↓

Was risk assessment positive? — Yes → Treat for *Chlamydia trachomatis*, gonococcal infection, bacterial vaginosis and *Trichomonas vaginalis*

No ↓

Treat for bacterial vaginosis and *Trichomonas vaginalis* →
Vulval edema/curd-like discharge erythema, excoriations present? — Yes → Treat for *Candida albicans*

No ↓

- Educate
- Counsel
- Promote and provide condoms
- Offer HIV counseling and testing, if both facilities are available

Risk factors need adaptation to local, social, behavioral and epidemiological situation.

Fig. 8.10: Summary of treatment of vaginal discharge

Choice of Antimicrobial Regimens

Efficacy

Efficacy is the most important criterion in choosing among available regimens. STI therapy regimens should, ideally, cure at least 95% of those infected with a bacterial STI. In order to reduce the risk of development and transmission of resistant strains of sexually transmitted pathogens to the general population, special programmes for effective case

Table 8.9: Recommended syndromic treatment—cervical infection

Drug options for gonorrhea	Drug options for chlamydia
Ciprofloxacin	Doxycycline
Azithromycin	Azithromycin
Ceftriaxone	
Cefixime	
Spectinomycin	
Alternatives	*Alternatives*
Kanamycin	Amoxycillin
Trimethoprim/sulfamethoxazole	Ofloxacin
	Erythromycin (if tetracyline is contraindicated)
	Tetracycline

• Tetracyclines are contraindicated in pregnancy.
• Trimethoprim/sulfamethoxazole should only be used in areas where this combination has been shown to be effective against uncomplicated gonorrhea.

Table 8.10: Vaginal infection

Drug options for BV	Drug options for TV	Drug options for candida
Metronidazole	Metronidazole	Miconazole
	Tinidazole	Clotrimazole
		Fluconazole
Alternatives		*Alternative*
Clindamycin		Nystatin
Metronidazole gel		
Clindamycin vaginal cream		

Patients taking metronidazole should be cautioned to avoid alcohol.

management should be designed for groups at high risk, such as sex workers and their clients. *Treatment regimens for these groups should be nearly 100% effective.*

Safety

Toxicity is a second major concern in STI treatments because of the frequency with which patients become reinfected and their consequent exposure to repeated courses of antimicrobials. Combination regimens further increase the risk of adverse drug reactions. Pregnancy, relatively common in sexually active groups with a high incidence of STI, represents a special situation in which additional considerations of fetal safety become important. The safety of the fluoroquinolones in pregnancy and adolescence is uncertain and limits their use in groups with a high level of sexual activity. In some areas, doxycycline is not used because of the danger of photosensitization. Tetracyclines are contraindicated in pregnancy and children under 8 years of age.

The prominence of third-generation cephalosporins in the recommended regimens results from their combination of high efficacy, even against relatively resistant organisms and low toxicity.

Compliance and Acceptability

Patient compliance with STI treatment regimens is a continuing problem seriously limiting the effectiveness of multidose regimens such as those involving erythromycin and tetracyclines. Single-dose or very short course regimens should, therefore, be given preference. Appropriate counseling and health education have been shown to increase compliance and should be a part of clinical management.

In view of the emergence and spread of HIV infection, preference should be given to oral regimens, in order to reduce risks associated with the reuse of non-sterilized injection equipment. Patient education on the efficacy of oral preparations must be part of STI management.

Coexistent Infections

When several STIs are prevalent in a population, co-infection may be a common occurrence. In most cases, dual therapy is now required for simultaneous gonococcal and chlamydial infections. Coincident chancroid and syphilis require a multi-drug regimen. The severity of disease caused by several sexually transmitted pathogens (e.g. herpes simplex virus, *H. ducreyi, T. pallidum*) may be increased in HIV infection and AIDS, and treatment must be intensified and prolonged.

Commonly Used Drugs

Cephalosporins

Several third-generation cephalosporins have been shown to be effective in the treatment of gonorrhea. Cefixime has the advantage of being an oral preparation. It is also likely to be effective against chancroid, but it has not yet been evaluated in this condition. The efficacy of ceftriaxone in the treatment of gonorrhea and chancroid has been well documented. There is a strong positive correlation between the minimum inhibiting concentrations of penicillins and cephalosporins.

Macrolides

Of the newer macrolides, azithromycin is currently considered the drug of choice for treating chamydial infection. The drug has a prolonged bioavailability that permits single-dose administration and it accumulates within cells. Azithromycin 1 gm single-dose therapy has been shown to be as effective as a week-long course of doxycycline 100 mg twice daily in the treatment of chlamydia.

Sulphonamides

The addition of trimethoprim to sulphonamides does not increase their antichlamydial activity. A three-day regimen of sulfamethoxazole and trimethoprim is inadequate for chlamydial infection.

Quinolones

The *in vitro* activity of individual fluoroquinolones against *N. gonorrhoeae* varies considerably. Ciprofloxacin is considered to be the agent with the greatest activity against *N. gonorrhoeae*.

Experience with treating chlamydial infection with fluoroquinolones is limited. Of the currently studied agents, ofloxacin has the greatest potential when given as 300 mg twice daily for 7 days.

Antimicrobial Resistance in *N. gonorrhoeae*

There are two main types of antibiotic resistance in *N. gonorrhoeae*: *Chromosomal resistance* involves penicillins and a wide range of other therapeutic agents such as tetracyclines, spectinomycin, erythromycin, quinolones, thiamphenicol, and cephalosporins; *Plasmid-mediated resistance* affects penicillins and tetracyclines. Chromosomally resistant *N. gonorrhoeae*, penicillinase-producing gonococci, and plasmid-mediated, tetracycline-resistant strains are all increasing and have had a major impact on the efficacy of traditional regimens for treating gonorrhea.

Comprehensive Case Management of STI

One of the essential components of the public health package is comprehensive case management of STI, which comprises:

Identification of the syndrome: This can be done through syndromic diagnosis or laboratory tests.

Educating the patient: Patients should be informed about the nature of the infection, the importance of taking the full course of medication, among other things.

Antibiotic treatment for the syndrome: Whichever means is used for diagnosis—flow charts or laboratory tests—the availability and use of effective antibiotics is an absolute requirement. The drugs must be available at the first point of contact with a patient with an STI. Effective treatment must also be available and used in the private sector.

Condom supply: With people being encouraged to use condoms, health authorities should ensure that there is an adequate supply of good-quality, affordable condoms at health facilities and at various other distribution points in the community. Social marketing of condoms is another way of increasing access to condoms.

Counseling: Counseling should be made available for cases where it is needed—for example, in chronic cases of genital herpes or warts—either for individuals or for couples in a sexual relationship.

Information on partner notification and treatment: Contacting sex partners of clients with STI, persuading them to present themselves to a site offering STI services, and treating them, promptly and effectively are essential elements of any STI control programe. These actions, should, however, be carried out with sensitivity, with social and cultural factors taken into account. This will avoid ethical problems, as well as practical problems such as rejection and violence, particularly against women.

Development of Female Genital Tract

Anatomic Relationship between Genital and Urinary Systems

The development of the genital apparatus accompanies that of the urinary system. It originates in the **intermediate mesoderm** and **urogenital sinus**. The **primordial germ cells** share in the formation of the gonads, but have an **ectodermal origin.** In males, the development of the testes is closely tied with that of the mesonephros. In females, on the other hand, the mesonephros plays no role at all. The intermediate mesoblast is the origin of an elongated structure, the urogenital ridge which lies on both sides of the midline between the lateral mesoderm and the root of the dorsal mesenterium of the embryo. It consists of two main components, the **nephrogenic cord** (Fig. 9.1), from

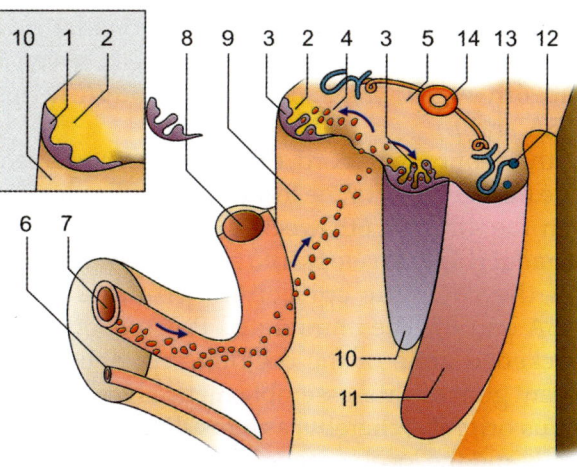

1. Coelomic epithelium	8. Intestine
2. Local mesenchyma (in proliferation)	9. Dorsal mesentery
3. Gonadal cord	10. Genital ridge
4. Primordial germ cells (PGC)	11. Nephrogenic cord
5. Mesenchyma	12. Mesonephric duct (Wolff)
6. Allantois	13. Mesonephric tubule
7. Omphalomesenteric duct	14. Aorta

Fig. 9.1: Development of the indifferent gonad with the migration of primordial germ cells (PGC) at around the 6th week

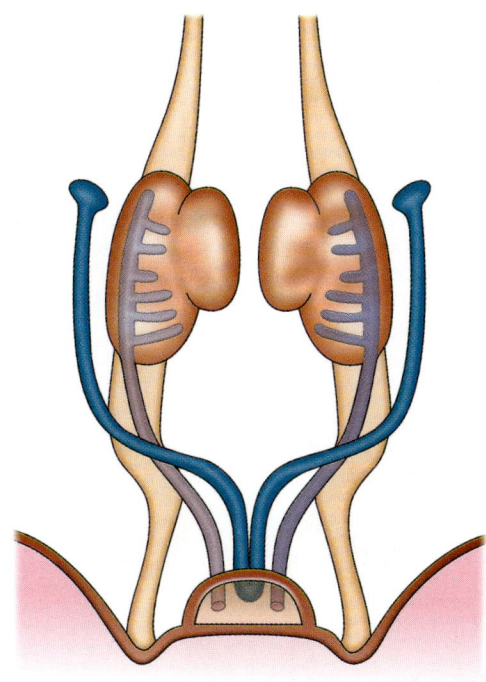

Fig. 9.2: In an embryo with indifferent gonads, two bands secure the gonads at the lower and upper poles

which the **urinary apparatus** arises and the **genital ridge.** The genital ridge extends from the upper thorax region to the level of the cloaca. The cranial and caudal parts of the urogenital ridge form the upper and lower gonadal bands, respectively, to secure the gonads cranially and caudally.

After the mesonephros has atrophied, the lower **gubernaculum** inserts at the lower pole of the gonad, extends to the inguinal region and, in **man**, thus forms the **gubernaculum** and, in **woman**, the **ovarian ligament and round ligament** (ligamentum teres uteri) (Fig. 9.2). After the atrophy of the mesonephros, the **upper gubernaculum** disappears in men while in women, the **suspensory ligament of ovary** is formed, which extends from the upper pole of the ovary towards the back and upwards into the lumbar region (Fig. 9.3A and B).

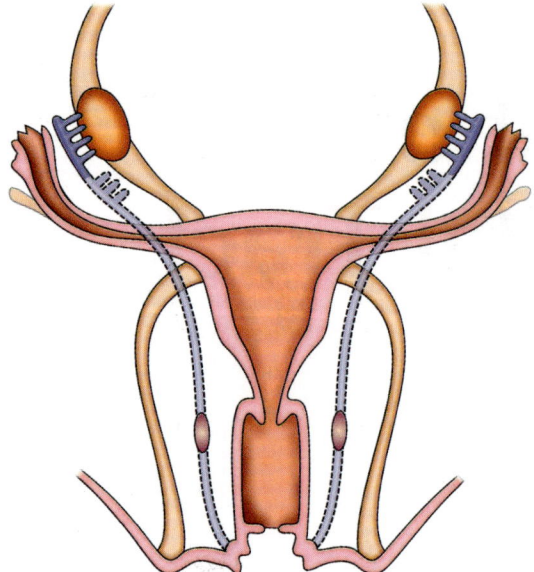

Fig. 9.3A: In a **woman**, the upper gubernaculum inserts at the upper pole of the ovary and forms the suspensory ligament of ovary. The lower gubernaculum inserts at the lower pole of the ovary and extends as the ovarian ligament to the uterine tube angle, where it continues as the round ligament of uterus (ligamentum teres uteri)

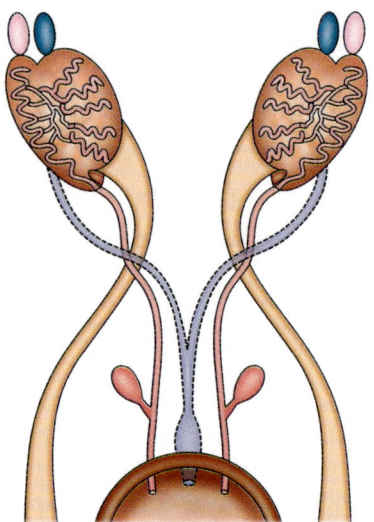

Fig. 9.3B: In a **man**, the upper gubernaculum disappears, while the gubernaculum testis forms from the lower portion

Gonads: Indifferent Stage

The gonads arise from **two very different kinds of cells** that originate in the embryo:

The **primordial germ cells (PGC)** will form the **gametes** (sperm cells and oocytes). These cells come from the **ectoderm**, but they separate themselves from it at a very early stage in the development (Fig. 9.4A and B).

The **somatic cells** with nourishing functions surround the primordial germ cells and form the

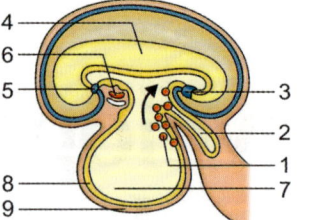
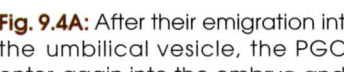
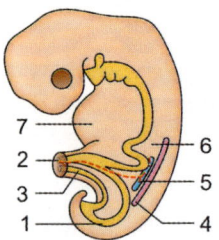

1. PGC	7. Umbilical vesicle (yolk sac)
2. Allantois	
3. Cloacal membrane	8. Endoderm
4. Epiblast	9. Mesoderm
5. Pharyngeal membrane	
6. Heart anlage	

| 1. Rectum |
| 2. Omphalomesenteric duct |
| 3. Allantois |
| 4. Nephrogenic cord (pink) |
| 5. Gonadal ridge (green) |
| 6. PGC |
| 7. Heart anlage |

Fig. 9.4A: After their emigration into the umbilical vesicle, the PGC enter again into the embryo and thence into the intestinal wall

Fig. 9.4B: From the intestine, they colonize the gonadal ridge in that they emigrate there via the mesentery

somatic gonadal blastema. In the testes, the **supporting cells are Sertoli** and the **interstitial cells of Leydig**. In the ovary, they are **follicle cells** and the **theca cells**.

The **primordial germ cells (PGC)** already appear at the time of gastrulation in the **epiblast** and complete an **emigration** out of the embryo into the wall of the **yolk sac** (umbilical vesicle) by collaboration of three factors—folding of the embryo, chemotactic factors and ameboid movements. The germ cells get from here into the wall of the intestinal tract within the embryo again and via the dorsal mesentery into the gonadal ridge. During their migration, which takes place between the 4th and 6th week, they multiply through mitosis (Fig. 9.5A and B).

Like the nephrogenic cord, the gonadal ridge extends from the heart region to the location near the cloaca. In between the 4th and 6th week, the middle section of this **gonadal ridge** develops into a **gonad anlage** in that cells of the coelomic epithelium proliferate there (Fig. 9.6A and B). The immigrated PGC penetrate into this thickened zone of the coelomic epithelium. The indifferent gonads thus assemble themselves from cells of various origins, whereby, as a result, the primordial germ cells and the local somatic blastema influence each other reciprocally.

The **local coelomic mesenchyma** underneath also multiplies. The **coelomic epithelium**, which now becomes multi-layered, loses for now its basal membrane. **Gonadal cords** arise that surround the PGC and extend into the depths. In the male, **mesonephric cells** are also involved, but it is unknown whether in females the cells immigrate as far as the gonadal ridge.

Up to the 6th week, **male** and **female** gonads cannot be distinguished. The gonadal cords and the PGC can

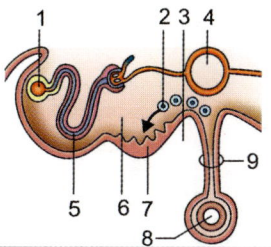

1. Mesonephric duct (Wolff)
2. PGC
3. Peritoneal cavity
4. Aorta
5. Mesonephric tubule
6. Local coelomic mesenchyme
7. Thickened coelomic epithelium
8. Intestine
9. Mesentery

Fig. 9.5A: Cells of the thickened coelomic epithelium leave the cellular envelope and migrate into the depths where they form the gonadal cords with the PGC and the local mesenchyme. The anlage of the paramesonephric duct (Müller) is now formed

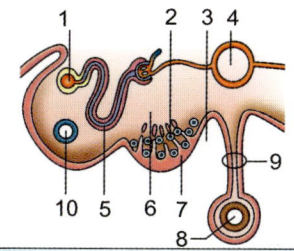

1. Mesonephric duct (Wolff)
2. PGC
3. Peritoneal cavity
4. Aorta
5. Mesonephric tubule
6. Local coelomic mesenchyme
7. Thickened coelomic epithelium
8. Intestine
9. Mesentery
10. Anlage of the para-mesonephric duct (Müller)

Fig. 9.5B: The PGC immigrate into the genital ridge. At this time, the mesonephros structures develop in the mesonephric ridge

Testes: Differentiation

The testes differentiate themselves **earlier** than the ovaries, namely in the course of the 7th week (44 days). This is because of the SRY gene on the Y chromosome that induces the development of the testes through the activation of a series of sex-determining genetic factors and hormones.

The **differentiation of Sertoli's supporting cells** forms the **first step in the organogenesis of the testes**. These cells originate most likely from pluripotent coelomic epithelial cells of the gonadal ridge. In the gonadal anlage, under the influence of SRY, they form intercellular membrane connections and in this way surround more and more the primordial germ cells, while growing at the same time as gonadal cords into the medulla (Fig. 9.7A and B). In addition, in a male embryo, cells of mesonephric origin are involved as well in forming the gonadal cords, by accumulating on the outside of the gonadal cords and forming the **peritubular myoblasts**. From the gonadal cords, the testicular cords form that then differentiate to become the **convoluted seminiferous tubules** and **straight seminiferous tubules** of the mature testicles.

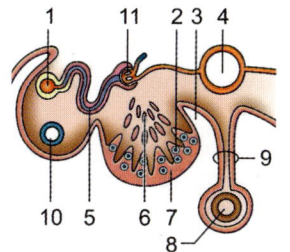

1. Mesonephric duct (Wolff)
2. PGC
3. Peritoneal cavity
4. Aorta
5. Mesonephric tubule
6. Degenerated gonadal cords
7. Thickened coelomic epithelium
8. Intestine
9. Mesentery
10. Anlage of the paramesonephric duct (Müller)
11. Atrophying mesonephric nephron

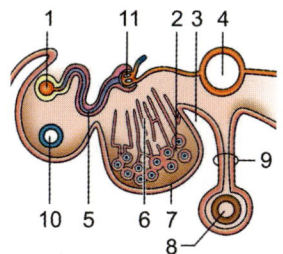

1. Mesonephric duct (Wolff)
2. PGC
3. Peritoneal cavity
4. Aorta
5. Mesonephric tubule
6. Gonadal cords
7. Coelomic epithelium
8. Intestine
9. Mesentery
10. Anlage of the paramesonephric duct (Müller)
11. Mesonephric nephron

Fig. 9.6A and B: Gonad at sex cords degenerates at medulla and settle at cortex

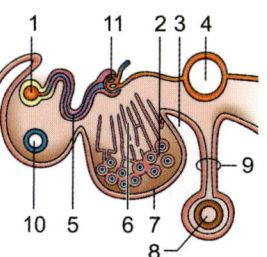

1. Mesonephric duct (Wolffian duct)
2. PGC
3. Peritoneal cavity
4. Aorta
5. Mesonephric tubule
6. Gonadal cords
7. Coelomic epithelium
8. Intestine
9. Mesentery
10. Anlage of the paramesonephric duct (Müller)
11. Mesonephric nephron

Fig. 9.7A: The gonadal cords (future testicular cords) increase in the depths while the nephrons of the meso-nephros slowly atrophy. Only the distal part of the meso-nephric tubules stays in existence in the male gonads

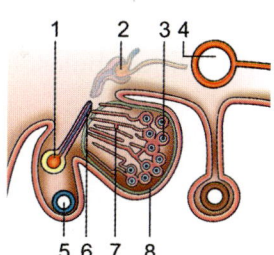

1. Mesonephric duct (Wolff)
2. Mesonephric nephron (atrophying)
3. Testicular cords surround the PGC
4. Aorta
5. Paramesonephric duct (Müller)
6. Mesonephric tubule
7. Testicular cords that grow into the medulla
8. Tunica albuginea

Fig. 9.7B: In the periphery, the testicular cords surround PGC and in the depths, take up contact with the mesonephric tubules

be found both in the cortical as well as in the medullar zones of the future gonads.

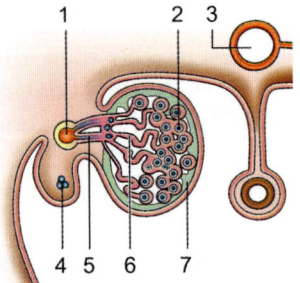

1. Mesonephric duct (Wolff)
2. Testicular cords surround the PGC
3. Aorta
4. Paramesonephric duct (Müller) (atrophying)
5. Mesonephric tubule (later efferent ductules)
6. Testicular cords
7. Tunica albuginea

Fig. 9.8A: Formation of Wolffian duct

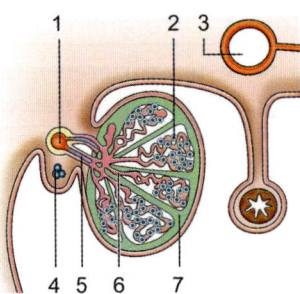

1. Mesonephric duct (Wolff)
2. Testicular cords surround the PGC
3. Aorta
4. Paramesonephric duct (Müller) (atrophying)
5. Mesonephric tubule (later efferent ductules)
6. Testicular cords
7. Tunica albuginea

Fig. 9.8B: Formation of the rete testis

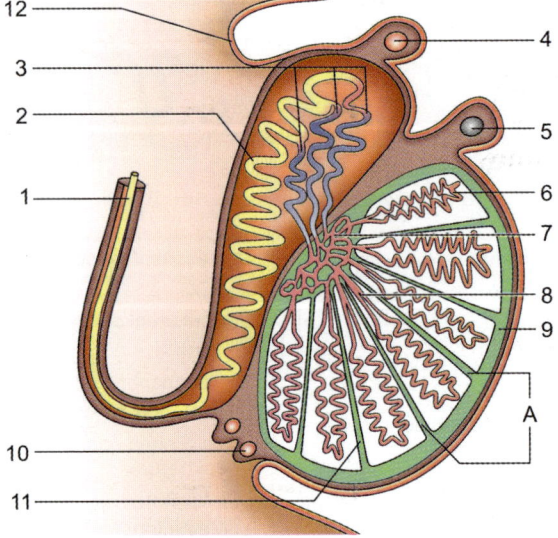

1. Deferent duct (Wolff)	8. Straight seminiferous tubules
2. Epididymis	9. Tunica albuginea
3. Efferent ductules	10. Paradidymis
4. Appendix epididymis	11. Interlobular septum
5. Appendix testis	12. Mesothelium
6. Convoluted seminiferous tubules	A. Lobule
7. Rete testis	

Fig. 9.9: Formation of testicular rete cords to open into mesonephric duct

The testicular cords penetrate into the medulla, branch within the tunica albuginea, and form anastomoses among themselves and with the mesonephric tubules, leading to the formation of the rete testis.

The deep portion of the testicular cords form the straight seminiferous tubules, which converge to the rete testis, from which the efferent ductules (mesonephric tubules) depart. Finally, they empty into the mesonephric duct (Wolffian duct) (Fig. 9.8A and B).

Until puberty, the coiled testicular cords are **filled**. During puberty, they form lumens and are from then on called **convoluted seminiferous tubules**. The germ cells on the other hand divide mitotically, but their meiosis begins only with puberty. The deep portions of the **coiled testicular cords**, which are delimited by septa, are stretched and are called **straight seminiferous tubules**. These go over into the rete testis, which is a **labyrinth** of small passages in the tunica albuginea. The thin wall possesses a cubic epithelium. During the 9th week, from 5–12 mesonephric tubules, the **efferent ductules** form that bind with the **rete testis** in the 3rd month (Fig. 9.9).

The deep medullary portions of the testicular cords are stretched and converge towards the rete testis, which on the other side goes over into the efferent ductules (mesonephric tubules) that go out from the mesonephric duct (Wolffian). From the 8th week, the latter form compact convolutions, the ductus epididymidis. Outside the epididymis, this continues

as the deferent duct. The tunica albuginea is now a taut connective tissue layer that envelops the testicles. Connective tissue septa subdivide the testicles into lobules.

The **efferent ductules** form the connection between the rete testis and mesonephric duct. Towards the end of the 8th week, under the influence of testosterone, the cranial part of the mesonephric duct gets to be tightly coiled and so forms the ductus epididymidis which, outside the epididymis, continues as the deferent duct.

After the 8th week certain mesenchymal cells between the testicular cords differentiate to become **interstitial cells (Leydig)**, which produce testosterone. The testes thus represent an endocrine gland that produces androgens. The origin of these cells is still unclear–one suspects that a steroid-producing population of cells in the ventral part of the mesonephros differentiate and form both the origin of the adrenal cortex cells and also interstitial cells (Leydig).

Development of the Stroma

The mesenchyma between the testicular cords dissolves and forms **connective tissue septa** that subdivide the testicles into lobules. This mesenchyma also forms a **taut connective tissue** layer between the testicular cords and the coelomic epithelium as well as the future **tunica albuginea**. Finally, the coelomic epithelium transforms itself into a mesothelium, just like the coelomic epithelium around the other serous cavities (peritoneum, pleura, pericardium).

Summary

- In the **testicular cords, primordial germ cells** (PGC—future spermatozoa) are to be found. The somatic cells differentiate themselves into **Sertoli's supporting cells**, responsible for nourishing the spermatozoa and secreting the **antimüllerian hormone (AMH)**, which promotes the **atrophy of the paramesonephric duct**.
- The **rete testis** forms the continuation of the centrally-lying testicular cords or the straight seminiferous tubules.
- The **efferent tubules** connect the rete testis with the **mesonephric duct**, the **future epididymis**, which continues with the **deferent duct**.
- The **interstitial mesenchymal cells** of the testes develop into **Leydig's interstitial cells**. They are responsible for the production of testosterone.
- The **stroma**, made of connective tissue, subdivides the testes into lobules and forms the **tunica albuginea**.

Ovaries: Differentiation

The differentiation of the ovaries happens **later** than that of the testes, taking place during the 8th week. Since females lack the Y chromosome, they have no SRY gene, except when a translocation of the gene on to the X chromosome occurs.

Histologically, two regions can be distinguished in an ovary:
- **Cortex**, containing all the elements of the **parenchyma**
- **Medulla**, which shares the elements of the **stroma** with the cortex.

Development of the Stroma

In an ovary, the majority of the **gonadal cords stay in contact** with the surface coelomic epithelium (Fig. 9.10). Those gonadal cords that go into the depths out of the thickened coelomic epithelium and **lose** contact with its atrophy. Some signals from the ovary actively prevent the differentiation into male gonads like **WNT-4** which functions partly as an **anti-testis gene** to suppress developmental steps of differentiation in the direction of the testes.

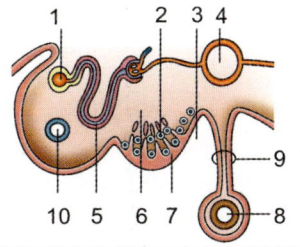

1. Mesonephric duct (Wolff)	1. Mesonephric duct
2. PGC	2. PGC
3. Peritoneal cavity	3. Peritoneal cavity
4. Aorta	4. Aorta
5. Mesonephric tubule	5. Mesonephric tubule
6. Local coelomic mesenchyme	6. Degenerated gonadal cords
7. Thickened coelomic epithelium	7. Thickened coelomic epithelium
8. Intestine	8. Intestine
9. Mesentery.	9. Mesentery
10. Anlage of the paramesonephric duct	10. Anlage of the paramesonephric duct
	11. Atrophy of the mesonephric nephron

Fig. 9.10: Formation of genital cords

The PGC immigrate into the genital ridge. Gonadal cords continue to develop and become infiltrated with PGC. At this time, the mesonephric structures develop into the mesonephric ridge. The paramesonephric duct is also formed. Those gonadal cords, which extend into the depths, atrophy. Only the gonadal cords, which stay in contact with the coelomic epithelium, remain.

In the **course of the 4th month,** the gonadal cords dissolve, also in the cortex, due to blood vessels that are sprouting from the medulla and isolated cell accumulations surround the oogonia that increasingly divide synchronously (mitosis). Like the spermatogonia, the oogonia form similar **cell clones**. The individual cells are connected with each other via cellular bridges. One can now distinguish various zones in the cortex: In the outermost zone, proliferating **oogonia** are found; somewhat further inward, one recognizes **oocytes** that have spontaneously entered into the **prophase of the first meiosis** (meiosis 1).

From the 5th month, a third zone becomes visible towards the medulla in which the oocytes have already completed the prophase of the first meiosis and are surrounded by a monolayer of cells that have differentiated out of the gonadal cord cells and now are called **follicle or granulosa cells**. The primary oocytes that are enveloped by follicle cells are now designated **primordial follicles** and then remain in this **stage of the first meiosis (diplotene stage)** (Fig. 9.11).

The gonadal cords in the center of the ovary degenerate and only those that are near the surface epithelium remain. Through blood vessels that grow

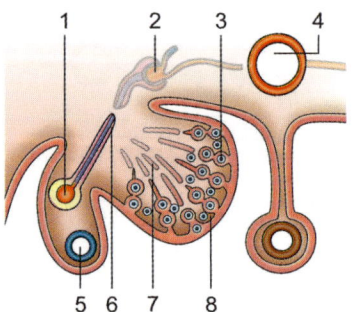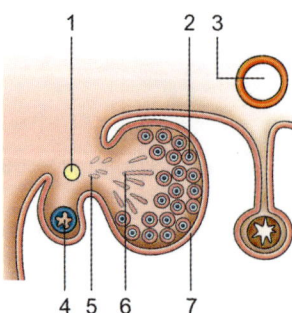

1. Mesonephric duct
2. Mesonephric nephron atrophying
3. Oogonia in the ovarian cortex
4. Aorta
5. Paramesonephric duct
6. Mesonephric tubules atrophying
7. Degenerated gonadal cords
8. Thickened coelomic epithelium in contact with the gonadal cords

1. Mesonephric duct atrophying
2. Primordial follicle in the ovarian cortex
3. Aorta
4. Paramesonephric duct
5. Mesonephric tubules atrophying
6. Degenerated gonadal cords
7. Mesothelium of the ovary

Fig. 9.11: Development of primary follicles in the cortex

into it and connective tissue stroma from the medulla, the gonadal cords in the cortex break up into small cell accumulations. These increasingly surround the PGC and the primary oocytes that also further develop in the cortex.

After approximately the middle of the pregnancy (20th week), the entire cortex is filled uniformly with primordial follicles. The rete ovarii receives no connection to the mesonephric tubules or the mesonephric duct.

During the early fetal period, millions of primordial follicles arise through intensive mitotic divisions of the oogonia during the follicular stages from primordial follicle to tertiary follicle.

The **number of the primordial follicles** at birth amount to between **300,000 and 2 million**, but they decrease massively from then till puberty. At the beginning of puberty, only **40,000** still remain. Of these, only **300** primary oocytes develop further between puberty and menopause into fertilizable oocytes.

It is to be noted that follicles only form in the presence of the PGC. Without them, **sterile gonadal cords** are formed that then further degenerate and as a consequence the ovary then consists only of stroma.

Summary

The development of the ovary is characterized by the following:

- Gonadal cords remain in existence only near the cortex; in the medulla they atrophy. The rete ovarii is only rudimentarily developed. Its cells probably come from the mesonephros, but a **connection between the rete testis and the mesonephros never comes into existence**.
- **Cortical gonadal cords** separate themselves from the others in order to make isolated cell accumulations around the oocytes and thus to form the **primordial follicles**.
- Coelomic epithelium, out of which a simple cubic **ovarian mesothelium** arises.

Phase A: A migration of the PGC into the genital ridge where they mitotically multiply through contact with the coelomic epithelium. Formation of the gonadal cords that partially degenerate (weeks 6–7).

Phase B: Active proliferation phase of the PGC and differentiation into oogonia (weeks 9–22). The maximal number of PGC (7 million) is attained with 20 weeks.

Phase C: The oogonia enter spontaneously into meiosis and become arrested in the diplotene of the prophase of the first meiosis. One now designates them as primary oocytes (weeks 12–25).

Phase D: Formation of primordial follicles (weeks 16–29).

Phase E: Follicular atresia continue from the 16th week onwards. Between 300,000 and 2 million primordial follicles remain up to birth and of these 300 primordial follicles develop further between puberty and menopause for fertilization. The rest of the follicles thus perish along the way.

Displacement of the Ovaries

The ovaries are also **moved slightly**—from the location where they are engendered in the middle of the abdomen to the pelvis. This migration results partially from the massive growth of the upper abdominal region in comparison with the pelvic area.

The influence of the **lower gubernaculum** in this process is not entirely clear.

The **mesonephros** atrophies in the 7th week. Only the ovary with its **mesovarium** medially and the paramesonephric duct with the **mesosalpinx lateral** to the mesoderm of the original urogenital tract remain. They are connected with the dorsal abdominal wall of the embryo via the mesoderm of the original urogenital tract.

Through atrophy of the mesonephros, the **upper gubernaculum** connects the ovary directly with the upper rear body wall and becomes designated as the **suspensory ligament of ovary**.

The **lower gubernaculum** has its origin in the bottom side of the ovary and forms the **ovarian ligament** and, further down, the **round ligament of uterus** that reaches the genital swelling (labia majora) through the inguinal canal.

The **nephrogenic cord** is originally **vertical** (Figs 9.12 and 9.13). The **fallopian tube**, which forms from the upper part of the paramesonephric duct, finally takes on a **horizontal** position in that it is drawn medially by the joining of the lower part of the paramesonephric duct as the uterus is being formed.

The **ovary**, which initially lies **medially** to the fallopian tube (paramesonephric duct) in front of the atrophying mesonephros, slides backwards as a result (Figs 9.14 and 9.15).

The peritoneal mesentery **passively** follow these movements. Finally the **broad ligament** of uterus forms with three sections:

1. Upper section: Mesosalpinx with the fallopian tube
2. Ventral section: Mesometrium with the round ligament of uterus
3. Dorsal section: Mesovarium with the ovarian ligament.

Up to the 7th week, the internal genital organs in both sexes on both sides consist of two canal systems:

1. The **mesonephric duct and the mesonephric tubules**, which first form on the dorsal side of the nephrogenic cord at the level of the 9th somite in the form of solid, **cellular mesenchymal cords**. They detach themselves from the nephrogenic cord and are located below the coelomic epithelium that is thickened at this place.

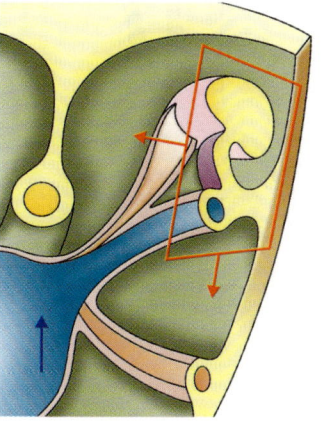

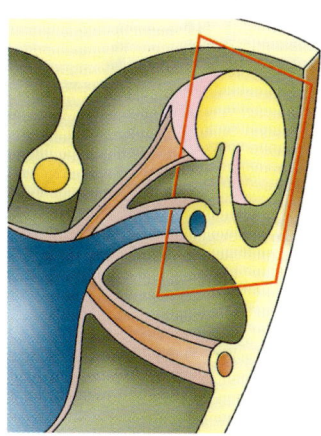

Fig. 9.14: Displacement of ovaries at start of 4th month

Fig. 9.15: Definitive position of ovaries at the end of 4th month

2. The **paramesonephric duct** is formed from a finger-shaped invagination of the coelomic epithelium on the upper pole of the mesonephros. It forms here a funnel that opens into the coelomic cavity (future ampulla of the fallopian tube).

The paramesonephric duct invades on both sides—**laterally** to the mesonephric duct—into the mesonephros and grows in the caudal direction. At the lower end of the mesonephros, the paramesonephric duct **crosses over** the mesonephric duct in order to grow further medially. There, the paramesonephric ducts meet on both sides and fuse to form a canal. They then push on the urogenital sinus, forming a small **protrusion**, the **paramesonephric tubercle**.

In Females: Differentiation of the Canal System in the Genital Organ

During the **7th week,** the canal system of the female sex organs differentiates. The **mesonephric duct** and its tubules atrophy and out of the **paramesonephric duct** arises the future fallopian tube, the uterus and the upper part of the vagina (Fig. 9.16).

Sometimes, a few embryonic remnants of the mesonephric duct remain in the form of the **epoöphoron**, the **paroöphoron** at the level of the mesovarium, and a row of small **cysts of Gartner**.

Out of the upper, non-fused portion of the **paramesonephric duct** arises the fallopian tube and its ampulla. The lower section fuses after it crosses medially on both sides of the inferior ovarian gubernaculum and forms the **uterovaginal canal**. The medial septum in between disappears at the **end of the 3rd month** (Figs 9.17 and 9.18).

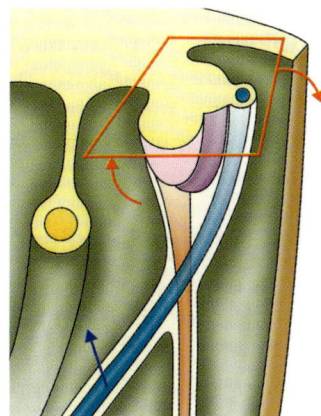

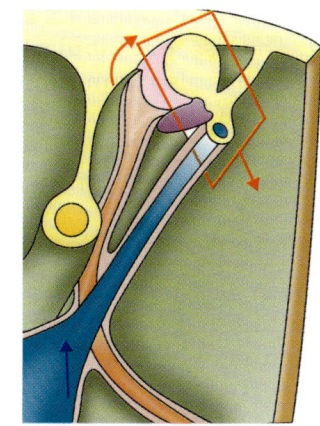

Fig. 9.12: Originally, the urogenital tract finds itself in a vertical position

Fig. 9.13: Through a sideways tipping displacement, the ovary finds itself temporarily above the atrophying mesonephros

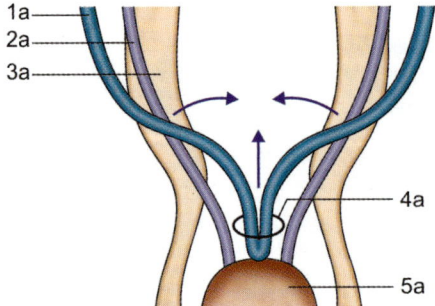

Fig. 9.16: Formation of the uterus, 7th–8th weeks

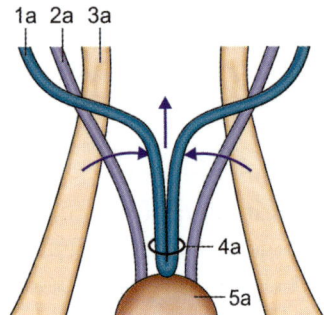

Fig. 9.17: Formation of the uterovaginal canal through fusion of the lower section of the two paramesonephric ducts. From the upper section, on both sides, arise the fallopian tubes with their ampullae

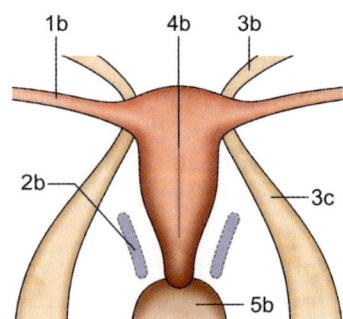

Fig. 9.18: At the end of the 3rd month, the separating wall dissolves in the uterus and the vagina. The uterus lengthens in that the solid lower end of the paramesonephric duct stretches in a downward direction and is subsequently canalized. Out of the lower section, arises the upper part of the vagina. It joins with the vaginal lamina, which arises from the urogenital sinus and forms the lower portion of the vagina

1a. Paramesonephric duct (Müller)	1b. Fallopian tube
2a. Mesonephric duct (Wolff)	2b. Atrophied mesonephric duct (Wolff)
3a. Lower gubernaculum	3b. Ovarian ligament
4a. Utero-vaginal canal	3c. Round ligament of uterus
5a. Urogenital sinus	4b. Uterus
	5b. Vagina

Development of the Ligaments

The ovarian gubernaculum gets attached on the developing uterovaginal canal there where it goes over into the fallopian tube. Above it forms the ovarian ligament and below the round ligament of uterus, which goes through the inguinal canal and inserts in the female genital swelling (labia majora).

If the separating wall beyond the fusion location of the two paramesonephric ducts is not resorbed, various uterovaginal anomalies result.

The blind end of the uterovaginal canal forms the **sinu–vaginal eminence** and ends at the back wall of the urogenital sinus.

The sinu–vaginal eminence becomes thicker due to epithelial proliferation and retracts, while the wall of the urogenital sinus (UGS) also thickens there. These epithelial layers, which form at the lower end of the **uterovaginal canal**, are known as the **vaginal plate**. At their **cranial end,** they form a circular protrusion, the location of the future vaginal fornix.

Through **canalization** of the vaginal plate, the uterovaginal canal opens itself towards the outside. The upper 3/4 of the vagina comes from the mesoderm and the lower fourth from the endoderm.

The **fibromuscular walling** forms from the **neighboring mesenchyma**. The vagina is separated from the urogenital sinus (UGS) by the hymen. Its origin is not entirely clear.

Differentiation of the Accessory Sex Glands in Females

The accessory glands arise from the **endoderm** of the UGS:
- The **greater vestibular glands (Bartholini)** are paired glands that form in the course of the 12th week from the endoderm of the UGS. The outflow canals empty sideways in the vaginal vestibule. They correspond to the bulbourethral gland (Cowper) in males.
- The **lesser vestibular glands (Skene)** or paraurethral glands also form from epithelial buds (endoderm) of the UGS and grow into the neighboring mesenchyma. They are distributed over the whole vaginal vestibule and in males correspond to the **prostate**.

Differentiation of the Urogenital Sinus in Females

In females, the **cranial portion of the pelvic part of the definitive UGS** remains narrow and forms the **female urethra**, which is very short.

With the progressing development, the **caudal portion of the pelvic part** shrinks and becomes included in the phallic part (vaginal vestibule). The **phallic part of the definitive UGS** enlarges to become the vaginal vestibule that is caudally closed off externally by the urogenital membrane. It then tears in the course of the 7th week (Figs 9.19–9.23).

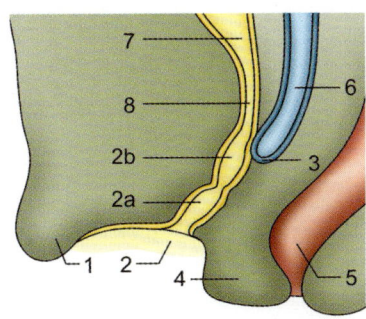

1. Genital tubercle	4. Perineum
2. Vestibule	5. Rectum
2a. Urovaginal sinus: Pelvic part	6. Uterovaginal canal
2b. Urovaginal sinus: Phallic part	7. Urinary bladder
3. Vaginal plate	8. Urethra

Fig. 9.19: The uterovaginal canal comes up against the urogenital sinus and forms the sinu–vaginal eminence

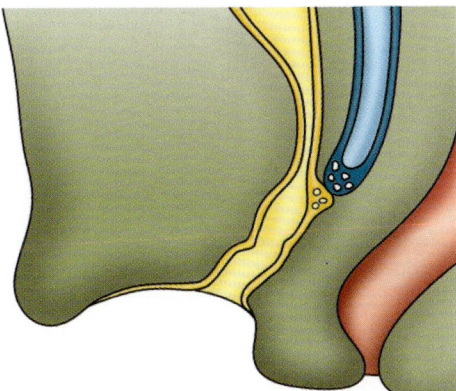

Fig. 9.20: This sinu–vaginal eminence becomes thicker due to epithelial proliferation. This also leads to an epithelial proliferation in the UGS epithelium. Together they form the vaginal plate

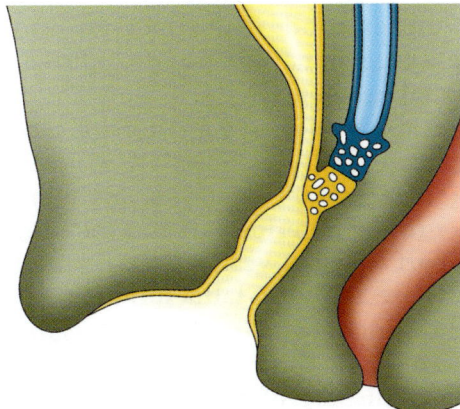

Fig. 9.21: The canalization of the vaginal plate begins in the 3rd month

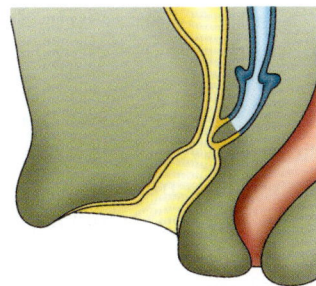

Fig. 9.22: In the 5th month, the vaginal canal is completely canalized, but the lumen is separated from the UGS by the hymen

Summary

From the paramesonephric duct (Müller) arise:
- Uterus
- Fallopian tube
- Vagina (3/4)

From the UGS endoderm arise:
- Vagina (1/4)
- Urethra
- Vaginal vestibule
- Urethral glands, paraurethral and vestibular glands

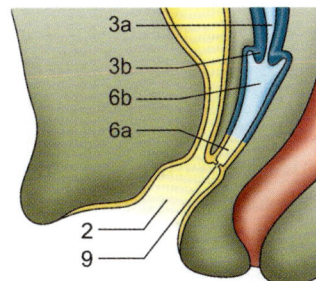

2.	Vaginal vestibule
3a.	Uterine cavity
3b.	Uterine cervix (neck)
6a.	Vagina: The lower fourth out of endoderm
6b.	Vagina: The upper 3/4 out of mesoderm
9.	Hymen

Fig. 9.23: Normally, the hymen tears open at the time of birth. The uterus and the vagina then have a connection to the vaginal vestibule

Development of the Internal Genital Organs

In **males,** the internal sex organs come from the **mesonephric duct** that differentiates itself into the epididymis, deferent duct, seminal vesicle and the ejaculatory duct. The paramesonephric duct atrophies. It leaves behind embryonic remnants such as the testicular appendage (hydatid) and parts of the prostatic utricle.

In **females,** the **paramesonephric duct** remains in existence and differentiates itself into the fallopian tube with its ampullae and, following its fusion at the caudal end, into the uterus and the upper part of the vagina. The mesonephric duct (Wolff) with its tubules atrophies and leaves embryonic remnants such as the ductus longitudinalis epoöphori (Gartner), epoöphoron and paroöphoron.

During the **third week,** the cloacal membrane is formed and lies below the **umbilical cord.**

In the **fourth week,** as the lower abdominal wall is being formed, the cloacal membrane is shifted caudally by immigrating mesenchyma coming from various sources.

It is now delimited in front by a prominent mesenchymatous eminence with an epithelial covering, the anlage of the future genital tubercle.

Development of External Female Genitalia

At the **end of the 5th week,** several **cloacal folds** (Fig. 9.24) form on both sides of the cloacal membrane. At their anterior end they join, delimited by the **genital tubercle.** During the **7th week,** the urorectal septum divides the cloacal membrane into **urogenital membrane** (ventrally) and **anal membrane** (dorsally). From the ventral section of the cloacal swellings around the urogenital sinus develop **urethral folds** and in the dorsal section around the anus **develop anal folds** (Figs 9.25 and 9.26). Lateral to the urethral folds develop another pair of swelling, the **genital swelling.**

The urogenital membrane dissolves during the 7th week so that the urogenital sinus communicates freely with the amniotic cavity.

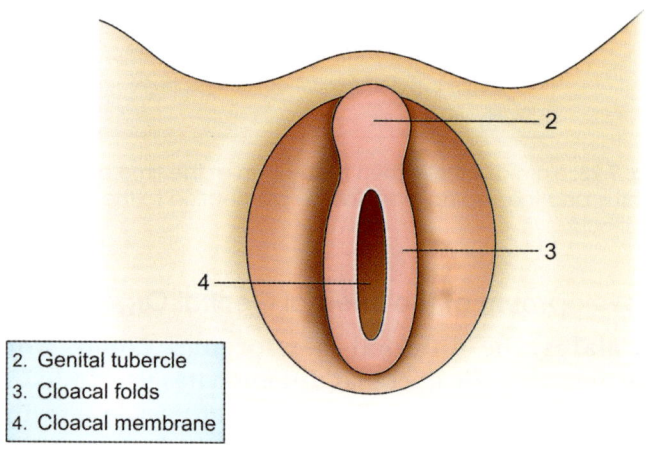

| 2. Genital tubercle |
| 3. Cloacal folds |
| 4. Cloacal membrane |

Fig. 9.24: In front, the cloacal membrane is delimited by a swelling, the future genital tubercle, that at the rear continues in the two cloacal folds

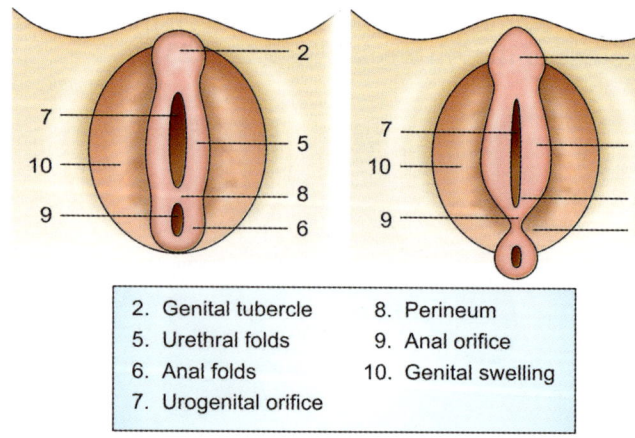

2. Genital tubercle	8. Perineum
5. Urethral folds	9. Anal orifice
6. Anal folds	10. Genital swelling
7. Urogenital orifice	

Fig. 9.25: Formation of female external genitals

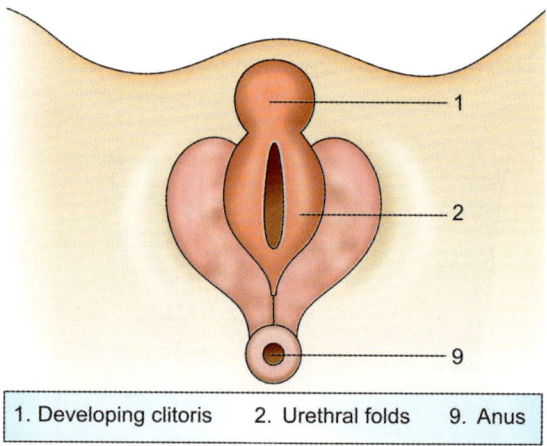

| 1. Developing clitoris | 2. Urethral folds | 9. Anus |

Fig. 9.26: In the female, the genital tubercle lengthens only a little and shrinks again while forming the clitoris. The urethral folds do not fuse and the urogenital sinus remains wide open

Differentiated Stage of the Female Genitalia

The mechanisms that are responsible for the development of the external female genitalia are still not well understood. The placenta and ovaries producing estrogen may contribute to this.

The **genital tubercle** lengthens only a little, retracts again and, after 14 weeks, the **clitoris** is recognizable. The **genital swellings** do not fuse and, for this reason, the urogenital sinus remains wide open with the **urethra in the anterior part** and the **vagina in the posterior part** (vaginal vestibule). The urethral folds also do not fuse and form **labia minora** (Fig. 9.27).

From the genital swellings arise the **labia majora.** They fuse only in the rear portion and form the posterior **commissure of the labia.** In the front they form the **mons pubis.** Towards the rear, the posterior labial commissure is continued by the **perineum.**

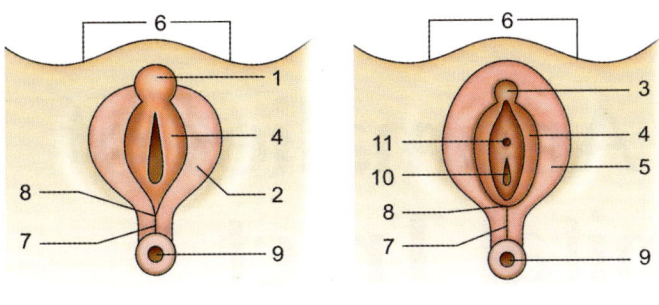

1.	Genital tubercle	7.	Perineum
2.	Genital swelling	8.	Posterior labial commissure
3.	Clitoris	9.	Anus
4.	Labia minora	10.	Hymen
5.	Labia majora	11.	External urethral orifice
6.	Mons pubis		

Fig. 9.27: The urethral folds do not fuse—the la bia minora arise from them. From the genital swellings arise the labia majora. They fuse only in the rear part and form the posterior labial commissure that is continued towards the rear by the perineum

Embryonic Development of the External Genitalia
(Table 9.1)

By the sixth week, a swelling called the genital tubercle is apparent in the groin of the embryo. The mesonephric and paramesonephric ducts open to the outside through the genital tubercle. The genital tubercle consists of a glans, a urethral groove, paired urethral folds, and paired labioscrotal swellings. As the glans portion of the genital tubercle enlarges, it becomes known as the phallus.

Early in fetal development from the 10th to 12th week, sexual distinction of the external genitalia becomes apparent. In the male, the phallus enlarges and develops into the glans of the penis. The urethral folds fuse around the urethra and become the erectile tissue that forms the body of the penis. The labioscrotal swellings fuse to form the scrotum, into which the testes will descend. In the female, the phallus gives rise to the clitoris, the urethral folds remain separated as the labia minora, and the urethral groove is retained as a longitudinal cleft known as the vestibule.

Table 9.1: Overview of development of female genitals in different gestational age

Gestational age	Development
3rd week	Primordial germ cells
4th week	Formation of the mesonephric duct (wolffian duct)
	Migration of the primordial germ cells
	Connection of the mesonephric duct with the cloaca
5th week	Subdivision of the cloaca into the rectum (dorsally) and the urogenital sinus (ventrally)
	The primordial germ cells colonize the genital ridge
	Formation of the paramesonephric duct (Müllerian)
7th week	Formation of the urethral groove
	The urorectal septum subdivides the cloacal membrane
	Formation of the anal and urogenital folds
	Rupture of the cloacal membrane
8th week	End of the indifferent gonads in the female
	Atrophy of the mesonephros
	Atrophy of the medullary gonadal cords as well as the rete ovarii and its connection to the mesonephric tubules
10th week	Feminine phenotypic sex is recognizable
	The paramesonephric ducts join at the distal end and form by SUG the sinovaginal bulb
	Labia minora and majora are formed from genital folds
	Formation of the posterior labial commissure

10 Congenital Anomalies of Female Genital Tract

Developmental anomalies of the müllerian duct system represent some of the most fascinating disorders that gynecologists encounter. The müllerian ducts are the primordial anlage of the female reproductive tract. They differentiate to form the fallopian tubes, uterus, the uterine cervix, and the superior aspect of the vagina. A wide variety of malformations can occur when this system is disrupted. They range from uterine and vaginal agenesis to duplication of the uterus and vagina to minor uterine cavity abnormalities. Müllerian malformations are frequently associated with abnormalities of the renal and axial skeletal systems.

Most müllerian duct anomalies (MDAs) are associated with functioning ovaries and age-appropriate external genitalia. These abnormalities are often recognized after the onset of puberty. In the prepubertal period, normal external genitalia and age-appropriate developmental milestones often mask abnormalities of the internal reproductive organs. After the onset of puberty, young women often present to the gynecologist with menstrual disorders. Late presentations include infertility and obstetric complications.

Incidence and Prevalence

The actual incidence and prevalence of müllerian anomalies in the general population are unknown. Incidence rates vary widely and most authors report incidences of 0.1–3.5%. In women with fertility problems, the incidence of müllerian duct anomalies is slightly higher at 3–6%. In general, women with recurrent abortions have an incidence of 5–10%, with the highest incidence of müllerian defects occurring in patients having third-trimester miscarriages. The most commonly reported müllerian duct anomalies are septate, arcuate, didelphys, unicornuate, or hypoplastic uteri.

The prevalence of müllerian duct anomalies also varies significantly, with reports ranging from 0.16 to 10%. When these data are obtained in women with recurrent pregnancy loss who are undergoing hysterosalpingography (HSG), the prevalence of müllerian anomalies is 8–10%.

Abnormal Development and Classifications

The vast array of structural anomalies seen in müllerian duct defects results from interruption or dysregulation in müllerian duct development at various stages of morphogenesis. Well-known factors, such as intrauterine and extrauterine elements, genetics, and teratogens (e.g. diethylstilbestrol [DES], thalidomide), have been associated with müllerian duct anomalies. The genetics of müllerian duct anomalies are complex.

The developmental stages when interruptions in development occur are well established, and müllerian defects are frequently grouped according to the failed developmental mechanism that gives rise to a given malformation. This form of classification, which includes agenesis or hypoplasia, lateral fusion defects, vertical fusion defects, and DES-related abnormalities, is not mutually exclusive. Indeed, many müllerian duct anomalies often coexist.

The most common müllerian duct defects involve the vagina and the uterus. Vaginal agenesis is a consequence of developmental failure of the sinovaginal bulbs. Without the sinovaginal bulbs, the vaginal plate cannot form. The uterus is usually absent in this condition because the uterovaginal plate (UVP) induces differentiation of the sinovaginal bulbs. Vaginal agenesis is frequently accompanied by urinary tract anomalies. Partial vaginal agenesis with a normal upper genital tract is uncommon and must be distinguished from vaginal atresia. Vaginal atresia is due to an interruption in urogenital sinus (UGS) development and is usually associated with normal müllerian-derived structures.

Agenesis of the uterine cervix is rare and usually occurs in association with complete or partial vaginal agenesis. Additional anomalies include cervical atresia as well as defects involving the length, width, and/or size of the cervix. Isolated cervical defects are also rare.

Fallopian tube agenesis is a rare condition and include accessory ostia, fallopian tube duplication, absent muscular layer, ectopic location, luminal atresia, and absent ampulla with blind fimbria.

Disorders of lateral (horizontal or longitudinal) fusion manifest the widest range of structural abnormalities among the müllerian duct anomalies. In the contemporary American Fertility Society (AFS) classification, they are included in classes II-VI. Lateral fusion defects are divided into symmetric and asymmetric groups and are further subdivided into obstructive or nonobstructive categories. These defects occur by means of arrests in different stages of müllerian duct development. In general, the arrested stages include incomplete fusion of the caudal müllerian ducts, failed septum resorption, and defective development of all or part of a duct.

Asymmetric, obstructive lateral fusion defects of the müllerian system are frequently associated with unilateral mesonephric agenesis and manifest as ipsilateral renal agenesis, ureter agenesis, or both. Horizontal vaginal septa are included in this classification because some experts maintain that they occur as a consequence of defective lateral fusion; however, others hypothesize that horizontal septa arise from mesodermal hyperproliferation or persistence of epithelium during canalization.

Disorders of vertical (transverse) fusion result from abnormal canalization of the vaginal plate and, in some cases, failure of the UVP and the sinovaginal bulbs to fuse. These disruptions can result in the formation of a transverse vaginal septum (TVS), an imperforate hymen, and, in extreme cases, vaginal atresia. The TVS is subdivided according to whether the defect is complete or partial. TVS can be accompanied by urinary tract anomalies. A partial septum may occur in females exposed to diethylstilbesterol (DES). Imperforate hymen and vaginal atresia result from structural defects involving derivatives of the UGS.

DES exposure *in utero* can influence the development of the female reproductive tract. Approximately one half the women exposed to DES *in utero* develop uterine cavity anomalies. *In utero* DES exposure is also associated with developmental defects of the lower genital tract. Uterine anomalies similar to those related to DES exposure have been reported in women without *in utero* DES exposure.

The most widely accepted method of categorizing müllerian duct anomalies is the AFS classification (1988). This system organizes müllerian anomalies according to the major uterine anatomic defect. The current AFS classification of müllerian duct anomalies includes 7 classes, as shown in Table 10.1.

Table 10.2 shows classification by European Society of Human Reproduction and Embryology (ESHRE).

Class I—Vaginal Agenesis (Fig. 10.1)

Vaginal agenesis is characterized by an absence or hypoplasia of the uterus, proximal vagina, and, in some cases, the fallopian tubes. It occurs in an estimated 1 in 5000 newborn females. In approximately 7–10% of women with müllerian aplasia, a normal but obstructed uterus, or a rudimentary uterus with functional endometrium, is present.

Table 10.1: AFS classification of anomalies of the müllerian duct

Clinical finding	Description
Segmental or complete agenesis or hypoplasia	Agenesis and hypoplasia may involve the vagina, cervix, fundus, tubes, or any combination of these structures. Mayer-Rokitansky-Küster-Hauser (MRKH) syndrome is the most common example in this category.
Unicornuate uterus with or without a rudimentary horn	When an associated horn is present, this class is subdivided into communicating (continuity with the main uterine cavity). The noncommunicating type is further subdivided on the basis of whether an endometrial cavity is present in the rudimentary horn. These malformations have previously been classified under asymmetric lateral fusion defects. They accompanied by ipsilateral renal and ureter agenesis.
Didelphys uterus	Complete or partial duplication of the vagina, cervix, and uterus characterizes this anomaly.
Complete or partial bicornuate uterus	Complete bicornuate uterus is characterized by a uterine septum that extends from the fundus to the cervical os. The partial bicornuate uterus demonstrates a septum, which is located at the fundus. In both variants, the vagina and cervix each has a single chamber
Complete or partial septate uterus	A complete or partial midline septum is present within a single uterus.
Arcuate uterus	A small septate indentation is present at the fundus.
DES-related abnormalities	A T-shaped uterine cavity with or without dilated horns is evident.

Table 10.2: ESHRE classification of female genital tract

Uterine anomaly	Main class	Sub-class	Coexisting class	Cervical/vaginal anomaly
U0	Normal uterus		C0	Normal cervix
U1	Dysmorphic uterus	a. T-shaped	C1	Septate cervix
		b. Infantilis		
		c. Others		
U2	Septate uterus	a. Partial	C2	Double 'normal' cervix
		b. Complete		
U3	Bicorporeal uterus	a. Partial	C3	Unilateral cervical aplasia
		b. Complete		
		c. Bicorporeal septate		
U4	Hemiuterus	a. With rudimentary cavity (communicating or not horn)	C4	Cervical aplasia
		b. Without rudimentary cavity (horn without cavity/no horn)	V0	Normal vagin
			V1	Longitudinal nonobstructing vaginal septum
U5	Aplastic	a. With rudimentary cavity (bi- or unilateral horn)	V2	Longitudinal obstructing
		b. Without rudimentary cavity (bi-/unilateral horn/aplasia)	V3	Transverse vaginal septum/
			V5	Vaginal aplasia
U6	Unclassified malformation			

Congenital Müllerian Anomalies

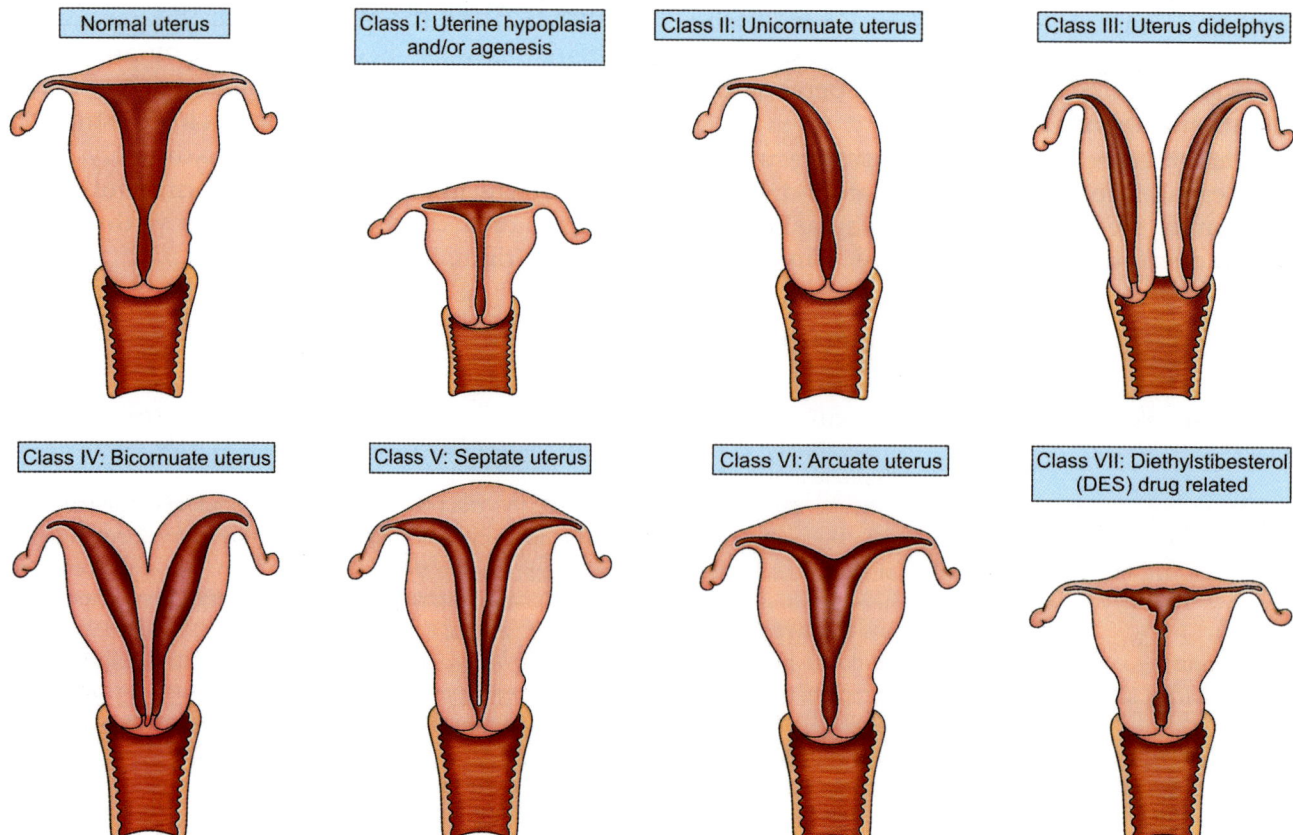

Fig. 10.1: Different uterine anomalies

Müllerian aplasia can be partial or complete. Partial müllerian aplasia is more rarely encountered and is characterized by a normal uterus and small vaginal pouch distal to the cervix. Complete müllerian aplasia (MRKH syndrome) is the most common variant encountered and it is characterized by congenital absence of the vagina and the uterus in 90–95% of cases. The fallopian tubes are normal, and the ovaries have normal endocrine and oocyte function.

The incidence of associated urologic abnormalities ranges between 15% and 40%, and skeletal anomalies, such as congenital fusion or absence of vertebra, occur in approximately 12–50% of cases. An association between MRKH syndrome and Klippel-Feil syndrome has been reported. This syndrome is characterized by congenital fusion of the cervical spine, a short neck, a low posterior hairline, and limited range of motion in the cervical spine. The **MURCS** association (i.e. **M**üllerian duct aplasia, **U**nilateral **R**enal aplasia, **C**ervicothoracic **S**omite dysplasia) is another variant.

The etiology of müllerian aplasia is unclear. Most cases occur sporadically, although the rising number of reported familial cases indicates a genetic etiology. The karyotype of females having müllerian aplasia is 46,XX. Approximately 4% of reported cases are familial, with affected siblings, and in some cases it is transmitted as an autosomal dominant trait.

Müllerian agenesis has been associated with variants of the galactose-1-phosphate uridyltransferase (GALT) enzyme deficiency; this finding suggests that increased exposure to galactose is responsible for abnormal vaginal development.

Other authorities have speculated that mutations in either the antimüllerian hormone or müllerian inhibitory substance (*MIS*) gene or its receptor gene are responsible for this disorder.

Diagnosis of Müllerian Aplasia (Vaginal Agenesis)

Müllerian aplasia is usually diagnosed at puberty when adolescents present to the gynecologist with primary amenorrhea. It is the second most common cause of primary amenorrhea in adolescents. Physical examination reveals normal growth and development with age-appropriate secondary sexual characteristics. External genitalia are normal. Pelvic examination often reveals a patulous urethra.

The vaginal vault can be either completely absent or a short vaginal pouch can be present. Occasionally, a short vaginal dimple is present, located 1–2 cm superior to the hymenal ring. Uterus is not palpated on rectal examination. On pelvic examination, a smooth band that crosses the pelvis is sometimes appreciated and

most likely represents a remnant of the uterosacral ligament.

Ultrasonographic findings can add support to the clinical findings suggesting the absence of uterus and fallopian tubes in the presence of normal ovaries. MRI is extremely useful but not routinely done as it is expensive. The hormonal profile is that of a normal female with age-appropriate luteinizing hormone, follicle-stimulating hormone, estradiol, and testosterone levels. This profile helps distinguish the MRKH syndrome from androgen insensitivity syndromes in which postpubertal testosterone is elevated.

Laparoscopy is not usually indicated unless the diagnosis cannot be determined from other studies or if the presence of a functioning uterus or rudimentary uterine tissue is a concern. Patients with these findings are not candidates for HSG (Fig. 10.2).

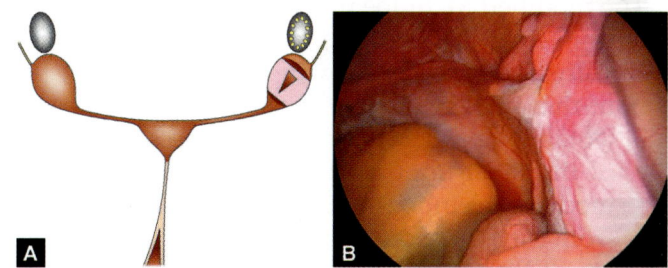

Fig. 10.2: (A) Schematic diagram of müllerian agenesis, (B) laparoscopic view

Preoperative Evaluation

Surgical and nonsurgical methods of treatment have been used. The nonsurgical approach relies on graduated dilators that progressively create a neovagina. This method may take several months or a few years before a functional vagina is formed. Surgery remains the most effective method of treatment for müllerian aplasia.

Choosing the proper time to perform a vaginoplasty is of paramount importance. Surgical treatment should be considered only when the patient can participate in the decision making wishes to become sexually active and is highly motivated to use a vaginal prosthesis for several months after surgery.

Since the ovaries are normal, oocyte harvesting can be conducted so that these women can have children with a surrogate and these young women should be counseled about various reproductive options.

Routine preoperative evaluation should include intravenous pyelography (IVP) and renal sonography to exclude urinary tract anomalies. Associated skeletal defects can be detected by reviewing images from IVP radiographic studies for vertebral abnormalities. If a pelvic mass is present, sonograms should help in differentiating hematometra, hematocolpos, ovarian cysts, and a pelvic kidney. Discovery of a pelvic kidney is important in planning corrective surgery because its presence may limit the potential space available for graft placement.

Surgical Techniques for Müllerian Aplasia (Vaginal Agenesis)

The aim of surgical treatment is to create a neovagina. The strategy for vaginoplasty is to develop a space between the bladder and the rectum. A stent or form is placed in the newly created space to ensure patency while healing occurs.

Skin grafting remains the most popular material used in vaginoplasties; however, scar formation at the graft site has been a concern.

The modified McIndoe procedure remains the most common surgical approach to vaginoplasty. The procedure involves the following steps.
- Split-thickness grafting
  - Obtaining a satisfactory split-thickness graft is one of the most important steps in performing the modified McIndoe procedure. The graft harvested from each buttock should measure 8 × 9 cm, and excised to a depth of 0.045 cm (0.018 in). In total, the graft dimensions should measure approximately twice the vaginal depth.
  - The graft is usually taken from the buttocks. After preparing the graft site with antiseptic solution, a single layer is removed avoiding any variation in graft thickness.
- After retrieval, the graft is placed between saline-moistened gauze and reserved for later use.

Creation of the Vaginal Space

- The goal is to create an adequate space between the urethra and/or bladder and the rectum without exposing too much peritoneum.
- A transverse incision is made in the mucosa at the apex of the vaginal dimple.
- The dissection is initiated along one side of the midline, creating a small space in the fibroconnective tissue between the bladder and the rectum using blunt dissection. This process is repeated on the opposite side. The median raphe is divided with scissors, joining the spaces. The dissection is continued up to the peritoneum. It is importantly not to expose too much peritoneum because an enterocele can develop postoperatively.

- Meticulous hemostasis is needed to avoid bleeding, which can cause the graft to separate from its bed and result in engraftment failure.

Prosthesis Assembly

- The stent should be made from material that can maintain the patency of the vaginal cavity. A foam-rubber form measuring 10 × 10 × 20 cm works well.
- The prosthetic device is sterilized, and the size is customized to fit the patient's vagina. The prosthetic material is cut to twice the desired size of the vagina, folded in half, and compressed by the placement of 2 condoms over the surface. The condoms are tied at the open end.

Graft Attachment to a Prosthesis (Fig. 10.3)

- The graft is placed over the stent with the epidermis approximating the surface of the stent and the dermis facing out. This graft is sutured over the form using 5-0 absorbable sutures.
- The graft-covered prosthesis is carefully inserted into the vaginal canal.
- The edges of the graft are sutured to the previously cut edges of the mucosal margins of the vaginal introitus. This contact is often adequate, rendering sutures unnecessary. If the contact between the graft and the vaginal space is too tight, serum may collect and compromise the engraftment.
- The labia minora are sutured around the stent using nonreactive sutures.
- To avoid applying too much pressure to the stented graft, the transurethral catheter is replaced with a suprapubic bladder catheter.

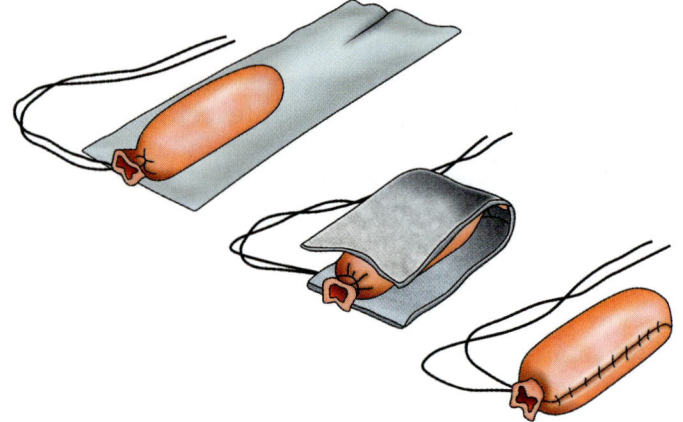

Fig. 10.3: Use of vaginal mold covered with graft

Postoperative Management

One week after surgery, the labial sutures are removed, and the stent is carefully removed. The neovagina is irrigated with warm sodium chloride solution and carefully inspected to determine whether the graft has taken satisfactorily. A new form covered with a sterile sheath is reinserted.

Patient is educated regarding the importance of continuous, prolonged dilatation and stent care during the healing phase. The form is worn continuously for 6 weeks and is removed only for urination and defecation. Tthe form is cleaned with a povidone-iodine solution, covered with a fresh condom, lubricated, and reintroduced into the neovagina. After 6 weeks, a silicone form that is inserted nightly for the next 12 months replaces the original stent. In most cases, the vagina is functional 6–10 weeks after surgery.

Class II—Unicornuate Uterus

The unicornuate uterus is formed when 1 müllerian duct completely or incompletely fails to elongate while the other develops normally. Unicornuate uterus accounts for approximately 2.4–13% of all müllerian anomalies. The unicornuate uterus may occur alone, but it is frequently associated with a rudimentary horn. The AFS classification divides this group into 4 categories based on the presence or absence of a rudimentary horn. The accessory horn can have a uterine cavity with functional endometrium, and, in some cases, a communication may exist with the main endometrial cavity and these associated urologic anomalies are frequent (44%), especially in the presence of an obstructed horn and these include ipsilateral renal agenesis (67%), horseshoe kidneys, and ipsilateral pelvic kidney (15%).

Noncommunicating accessory horns that have an endometrial cavity are the most common unicornuate subtype and are the most clinically significant. This subtype is associated with hematometra of the obstructed horn and there is also an increased risk of developing endometriosis, which usually resolves after excision of the horn.

Although normal pregnancies can occur, obstetric outcomes are generally poor in this group. Unicornuate uterus is associated with the poorest fetal survival among all müllerian anomalies. Cesarean delivery rates are high. Common obstetrical complications include malpresentation, intrauterine growth retardation, and preterm birth.

Adverse obstetric complications can also involve the accessory horn and include ectopic pregnancy, missed abortion, and uterine rupture. For these reasons, the horn should be excised prior to pregnancy as a preventative measure. Pregnancy in a non-communicating horn is uncommon and is thought to be due to transperitoneal sperm migration into the fallopian tube of the rudimentary horn. Most obstetric complications occur in the first 20 weeks and can result in abortion, uterine rupture and even maternal death (0.5%).

Diagnosis of Unicornuate Uterus

Women with non-communicating, functioning rudimentary horns may present with pelvic pain usually secondary to hematometra or endometriosis. Although HSG is useful in diagnosing a unicornuate uterus, it does not help in detecting a non-communicating horn. High-resolution ultrasonography is useful for identifying rudimentary horns and is more reliable than laparoscopy for determining whether the horn is communicating.

MRI reliably helps in making this distinction and should be one of the first diagnostic tools used in evaluating such patients. MRI reveals a slender, laterally deviated banana-shaped uterus.

Only 1 fallopian tube is identified. The zonal anatomy is normal, though the uterine volume is reduced. The accessory horn can appear solid because it is not opacified when endometrium is absent. It is located adjacent to the main uterine cavity. It can also be observed as a soft tissue mass. When endometrium is present, a small cavity can be detected; this may or may not communicate with the main endometrial cavity.

Laparoscopy is rarely indicated in the workup of an obstructed, noncommunicating horn.

Additional studies should include IVP or renal ultrasonography to help evaluate for ipsilateral renal agenesis, horseshoe kidney, and ipsilateral pelvic kidney.

Surgical Technique for Rudimentary Horn Excision

Excision of an accessory horn is accomplished by means of laparoscopic hemihysterectomy. Anatomic variations of horn attachment to the unicornuate uterus exist. A fibromuscular band often connects the 2 horns. In this setting, the uterine artery courses inferior to the band and can be easily coagulated. The band is desiccated by using bipolar cautery and transected. On occasion, the horn can be firmly attached to the unicornuate uterus. In this setting, the uterine artery courses inferior to the horn and lateral to the unicornuate uterus.

The pedicle of the rudimentary horn is coagulated using bipolar coagulation. Scissor division is performed close to the desiccation line to ensure that the compressed pedicle remains intact. The mesosalpinx is cauterized and cut, allowing removal of the fallopian tube. The peritoneum of the vesicouterine space can be grasped and elevated with forceps, while the vesicouterine space is dissected by using scissors. Aquadissection may be used to separate the leaves of the broad ligament. The vesicouterine space is distended, and the bladder attachments are coagulated and cut. The tube and rudimentary horn are removed, leaving the functional ovary.

In the event, a pregnancy occurs in a noncommunicating horn, laparoscopic excision of the pregnant horn is advocated. Successful pregnancy in the major horn has been reported after laparoscopic removal of accessory horn.

Endometrial ablation of accessory horn through a hysteroscopic approach is reported for treatment of symptomatic hematometra. Hysteroscopic drainage of a hematometra in a noncommunicating accessory horn by using electrocautery to create a communication between the horns has also been described.

Class III—Uterus Didelphys

Didelphys uterus arises when midline fusion of the müllerian ducts is arrested, either completely or incompletely. Approximately 11% of uterine malformations are didelphys uterus. The complete form is characterized by two hemiuteri, two endocervical canals with cervices fused at the lower uterine segment. Each hemiuteri is associated with one fallopian tube. Ovarian malposition may also be present. The vagina may be single or double, with duplication a frequent component. The double vagina manifests as a longitudinal (horizontal) septum that extends either completely (complete septum) or partially (partial septum) from the cervices to the introitus.

Patients with a uterine didelphys are usually asymptomatic, unless an obstruction is present. In such cases, hematometrocolpos, hematometra, and hematosalpinx may develop.

Renal agenesis most commonly occurs in association with uterine didelphys than with any other type of müllerian anomaly. The reported incidence of renal anomalies in this group is 20%. Obstructed unilateral vagina in patients with uterus didelphys is frequently associated with ipsilateral renal and ureter agenesis; this is known as Wunderlich-Herlyn-Werner syndrome, a rare but well-established anomaly.

Renal agenesis is thought to be due to developmental arrest in one wolffian duct that in turn affects induction of nephrogenesis and positioning of the ipsilateral müllerian ducts. The malpositioned müllerian duct is incapable of successful fusion, and two hemiuteri develop. Familial occurrences are reported, though definitive genetic associations have not been identified.

Diagnosis of Uterine Didelphys

Nonobstructive uterus didelphys is usually asymptomatic until menarche. The most frequent complaint is failure of tampons to obstruct menstrual flow. The diagnosis is often rendered during the initial pelvic examination, when two cervices are identified. A history of second-trimester spontaneous abortion is often a clue to this condition.

In hemivaginal obstruction, the clinical presentations are variable and depend on the degree of obstruction and whether the obstruction has an opening. The most common presenting symptoms are onset of dysmenorrhea within the first years following menarche and progressive pelvic pain. A unilateral pelvic mass is detected on examination with the right affected nearly twice as frequently as the left.

Diagnostic modalities are similar to those used for unicornuate uterus. Workup should include HSG, MRI, and IVP to confirm or exclude associated urinary tract anomalies. MRI reveals two widely separated uterine horns, and two cervices are typically identified. The intercornual angle is >60°. The zonal anatomy is preserved within each hemiuterus. A TVS usually observes variable dilation of the vaginal component and diminished endometrial dilatation.

Preoperative Evaluation

The obstructed unilateral vagina is an indication for resection of the vaginal septum. Surgery is necessary to preserve reproductive capacity and to prevent impairment of the uterus and tubes. Unless readily removed after diagnosis, retrograde menstruation continues and hematometra and hematosalpinx may develop. Endometriosis and pelvic adhesions also may occur.

When the vagina is not obstructed the indications for surgical correction are limited and may be done, if dysparunia is a distressing problem. Selected patients with a long history of recurrent spontaneous abortions or preterm births may benefit from metroplasty. Indeed, unification surgery for the didelphys uterus has few indications and the results may be disappointing.

The management of a nonobstructed longitudinal septum in pregnancy is not clear. Some authors advocate excision, whereas others recommend leaving it undisturbed unless it becomes obstructed during labor.

Surgical Techniques

- Uterine didelphys with obstructed unilateral vagina:
  - Full excision and marsupialization of the vaginal septum is the preferred approach and is performed as a single procedure. After the septum has been excised, laparoscopy can be performed for potential treatment of associated endometriosis, adhesions, or both.
  - Hemihysterectomy with or without salpingo-oophorectomy is rarely indicated.
- Uterus didelphys, nonobstructed:
  - The indications for septum resection in the nonobstructed didelphys uterus are limited. These patients are not candidates for surgical unification. If the woman carries a pregnancy, obstetric complications are usually minimal.
  - The decision to perform metroplasty should be individualized, and only selected patients may benefit from surgical reconstruction. The recommended procedure is the Strassmanns metroplasty. This method unifies the uterine cavities at the fundus, while the cervices are left intact.

Class IV—Bicornuate Uterus

The bicornuate uterus is formed when the müllerian ducts incompletely fuse at the level of the uterine fundus. In this anomaly, the lower uterus and cervix are completely fused, resulting in 2 separate but communicating endometrial cavities, a single-chamber cervix and vagina. A muscular intrauterine septum is also present, and this defect corresponds externally to an indentation or groove at the fundus. The depth of the groove and length of the uterine septum depend in the adult uterus on the length of the incompletely fused müllerian ducts in the fetus.

Subclassification into complete or partial categories depends on septum length. Complete uterine septa that extend either to the internal or external os are known as bicornuate unicollis uterus and bicornuate bicollis uterus, respectively. When the septum is confined to the fundal region, it is considered a partial bicornuate uterus.

Women with this anomaly usually have few reproductive-associated problems. The condition usually remains undiagnosed until cesarean delivery or other procedures reveal its existence. Approximately 60% of patients can expect to deliver a viable infant, though they may present with late abortion or premature labor.

Diagnosis of Bicornuate Uterus

The most important step is to distinguish the bicornuate uterus from the septate uterus. An accurate, definitive diagnosis must be rendered because their treatment strategies and reproductive outcomes markedly differ. Indeed, uterine bicornuate does not usually require surgery and is associated with minimal reproductive problems, while the septate uterus can be surgically corrected and has a high association with reproductive failure.

Evaluation of bicornuate uterus should begin with ultrasonography during the luteal phase of the menstrual cycle, when the endometrial echo complex is better identified. Sonographic studies based on the intercornual angle do not help in accurately distinguishing a septate uterus from a bicornuate uterus.

The cornerstone of the diagnostic evaluation for most uterine structural anomalies is HSG; however, HSG cannot reliably distinguish bicornuate from septate uteri because their uterine cavity images are similar (i.e. double uterus). The reported accuracy of HSG in differentiating bicornuate from septate is 55%.

Further evaluation by MRI can help make this distinction. On MRI, 2 uterine bodies and a single cervix characterize the bicornuate uterus. The intercornual distance is increased to >105°. The myometrial tissue that separates the 2 horns has a signal intensity identical to that of the myometrium. The external contour is outward concave, which contrasts with the outward convexity of normal and septate uteri. MRI findings of the septate uterus reveal a persistent longitudinal septum partially dividing the uterine cavity with intercornual angle ≤75°. The gray area is when the intercornual angle is >75° but <105°. In this condition, other diagnostic modalities, such as laparoscopy, must be considered.

Laparoscopic examination of the fundal contour can readily distinguish the bicornuate uterus from the septate uterus. The major difference between the two is the anatomic appearance of the external uterine fundus. The bicornuate uterus has 2 horns, whereas the appearance of external fundus of the septate uterus is normal (Fig. 10.4).

Preoperative Evaluation

Bicornuate uterus seldom requires surgical reconstruction. Metroplasty should be reserved for women who

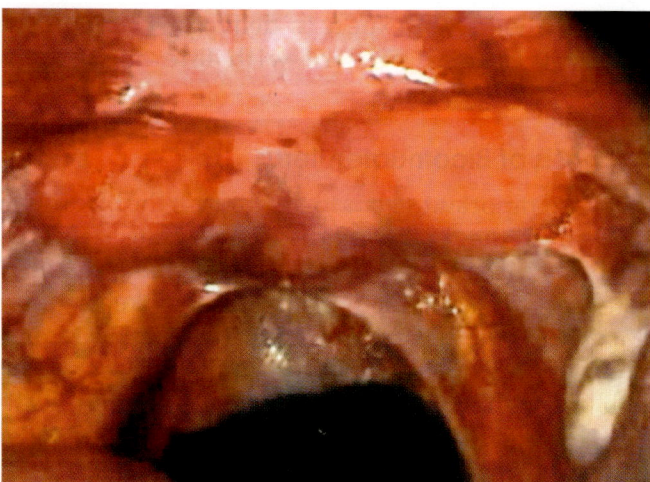

Fig. 10.4: Laparoscopy view of bicornuate uterus

have experienced recurrent spontaneous abortions, midtrimester loss, premature birth, and in whom no other etiologic factor has been identified.

Surgical Techniques for Bicornuate Uterus

Although a number of metroplasty procedures are available, the Strassmann procedure is the surgical treatment of choice for unifying the bicornuate and didelphys uteri. Transcervical lysis used in other anomalies is contraindicated in this setting because it can result in uterine perforation. The Strassmann procedure removes the septum by wedge resection with subsequent unification of the two cavities.

A Pfannenstiel incision is made, and the pelvic organs, vessels, and ureters are examined. The rectovesical ligament is frequently present and should be completely excised prior to performing the wedge resection. It is identified anteriorly by its attachment to the bladder and courses between both uterine horns, where it is also attached. It continues posteriorly in the cul-de-sac to terminate at its attachment to the anterior surface of the sigmoid and rectum.

- *Wedge resection of the uterine horns:*
  - Tourniquets are applied similar to the modified Jones procedure to promote hemostasis. A wedge-shaped incision, deep enough to enter the endometrial cavity, is made on the medial aspect of each uterine horn.
  - The incision extends from the superior aspect of each horn, near the interstitial region of the fallopian tubes, to the inferior aspect of the uterus.
  - The goal is to achieve a single endocervical canal. If two cervices are present, their unification is not recommended.

- *Apposition of the myometrium:*
  - After resecting the wedge, the myometrial edges naturally evert. Apposition of the opposing myometrium is achieved using interrupted vertical figure-8 sutures along the posterior and anterior uterine walls.
  - When suturing the fundal region, one must be mindful in placing the sutures too close to the tubal ostia. The opposing myometrium merges as the sutures are tied forming a united uterine cavity.
  - The final layer is closed using continuous subserosal sutures, without exposing any suture material to the peritoneal cavity.
  - After tourniquet removal, broad ligament incisions are repaired using very fine sutures. Transvaginal dilatation of the cervix is performed, assuring proper endometrial cavity drainage.

Class V—Septate Uterus

Septate uterus is the most common structural abnormality of all müllerian duct defects. It results from incomplete resorption of the medial septum after complete fusion of the müllerian ducts has occurred. The septum, located in the midline fundal region, is composed of poorly vascularized fibromuscular tissue. Numerous septal variations exist. The complete septum extends from the fundal area to the internal os and divides the endometrial cavity into two components. This anomaly is often associated with a longitudinal vaginal septum. The partial septum does not extend to the os.

A variant septate anomaly characterized by the triad of complete septate uterus, duplicated cervix, and vaginal septum exist. The most common presenting symptoms are dyspareunia, dysmenorrhea and primary or secondary infertility. Because of the presence of two cervices, this entity should be distinguished from the didelphys uterus. In general, a complete septum would be removed hysteroscopically while no surgical intervention would be recommended for the uterine didelphys. On laparoscopy, the uterine fundus has a normal, smooth contour.

A rare variant septate uterus is the Robert uterus. This entity is characterized by a complete septum and noncommunicating hemiuteri with a blind horn. Patients usually present with unilateral hematometra and dysmenorrhea.

Diagnosis of the Septate Uterus

In general, a combination of diagnostic modalities is needed to arrive at a definitive diagnosis. The most frequently used approaches are HSG, hysteroscopy, and laparoscopy. Ultrasonography and MRI are also useful. MRI provides excellent tissue characterization and helps in reliably differentiating a septate uterus from a bicornuate uterus. MRI reveals low signal intensity for the septum, a normal fundal contour with outward fundal convexity.

HSG reveals a 2-chambered uterus. The length and thickness of the septum can be assessed, and tubal patency can be concomitantly assessed. However, neither HSG nor hysteroscopy help in distinguishing a septate uterus from a bicornuate uterus. Laparoscopy aimed at determining normal fundal contour is best for distinguishing these entities.

Surgical Techniques (Fig. 10.5)

The surgical procedure of choice is hysteroscopic metroplasty with concurrent laparoscopy. Laparoscopy helps reduce the risk of uterine perforation during septal incision.

Laparoscopy

Examination of the uterus can help verify the concave external shape of the septate uterus, further distinguishing it from a bicornuate uterus. It can also help in detecting unexpected pelvic disease.

Hysteroscopy

- The laparoscope is placed, and hysteroscopy commences. The cervix is dilated to 6 mm, and the hysteroscope is inserted to the level of the external os. It is advanced into the uterine cavity under direct vision. Distention media depends on the instruments used to dissect the septum.
- Operative hysteroscopic metroplasty can be performed by using microscissors, electrosurgery, or a laser. The following approach uses microscissors. Flexible microscissors are passed through the operating channel of the hysteroscope. The inferior aspect of the septum is identified, and the septum is progressively dissected until a cavity with a normal-appearing contour is achieved. The laparoscopist observes the serosal surface of the uterus to detect any tissue blanching and localized light emanating from the hysteroscope. When this occurs, the procedure is too close to the surface.
- Dissection of the septum is complete when the hysteroscope can be moved freely from 1 tubal ostium to the other without obstruction, the tubal ostia are visualized simultaneously, and bleeding occurs from small vessels at the fundal myometrium.
- Abdominal Modified Jone's metroplasty was done on laparotomy/laparoscopy with V-shape cut in the septofundal junction to remove the septal tissue and unifying the two cavity to restore normal cavity of the uterus.

Postoperative Management

Postoperative placement of an intrauterine device for a month is controversial. Some think that it may prevent intrauterine adhesion formation, whereas most experts maintain that this procedure is unnecessary and may provoke local inflammation with subsequent synechiae.

Conjugated estrogens 1.25 mg/day for 25 days and progesterone 10 mg/day added on days 21–25 are frequently prescribed after surgery to assist with epithelialization.

The postoperative follow-up examination is recommended after one month with either hysteroscopy or HSG to assess the status of the uterine cavity. When findings on postoperative follow up examination are normal, pregnancy can be attempted.

Hysteroscopic metroplasty with concurrent laparoscopy is the treatment of choice for symptomatic septate uterus. This approach is a safe and effective method of achieving normal or near-normal uterine architecture and is superior to the transabdominal approach. The risk of pelvic adhesions is limited, and recovery is rapid, with no prolonged postoperative delay in conception. Moreover, it allows for vaginal delivery, obviating subsequent cesarean delivery, as was recommended after the transabdominal approach.

Class VI—Arcuate Uterus

The arcuate uterus results from near-complete resorption of the uterovaginal septum. It is characterized by a small intrauterine indentation shorter than 1 cm and located in the fundal region. It is the most commonly observed uterine anomaly detected by HSG. The arcuate uterus is clinically benign despite an infrequent association with adverse obstetric outcomes, and may not affect reproductive outcomes.

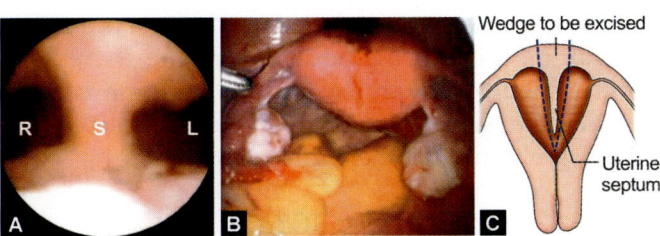

Fig. 10.5: (A) Hysteroscopy picture of septum, (B) Laparoscopy view of fundus of septate uterus, (C) schematic diagram of septum

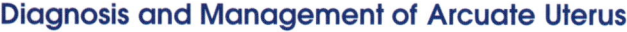

Diagnosis and Management of Arcuate Uterus

HSG reveals a single uterine cavity with a saddle-shaped fundal indentation. MRI findings show convex or flat external uterine contour. The indentation is broad and smooth. The signal intensity is myometrial in composition.

Defects Not Classified by the AFS

Transverse Vaginal Septum (TVS)

TVS is formed when the tissue between the vaginal plate and the caudal aspect of the fused müllerian ducts fails to reabsorb. This anomaly divides the vagina into two segments, reducing its functional length. TVS can be perforate or imperforate, and can occur at nearly all levels in the vagina. Most of these septa are located in the superior vagina at the junction between the vaginal plate and caudal aspect of the UVP (46%). The next most common locations are the mid-vagina, at a rate of 40%, and the inferior vagina, at a rate of 14%.

TVS is one of the most rare müllerian duct anomalies, with an approximate frequency of 1 case in 70,000 females. TVS has been associated with other structural anomalies, including imperforate anus, bicornuate uterus, coarctation of the aorta, atrial septal defect, and malformation of the lumbar spine.

Diagnosis of TVS—Fetuses, Neonates, and Infants

TVS is rarely diagnosed in the neonate or infant unless the obstruction causes a significant hydromucocolpos. In rare cases, copious amounts of fluid may collect in the vagina above the obstructing septum and create a mass effect in which the surrounding organs are compressed. Hydromucocolpos can be diagnosed *in utero* during third trimester transabdominal sonography. In these cases, fetal abdominal distension is noted secondary to an abdominal or pelvic mass.

Diagnosis of hydromucocolpos in the neonate and infant can be challenging. A large mass is often palpated in the lower abdomen. MRI can also be useful to depict pelvic anatomy and determine the thickness of the vaginal septum.

Surgical Management of TVS— Fetuses, Neonates, and Infants

When third-trimester ultrasonographic findings lead to the diagnosis, early delivery and drainage of the obstructed vagina and uterus are indicated when other organs are compromised.

In infants, the vaginal septum is usually thin and can be corrected without extensive procedures. Surgical excision of the obstructed septum through a perineal approach is most efficacious. Bilateral incisions may be required to ensure complete removal.

Postoperative Management

Clinical follow-up is necessary because vaginal stenosis with subsequent accumulation of fluid may develop postoperatively. Vaginal reconstruction may be required to allow satisfactory menstruation and coitus.

Diagnosis of TVS—Postmenarche

In general, TVS remains undetected until the time of menarche. Presentation after menarche varies depending on whether the septum is complete or incomplete. If the TVS is complete, the patient commonly presents with primary amenorrhea and cyclic pelvic pain. Like an imperforate hymen, symptoms are caused by obstructed menstrual flow with retention of mucus, blood, or both. Physical examination frequently reveals a palpable central lower abdominal or pelvic mass secondary to hematocolpos, hematometra, hematosalpinx, and even hemoperitoneum. However, unlike an imperforate hymen, examination of the genitalia reveals no evidence of bulging at the introitus.

Incomplete TVS allows menstrual flow to escape periodically, but hematocolpos and hematometra often develop over time. Complaints include foul-smelling vaginal discharge, dyspareunia secondary to a short vagina, and infertility. In addition, TVS can cause soft tissue dystocia in patients who eventually become pregnant.

Preoperative Evaluation

Preoperative evaluation includes preliminary ultrasonography, MRI to determine the thickness of the vaginal septum, and IVP and renal sonography to help detect the occasional urinary tract anomaly.

Surgical Management of TVS—Adults

The surgical approach to TVS excision depends on the character, thickness, and location of the septum. The TVS can be thick in the adult, rendering its removal more difficult than in the infant. In some cases, a considerable length of vagina is underdeveloped, and it may rarely involve the entire vagina.

Surgical Techniques (Fig. 10.6)

The approach to surgical correction of TVS depends on its location within the vagina and its thickness.

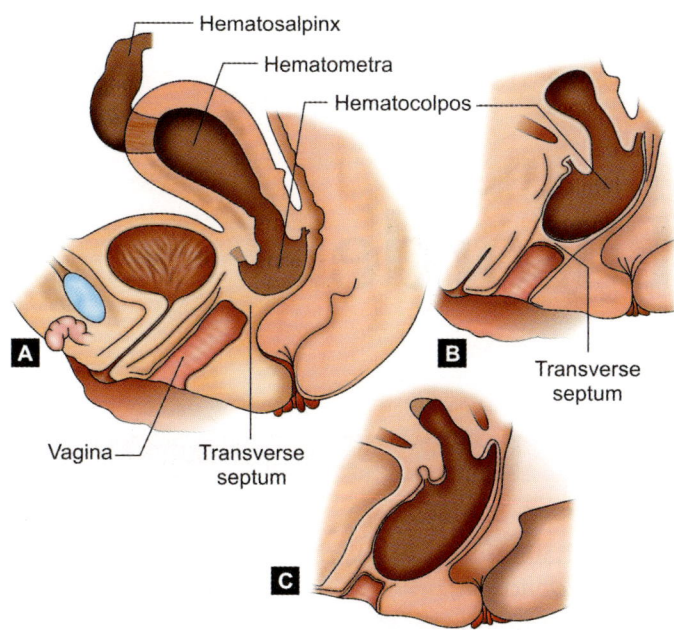

Fig. 10.6: Different levels of obstruction in TVS

- **High TVS**
  - Surgical correction of high TVS is more difficult because the septum is usually thick and extensive; dissection between the bladder and the rectum is required. The bladder and anteriorly associated structures are distinguished from the posterior rectum. A transurethral catheter is placed to provide the anterior boundaries.
  - A transverse incision is then made through the vaginal vault. If the TVS is imperforate, a portion of the septum is separated using blunt and sharp dissection. A probe is then introduced through the septum. Palpation of the urethral catheter anteriorly and a gloved rectal finger posteriorly provide identification of surgical landmarks so that neither the bladder nor the rectum is compromised. Blind dissection is continued until the cervix is palpated. The lateral margins of the septum are excised with a scalpel.
  - When a high hematocolpos cannot be drained vaginally, it may be necessary to perform an exploratory laparotomy. A probe is introduced through the uterine fundus and cervix to serve as a guide in locating the high hematocolpos. If a considerable amount of blood has accumulated in the obstructed upper vagina, an aspiration needle is used as a probe to identify it. The upper vagina is then entered.

  When excision of a wide septum leaves an area too large to be closed using the available tissue,

an indwelling stent is placed in the vagina to assist in epithelialization. If the septum is quite thick, excision may require the implantation of a split-thickness skin graft in a fashion similar to the McIndoe procedure.

- **Low, mid, and thin TVS**
  - Thin, low, and mid-vaginal septa are best excised with multiple radial incisions. The edges of the upper and lower vaginal mucosa are undermined and mobilized enough to permit anastomosis.
  - Joining of the upper and lower vaginal segments using interrupted delayed absorbable sutures follows this procedure. When the septal opening is small, manual dilatation can be used.

Postoperative Management

The stent is left in place for 4–6 months. Daily dilatation for the next 2–4 months is required to ensure continued vaginal patency. It is often necessary to make lateral incisions along the sides of the stent during removal. Coitus can be initiated, or, if the patient is not sexually active, a silicone vaginal form is inserted nightly until the constrictive phase of healing is complete. Care must be taken to maintain good hemostasis, which avoids sloughing of the graft.

Vaginal Atresia

Vaginal atresia occurs when the UGS fails to contribute to the inferior portion of the vagina. The müllerian structures are usually normal, but fibrous tissue completely replaces the inferior segment of the vagina. Although not müllerian in origin, vaginal atresia can clinically mimic vaginal agenesis and imperforate hymen and may be another anomaly in the continuum of segmental vaginal defects. Surgical management is similar to that of vaginal agenesis.

Conclusion

Müllerian anomalies are a morphologically diverse group of developmental disorders that involve the internal female reproductive tract. Establishing an accurate diagnosis is essential for planning treatment and management strategies. The surgical approach for correction of müllerian duct anomalies is specific to the type of malformation and may vary in a specific group. For most surgical procedures, the critical test of the procedure's value is the patient's postoperative ability to have healthy sexual relations and achieve successful reproductive outcomes.

11 Menstrual Disorders

11A. AMENORRHEA

Definition

This is the absence of menstruation.

It may be physiological as before the menarche, after the menopause or in pregnancy, or it may be post-operative, if the patient has had a hysterectomy.

Amenorrhea can be divided into primary and secondary:

- **Primary amenorrhea** is when menses have not occurred by the time of the expected menarche. This may be taken as age of 14 years in the absence of secondary sexual characteristics, but it is worth waiting until age of 16 years, if other features are developing normally.
- Very recently it is defined as absence of menses at the age of 13 years in absence of secondary sex characters or age of 15 years in presence of normal secondary sex characters.
- **Secondary amenorrhea** is when menstruation has previously occurred but it has stopped for at least six consecutive months.

WHO defined **three** classes of amenorrhea:

- *WHO group I:* Women with no evidence of endogenous estrogen production, normal or low FSH levels, normal prolactin levels and no lesion in hypothalamic–pituitary region (hypogonadotropic hypogonadism).
- *WHO group II:* Women with evidence of estrogen production and normal levels of prolactin and FSH like in PCOS.
- *WHO group III:* Women with elevated serum FSH indicating gonadal insufficiency or failure (hypergonadotropic hypogonadism).

Incidence

- The incidence of primary amenorrhea is 0.3% and secondary amenorrhea is 3%.
- The prevalence is higher in college students (3–5%), competitive athletes (5–60%), and ballet dancers (19–44%).
- Between 10 and 20% of women presenting with infertility have amenorrhea.

Primary Amenorrhea

There are five basic factors involved in the onset and continuation of normal menstruation. These are (Table 11.1):

a. Anatomical patency of the genital tract
b. Normal female chromosomal pattern

Table 11.1: Etiological background in primary amenorrhea

1. Developmental defect of genital tract	
a. Complete absence of vagina (true amenorrhea)	Müllerian agenesis, testicular feminization syndrome (complete variety)
b. Short blind vagina (cryptoamenorrhea)	Imperforate hymen, transverse vaginal septum, partial absence of upper part of vagina.
c. Blind vagina (true amenorrhea)	Annular constriction of upper part of vagina with cervical stenosis
2. Abnormal chromosomal pattern	Turner's syndrome and other varieties of gonadal dysgenesis
3. Hypothalamic–pituitary–ovarian dysfunction	CNS defect, hypopituitarism, PCOS, androgen producing tumor of ovary, delayed menarche
4. Dysfunction of thyroid and adrenal cortex	Androgenital syndrome, Cushing disease, cretinism
5. Unresponsive or absent endometrium	Congenital receptor defect, uterine synechiae

c. Co-ordinated hypothalamic–pituitary–ovarian axis
d. Active support by two endocrine glands, thyroid and adrenal cortex
e. Responsive endometrium.

Primary amenorrhea can be divided into anatomical, endocrine or constitutional.

For the purpose of investigation, it is useful to divide it into those with and those without normal development of secondary sexual characteristics.

I. **Amenorrhea without secondary sex characters can be:**
   a. Hypergonadotropic hypogonadism within which main causes are: (i) Different varieties of gonadal dysgenesis, (ii) FSH receptor defect, (iii) sex chromosome mosaicism, and (iv) 17-hydroxylase deficiency in XX individual.
   b. Hypogonadotropic hypogonadism which include: (i) Physiological delay, (ii) Kallmann syndrome, and (iii) CNS tumors.
II. **Amenorrheas with secondary sex characters** include: (i) Anatomical defects, (ii) pelvic infections including tuberculosis, schistosomiasis, etc. (iii) PCOS, hyperprolactinemia, premature ovarian failure, etc.

Conventionally amenorrhea is divided into primary and secondary types as the etiological factors are entirely different in these two types and treatment of most of the secondary amenorrhea cases are satisfactory whereas those of primary amenorrhea are not.

Similarly, American Society of Reproductive Medicine classifies causes of primary amenorrhea into three distinct groups:
1. Primary amenorrhea with breast development (30%)
2. Primary amenorrhea with no breast development and high FSH (40%)
3. Primary amenorrhea with no breast development and low FSH (30%).

Incidence

Amongst the primary amenorrhea cases, the overall incidence of gonadal dysgenesis is found in 33%, Müllerian duct anomalies in 25%, testicular feminization in 2.3%, genital tuberculosis in 2.3%, hypogonadotropic hypogonadism including delayed puberty in rest of the cases.

Genital Tract Anomalies

A definite correlation exists between type of uterine anomalies and defect in the vagina. Therefore, vaginal malformation can be graded into four types on the basis of their prognosis to surgical correction (Table 11.2).

Complete Absence of Vagina

This condition is also termed as **Mayer-Rokitanski-Kuster-Hausen syndrome**. They have the following characters:
1. Phenotypically female.
2. Chromosomal karyotype is 46XX.
3. There is a complete absence of vaginal opening.
4. There are remnants of müllerian tissue with two solid müllerian knobs connected in the middle by a fibromuscular band in place of the normal uterus indicating two müllerian halves which may sometimes contain functioning endometrial tissue. There are sometimes a third müllerian knob seen behind the bladder which denotes the lower fused portion of the müllerian ducts, embryological remnant of adult cervix.
5. At the lateral ends, there are presence of ovaries and some portion of the fallopian tubes.
6. Urinary tract malformation like pelvic kidney is present in about 30% of cases and bony abnormality like split pelvis, spinal anomalies, absent digits, webbed fingers, toes is detected in 5–12% cases.
7. Sometimes it is associated with abnormal galactose metabolism.
8. Normal breast development, secondary sex characters.
9. Normal LH, FSH.

Treatment

Nonsurgical methods:
- By dilators (Frank and Ingram) (Fig. 11.1).

	Types of vaginal development	Clinical diagnosis	Co-existing abnormality
Grade I	Complete absence of vagina	True amenorrhea	Uterus absent, replaced by two müllerian knobs, normal fallopian tubes, ovaries
Grade II	Transverse vaginal septum	Hematocolpos and hematometra	Functioning uterus normal or malformed
Grade III	Partial agenesis of upper part of vagina	Hematometra only	Functioning uterus normal or malformed, cervix ill-developed, cord-like, non-vanalized
Grade IV	Annular constriction of upper part of vagina	Functional amenorrhea	Isthmial stenosis

Table 11.2: Levels in vaginal obstruction

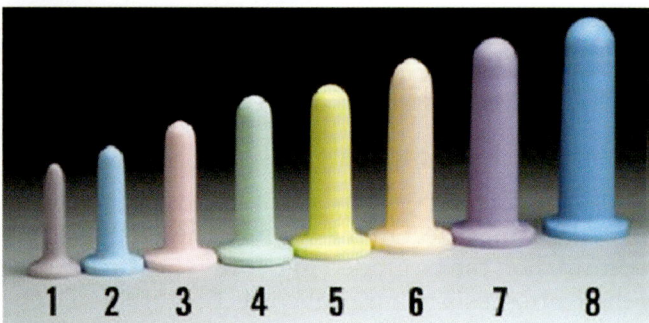

Fig. 11.1: Serial vaginal dilators

- Dilate at a 15° angle daily after warm bath for 20 minutes.
- Progressively work up to larger dilators.
- Success is defined as non-painful intercourse or vaginal length of 7 cm.
- Studies demonstrate up to an 88% success rate at 19 months of use.

Surgical Treatment

The whole purpose of treatment is to provide them coital function only; there is no possibility of restoring menstrual and reproductive function though in rare cases hysteroplasty is attempted without much favorable results.

Management of Vaginal Agenesis by Modified McIndoe Operation and Mold Made of Sponge and Condom

Vaginoplasty is a surgical procedure whose purpose is to treat vaginal structure defect (Fig. 11.2). Vaginal agenesis is estimated to occur in 1 in 4,000–5,000 live female births. Among various methods, McIndoe technique has remained most popular, here split thickness skin graft is used to line the neovagina. The main advantages are its simplicity and low morbidity. The disadvantages are graft contraction, fistula formation and need for long-term use of vaginal retainer.

The modified McIndoe method is where instead of skin graft a mold made by sponge and condom has been used for long period to maintain the space and to allow epithelialization. A transverse incision is given on the introitus and then a space is created in between the urethra and bladder in front and rectum behind by blunt finger dissection (Fig. 11.3). The created space is about 12 cm in length and 5 cm in diameter. A mold made by sponge and condom is placed in the newly created space (Figs 11.4–11.6). 3/4 stitches are given

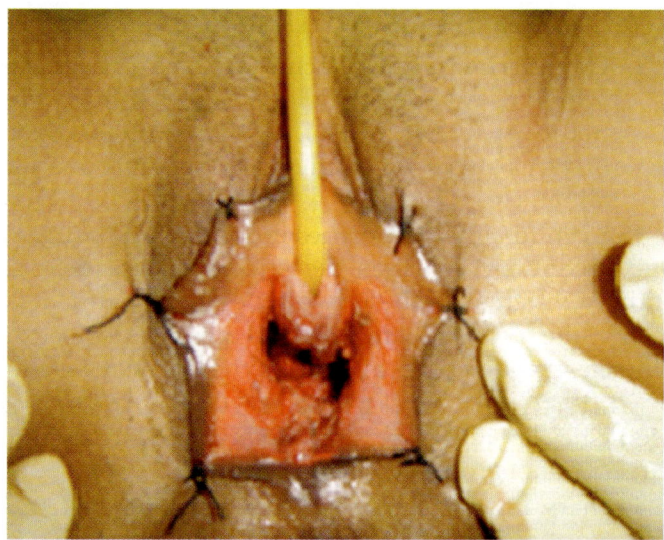

Fig. 11.3: Potential space created between vagina and rectum

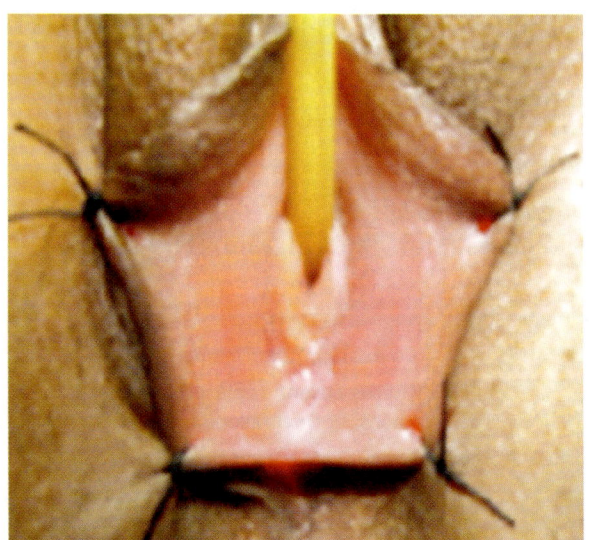

Fig. 11.2: Complete agenesis of vagina

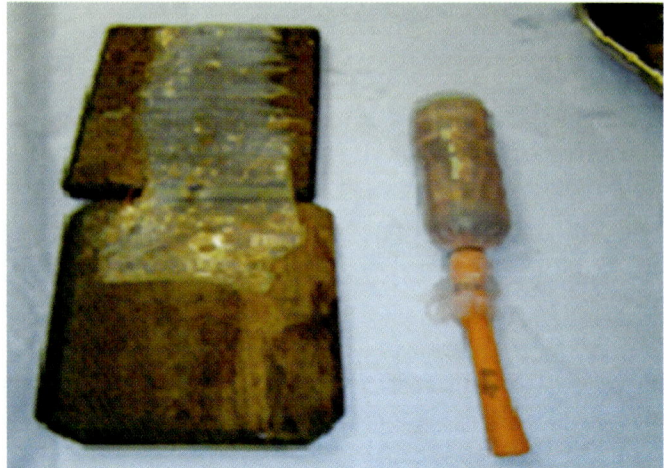

Fig. 11.4: Mold being prepared

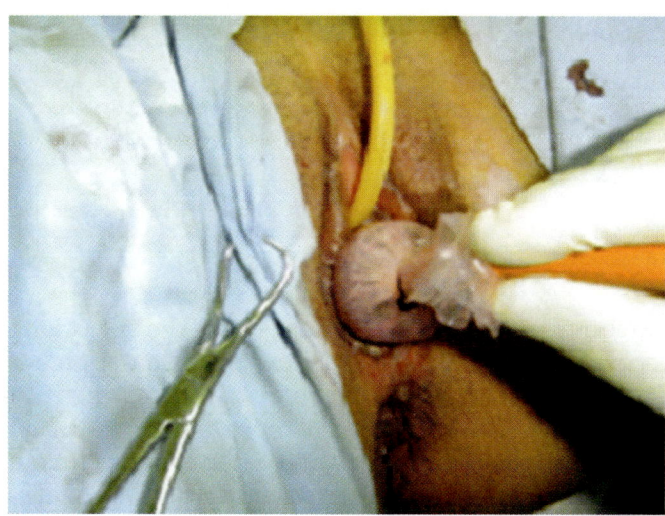

Fig. 11.5: Placement of vaginal mold with graft

Table 11.3: Different grafts for vaginoplasty
1. Abbe-McIndoe skin graft
2. Constructing neovagina from bowel segments
3. Fasciocutaneous flaps
4. Labia minora flaps (flaps raised following tissue)
5. Interceed absorbable adhesion barrier
6. McIndoe and Bannister procedure
7. Pudendal-thing flaps
8. Gracilis myocutaneous flaps
9. Peritoneum and bladder mucosa expansion of the labial pocket
10. Amnion from recently performed CS
11. Autologous buccal mucosa graft

The amnion is often used as a homograft but failure rate is high. Sigmoid neovaginoplasty offers some advantages as the gut is distensible and self-lubricating but procedure is complicated.

I. *Imperforate Hymen* (Fig. 11.7)

This presents with cryptomenorrhoea due to obstructing membrane at the level of introitus. There may be additional symptoms of periodic lower abdominal pain and retention of urine. A bluish bulge on the obstructive membrane is visible at the introitus due to retained blood behind the membrane. Abdominopelvic examination reveal a lump due to hematocolpos and hematometra (Table 11.4).

Treatment is by cruciate incision and excision of the membrane to restore the opening of the introitus. The old collected dark-colored menstrual blood starts coming out. While blood is draining, external abdominal pressure is avoided to prevent backward spill of menstrual blood into the abdomen to prevent endometriosis. The internal genital organs, like uterus,

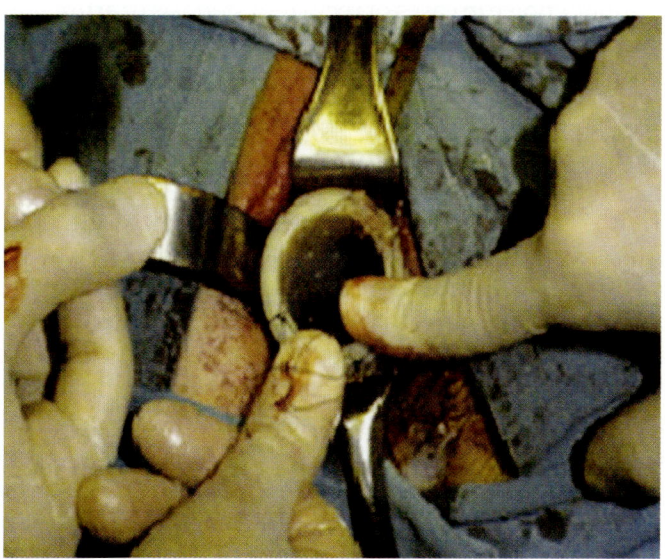

Fig. 11.6: Mold replaced by new one

through the inner aspect of the labia over the mold so the mold does not come out. After 7 days, mold is removed. Another freshly prepared mold is placed in the space as before. All the process is repeated weekly for another two/three times. Then the patient is asked to wear the mold continuously for three months and then at night for another three months. Thereafter, they are advised for daily dilatation with the mold or practice regular coitus. Married women are allowed to perform physical relation after 6 weeks.

There are various methods for surgically constructing neovaginas and the difference among the various surgical approaches lies in the tissues used to line the neovagina (as mentioned in Table 11.3).

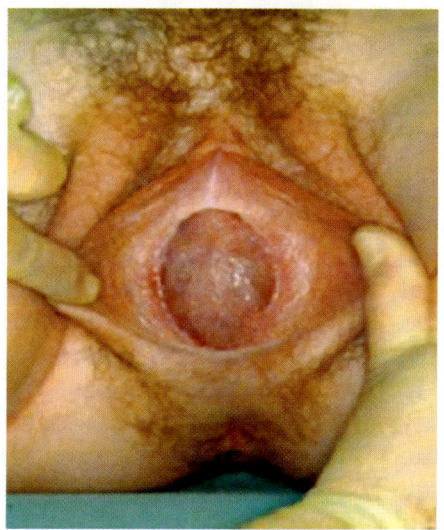

Fig. 11.7: Imperforate hymen

Findings	Imperforate hymen	Müllerian agenesis
Table 11.4: Clinical differential diagnosis between imperforate hymen and Müllerian agenesis		
Color of obstructing membrane	Pearly white, smooth	Pinkish with rugosity of vaginal mucosa
Surface of obstructing wall	Convex outwards	Concave inwards
Syringing and needle puncture test	Saline introduced can be aspirated	Saline cannot be aspirated
Rectal examination	Uterus palpable	Uterus not palpable
USG	Hematocolpos, hematometra	Absent uterus

tubes, ovary, are healthy. Chromosomal karyotype is 46XX.

II. *Transverse Vaginal Septum* (Fig. 11.8)

There is a transverse partition in the middle third of the vagina. This results in hematometra and hematocolpos since the uterus and cervix is functionally normal. This is characterized by cyclical pain, abdominopelvic lump and retention of urine. The treatment is surgical excision of the septum by transverse incision and mobilization of the vaginal septa to fix it with posterior vaginal wall to avoid restenosis.

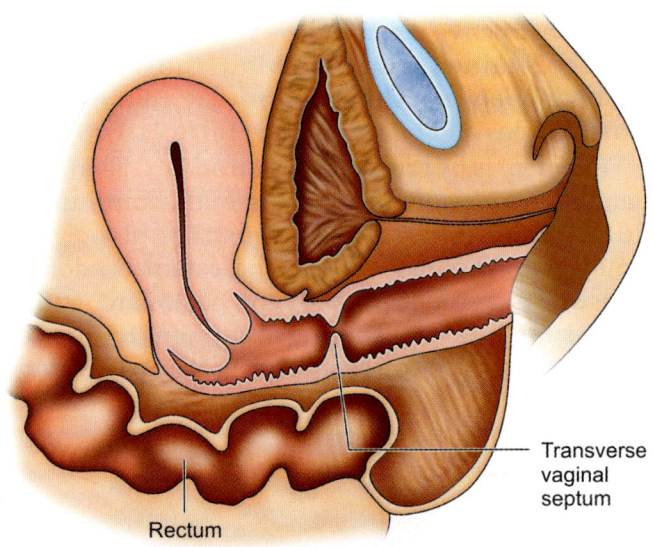

Fig. 11.8: Transverse vaginal septum

III. *Agenesis of Upper One-third of Vagina*

This reveal same clinical picture of increasing hematocolpos and hematometra. But from embryological and therapeutic point of view, it is more complicated. Here in addition to vaginal agenesis, the cervix is rudimentary and non-canalized while uterus is found normally functioning. This makes the surgical treatment very difficult. The procedure involves reconstruction of upper part of vagina using graft and canalization from abdominal route to communicate with uterocervical canal

above and newly created vagina below. The operation is performed by simultaneous abdominovaginal approach. One copper-T or pediatric Foley catheter is kept for 2 weeks. Success rate is good, if the patency of the tract is well-epithelialized and the patient starts normal menstrual and reproductive function. There is always a risk of restenosis after the prosthesis is removed. Repeat vaginal dilatations are essential to maintain the patency of the uterovaginal canal. Hysterectomy remains the ultimate choice in cases of recurrent stenosis of artificially constructed cervicovaginal canal, recurrent dysmenorrhea, endometriosis, endosalpingiosis, hematometra and infection.

IV. *Annular Constriction at Upper Part of Vagina*

This is a rare cause of primary amenorrhea. Here along with annular narrowing of upper part of vagina, there is presence of congenital isthmial stenosis with true amenorrhea. There is no cryptomenorrhea because of reflex hypothalamic dysfunction. Retrograde dilatation of cervical canal by abdominal route is done with a prosthesis left behind for a period of 3–6 months to maintain patency.

Differential Diagnosis of Absence of Vaginal Opening

1. ***Müllerian agenesis:*** Defect at vestibule; presents with true amenorrhea.
2. ***Labial agglutination:*** Obstruction is at level of labia majora. This is due to local vulvitis with a small opening at upper end of fused labia for urine to escape. This is very common in young girls with repeated infection.
3. ***Labial fusion associated with congenital adrenal hyperplasia:*** Defect is in labia minora. This is a problem encountered in prepubertal age. Ambiguity of external genitalia may raise the suspicion of intersex. Internal genital organs (uterus, tubes, ovary) remain unaffected, even if adrenal cortex becomes hyperactive. This is diagnosed by elevated urinary 17-ketosteroids and 17-hydroxycorticosteroids with 46XX karyotype. The treatment consists of corticosteroids and surgical correction of labioscrotal fusion.

Androgen Insensitivity Syndrome

The syndrome was first documented by Morris in 1953. The incidence is 1/60,000 although is responsible for 9% of causes of primary amenorrhea.

This is a genetic condition where affected people have male chromosomes and male gonads with complete or partial feminization of the external genitals. It is an inherited X-linked recessive disease with a mutation in the androgen receptor (AR) gene resulting in: (a) Functioning Y sex chromosome (b) abnormality on X sex chromosome. This is of the following types:

i. *CAIS (completely insensitive to AR gene):* External female genitalia lacking female internal organs.
ii. *PAIS (partially sensitive-varying degrees):* External genitalia appearance on a spectrum of male to female type.
iii. *MAIS (mildly sensitive, rare):* Impaired sperm development and/or impaired masculinization.

Genetic Basis

AIS results from mutations in the androgen receptor gene, located on the long arm of the X-chromosome (Xq11-q12). The AR gene provides instructions to make the protein called androgen receptor, which allows cells to respond to androgens, such as testosterone, and directs male sexual development. Androgens also regulate hair growth and sex drive. Mutations include complete or partial gene deletions, point mutations and small insertions or deletions.

In AIS, the chromosome sex and gonad sex do not agree with the phenotypic sex. Phenotypic sex results from secretions of hormones from the testicles. The two main hormones secreted from the testicles are testosterone and müllerian duct inhibitor. (a) Testosterone is converted into dihydrotestosterone, (b) Müllerian duct inhibitor suppresses the mullerian ducts and prevents the development of internal female

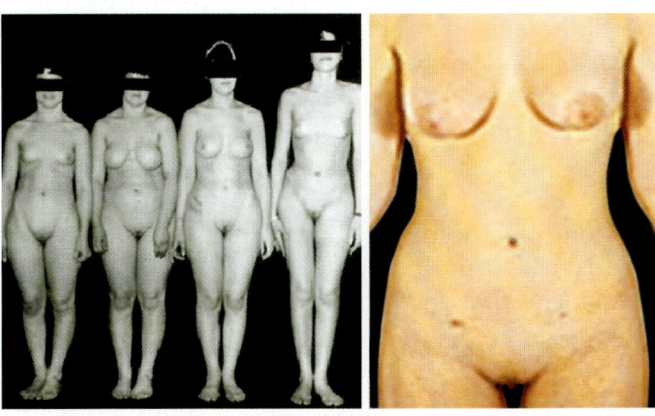

Fig. 11.9: Androgen insensitivity syndrome

sex organs in males. Wolffian ducts help develop the rest of the internal male reproductive system and suppress the müllerian ducts. Defective androgen receptors cause the wolffian ducts and genitals to be unable to respond to the androgens, testosterone and dihydrotestosterone (Fig. 11.9).

Classification of AIS Forms

Exists along continuum depending on degree of mutation in AR gene.

Grade 1 PAIS	Male genitals, infertile
Grade 2 PAIS	Male genitals but mildly 'undermasculinized'
Grade 3 PAIS	Male genitals more severely undermasculinized
Grade 4 PAIS	Ambiguous genitals
Grade 5 PAIS	Essentially female genitalia, with enlarged clitoris.
Grade 6 PAIS	Female genitalia with pubic/underarm hair
Grade 7 CAIS	Female genitalia with little to no pubic/underarm hair

The characteristic clinical features are:
- *Genetics:* X-linked recessive.
- *Phenotype:* Female; Genotype: XY.
- *Cause:* Mutations in the androgen receptor.

Physical Examination (Table 11.5)

- Slim and taller than average female.
- Large breasts with juvenile nipples.
- Absent pubic/axillary hair, no acne or other signs of androgen action.
- May have inguinal hernia.

Bilateral testes may be in the (a) intra-abdominal cavity, (b) labioscrotal folds, (c) inguinal region. Gonads on histology reveal normal testicular tissue with immature germ cells, Sertoli cells, but prominent Leydig cells.

- The condition is familial, therefore, sisters may be affected with the same condition.
- The testes are hormonally competent and produce normal testosterone. But due to total andorgen receptor sensitivity, the phenotype remains female. The defect is deficiency of cytosol androgen receptor in the target organs. This defect at the receptor level is genetically determined and defect primarily involves the male determining gene which is located on the short arm of Y chromosome.
- Müllerian inhibitory factor of testes is normal and therefore, there is suppression of mullerian tissue

Table 11.5: Difference between müllerian agenesis and complete TFS

Issue	Mullerian agenesias	Complete TFS
1. Type of amenorrhea	True primary amenorrhea	True primary amenorrhea
2. Phenotype	Feminine in type	Feminine in type
3. Chromosomal karyotype	46XX	46XY
4. Height	Normal	Lanky and tall
5. Breast development	Normal adult type	Developed but without functioning glands
6. Axillary and pubic hairs	Normal female type	Scanty or absent
7. External genitalia	Female type	Female type
8. Vagina	Complete absence of vagina	Short blind vagina
9. Gonads	Ovary in normal position	Testis in inguinal region or in labia majora
10. Internal genitalia	Uterus/cervix absent	Uterus and cervix absent by PR examination
11. Associated anomaly	Renal and skeletal anomaly	No other anomaly
12. Treatment	Vaginal reconstruction	Late pubertal gonadectomy and vaginoplasty

(absence of uterus, fallopian tubes, upper part of vagina).

- The short blind vagina present in the testicular feminization syndrome develops from remnants of urogenital sinus.
- Feminine development at puberty is due to normal adrenal and testicular estrogen levels acting on end organs which are resistant to androgens.
- These individuals are male intersex and reared up as females.
- Gonadectomy is indicated because these gonads situated in ectopic sites are vulnerable to undergo malignant change (22%). Most common histology is though Leydig cell hyperplasia. This is done after pubertal development is complete so that feminine development is complete by estrogen developed from peripheral conversion of androgens. Therefore, it is recommended at age 16–18 years. But it is not true for 'incomplete variety of testicular feminization syndrome' when there is partial response of testosterone to target organs resulting in growth of axillary and pubic hairs and phallic enlargement. Therefore, gonads are removed at the onset of puberty.
- Once testes are removed, patient will be treated with hormone replacement therapy.

Total treatment in case of true TFS is late gonadectomy, vaginal reconstruction followed by ET and in case of incomplete TFS, it is early gonadectomy, excision of enlarged phallus followed by ET. In both the cases, they are reared up as females.

Primary Amenorrhea associated with Lack of Secondary Sex Characters

I. *Hypergonadotropic hypogonadism*
a. Gonadal dysgenesis—Turner syndrome, pure gonadal dysgenesis, mixed gonadal dysgeneis.

b. Rare enzyme deficiency—congenital lipoid adrenal hyperplasia, 17alfa-hydroxylase and 17, 20-lyase deficiency, aromatase deficiency, galactosemia.
c. Rare gonadotropin receptor mutation—LH receptor mutation, FSH receptor mutation.

II. *Hypogonadotropic hypogonadism*
Physiologic delay, Kallmann syndrome, CNS tumors, other causes of GnRH deficiency.

III. *Genetic disorders*
5-alfa reductase deficiency, GnRH receptor mutations, FSH deficiency, functional gonadotropin deficiency.

Turner's Syndrome

Turner described in 1938 a series of females with sexual infantilism, webbing of neck, retardation of growth and bilateral cubitus valgus. These girls usually present with primary amenorrhea though they initially have normal ovarian development in utero. The amenorrhea is due to accelerated atresia of the follicles making the ovaries fibrotic and hence called streak ovaries.

Turner syndrome is a chromosomal condition that alters development in females. Women with this condition tend to be shorter than average and are usually infertile because of an absence of ovarian function. Other features include webbed neck, lymphedema of the hands and feet, skeletal abnormalities, heart defects and kidney problems (Fig. 11.10).

Incidence

This condition occurs in about 1 in 2,500 female births worldwide, but is much more common among pregnancies that end in miscarriages and stillbirths.

Chromosomal Background

Turner syndrome is a chromosomal condition related to the X chromosome. The main chromosomal defect

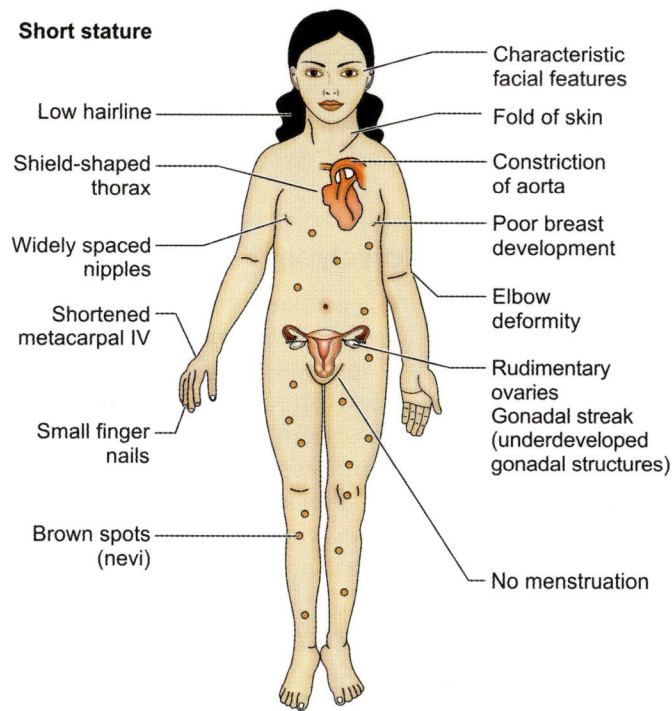

Short stature

Low hairline

Shield-shaped thorax

Widely spaced nipples

Shortened metacarpal IV

Small finger nails

Brown spots (nevi)

Characteristic facial features

Fold of skin

Constriction of aorta

Poor breast development

Elbow deformity

Rudimentary ovaries
Gonadal streak (underdeveloped gonadal structures)

No menstruation

Fig. 11.10: Turner's syndrome

is 45XO; though there may be mosaics of 45XO/ 46XX in about 10–15% cases where some ovarian differentiation and secondary sex characters are developed. The ovarian development in Turner girl is normal until 20 weeks of pregnancy and oocytes are formed in the ovaries until this stage. Thereafter, there is failure of the oocyte to undergo further maturation which requires the influence of both sex chromosomes and oocytes begin to undergo a process of atresia.

Researchers have not yet determined which genes on the X chromosome are responsible for most signs and symptoms of Turner syndrome. They have, however, identified one gene called SHOX that is important for bone development and growth. Missing one copy of this gene likely causes short stature and skeletal abnormalities in women with Turner syndrome. Therefore, the loss of short or long arm of a chromosome may be complete or partial and the genetic material lost determines the impact of turner features on the patients.

Features of Turner Syndrome

- *Growth and height:* Turner girls are usually shorter than average but they may be normal with deletion of long arm of X chromosome. They have normal height for the first three years of life, but then statrt growing slow without any growth spurt.
- *Breasts:* Poorly developed due to lack of ovarian estrogen. Normally, a girl's ovaries begin to produce

estrogen and progesterone at puberty. This does not happen in girls with Turner syndrome. They do not start periods or develop breasts without hormone treatment at the age of puberty.

- Axillary and pubic hairs are developed but scanty due to less ovarian androgens.
- *External genitalia:* Female in type but infantile in nature.
- *Internal genitalia:* Uterus, tubes, vagina are developed but remain infantile due to lack of estrogen.
- Girls with Turner syndrome are usually of normal intelligence with good verbal skills and reading skills. Some girls, however, have problems with memory and fine finger movements.

Additional symptoms of Turner syndrome include the following:

- An especially wide neck (webbed neck) and a low or indistinct hairline.
- A broad chest and widely spaced nipples.
- Arms with wide carrying angle at the elbow (>135°).
- *Cardiac anomalies:* Coarctation of aorta in 30% of patients, also bicuspid aortic valve, mitral valve prolapse.
- A tendency to develop high blood pressure.
- Renal anomalies: Horseshoe kidney may be present.
- Minor eye problems that are corrected by glasses.
- Scoliosis occurs in 10% of adolescent girls who have Turner syndrome.
- Features of hypothyroidism (10%).
- Older or over-weight women with Turner syndrome are slightly more at risk of developing diabetes.
- Osteoporosis can develop because of lack of estrogen, but this can largely be prevented by hormone replacement therapy.
- Sometimes diagnosis is made at birth because of heart problems, lymphedema of hands and feet, short 4th metacarpals and metatarsals and cystic hygroma in neck.

Treatment

- During childhood and adolescence, girls may be under the care of a pediatric endocrinologist.
- Growth hormone injections are beneficial in some individuals with Turner syndrome. Injections often begin in early childhood and may increase final adult height by a few inches.
- Estrogen replacement therapy is usually started at the time of normal puberty, around 12 years to start breast development. Progesterone is added little later along with estrogens to begin monthly period. Estrogen is also given to prevent osteoporosis.

- Babies born with a heart murmur or narrowing of the aorta may need corrective surgery.
- Repeated middle ear infections may lead to hearing loss and should be evaluated.
- Hypertension may be present due to narrowing of the aorta or a kidney abnormality.
- Women with Turner syndrome have a slightly higher risk of having an under active thyroid or developing diabetes.
- Almost all women are infertile, but pregnancy with donor embryos may be possible.

Gonadal Dysgenesis: 46XX

- Refers to a number of conditions in which abnormal development leads to streak gonads (Fig. 11.11).
- Incidence: <1/10,000 in women less than 30.
- Familial inheritance 7–30%.
- Premutations in the FMR1 gene (Fragile X syndrome)
- 15% of carriers have POF.
- Associated with autoimmune diseases (18–30%)
- Hashimoto's thyroiditis, Addison's disease, hypoparathyroidism, vitiligo.
- Acquired due to exposure to radiation, chemotherapy, childhood viruses.

Diagnosis

- May present with secondary amenorrhea.
- Increased FSH in the menopausal range (>40 u/mL).
- Ultrasound: >60% of patients have undetectable ovaries by ultrasound. Majority show no follicular growth.
- DEXA scan in addition to screening for autoimmune diseases.

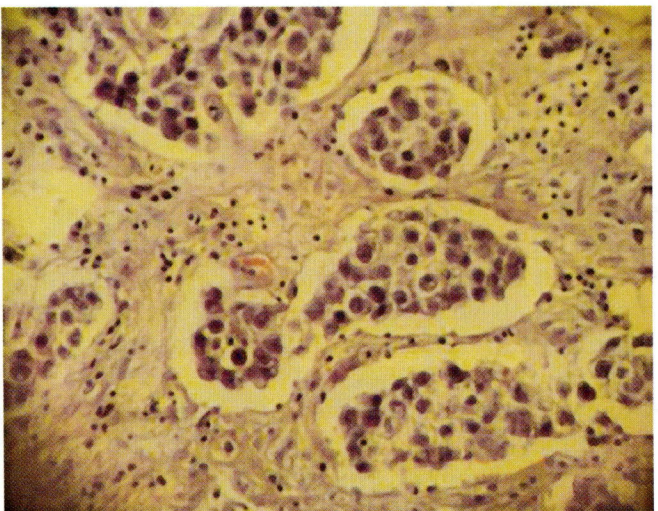

Fig. 11.11: Dysgerminoma in 46XY streak gonad

- Hormone replacement with low-dose estradiol (1–2 mg/day) for 12–18 months before addition of progestogenic agent for regular menstruation.
- Fertility: 5–10% may have spontaneous pregnancy as patients with gonadal dysgenesis may ovulate inconsistently.

Turner with Mosaic Karyotype

In classic Turner, there is a missing sex chromosome which may be either X or Y. However, there are many cases of gonadal dysgenesis associated with mosaic karyotype. Here two cell lines coexist within one individual—the commonest being 45X/46XX and 45X/46XY. The 45X/46XY group is sometimes designated as 'male female Turner' and has an increased predisposition to malignant tumors of the dysgerminoma/seminoma type. Therefore, these gonads are to be removed.

Tall Turner (Pure Gonadal Dysgenesis with 46XX)

- These girls are relatively tall (>63 inches) with absence of secondary sex characters. Tallness is due to delayed epiphyseal fusion because of unopposed action of growth hormone in the absence of ovarian estrogens.
- They have genital hypoplasia and streak gonads.
- They have normal chromosomal complement of 46XX.
- Diagnosed by elevated LH/FSH in menopausal range.
- Treatment is estrogen replacement therapy after pubertal growth is complete for regular withdrawl bleeds.

Pure Gonadal Dysgenesis with 46XY: Swyer Syndrome

- Cause: Associated with mutations in the SRY gene located at Yp11.
- Streak gonads present; no testes formation.
- Therefore, anti-müllerian hormone and testosterone are not produced. Thus normal uterus and fallopian tubes, female external genitalia is formed.
- Estrogen also is not produced from streak gonads, therefore, breast development does not occur.
- Elevated FSH/LH.
- Streak gonads need removal as they are at increased risk (25%) for germ cell tumors—most common is gonadoblastoma.

Mixed Gonadal Dysgenesis

Most patients are XY and have ambiguous genitalia with a streak gonad on one side and a malformed testis on the opposite. A small proportion of these patients have mutation in the SRY gene.

Some Rare Causes of Hypergonadotropic Hypogonadism

1. Aromatase Deficiency

- This is a very rare autosomal recessive disorder which prevents aromatization of androgens in the ovary for estrogen production. This condition may be suspected even before birth because most mothers of affected children become virilized during pregnancy. This occurs because placenta cannot convert fetal androgens to estrogen as they diffuse into maternal secretion.
- At birth, a female child has clitoromegaly and labioscrotal fusion. At puberty, there is no breast development, primary amenorrhea, worsening virilization, absent growth spurt, delayed bone age, multicystic ovaries.
- Diagnosis consists of elevated LH/FSH, testosterone, DHEAS and undetected level of estrogen.
- Treatment is by estrogen therapy to improve feminine build and prevent bony abnormality.

2. 17alfa-hydroxylase and 17,20-lyase Deficiency

- Mutation in the CYP17 gene cause abnormality in both the enzyme functions in adrenal and gonadal steroidogenic pathways. More than 20 mutations are identified.
- Patients have either 46XX or 46XY karyotype.
- Girls will have no secondary sex characters, but with female phenotype, hypertension and hypokalemia.
- Girls with XY do not have uterus.
- Diminished level of 17OH lase produce decreased cortisol production which lead to rise of ACTH. This lead to increase in mineralocorticoid production as 17OH lase is not required for its production. This causes sodium retention, hypertension and loss of potassium.
- Diagnosed by elevated LH/FSH and low cortisol and raise ACTH and disturbed electrolytes.
- Treatment is by corticosteroids and estrogen. Progesterone is added every 3 months to protect the endometrium

Hypogonadotropic Hypogonadism

a. *Delayed puberty:* Physiological or constitutional delay results from physiological delay in maturation of hypothalamic–pituitary–gonadal axis as there is delayed reactivation of GnRH pulse generator. Levels of GnRH are functionally deficient in relation to chronological age but normal in terms of physiological development.

b. *Kallmann syndrome:* This is due to insufficient pulsatile secretion of GnRH leading to deficiency of LH, FSH. This condition is because of X-linked recessive mutation in the KAL gene. It is often associated with anosmia because of failure of proper neuronal migration in olfactory region. It may also have midline facial defects and occasional renal agenesis. Treatment is by hormone replacement therapy to promote sexual maturation and fertility is possible using gonadotropins

Genetic Disorders: 5-alfa Reductase Deficiency

a. Patients are genetically 46XY. This induces virilization at puberty.

b. These girls have testes because of functioning XY chromosomes.

c. They have no uterus, cervix and tubes as a result of functioning AMH.

d. 5-alfa reductase converts testosterone to its more potent form dihydrotestosterone which is required for differentiation to male external genitalia. In absence of this enzyme, these girls have female external genital development and girls are reared up as females.

e. They do not develop breast at puberty as in complete variety of TFS but because of effect of testosterone.

f. They have normal internal genitalia of male type which includes vas deference, epididymis, prostate and seminal vesicles as testosterone can act on wolffian duct.

g. Male pattern of hair growth, muscle mass and voice deepening occurs as these are testosterone dependent.

h. Treatment is orchidectomy before virilization starts. This is followed by estrogen therapy as they are reared up as females.

Amenorrhea with Secondary Sex Characters with Normal Pelvic Anatomy

Hyperprolactinemia

Most common cause of pituitary related amenorrhea. It mostly present with secondary amenorrhea.

Mechanism: Elevated PRL levels can suppress hypothalamic GnRH secretion.

Table 11.6: Etiological factors with Frequency

Category	Approximate frequency (%)
No breast development low FSH	30
Constitutional delay	10
Prolactinomas	5
Kallmann syndrome	2
Other CNS	3
Strees, weight loss, anorexia	3
PCOS	3
Other	4

Prolactin (PRL)

Prolactin, also known as lactotrope, is a protein that in humans is encoded by the PRL gene. Prolactin is a peptide hormone discovered by **Oscar Riddle.** In humans, prolactin is produced in the pituitary, decidua, myometrium, breast, lymphocytes, leukocytes and prostate. The structure of prolactin is similar to that of growth hormone and placental lactogen. The molecule is folded due to the activity of three disulfide bonds. There are mainly three different forms of prolactin in regard to size:

- *Little prolactin* is the predominant form. It has a molecular weight of approximately 22-kDa. It is a single-chain polypeptide of 198 amino acids, and is apparently the result of removal of some amino acids.
- *Big prolactin* of approximately 48 kDa. It may be the product of interaction of several prolactin molecules. It appears to have little, if any, biological activity.
- *Big big prolactin* of approximately 150 kDa. It appears to have a low biological activity.

Prolactin synthesis and secretion by pituitary lactotroph cells is tonically suppressed by hypothalamic dopamine traversing the portal venous system to impinge on lactotroph D_2 receptors. Factors inducing prolactin synthesis and secretion include estrogen, thyrotropin-releasing hormone, epidermal growth factor, and dopamine receptor antagonists.

Nonpuerperal hyperprolactinemia is caused by lactotroph adenomas (prolactinomas), which account for approximately 40% of all pituitary tumors. Hyperprolactinemia may also develop due to pharmacological or pathological interruption of hypothalamic–pituitary dopaminergic pathways and is sometimes called idiopathic. Regardless of etiology, hyperprolactinemia may result in hypogonadism, infertility, and galactorrhea, or it may remain asymptomatic. Bone loss occurs secondary to hyperprolactinemia-mediated sex steroid attenuation. Spinal bone density is decreased by approximately 25% in women with hyperprolactinemia and is not necessarily restored with normalization of prolactin levels. The reported population **prevalence** of clinically apparent prolactinomas is approximately 30 per 100,000 in women, with a peak prevalence for women in aged 25–34 years (Table 11.7).

Causes of Hyperprolactinemia

A number of physiological states including **pregnancy, breastfeeding, stress, exercise, and sleep** can cause prolactin elevation, as well as some medications).

Patients with **renal insufficiency** may have moderate hyperprolactinemia caused by impaired renal degradation of prolactin and altered central prolactin regulation. Dialysis does not alter serum levels, but prolactin levels normalize after renal transplantation.

Some patients with **hypothyroidism** have moderate hyperprolactinemia . Long-term or inadequately treated primary hypothyroidism can cause pituitary hyperplasia that may mimic pituitary tumor.

Table 11.7: Etiology of hyperprolactinemia

Physiological	Pharmacological	Pathological	Pathological	Pathological
Coitus	Anesthetics	Hypothalamic-pituitary stalk	Acromegaly	Systemic disorders
	Anticonvulsants	Granulomas		
Exercise	Antidepressants	Infiltrations	Idiopathic	Chest-neurogenic
	Antihistamines (H2)	Irradiation		
Lactation	Antihypertensives	Rathke's cyst	Lymphocytic	Herpes zoster
Pregnancy	Cholinergic agonist	Trauma: pituitary stalk section	Parasellar mass	Chronic renal failure
	Catecholamine depletors			
Sleep	Dopamine receptor	Tumors: craniopharyngioma, hypothalamic metastases	Macroadenoma	Cirrhosis
Stress	Dopamine synthesis	Pituitary mass extension	Macroprolactinemai	Cranial radiation
	Estrogens: oral		Prolactinoma	Epileptic seizures
			Surgery	Polycystic ovarian
			Trauma	Pseudocyesis

Hyperprolactinemia and enlargement of the pituitary gland due to hypothyroidism can be reversed by treatment with L-thyroxine.

Because prolactin secretion is tonically inhibited by hypothalamic dopamine, disruption or compression of the pituitary stalk by a **non-prolactin-secreting pituitary tumor or other parasellar mass** will lead to hyperprolactinemia. Patients with large non-functioning pituitary tumors, **craniopharyngiomas, or granulomatous infiltration of the hypothalamus** can develop hyperprolactinemia because of pituitary stalk compression or dopaminergic neuronal damage. **Prolactin level greater than 94 µg/liter reliably distinguishes between prolactinomas and non-functioning adenomas**.

Fewer than 10% of patients with idiopathic hyperprolactinemia are found to harbor a microadenoma, and progression from a microadenoma to a macroadenoma is rare. Spontaneous normalization of prolactin levels occurs in approximately 30% of patients with idiopathic hyperprolactinemia. It is important to determine whether patients with hyperprolactinemia also have **acromegaly** because prolactin is elevated in up to 50% of patients with GH-secreting tumors.

The most frequent cause of nontumoral hyper-prolactinemia is medications. **Neuroleptics/ antipsychotic** agents are the ones most commonly cause hyperprolactinemia

Among patients taking typical antipsychotics (*e.g.* **phenothiazines or butyrophenones),** 40–90% have hyperprolactinemia, as do 50–100% of patients on **risperidone**. With drug-induced hyperprolactinemia, prolactin levels increase slowly after oral administration and it usually takes 3 days for levels to return to normal after drug discontinuation. Although some patients with medication induced hyperprolactinemia remain asymptomatic, women may develop galactorrhea and amenorrhea and men may present with low libido and erectile dysfunction. Medication-induced hyper-prolactinemia is usually associated with prolactin levels ranging from 25 to 100 µg/liter, but metoclopramide, risperidone, and phenothiazines can lead to prolactin levels exceeding 200 µg/liter.

Verapamil causes hyperprolactinemia in 8.5% of patients, presumably by blocking hypothalamic dopamine acting through the receptor to cause mild hyperprolactinemia. The role of estrogen in causing hyperprolactinemia is controversial. 12 to 30% of women taking higher estrogen containing oral contraceptives may have a small increase in serum prolactin, but this is rarely an indication for therapy.

The first step in treatment of medication-induced hyperprolactinemia is to stop the drug and change to an alternative drug with a similar action that does not cause hyperprolactinemia. If this is not feasible, administration of a dopamine agonist is considered.

Diagnosis of Hyperprolactinemia

To establish the diagnosis of hyperprolactinemia, a single measurement of serum prolactin is recommended; a level above the upper limit of normal confirms the diagnosis as long as the serum sample was obtained without excessive venipuncture stress.

Tests

Normal values of prolactin are higher in women than in men and is generally lower than 25 µg/liter. A prolactin level greater than 500 µg/liter is diagnostic of a macroprolactinoma. Although a prolactin level greater than 250 µg/liter usually indicates the presence of a prolactinoma. Larger prolactin forms (macro-prolactin) are less bioactive, and macroprolactinemia should be suspected when typical symptoms of hyperprolactinemia are absent.

Patients with macroprolactinemia has galactorrhea present in 20%, oligo/ amenorrhea in 45%, and pituitary adenomas in 20%. Because macroprolactinemia is a common cause of hyperprolactinemia, routine screening for macroprolactin can eliminate unnecessary diagnostic testing and treatment.

When there is a discrepancy between a very large pituitary tumor and a mildly elevated prolactin level, serial dilution of serum samples (up to 1/100) is recommended to eliminate an artifact that can occur with some immune-radiometric assays leading to a falsely low prolactin value ("hook effect").

Treatment (Endocrine Society Clinical Practice Guideline)

Dopamine agonist therapy is recommended to lower prolactin levels, decrease tumor size, and restore gonadal function for patients harboring symptomatic prolactin-secreting microadenomas or macroadenomas. **Cabergoline** is mostly preferred to other dopamine agonists because it has higher efficacy in normalizing prolactin levels, as well as a higher frequency of pituitary tumor shrinkage. It is unclear why cabergoline is more effective than bromocriptine, but the greater efficacy may be explained by the fact that cabergoline has a higher affinity for dopamine receptor binding sites. Because the incidence of unpleasant side effects is lower with cabergoline, drug compliance may be superior for this medication.

Prolactinomas are associated with galactorrhea, sexual dysfunction and decreased bone density, if gonadal steroids are reduced. When a prolactinoma is present, serum prolactin levels generally parallel the size of the tumor. However, a prolactinoma may be associated with any level of prolactin.

Dose

- *Bromocriptine:* 2.5 mg/day; increase to 7.5 mg/day.
- *Cabergoline:* 0.25 mg/0.5 mg twice a week

In patients who begin dopamine agonist therapy, follow-up includes: (1) periodic prolactin measurement starting 1 month after therapy to guide treatment; (2) repeat MRI every year (or in 3 months in patients with macroprolactinoma, rising prolactin levels or with new symptoms, *e.g.* galactorrhea, visual disturbances, headaches; (3) visual field defects; (4) persistent galactorrhea. With careful clinical and biochemical follow-up, therapy may be tapered and perhaps discontinued in patients who have been treated with dopamine agonists for at least 2 years who no longer have elevated serum prolactin, and who have no visible tumor remnant on MRI.

But follow-up continues which includes: (1) measurement of serum prolactin levels every 3 months for the first year and then annually thereafter; (2) MRI brain, if prolactin increases above normal levels. In women with microprolactinomas, it may be possible to discontinue dopaminergic therapy when menopause occurs.

Microadenomas are less resistant to dopamine agonists than are macroadenomas. 10% of patients with microadenomas and 18% of patients with macroadenomas do not achieve normal prolactin levels on cabergoline. Increasing the cabergoline dose to as much as 11 mg/wk may be necessary to overcome resistance. Caution must be exercised with use of high-dose cabergoline because of the potential risk of cardiac valvular regurgitation.

Clinicians offer transsphenoidal surgery to symptomatic patients with prolactinomas who cannot tolerate high doses of cabergoline or who are not responsive to dopamine agonist therapy. For patients who are intolerant of oral bromocriptine, intravaginal administration may be attempted. For patients who fail surgical treatment or who harbor aggressive or malignant prolactinomas, radiation therapy is advocated. A malignant prolactinoma is defined as one that exhibits metastatic spread within or outside the central nervous system.

Management of Prolactinoma in Pregnancy

Women with prolactinomas may be instructed to discontinue dopamine agonist therapy as soon as they become pregnant. In selected patients with macroadenomas who become pregnant on dopaminergic therapy and who have not had prior surgical or radiation therapy, it may be prudent to continue dopaminergic therapy throughout the pregnancy, especially if the tumor is invasive or is abutting the optic chiasm.

Because bromocriptine crosses the placenta, fetal drug exposure is likely in the first 4 week after conception, a critical period for early organogenesis. It is, therefore, recommended to discontinue bromocriptine or cabergoline therapy in women who become pregnant.

In pregnant patients with prolactinomas, **serum prolactin measurements is not routinely recommended during pregnancy**. During pregnancy, serum prolactin levels increase 10-fold reaching levels of 150 to 300 µg/liter by term. Moreover, the pituitary gland increases in volume more than 2-fold, primarily due to estrogen stimulated increase in the number of lactotrophs. When dopamine agonists are discontinued at the start of pregnancy, serum prolactin levels increase, and subsequent increases in prolactin levels do not accurately reflect changes in tumor growth or activity. Moreover, serum prolactin levels may not increase during pregnancy in all patients with prolactinomas. In some patients, hyperprolactinemia may resolve entirely after pregnancy.

Routine use of pituitary MRI during pregnancy is not advised in patients with microadenomas or intrasellar macroadenomas unless there is clinical evidence for tumor growth such as visual field compromise. There is a concern that macroprolactinomas may grow during pregnancy. Microadenomas are unlikely to expand during pregnancy. Because the risk of symptomatic tumor growth is low, pregnant patients with microadenomas may be followed by clinical examination during each trimester. The risk of symptomatic tumor growth in pregnant patients with macroadenomas is only 2.8%.

The onset of new or worsening headache, or a change in vision, or both mandates the urgent performance of formal visual field testing and a pituitary MRI without the use of gadolinium.

Although some endocrinologists may recommend pituitary surgery to all patients with macroprolactinomas before attempting pregnancy, surgery can cause hypopituitarism, which may lead to the need for advanced reproductive technologies to achieve

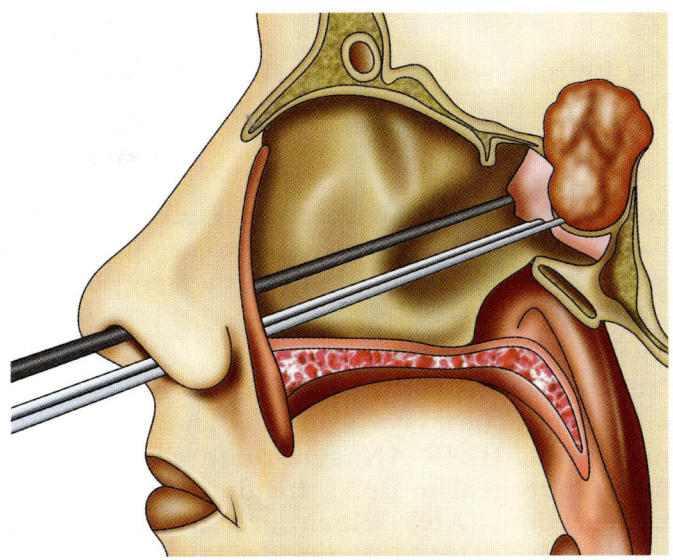

Fig. 11.12: Transsphenoidal approach

pregnancy, as well as lifelong hormone replacement therapy. Pituitary surgery is of the following types:

- Transsphenoidal approach (Fig. 11.12): Used for 95% of pituitary tumors.
- Endonasal submucosal transseptal approach.
- Septal pushover/direct sphenoidotomy.
- Endoscopic approach.

If the fetus is near term, it may be reasonable to induce delivery before neurosurgical intervention is undertaken. It is otherwise always recommended to use dopamine agonists to treat a growing prolactinoma during pregnancy to avoid the potential risk of surgery during pregnancy.

PCOS

Introduction

Stein and Leventhal were the first to recognize an association between the presence of polycystic ovaries and signs of hirsutism and amenorrhea (e.g. oligomenorrhea, obesity). After women diagnosed with Stein-Leventhal syndrome underwent successful wedge resection of the ovaries, their menstrual cycles became regular, and they were able to conceive. As a consequence, a primary ovarian defect was thought to be the main culprit, and the disorder came to be known as polycystic ovarian disease. Further biochemical, clinical, and endocrinologic studies, however, reveal array of underlying abnormalities; hence, the condition is now referred to as polycystic ovary syndrome (PCOS), though it may occur in women without ovarian cysts.

Incidence

PCOS is one of the most common endocrine disorders of women in the reproductive age group, with a prevalence of 4–12%.

Pathophysiology

Women with PCOS have abnormalities in the metabolism of androgens and estrogen and in the control of androgen production. High serum concentrations of androgenic hormones, such as testosterone, androstenedione, and dehydroepiandrosterone sulfate (DHEA-S), may be encountered in these patients.

PCOS is also associated with peripheral insulin resistance and hyperinsulinemia, and obesity amplifies the degree of both abnormalities. Insulin resistance in PCOS can be secondary to a postbinding defect in insulin receptor signaling pathways and elevated insulin levels may have gonadotropin-augmenting effects on ovarian function.

In addition, insulin resistance in PCOS has been associated with **adiponectin**—a hormone secreted by adipocytes that regulates lipid metabolism and glucose levels; both lean and obese women with PCOS have lower adiponectin levels than women without PCOS.

A proposed mechanism for anovulation and elevated androgen levels suggests that, under the increased stimulatory effect of luteinizing hormone (LH) secreted by the anterior pituitary, stimulation of the ovarian theca cells is increased. In turn, these cells increase the production of androgens (e.g. testosterone, androstenedione). Because of a decreased level of follicle-stimulating hormone (FSH) relative to LH, the ovarian granulosa cells cannot aromatize the androgens to estrogens, which leads to arrest of further follicular developement and consequent anovulation. Growth hormone (GH) and insulin-like growth factor-1 (IGF-1) may also augment the effect on ovarian function.

Hyperinsulinemia is also responsible for dyslipidemia and for elevated levels of plasminogen activator inhibitor-1 (PAI-1) in patients with PCOS. Elevated PAI-1 levels are a risk factor for intravascular thrombosis.

Polycystic ovaries are enlarged bilaterally and have a smooth thickened capsule that is avascular. On cut sections, subcapsular follicles in various stages of atresia are seen in the peripheral part of the ovary. The most striking ovarian feature of PCOS is hyperplasia of the theca stromal cells surrounding arrested follicles (Flowchart 11.1).

Flowchart 11.1: Pathogenesis of PCOS

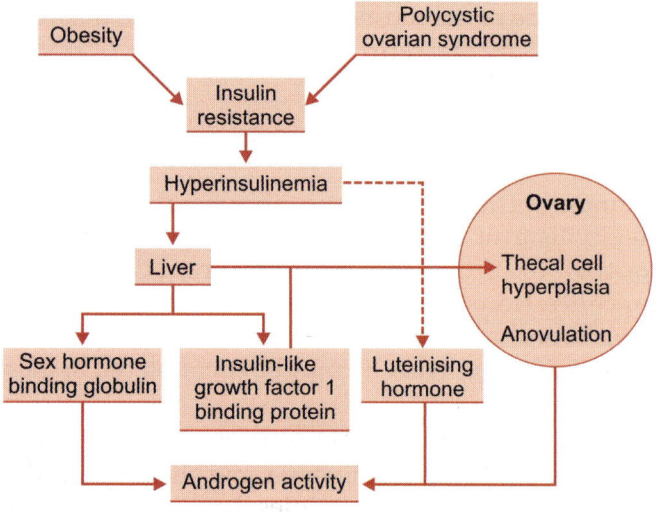

History

Patients with PCOS may present with various clinical features.

Menstrual Abnormalities

- This is mainly attributed to chronic anovulation.
- Some women have oligomenorrhea (i.e. menstrual bleeding that occurs at intervals of 35 days to 6 months, with <9 menstrual periods per yr) or secondary amenorrhea (an absence of menstrual for 6 months).
- Dysfunctional uterine bleeding and infertility are the other consequences of anovulatory menstrual cycles.
- The menstrual irregularities in PCOS usually manifest around the time of menarche and may present with primary amenorrhea.

Hyperandrogenism

- Hyperandrogenism clinically manifests as excess terminal body hair in a male distribution pattern. Hair is commonly seen on the upper lip, chin, around the nipples, and along the linea alba of the lower abdomen.
- Some patients have acne and/or male-pattern hair loss (androgenic alopecia).
- A few patients may also have increased muscle mass, deepening voice, and/or clitoromegaly due to excessive androgens.

Infertility

A subset of women with PCOS are infertile, since most women with PCOS anovulate or ovulate intermittently.

Obesity

Obesity is present in nearly half of all women with PCOS.

Diabetes Mellitus

Approximately 10% of women with PCOS have type 2 diabetes mellitus, and 30–40% of women with PCOS have impaired glucose tolerance by the age of 40 years.

Acanthosis Nigricans

Patients with PCOS may have dark, pigmented skin on the nape of their neck, skin folds, knuckles, and/or on elbows. **HAIR-AN syndrome** comprises of **H**yperandrogenism (HA), **I**nsulin resistance(IR), **A**novulation (AN) which are the composite manifestation of established case of PCOS.

Metabolic Syndrome

- In women, metabolic syndrome is characterized by abdominal obesity (waist circumference >35 in.), dyslipidemia (triglyceride level >150 mg/dL, high-density lipoprotein cholesterol [HDL-C] level <50 mg/dL), elevated blood pressure, a proinflammatory state characterized by an elevated C-reactive protein level, and a prothrombotic state characterized by elevated PAI-1 and fibrinogen levels.
- Prevalence of metabolic syndrome may be around 43% in women with PCOS.
- Women with PCOS have increased prevalence of coronary artery calcification and a thickened carotid intima media, which may be responsible for subclinical atherosclerosis.

Physical

- *Hirsutism:* Patients may have excessive body hair in a male distribution pattern and acne. Some patients have virilizing signs, such as male-pattern balding or alopecia, increased muscle mass, deepening voice, or clitoromegaly.
- *Obesity:* Approximately 50% of women with PCOS have abdominal obesity characterized by a waist circumference of greater than 35 inch (>88 cm).
- *Acanthosis nigricans:* This is a diffuse, velvety thickening and hyperpigmentation of the skin. It may be present at the nape of the neck, axillae, area beneath the breasts, and exposed areas (e.g. elbows, knuckles). In patients with PCOS, acanthosis nigricans is thought to be the result of insulin resistance.
- *Blood pressure:* Patients with signs and symptoms of metabolic syndrome may have elevated blood

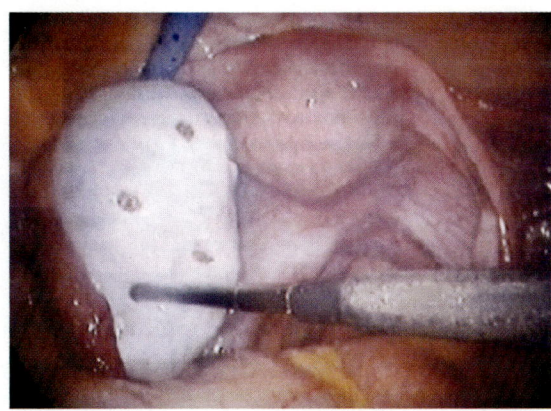

Fig. 11.13: Pearly-white polycystic ovary in laparoscopy

pressure with a systolic blood pressure of 130 mm Hg or higher and diastolic blood pressure of 85 mm Hg or higher.

Laboratory Studies (Table 11.8)

A 1990 expert conference sponsored by National Institute of Child Health and Human Disease (NICHD) of the United States National Institutes of Health (NIH) proposed the following criteria for the diagnosis of PCOS:

- Oligo-ovulation or anovulation manifested by oligomenorrhea or amenorrhea.
- Hyperandrogenism (clinical evidence of androgen excess) or hyperandrogenemia (biochemical evidence of androgen excess).
- Exclusion of other disorders that can result in menstrual irregularity and hyperandrogenism.

The European Society for Human Reproduction and Embryology (ESHRE) and the American Society for Reproductive Medicine (ASRM) recommended that at least 2 of the following 3 features are required for PCOS to be diagnosed (**Rotterdam criteria**).

- Oligo-ovulation or anovulation manifested as oligomenorrhea or amenorrhea.
- Hyperandrogenism (clinical evidence of androgen excess) or hyperandrogenemia (biochemical evidence of androgen excess).
- Polycystic ovaries (as defined on ultrasonography): Polycystic ovaries are defined as 12 or more follicles in at least 1 ovary measuring 2–9 mm in diameter or a total ovarian volume of >10 cm^3.

The diagnosis of PCOS requires the exclusion of all other disorders that can result in menstrual irregularity and hyperandrogenism. Biochemical and/or imaging studies must be done to rule out these other possible disorders and ascertain the diagnosis.

Samples for laboratory studies should be drawn early in the morning, with the patient in a fasting state, and, in women with regular menses, between days 5 and 9 of the menstrual cycle.

- Androgen excess can be tested by measuring total and free testosterone levels or a free androgen index. An elevated free testosterone level is a sensitive indicator of androgen excess.
- Other androgens, such as dehydroepiandrosterone-sulfate (DHEA-S), may be normal or slightly above the normal range in patients with PCOS.
- Levels of sex hormone-binding globulin (SHBG) are usually low in patients with PCOS.

A serum hCG level should be checked to rule out pregnancy in women with oligomenorrhea or amenorrhea.

Patients with androgen-secreting ovarian or adrenal tumors can present with hirsutism, amenorrhea, and signs of virilization. However, these tumors are rapidly

Table 11.8: Definitions of PCOS (diagnostic criteria)		
NIH criteria (1999)	*Rotterdam criteria (2003)*	*AES criteria (2006)*
All three of the following:	At least two of the following:	All three of the following:
1. Clinical or biochemical evidence of hyperandrogenism	1. Oligomenorrhea and/or anovulation	1. Hyperandrogenism (clinical or biochemical)
2. Oligomenorrhea and/or anovulation	2. Clinical and/or biochemical signs of hyperandrogenism	2. Ovarian dysfunction (oligomenorrhea or anovulation and/or polycystic ovarian morphology)
3. Exclusion of other disorders	3. Polycystic ovaries	3. Exclusion of other androgen excess or related disorders
	4. PCOS can be diagnosed only after the exclusion of related disorders (e.g. severe insulin resistance, androgen secreting neoplasms, Cushing's syndrome, hyperprolactinemia and thyroid abnormalities)	4. PCOS is predominantly a disorder of androgen excess

progressive, and patients have high androgen levels. Their testosterone level may be greater than 150 ng/dL, and their DHEA-S level may be above 800 µg/dL.

Late-onset congenital adrenal hyperplasia due to 21-hydroxylase deficiency can be ruled out by measuring serum 17-hydroxy-progesterone levels after a **cosyntropin stimulation test**. A 17-hydroxy-progesterone level of less than 1000 ng/dL, as measured 60 minutes after cosyntropin stimulation, rules out late-onset congenital adrenal hyperplasia.

Cushing syndrome can be ruled out by checking a 24-hour urine sample for free cortisol and creatinine. Levels of urinary free cortisol that are 4-fold the upper limit of normal are diagnostic for Cushing syndrome.

Hyperprolactinemia can be excluded by checking a fasting serum prolactin concentration.

Because the prevalence of impaired glucose tolerance and type 2 diabetes mellitus is high in women with PCOS, a 75 g oral glucose-tolerance test (OGTT) can be performed. A 2-hour postload glucose value of less than 140 mg/dL indicates normal glucose tolerance, a value of 140–199 mg/dL indicates impaired glucose tolerance, and a value of 200 mg/dL or higher indicates diabetes mellitus.

The fasting lipid profile is often abnormal and shows elevated triglyceride and low-density lipoprotein cholesterol (LDL-C) levels and a decreased HDL-C level.

The thyroid-stimulating hormone (TSH) should be measured to rule out hypothyroidism, and the FSH level should be checked to rule out primary ovarian failure.

A serum IGF-1 level should be checked to rule out acromegaly. Serum IGF-1 is a sensitive and specific marker of GH excess. Normal levels rule out GH excess.

Imaging Studies (Fig. 11.14)

- Ovarian ultrasonography, preferably accomplished by using a transvaginal approach, can be performed to assess ovarian morphology (**Adam's criteria**).
- Polycystic ovaries are defined as 12 or more follicles in at least 1 ovary measuring 2–9 mm in diameter or a total ovarian volume of >10 cm^3.

Treatment

Medical management is aimed at the treatment of metabolic derangements, anovulation, hirsutism, and menstrual irregularity.

Metabolic Derangements

- *Diet and exercise:* In patients with PCOS who are obese, endocrine-metabolic parameters markedly

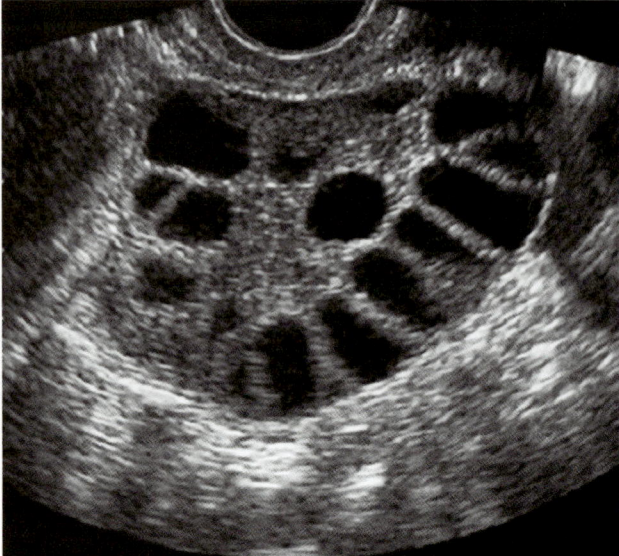

Fig. 11.14: PCO on USG

improve after 4–12 weeks of dietary restriction. Their SHBG levels rise and free testosterone levels fall by 2-fold. Serum insulin and IGF-1 levels also decrease. Weight loss in patients with PCOS who are obese is associated with a reduction of hirsutism and a return of ovulatory cycles in 30% of women. A moderate amount of daily exercise increases levels of IGF-1 binding protein and decreases IGF-1 levels by 20%. Modest weight loss of 2–5% of total body weight can help restore ovulatory menstrual periods in obese patients with PCOS.

- *Metformin:* This antidiabetic drug improves insulin resistance and decreases hyperinsulinemia in patients with PCOS. Metformin also has a small but beneficial effect on metabolic syndrome.

The usual starting dose is 500 mg given orally twice a day and can be increased to 1500 mg/day. Common adverse effects are nausea, vomiting, and diarrhea. Patients who develop these adverse effects can reduce the dose to once a day for a week and then gradually increase the dosage. They should continue the drug as the drugs initiate ovulatory cycles while taking metformin.

Anovulation

- Evidence suggests that metformin frequently, but not in all improves ovulation rates in women with PCOS. In addition, pretreatment with metformin enhance the efficacy of clomiphene for inducing ovulation. Whether short-course metformin pretreatment (less than 4 weeks) is as effective as conventional long-course metformin remains uncertain. N-acetylcysteine may also enhance the effect of clomiphene for ovulation induction in case of infertility.

- *Management of infertility:* Weight reduction, life-style changes, metformin, clomiphene and gonadotropins are useful drugs for management of infertility.

Use of metformin in PCOS

- Lowers hepatic glucose production by reducing gluconeogenesis.
- Increases peripheral glucose uptake by skeletal muscle and adipose tissue.
- Reduces intestinal glucose absorption

Outcomes

- Estimated 31% reduction in development of type II DM over mean period 3 years.
- Taken during pregnancy, reduction in gestational diabetes and major fetal complications.
- Associated with 10-fold reduction in GDM.
- Continuous use during pregnancy significantly reduces the rate of miscarriage.
- Pretreatment with metformin improves *in vitro* maturation in terms of embryo quality and clinical pregnancy rate as well as implantation rate in IVF cycle; reduces risk of OHSS.

Metformin in PCOS: Action on insulin resistance

- One of the major effect of metformin in PCOS is due to its insulin sensitizing action through activation of the AMPK pathway.
- Metformin reduce basal hepatic glucose production by 9 to 30% in patients with T2DM through multiple effects such as:
  - Enhanced glycogenesis
  - Inhibition of hepatic gluconeogenesis through AMPK-dependent regulation of the orphan nuclear receptor SHEP.
  - Decreased FFA oxidation which contributes to reduction in gluconeogenesis.
  - Increase in glucose uptake and oxidation in skeletal muscle thus improving insulin sensitivity.
- It has been hypothesized that metformin can act directly on the ovary thus improving abnormal steroidogenesis (systemic and/or local on ovarian) and subsequently the follicular function.
- Metformin can act on hypothalamic AMP, exerting both a direct and an indirect effect via a paracrine / endocrine action of adipokines and ghrelin, low in PCOS. Thus metformin exerts a favorable effect also by other parallel mechanisms involved in PCOS but not necessarily implicated with insulin resistance.

Metformin in gestational diabetes (MiG study)

- Advocates use of metformin throughout all trimesters in pregnancy.
- Analyses perinatal complications with metformin use in 2nd and 3rd trimesters of pregnancy.
- No difference in pre-eclampsia, perinatal loss and neonatal morbidity in mothers with T2DM and GDM on metformin.
- This study did a 2-year follow-up of the babies and did not find any adverse effect.

Ideal PCOS women who will benefit most from metformin are:

- Women with IGT or diabetes.
- Women with risk of developing metabolic syndrome.
- Women with clomiphen citrate resistant infertility.
- Obese adolescent girl with features of hyperandro-genism.
- In pregnancy following treatment with metformin.

Hirsutism

- *Hair removal:* Short-term non-pharmacologic treatment of hirsutism includes shaving and use of chemical depilatories and/or bleaching cream. Plucking or waxing unwanted hair can result in folliculitis and ingrown hairs. Long-term measures include techniques such as electrolysis and laser treatment of unwanted hairs.
- *Weight reduction:* Weight reduction decreases androgen production in women who are obese; therefore, losing weight can slow hair growth.
- *Oral contraception:* Women who do not wish to become pregnant can be effectively treated for hirsutism with oral contraceptives. Oral contraceptives slow hair growth in 60–100% of women with hyperandrogenemia. Therapy can be started with a preparation that has a high dose of estrogen and a nonandrogenic progestin. Preparations that have norgestrel and levonorgestrel should be avoided because of their androgenic activity.
- *Spironolactone:* Antiandrogens, such as spirono-lactone, are effective for hirsutism. Spironolactone 50–100 mg twice daily is an effective primary therapy for hirsutism. Adverse effects of spironolactone include GI discomfort, and irregular menstrual bleeding.
- *Eflornithine:* Eflornithine is a topical cream that can be used to slow hair growth. Eflornithine works by inhibiting ornithine decarboxylase, which is essential for the rapidly dividing cells of hair follicles.

Menstrual Irregularity

Many women present with secondary but occasional primary amenorrhea. This often is clinically confirmed by progesterone challenge test when 10 mg medroxy-progesterone daily for 7–10 days will induce withdrawl bleeding. This is followed by treatment with an oral contraceptive, which not only inhibits ovarian androgen production but also increases SHBG production.

Surgical Care

Surgical management is aimed mainly at restoring ovulation.

- *Ovarian wedge resection:* This procedure has fallen out of favor because of postoperative adhesion formation and the introduction of ovulation-inducing medications.
- *Laparoscopic surgery:* Various laparoscopic methods, including electrocautery, laser drilling have been used with the goal of creating focal areas of damage in the ovarian cortex and stroma. The recommendation is to drill not more than 4 sites with depth of 3–4 mm and with a current of 30 watts for 4 seconds to avoid potential complications like formation of adhesions and ovarian atrophy. It decreases mechanical crowding of the cortex by cysts which can enable the process of normal graafian follicle movement to the surface of the ovary. After surgery, ovulation occurs spontaneously in 70–90% of women and cumulative pregnancy in the range of 40–60% after 12 months of use. Ovarian drilling results in a transient increase followed by a significant reduction in ovarian volume from a preoperative volume of 12.2 to 6.9 mL in three weeks after surgery and the effect is sustained for 9 years.
- Multiple pregnancy rates are lower with ovarian drilling than with gonadotropin treatment (1% versus 16%), but there are ongoing concerns about the long-term effects on ovarian function.

RCOG Guidelines on PCOS

1. How is PCOS Diagnosed?

Diagnosis of PCOS can only be made when other etiologies have been excluded (thyroid dysfunction, congenital adrenal hyperplasia, hyperprolactinemia, androgen-secreting tumors and Cushing syndrome).

The National Institutes of Health (NIH) 1990 preliminary consensus definition has now been replaced by a more recent definition by the Rotterdam European Society for Human Reproduction and Embryology (ESHRE) and the American Society of Reproductive Medicine (ASRM) PCOS Consensus Workshop Group. This has suggested a broader definition for PCOS, with two of the three following criteria being diagnostic of the condition:

- Polycystic ovaries (either 12 or more peripheral follicles or increased ovarian volume greater than 10 cm^3).
- Oligo- or anovulation.
- Clinical and/or biochemical signs of hyperandrogenism

2. What is the risk of developing type II diabetes in women with PCOS?

Women presenting with PCOS, particularly if they are obese (body mass index greater than 30), have a strong family history of type 2 diabetes or are over the age of 40 years, are at increased risk of type 2 diabetes and should be offered a glucose tolerance test.

3. What is the risk of developing sleep apnea in women with PCOS?

Women diagnosed with PCOS should be asked about daytime fatigue/somnolence and informed of the possible risk of sleep apnea, and offered investigation and treatment when necessary. Sleep apnea is an independent cardiovascular risk factor and has been found to be more common in PCOS.

4. What is the risk of developing cardiovascular disease in women with PCOS?

Clinicians need to be aware that conventional cardiovascular risk calculators have not been validated in women with PCOS. In clinical practice, hypertension should be treated but lipid-lowering treatment is not recommended routinely.

5. What are the implications of PCOS for pregnancy?

Women who have been diagnosed as having PCOS before pregnancy (such as those requiring ovulation induction for conception) should be screened for gestational diabetes before 20 weeks of gestation.

Metformin is currently not licensed for use in pregnancy in the UK and is not recommended for use in pregnancy.

6. What are the risks of cancer in women with PCOS?

Oligo- or amenorrhea in women with PCOS may predispose to endometrial hyperplasia and later

Table 11.9: Causes of primary amenorrhea

Breast development	No breast development: High FSH (40%)	No breast development: Low FSH (30%)
Müllerian agenesis (10%)	Turner's syndrome and variants (20%)	Constitutional delay (10%)
Androgen insensitivity (9%)	Gonadal dysgenesis (46XX) (15%)	Prolactinomas (10%)
Vaginal septum (2%)	Gonadal dysgenesis (46XY) (5%)	Kallmann syndrome (8%)
Imperforate hymen (1%)		Other CNS lesions (3%)
Constitutional delay (8%)		Stress, weight loss, anorexia (3%)
PCOS (3%)		
Other (4%)		

Flowchart 11.2: Diagnostic workup of primary amenorrhea

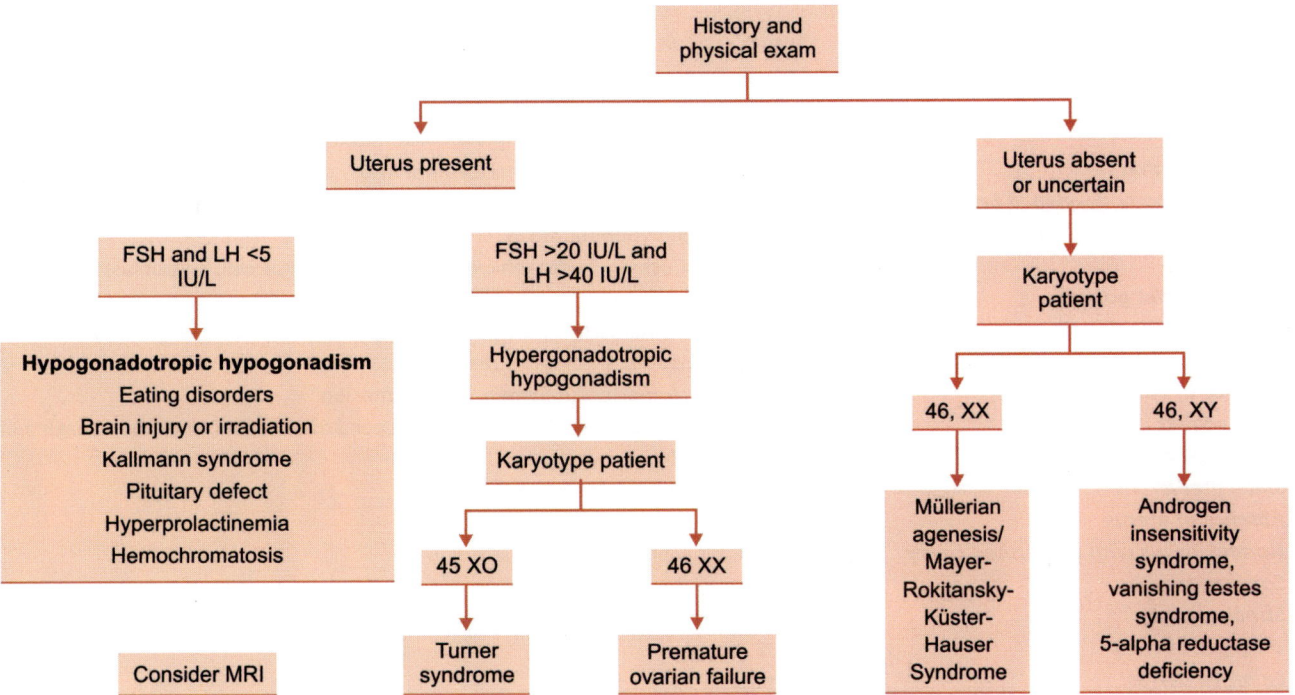

carcinoma. It is good practice to recommend treatment with progestogens to induce a withdrawal bleed at least every 3–4 months.

There does not appear to be an association with breast or ovarian cancer and no additional surveillance is required.

7. Is drug therapy appropriate for women with PCOS?

Insulin-sensitizing agents have not been licensed in the UK for use in women who are not diabetic.

Use of weight-reduction drugs may be helpful in reducing insulin resistance through weight loss.

8. What is the prognosis following surgery?

Ovarian electrocautery should be reserved for selected anovulatory women with a normal BMI.

9. How should women with hirsutism and acne be advised?

Women should be advised that there is insufficient evidence in favor of either metformin or the oral contraceptive pill in treating hirsutism or acne.

Secondary Sexual Characteristics Present with Normal Pelvic Anatomy

Constitutional delay: This is when there is no abnormality but girl is a little later than her peers in reaching her menarche. There may be history of delayed menarche in her mother and any older sisters. Reassure that the menarche is the last of the characteristics to develop.

Hyperprolactinemia: Elevation of prolactin produces abnormal GnRH secretion leading to menstrual disturbance. It is raised in many CNS lesions like

Clinical Approach to Diagnosis of Amenorrhea

i. **History**	**Probable diagnosis**
• Periodic pain with retention of urine	Cryptomenorrhea
• Headache, visual disturbance	Intracranial lesion
• Galactorrhea	Hyperprolactinemia
• Anosmia	Kallmann syndrome
• Weight loss, anorexia	Tuberculosis, anorexia nervosa
ii. **Family history**	
• Tuberculosis	Genital tubrculosis
• Primary amenorrhea	Testicular feminization syndrome
	Delayed menarche
iii. **Stature**	
• Short	Turner's, pituitary, thyroid dwarf
• Tall	Mosaic Turner's, TFS
• Abnormally tall, gigantic	Acromegaly
iv. **Obesity**	PCOS, hypothyroidism, Cushing's disease, pituitary and hypothalamic obesity
iv. **Abnormally thin**	Tuberculosis, malnutrition, anorexia nervosa
v. **Absent or poorly developed breasts**	Turner's, hypopituitarism, cretin, Cushing,
vi. **Absent or scanty pubic and axillary hairs**	TFS, Turner's, hypopituitarism, cretinism
vii. **Hirsutism**	PCOS, CAH, Cushing, androgenic ovarian tumors (Hilus cell, androblastoma)
vii. **Inguinal/labial gonads**	TFS
ix. **Lower abdominal lump**	Hematometra, hematocolpos, pelvic kidney
	Distended bladder, encysted tuberculosis
x. **Absence of vaginal opening**	MRKH, CAH, imperforate hymen, labial adhesion
xi. **Blind vagina**	Transverse vaginal septum, agenesis of upper 3rd of vagina, short blind vagina of TFS
xii. **Clitoromegaly**	Congenital adrenal hyperplasia, PAIS
xiii. **Small uterus**	Turner's, hypopituitarism, cretin
xiv. **Absence of uterus**	MRKH, TFS
xv. **Normal uterus with obliterated cavity**	Uterine synechiae of tubercular origin
xvi. **Small ovaries**	POF, gonadal agenesis
xvii. **Streak gonads**	Turner's, gonadal dysgenesis
xviii. **Enlarged ovaries**	PCOS, neoplasm
xiv. **Enlarged uterus**	Hematometra
xv. **Tubo-ovarian lump**	Tubercular infection

pituitary adenoma, in different stress situations, in hypothyroidism and on exposure to drugs which interfere with dopamine secretion like antidepressants, antipsychotics, antihypertensives, H_2 receptor bockers.

Hypothalamic failure: This can be due to chronic illness, stress or being significantly underweight. Anorexia nervosa usually develops after the menarche and represents a regression. Obesity is also more likely to cause secondary amenorrhea.

Other causes of failure of the hypothalamic-pituitary axis include:

Kallmann's syndrome: Characterized by failure of secretion of gonadotropin-releasing hormone (GnRH), tumors of the hypothalamus or pituitary along with other causes of hypopituitarism and hydrocephalus.

Hyperprolactinemia: This can be due to many causes including hypothyroidism and drugs, especially phenothiazines. If it is due to a pituitary tumor, the level of prolactin (PRL) is usually very high. Hyperprolactinemia occurs in 60% of secondary amenorrhea.

Premature ovarian failure: This is a poorly understood condition that may represent an autoimmune phenomenon. It can also follow radiotherapy or chemotherapy. Menstruation and fertility can sometimes resume spontaneously when causes are withdrawn. Ovarian failure will cause elevation of gonadotropins and so hot flushes are likely. Premature menopause is defined as occurring before the age of 40.

Depot and implant contraception: This often produces amenorrhea and the progestogen-only pill can do so less often. Intrauterine contraceptive devices usually increase menstrual flow but Mirena reduces it and may stop it.

Cervical stenosis and intrauterine adhesions: These are known as Asherman's syndrome and should be considered.

Loss of weight: This can cause amenorrhea, especially if rapid. Body mass index (BMI) is rarely above 19 and at least 10% of normal body weight has been lost. Anorexia nervosa and other eating disorders including bulimia nervosa should be considered.

Pituitary disease and hyperprolactinemia: Drugs, especially phenothiazines and metoclopramide, raise PRL. Prolonged amenorrhea is very common in heroin abusers. They are usually underweight but there may also be a pharmacological effect.

Sheehan's syndrome: The pituitary may be damaged by tumors, trauma, cranial irradiation, sarcoidosis or tuberculosis.

"Post-pill amenorrhea": This is when stopping oral contraceptives do not lead to a resumption of a normal menstrual cycle. It usually settles spontaneously in around three months but, if not, it requires investigation. The condition is probably not a true entity but the cause of amenorrhea is hypothalamic in origin.

Signs of Androgen Excess

Polycystic ovarian syndrome (PCOS): PCOS accounts for as many as 30% of cases of amenorrhea. Both androgens and estrogens may be normal or slightly raised so that, whilst there are signs of virilization, there is no evidence of estrogen deficiency. They are usually, but not always, overweight and may have insulin resistance. Fat is very important in the metabolism of the steroid sex hormones and it accounts for both the excess in PCOS and the deficiency in anorexia.

Cushing's syndrome: This may be spontaneous or iatrogenic.

Late onset **congenital adrenal hyperplasia:** Produces androgens.

Adrenal or ovarian carcinoma: These also produce androgens.

11B. ABNORMAL UTERINE BLEEDING (AUB)

Introduction

- The average woman experience approximately 400 cycles in contrast to 40 cycles she would have experienced 50 years ago. This is due to smaller family size, availability of effective contraception, early menarche and late menopause. AUB includes all menstrual pattern which are not normal and affects physical health of the woman. HMB means when menstrual blood loss is heavy in a particular cycle or throughout.

- HMB is defined as excessive menstrual blood loss which interferes with the woman's physical, emotional, social wellbeing and quality of life, and which can occur alone or in combination with other symptoms. Therefore, HMB includes:
  - DUB
  - Pelvic pathology
  - Medical disorders
  - Coagulation disorders

Dysfunctional uterine bleeding (DUB) is defined as abnormal uterine bleeding in the absence of organic disease. It is the most common cause of abnormal vaginal bleeding during a woman's reproductive years. Novak defined it as abnormal uterine bleeding due to causes other than tumor, inflammation and pregnancy.

Characters of Menstrual Blood Loss (Table 11.10)

Terms frequently used to describe abnormal uterine bleeding:

- Menorrhagia—prolonged (>8 days) or excessive (>80 mL daily) uterine bleeding occurring at regular intervals.
- Metrorrhagia—uterine bleeding occurring at irregular and more frequent than normal intervals.
- Menometrorrhagia—prolonged or excessive uterine bleeding occurring at irregular and more frequent than normal intervals.
- Intermenstrual bleeding—uterine bleeding of variable amounts occurring between regular menstrual periods.
- Midcycle spotting—spotting occurring just before ovulation, typically from declining estrogen levels.
- Postmenopausal bleeding—recurrence of bleeding in a menopausal woman at least 6 months to 1 year after cessation of cycles.
- Amenorrhea—no uterine bleeding for 6 months or longer.

Table 11.10: Characters of menstrual patterns

Characters	Description	Normal value
Frequency	Frequent	<24 days
	Normal	24–38 days
	Infrequent	>38 days
Duration of flow	Prolonged	>8 days
	Normal	4–8 days
	Short	<4 days
Volume of monthly blood loss	Heavy	>80 mL
	Normal	5–80 mL
	Light	<5 mL

Dysfunctional uterine bleeding is a diagnosis of exclusion. It is ovulatory or anovulatory bleeding, diagnosed only after pregnancy, medications, iatrogenic causes, genital tract pathology, malignancy, and systemic disease have been ruled out by appropriate investigations. Approximately 90% of dysfunctional uterine bleeding cases result from anovulation and 10% of cases occur with ovulatory cycles.

Types of DUB

I. (1) Primary DUB, (2) Secondary DUB
Primary DUB is related to dysfunction of HPO axis. Secondary DUB includes:
a. Bleeding from hematological diseases like ITP, von Willebrand disease.
b. Bleeding due to IUD, Depo-Provera, progesterone only pill.

II. (1) Ovulatory DUB, (2) Anovulatory DUB
Incidence: An estimated 5–10% of women aged 15–49 years will consult a physician each year for treatment of menorrhagia.

Mechanism of normal menstrual flow: Endometrial surface area is 10–45 cm². Withdrawal of progesterone from estrogen-endometrium results in shedding. Many local substances like MMP 1,2,9, TGFβ are stimulated. Spiral arterioles are cleaved at junctional zone between endometrial functionalis and basalis. This is followed in next 20 hours by hemostasis, vasoconstriction, endometrial repair which involves stimulation of different local substances like **vascular endothelial growth factor, fibroblastic growth factor, and epidermal growth factor.**

Pathophysiology

Dysfunctional uterine bleeding is most common at the extreme ages of a woman's reproductive years, either at the beginning or near the end, but it may occur at any time during her reproductive life.

- Most cases of dysfunctional uterine bleeding in adolescent girls occur during the first 2 years after the onset of menstruation, when their immature hypothalamic-pituitary axis may fail to respond to estrogen and progesterone, resulting in anovulation.

- Abnormal uterine bleeding affects up to 50% of perimenopausal women. In the perimenopausal period, dysfunctional uterine bleeding may be an early manifestation of ovarian failure causing decreased hormone levels or responsiveness to hormones, thus also leading to anovulatory cycles. In patients who are 40 years or older, the number and quality of ovarian follicles diminishes. Follicles continue to develop but do not produce enough estrogen in response to FSH to trigger ovulation. The estrogen that is produced usually results in late-cycle estrogen breakthrough bleeding.

- Anovulatory dysfunctional uterine bleeding results from a disturbance of the normal hypothalamic-pituitary-ovarian axis. When ovulation does not occur, no progesterone is produced to stabilize the endometrium; thus, proliferative endometrium persists. Bleeding episodes become irregular, and amenorrhea, metrorrhagia, and menometrorrhagia result. Bleeding from anovulatory dysfunctional uterine bleeding may result from changes in prostaglandin concentration, increased endometrial responsiveness to vasodilating prostaglandins (PGE_2 and PGI_2) and changes in endometrial vascular structure.

- In ovulatory dysfunctional uterine bleeding, bleeding occurs cyclically, and menorrhagia is thought to originate from defects in the control mechanisms of menstruation. It is thought that, in women with ovulatory dysfunctional uterine bleeding, there is an increased rate of blood loss resulting from vasodilatation of the vessels supplying the endometrium due to decreased vascular tone, and delay in vasoconstriction of denuded vessels and poor regeneration of the basal endometrium. Therefore, these women lose blood at rates about 3 times faster than women with normal menses.

- Local causes appear to be responsible for excess bleeding:
  a. Altered balance between vasoconstrictors $PGF_{2\alpha}$ and vasodilators PGE_2 when prostaglandin E_2 dominates and vessel remains dilated and bleeds heavily.
  b. Predominance of PGI_2, another vasodilator over thrombaxane A_2, a vasoconstrictor liberated from platelets
  c. Increased lysosomal activity
  d. Increased relaxin activity
  e. Decreased regeneration of basal layers of endometrium

History

- Patients often present with complaints of menorrhagia, metrorrhagia, or menometrorrhagia. The amount and frequency of bleeding and the duration of symptoms, as well as the relationship to the menstrual cycle, should be established. Patients are asked to compare the number of pads or tampons used per day in a normal menstrual cycle to the number used at the time of presentation. The average tampon or pad absorbs 20–30 mL of vaginal effluent. Personal habits vary greatly among women; therefore, the number of pads or tampons used is unreliable. The patient should also be questioned about the possibility of pregnancy.

- A reproductive history should always be obtained, including the following:
  - Age of menarche and menstrual history and regularity.
  - Last menstrual period (LMP), including flow, duration, and presence of dysmenorrhea
  - Postcoital bleeding
  - Gravida and para
  - Previous abortion or recent termination of pregnancy.
  - Contraceptive use, use of barrier protection, and sexual activity (including vigorous sexual activity or trauma).
  - History of sexually transmitted diseases (STDs) or ectopic pregnancy.

Questions about medical history should include the following:
- Signs and symptoms of anemia or hypovolemia (including fatigue, dizziness, and syncope).
- Diabetes mellitus.
- Thyroid disease
- Endocrine problems or pituitary tumors
- Liver disease
- Recent illness, psychological stress, excessive exercise, or weight change.
- Medication usage, including exogenous hormones, anticoagulants, aspirin, anticonvulsants, and antibiotics.

An underlying bleeding disorder should be considered when a patient has any of the following:

- Menorrhagia since menarche
- Family history of bleeding disorders
- Personal history of 1 or several of the following:
  - Notable bruising without known injury
  - Bleeding of oral cavity or GI tract without obvious lesion.
  - Epistaxis >10 min duration

Physical Examination

- Vital signs, including postural changes, should be assessed. Initial evaluation should be directed at assessing the patient's general status and degree of anemia.
- An abdominal examination should be performed. Any suprapubic mass should be identified which may be uterine, ovarian or tubo-ovarian in origin. Femoral and inguinal lymph nodes should be examined. Stool should be evaluated for the presence of blood.
- Patients also require speculum, bimanual, and rectovaginal examination to define the etiology of vaginal bleeding. The examination should look for the following:
  - The vagina should be inspected for signs of trauma, lesions, infection, and foreign bodies by Sim's speculum.
  - The cervix should be visualized and inspected by Cusco's speculum for lesions like polyps, erosion, infection, intrauterine device (IUD) or growth.
  - **PV examination**—to assess the size, shape, position, feel, mobility, tenderness of uterine, cervical or adnexal mass.
  - **Rectovaginal examination** should be performed to evaluate the cul-de-sac, posterior wall of the uterus, and uterosacral ligaments.
- Patients with hematologic pathology may also have cutaneous evidence of bleeding diathesis like petechiae, purpura, and mucosal bleeding in gums in addition to vaginal bleeding.
- Patients with liver disease that has resulted in abnormal coagulopathy may manifest spider angioma, palmar erythema, splenomegaly, ascites, jaundice, and asterixis.
- Women with polycystic ovary disease present with signs of hyperandrogenism, including hirsutism, obesity, acne, palpable enlarged ovaries, and acanthosis nigricans (hyperpigmentation typically seen in the folds of the skin in the neck, groin, or axilla).

- Hyperactive and hypoactive thyroid can cause menstrual irregularities. Patients may have varying degrees of characteristic vital sign abnormalities, eye findings, tremors, changes in skin texture and goiter.

Causes of Bleeding in Pubertal Girls

- DUB
- PCOS
- Hematological-ITP, coagulation disorders like von Willebrand disease, Bernard-Soulier disease, etc.
- Early endometrial Koch's
- Pregnancy related bleeding
- Thyroid dysfunction
- Local causes like polyps, fibroids, sarcoma, boytrioids

Laboratory Study

- Blood for Hb, TC, DC, platelets, BT, CT, PPBS, LFT, RFT.
- PT, APTT, coagulation study.
- *Hormone profile in PCOS:* Insulin, testosterone, thyroid dysfunction
- Pap smear.
- Investigate for Koch:
  - Endometrium for typical Koch's histological lesion or Bactec culture.
  - DNA or RNA PCR of menstrual blood or endometrium for *Mycobacterium tuberculosis*.

USG (Fig. 11.15)

- TVS for endometrial thickness >12 mm need histological study.
- Endomtrial polyps
- Endometrial cancer
- Submucus fibroid
- Asherman's syndrome of Koch's in hyperemic stage
- Ovarian SOL-PCOS, feminizing tumor
- Chronic tubo-ovarian mass

USG picture of PCOS includes:

- Peripheral arranged follicle of 4–8 in number and 6–12 mm in size.
- Ovarian volume >12 cc
- Increased stromal thickness

Hysteroscopy and Hysteroscopy-guided Endometrial Biopsy (Fig. 11.16)

Hysteroscopy is done to locate and evaluate the cause of uterine bleeding, such as uterine fibroids, when blood loss is severe. Results of hysteroscopy may include the following (Fig. 11.17):

    i. ***Normal:*** No abnormalities are found.

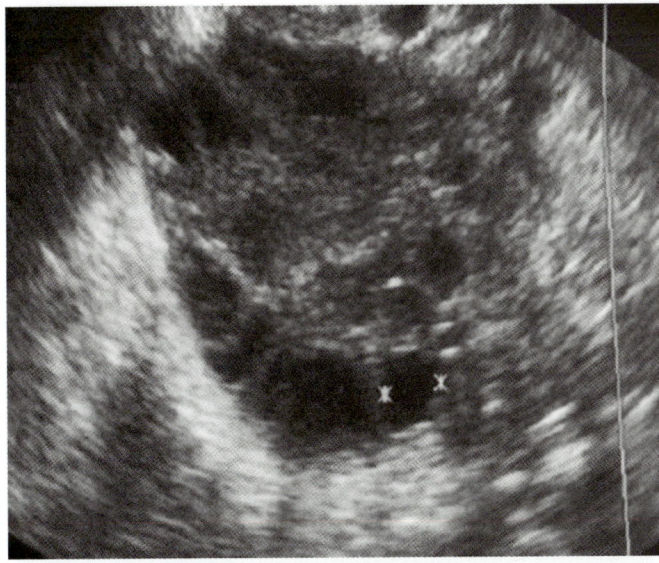

I. USG picture of PCOS

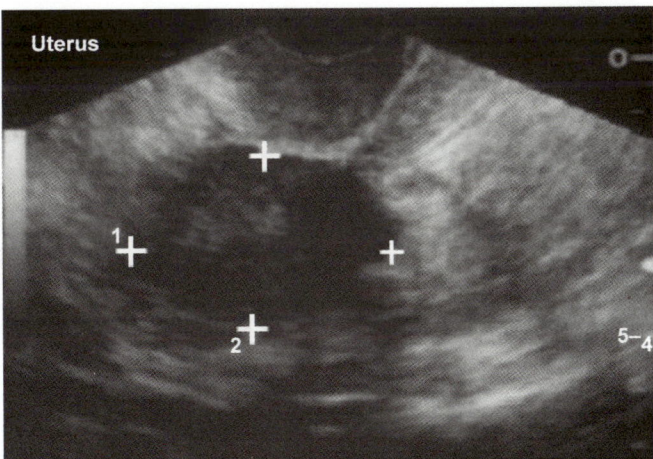

III. USG picture of endometrial hyperplasia

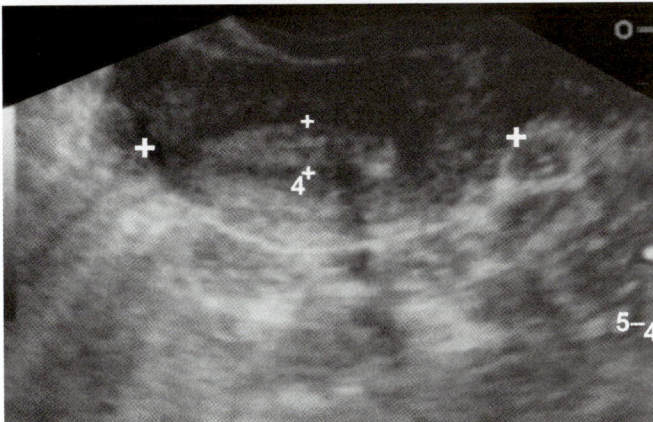

II. USG picture of fibroid

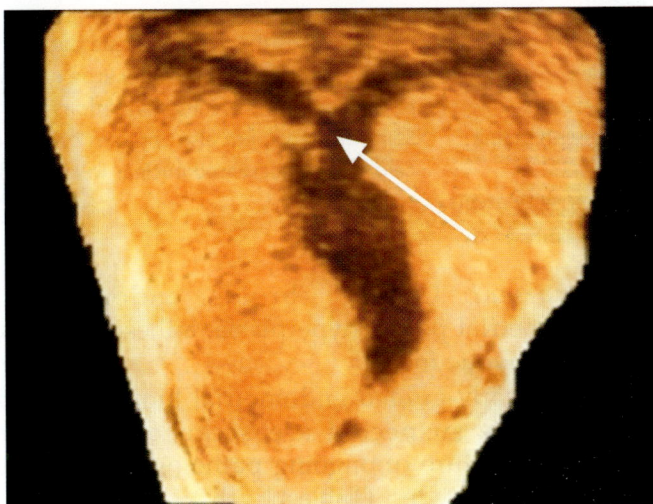

IV. USG picture of early Asherman syndrome

Fig. 11.15: USG picture of PCOS

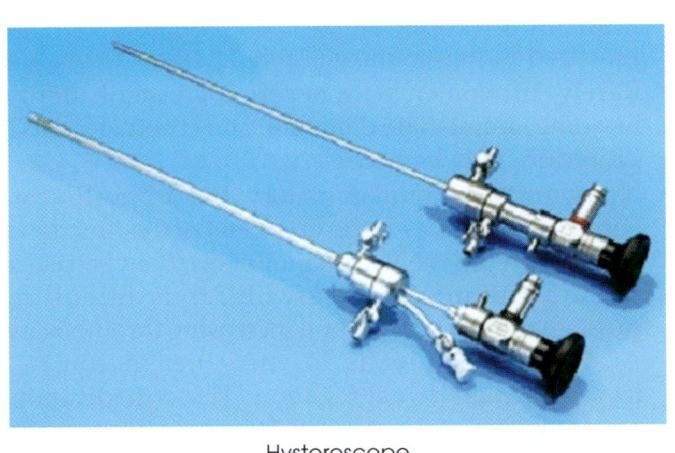

Hysteroscope

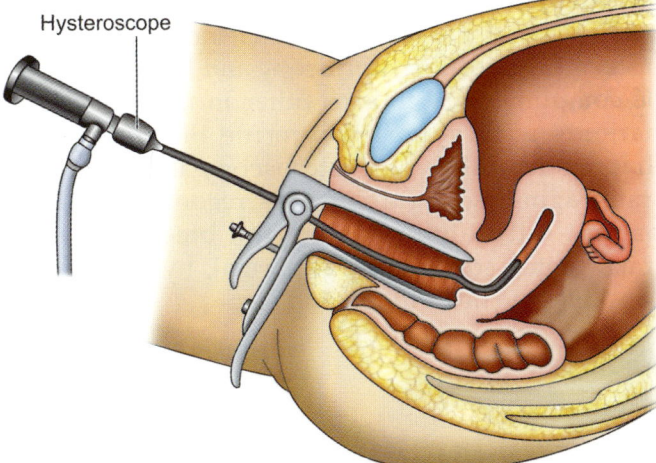

Hysteroscope

Fig. 11.16: Hysteroscopic procedure

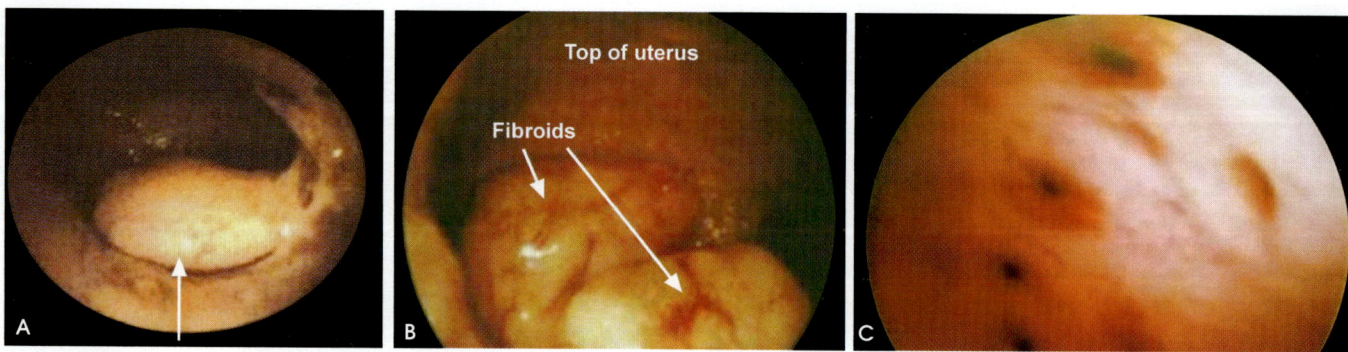

Fig. 11.17A–C: (A) Uterine polype; (B) Submucus fibroid in uterine cavity; (C) Hysteroscopy picture of adenomyosis

Table 11.11: Different endometrial pathology on endometrial biopsy

Type	Description	Risk of progression to endometrial cancer
Simple	Dilated glands that contain some outpouching and abundant endometrial stroma	1%
Complex	Glands are crowded with very little endometrial stroma, and a very complex gland pattern and outpouching formations	3–5%
Simple with atypia	Same as above, but also contains cytologic atypia. Hyperchromatic, enlarged epithelial cells with an increased nuclear to cytoplasmic ratio	3–5%
Complex with atypia	—Do—	25–30%

ii. **Abnormal:** Uterine fibroids, endometritis, endometrial polyp, hyperplasia, adhesive bands, adenomyotic foci.

Hysteroscopy-guided endometrial biopsy carried out from the suspected areas can confirm the histological picture of ongoing pathology and is the most confirmatory test (Table 11.11).

Hysteroscopy is not a substitute for tissue diagnosis, hysteroscopy along with curettage improves the accuracy of clinical diagnosis, the procedures being complimentary. Though there is not sufficient evidence to recommend liberal use of diagnostic laparoscopy in women with abnormal uterine bleeding, it should be considered in women who do not respond to initial medical therapy or have additional indications in their history. Diagnostic hysteroscopy and laparoscopy can be complimentary to each other in management of patients with abnormal uterine bleeding. Since diagnostic ability of hysteroscopy is higher than transvaginal sonography, it is recommended that patient with abnormal uterine bleeding whose transvaginal sonography is normal, hysteroscopy is considered to be as the second step.

Treatment

Medical Treatment

This is suitable for puberty menorrhagia and DUB for reproductive age group. Endometrial biopsy is indicated for DUB in perimenopausal group before deciding any treatment for them.

Emergency care

- Hemodynamically unstable patients with uncontrolled bleeding and signs of significant blood loss should have aggressive resuscitation with saline and blood as with other types of hemorrhagic shock.
- Evaluate ABCs
- Initiate two large-bore intravenous lines (IVs), oxygen, and cardiac monitor.
- If bleeding is profuse and the patient is unresponsive to initial fluid management, conjugated estrogen (premarin) 25 mg IV is administered every 4–6 hours until the bleeding stops are advocated but not practised in this country (Table 11.12).
- Rarely, in women with severe, persistent uterine bleeding, immediate dilatation and curettage (D&C) procedure may be necessary.
- Nonsteroidal anti-inflammatory drugs (NSAIDs) are generally effective for the treatment of dysfunctional uterine bleeding. NSAIDs inhibit cyclooxygenase in the arachidonic acid cascade, thus inhibiting prostaglandin synthesis and increasing thromboxane A2 levels. This leads to vasoconstriction and increased platelet aggregation. These medications may reduce blood loss by 20–50%. NSAIDs are most effective, if used with the onset of menses or just prior to its onset and continued throughout its duration.

Table 11.12: Use of estrogens in AUB	
Use of estrogens	*Indications*
Intravenous estrogen 25 mg 4 hourly for maximum of 3 doses or until bleeding stops	For acute, heavy, uncotrolled bleeding
Oral conjugated estrogen in divided doses up to 10 mg/day	For less severe bleeding. Should be followed by 10 mg of medroxyprogesterone per day for about 10 days
Oral conjugated estrogen in dose of 2.5 to 5 mg/day	Used for DUB and patients with low-dose OCPS with midcycle spotting
Conjugated estrogen 1.25 mg/day	Used in treatment of peri- or postmenopausal women

- Tranexamic acid is an antifibrinolytic drug that exerts its effects by reversibly inhibiting plasminogen. It diminishes fibrinolytic activity within endometrial vessels to prevent bleeding. It has been shown effective in reducing bleeding in 50% of women with dysfunctional uterine bleeding. Dose is maximum 500 mg tablets 6 tablets a day (total—3000 mg/day).

- Combined oral contraceptive pills may be used in women who are not pregnant and have no anatomic abnormalities. An oral contraceptive with 35 μg of ethinyl estradiol and 1.5 mg. Norethisterone acetate can be taken twice a day until the bleeding stops for up to 7 days, at which time the dose is decreased to once a day until the pack is completed. They provide the additional benefits of reducing dysmenorrhea and providing contraception. Low dose OC pill is beneficial for perimenopausal DUB.

- Progesterone alone can be used to stabilize an immature endometrium. It is usually successful in the treatment of women with anovulatory dysfunctional uterine bleeding (DUB) because these women have unopposed estrogen stimulation. Three types of modalities exist:
  a. Norethisterone acetate in high doses of 30 mg/day is started to stop the bleeding.
  b. Maintenance therapy is continued as 15 mg/day from day 5 to day 25 cyclically.
  c. To stabilize the luteal phase, often medroxyprogesterone acetate 10 mg or 200–400 mg Micronised progesterone is taken orally from day 16–day 25 to regularize the cycle particularly for ovulatory DUB though oral estrogen-progesterone pills act better for them.

- Danazol creates a hypoestrogenic and hyperandrogenic environment, which induces endometrial atrophy resulting in reduced menstrual loss. Side effects include musculoskeletal pain, breast atrophy, hirsutism, weight gain, oily skin, and acne. Because of the significant androgenic side effects, this drug is usually reserved as a second-line treatment for short-term use prior to surgery.

- Gonadotropin-releasing hormone agonists may be helpful for short-term use in inducing amenorrhea and allowing women to rebuild their red blood cell mass. They produce a profound hypoestrogenic state similar to menopause. Side effects include menopausal symptoms and bone loss with long-term use.

- Thyroxin replacement is essential for secondary DUB in hypothyroidism.

- Anti-Koch's therapy for endometrial tuberculosis.

- Clomiphene citrate is used for treatment of anovulatory DUB in reproductive women

Surgical Treatment

Conservative surgical treatment: Endometrial curettage has got some therapeutic value to destroy the proliferating endometrium. This is to be followed up by progesterone.

Endoscopic Ablation Therapy

Endoscopic ablation therapy is of the following types:

a. Thermal Balloon Ablation (Fig. 11.18)

- A silicon balloon is inserted into the endometrial cavity and filled with hot water for eight minutes.

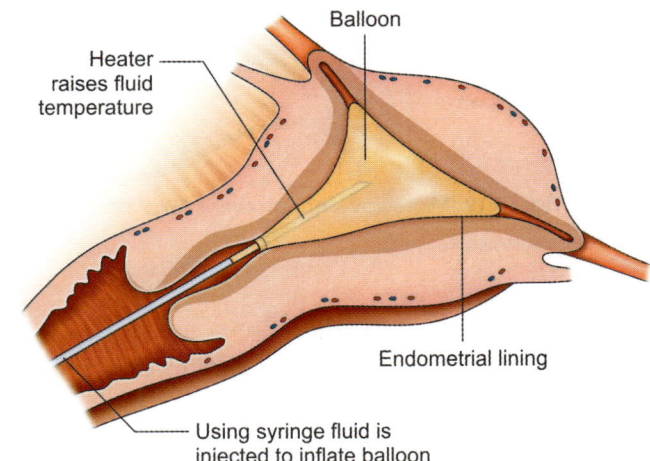

Fig. 11.18: Thermal balloon ablation

- This thermally destroys the lining of the uterus.
- Ablation is indicated for heavy bleeding with a normal uterus—no fibroids or polyps or when hormones offer no help.
- Ablation should not be done in women who want pregnancy in future.
- Thermal ablation is an outpatient procedure.
- The procedure is safe and effective and half the cost of hysterectomy.

b. Microwave Endometrial Ablation (Fig. 11.19)

- It applies very low-power microwaves to the uterus.
- It limits tissue destruction only to the lining without causing any unnecessary harm to other tissues.
- It completely destroys endometrium regardless of uterine shape or size and without the use of a hysteroscope or distension fluids.
- The microwave energy is delivered by means of an applicator that is gently inserted into the uterus via the cervix.

When the applicator is inside the uterus, the microwave energy is applied while the applicator is slowly withdrawn with a sweeping movement to ensure that all of the endometrium is treated.

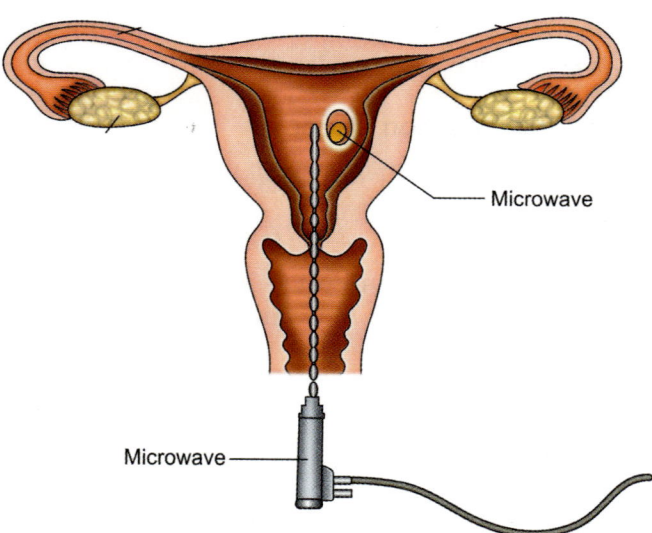

Fig. 11.19: Microwave endometrial ablation

c. Hydrothermablation (Fig. 11.20)

- Water is circulated at 90°C for 10 minutes to remove the lining.
- This can treat submucus myomas up to 3–6 cm; irregular cavities and cavities larger than 10 cm.
- It is FDA approved in 2001.

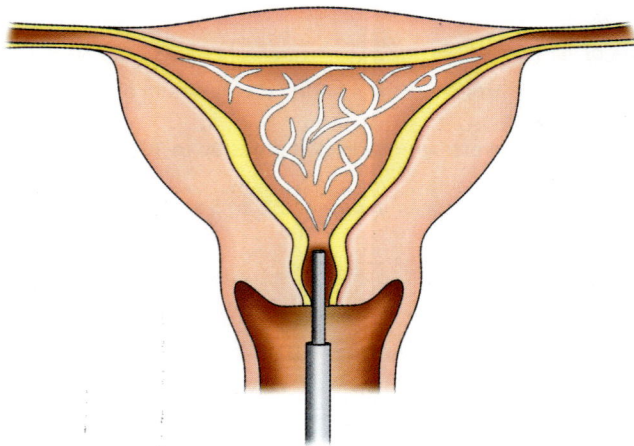

Fig. 11.20: Hydrothermablation

d. Cryoablation (Fig. 11.21)

- This freezes the uterine lining to –100 to –120°C at tip.
- It requires 2 treatment cycles, 4–6 minutes each; requires little anesthesia.

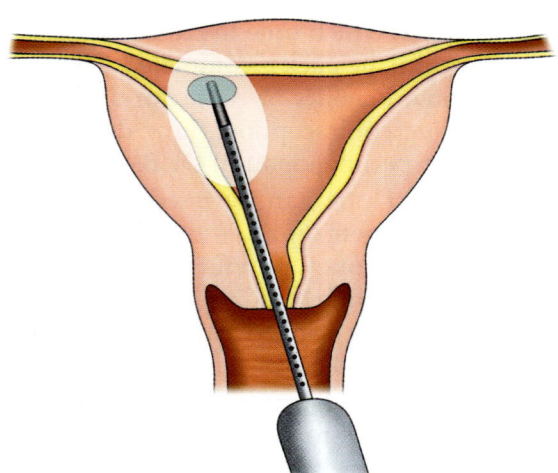

Fig. 11.21: Cryoablation

e. NovaSure System (Fig. 11.22)

- The NovaSure electrode array expands to conform to the contours of each patient's uterine cavity.
- The NovaSure endometrial ablation procedure delivers radiofrequency energy until tissue impedance reaches 50 ohm; on average, the procedure is completed in approximately 90 seconds.
- The electrode array is retracted for easy removal, leaving the uterine lining desiccated down to the superficial myometrium.
- Success rate of conversion to NMB is 90%.

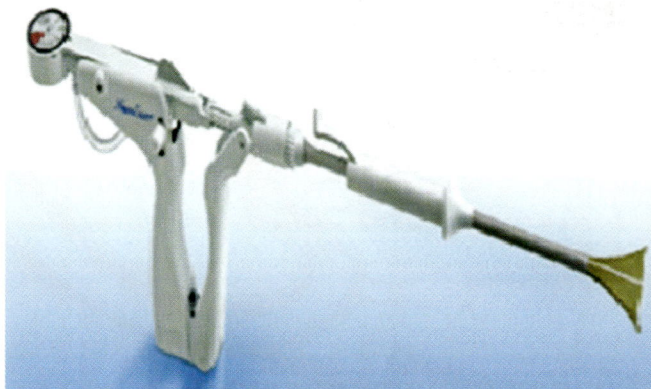

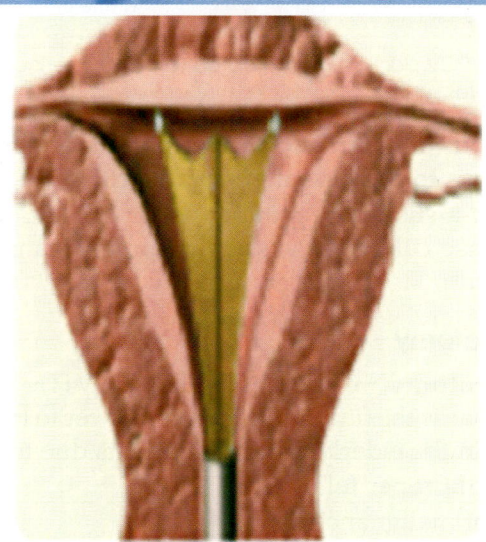

Fig. 11.22: NovaSure system

How Successful are Ablation Procedures?

- Ninety percent of women remain asymptomatic for at least five years.
- In women 45 years or over, 50% will have no periods after an ablation procedure. About 30% will have significantly reduced bleeding.
- But about 10–20% of women will continue to have heavy periods after an ablation procedure, depending on the original cause of their bleeding.

Endometrial Resection (TCRE)

Transcervical resection of endometrium is done in those cases in relatively younger patients where medical treatment is not very effective and biopsy is of benign in nature and the pregnancy is desired (Figs 11.23 and 11.24).

Procedure

- Glycin media is used.
- Help of laparoscopy is needed.

- Loop electrode is used to resect the endometrium.
- 3-month course of danazol or GnRH analogue is used before surgery.

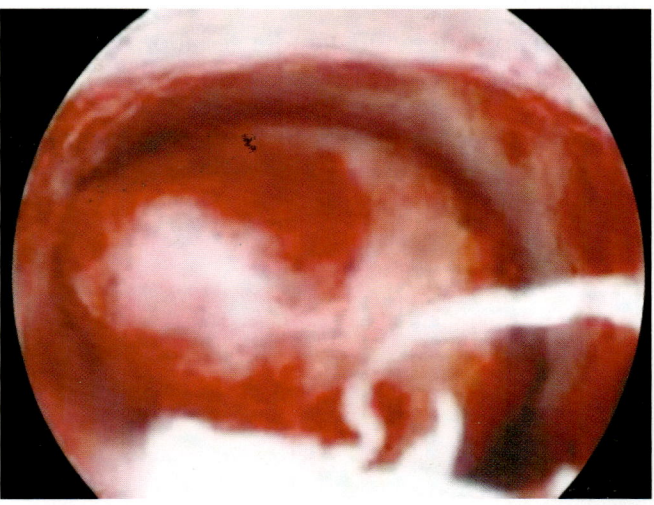

Fig. 11.23: TCRE for endometrial polyp

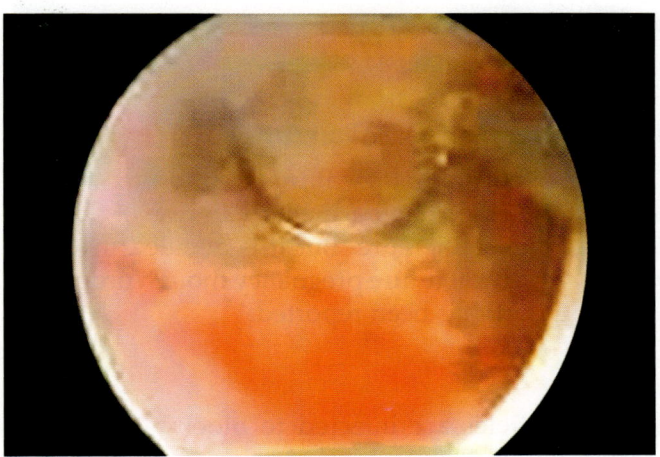

Fig. 11.24: Hysteroscopic endometrial resection

- Experience is required to determine the endpoint of the resection under laparoscopic guidance.
- Resected material is removed in between to improve the visibility and sent for biopsy.

Mirena (Fig. 11.25)

This is a levonorgestrel IUD. It contains 56 mg of progesterone in a 1:1 mixture with polydimethyl-siloxane.

- Effective treatment for endometrial hyperplasia in AUB as well as for concurrent contraception.
- Effective also in endometrial hyperplasia in interstitial fibroid uterus.
- It reduces blood loss by 80%.

- Its main advantage over ablative techiniques is that it is reversible.
- It releases 20 µg of levonorgestrel daily into the uterine cavity.
- It can be applied in OPD under sedation.
- The procedure hardly takes 5 minutes.

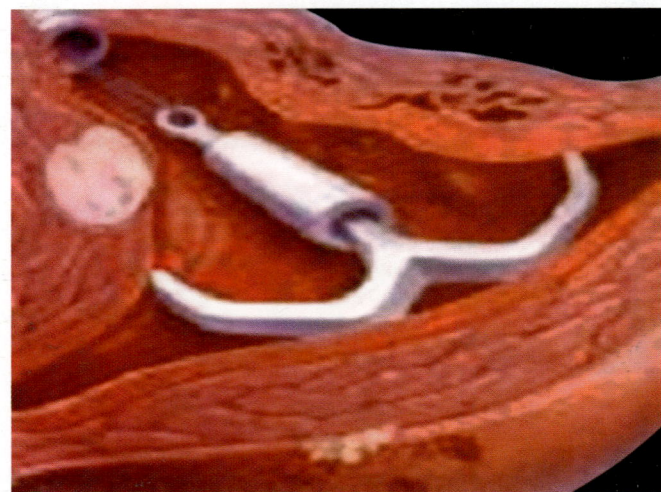

Fig. 11.25: Mirena

Uterine Artery Embolization (UAE)

This is a useful radiological intervention to stop the heavy uterine bleeding particularly in case of fibroids. It has a long-lasting cure. But it is avoided in young patients who want future pregnancy though pregnancy following UAE has been reported.

How is it useful?

- PVC particles are injected to block both uterine arteries (Fig. 11.26).

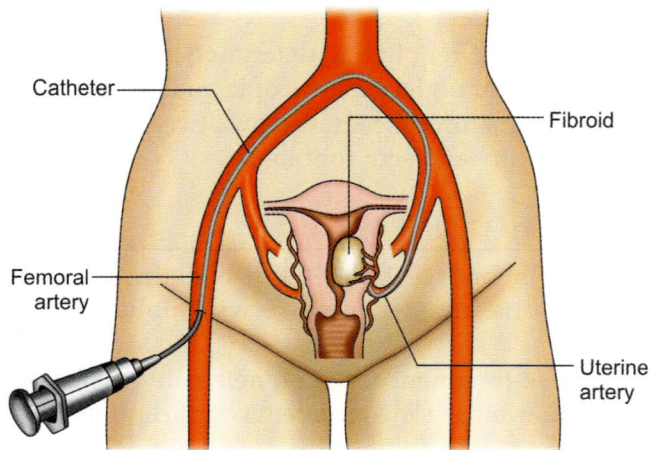

Fig. 11.26: Catheter inserted through femoral artery into uterine artery

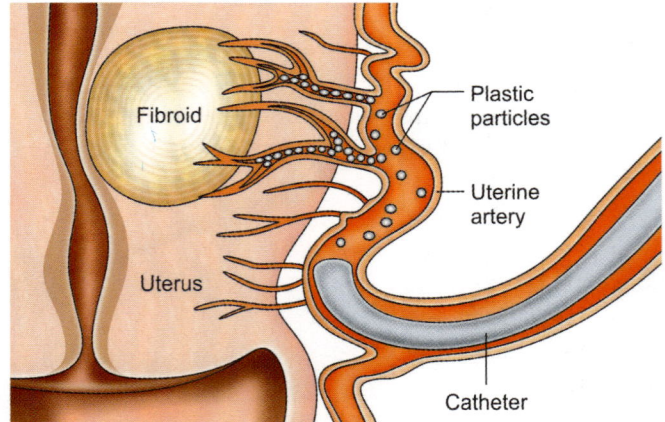

Fig. 11.27: PCV particles are injected to bloc k uterine vessels in fibroid uterus

- It is considered in HMB when fibroids >3 cm in size desirous to preserve uterus and fertility (Fig. 11.27).
- GnRH-a should be stopped prior to UAE as they decrease caliber of vessels and make cannulation difficult.

Hysterectomy

Hysterectomy, either NDVH, LAVH, TLH or abdominal is the final and ultimate answer to treatment of DUB in the elderly group of patients due to:
- Lack of proper follow-up
- Fear of malignancy
- Medical and surgical conservative failing
- Coincidental ovarian or cervical lesion warrents it.
- On patients' demand.

SOGC Guidelines Recommendations

1. Women with irregular menstrual bleeding should be investigated for endometrial polyps and/or submucus fibroids. (II-2B)
2. Women presenting with menorrhagia should have current cervical cytology and complete blood count. It is useful to delineate if the bleeding results from ovulatory or anovulatory causes in order to choose the appropriate treatment. (IIIB)
3. An office endometrial biopsy should be obtained in all women presenting with abnormal uterine bleeding over 40 years of age or weighing more than or equal to 90 kg. (IIB)
4. Hysteroscopically-directed biopsy is indicated for women with persistent abnormal menstrual bleeding, failed medical therapy, or transvaginal saline sonography suggestive of focal intrauterine pathology such as polyps or myomas. Women with persistent symptoms but negative tests should be reevaluated. (IIB).

5. Progestogens given in the luteal phase of the ovulatory menstrual cycles are not effective in reducing regular heavy menstrual bleeding. (IA)
6. While dilatation and curettage (D&C) may have a diagnostic role, it is not effective therapy for women with heavy menstrual bleeding. (IIB)
7. The endometrium can be destroyed by several different techniques but reoperation rates at 5 years may be up to 40% with roller ball ablation. This should be reserved for the women who has finished her childbearing and is aware of the risk of recurrent bleeding. (IA)

Interventions for Uterine Fibroids associated with HMB: NICE, 2007

- Myomectomy is recommended for women with HMB associated with uterine fibroids and who want to retain their uterus. [D]
- UAE is recommended for women with HMB associated with uterine fibroids and who want to retain their uterus and/or avoid surgery. [B]
- Prior to scheduling of UAE or myomectomy, the uterus and fibroid(s) should be assessed by ultrasound.
- If further information about fibroid position, size, number and vascularity is required, MRI should be considered. [D(GPP)]
- Pre-treatment before hysterectomy and myomectomy with a gonadotropin-releasing hormone analogue for 3 to 4 months should be considered where uterine fibroids are causing an enlarged or distorted uterus. [A]
- If a woman is being treated with gonadotropin-releasing hormone analogue and UAE is then planned, the gonadotropin-releasing hormone analogue should be stopped as soon as UAE has been scheduled. [D(GPP)]

NICE Recommendations

- If appropriate, a biopsy should be taken to exclude endometrial cancer or atypical hyperplasia.
- Indications for a biopsy include:
  a. Persistent intermenstrual bleeding
  b. In women aged 45 and over
  c. Treatment failure or ineffective treatment. [D(GPP)]
- Ultrasound is the first-line diagnostic tool for identifying structural abnormalities/endometrial thickness. [A] If history and investigations indicate that pharmacological treatment is appropriate and either hormonal or non-hormonal treatments are

acceptable, treatment should be considered in the following order:
1. Levonorgestrel-releasing intrauterine system (LNG-IUS) provided long-term (at least 12 months) use is desired. [A]
2. Tranexamic acid [A] or nonsteroidal anti-inflammatory drugs (NSAIDs) [A] or combined oral contraceptives [B] are alternative options.
3. Norethisterone (15 mg) daily from days 5 to 26 of the menstrual cycle, or injected long-acting progestogens are often used. [A]

- In women with HMB alone, with uterus no bigger than a 10-week pregnancy, endometrial ablation should be considered preferable to hysterectomy. [A]
- Taking into account the need for individual assessment, the route of hysterectomy should be considered in the following order: first-line vaginal; second-line abdominal. [A]

Conclusion

- AUB—not synonymous to DUB; it includes many more.
- DUB is a diagnosis of exclusion. Spectrum of DUB has become very narrow. Endoscopy, USG, CT, MRI helps in organic diagnosis.
- Medical treatment is the mainstay of treatment.
- Conservative surgery is the recent modality of treatment.
- Hysterectomy is final and a definitive option for the elderly.
- Ovarian preservation is a good thinking step.

Current Recommendations according to PALM-COEIN System

The current recommendations are organized etiology-wise according to the PALM-COEIN system.

Diagnosis of AUB

Recommendations Regarding History and Initial Examination

1. It is suggested to abandon the old overlapping terminology and to use PALM-COEIN classification for the diagnosis of AUB (Grade A; Level 4)
2. It is recommended to obtain a thorough history and to conduct a physical examination to direct the need for further investigations and treatment (Grade A; Level 4)
3. It is recommended to obtain information about the concomitant use of any medications which may likely be the cause of AUB (Grade B; Level 4)

4. In patients with AUB, any of the following criteria should be considered a positive screen for coagulopathies (Grade B; Level 4)
   - History of heavy bleeding starting at menarche
   - One of the following:
     – Postpartum hemorrhage
     – Bleeding associated with dental surgery
     – Surgery related bleeding
   - At least two of the following symptoms:
     – At least one episode of bruising per month
     – At least one episode of epistaxis per month
     – Frequent gum bleeding
     – Family history of bleeding symptoms
   - Examination including assessment of weight, BMI, pallor, thyroid, breasts, acne, FG score (if hirsutism is present), abdominal, P/S, PV examination (Grade A, Level 4)

Investigations

Recommendations on Laboratory Testing

1. A complete blood count (CBC) is recommended for all women with AUB
2. It is recommended to perform a sensitive urine pregnancy test if pregnancy is suspected.
3. Bleeding time, platelet count, prothrombin time, and partial thromboplastin time, are recommended in all adolescents and in adults with a positive screen for coagulopathies. Further testing for Von Willebrand disease, Ristocetin cofactor activity, factor VIII activity, and Von Willebrand factor antigen is recommended in consultation with a hematologist.
4. TSH test is done when clinically indicated.

Imaging

Recommendations on Investigations

1. *USG* should be done in AUB to evaluate uterus, adnexae and endometrial thickness (Grade A, Level 1)
2. *Doppler USG:* In suspected arteriovenous malformation, malignancy, and to differentiate between fibroid and adenomyomas (Grade B, Level 3)
3. *3D-USG:* For evaluating intracavitary and myometrial lesions in suspected patients and for mapping and typing of myomas. 3D-USG is a non-invasive alternative to hysteroscopy (Grade B; Level 4)
4. *SIS:* If intracavitary lesion is suspected and hysteroscopy is not available (Grade A; level 1)
5. *Hysteroscopy:* For diagnosis of intracavitary lesions and type of myomas (Grade A; Level 1)
6. *MRI:* To differentiate between fibroids and adenomyomas, for mapping exact location of fibroids while planning conservative surgery and prior to therapeutic embolization for fibroids (Grade A; level 3)

Recommendations on Endometrial Histopathology

1. Endometrial histopathology is recommended in AUB
   - In women >40 years (Grade A; Level 2)
   - In women <40 years who have high risk factors for carcinoma endometrium such as irregular bleeding, obesity, hypertension, PCOS, diabetes, endometrial thickness >12 mm on ultrasound, family history of malignancy of ovary/breast/endometrium/colon, use of tamoxifen for HRT or breast cancer, HNPCC, AUB unresponsive to medical treatment (Grade A; Level 2)
2. Endometrial aspiration should be the preferred procedure for obtaining endometrial sample for histopathology. If endometrium is thick on imaging, but where HPE is inadequate or atrophic, hysteroscopy should be performed to rule out polyps (Grade A; Level 2)
3. Dilatation and curettage should not be the procedure of choice for endometrial assessment (Grade A, Level 3)

Recommendations for Management of Patients with AUB

AUB-P (Polyps)

1. Hysteroscopic polypectomy is recommended for younger women who wish to preserve fertility (Grade A; Level 1).
2. In women with multiple endometrial polyps and not desirous of continued fertility, it is suggested to perform hysteroscopic polypectomy followed by LNG-IUS insertion after confirmation of benign lesion on histopathology (Grade A, Level 2)
3. Polyp should be sent for histopathology. If histopathology suggests malignancy, further management should be as AUB-M.

AUB-A (Adenomyosis)—Recommendations for Management

1. It is suggested to consider age, symptomatology, (AUB, pain, infertility) and association with other conditions (leiomyomas, polyps, and endometriosis).
2. In AUB-A women desirous of preserving fertility but not wishing immediate conception, progestogens especially LNG-IUS is recommended as firstline therapy (Grade A; Level 1)

3. In AUB-A patients desirous of preserving fertility and resistant to LNG-IUS/unwilling to use LNG-IUS, GnRh-agonists with add-back therapy is recommended as second-line therapy (Grade A, Level 1)

4. In AUB-A patients not desirous of preserving fertility, medical management with LNG-IUS or GnRH agonists with Add-back therapy can be initiated.

5. Combined oral contraceptives, danazol, NSAIDs and progestogens can be offered for symptomatic relief where LNG-IUS and GnRH agonists cannot be indicated. (Grade B, Level 4)

6. Adenomyomectomy is the conservative surgery that may be offered in selected cases presenting with infertility or with strong desire to retain uterus (Grade A, Level 2).

7. In case of failure/refusal for medical management, vaginal or laparoscopic hysterectomy is indicated (Grade A, Level 1).

Recommendations for AUB-L (Leiomyoma)

The treatment for AUB-L should be individualized as any variables such as age, parity, symptoms, and fertility desire may affect the treatment preference. Various options can be generalized as follows:

1. Women with intramural or subserous myommas (type 2–6) causing symptoms and desirous of preserving fertility can be managed with tranexamic acid, COCs, or NSAIDs (Grade A, Level 2).

2. Women with intramural or subserous myomas (type 2–6) causing symptoms and desirous of preserving fertility/uterus can be offered LNG-IUS if above medical treatment fails.

3. If medical treatment fails or if myoma is causing infertility, myomectomy is recommended by conventional laparotomy/laparoscopic or hysteroscopic route depending on myoma location, size and number (Grade A, Level 3).

4. For submucosal myomas(type 0–1), hysteroscopic resection (for <4 cm diameter myomas) or abdominal myomectomy(>4 cm diameter) is the recommended treatment. (Grade B, Level 4)

5. In women >40 yrs of age with symptomatic leiomyomas, not desirous of continued fertility, hysterectomy is the definitive treatment; however, medical management or LNG-IUS may be recommended in small fibroids (<4 cm diameter) before resorting to definitive surgery in case of failure or relief (Grade B; Level 3)

6. For short-term management (up to 6 months), GnRH agonists is an option in the following situations:

- For improving general condition, anemia
- In selected patients prior to myomectomy
- In younger patients to delay/avoid early surgical interventions
- In selected perimenopausal women so that they can tide over to menopause (Grade A; Level 1)

7. For long-term management of symptomatic leiomyomas, LNG-IUS can be recommended except in AUB-L, type 0 and 1. LNG-IUS can be advised in selected cases of AUB-1, type 2 also.

8. Newer promising options are progesterone receptor modulators such as Uripristal acetate (grade A; level 1). Low dose mifepristone (daily 5–10 mg) although effective (Grade A; Level 1), is not available in India in tablets containing required strength.

Recommendations for AUB-M (Malignancy and Endometrial Hyperplasia)

1. In AUB-M with endometrial malignancy, standard protocol for management of malignancy should be followed. (Grade B; Level 4)

2. In AUB-M with endometrial hyperplasia with atypia, hysterectomy is the standard treatment (Grade B; Level 2). Conservative treatment with high-dose progestins and close histological monitoring should only be considered in exceptional cases (when the patient wants to have children and compliance is satisfactory).

3. In AUB-M with endometrial hyperplasia without atypia, LNG-IUS can be considered as first-line therapy; alternatively oral progestins can be used (Grade A; Level 1). Preventive hysterectomy should only be considered in exceptional cases (e.g. extreme obesity without any prospect of weight loss).

Recommendations for AUB-C (Coagulopathy)

1. In patients with AUB-C, nonhormonal treatment with tranexamic acid (1 gm four times daily) as primary option and hormonal treatment with COCs,/LNG-IUS as secondary option are recommended in consultation with a hematologist with the following considerations (Grade A; Level 2):

a. For refractory patients of vWD with uncontrolled uterine bleeding with above medical management, specific factor replacement where possible or desmopressin to be given in refractory cases of Von Willebrand disease in consultation with hematologists.

b. When surgical interventions are indicated, appropriate pre-, intra-, and postoperative management of bleeding should be done.

c. NSAIDs are contraindicated as they can alter platelet function and interact with drugs that might affect liver function and production of clotting factors.

d. Intramuscular injectable preparations are contraindicated except in mild coagulation abnormalities. When administered, prolonged pressure should be applied at injectionsite.

Recommendations for Management of AUB-O (Ovulatory Dysfunction)

1. In women not desiring conception presently, COCs can be used as first-line therapy for 6–12 months (Grade A; Level 1).
2. Cyclic luteal phase progestins for 10–14 days can be used as as a specific treatment with AUB-O (Grade A; Level 1).
3. Norethisterone cyclically for 21 days is given as initial therapy in acute episodes of bleeding for short-term management of 3 months (Grade B; Level 4).
4. It is suggested to assess response after 1 year of medical management and judge to continue/discontinue existing therapy (Grade B; Level 4).
5. Surgical intervention is not recommended unless, there is evidence of persistent AUB or failure of medical management to alleviate the condition (Grade A; Level 4).
6. If COCs are contraindicated or patient is unwilling for COCs, LNG-IUS is recommended if she wishes to use it for at least one year (Grade A; Level 1).
7. In adolescents with AUB-O, both hormonal and nonhormonal therapies can be prescribed (Grade A; Level 4).

Recommendations for AUB-E (Endometrial)

Management of AUB-E is similar to management of AUB-O (Grade A; Level 4)

Recommendations for AUB-I (Iatrogenic)

1. Whenever feasible, medications causing AUB should be changed to other alternatives if no alternatives are available.
2. LNG-IUS is recommended for treatment (Grade A; Level 1).

Recommendations for AUB-N (Not defined)

1. In patients with AUB-N who desire effective contraception, LNG-IUS is recommended as first-line therapy to reduce menstrual bleeding (Grade A; Level 1), and COCs are recommended as second-line therapy (Grade A; Level 1)
2. For AUB that is cyclic or predictable in timing, non-hormonal options such as NSAIDs and tranexamic acid are recommended (Grade A; Level 1)
3. When medical or conservative surgical treatments (e.g. ablation of endometrium) have failed or are contraindicated, GnRH agonists along with add-back hormone therapy are recommended to reduce idiopathic AUB.
4. Uterine artery embolization is recommended for A-V malformations
5. Hysterectomy is the last resort (Grade B; Level 4)

General Management Guidelines on PALM-COEIN

Recommendations

1. Tranexamic acid is the first-line therapy. Other non-hormonal option is NSAIDs (Grade B; Level 1).
2. In women desiring effective contraception, LNG-IUS is recommended (Grade A; Level 1).
3. COCs are recommended as second-line therapy in patients desiring effective contraception, but unwilling or unsuitable for LNG-IUS (Grade A; Level 4).
4. Cyclic oral progestins from day 5 to 2 are recommended if COCs are contraindicated (Grade B; Level 1).
5. For AUB-O, cyclic luteal phase progestins from day 15–25 are recommended (Grade A; Level 4).
6. Centchroman (Formeloxifene) is an option when steroid hormones are not suitable (Grade B; level 3).
7. GnRH agonists with add-back hormone therap is an option when steroid hormones are not suitable (Grade B; level 3).
8. GnRH agonists with add-back hormone therapy are recommended as a last resort when medical treatment for AUB have failed and surgical treatment is contraindicated (Grade B; Level 4).
9. Role of conservative surgery such as ablation has decreased due to availability of LNG-IUS which works like medical ablation.

11C. DYSMENORRHEA

Dysmenorrhea is defined as painful menstruation. It is one of the most common gynecologic complaints in young women. Optimal management of this symptom depends on an understanding of the underlying cause. Dysmenorrhea can be divided into two broad categories—primary (spasmodic) and secondary (congestive).

Primary dysmenorrhea is defined as menstrual pain that is not associated with organic pelvic pathology (i.e. occurs in the absence of pelvic disease). It typically occurs in the first few years after menarche and affects as many as 50% of postpubertal females.

Secondary dysmenorrhea is defined as menstrual pain resulting from anatomic or macroscopic pelvic pathology as is seen in women with endometriosis or chronic pelvic inflammatory disease. It is most often observed in women aged 30–45 years.

The following risk factors are associated with severe episodes of dysmenorrhea:

- Earlier age at menarche
- Long menstrual periods
- Heavy menstrual flow
- Smoking
- Positive family history

Some studies have found obesity and alcohol consumption to be associated with dysmenorrhea. Physical activity and the duration of the menstrual cycle do not appear to be associated with increased menstrual pain.

Although dysmenorrhea is not life-threatening, it can be debilitating and psychologically taxing for many women. Dysmenorrhea is responsible for significant absenteeism from work, and it is the most common reason for school absence among adolescents.

The history is critical in establishing the diagnosis of dysmenorrhea and should include an assessment of the onset, duration, type, and severity of pain. A thorough menstrual history is also essential. A complete physical examination should be performed. For younger adolescents who have never been sexually active, a careful abdominal examination is appropriate. In older adolescents or those known to be sexually active, a pelvic examination is crucial.

Epidemiology

Dysmenorrhea may affect more than 50% of menstruating women, and its reported prevalence has been highly variable.

Primary dysmenorrhea peaks in late adolescence and the early 20s. The incidence falls with increasing age and with increasing parity. The prevalence of this condition is estimated to be 25% among adult women and as high as 90% among adolescents.

Pathophysiology

Primary Dysmenorrhea

Current evidence suggests that the pathogenesis of primary dysmenorrhea is due to **prostaglandin $F_{2\alpha}$**, a potent myometrial stimulant and vasoconstrictor in the secretory endometrium. Substantial evidence attributes dysmenorrhea to prolonged uterine contractions and decreased blood flow to the myometrium.

Leukotrienes heighten the sensitivity of pain fibers in the uterus. Substantial amounts of leukotrienes have been demonstrated in the endometrium of women with primary dysmenorrhea that does not respond to treatment with prostaglandin antagonists.

The posterior pituitary hormone **vasopressin** may be involved in myometrial hypersensitivity, reduced uterine blood flow, and pain in primary dysmenorrhea. Vasopressin's role in the endometrium may be related to prostaglandin synthesis and release.

In addition, a neuronal hypothesis has been advocated for the pathogenesis of primary dysmenorrhea. Type C pain neurons are stimulated by the anaerobic metabolites generated by an ischemic endometrium.

Primary dysmenorrhea has also been attributed to behavioral and psychological factors. Although these factors have not been convincingly demonstrated to be causative, they should be considered, if medical treatment fails.

In primary dysmenorrhea, there is a highly complex interplay between hormones and mediators, basal body temperature, sleep patterns, and the central nervous system (CNS), the extent of which is not completely understood.

Secondary Dysmenorrhea

Elevated prostaglandins may also play a role in secondary dysmenorrhea, but by definition, concomitant pelvic pathology must be present. A number of factors may be involved in the pathogenesis of secondary dysmenorrhea which include the following:

- Endometriosis

- Pelvic inflammatory disease
- Ovarian cysts and tumors
- Cervical stenosis
- Adenomyosis
- Fibroids
- Uterine polyps
- Intrauterine adhesions
- Congenital malformations (e.g. bicornuate uterus or subseptate uterus)
- Intrauterine contraceptive device
- Transverse vaginal septum
- Pelvic congestion syndrome

Risk factors for primary dysmenorrhea include the following:
- Early age at menarche (< 12 years)
- Nulliparity
- Heavy or prolonged menstrual flow
- Smoking
- Positive family history
- Obesity

Risk factors for secondary dysmenorrhea include the following:
- Fibroids
- PID
- Tubo-ovarian abscess
- Ovarian torsion
- Endometriosis

The common causes of secondary dysmenorrhea are briefly summarized below.

Uterine leiomyoma: Uterine leiomyomata are benign tumors of the uterine musculature that are a common cause of dysmenorrhea because they stretch the walls of the uterus or when in uterine cavity as submucus fibroid uterus produces spasmodic contraction to expel the tumor or fibroid can undergo torsion or degeneration which produces pain.

Pelvic inflammatory disease: PID is an infection of the uterus and fallopian tubes, with or without ovarian or parametrial involvement. It is an ascending infection that develops during or immediately after menses; if chronic, it can lead to dysmenorrhea. The most common causative pathogens are *Chlamydia trachomatis* and *Neisseria gonorrhoeae*, though PID also can be caused by other organisms, such as *Gardnerella vaginalis*, anaerobes, gram-negative rods and *Mycobacterium tuberculosis*. The diagnosis of PID, though primarily clinical, is based on the presence of 3 major criteria (abdominal pain, adnexal pain, and cervical motion tenderness), and 1 minor criterion (fever, vaginal discharge, leukocytosis, positive cervical cultures for gram-negative intracellular diplococci, or white blood cells on vaginal smear).

Tubo-ovarian abscess: Tubo-ovarian abscess is a loculated infection within the fallopian tubes or ovaries, usually occurring as a sequela of PID. It is often polymicrobial. Most commonly, patients present with fever and gradually worsening pelvic pain and tenderness; nausea, vomiting, and vaginal bleeding or discharge may be present as well. Examination may elicit tenderness on cervical motion and in the adnexal area. A pelvic mass may be present, though it is often difficult to palpate.

Ovarian torsion: Ovarian torsion involves twisting of the adnexal structures, which leads to ischemia and ultimately necrosis, if the process is not reversed in time. It, therefore, produces acute abdomen which needs urgent laparotomy.

Ovarian cyst rupture or hemorrhage: A hemorrhagic ovarian cyst comes from an ovarian follicle in the absence of ovulation. Patients often present with the acute onset of pelvic or abdominal pain, along with nausea and vomiting. Examination may reveal an adnexal mass, but almost all patients with ruptured ovarian cysts have some level of adnexal tenderness and signs of peritoneal irritation.

Endometriosis: Endometriosis is the presence of endometrium like tissue found outside of the uterus, most commonly in the ovaries. Women often present with dyspareunia and pelvic and back pain. Although endometriosis is a diagnosis of exclusion, patients may give a history of dysmenorrhea that was cyclic with menses

Adenomyosis: Adenomyosis is defined as an invasion of myometrium by uterine glands which bleeds on hormone withdrawal during periods producing uterine stretch and pain.

Intrauterine contraceptive device: IUCDs may cause uterine spasm and pain particularly if it is displaces inside or invites uterine infection and rarely uterine wall penetration or perforation.

Premenstrual dysphoric disorder: Besides dysmenorrhea, patients with premenstrual dysphoric disorder (formerly called premenstrual syndrome) may have bloating, body aches, migraine headaches, breast tenderness, and emotional complaints. Aside from possible vaginal brownish discharge or bleeding, pelvic examination findings are normal.

History

A complete history should include the following:

- Age at menarche
- Menstrual frequency, length of period, estimated menstrual flow, and presence or absence of intermenstrual bleeding
- Associated symptoms
- Onset, duration, type, and severity of pain, as well as its relation to the menstrual cycle
- External factors affecting the pain
- Impact of dysmenorrhea on physical and social activity
- Progression of symptom severity
- Sexual and obstetric history

Primary dysmenorrhea should be distinguished from secondary dysmenorrhea on the basis of clinical features. Clinical features of primary dysmenorrhea include the following:

- Onset shortly after menarche (typically within 6 months)
- Usual duration of 48–72 hours (often starting several hours before or just after the menstrual flow)
- Cramping pain
- Background of constant lower abdominal pain, radiating to the back or the anterior or medial thigh
- Often unremarkable pelvic examination findings (including rectal)

Associated general symptoms, such as malaise, fatigue (85%), nausea and vomiting (89%), diarrhea (60%), lower backache (60%), and headache (45%), may be present with primary dysmenorrhea. Dizziness, nervousness, and even collapse are also associated with dysmenorrhea.

A different pattern of pain is observed with secondary dysmenorrhea that is not limited to the onset of menses; this is usually associated with abdominal bloating, pelvic heaviness, and back pain. Typically, the pain progressively increases during the luteal phase until it peaks around the onset of menstruation.

The following may indicate secondary dysmenorrhea:

- Dysmenorrhea beginning in the 20s or 30s, after relatively painless menstrual cycles in the past
- Heavy menstrual flow or irregular bleeding
- Dysmenorrhea occurring during the first or second cycles after menarche, which may indicate congenital outflow obstruction
- Pelvic abnormality with physical examination (consider endometriosis, pelvic inflammatory disease [PID], pelvic adhesions, and adenomyosis)

- Little or no response to nonsteroidal anti-inflammatory drugs (NSAIDs) or OCs
- Infertility
- Dyspareunia
- Vaginal discharge

Physical Examination

A complete physical examination should be performed. For younger adolescents who have never been sexually active, a careful abdominal examination is appropriate. In older adolescents or those known to be sexually active, a pelvic examination is crucial for excluding uterine irregularities, cul-de-sac tenderness, or suggestive nodularities. This examination includes the following:

- Inspection of the external genitalia for rashes, swelling, or discoloration.
- Inspection of the vaginal vault for discharge, blood, or foreign bodies.
- Inspection of the cervix for the above, plus any masses or signs of infection.
- Bimanual examination to assess cervical motion tenderness, uterine or adnexal tenderness, or any masses in the pelvis.

Women with primary dysmenorrhea usually have normal findings on pelvic examination. Lower abdominal or uterine tenderness may be present. Cervical stenosis may contribute to retrograde flow.

Women with secondary dysmenorrhea may have pelvic pathology. Women with endometriosis who present with secondary dysmenorrhea have palpable ovarian cysts or peritoneal lesions. Presence of enlarged uterine mass and cervical motion tenderness is diagnostic of organic cause. There may be adnexal tenderness or a palpable mass. Vaginal or cervical discharge may be seen. Visible vaginal pathology (e.g., mucosal tears, masses, or prolapse) may be visible.

Differential Diagnosis of Dysmenorrhea

The key diagnostic issue in dysmenorrhea is differentiating primary dysmenorrhea from secondary dysmenorrhea and in the differential diagnosis of different causes of secondary dysmenorrhea. Besides these, others are:

- Cystitis in females
- Ectopic pregnancy
- Abortion
- Pelvic infections
- Worm infestations
- Inflammatory bowel disease
- Irritable bowel syndrome

- Appendicitis
- Pelvic inflammatory disease

Dysmenorrhea Workup

I. Approach Considerations

No tests are specific to the diagnosis of primary dysmenorrhea. The diagnosis is made on the basis of clinical findings. Laboratory studies may be indicated to elucidate the cause of secondary dysmenorrhea. Noninvasive studies may include abdominal and transvaginal ultrasonography. Other more invasive studies, including hysterosalpingography, may be required. Further investigation includes hysteroscopy or laparoscopy; the latter is usually indicated when initial interventions fail to relieve symptoms.

II. Laboratory Studies

The following laboratory studies may be performed to identify or exclude organic causes of secondary dysmenorrhea:

- Complete blood count (CBC) with differential to search for evidence of infection or a neoplastic process.
- Gonococcal and chlamydial cultures, enzyme immunoassay (EIA), and DNA probe testing to exclude sexually transmitted infections (STIs) and pelvic inflammatory disease (PID).
- Quantitative human chorionic gonadotropin level to exclude ectopic pregnancy.
- Erythrocyte sedimentation rate (ESR) for subacute salpingitis.
- Urinalysis to exclude urinary tract infection.
- Stool test to rule out worm infestation and GI bleeding.
- Cancer antigen 125 (CA-125) assay: This test has relatively low negative predictive value and thus is of limited clinical utility for evaluating dysmenorrheal women.

Although these tests can be useful adjuncts in the workup of dysmenorrhea, but for diagnosing dysmenorrhea and its underlying cause, laboratory testing should play an ancillary rather than a primary role and should not be allowed to replace a sound clinical basis for the diagnosis.

Ultrasonography and other Imaging Studies

In cases of well-established primary dysmenorrhea, imaging studies are of little value. However, if pelvic pathology is suspected, abdominal and transvaginal ultrasonography is done. It is indicated for evaluating situations like endometriosis, abortions, ectopic pregnancy, ovarian cysts, fibroids, comlex mass in chronic PID and intrauterine contraceptive devices (IUCDs).

Hysterosalpingography is used to exclude endometrial polyps, leiomyomas, and congenital abnormalities of the uterus. Intravenous pyelography is indicated, if uterine malformation is confirmed as a cause or contributing factor for the dysmenorrhea.

Although computed tomography (CT) is not routinely performed for patients with dysmenorrhea, it does have some utility, particularly in identifying ovarian torsion. Magnetic resonance imaging (MRI) is also effective in differentiating adenomyosis and submucous myomas that might otherwise be missed by other imaging modalities.

Laparoscopy, Hysteroscopy and Biopsy

On occasion, other more invasive studies, including laparoscopy, hysteroscopy, and dilatation and curettage (D&C), may be required.

Laparoscopic examination is the single most useful procedure. It involves a complete diagnostic survey of the pelvis and reproductive organs to ascertain the presence of any pathology that may account for the clinical symptoms. Hysteroscopy and D&C may be indicated to evaluate intrauterine pathology found on imaging. An endometrial biopsy may be indicated, if endometritis is considered likely.

Treatment and Management

Treatment of dysmenorrhea is aimed at providing symptomatic relief as well as inhibiting the underlying processes that cause symptoms. Grading dysmenorrhea according to the severity of pain and the degree of limitation of daily activity may help guide the treatment strategy. Medications used may include NSAIDs and opioid analgesics, as well as oral contraceptives (OCs). In addition to pain relief, mainstays of treatment include reassurance and education.

Pharmacologic Therapy

Treatment of primary dysmenorrhea is directed at providing relief from the cramping pelvic pain and associated symptoms (e.g. headache, nausea, vomiting, flushing, and diarrhea) that typically accompany or immediately precede the onset of menstrual flow. The pelvic pain can be distressing and occasionally radiates to the back and thighs, often necessitating prompt intervention.

Currently, pharmacotherapy has been the most reliable and effective treatment for relieving dysmenorrhea. Because the pain results from uterine vasoconstriction, anoxia, and contractions mediated by prostaglandins, symptomatic relief can often be obtained by using agents that inhibit prostaglandin synthesis and possess anti-inflammatory and analgesic properties.

NSAIDs and combination OCs are the most commonly used therapeutic modalities for the management of primary dysmenorrhea. These agents have different mechanisms of action and can be used adjunctively in refractory cases. Lack of response to NSAIDs and OCs (or a combination thereof) may increase the likelihood of a secondary cause for dysmenorrhea.

Treatment of secondary dysmenorrhea involves correction of the underlying organic cause. Specific measures (medical or surgical) may be required to treat pelvic pathologic conditions (e.g., endometriosis) and to ameliorate the associated dysmenorrhea. Periodic use of analgesic agents as adjunctive therapy may be beneficial.

Nonsteroidal Anti-inflammatory Drugs

NSAIDs are the most common treatment for both primary and secondary dysmenorrheas. They decrease menstrual pain by decreasing intrauterine pressure and lowering prostaglandin $F_{2\alpha}$ levels in menstrual fluid. NSAIDs that inhibit type I prostaglandin synthetase and suppress production of cyclic endoperoxides (e.g. fenamates, cyclooxygenase [COX]-2-selective agents, propionic acids, and indole acetic acids) alleviate symptoms by decreasing endometrial and menstrual fluid prostaglandin concentrations.

If taken early enough and in sufficient quantity, NSAIDs are extremely successful in alleviating menstrual pain. Because they are used for short periods in otherwise healthy young women, they are generally well tolerated and free of serious toxicity. Gastrointestinal (GI) upset is the most common adverse effect associated with NSAIDs, and patients receiving these medications should be monitored for more serious adverse effects, including GI bleeding and renal dysfunction.

Patients should also be monitored for potential pharmacokinetic and pharmacodynamic drug interactions and possible effects on platelet aggregation. NSAIDs are contraindicated in patients with renal insufficiency, peptic ulcer disease, gastritis, bleeding diatheses, or aspirin hypersensitivity. NSAIDs should be started at the onset of menstrual bleeding.

The NSAIDs specifically approved by the US Food and Drug Administration (FDA) for treatment of dysmenorrhea are as follows:
- Diclofenac
- Ibuprofen
- Meclofenamate
- Mefenamic acid
- Naproxen

NSAIDs that achieve peak serum concentrations within 30–60 minutes and have a faster onset of action (e.g. ibuprofen, naproxen, and meclofenamate) may be preferred.

COX-2 specific inhibitors have also proven effective in relieving menstrual pain. Their selectivity reduces the GI symptoms caused by inhibition of the COX-1 receptor. Despite some preliminary data suggesting efficacy in patients with primary dysmenorrhea, COX-2 inhibitors have not been demonstrably superior to conventional NSAIDs.

Other Analgesic Agents

In an emergency setting, patients who do not respond to NSAIDs may require treatment with narcotics for pain control.

Oral Contraceptives

OCs, which block monthly ovulation and may decrease menstrual flow, may also relieve dysmenorrhea though these agents are not approved by the FDA for this indication.

OCs may be an appropriate choice for patients who do not wish to conceive. Combination OCs suppress the hypothalamic-pituitary-ovarian axis, thereby inhibiting ovulation and preventing prostaglandin production in the late luteal phase. This generally reduces the amount of menstrual flow and alleviates primary dysmenorrhea in most patients.

Combination OCs, the levonorgestrel intrauterine device, and depot medroxyprogesterone acetate provide effective pain relief and are associated with reduced menstrual flow. It may be necessary to add an NSAID to the OC, especially during the first few cycles after initiation of the OC. The ethinyl estradiol dose should generally be less than 50 µg; a monophasic OC containing 30 µg is a reasonable choice.

Dietary and Other Therapies

Other therapies for dysmenorrhea have been proposed, but most are not well studied. A low-fat vegetarian diet has been reported to reduce menstrual pain in some women. Certain dietary supplements like thiamine, fish oil, pyridoxine, magnesium, and vitamin E may be

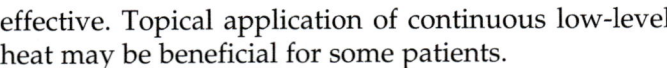

effective. Topical application of continuous low-level heat may be beneficial for some patients.

Prevention

Various measures have been used to manage dysmenorrhea in the outpatient setting, including the following:

- Lifestyle modification seems to be helpful.
- Smoking cessation should be encouraged, in that smoking may be a risk factor for dysmenorrhea.

Exercise has been shown to alleviate symptoms of dysmenorrhea, though the mechanism is not well understood.

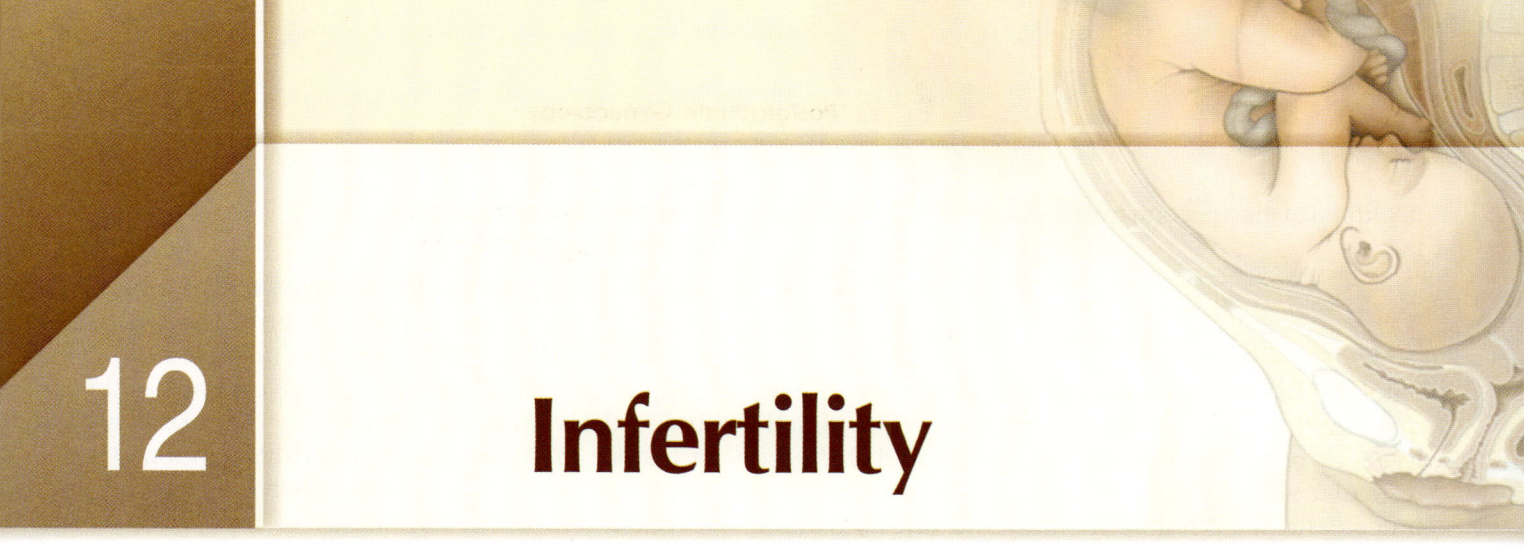

12 Infertility

Introduction

Infertility is the failure to conceive (regardless of cause) after 1 year of unprotected intercourse. Infertility affects approximately 10–15% of reproductive-aged couples. Its overall prevalence has been stable during the past 50 years; however, a shift in etiology and patient age has occurred. As a woman's age increases, the incidence of infertility also increases.

Fertility is defined as the capacity to reproduce or the state of being fertile. This term should be differentiated from **fecundability,** which is the probability of achieving a pregnancy each month, and **fecundity**, which is the ability to achieve a live birth within 1 menstrual cycle. The fecundability rate in the general reproductive-aged population is fairly constant and is approximately 0.22 per month. The estimated fecundity rate is 0.15–0.18 per month, representing a cumulative pregnancy rate of 90% per year.

In societies where family planning and professional career development are prioritized, some women postpone childbearing until their 30s and beyond. As a result, these women may have more difficulty conceiving and have an increased risk of miscarriage. Because fecundability rates are higher in younger women and lower in older women, counselling a 40-year-old woman to wait a year before seeking fertility services is inappropriate. In women older than 35 years, a complete evaluation after 4–6 months of trying to conceive is prudent because their response to treatment may be suboptimal due to diminished ovarian reserve.

Etiology of Infertility

Reproduction requires the interaction and integrity of the female and male reproductive tracts, which involves (1) the release of a normal preovulatory oocyte, (2) the production of adequate spermatozoa, (3) the normal transport of the gametes to the ampullary portion of the fallopian tube where fertilization occurs, and (4) the subsequent transport of the cleaving embryo into the endometrial cavity for implantation and development.

Infertility is caused by male and/or female factors. Male and female factors each account for approximately 35% of cases. Often, there is more than one factor, with male and female factors combined causing 20% of infertility. In the remaining 10% of cases, the etiology is unknown.

Couples with unknown etiology can be categorized as unexplained infertility or normal infertile couples (NICs), indicating that all findings from standard tests used in the infertility workup are normal. In normal infertile couples, the actual cause for infertility cannot be detected; perhaps there is dysfunctional interaction between the sperm and the oocyte, poor quality of the embryo, or a disruption at the implantation site.

Other lifestyle factors that have been associated with an increased risk of infertility include environmental and occupational factors; toxic effects related to tobacco, marijuana, or other drugs; excessive exercise; inadequate diet associated with extreme weight loss or gain; and advanced age.

Factors Affecting Both Sexes

Environmental and Occupational Factors

Concern regarding the impact of environmental factors on fertility is increasing.

Excessive radiation damages the germinal cells. Exposure to lead, other heavy metals, and pesticides has also been associated with male infertility. Many other factors, such as excessive heat exposure, microwave radiation, ultrasonography, and other health hazards are controversial as infertility-inducing factors.

Toxic Effects Related to Tobacco, Marijuana, and Other Drugs

Smoking has been associated with infertility in both males and females. Nicotine and polycyclic aromatic hydrocarbons block spermatogenesis and decrease testicular size. In women, tobacco alters the cervical mucus and the cilial epithelium and affects gamete transport.

Marijuana and its metabolite, delta-9-tetra-hydrocannabinol, inhibit the secretion of LH and FSH, thus inducing ovulatory disorders and luteal phase dysfunction in women. Marijuana use affects males by decreasing the sperm count and the quality of the sperm.

Chronic alcoholism may induce ovulatory dysfunction, therefore, impacting fertility. Alcohol use by males interferes with the synthesis of testosterone and has an impact on sperm concentration. Alcoholism may inhibit sexual response and cause impotence.

Exercise

Exercise should be encouraged as part of normal activity. However, compulsive exercise is deleterious, especially for long-distance runners. Jogging stimulates the secretion of endorphins; excessive secretion of endorphins interferes with the normal production of FSH and LH, in turn inducing ovulatory disorders and luteal phase dysfunction, which accounts for lack of embryo implantation and first-trimester miscarriages. In males, exercise has been associated with oligospermia.

Inadequate Diet associated with Extreme Weight Loss or Gain

Although weight loss associated with anorexia nervosa or bulimia induces hypothalamic amenorrhea, obesity may be associated with anovulation and oligo-menorrhea. In men, obesity has been associated with decreased sperm quality.

Causes of Infertility

- Sperm disorders—30.6%
- Anovulation/oligoovulation—30%
- Tubal disease—16%
- Unexplained—13.4%
- Cx factors—5.2%
- Peritoneal factors—4.8%

General Guidance on Evaluation of Infertility

Infertility is a problem that involves both partners. The consultation is incomplete, if only the woman is evaluated. Diagnostic testing is unnecessary, if the couple has not attempted to conceive for at least 1 year, unless the woman is 35 years old or older, or they have a history of a male factor infertility, endometriosis, pelvic inflammatory disease, or pelvic surgery. A brief explanation of the physiology of reproduction and reassurance are usually enough to lessen the anxiety of the couple.

History

The couple should provide a copy of their previous medical records and complete a medical history questionnaire. This is important for the following purpose:

- To obtain a detailed medical history regarding the type of infertility (primary or secondary) and its duration.
- To obtain a history of previous pregnancies and their outcomes; interval between pregnancies; and detailed information about pregnancy loss, duration of pregnancy, ultrasonographic data, etc.
- Take the history of previous infertility evaluation and treatment, specific questions should address the issues of frequency of intercourse, use of lubricants (e.g. K-Y gel) that could be spermicidal, use of vaginal douches after intercourse, and the presence of any sexual dysfunction such as anorgasmia or dyspareunia.
- Question female patients about their menstrual history, frequency, and patterns since menarche. A history of weight changes, hirsutism, frontal balding, and acne should also be addressed.
- Male patients are asked about previous semen analysis results, history of impotence, premature ejaculation, erectile dysfunction, change in libido, history of testicular trauma, previous relationships and the existence of offspring from previous partners.
- The couple is questioned about history of sexually transmitted infections (STIs); lifestyle; consumption of alcohol, tobacco, and recreational drugs, occupation; and physical activities.
- Enquiry is done about current use of any medical treatment, whether they have a history of allergies.
- A complete review of any known endocrinological or immunological problem that may be associated with infertility.

Physical Examination

A physical examination should be completed:

- Routine records of blood pressure, pulse rate, and temperature (if applicable) are needed.
- Measure height and weight to calculate the body mass index, and measure arm span when indicated.
- Perform an eye examination to establish the presence of exophthalmos, which can be associated with hyperthyroidism.
- The presence of epicanthus, lower implantation of the ears and hairline, and webbed neck can be associated with chromosomal abnormalities.
- Carefully evaluate the thyroid gland to exclude gland enlargement or thyroid nodules.
- Perform breast examination to evaluate breast development and to seek abnormal masses or secretions, especially galactorrhea.

The abdominal examination should be directed to the presence of abnormal masses at the hypogastrium level.

- A thorough gynecologic examination should include an evaluation of hair distribution, clitoris size, Bartholin glands, labia majora and minora, and any condylomata acuminata or other lesions that could indicate the existence of venereal disease.
- The inspection of the vaginal mucosa may indicate a deficiency of estrogens or the presence of infection.
- The evaluation of the cervix should include a Papanicolaou test and cultures for gonorrhea, chlamydia, *Ureaplasma urealyticum*, and *Mycoplasma hominis*.
- Bimanual examination should be performed to establish the direction of the cervix and the size and position of the uterus to identify the presence of uterine fibroids, adnexal masses, tenderness, or pelvic nodules indicative of infection or endometriosis.
- The examination of the extremities is important to rule out malformation, such as shortness of the fourth finger or cubitus valgus, which can be associated with chromosomal abnormalities and other congenital defects. Examine the skin to establish the presence of acne, hypertrichosis and hirsutism.
- The urologist usually examines the male partner, if the patient's history of semen analysis produces any abnormal finding.
  a. Attention should be directed to congenital abnormalities of the genital tract (e.g. hypospadias, cryptorchidism, congenital absence of the vas deferens).
  b. Testicular size, urethral stenosis, and presence of varicocele are also determined.
  c. A history of previous inguinal hernia repair can indicate an accidental ligation of the spermatic artery

MALE INFERTILITY

Male infertility refers to the inability of a male to contribute to conception with a fertile female.

Among couples with infertility, approximately 55% have a female problem, about 45% have a male factor problem and 25% have issues on both sides. The ability to treat female and male infertility in parallel is, therefore, crucial.

Male Reproductive Physiology

The Hypothalamic–Pituitary–Gonadal Axis

The hypothalamus is the integrated center of the reproductive axis and receives messages from both the central nervous system and the testes to regulate the production and secretion of gonadotropin-releasing hormone (GnRH). Neurotransmitters and neuro-peptides have both inhibitory and stimulatory influence on the hypothalamus. The hypothalamus releases GnRH in a pulsatile nature which appears to be essential for stimulating the production and release of both luteinizing hormone (LH) and follicle-stimulating hormone (FSH). Interestingly and paradoxically, after the initial stimulation of these gonadotropins, the exposure to constant GnRH results in inhibition of their release. LH and FSH are produced in the anterior pituitary and are secreted episodically in response to the pulsatile release of GnRH. LH and FSH both bind to specific receptors on the Leydig cells and Sertoli cells within the testis. Testosterone, the major secretory product of the testes, is a primary inhibitor of LH secretion in males. Testosterone may be metabolized in peripheral tissue to the potent androgen dihydrotestosterone or the potent estrogen estradiol. These androgens and estrogens act independently to modulate LH secretion. The mechanism of feedback control of FSH is regulated by Sertoli cell product called inhibin. Decreases in spermatogenesis are accompanied by decreased production of inhibin and this reduction in negative feedback is associated with reciprocal elevation of FSH levels. Isolated increased levels of FSH constitute an important, sensitive marker of the state of the germinal epithelium.

Prolactin also has a complex inter-relationship with the gonadotropins, LH and FSH. In males with hyperprolactinemia, prolactin tends to inhibit the production of GnRH. Besides inhibiting LH secretion and testosterone production, elevated prolactin levels may have a direct effect on the central nervous system. In individuals with elevated prolactin levels, libido and sexual function do not return to normal with testosterone as long as the prolactin levels are elevated.

The Testes

I. Leydig Cells

Testosterone is secreted episodically from the **Leydig cells** in response to LH pulses and has a diurnal pattern, with the peak level in the early morning and the trough level in the late afternoon or early evening. In the intact testis, LH receptors decrease or downregulate after exogenous LH administration. Large doses of GnRH or its analogs can reduce the numbers of LH receptors and, therefore, inhibit LH secretion. There appears to be an intratesticular ultrashort loop feedback where exogenous testosterone will override the effect of LH and inhibit testosterone production. In normal males, only 2% of testosterone is free or unbound. 44% is bound to testosterone-estradiol-binding globulin or TeBG. 54% of testosterone is bound to albumin and other proteins. These steroid-binding proteins modulate androgen action.

TeBG has a higher affinity for testosterone than for estradiol, and changes in TeBG alter or amplify the hormonal milieu. TeBG levels are increased by estrogens, thyroid administration and cirrhosis of the liver and may be decreased by androgens, growth hormone and obesity.

The biological actions of androgens are exerted on target organs that contain specific androgen receptor proteins. Testosterone leaves the circulation and enters the target cells where it is converted to the more potent androgen dihydrotestosterone by an enzyme 5-alpha-reductase. The major functions of androgens in target tissues include:

1. Regulation of gonadotropin secretion by the hypothalamic–pituitary axis
2. Initiation and maintenance of spermatogenesis
3. Differentiation of the internal and external male genital system during fetal development; and
4. Promotion of sexual maturation at puberty.

II. Seminiferous Tubules (Fig. 12.1)

The seminiferous tubules contain all the germ cells at various stages of maturation and their supporting Sertoli cells. These account for 85–90% of the testicular volume. **Sertoli cells** are a fixed-population of non-dividing support cells. They rest on the basement membrane of the seminiferous tubules. They are linked by tight junctions. These tight junctions coupled with the close approximation of the myoid cells of the peritubular contractile cell layers serve to form the blood–testis barrier. This barrier provides a unique microenvironment that facilitates spermatogenesis and maintains these germ cells in an immunologically privileged location. This isolation is important because spermatozoa are produced during puberty, long after the period of self-recognition by the immune system.

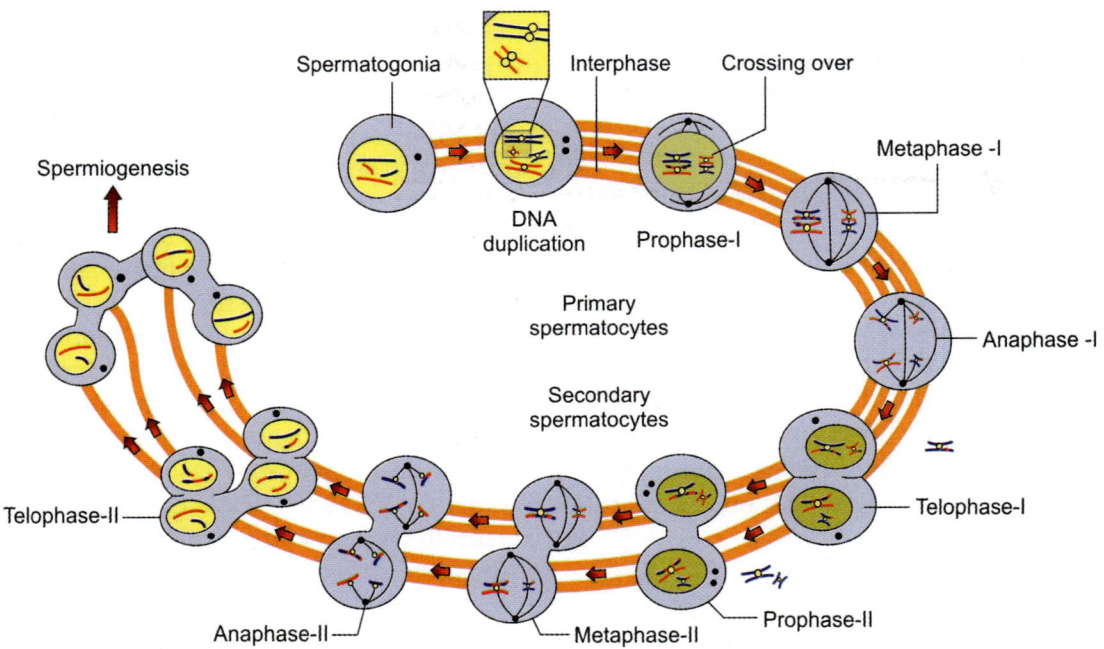

Fig. 12.1: Male gametogenesis

If these developing spermatozoa are not immuno-logically protected, they will be recognized as foreign and attacked by the body's immune system. Sertoli cells appear to be involved with the nourishment of developing germ cells as well as the phagocytosis of damaged cells. Spermatogonia and young spermatocytes are lower down in the basal compartment of the seminiferous tubule, whereas mature spermatocytes and spermatids are sequestered higher up in the adluminal compartment.

Sertoli cells serve a number of functions during spermatogenesis, they support the developing gametes in the following ways:

- Maintain the environment necessary for development and maturation, via the blood–testis barrier
- Secrete substances initiating meiosis.
- Secrete supporting testicular fluid.
- Secrete androgen-binding protein (ABP), which concentrates testosterone in close proximity to the developing gametes.
- Secrete hormones affecting pituitary gland control of spermatogenesis, particularly the polypeptide hormone, inhibin.
- Phagocytose residual cytoplasm left over from spermiogenesis.
- They release anti-müllerian hormone which prevents formation of the müllerian duct.
- Protect spermatids from the immune system of the male, via the blood–testis barrier.

The intercellular adhesion molecules ICAM-1 have antagonistic effects on the tight junctions forming the blood–testis barrier. ICAM-2 molecules regulate spermatid adhesion on the apical side of the barrier (towards the lumen).

The **germinal cells** or the spermatogenic cells are arranged in an orderly manner from the basement membrane up to the lumen. Spermatogonia lie directly on the basement membrane, and next in order, progressing up to the lumen, are found the primary spermatocytes, secondary spermatocytes and spermatids. There are 13 different germ cells representing different stages in the developmental process.

Spermatogenesis is a complex process whereby primitive stem cells or spermatogonia, either divide to reproduce themselves for stem cell renewal or they divide to produce daughter cells that will later become spermatocytes. The spermatocytes eventually divide and give rise to mature cell lines that eventually give rise to spermatids. The spermatids then undergo transformation into a spermatozoa. This transformation includes nuclear condensation, acrosome formation,

loss of most of the cytoplasm, development of a tail and arrangement of the mitochondria into the middle piece of the sperm which basically power the tail for its movement. There are six stages of seminiferous epithelium development. The progression from stage one through stage six constitutes one cycle. In humans the duration of each cycle is approximately 16 days and 4.6 cycles are required for a mature sperm to develop from early spermatogonia. Therefore, the duration of the entire spermatogenic cycle in humans is 4.6 cycles times 16 days equal to 74 days.

Hormonal Control of Spermatogenesis

An intimate structural and functional relationship exists between the two separate compartments of the testis, i.e. the **seminiferous tubule** and the **interstitium** between the tubules. LH affects spermatogenesis indirectly in that it stimulates androgenous testosterone production. FSH targets Sertoli cells. Therefore, testosterone and FSH are the hormones that are directed at the seminiferous tubule epithelium. Androgen-binding protein which is a Sertoli cell product carries testosterone intracellularly and may serve as a testosterone reservoir within the seminiferous tubules in addition to transporting testosterone from the testis into the epididymal tubule. The physical proximity of the Leydig cells to the seminiferous tubules and the elaboration by the Sertoli cells of androgen-binding protein, cause a high level of testosterone to be maintained in the microenvironment of the developing spermatozoa. The hormonal requirements for initiation of spermatogenesis appear to be independent but for maintenance of spermatogenesis, testosterone is required. However, if spermatogenesis is to be re-initiated after the germinal epithelium has been allowed to regress completely, then both FSH and testosterone are required.

Transport–Maturation–Storage of Sperm

Although the testis is responsible for sperm production, the epididymis is intimately involved with the maturation, storage and transport of spermatozoa. Testicular spermatozoa are non-motile and are incapable of fertilizing ova. Spermatozoa gain progressive motility and fertilizing ability after passing through the epididymis. The coiled seminiferous tubules terminate within the rete testis, which in turn coalesces to form the efferent ductules. These efferent ductules conduct testicular fluid and spermatozoa into the head of the epididymis. The epididymis consists of a single convoluted tubule that is 5–6 meters in length. The epididymis is divided into the head, body, and tail.

Although epididymal transport time varies with age and sexual activity, the estimated transit time of spermatozoa through the epididymis in healthy males is approximately four days. It is during the period of maturation in the head and body of the epididymis, the sperm develop the increased capacity for progressive motility and also acquire the ability to penetrate oocytes during fertilization. The epididymis also serves as a reservoir or storage area for sperm. It is estimated that the extragonadal sperm reservoir is 440 million spermatozoa and that more than 50% of these are located in the tail of the epididymis. The sperms that are stored in the tail of the epididymis enter the vas deferens which is a muscular duct 30–35 cm in length. The contents of the vas are propelled by peristaltic motion into the ejaculatory duct. Sperms are then transported to the outside of the male reproductive tract by emission and ejaculation.

During emission, secretions from the seminal vesicles and prostate are deposited into the posterior urethra. Prior to ejaculation, peristalsis of the vas deferens and bladder neck occurs under sympathetic nervous control. During ejaculation, the bladder neck tightens and the external sphincter relaxes with the semen being propelled through the urethra via rhythmic contractions of the perineal and bulbourethral muscles. It is true that the first portion of the ejaculate contains a small volume of fluid from the vas deferens which is rich in sperm. The major volume of the seminal fluid comes from the seminal vesicles and secondarily the prostate. The seminal vesicles provide the nourishing substrate fructose as well as prostaglandins and coagulating substrates. A recognized function of the seminal plasma is its buffering effect on the acidic vaginal environment. The **coagulum** formed by the ejaculated semen liquefies within 20 to 30 minutes as a result of prostatic proteolytic enzymes. The prostate also adds zinc, phospholipids, spermine, and phosphatase to the seminal fluid. The first portion of the ejaculate characteristically contains most of the spermatozoa and most of the prostatic secretions, while the second portion is composed primarily of seminal vesicle secretions and fewer spermatozoa.

FERTILIZATION

Fertilization normally takes place within the uterine tubes after ovulation has occurred. During the menstrual mid-cycle, the cervical mucus changes to become more abundant, thinner and more watery. These changes serve to facilitate entry of the sperm into the uterus and to protect the sperm from the highly acidic vaginal secretions. Physiologic changes in the spermatozoa known as **capacitation** occur within the female reproductive tract in order for fertilization to occur. As the sperm cell interacts with the egg, there is initiation of new flagellar movement called hyperactive motility and morphologic changes in the sperm that result in release of lytic enzymes and exposure of parts of the sperm's structure known as the **acrosome reaction**. As a result of these changes, the fertilizing sperm cell is able to reach the oocyte, traverse its various layers, and become incorporated into the ooplasm of the egg.

Clinical Findings

History

The cornerstone of the evaluation of infertile man is a careful history and physical examination.

a. **Specific childhood illnesses** should be sought including cryptorchidia, postpubertal mumps orchitis and testicular trauma or torsion. Precocious puberty may indicate the presence of an adreno-genital syndrome, whereas delayed puberty may indicate Klinefelter's syndrome or idiopathic hypogonadism.

b. Prenatal exposure to diethylstilbesterol should be ascertained because this may cause an increased incidence of epididymal cysts or a slightly increased frequency of cryptorchidism.

c. A detailed history of exposure to occupational and environmental toxins, excessive heat, or radiation should be elicited. Cancer chemotherapy has a dose-dependent and potentially devastating effect on the testicular germinal epithelium.

d. The drug history should be reviewed for anabolic steroids, cimetidine and spironolactone which can affect the reproductive cycle. Medications like sulfasalazine and nitrofurantoin may affect sperm motility. Illicit drugs and excessive alcohol consumption are associated with a decrease in sperm count and hormonal abnormalities.

e. **Previous medical diseases** and their treatment may occasionally compromise reproductive function. Men with unilateral undescended testes will have overall semen quality of considerably less than normal. Diabetic neuropathy may result in either retrograde ejaculation or impotence. In patients with cystic fibrosis, the vas deferens or epididymis and seminal vesicles are usually absent. The ejaculate may be affected for three months after the event, as spermatogenesis takes about 74 days from initiation to the appearance of mature sperm.

f. Previous surgical procedures such as bladder neck operations or retroperitoneal lymph node dissection for testicular cancer may cause retrograde ejaculation or absent emission. Both the vas deferens and the testicular blood supply can easily be injured during hernia repair.

g. Sexual habits including frequency of intercourse, frequency of ejaculation, use of coital lubricants and the patient's understanding of the ovulatory cycle should be discussed.

h. Previous infertility evaluation and treatment and the reproductive history from previous marriages should be ascertained.

i. A history of recurrent respiratory infections and infertility may be associated with the immotile cilia syndrome, in which the sperm count is normal but the spermatozoa are completely non-motile due to ultrastructural defects. **Kartagener's syndrome**, which is a variant of immotile cilia syndrome, consists of chronic bronchiectasis, sinusitis, situs inversus and immotile spermatozoa. In **Young's syndrome**, also associated with pulmonary disease, the cilia ultrastructure is normal but the epididymis is obstructed due to inspissated material and these patients present with azoospermia.

j. Loss of libido associated with headaches, visual abnormalities and galactorrhea may suggest a pituitary tumor.

h. Other medical problems that have been associated with infertility include thyroid disease, seizure disorders (use of phenytoin which suppress FSH), and liver disease. Chronic systemic diseases, such as renal disease and sickle cell disease, are associated with abnormal reproductive hormonal parameters.

Physical Examination

During the physical examination, particular attention should be paid to discerning features of hypogonadism. Typically this would be viewed as poorly developed secondary sexual characteristics, eunuchoidal skeletal proportions, i.e. arm span two inches greater than height, ratio of upper body segment (crown to pubis) to lower body segment (pubis to floor) less than 1, and the lack of normal male hair distribution, i.e. sparse axillary, pubic, facial, and body hair in conjunction with lack of temporal hair recession. One should also lookout for infantile genitalia, i.e. small penis, testes, and prostate with underdeveloped scrotum.

A careful examination of the testes is an essential part of the examination. Normal adult testes are on the average about 4.5 cm long and 2.5 cm wide with a mean volume of about 20 cc. A caliper or orchidometer may be used to measure testicular size. If the seminiferous tubules are damaged before puberty, the testes are small and firm. With postpubertal damage, they are usually small and soft.

Gynecomastia is a consistent feature of a feminizing state. Men with congenital hypogonadism may have associated midline defects such as anosmia, color blindness, cerebellar ataxia, hair lip, and cleft palate. Hepatomegaly may be associated with problems of hormonal metabolism. Proper neck examination may help rule out thyromegaly, a bruit or nodularity associated with disease. Neurologic examination should test the visual fields and reflexes.

Irregularities in the epididymis suggest a previous infection and possible obstruction. Examination may reveal a small prostate with androgen deficiency or slight tenderness (bogginess) in men with prostatic infection. Any penile abnormalities like hypospadias, abnormal curvature, phimosis, should be looked for. The scrotal contents should be carefully palpated with the patient in both the supine and standing positions. Many varicoceles are not visible and may only be discernible when the patient stands or performs the Valsalva maneuver. Varicoceles can often result in a smaller left testis, and a discrepancy in size between the two testes should arouse suspicion. Both vas deferens should be palpated, as 2% of infertile men have congenital absence of the vas and seminal vesicles.

Pretesticular Causes of Infertility

Hypothalamic disease
- Isolated gonadotropin deficiency (Kallmann's syndrome)
- Isolated LH deficiency ("Fertile eunuch") Isolated FSH deficiency
- Congenital hypogonadrotropic syndromes

Pituitary disease
- Pituitary insufficiency (tumors, infiltrative processes, operation, radiation)
- Hyperprolactinemia
- Hemochromatosis
- Exogenous hormones (estrogen–androgen excess, glucocorticoid excess, hyper- and hypothyroidism).

Hypothalamic Disease

Kallmann's syndrome which is an **isolated gonadotropin (LH and FSH) deficiency** occurs in both a sporadic and familial form and although uncommon, i.e. 1 in 10,000 men, it is second to Klinefelter's syndrome as a cause of hypogonadism. The syndrome is often associated with anosmia, congenital deafness, hair lip, cleft palate, craniofacial asymmetry, renal abnormalities, color blindness with testes less than 2 cm in diameters. The hypothalamic hormone GnRH appears to be absent. If exogenous GnRH is administered, both LH and FSH are released from the pituitary. Except for the gonadotropin deficiency, anterior pituitary function is intact. The syndrome appears to be inherited either as an autosomal recessive trait or an autosomal dominant trait with incomplete penetrance.

"**Fertile eunuchs**" are individuals with **isolated LH deficiency.** They have eunuchoid proportions with variable degrees of virilization and gynecomastia. They characteristically have large testes and semen containing a few sperm. Plasma FSH levels are normal but both the serum LH and testosterone concentrations are low normal. The cause appears to be a partial gonadotropin deficiency in which there is adequate FSH to stimulate testosterone production with resultant spermatogenesis but insufficient testosterone to promote virilization.

In **isolated FSH deficiency** which is rare, patients are normally virilized and have normal testicular size and baseline levels of LH and testosterone. Sperm counts range from zero to a few sperm. Serum FSH levels are low and do not respond to GnRH stimulation.

Congenital hypogonadotropic syndromes are associated with secondary hypogonadism and a multitude of other somatic findings. **Prader-Willi syndrome** is characterized by hypogonadism, hypomentia, hypotonia at birth and obesity. **Laurence-Moon-Bardet-Biedel syndrome** is an autosomal recessive trait characterized by mental retardation, retinitis pigmentosa, polydactyly and hypogonadism. These syndromes are felt to be due to a defect in hypothalamic deficiency of GnRH.

Pituitary Disease

Pituitary insufficiency may result from tumors, infarctions, iatrogenic causes like surgery and radiation or one of several infiltrative processes. If pituitary insufficiency occurs prior to puberty, growth retardation associated with adrenal and thyroid deficiency is the major clinical presentation. Hypogonadism that occurs in sexually mature male usually has its origin in a pituitary tumor. Decreasing libido, impotence and infertility may occur years before symptoms of an expanding tumor, i.e. such as headaches, visual abnormalities, or thyroid/adrenal hormone deficiency is manifested. Once an individual has passed through normal puberty, it takes a long time for secondary sexual characteristics to disappear unless adrenal insufficiency is present. The testes will eventually become small and soft. The diagnosis is made by low serum testosterone levels with low or low normal plasma gonadotropins concentrations. Depending on the degree of panhypopituitarism, plasma corticosteroids will be reduced with plasma TSH and growth hormone levels.

Hyperprolactinemia can cause both reproductive and sexual dysfunction. Prolactin-secreting tumors of the pituitary gland whether from a microadenoma (less than 10 mm) or a macroadenoma, can result in loss of libido, impotence, galactorrhea, gynecomastia and alter spermatogenesis. Patients with a macroadenoma usually first present with visual field abnormalities and headaches. They should undergo CT or MRI scanning of the pituitary and laboratory testing of anterior pituitary, thyroid and renal function. These patients have low serum testosterone levels but basal serum levels of LH and FSH are either low or low normal and reflect an inadequate pituitary response to depressed testosterone.

Approximately 80% of men with **hemochromatosis** have testicular dysfunction. Their hypogonadism may be secondary to iron deposition in the liver or may be primarily testicular as a result of iron deposition in the testes. Iron deposits have also been found in the pituitary, implicating this gland as the major site of abnormality.

Tumors, like *adrenocortical tumors, Sertoli cell tumors, interstitial cell tumors* of the testes, may at times be estrogen-producing. **Androgens** can also suppress pituitary gonadotropin secretion thereby leading to secondary testicular failure. The current use of *anabolic steroids* by certain athletes may result in temporary sterility. Endogenous androgen excess may be due to an androgen-producing adrenocortical tumor or testicular tumor but more likely to congenital adrenal hyperplasia. As a consequence of this disease, the production of androgenic steroids by the adrenal cortex is increased, resulting in premature development of secondary sexual characteristics and abnormal phallic enlargement. The testes fail to mature because of gonadotropin inhibition and are characteristically small. Careful laboratory evaluation is essential. Infertility caused by documented congenital adrenal hyperplasia is treatable with corticosteroids.

Sometimes **glucocorticoid excess** (prednisolone usage) is exogenous in the therapy of ulcerative colitis, asthma, or rheumatoid arthritis. The result is decreased spermatogenesis. The elevated plasma cortisone levels depress LH secretion and can cause secondary testicular dysfunction. Correction of the glucocorticoid excess results in improvement in spermatogenesis.

Hyper- and hypothyroidism can alter spermatogenesis. Hyperthyroidism affects both pituitary and testicular function with alterations in the secretion of releasing hormones and increased conversion of androgens to estrogens.

Testicular Causes of Infertility

- Chromosomal abnormalities (Klinefelter's syndrome, XX disorder (sex reversal syndrome), XYY syndrome)
- Noonan's syndrome (male Turner's syndrome)
- Myotonic dystrophy
- Bilateral anorchia (vanishing testes syndrome)
- Sertoli-cell-only syndrome (germinal cell aplasia)
- Gonadotoxins (drugs, radiation)
- Orchitis
- Trauma
- Systemic disease (renal failure, hepatic disease, sickle cell disease)
- Defective androgen synthesis or action
- Cryptorchidism
- Varicocele

Klinefelter's syndrome is a genetic disorder due to the presence of an extra X chromosome in the male, the common karyotype being either 47XXY which is the classic form or 46XY/47XXY the mosaic form. The incidence is about 1:500 males. Characteristically, these individuals have small, firm testes, delayed sexual maturation, azoospermia and gynecomastia. Because the features of hypogonadism are not evident until puberty, the diagnosis is delayed. The decrease in testicular mass is usually due to sclerosis and hyalinization of the seminiferous tubules. The testes characteristically have a length of less than 2 cm and 12 cc volume. LH and FSH levels are characteristically elevated. Testosterone levels can range from normal to low and decrease with age. Serum estradiol levels are often increased. The higher estrogen levels relative to testosterone cause the feminized appearance in gynecomastia. About 10% of these patients have chromosomal mosaicism. The mosaics have less severe features of Klinefelter's syndrome and may be fertile. Mild mental deficiency and restrictive pulmonary disease occur more frequently in these patients. The infertility is irreversible and later in life most of these men will require androgen replacement therapy for optimal virilization and normal sexual function.

XX disorder or *sex reversal syndrome* is a variant of Klinefelter's syndrome. The signs are similar except for the average height is less than normal, hypospadias is common and a decreased incidence of mental deficiency. These patients have a 46,XX chromosome complement. This paradox is explained by the fact that their cells express H-Y antigen and are presumed to have a Y chromosome somewhere in their genomes. The incidence of the **XYY syndrome** is the same as that of Klinefelter's syndrome but its phenotypic expression is more variable. Semen from these subjects may vary from azoospermia to normal. These patients are excessively tall. A percentage have anti-social behavior. Most have a normal LH and testosterone level with the FSH level dependent on the extent of germ cell damage. There is no treatment for their infertility.

Noonan's syndrome is the male counterpart of Turner's syndrome (X0) and these individuals typically have similar features, i.e. short stature, web neck, low-head ears, cubitus valgus, ocular abnormalities and cardiovascular abnormalities. Most males with Noonan's syndrome have cryptorchidism and diminished spermatogenesis and are infertile. Those with diminished testicular function will have elevated serum FSH and LH levels. They demonstrate on chromosomal analysis a sex chromosome abnormality such as X0/XY mosaicism. There is no treatment for their infertility.

Patients with **myotonic dystrophy** suffer from delayed muscle relaxation after initial contraction. The major clinical features also include lenticular opacities, frontal baldness and testicular atrophy. By inheritance it is autosomal dominant and the expression is variable though 80% develop testicular atrophy. Pubertal development is usually normal and testicular damage occurs later in adult life. Leydig cell function remains normal and there is no gynecomastia.

Bilateral anorchia or *vanishing testes syndrome* is an extremely rare disorder affecting about 1 in 20,000 males. Patients will present at birth with non-palpable testes and sexual immaturity later in life because of the absence of testicular androgens. The karyotype is normal, but LH and FSH levels are elevated and testosterone is extremely low. *In utero,* the testes may have been lost due to torsion, trauma, vascular injury or infection. However, functioning testicular tissue must have been present at least for the first trimester of fetal life in order for the male reproductive ducts and for the external genitalia to differentiate along male lines. These patients have eunuchoid proportions but no gynecomastia. Therapy is directed at replacement of testosterone deficiency by androgenic steroids.

Sertoli-cell-only syndrome or germinal cell aplasia may have several causes including congenital absence of the germ cells, genetic defects, or androgen resistance. Upon testicular biopsy, there will be complete absence of germinal elements. Clinical findings include azoospermia in association with normal virilization, testes of normal consistency but slightly smaller in size, and no gynecomastia. Testosterone and LH levels are normal but FSH levels are usually elevated. Sometimes in patients who have had other testicular disorders like mumps, cryptorchidism or radiation/toxin damage, the seminiferous tubules may also contain only Sertoli cells, but in these men the testes are small and the histologic pattern is more likely to have severe sclerosis and hyalinization as prominent features. There is no treatment for their infertility.

Gonadotoxins like *drugs* and *radiation* can affect the germinal epithelium because it is a rapidly dividing tissue and susceptible to interference of cell division. Cancer chemotherapy has a dose-dependent effect on testicular germinal epithelium. The germinal epithelium appears to be more resistant to toxic drugs before puberty than in adulthood. The alkylating agents, like cyclophosphamide and nitrogen mustard, are toxic to the testes. In some patients, cryopreservation of semen can be performed before cancer chemotherapy is begun. Cyproterone, ketoconazole, spironolactone and alcohol all interfere with testosterone synthesis. Cimetidine is a testosterone antagonist, blocking peripheral testosterone action. These men will often present with gynecomastia and decreased sperm counts.

Germ cells are particularly sensitive to radiation while the Leydig cells are relatively resistant. At exposures below 600 rads, germ cell damage is reversible but above this level of exposure permanent damage is likely. Recovered spermatogenesis may take up to 2–3 years even in men who receive low doses of radiation. Elevated FSH levels reflect the impaired spermatogenesis, with return to normal once the testes recover.

Orchitis: About 15–25% of adult men who contract mumps can develop **orchitis** which is more commonly unilateral though bilateral involvement occurs in about 10% of affected men. Testicular atrophy can develop within 1 to 6 months or may take years. Fewer than one-third of men with bilateral orchitis recover normal semen parameters.

Trauma: The exposed position of the testicles make them susceptible to **trauma** and subsequent atrophy. Iatrogenic injury may occur during inguinal surgery and interfere with testicular blood supply or damage the vas deferens.

Systemic diseases, like **renal failure** resulting in uremia in males, are associated with decreased libido, impotence and altered spermatogenesis and gynecomastia. LH and FSH levels are elevated and testosterone levels are decreased. The cause of hypogonadism in uremia is probably multifactorial. It has been found that serum prolactin levels are elevated in one-fourth of the patients. An excess in estrogen may be responsible. Antihypertensive drugs and uremic neuropathy may also play a role in uremic impotence and hypogonadism. After successful renal transplantation, uremic hypogonadism improves. A large percentage of males with **cirrhosis of the liver** have testicular atrophy, impotence and gynecomastia. Testosterone levels are decreased. Estradiol is increased as a result of decreased hepatic extraction of androgens with increased conversion to estrogen peripherally. LH and FSH levels are only moderately elevated relative to the low serum testosterone levels. Ethanol also acutely reduces testosterone levels by inhibiting testicular testosterone synthesis.

Many men with **sickle cell disease** have evidence of hypogonadism. Even though LH and FSH levels may be variable, testosterone levels are low. Hypogonadism of sickle cell disease is likely secondary to a mixture of testicular and pituitary-hypothalamic causes.

Rare heredity disorders due to enzymatic defects can result in **defective testosterone synthesis** and are associated with inadequate virilization that is evident at birth as ambiguous genitalia. Several forms of **androgen resistance** result in under masculinization and infertility in males with otherwise normally developed external genitalia. Diagnosis is made by the finding of abnormal androgen receptors in a culture of genital skin fibroblasts. Characteristically, there is an elevation of testosterone and LH levels and there is no treatment for their infertility.

Cryptorchidism is a common developmental defect with incidence of 0.8% in adult males. The undescended testes become morphologically abnormal after age of 2 years. Though in spite of prophylactic orchidopexy, unilateral cryptorchid patients have reduced fertility potential. It appears that in the cryptorchid individual, there is dysgenesis of both the normally and abnormally descended testis. Semen quality is particularly poor in patients with bilateral undescended testicles though baseline serum FSH, LH and testosterone levels may be high or normal.

A scrotal varicocele is the most common causative finding in infertile men. It results from backflow of blood secondary to incompetent or absent valves in the spermatic veins. This valvular deficiency combined with the long vertical course of the internal spermatic vein on the left side, leads to the formation of most varicoceles on the left side (90%). Varicoceles are not commonly seen on the right side because of the oblique course of the right internal spermatic vein from the vena cava. A unilateral right-sided varicocele suggests venous thrombosis/tumor or situs inversus. Newer diagnostic tests have shown the incidence of bilateral varicoceles to be greater than 40%. The incidence of varicoceles in the adult male population is approximately 20% and in the infertile population approximately 40%. 50% of men with varicoceles will have impaired semen quality.

To explain the abnormalities in spermatogenesis with varicocele, the following theories have been proposed:
1. Elevation of testicular temperature due to venous stasis
2. Etrograde flow of toxic metabolites from the adrenal or kidney
3. Blood stagnation with germinal epithelial hypoxia
4. Alterations in the hypothalamic-pituitary-gonadal axis.

Unfortunately, at least 25–40% of infertile men have idiopathic infertility for which no cause can be identified.

Post-testicular Causes of Infertility

Disorders of sperm transport
- Congenital disorders
- Acquired disorders
- Functional disorders

Disorders of sperm motility or function
- Congenital defects of the sperm tail
- Maturation defects
- Immunologic disorders
- Infection

Sexual dysfunction

Disorders of Sperm Transport

Congenital disorders of sperm transport are rarely due to absence or atresia of portions of the male ductal system. Males with cystic fibrosis have a high incidence of congenital hypoplasia or absence of the major portion of the epididymis, vas deferens, and seminal vesicles. Absence of the seminal vesicles is always associated with azoospermia, and absence of fructose. In Young's syndrome which is associated with pulmonary disease, the ultrastructure of the cilia is normal but the epididymis is obstructed due to inspissated material leaving these patients azoospermic.

Acquired disorders of sperm transport are usually due to bacterial infections which may acutely or chronically involve the epididymis with subsequent scarring and obstruction. Apart from vasectomy, the vas may accidentally be ligated during hernia repair, orchidopexy, and even during varicocelectomy.

Functional obstruction of sperm transport results from **neuropathic** insults like injuries to the sympathetic nerves during retroperitoneal lymph node dissection or pelvic surgery. This may cause lack of peristalsis of the vas deferens with resultant lack of emission and/or failure of the bladder neck to close at the time of ejaculation leading to retrograde ejaculation. **Diabetic males with autonomic neuropathy** frequently present with both erectile dysfunction and/or retrograde ejaculation. **Spinal cord injury** can result in paraplegia or quadriplegia with resultant erectile dysfunction and lack of emission and ejaculation. There are many medications such as tranquilizers, antidepressants, and antihypertensives that may interfere with the sympathetic nervous system as well.

Disorders of Sperm Motility or Function

Disorders of sperm motility and function exist secondary to problems that include congenital defects of the sperm tail, maturation defects and immunologic defects.

Immotile cilia syndrome is a group of disorders characterized by immotility or poor motility of spermatozoa (Kartagener syndrome). In these disorders, testicular biopsy is normal and the sperm count is adequate but sperm motility is either markedly reduced or absent. The defective structural abnormality leading to impairment of both the cilia and spermatozoa is seen only with the electron microscope. The defects known to cause immotile cilia syndrome include absent dynein arms, short or absent spokes with no central sheath and missing central microtubules. Motility problems may also be associated with deficiency of the protein carboxylmethylase in the tail of the sperm. Normal sperm counts with poor motility following vasectomy reversal may be a result of **epididymal dysfunction**. Chronic intratubular pressure following vasectomy may have a deleterious effect on the epididymis such that spermatozoa may not gain their usual maturation and capacity for motility. Breakdown of the blood–testes barrier by infection, trauma or operation allows sensitization of the spermatozoa antigens. **Sperm antibodies** may be a relative cause of infertility in about 3–7% of infertile males. Immunity does not appear to be an all-or-none phenomenon but may contribute to reduced fertility potential.

Infections: High concentrations of gram-negative bacteria like *E. coli* in the semen can impair sperm motility. Sexually transmitted organisms such as *Chlamydia trachomatis, Mycoplasma hominis* and *Ureaplasma urealyticum* have rarely been implicated in reproductive failure though there is no convincing evidence to support the use of routine cultures or empirical therapy in asymptomatic infertile males.

Sexual dysfunction has been reported in 20% of infertile males. Decreased sexual drive, erectile dysfunction, premature ejaculation, performance anxiety and failure of intromission are all potentially correctable causes of reproductive failure. Decreasing libido and erectile dysfunction may reflect low serum testosterone levels with an organic cause.

Diagnostic Testing

Semen Analysis (Table 12.1)

A carefully performed semen analysis is highly predictive indicator of the functional status of the male reproductive hormonal cycle, spermatogenesis and the patency of the reproductive tract. Clinical studies of infertile patients have established ″**limits of adequacy**″ below which the chance of spontaneous pregnancy becomes more difficult. These parameters are not absolute because some fertile men may have values below these ″limits of adequacy″. Conversely, infertile men may have normal semen parameters by standard analysis techniques but standard evaluation does not assess the functional integrity of the sperm.

The semen specimen is best obtained by masturbation after a two to three day period of abstinence. The specimen should be assessed within 30 minutes of collection. Samples obtained by coitus interruptus or from silastic condoms devoid of spermatocidal agents are less desirable but satisfactory. Therefore, collection at the site of analysis is ideal. Besides laboratory error, there are variations in sperm density, motility and morphology among multiple samples from a given man. Abstinence intervals give large source of variability. With each day of abstinence (up to one week), semen volume increases by 0.4 cc, sperm concentration by 10–15 million per cc, and total sperm count by 50–90 million. Sperm motility and morphology appear to be unaffected by 5–7 days of

abstinence, but longer periods lead to impaired motility. The minimum number of specimens to define good or poor quality of semen is three samples over a 6–8-week interval with a consistent period of abstinence of 2–3 days.

Semen volume assesses total sperm production by the testes. Semen volume per se, however, affects fertility only when it falls below 1.5 cc due to the inadequate buffering of vaginal acidity or when the volume is greater than 5 cc. Low volumes may be associated with incomplete collection, retrograde ejaculation, ejaculatory duct obstruction, or androgen deficiency. For most clinicians, a sperm concentration of less than 20 million per cc is the lower limit of normal.

Sperm motility is the single most important measure of semen quality and can be a compensatory factor in men with low sperm counts. Sperm motility is usually rated in two ways—the number of motile sperm as a percentage of the total, and the quality of forward progressive sperm movement, i.e. how fast and how straight the sperm swims. The degree of forward progression is a classification based on the pattern displayed by the majority of motile sperm. It ranges from zero (no movement) to 4 (excellent forward progression). Typically, normal good sample have at least 50% of the sperm with good forward progression. Microscopic evaluation of the liquefied semen may reveal agglutination (clumping) of sperm. Agglutination may be head-to-head, head-to-tail, or tail-to-tail and may suggest an inflammatory or immunologic process.

Sperm Morphology

Morphology is assessed on stained seminal smears and is scored; after viewing at least 100 cells. Typically, at least 30% of the sperm should have normal oval heads, mid-piece and tail. The increased numbers of tapered, amorphous and immature cells represent altered testicular function. Semen from normal men coagulates and then after 20–30 minutes liquefies. Delayed liquefaction of semen greater than 60 minutes may indicate disorders of accessory gland function. Diagnosis of the liquefaction problem should be made, if there is absence of sperm in the post-coital test. If sperms are capable of reaching the cervical mucus, problems of semen liquefaction are not clinically relevant. Increased semen viscosity signifies a disorder of accessory gland function and may affect the accuracy of assessment of both sperm density and motility. It is only clinically relevant when there are very few sperm in the post-coital test.

Table 12.1: Understanding semen analysis (WHO criteria)

Macroscopic semen characteristics (Table 1)

	Source	Volume characteristics
Urethral and bulbourethral glands	0.1–0.2 cc	Viscous, clear
Testes, epididymides, vasa deferentia	0.1–0.2 cc	Sperm present
Prostate	0.5–1.0 cc	Acidic, watery
Seminal vesicles	1.0–3.0 cc	Gelatinous, fructose positive
Complete ejaculate	2.0–5.0 cc	Liquefies in 20–25 min

Commonly used normal semen paramenters (WHO) Table 2

Volume	>2.0 mL
pH	7.2–7.8
Concentration	$>20 \times 10^5$/mL
Mobility	>50%
Morphology	>30% with normal morphology
WBC	$<1 \times 10^5$/mL

Gradation of sperm motility (WHO) Table 3

Type of motility	Score	Classes of spermatozoa motility	Normal value
No movement	0	Rapid progressive class A	>25%
Movement, none forward	1	Progressive class B	>25%
Occasional movement of a few sperm	1+	Class A + B	>50%
Slow, undirected	2	Non-progressive class C	<50%
Slow, directly forward movement	2+	Immotile or static class D	<50%
Fast, but undirected movement	3–		
Fast, direct forward movement	3		
Very fast forward movement	3+		
Extremely fast forward movement	4		

Nomenclature for semen variables (WHO)

Normozoospermia	Normal ejaculate as defined in tables 1, 2 and 3
Oligozoospermia	Sperm concentration fewer than 20×10^6/mL
Asthenozoospermia	Fewer than 50% spermatozoa with forward progression (categories A and B) or fewer than 25% spermatozoa with category A movement
Teratozoospermia	Fewer than 30% spermatozoa with normal morphology
Oligoasthenoteratozoospermia	Signifies disturbance of all three variables (combination of only two prefixes can be used)
Azoospermia	No spermatozoa in the ejaculate
Aspermia	No ejaculate

The presence of **white blood cells** in semen should be noted. It is difficult to differentiate between white blood cells and immature spermatozoa on routine analysis, because both may appear as round cells in the semen. Peroxidase stain and, more recently monoclonal antibodies have been utilized to aid in this differentiation. Excessive white cells (>1 million/cc) may indicate an infection that may contribute to subfertility. If no spermatozoa are observed, a qualitative test for **fructose** should be performed. A low ejaculate volume and lack of fructose, along with failure of the semen to coagulate suggest congenital absence of the vas deferens and seminal vesicles or obstruction of the ejaculatory ducts. Fructose is androgen-dependent and is produced in the seminal vesicles.

Computer-assisted semen analysis (CASA) systems couple video technology and sophisticated microcomputers for automatic image digitalization and processing. CASA permits the measurement of additional motility parameters such as curvalinear velocity, straight-line velocity, linearity, and flagellar beat frequency.

WHO Modified Semen Parameters (2010)
(Table 12.2)

Volume: Lower reference limit for semen volume is 1.5 mL. This is a change from previous cut-off value of 2 mL. Low semen volume can be an indicator of obstruction/absence of vas deferens/incomplete collection or ejaculatory dysfunction or androgen deficiency. High semen volume may reflect inflammation of accessory glands.

Table 12.2: Lower reference limits for semen analysis WHO 2010	
Parameter	Lower reference limits (WHO 2010)
Volume (mL)	1.5
Total sperm number (10^6 per ejaculate)	39
Sperm concentration (10^6 per mL)	15
Total motility (%)	40
Progressive motility (%)	32
Vitality (live spermatozoa, %)	58
Sperm morphology (normal forms, %)	4
pH	>7.2
Peroxidase-positive leukocytes (10^6 per mL)	<1.0

Sperm concentration denotes total number of sperm per ejaculate. The lower reference value for sperm concentration is **15 × 10^6 sperm per mL.** This replaces the current limit of 20 × 10^6 per mL. The lower reference value for total sperm number is 39 × 10^6 sperm per ejaculate.

Motility: The percentages of progressive motile sperms (PR), nonprogressive motile (NP) sprems and immotile sperms are calculated. The lower reference range for total motility (PR+NP) is 40% and progressive motility is 32%. This replaces the existing limit of 50%.

Morphology: Spermatozoa consist of head, neck, middle piece, principal piece and endpiece. For spermatozoa to be considered normal, both its head and tail must be normal. All borderline forms should be considered abnormal. **The lower reference value for normal is 4%.** This replaces the current limit of 15%.

Hormone Evaluation

Most cases of male infertility are non-endocrine in origin. Routine evaluation of hormonal parameters is not warranted unless sperm density is extremely low or there is clinical suspicion of an endocrinopathy. The incidence of primary endocrine defects in infertile men is **less than 3%.** Such defects are rare in men with a sperm concentration of greater than 5 million per cc.

Because of the episodic nature **of LH** secretion and its short half-life, a single LH determination has an accuracy of ±50%.

Similarly, **testosterone** is secreted episodically in response to LH pulses and has a diurnal pattern with an early morning peak.

Serum FSH has a longer half-life, and these fluctuations are less obvious. A low testosterone level is one of the best indicators of hypogonadism of hypothalamic or pituitary origin. Low LH and FSH values concurrent with low testosterone levels indicate hypogonadotropic hypogonadism. Elevated FSH and LH values distinguish primary testicular failure (hypergonadotropic hypogonadism) from secondary testicular failure (hypogonadotropic hypogonadism). Most patients with primary hypogonadism have severe, irreversible testicular defects. On the other hand, secondary hypogonadism has a hypothalamic or pituitary origin and infertility may be correctable. Elevated FSH levels are usually a reliable indicator of germinal epithelial damage and are usually associated with azoospermia or severe oligospermia, depicting significant and usually irreversible germ cell damage. In azoospermic and severely oligospermic patients with normal FSH levels, primary spermatogenic defects cannot be distinguished from obstructive lesions by hormonal investigation alone. Therefore, scrotal exploration and testicular biopsy should be considered. An elevated FSH level associated with small, atrophic testes implies irreversible infertility and a biopsy is not warranted.

The diagnostic value of **prolactin** measurement is extremely low in men with semen abnormalities unless these are associated with decreased libido, erectile dysfunction, and evidence of hypogonadism.

Individuals with gynecomastia, obesity, history of alcohol abuse, or suspected androgen resistance should have a serum estradiol level. In men with a history of precocious puberty, one should consider **congenital adrenal hyperplasia**. In the common variant (21-hydroxylase deficiency), serum levels of 17-hydroxyprogesterone are elevated. In 11-hydroxylase deficiency, serum 11-deoxycortisol levels are elevated.

In patients with hypogonadotropic hypogonadism, the other pituitary hormones like ACTH, TSH, GH should also be assessed. **Thyroid dysfunction is a rare cause of male infertility and, therefore, routine screening for thyroid abnormality should be discouraged.**

Chromosomal Studies

Subtle genetic studies can be considered in men with severe oligospermia and azoospermia to look for both autosomal and sex chromosomal abnormalities. The diagnostic yield is greatest in men with small testes, azoospermia, and elevated FSH levels.

Immunologic Studies

Antisperm antibodies, although not an absolute cause of infertility, is capable of reducing the likelihood of pregnancy. The concentration of antisperm antibodies in the semen influences the degree of impairment.

Antisperm antibodies do not lyse or immobilize sperm. They interfere with sperm function by simply attaching to the plasma membrane of the spermatozoa. Antisperm antibodies should be suspected in couples with repeated abnormal post-coital tests. Antisperm antibodies, therefore, interfere with normal penetration and transit of sperm through normal cervical mucus.

Immunological factors may also play a role in the pathogenesis of 10–20% cases of "unexplained infertility". The presence of humoral antibodies directed against sperm is not relevant to fertility unless these circulating antibodies are also present within the reproductive tract. The immunobead binding test (IBT) is one of the most informative and specific of all assays currently available to detect antisperm antibodies bound to the surface of sperm.

Sperm Function Tests

Sperm–Cervical Mucus Interaction

The post-coital test assesses the ability of sperm to penetrate and progress through cervical mucus. Cervical mucus is examined 2–8 hours after intercourse at the time of expected ovulation. The presence of greater than 10–20 motile sperm per high power field is generally accepted as a normal post-coital test. Post-coital testing is a bioassay that provides information concerning sexual function, motility of the sperm, and the sperm–mucus interaction. A positive result implies normal semen and mucus. A poor result in an individual with normal semen parameters implies either cervical abnormality or the presence of sperm antibodies.

Sperm Penetration Assays

Penetration of an oocyte requires sperm capacitation, acrosome reaction, fusion and incorporation into the oocyte. Cross-species fertilization is normally prevented by the zona pellucida. Hamster eggs stripped of the zona pellucida can be penetrated by human sperm. This *in vitro* functional test measures the penetration ability of the sperm. The end point of this assay is penetration of the ovum and decondensation of sperm heads. The percentage of oocytes penetrated and the number of sperm penetrating each oocyte are measured. Sperm that are capable of penetrations per oocyte have greater fertilizing potential than sperm that do not penetrate. The results of the sperm penetration assay (SPA) have primarily been used to predict the results of assisted reproductive techniques, in particular, *in vitro* fertilization. Men with sperm of low SPA score are less likely to achieve a spontaneous pregnancy than those

with a high SPA score. It must be emphasized that the abnormal penetration does not indicate that fertilization cannot occur, nor does good penetration assure fertilization. The general consensus is that less than 10% penetration is evidence of sperm dysfunction and male infertility. Indications for SPA include unexplained infertility, and its use is also recommended prior to assisted reproductive techniques. Although SPA is a reliable indicator of the fertilizing capacity of human spermatozoa, it does not predict the ability of sperm to bind to and penetrate zona pellucida or the sperm's motility and progression in the female reproductive tract.

As SPA with zona free hamster eggs can demonstrate completion of the human sperm acrosome reaction and sperm oocyte plasma membrane fusion, only tests with human zona pellucida can assess the capability of human sperm to bind to the human oocyte. The **hemizona assay** uses zona pellucida from non-living human oocytes that have been microsurgically bisected. Sperm are allowed to interact and bind with the hemizona. The patient's sperm and fertile sperm are compared utilizing the identical halves of hemizona. The results are expressed as the **hemizona index**, i.e. bound sperm by the subfertile man divided by bound sperm from the fertile donor multiplied by 100. This assay requires significant expertise in micro-manipulation. The hemizona assay is not indicated in the routine evaluation of the subfertile man.

Acrosome Evaluation

The acrosome reaction is necessary for fertilization to take place. Evaluating the ability of sperm to undergo the acrosome reaction may provide an additional assessment of sperm function. It is possible to determine the acrosomal status of sperm by utilizing electron microscopy, staining, immunofluorescent techniques and monoclonal antibodies.

Hypo-osmotic Swelling

It has been found that when sperm from normal fertile men are exposed to a known solution of fructose and sodium citrate, 33–80% of the spermatozoa will exhibit tail swelling. Sperm that are not viable or sperm with non-functioning membranes do not swell. This appears to be explained by the ability of the normal cell membrane to maintain an osmotic gradient. Attempts have been made to correlate this finding with the fertilization potential for semen samples. Samples with greater than 62% swelling are able to fertilize ova, whereas less than 60% swelling is observed in samples of infertile semen.

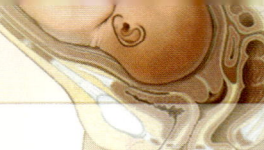

Bacteriological Investigation

If urinalysis is abnormal or bacterial prostatitis is implicated by either the history or physical examination, appropriate cultures are indicated. The common sexually transmitted organisms such as *Chlamydia trachomatis*, *Mycoplasma hominis* and *Ureaplasma urealyticum* have been implicated in reproductive failure in humans. Without evidence of inflammation, there is no indication for routine culture or antibiotic treatment of infertile men.

Testicular Biopsy and Vasography

In azoospermic patients or selected cases of severe oligospermia with normal FSH levels, primary spermatogenic defects cannot be differentiated from obstructive lesions by hormonal investigation alone, and testicular biopsy and sometimes vasography should be considered. When patients have azoospermia or severe oligospermia in conjunction with markedly shrunken testes and serum FSH levels twice normal, testicular biopsy can be avoided as it will indicate untreatable testicular pathology. The exception is the patient who has undergone chemotherapy in whom the elevated FSH level may normalize with return of spermatogenesis. Before biopsy, at least two semen analyses should reveal azoospermia and retrograde ejaculation should be ruled out by examining a post-ejaculatory urine specimen. In men with acidic semen, i.e. pH of less than 7.0 and a volume of less than 1 cc, suspect ejaculatory duct obstruction or congenital absence of the seminal vesicles and vas deferens. For confirmation, seminal fructose levels should be determined. The presence of fructose rules out obstruction or atresia of the ejaculatory ducts but does not verify total ductal patency. The testicular tissue is always placed atraumatically into a container of Bouin's or Zenker's solution. **Formalin should be avoided as it distorts the testicular architecture.**

Vasography (not practised currently) can be used to rule out obstruction of the vas deferens, seminal vesicles, and ejaculatory ducts. Vasography should be performed only at the time of definitive reconstructive surgery. A vasotomy is generally performed at the junction of the straight and convoluted portions of the vas. Any fluid obtained from the vasotomy is evaluated for the presence of sperm. Patency of the ductal structures distal to this point is assessed by the injection of radiopaque contrast solution. Injection of 3–5 cc of 50% Hypaque or Renografin-60 will provide adequate films of the vas, seminal vesicles and ejaculatory ducts. Methylene blue may also be instilled as the bladder is catheterized. The presence of blue or green urine documents patency distal to the instillation site. Retrograde injection of solution towards the testis makes images of the epididymal anatomy that are extremely difficult to interpret. There is also significant risk of causing epididymal injury and should be avoided.

Radiologic Investigation

Both clinical and laboratory investigations have provided convincing evidence that varicoceles are detrimental to spermatogenesis in some men. Because small but clinically significant varicoceles may be missed even on careful physical examination, several diagnostic techniques have been tried.

Color flow duplex ultrasonography measures the diameters of the spermatic cord veins by imaging these vessels, at rest and during a Valsalva maneuver, as well as to quantify and qualify the flow of blood through these veins.

Venography seems to be the most specific method of identification of varicoceles but it is invasive and associated with some morbidity. It is also expensive and so should be reserved for use in recurrent varicoceles for postoperative detection of aberrant veins.

Transrectal ultrasonography (TRUS) is ideally suited now for evaluation of the prostate, seminal vesicles and ejaculatory ducts in patients with azoospermia or low ejaculate volumes. It is accurate, inexpensive and relatively non-invasive. It can provide detailed images of the seminal vesicles and ejaculatory ducts. Vasography and testicular biopsy may be necessary to rule out testicular failure or proximal obstruction, if the transrectal ultrasound study is normal in the azoospermic patient. It may be used in place of vasography to identify obstruction or congenital anomalies of the ejaculatory ducts or seminal vesicles.

Treatment

Surgical Measures

I. *Varicocelectomy:* The relationship between varicocele, altered spermatogenesis, and infertility is widely accepted. Therefore, varicocelectomy is the most common surgical procedure for infertility in males. The term varicocelectomy is actually a misnomer. The procedure should be termed internal spermatic vein ligation, as in varicocelectomy the veins are not actually removed but ligated. This operation improves semen quality in about two-thirds of men and basically doubles the chance of conception. Ligation of varicoceles eliminates testicular venous reflux by interruption of the internal spermatic veins. The operation is usually performed through a small **inguinal** incision though modification of the older **Palomo procedure,** which is a retroperitoneal approach, is certainly acceptable. The **scrotal approach** is not recommended because of the numerous small veins encountered and risk of arterial injury is greater.

Percutaneous venographic occlusion is also an alternative to surgery but small veins outside the spermatic cord that are visualized during an open surgical procedure are not easily embolizable with the percutaneous approach.

Laparoscopic techniques to treat varicoceles are also currently utilized though do not have clear cut advantage over a small inguinal incision. Complications may occur in 3–5% following varicocelectomy which include hydrocele formation, epididymitis, injury to the internal spermatic artery and persistent or recurrent scrotal varicoceles.

II. *Vasovasostomy and epididymovasostomy:* With the application of microsurgical techniques along with the technical advances in magnification and microvascular sutures and needles, the rate of successful reapproximation with sperm present in the ejaculate is 80–90% with a functional success rate/pregnancy rate of 50–60%. Intraoperative predictors of success revolve around the quality of the vasal fluid at the time of vasovasostomy. When clear copious fluid with motile sperm is found, the prognosis for postoperative pregnancy is in the 60–70% range. If no fluid is found or it is thick an epididymovasostomy should preferentially be performed though postoperative pregnancy rate is reduced to 20–30%.

Failures of vasovasostomy may be attributed to anastomotic stenosis in about 10% of patients, antisperm antibodies, epididymal dysfunction, or an unrecognized epididymal tubule "blow-out" with subsequent obstruction.

Epididymal obstruction can be the result of 1) congenital anatomical abnormalities of the vas/epididymis; 2) inflammatory process, and 3) vasal obstruction. It is apparent that the results of microsurgical reconstruction procedures indicate that sperm which traverse greater portions of the epididymis are functionally superior. Therefore, the greater the length of epididymis that the sperm traverse, the better the pregnancy rate.

III. *Transurethral resection of ejaculatory duct (TURE):* Patients who present with azoospermia and even sometimes oligo-asthenospermia, normal sized testes,

and a normal testicular biopsy in conjunction with transrectal ultrasound findings of dilated ejaculatory ducts are good candidates for transurethral resection of the ejaculatory ducts. The orifices of the ejaculatory ducts exit within the prostatic urethra just lateral to the verumontanum. Under anesthesia, they are inspected endoscopically and then can be incised or unroofed. In select cases, transurethral resection of the ejaculatory ducts has resulted in marked improvement in semen parameters, and pregnancies have been achieved.

IV. *Microsurgical epididymal sperm aspiration (MESA):* MESA is an alternative treatment method for obstructive azoospermia in order to obtain sperm from the epididymis with the use of an operating microscope. Its indications include congenital bilateral absence of the vas deferens, bilateral ejaculatory duct obstruction not corrected by transurethral surgery, obstructive azoospermia secondary to surgical removal of the vasal ampullae and seminal vesicles during cystoprostatectomy or radical prostatectomy. MESA is performed in conjunction with either IVF or GIFT and/or assisted fertilization through gamete micromanipulation. Pregnancy rates vary widely ranging from 0 to 20% per attempt.

V. *Ablation of pituitary adenomas:* In selected cases, transsphenoidal surgical ablation of pituitary micro- or macroadenoma may be required in individuals with impotence and a spermatogenic defect associated with elevated prolactin levels.

Prophylactic Surgical Measures

Few undescended testes descend spontaneously after nine months of age. Histological data has shown a progressive decrease in the number of spermatogonia per tubule beginning before the age of two years. Therefore, **orchidopexy** is recommended prior to this age. If undescended testes have failed to respond to medical therapy with hCG injections or intranasal GnRH, then orchidopexy should be performed.

It is certainly important to **detorse a testicular torsion** as soon as possible. A deleterious effect of an infarcted testis on the contralateral healthy testicle is thought to be mediated through an autoimmune process resulting from the breakdown of the intact blood–testis barrier. It is recommended that the non-viable testicle be removed at the time of diagnosis of torsion.

Electroejaculation and Vibratory Stimulation

Ejaculatory dysfunction can result from either a spinal cord injury, retroperitoneal lymph node dissection and other types of retroperitoneal or pelvic surgery, diabetes mellitus, transverse myelitis, multiple sclerosis or psychogenic disorders. Through a rectal probe, an electrical current stimulates the post-ganglionic sympathetic nerve endings that innervate the structures involved in seminal emission and ejaculation. The semen recovered has variable parameters. The specimens are processed and then utilized for either intrauterine insemination or in conjunction with the various assisted reproductive techniques. Reported pregnancy rates approach 30–35%.

It is recommended that **vibratory stimulation** be attempted prior to enrolling a patient in an electroejaculation protocol. This technique involves the use of a high frequency vibrator placed along the glans penis for variable amounts of time ranging from a few minutes to 20 minutes until an ejaculate is produced.

Medical Measures

I. Endocrine Therapy

Infertile men with hypogonadotropic hypogonadism (secondary hypogonadism) are the most appropriate candidates for exogenous gonadotropin therapy. For initiation of spermatogenesis, LH must be given to stimulate the Leydig cells to produce high intratesticular testosterone levels. Therefore, inj. hCG 2,000 IU intramuscularly three times a week is usually effective in stimulating adequate production of testosterone for full virilization. After 8–12 months of hCG therapy, inj. HMG containing 75 IU of FSH and 75 IU of LH is given intramuscularly three times weekly. It takes months for sperm to appear in the ejaculate after initiation of FSH therapy. With the normal response, most patients achieve a sperm count of between 2 and 5 million sperm per ejaculate and then impregnation is possible.

An alternative to exogenous gonadotropin usage is the use of GnRH to stimulate LH and FSH endogenously. GnRH must be given in a pulsatile manner as continuous administration downregulates the pituitary. The initial dosage is 25–50 ng/kg every two hours by a small infusion pump. Pituitary disease is not amenable to GnRH therapy, and combined treatment with hCG and HMG will be necessary.

II. Therapy for Immunologic Infertility

When detectable antisperm antibodies are clinically relevant, treatment is difficult. Results are still unclear as to whether any recommended regimen of **steroid therapy** really lessens either the production or the clinical effects of antisperm antibodies in the male. The risks of this therapy must be weighed against its benefits. Even though complications are generally mild and self-limited, aseptic necrosis of the femur has been reported.

Several methods of semen manipulation have been advocated. The best method is superovulation with **sperm washing** followed by intrauterine insemination with a success rate of 20%. Simple processing methods rely on dilution of the semen and centrifugation followed by resuspension of the sperm pellet in culture medium such as Ham's F10. More elaborate methods of sperm processing include **swim-up procedures**, centrifugation through Percoll **density gradients**. On occasion, the patient's sperm may survive poorly in these procedures and it is desirable to test the semen in advance for the most appropriate preparative method. This is followed by intrauterine insemination.

ART (assisted reproductive techniques): In vitro fertilization (IVF) was originally intended for individuals with tubal disease and female factor unexplained infertility. It has now been expanded to include couples with male factor infertility. Human ova can be fertilized using this technique with concentrations of 20,000 to 100,000 motile sperm. Although male factor patients have a lower fertilization rate compared to non-male factor groups, once fertilization has taken place in male factor couples, the pregnancy rate is as high as in non-male factor couples.

The different techniques followed are:

a. Gamete intrafallopian transfer (GIFT) is a technique in which ova are retrieved in a manner similar to IVF but then the sperm are mixed together with the ova and injected directly into the fallopian tube for fertilization to occur. This technique has a theoretical advantage of allowing fertilization to occur in the fallopian tube.

b. There are other techniques also which include pronuclear stage tubal transfer (PROST), zygote intrafallopian transfer (ZIFT), tubal embryo transfer (TET) and tubal embryo stage transfer (TEST). They all involve the in vitro fertilization of human eggs followed by transfer of the early-stage embryo back into the fallopian tube.

Overall, the pregnancy rate for male factor patients has been reported to range from 10–35%.

III. Therapy for Retrograde Ejaculation

Antegrade ejaculation may be induced by treatment with alpha-adrenergic stimulation using sympathomimetic agents like pseudoephedrine or imipramine. Alkalinization of the bladder urine with oral sodium bicarbonate or citrate and retrieval of sperm from the bladder after ejaculation have been used successfully for artificial insemination.

IV. Treatment of Infection

Individuals with symptomatic or documented genitourinary tract infection should be treated with the appropriate antibiotics. Tetracycline is often the first-line drug of choice.

V. Artificial Insemination

By definition, artificial insemination involves the use of the husband's sperm for insemination. It is particularly useful with low semen volumes or in cases where repeated post-coital tests have shown cervical hostility. There really is no advantage in individuals with oligospermia or asthenospermia. Therapeutic **donor insemination** is by far the most successful and cost-effective form of therapy for couples with male infertility.

Micromanipulation

Despite the success that has been made available with IVF and GIFT, additional refinements have been necessary for patients whose concentration of functional sperm is extremely poor. Micromanipulation of gametes and assisted fertilization allows the surgical manipulation of sperm and ova. The methods of micromanipulation currently utilized include partial zone dissection (PZD), subzonal sperm injection (SZI) and intracytoplasmic sperm injection (ICSI). Overall, fertilization rates range from about 20–40%, with clinical pregnancy rates reported between 10 and 30%.

12B. FEMALE INFERTILITY

Female Factor Infertility

80% of couples will conceive within 1 year of unprotected intercourse whereas 86% conceive within 2 years.

Factors Responsible for Infertility

- Female factor ~40%
- Male factor ~30%
- Combined ~30%

Apart from male factors, female factor infertility can be divided into several categories: Cervical or uterine, ovarian, tubal, and other in the following proportions:

- Sperm disorders 30.6%
- Anovulation/oligoovulation 30%
- Tubal disease 16%
- Unexplained 13.4%
- Cervical factors 5.2%
- Peritoneal factors 4.8%

Detailed History

- Previous pelvic surgery
- PID
- Appendicitis
- IUD use
- Past ectopic pregnancy
- Irregular menses, amenorrhea, detailed menstrual history
- Vasomotor symptoms
- Weight changes
- Exercise
- Cervical and uterine surgery

Physical Examination

- Evidence of Koch's lymphadenopathy
- Thyroid enlargement
- Abdominopelvic/pelvic masses
- Uterine enlargement, tenderness
- Endometriotic cysts
- Uterine mobility, fixed retroversion
- Cervical abnormalities
- Uterosacral nodularity

Cervical Factor Infertility

Cervical factor infertility can be caused by stenosis or abnormalities of the mucus–sperm interaction. The cervix plays a pivotal role in the transport and capacitation of the sperm after intercourse. Cervical factors account for 5–10% of infertility.

At the beginning of the menstrual cycle, cervical mucus is scanty, viscous, and very cellular. The mucus forms a net-like structure that does not allow the passage of sperm. Mucus secretion increases during the mid-follicular phase and reaches its maximum approximately 24–48 hours before ovulation.

The water and salt concentration increases, changing the physical characteristics of the mucus. The mucus becomes thin, watery, alkaline, acellular, and elastic (spinnbarkeit) because of the increased concentration of sodium chloride, despite a fern-like pattern when the mucus is allowed to dry on a cover slide under the microscope (Fig. 12.2).

At this point, the mucus organizes itself, forming multiple microchannels so the spermatozoa can travel through. During this journey, the spermatozoa simultaneously undergo activation and capacitation. In addition, the mucus acts as a filter for abnormal spermatozoa and cellular debris present in the semen.

Mucus secretion may be altered by hormonal changes and medications, especially drugs like clomiphene citrate, which decrease the production. Hypoestrogenism may cause thickened cervical mucus, which impairs the passage of sperm.

Cervical stenosis can cause infertility by blocking the passage of sperm from the cervix to the intrauterine cavity. Cervical stenosis can be congenital or acquired in etiology, resulting from surgical procedures, infections, hypoestrogenism, and radiation therapy.

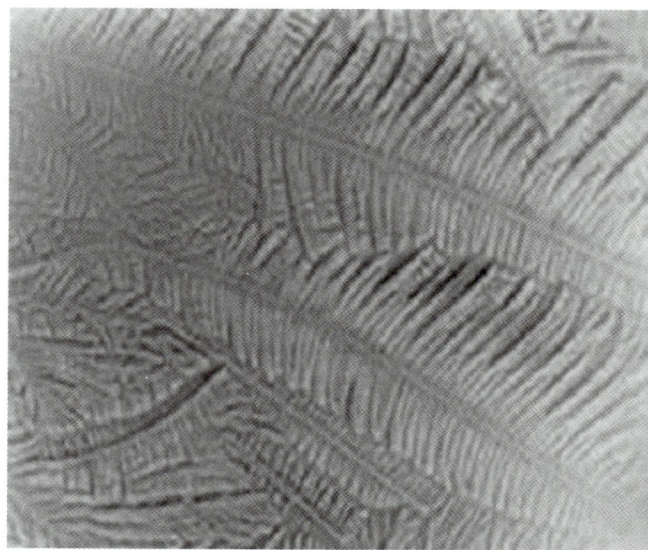

Fig. 12.2: Fern pattern of preovulatory mucus

Uterine Factor Infertility

Uterine factors can be congenital or acquired. They may affect the endometrium or myometrium and are responsible for 2–5% of infertility cases.

Physiology of Implantation

In humans, implantation of a fertilized ovum is most likely to occur about 9 days after ovulation, ranging between 6 and 12 days.

Implantation Window

The reception-ready phase of the endometrium of the uterus is usually termed the "implantation window" and lasts about 4 days. The implantation window follows around 6 days after the peak in luteinizing hormone levels or days 6–10 postovulation. On average, it occurs during the 20th to 23rd day after the last menstrual period.

Adaptation of Uterus

To enable implantation, the uterus goes through changes in order to be able to receive the embryo.

Predecidualization

The endometrium increases thickness, becomes vascularized and its glands grow to be tortuous and boosted in their secretions. These changes reach their maximum about 7 days after ovulation.

Decidualization

Decidualization further develops the uterine glands, the zona compacta and the epithelium of decidual cells lining it. The decidual cells become filled with lipids and glycogen and take the polyhedral shape characteristic for decidual cells. It is likely that the blastocyst itself makes the main contribution to this additional growing and sustaining of the decidua.

Parts of Decidua

The decidua can be organized into following layers, although they have the same composition.

- *Decidua basalis:* This is the part of the decidua which is located basolateral to the embryo after implantation.
- *Decidua capsularis:* Decidua capsularis grows over the embryo on the luminal side, enclosing it into the endometrium. It surrounds the embryo together with decidua basalis.
- *Decidua parietalis:* All other decidua on the uterine surface belongs to decidua parietalis.

After implantation, the decidua remains, at least through the first trimester. Its function is later replaced by the definitive placenta.

Pinopodes

Pinopodes are small, finger-like protrusions from the endometrium. They appear between day 19 and day 21 of gestational age. This corresponds to a fertilization age of approximately 5 to 7 days, which corresponds well with the time of implantation. They only persist for 2 to 3 days. The development of pinopods is enhanced by progesterone but inhibited by estrogens. Pinopodes endocytose uterine fluid and macro-molecules in it. By doing so, the volume of the uterus decreases, taking the walls closer to the embryoblast floating in it.

Adaptation of Secretions (Fig. 12.3)

Apart from structural transformation within the uterus, the secretion from its epithelial glands also changes. This change is induced by increased levels of progesterone from the corpus luteum. This is to provide nourishment to the embryoblast. The embryoblast spends approximately 72 hours in the uterine cavity before implanting. During this time, it cannot receive nourishment directly from the blood of the mother, and must rely on secreted nutrients into the uterine cavity, e.g. iron and fat-soluble vitamins.

Growth and Implantation

In addition to nourishment, the endometrium secretes several steroid-dependent proteins, important for growth and implantation. Implantation is further facilitated by synthesis of matrix substances, adhesion molecules and surface receptors for the matrix substances (Fig. 12.3).

Mechanism of Implantation

Implantation is initiated when the blastocyst comes into contact with the uterine wall.

Zona Hatching

To be able to perform implantation, the blastocyst first needs to get rid of its zona pellucida. This process is called "hatching". Lytic factors in the uterine cavity, as well as factors from the blastocyst itself are essential for this process. The substance probably involved is plasmin. Plasminogen, the plasmin precursor, is found in the uterine cavity and blastocyst factors contribute to its conversion to active plasmin.

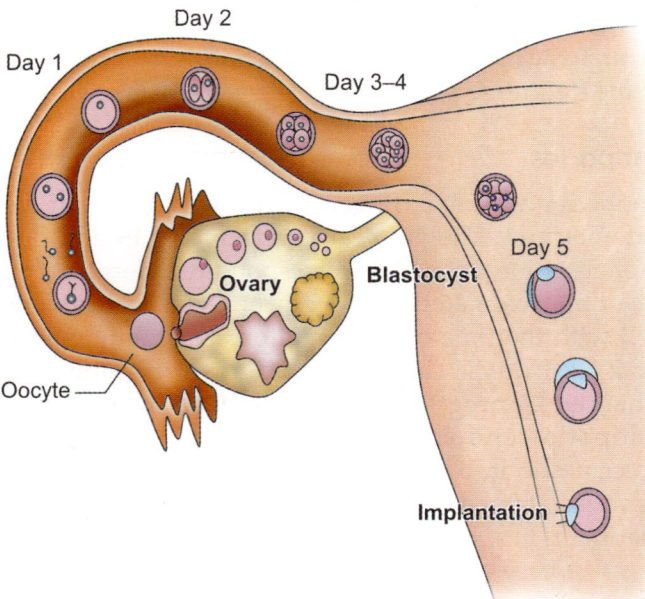

Fig. 12.3: Implantation of blastocyst

Apposition

The very first, but loose, connection between the blastocyst and the endometrium is called the apposition. The apposition is usually made on the endometrium where there is a small crypt in it which increases the area of contact with the spherical blastocyst. On the blastocyst, it occurs at a location where there has been enough lysis of the zona pellucida to have created a rupture to enable direct contact between the underlying trophoblast and the decidua of the endometrium. However, ultimately, the inner cell mass, inside the trophoblast layer, is aligned closest to the decidua. The inner cell mass rotates inside the trophoblast to align to the apposition. In fact, the entire surface of the blastocyst has a potential to form the apposition to the decidua.

Adhesion

Adhesion is a much stronger attachment to the endometrium than the loose apposition. The trophoblasts adhere by penetrating the endometrium, with protrusions of trophoblast cells. The blastocyst signals to the endometrium to adapt further to its presence, e.g. by changes in the cytoskeleton of decidual cells. This, in turn, dislodges the decidual cells from their connection to the underlying basal lamina, which enables the blastocyst to perform the succeeding invasion. This communication is conveyed by receptor–ligand interactions, both integrin-matrix and proteoglycan ones.

Invasion

Invasion is an even further establishment of the blastocyst in the endometrium. The protrusions of trophoblast cells that adhere into the endometrium continue to proliferate and penetrate into the endometrium. As these trophoblast cells penetrate, they differentiate to become a new type of cells, syncytiotrophoblast which refers to the transformation that occurs as the boundaries between these cells disappear to form a single mass of many cell nuclei (a syncytium).

Invasion continues with the syncytiotrophoblasts reaching the basal membrane beneath the decidual cells, penetrating it and further invading into the uterine stroma. Finally, the whole embryo is embedded in the endometrium. Eventually, the syncytiotrophoblasts come into contact with maternal blood and form chorionic villi. This is the initiation of forming the placenta.

Secretions

The blastocyst secretes several autocrine factors which stimulate it to further invade the endometrium.

Autocrine

Human chorionic gonadotropin is an autocrine growth factor for the blastocyst. Insulin-like growth factor 2, on the other hand, stimulates the invasiveness of blastocyst.

The syncytiotrophoblast dislodges decidual cells, both by degradation of cell adhesion molecules linking the decidual cells together as well as degradation of the extracellular matrix between them.

Cell adhesion molecules are degraded by syncytiotrophoblast secretion of **tumor necrosis factor-alpha.** This inhibits the expression of cadherins and beta-catenin. Cadherins are cell adhesion molecules and beta-catenin anchors them to the cell membrane. Inhibited expression of these molecules thus loosens the connection between decidual cells, permitting the syncytiotrophoblasts and the whole embryo with them to invade into the endometrium.

The extracellular matrix is degraded by serine endopeptidases and metalloproteinases. Examples of such metalloproteinases are **collagenases, gelatinases and stromelysins**. These collagenases digest Type-I collagen, Type-II collagen, Type-III collagen, Type-VII collagen and Type-X collagen. The gelatinases exist in two forms; one digest Type-IV collagen and the other one digest gelatin.

The process of trophoblast cell invasion is associated with the degradation of extracellular matrix (ECM) proteins mainly by the action of **matrix metalloproteinases (MMPs),** a family of zinc-dependent proteolytic enzymes. So far, more than 20 isoforms of MMPs have been identified. Based on the substrate specificities, MMPs can be classified into four groups—gelatinases, collagenases, stromelysins and membrane-type MMPs (MT-MMPs). Gelatinases A and B, which are also called MMP-2 and MMP-9 respectively, mainly degrade collagen IV and a number of other ECM proteins, such as Col I, V, VII, IX and X, fibronectin (FN), laminin (LN), elastin and vitronectin.

During early implantation, the placental villi undergo dramatic development, involving villous tissue remodeling. MMP-2, -9 and -14, as well as tissue inhibitors of MMPs (TIMP-1, -2 and -3), are produced by villous CT cells during pregnancy. MMP-2 and -9 are the main proteases responsible for degradation of the basement membranes whereas MMP-14, TIMP-2 and -3 coordinate the reconstruction of the basement membranes beneath the trophoblast epithelium during villous development.

Immunosuppressive

The embryo differs from the cells of the mother, and will be rejected as a parasite by the immune system of the mother, if it does not secrete immunosuppressive agents. Such agents are platelet-activating factor, human chorionic gonadotropin, prostaglandin E₂, Interleukin 1-alpha, Interleukin 6, interferon-alpha, leukemia inhibitory factor and colony-stimulating factor.

Clinical Causes of Implantation Failure

Congenital Defects

- The development of the müllerian ducts accounts for the normal anatomic configuration of the uterus, fallopian tubes, cervix, and upper vagina. The full spectrum of congenital/müllerian abnormalities varies from total absence of the uterus and vagina (Rokitansky-Küster-Hauser syndrome) to minor defects such as arcuate uterus and vaginal septa (transverse or longitudinal).

- Until the early 1970s, diethylstilbestrol (DES) was used to treat patients with a history of recurrent miscarriages. DES was found to be responsible for inducing malformations of the uterine cervix, irregularities of the endometrial cavity (e.g. T-shaped uterus), malfunction of the fallopian tubes, menstrual irregularities, and the development of clear cell carcinoma of the vagina.

- The relationship between müllerian anomalies and infertility is not entirely clear as it does not inhibit fertilization but may be largely responsible for implantation failure and spontaneous miscarriages like in septate and bicornuate uterus.

Acquired Defects

- *Endometritis* associated with a traumatic delivery, dilatation and curettage, intrauterine device, or any instrumentation (e.g. myomectomy, hysteroscopy) of the endometrial cavity may create intrauterine adhesions or synechiae (i.e. Asherman syndrome), with partial or total obliteration of the endometrial cavity.

- *Uterine polyps* may develop from biazzare endometrial proliferation.

- *Submucosal fibroids* may cause distortion of the cavity and compromise the blood supply. They may also be implicated in implantation failure, early miscarriages, premature delivery, and abruptio placentae.

Ovarian Factor Infertility

Oogenesis occurs in the ovary from the first trimester of embryonic life and is completed by 28–30 weeks of gestation. By then, approximately 7 million oocytes are present. They are arrested at the prophase stage of the first meiosis division. Subsequently, the number of oocytes decreases because of a continuous process of atresia. At birth, the pool of oocytes is reduced to approximately 2 million. By menarche, approximately 500,000 oocytes are present. Those oocytes are used throughout the reproductive years until menopause.

The ovulatory process is initiated once the hypothalamus-pituitary-ovarian axis matures and follicle-stimulating hormone (FSH) and luteinizing hormone (LH), under the regulation of gonadotropin-releasing hormone (GnRH), acquire their normal secretory patterns.

Ovulatory dysfunction is defined as an alteration in the frequency and duration of the menstrual cycle. A normal menstrual cycle lasts 25–35 days, with an average of 28 days. Failure to ovulate is the most common infertility problem. Anovulation or oligo-ovulation is often associated with primary amenorrhea, secondary amenorrhea, or oligomenorrhea.

Ovulatory dysfunction can be divided into 2 categories—hypergonadotropic hypogonadism and hypogonadotropic hypogonadism.

Hypergonadotropic hypogonadism is often related to early gonadal development failure, as in Turner syndrome, where the karyotype 45,XO or other chromosomal abnormalities like 46,XX (associated with partial deletions of the short or long arm of one of the X chromosomes) and mosaicism (e.g. 45X/XX); pure gonadal dysgenesis (46,XX; 46,XY). These patients present with a small uterus and normal fallopian tubes and vagina. This condition is associated with elevated FSH and LH levels and low estrogen levels. Hypergonadotropic hypogonadism is also seen in patients with a history of treatment with certain alkylating chemotherapy or pelvic radiation.

Ovulatory dysfunction also occurs in patients with hypothalamic failure (hypogonadotropic hypogonadism) secondary to inadequate GnRH synthesis, neurotransmitter defects, or isolated gonadotropin insufficiency. Chronic disease conditions, high levels of stress, and starvation or malnutrition are other possible etiologies.

Secondary amenorrhea is the absence of menses for more than 6 months in a woman who has previously menstruated. Pregnancy should always be ruled out first. In the absence of pregnancy, this condition is related to dysfunction of the endocrine system and can be related to thyroid, adrenal, and pituitary disorders, including tumors. One common cause of secondary amenorrhea is premature ovarian failure, which is the loss of ovarian function by the age of 40.

Oligomenorrhea is dysfunction of the hypothalamus-pituitary-ovarian axis and is the most common ovulatory disorder associated with infertility. Patients with this disorder present with a history of irregular menstrual cycles that fluctuate from 35 days to 2–5 months sometimes associated with a history of dysfunctional uterine bleeding or prolonged periods of breakthrough bleeding. Patients may have symptoms of hyperandrogenism, acne, hirsutism, and baldness. Obesity is frequently associated and aggravates the prognosis. Many of these women have polycystic ovarian syndrome.

Advanced Age

The prevalence of infertility rises dramatically as age increases. Furthermore, fertility decreases with marriage duration because of less frequent intercourse. Fertility appears to be stable until age 35 years, declines slightly until age 40 years, and is followed by a sharp decline after age 42 years. Infertility rates are 11% after age 34, 33% after age 40 and 87% at age 45.

Tubal Factors

Tubal disease is responsible for 25–35% of female infertility. It may involve the proximal, distal or the entire tube and may be transient (obstruction), or permanent (occlusion). Pelvic inflammatory disease is the most common cause of tubal disease representing more than 50% cases and may affect fallopian tube at multiple sites. After one episode of PID rate of infertility is 11% which increases to 23% and 54% after two and three episodes, respectively.

Proximal Tubal Disease

The causes of proximal tubal disease include intratubal debris, congenital malformation, endometriosis and salpingitis ischemica nodosa (SIN). With SIN, diverticulae of the intramural or proximal ischemic endosalpinx enlarge and obliterate the tubal lumen. SIN is bilateral in most affected patients. Tubal polyps also can cause transient proximal tubal blockage whereas tubal endometriosis may affect the intramural portion of the tube and is present in 7–14% of patients with tubal factor infertility.

Distal Tubal Disease

This is usually caused by multiple factors including salpingitis, adhesion from previous surgery and endometriosis. It is classified as mild, moderate and severe categories based on the size of hydrosalpinx, extent of adhesions, degree of fimbrial preservation and appearance of endosalpinx on HSG.

Peritoneal Factors

The uterus, ovaries, and fallopian tubes share the same space within the peritoneal cavity. Anatomical defects or physiologic dysfunctions of the peritoneal cavity, including infection, adhesions, and adnexal masses, may cause infertility. Pelvic inflammatory disease, peritoneal adhesions secondary to previous pelvic surgery, endometriosis, and ovarian cyst rupture all compromise the motility of the fallopian tubes or produce blockage of the fimbriae with development of hydrosalpinx. Large myomas, pelvic masses, or blockage of the cul-de-sac interferes with peritoneal fluid current and normal oocyte pickup mechanism. Periovarian adhesions that encapsulate the ovary interfere with the normal oocyte release at ovulation to become a mechanical factor for infertility. Pelvic inflammatory disease and endometriosis are the two most important peritoneal factors for infertility.

I. Pelvic Inflammatory Disease

Pelvic inflammatory disease (PID) is associated with gonorrhea, chlamydia and tuberculosis infection. The rate of damage to the fallopian tubes increases with subsequent PID episodes, from 34% for the first episode to 54% in women with second and third episodes. PID can be diagnosed clinically and confirmed by results from cervical culture and serologic antibody assays for gonorrhea and chlamydia.

II. Endometriosis

- Endometriosis remains an enigmatic disease that affects women during their reproductive years. The incidence increases with patient age and low parity.
- Classically, endometriosis appears as bluish-black pigments (i.e. "powder-burn lesions") that affect the peritoneal surfaces of the bladder, ovary, fallopian tubes, cul-de-sac, and bowel. Nonclassic endometriosis may appear as red, or white lesions and vesicles. The final diagnosis should be confirmed by demonstrating endometrial stroma and glands in biopsy tissue.
- The incidence of endometriosis in primary and secondary infertility is around 26% and 13%, respectively.
- Severe endometriosis with damage to the fallopian tubes and ovaries due to permanent block in adhesions or the presence of endometriomas is an obvious cause of infertility.
- Minimal and mild endometriosis is hypothesized to reduce fertility despite anatomical normalcy by the following mechanisms:
  - Increased peritoneal macrophages that increase phagocytosis of the sperm.
  - Decreased sperm binding to the zona pellucida.
  - Abnormal peritoneal currents.
  - Failure in ovum pick up by fimbria due to periadnexal adhesion.
  - Increased immunoglobulin production.
  - Defective natural killer activity.
- Endometriosis is associated with ovulatory disorders such as luteal phase deficiency (LPD), oligo-ovulation, and luteinized unruptured follicle (LUF) syndrome.

Evaluation of the Female Partner

A complete evaluation of the female reproductive tract must include cervical, uterine, endometrial, tubal, peritoneal, and ovarian factors.

Cervical Factors

The postcoital test (PCT), also known as the Sims-Huhner test, consists of evaluating the amount of spermatozoa and its motility within the cervical mucus during the preovulatory period. This test is no longer routinely performed in the standard infertility workup because it has limited diagnostic potential and poor predictive value. The mere presence of sperms within the cervical mucus does not predict its fertilizable quality.

Cervical stenosis can be diagnosed during a speculum examination. Complete cervical stenosis is confirmed by the inability to pass a 1–2 mm probe into the uterine cavity.

Uterine Factors

Many defects can be detected during the pelvic examination. These include absence of the vagina and uterus, vaginal septum, and the presence of fibroids. Detection of most defects requires ancillary studies such as HSG, pelvic ultrasonography, hysterosonogram, and MRI. Operative procedures, such as laparoscopy and hysteroscopy, are often necessary for confirmation of the final diagnosis.

Saline Infusion Sonography

Saline infusion sonography (SIS) provides a simple and inexpensive means to evaluate the uterine cavity and assess tubal patency. It is well-tolerated by patients and can be done in the office. Additionally, it eliminates the risks associated with the use of dye and radiation required by the HSG. SIS can reveal intracavitary abnormalities and uterine anomalies in infertile patients (Fig. 12.4).

Procedure

- SIS should be performed during cycle days 6–12 so that the endometrium is thin, allowing better detection of intrauterine lesions. In addition, this ensures that an undiagnosed pregnancy is not disrupted.

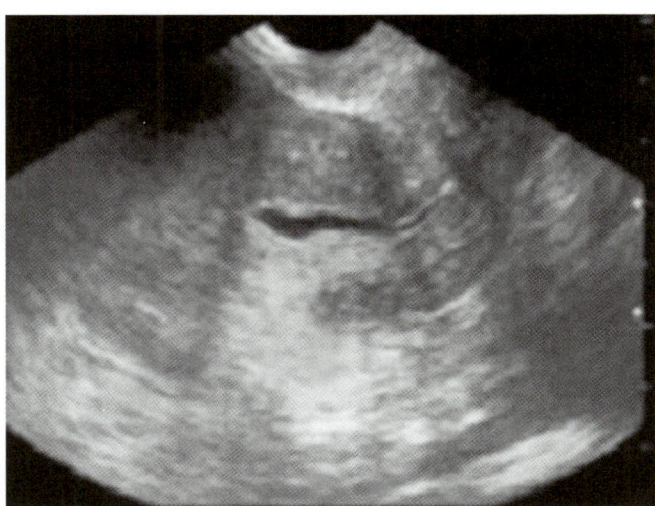

Fig. 12.4: Saline infusion sonography

- A speculum is placed and the cervix is cleansed with betadine solution. A transcervical Foley catheter with balloon is placed. The speculum is removed and saline is injected under ultrasonographic visualization. Longitudinal and transverse views of the cavity are evaluated for filling defects. Finally, a small amount of air bubbles are injected to assess tubal patency.
- If the patient has a history of genital tract infection or pelvic inflammatory disease, antibiotics may be given before and after the procedure particularly, if hydrosalpinges are noted.
- While the SIS can confirm tubal patency, it does not provide information about the contour of the tubes. Thus, if a patient has a history of endometriosis or other tubal disease, HSG would be preferred.

Hysteroscopy (Figs 12.5 to 12.8)

Hysteroscopy is a method of direct visualization of the endometrial cavity. Carbon dioxide and saline hysteroscopy is used for diagnostic purposes only. It does not require cervical dilatation and allows a rather easy evaluation of the endometrial cavity. The operative hysteroscope with resectoscope allows both the diagnosis and treatment of endometrial pathology. The instruments (e.g. scissors, cautery loops, lasers) facilitated the treatment of pathologies such as uterine synechiae, endometrial polyps, submucous myomas, and the removal of foreign bodies (e.g. intrauterine devices). In combination with specially designed catheters, it can be used to perform tubal cannulation.

Endometrial Biopsy

- This was a usual practice to determine the functional status of the endometrium in relation to the menstrual cycle. The diagnosis of luteal phase dysfunction is based on the finding of more than 2 days 'out of phase' endometrium on histology in 2 successive cycles though the importance of 'LPD' is not very clear.
- Endometrial sample for evaluation of endometrial tuberculosis by BACTEC test, AFB culture and DNA/RNA PCR for Myc. TB antigen has currently gained importance.

Magnetic Resonance Imaging

The use of MRI has increased in recent years, although it should be limited to those patients in whom a definitive diagnosis cannot be ascertained by conventional HSG, ultrasonography, and hysteroscopy findings. MRI is useful for delineating complex pelvic masses.

Tubal and Peritoneal Factors

The two most frequent tests used for diagnosis of tubal pathology are laparoscopy and hysterosalpingogram.

Hysterosalpingogram

- HSG is the most frequently used diagnostic tool to evaluate the endometrial cavity. A meticulous and well-executed procedure, performed under fluoroscopy, provides accurate information about the (1) endocervical canal, (2) diameter and configuration of the internal os, (3) endometrial cavity, (4) uterine/tubal junction (cornual ostium), (5) diameter, location, and direction of the fallopian tubes, (6) status of the fimbriae, and (7) spill into the endometrial cavity. Furthermore, HSG provides indirect evidence of pelvic adhesions and uterine, ovarian, or adnexal masses.
- HSG should be performed during the early follicular phase. At this time, the endometrium is thin and HSG provides better delineation of minor defects. In addition, the possibility of accidental irradiation to the fetus in an undiagnosed pregnancy is eliminated.
- The cervix is cleansed with a povidone-iodine solution (Betadine) to avoid the transfer of bacteria to the endometrial cavity during the procedure. A vaginal speculum is used to retract the vagina and a single-tooth tenaculum is used to apply traction of the uterus and to correct any anteflexion or retroflexion that yields suboptimal images. Radiocontrast media of about 10–15 mL is instilled through a metallic cannula tightly fitted in the cervical canal. The use of water-based contrast media is preferable to oil-based media to avoid the risks of oil embolism and granuloma formation. Figures 12.9 to 12.19) depict HSG findings in different intrauterine defects.

Laparoscopy (Fig. 12.20)

- Laparoscopy though is an useful modality for infertility evaluation when abnormalities are found on ultrasonography, HSG or suspected by clinical examination. Because of the added risks of surgery, need for anesthesia, and operative cost, it is only used when clearly indicated.
- Laparoscopy is contraindicated in patients with probable bowel obstruction and bowel distention, cardiopulmonary disease. Relative contraindications include massive obesity, large abdominal mass or advanced pregnancy, severe pelvic adhesions, and peritonitis. Figures 12.21 to 12.26 show laparoscopic findings in different clinical situations.

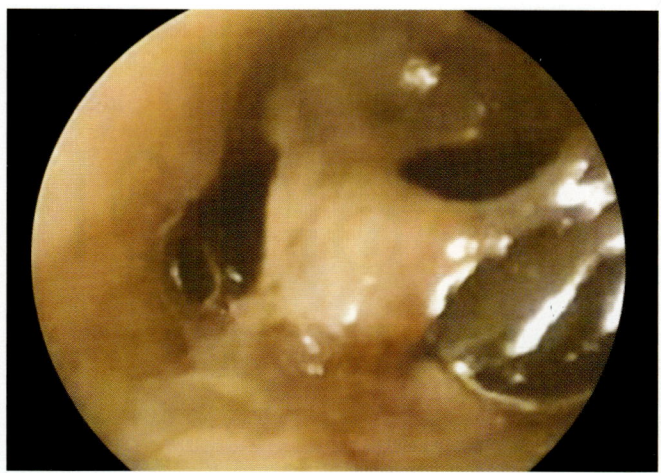

Fig. 12.5: Hysteroscopy—uterine synechiae

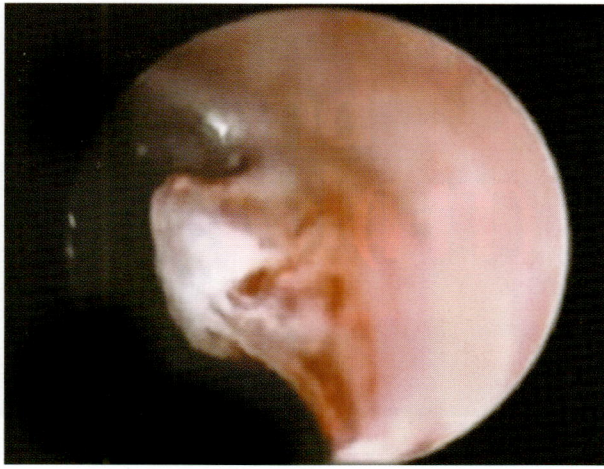

Fig. 12.8: Hysteroscopy—submucous fibroid

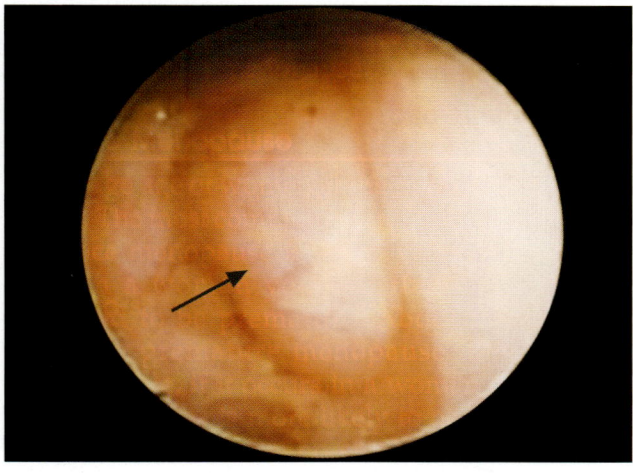

Fig. 12.6: Hysteroscopy—endometrial polyp

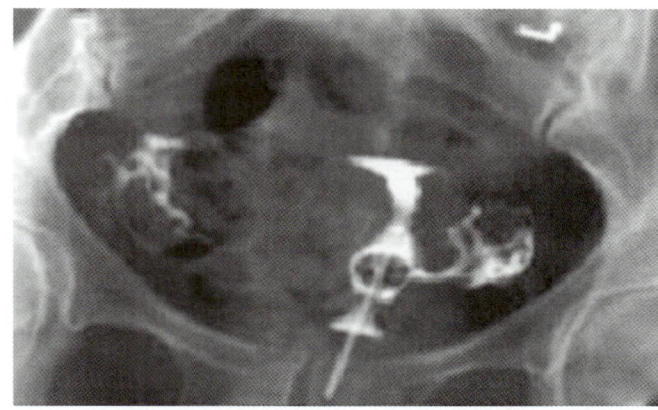

Fig. 12.9: Hysterosalpingogram image demonstrating normal findings with normal spillage

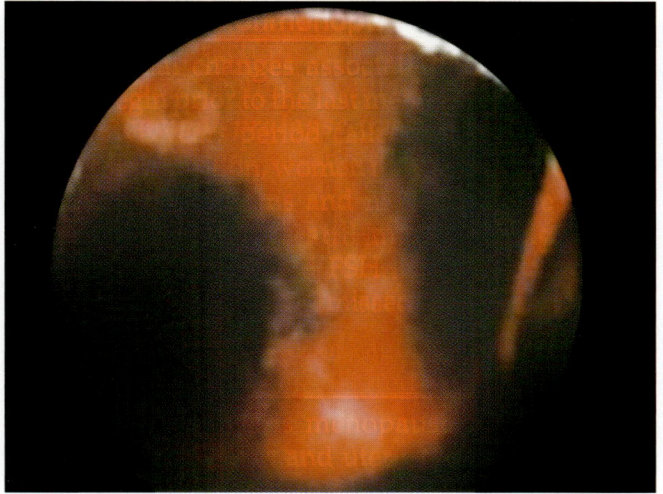

Fig. 12.7: Uterine septum

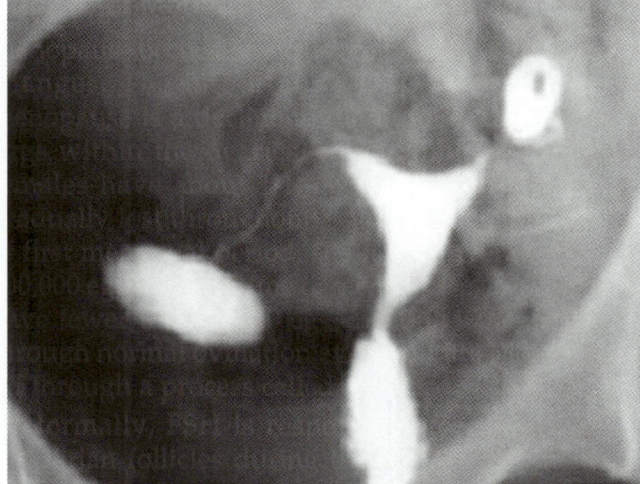

Fig. 12.10: Hydrosalpinx on HSG

Ovarian Factors

Ovulation

- Ovulation is usually inferred when a woman reports regular cycles, a progesterone value greater than 4 ng/mL and sonographic confirmation of follicle rupture with serial ultrasonography is established.

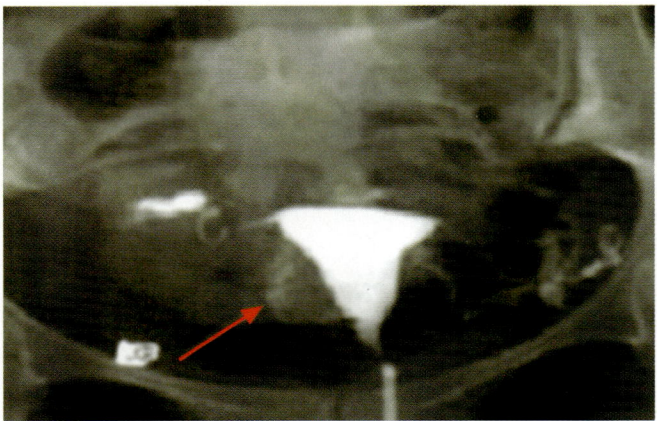

Fig. 12.11: Extravasation or lymphatic penetration of the contrast medium

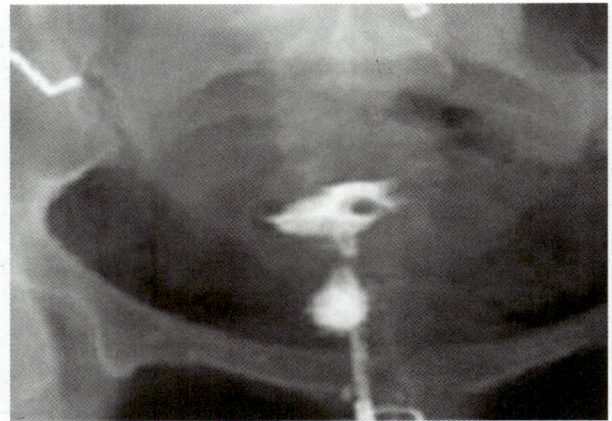

Fig. 12.14: Irregular cavity due to intr amural fibroids intruding into the cavity

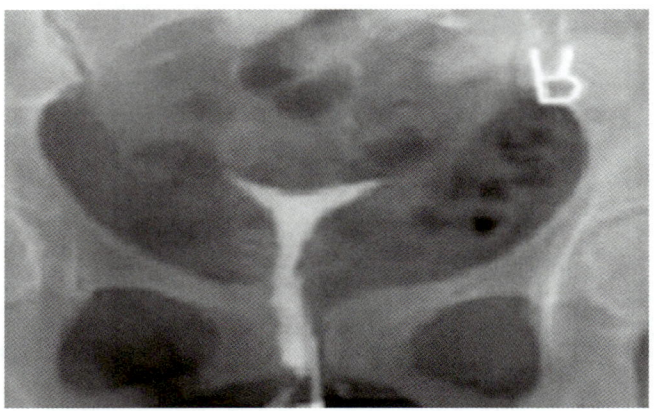

Fig. 12.12: Bilateral corneal obstruction

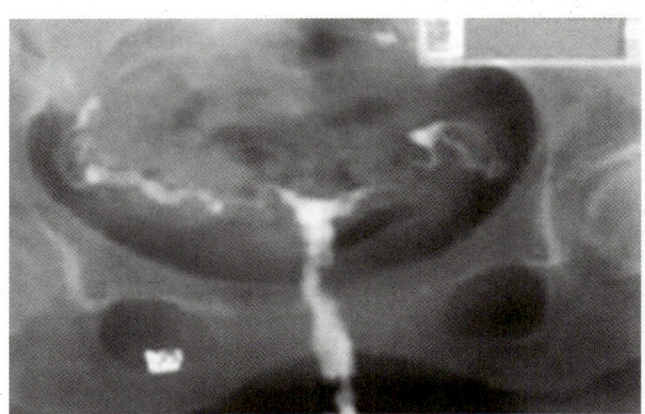

Fig. 12.15: Intrauterine synechiae

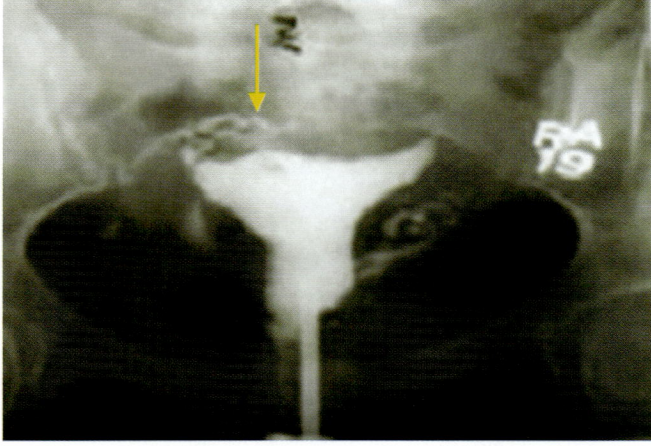

Fig. 12.13: Intravasation of the contrast medium due to myoma

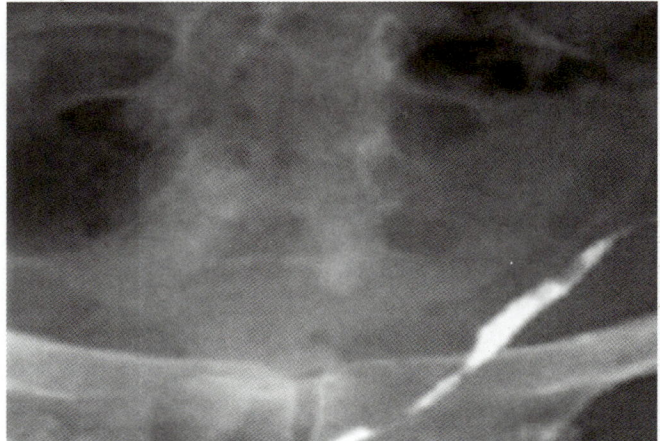

Fig. 12.16: Unicornuate uterus

- Basal body temperature charts, endometrial biopsy are not done nowadays for diagnosis of ovulation.

However, urinary ovulation predictor kits are favored by many as they are more accurate and easier to do.

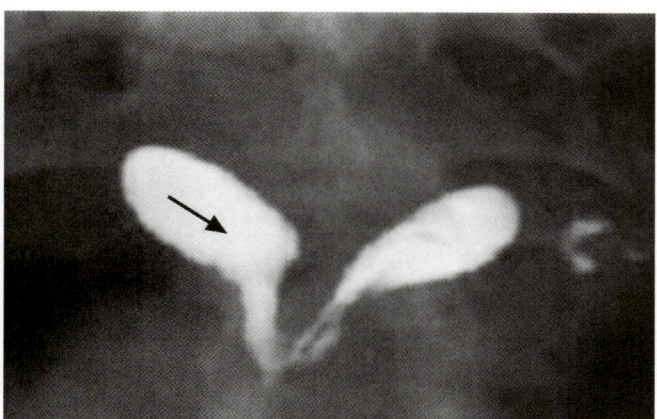

Fig. 12.17: Didelphys uterus on HSG

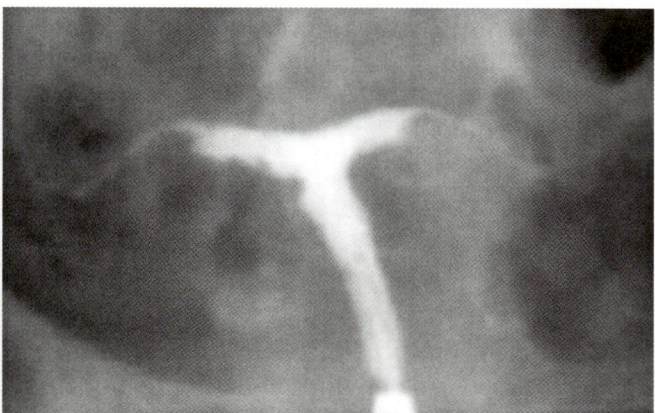

Fig. 12.18: T-shaped uterus

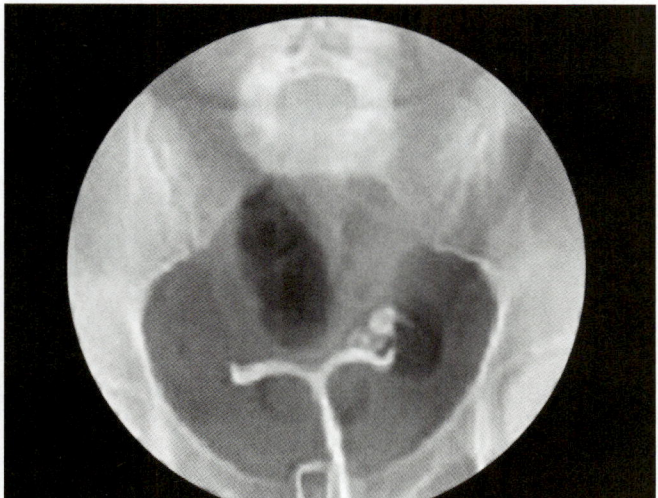

Fig. 12.19: Bicornuate uterus

Assessment of Ovarian Reserve

The level of ovarian reserve and the age of the female partner are the most important prognostic factors in the fertility workup.

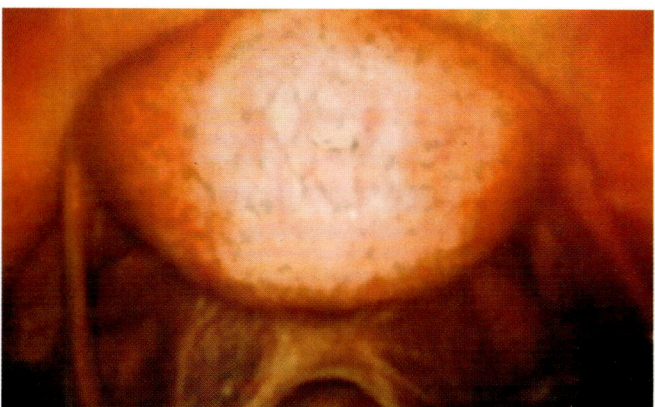

Fig. 12.20: Normal anatomy on laparoscopy

- Ovarian reserve is most commonly evaluated by checking a cycle day 3 FSH and estradiol level. Normal ovarian function is indicated when the FSH level is less than 10 mIU/mL and the estradiol level is less than 65 pg/mL.
- In cases where the patient is 35 years or older, dynamic ovarian reserve testing may be indicated. The most common test used is the clomiphene citrate challenge test (CCCT). A serum FSH and estradiol level is drawn on cycle day 3. Clomiphene citrate 100 mg by mouth is administered on cycle days 5–9 and a serum FSH level is drawn again on day 10. An FSH level greater than 10 is associated with decreased fertility and lower pregnancy rates.
- Other tests of ovarian reserve include antral follicle counts, ovarian volume, inhibin B, and anti-müllerian hormone. However, most of these are not found to be of adequate sensitivity, specificity and must be interpreted within the clinical context of the patient.
- A serum **AMH** assay can be used to identify patients with decreasing ovarian reserves and polycystic ovarian insufficiency. AMH is mainly secreted by small nonselected follicles because follicular granulosa cells are AMH-positive and serum AMH levels are normal/low-normal among women with FSH-resistant ovaries who lack follicle development beyond the small antral stage and it is high in PCOS.
- Since thyroid disease and hyperprolactinemia can cause menstrual abnormalities and infertility, a serum TSH and prolactin should always be checked and corrected prior to instituting therapy.

Ultrasonography (Figs 12.27 to 12.30)

Pelvic sonograms also help in the early detection of uterine fibroids, endometrial polyps, ovarian cysts, adnexal masses, and endometriomas. Ultrasonography can also assist in the diagnosis of anovulation, polycystic ovaries, and persistent corpus luteum cysts.

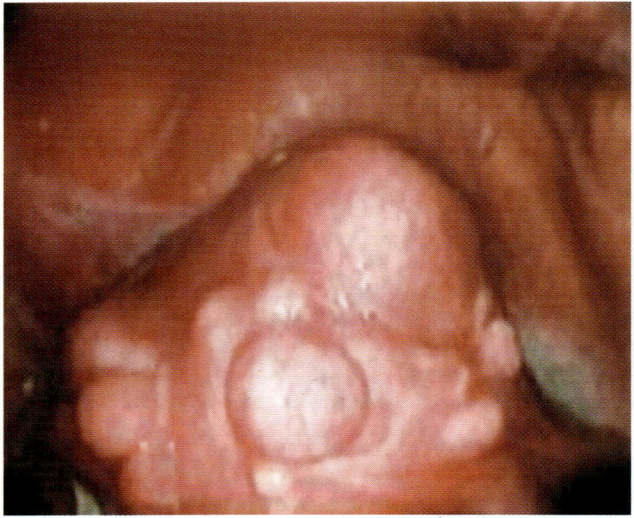

Fig. 12.21: Uterine fibroids

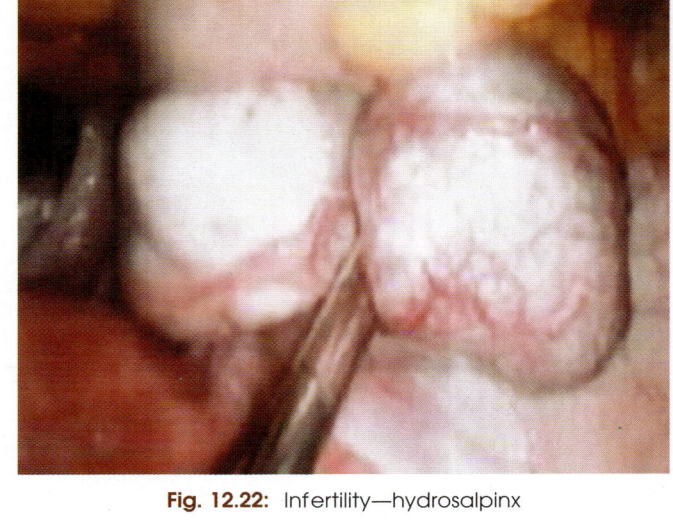

Fig. 12.22: Infertility—hydrosalpinx

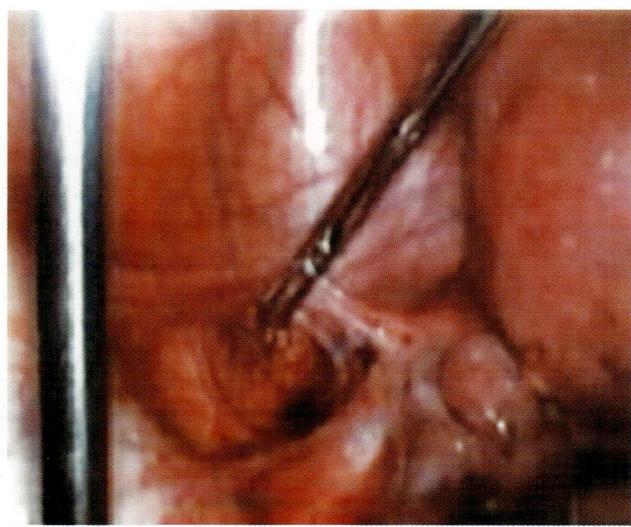

Fig. 12.23: Peritubal and ovarian adhesions

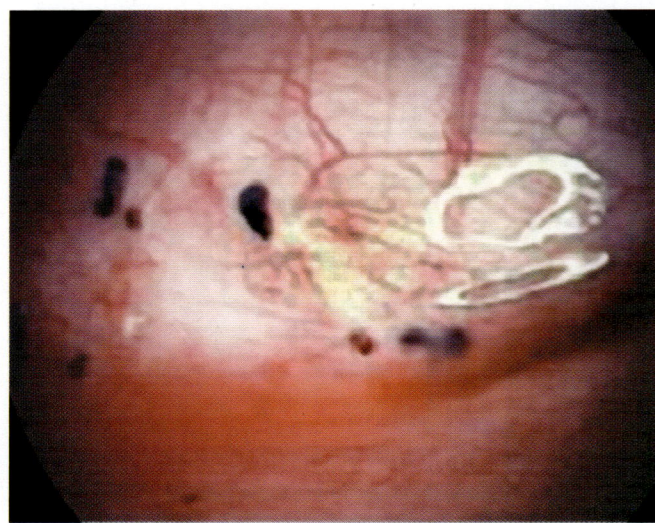

Fig. 12.24: Powder burn lesion in pelvic endometriosis

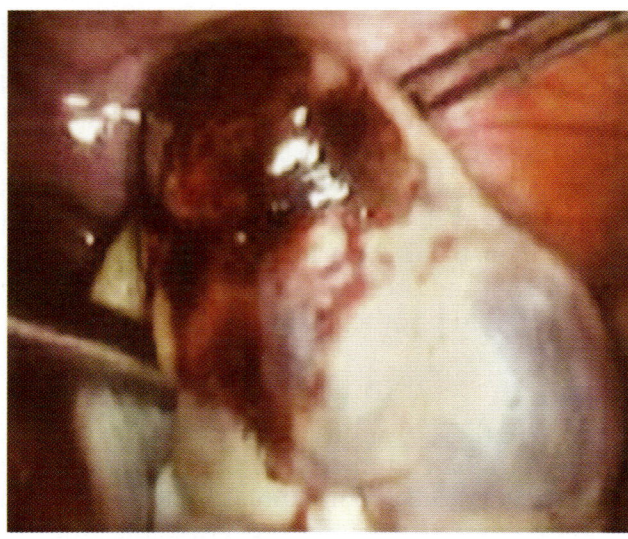

Fig. 12.25: Ovarian—endometrioma

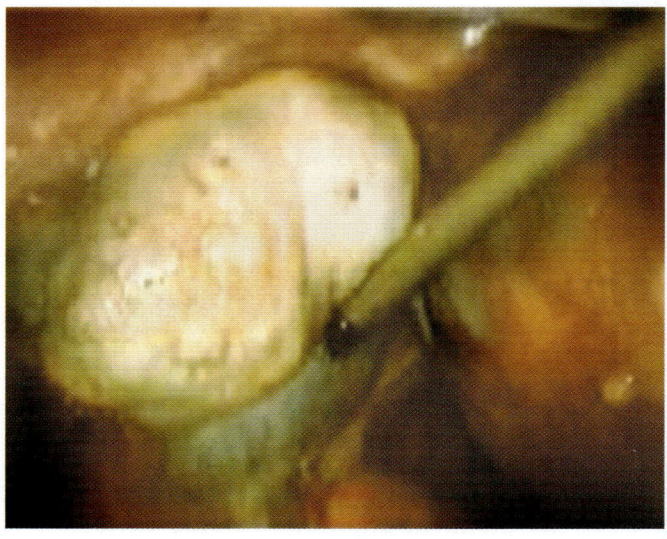

Fig. 12.26: Polycystic ovaries

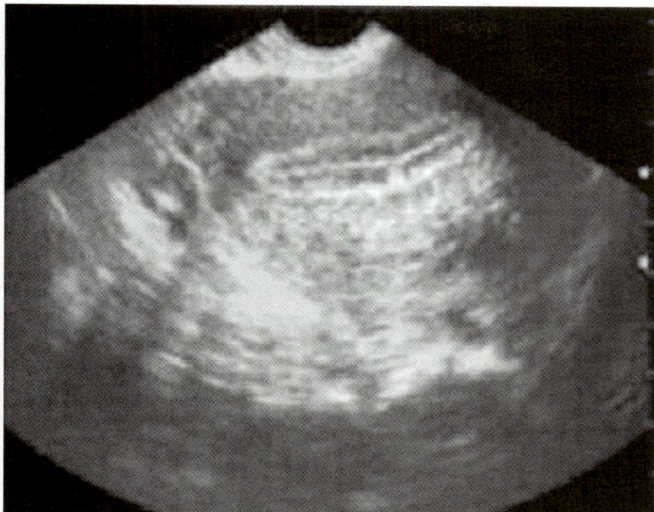

Fig. 12.27: Sonogram: Sagittal view showing three laminar pattern of endometrium

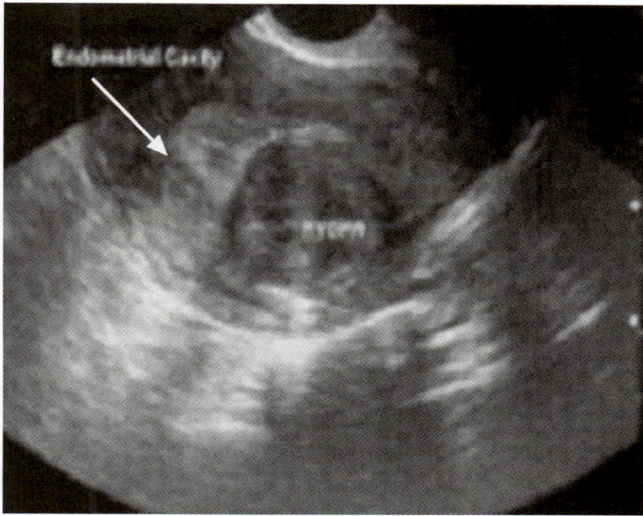

Fig. 12.29: Submucous myoma

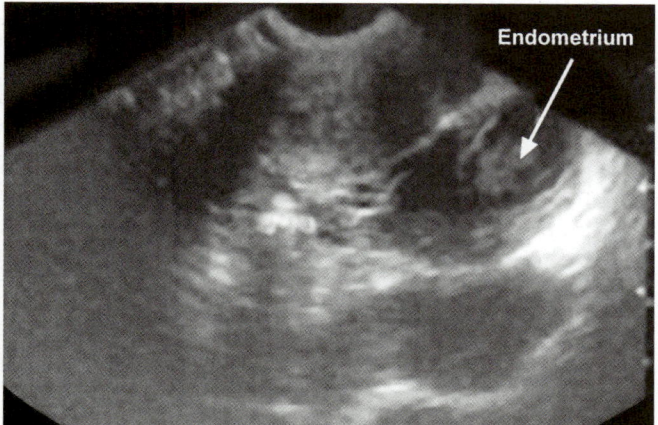

Fig. 12.28: Endometrioma of ovary

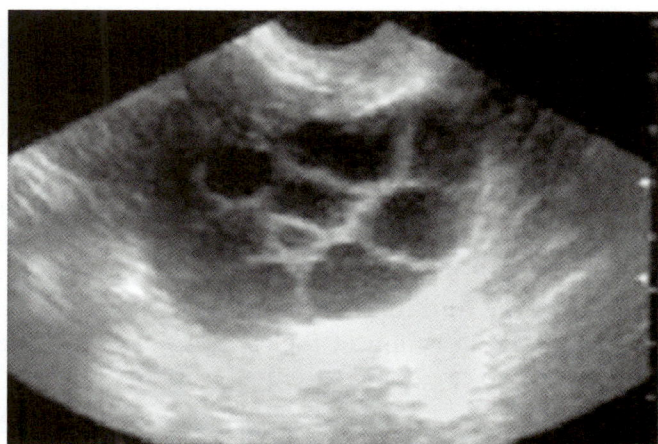

Fig. 12.30: Multiple follicles during ovulation induction

Infertility Treatment

A treatment plan should be generated according to the diagnosis, duration of infertility, and the woman's age. If pregnancy has not been established within a reasonable time, further evaluation and/or an alternative treatment plan should be considered.

Treatment of Cervical Factors

Chronic cervicitis may be treated with antibiotics like doxycycline and metronidazole for 7–14 days along with local antifungal therapy to eradicate all types of infective organisms. Reduced secretion of cervical mucus due to destruction of the endocervical glands by previous cervical conization, freezing, or laser vaporization responds poorly to low-dose estrogen therapy. The easiest and most successful treatment is intrauterine insemination (IUI).

The average pregnancy rate achieved after a natural-cycle intrauterine insemination is 8%. The rate increases to 10–15% after ovulation induction. Of the successful pregnancies, 85% are achieved within the first 4 cycles of intrauterine inseminations.

Treatment of Uterine Factors

The treatment of **uterine malformation**s depends on the severity of the problem. Fertility is not an issue for some patients affected by DES, and they remain undiagnosed until they have an abnormal Papanicolaou test result. Those who do have fertility problems are treated according to the following guidelines:

- Chronic cervical factor of absence of mucus—intrauterine insemination.
- Cervical incompetence—cerclage.
- Damage/absence of fallopian tubes—*in vitro* fertilization

Unicornuate uterus: A unicornuate uterus remains undetected unless fertility is compromised. Most problems are related to premature labor and pregnancy loss. Unicornuate uterus is associated with renal abnormalities including absence of a kidney or presence of a pelvic kidney; this occurs in 15% of cases. Thus, an intravenous pyelogram must be performed once this diagnosis is made. Whether interventions like resection of the rudimentary horn before conception or prophylactic cervical cerclage early in pregnancy improve obstetrical outcomes is uncertain; however, current practice suggests that such interventions may be helpful.

Bicornuate uterus: A bicornuate uterus causes minimal problems with infertility. It is more associated with malpresentation and preterm birth. A bicornuate uterus can be associated with a history of recurrent miscarriages and its repair or prophylactic encirclage is indicated, only if other etiologies for the miscarriage have been excluded.

Arcuate uterus: In general, an arcuate uterus does not cause infertility and, therefore, does not need correction.

Septate uterus: A uterine septum causes recurrent pregnancy loss more than infertility though the avascular nature of the septum can interfere with implantation and maintenance of the embryo. Hysteroscopic resection of the septum to restore the normal uterine cavity increase the fertility potential.

Uterine synechiae: Uterine synechiae are corrected using operative hysteroscopy. The surgery is performed during the early follicular phase. Once the synechiae have been resected, the patient receive high-dose estradiol (50 μg daily for 21 days) followed by medroxyprogesterone (10 mg for 10 days). A postoperative HSG should be performed 2 months later. Occasionally, more than one hysteroscopy is required for total resection.

Endometrial polyps: Endometrial polyps are removed through operative hysteroscopy followed by immediate ovulation induction for pregnancy associated with a dilatation and curettage, if necessary. An HSG follow-up procedure is not necessary.

Treatment of Myoma

In general, small and asymptomatic myomas do not require treatment, but the patient should be periodically monitored. Fibroids should be treated, if they are associated with abnormal uterine bleeding or if they are thought to be the cause of infertility. Three modalities are used to treat myomas—(a) medical treatment, (b) surgical treatment, and (c) embolization.

a. *Medical treatment* can be used to reduce the myoma size prior to removal. GnRH analog, like leuprolide acetate, nafarelin acetate, goserelin acetate, causes downregulation of the pituitary, inducing chemical menopause after injections of 3.75 mg intramuscularly every 4 weeks for a period of up to 6 months.

b. *Surgical treatment* of myomas is indicated in cases of abnormal uterine bleeding, when the myoma is implicated in recurrent miscarriages or when it is thought to interfere with embryo implantation. The 3 classes of surgical techniques are conventional laparotomy, operative laparoscopy, and operative hysteroscopy:
   - *Laparotomy* is indicated for large myomas, for submucous myomas larger than 3 cm in diameter or with a portion of the myoma deep inside the myometrium.
   - *Operative laparoscopy:* This technique is indicated for pedunculated and superficial intramural myomas. This technique should be reserved for myomas with a diameter less than 6 cm though many big myomas are now removed by morcellation. The reconstruction of the uterus after laparoscopic myomectomy is also improved now with good electrosurgical machine and Barbed sutures.
   - *Operative hysteroscopy:* The removal of a submucous fibroid using hysteroscopy should be limited to small fibroids (<3 cm) with minimal compromise of the myometrium. Very recently hysteroscopic morcellation device is also introduced by which bigger myomas can be removed.

c. *Embolization:* Pregnancy is reported after uterine embolization.

Treatment of Tubal and Peritoneal Factors

The treatment of tubal factor infertility has undergone major changes with the availability of microsurgerical tubal reconstruction and assisted reproductive therapy.

Tubal obstruction and lysis of adhesions can be corrected through laparotomy, operative laparoscopy, and, in special circumstances, through operative hysteroscopy and tubal cannulation.

Laparotomy is indicated in patients with severe pelvic adhesions that compromise the bowel, ovaries, and tubes, with obliteration of the cul-de-sac. The aim of the procedure is adequate restoration of the anatomy. Lysis of adhesions should be meticulous, using hydro-dissection and fine instruments with meticulous hemostasis. Constant irrigation with heparinized Ringer lactate solution prevents fibrin formation.

Operative hysteroscopy associated with tubal cannulation is helpful to treat cornual obstruction.

Operative laparoscopy currently allows surgical treatment of multiple tuboperitoneal pathologies through, electrocautery, endocoagulation, lasers, and Harmonics ultrasonography scalpels. Fimbrial phimosis and periadnexal disease can be treated with laparoscopy. The pregnancy rate after salpingolysis is 50–60% during the first year after treatment. Fimbrioplasty for fimbria agglutination or phimosis without destruction of the cilial epithelium is equally successful. The incidence rate of ectopic pregnancy after surgery is 5%.

Treatment of hydrosalpinx (distal tubal obstruction) with salpingostomy can be performed through microsurgery or operative laparoscopy. No difference in the pregnancy rate occurs, if a skillful microsurgeon or laparoscopist performs the salpingostomy. The success of the procedure is related to the diameter of the hydrosalpinx and to the damage to the cilial epithelium. If the cilial epithelium has been destroyed, the outcome of the procedure is poor, and it is better to perform a salpingectomy in preparation for future IVF. The pregnancy rate fluctuates from 20 to 35%, and the expected ectopic pregnancy rate is as high as 20%.

Before treating cornual obstruction, the diagnosis should be confirmed. In many cases, cornual obstruction diagnosed on HSG represents simple cornual spasm. Before performing a tubocornual anastomosis, the patient should have a diagnostic laparoscopy associated with tubal cannulation by hysteroscopy. If one tube remains open, anastomosis is not needed because pregnancy can be achieved in 50% of cases. The success rate of tubocornual anastomosis ranges from 20 to 58%. The ectopic pregnancy rate is 5–7%. If the obstruction is caused by salpingitis isthmica nodosa or fibrosis, the best results are achieved through IVF.

Surgical Preparation for IVF

It is always better with a single well-functioning fallopian tube than with two defective tubes, which elicit an increased risk for ectopic pregnancy or recurrence of pelvic adhesions. If the fallopian tubes are beyond repair, bilateral salpingectomy with destruction of the cornual area is recommended in preparation for IVF.

Tubal obstruction due to elective sterilization is better repaired with microsurgery or using operative laparoscopy. In either event, knowing in advance what type of tubal ligation technique was used is important. Unfortunately, tubal cauterization destroys a large amount of tissue, so the amount of fallopian tube remaining is often not long enough to facilitate a successful reanastomosis.

Before anastomosis, evaluate the patient using HSG and laparoscopy findings to measure how far proximal and distal fragments of the fallopian tubes remain from the tubal ligation. To have a successful reanastomosis, the final tube should measure at least 4.5 cm. If fimbriectomy was performed, no treatment is available other than IVF. The best candidates for tubal reanastomosis are patients who had tubal ligation by fallopian ring, Filshie clip, or Pomeroy method. The pregnancy rate following a tubal reanastomosis performed by a skilled surgeon varies from 70 to 80%. The ectopic pregnancy rate is approximately 7%.

Treatment of Endometriosis

Endometriosis treatment may be divided according to the severity of the disease and patient needs. Four alternatives are currently available to treat endometriosis—expectant therapy, surgical intervention, medical treatment, and combined therapy including ART.

Expectant Therapy

Expectant therapy should be based on a complete workup with diagnosis of very early stages of the disease (minimal) in patients without clinical symptoms, i.e. an incidental finding. If diagnosed on laparoscopy it is desired to cauterize and destroy small powder burn lesions, periadnexal adhesiolysis so that the disease does not progress to advanced stage, if pregnancy is not achieved though fertility prospect remains same if nothing is done at this stage.

A second-look laparoscopy is required for follow-up observation within 6–18 months.

Surgical Treatment

- Surgical treatment should be directed at destroying the disease using electrocoagulation, laser vaporization, endocoagulation, or excision. Removal of endometriomas >4 cm and lysis of adhesions complete the treatment.

- Most surgical treatment for endometriosis is currently performed through operative laparoscopy. Laparotomy is done to treat severe disease (III & IV) or with deep-seated bowel adhesions.

Medical Treatment

- Medical treatment is directed toward suppressing estrogen production by the ovary which delays the pregnancy but relieves the symptoms. Different modalities of treatment are available. Endometriosis can be treated with oral contraceptives, progestins, androgens, or GnRH agonists.
- The GnRH agonists are used mostly immediate post-surgery or pre-IVF but not more than 6 months. These are as follows:
  - Leuprolide acetate (3.75 mg IM every 4 wk or 11.25 mg IM every 3 months).
  - Nafarelin acetate (400 µg intranasal daily).
  - Goserelin acetate (3.6 mg SC every 4 wk or 10.8 mg SC every 3 months).

Combined Therapy

- Medical and surgical treatments are usually combined for the treatment of severe endometriosis. No consensus exists as to whether the medical treatment should precede surgery or vice versa.
- For patients wishing to conceive, the medical approach is not indicated, as it delays treatment for infertility. Medical treatment for minimal to mild disease has not been shown to be of benefit. However, for women with moderate to severe endometriosis, surgical treatment is followed by GnRH treatment for 3 months before assisted reproductive therapy can be offered.
- A more proactive approach now exists. Ovulation induction and intrauterine insemination are used after completion of the treatment in hopes of expediting the establishment of a pregnancy before relapse of the disease.

Treatment of Ovarian Factors

Ovulation induction is the appropriate treatment for infertile patients who have dysfunction of the hypothalamic-pituitary-ovarian axis. The ovulation induction agents used include clomiphene citrate, HMG, hCG, recombinant FSH, and recombinant LH.

Clomiphene Citrate (CC)

The chemical formula for CC is 2-phenoxy-triethylamine dihydrogen citrate. It is a nonsteroidal estrogen capable of interacting with estrogen receptor–binding proteins in a manner similar to estrogen but in a more prolonged way. Therefore, it behaves similar to an antiestrogen. Clomiphene is a selective estrogen receptor modulator (SERM) that increases production of gonadotropins by inhibiting negative feedback on the hypothalamus.

Chemistry: Clomiphene is a mixture of two geometric isomers, enclomifene (*E*-clomifene) and zuclomifene (*Z*-clomifene).

Enclomiphene   Zuclomiphene

The commercially available form of clomiphene is the dihydrogen citrate salt (clomiphene citrate). It contains two stereoisomers: zu-clomiphene (38%) and en-clomiphene (62%), which were originally called the *cis*-isomer and *trans*-isomer, respectively. En-clomiphene is cleared rapidly, while zu-clomiphene has a long half-life. The two clomiphene isomers have mixed estrogenic and antiestrogenic effects. Zu-clomiphene appears to have greater estrogenic activity than en-clomiphene.

Clomiphene citrate is absorbed by the gastrointestinal tract. Fifty percent of the oral dose is excreted after five days. It competes for the estrogen receptor at the hypothalamus, pituitary, and ovarian levels. Because of the action at the estrogen-receptor level within the hypothalamus, clomiphene citrate alleviates the negative feedback effect exerted by endogenous estrogens. As a result, CC normalizes the GnRH release; therefore, the secretion of increased FSH and LH is increased which normalizes follicular recruitment, selection, and induces ovulation.

The standard dose of clomiphene citrate is 50 mg oral daily for 5 days, starting on the menstrual cycle day 3–7 or 2–6 or after progestin-induced bleeding. As an antiestrogen, it requires that the patient have some circulating estrogen levels and intact HPO axis; otherwise, the patient will not respond to the treatment. The follicle should develop to a diameter of 23–24 mm before a spontaneous LH surge occurs.

Urinary monitoring of the LH surge (with an LH predictor kit): The patient can start monitoring the urinary LH secretion daily starting on menstrual cycle day 12. Ovulation usually occurs within 32–40 hours after the indicative color change.

Because of the antiestrogenic effect, clompiphene citrate may thicken the cervical mucus, creating an iatrogenic cervical factor that can be responsible for the lack of pregnancy in a patient who has otherwise ovulated. Other adverse effects associated with clomiphene are hot flashes, scotomas, dryness of the vagina, headache, and ovarian hyperstimulation, which, although rare, has been reported in patients who are sensitive. Whether the use of CC increases the risk of ovarian cancer is doubtful, although these are reported in literature.

The principal indications for use of clomiphene citrate are anovulation or oligo-ovulation with a minimum functional HPO axis especially in polycystic ovarian syndrome (PCOS), and for patients with slight menstrual irregularities. Its use has been extended to assisted reproductive technologies.

However, its use is contraindicated in cases of ovarian cyst, pregnancy, and liver disease. Its use is controversial in patients with a history of breast cancer.

Polycystic ovarian syndrome is the most frequent indication for ovulation induction. Clomiphene citrate is the drug of choice. However, the treatment is restricted to 6 ovulatory cycles because 85% of patients conceive by the sixth ovulatory cycle. If pregnancy is not achieved, further evaluation is required. If ovulation does not occur with the 50 mg dose, the dose must be increased in subsequent cycles to 100 mg for 5 days. The maximum recommended dosage is 150 mg/day for 5 days.

Clomiphene resistant cases are those who are failing to ovulate with clomiphene used for 3–6 consecutive cycles of use. **Clomiphene failure** cases are those who are not achieving pregnancy with use of clomiphene for 3–6 consecutive cycles of uses.

Aromatase Inhibitors

Aromatase inhibitors (letrozole, anastrozole) inhibit the action of the enzyme aromatase, which converts androgens into estrogens by a process called aromatization. As a result, estrogen levels are dramatically reduced, releasing the hypothalamic-pituitary axis from its negative feedback. **Unfortunately, aromatase inhibitors are not FDA approved for treatment of ovulation induction.**

When used in the early follicular phase, letrozole inhibits estrogen synthesis, thereby causing enhanced GnRH pulsatility and consequent FSH and inhibin stimulation. This results in normal or enhanced follicular recruitment without the risk of multiple ovulation and ovarian hyperstimulation syndrome. Letrozole has half-life of 45 hours and, therefore, is quickly cleared from the body. For this reason, it is less likely to adversely affect the endometrium and cervical mucus.

The usual dose for letrozole ovulation induction is 2.5 mg on cycle days 3–7. However, the optimal dosage and length of administration is under investigation. Aromatase inhibitors are generally well tolerated. The main side effects are hot flushes, gastrointestinal events (nausea and vomiting), headache, back pain, and leg cramps. These adverse effects are reported in older women with advanced breast cancer who were given the drugs on a daily basis over several months. In younger women taking them at lower doses for a short period of time, these adverse effects are rarely noted.

The use of aromatase inhibitors for ovulation induction in premenopausal women is controversial due to the possibility of fetal toxicity and fetal malformations raised by one abstract. However, 2 subsequent publications have shown no evidence of fetal malformations with the letrozole and no difference in birth weight compared with spontaneous conceptions. Furthermore, based on the half-life of each drug, administration in the early follicular phase should result in clearance of the aromatase inhibitors before implantation takes place.

Human Menopausal Gonadotropins

HMG contains 75 U of FSH and 75 U of LH per mL, although the concentration may vary among batches (ranges from FSH at 60–90 U and LH at 60–120 U). In the 1980s, a pure form of FSH containing 75 U FSH became available. The new generations of available gonadotropins are produced by genetically engineered mammalian cells (i.e. Chinese hamster ovary cells), in which the gene coding for the alpha and beta FSH subunits has been inserted. Recombinant LH may be added to recombinant FSH protocols as an alternative, particularly useful in patients with hypothalamic amenorrhea.

Treatment protocol of HMG: HMG is the treatment of choice for patients with amenorrhea due to hypopituitarism. The risk of ovarian hyperstimulation syndrome and multiple pregnancy is heightened; therefore, HMG should be started at the minimal dose (75 IU SC daily for 7 days). On the seventh day, E_2 measurement and ultrasonography are performed. If the E_2 level is below 100 pg/mL and the sonogram shows small follicular development, HMG is increased to 150 IU/day for an additional 5 days. However, if the E_2 level is greater than 100 pg/mL and the follicles are 10 mm in diameter, HMG should be continued at the same dose. Once the follicular diameter reaches 18 mm and the E_2 level is below 2000 pg/mL, ovulation is triggered by the administration of hCG (10,000 IU IM).

The ideal response is one in which only 2–3 follicles develop. If the response is exaggerated, with more than 5 sizable follicles (18 mm in diameter), and the E_2 level is greater than 2500 pg/mL, cancelling the ovulation is better to avoid the risk of ovarian hyperstimulation syndrome and a high order of multiple pregnancy. In current practice, an alternative for patients with more than 5 sizable follicles is to convert the treatment to IVF.

Multiple adverse effects and complications may occur during the use of the gonadotropins, including (1) multiple pregnancy (24–33%), (2) ectopic pregnancy (5–8%), (3) miscarriages (15–21%), (4) ovarian torsion and rupture, (5) ovarian hyperstimulation syndrome, which is most severe.

HMG, therefore, is indicated for ovulation induction in patients with primary amenorrhea due to hypopituitarism and in patients with secondary amenorrhea who did not respond to clomiphene citrate ovulation induction.

Gonadotropin-releasing Hormone

Synthetic GnRH has a chemical composition similar to native GnRH and is indicated for patients with hypothalamic dysfunction, especially those who do not respond to clomiphene. This drug is administered in a pulsatile fashion every 60–120 minutes, intravenously or subcutaneously using a delivery pump. The starting dose is 5–25 µg subcutaneously. The administration of GnRH should be extended throughout the luteal phase before gonadotropin stimulation.

Usually ovarian hyperstimulation syndrome does not occur. In most cases, only 1 follicle is recruited and develops until ovulation. Urinary LH kit is a practical way to monitor these patients.

Lack of Ovulation

Patients with anovulation who do not ovulate after several cycles of clomiphene at different doses are clomiphene resistant. This situation can be related to the presence of other endocrine disorders such as hyperprolactinemia, congenital adrenal hyperplasia, adrenal tumors, Cushing syndrome, thyroid dysfunction, and extreme obesity.

A subgroup of patients has PCOS with hyper-insulinism, hyperandrogenism associated with acanthosis nigricans, and resistance to clomiphene. This group is amenable to metformin treatment. Metformin improves insulin sensitivity and decreases hepatic gluco-neogenesis and, therefore, reduces hyperinsulinism, basal LH levels, and free testosterone concentration. Consequently, the patient with PCOS becomes responsive to clomiphene.

Adverse effects of metformin include GI intolerance, nausea, vomiting, and abdominal cramps. The initial dose is 500 mg daily for 7 days, then 500 mg twice daily for another 7 days, and, finally, 500 mg three tmes daily. Clomiphene is started at the initial dose of 50 mg/day for 5 days. In many instances, patients can ovulate while on metformin treatment.

Gonadotropin Stimulation

Treatment with pure FSH or HMG is another alternative for patients with PCOS who are clomiphene resistant. It is started at 37.5 IU/day subcutaneously. The dose is increased slowly (i.e. by 37.5 IU for 5 days) until follicle development is detectable based on an elevation of the E_2 levels and the presence of follicle development on sonograms. Using this small amount of FSH, the patient generally develops 1–2 follicles, decreasing the risk for multiple pregnancy and eliminating the risk of ovarian hyperstimulation syndrome.

Lack of Pregnancy

Lack of pregnancy can be related to disruption of the cervical mucus, inadequate follicular development, presence of luteinized unruptured follicle syndrome, progesterone deficiency, implantation failure and premature administration of hCG to trigger ovulation.

Luteinized unruptured follicle syndrome can be prevented by the administration of hCG (10,000 IU IM) once the follicle reaches 23–24 mm in diameter. Progesterone deficiency can be corrected by the administration of progesterone during the luteal phase, starting 48 hours after ovulation.

Patients with **hyperprolactinemia** need a thorough evaluation to exclude a pituitary microadenoma. The patient must be treated with bromocriptine at an initial dose of 2.5 mg once daily and increased to 5 mg once tolerance is built. If the GI symptoms persist, the medication can be administered intravaginally. Alternatively, cabergoline can be used orally or vaginally weekly at a starting dose of 0.5 mg/wk. Cabergoline is associated with fewer side effects but is more expensive. Patients with adrenal hyperplasia and other disorders must be treated with prednisone. Patients with hyperthyroidism or hypothyroidism must be treated with antithyroid drugs or thyroid replacement therapy, respectively. Weight reduction should be part of the treatment because it helps the patient's response to ovulation induction.

Ovarian Hyperstimulation Syndrome

Ovarian hyperstimulation syndrome (OHSS) is a rare, iatrogenic complication for ovarian stimulation by assisted reproductive technology and other infertility treatments. Following gonadotropin therapy, OHSS usually develops several days after oocyte retrieval or assisted ovulation. This syndrome is characterized by ovarian enlargement due to multiple ovarian cysts and an acute fluid shift into the extravascular space. Complications of OHSS include ascites, hemoconcentration, hypovolemia, and electrolyte imbalances.

Classification

To understand OHSS and its management, one must first be aware of its various grades of severity: (1) mild OHSS, (2) moderate OHSS, and (3) severe OHSS.

Mild OHSS is classified as follows:
- Grade 1—Abdominal distention and discomfort.
- Grade 2—Grade 1 disease plus nausea, vomiting, and/or diarrhea, as well as ovarian enlargement of 5–12 cm.

Moderate OHSS is classified as follows:
Grade 3—Features of mild OHSS plus ultrasonographic evidence of ascites.

Severe OHSS is classified as follows:
- Grade 4—Features of moderate OHSS plus clinical evidence of ascites and/or hydrothorax and breathing difficulties.
- Grade 5—All of the above plus a change in the blood volume, increased blood viscosity due to hemoconcentration, coagulation abnormalities, and diminished renal perfusion and function.

Pathophysiology

a. *Abdominal pain, nausea, and vomiting:* These are due to gross enlargement of the ovaries. The enlargement is sometimes as much as 25 cm.

b. *Ascites and tense distention:* This occurs because of extravasation and increased leakage of protein-rich fluid from the intravascular space into the abdominal cavity, owing to an osmolar differential. Leakage of fluid from large follicles, increased capillary permeability (due to the release of vasoactive substances), or frank rupture of follicles can all contribute to ascites.

c. *Localized or generalized peritonitis:* This is caused by peritoneal irritation secondary to blood from ruptured cysts, protein-rich fluid, and inflammatory mediators.

d. *Acute abdominal pain:* This may be due to ovarian torsion, intraperitoneal hemorrhage, or rupture of cysts secondary to enlarged ovaries with fragile walls.

e. *Hypotension and/or hypovolemia:* Follicular fluid and perifollicular blood containing large amounts of vascular endothelial growth factor (VEGF), which is thought to increase vascular permeability, escape into the peritoneal cavity. Blood vessels within and outside the ovary become functionally impaired, resulting in the leakage of fluid through those vessels and a massive fluid shift from the intravascular to the extravascular compartment. This process results in intravascular hypovolemia with the concomitant development of edema, ascites, hydrothorax, and/or hydropericardium.

Hypotension and/or hypovolemia are also caused by compression of the inferior vena cava because of enlarged cysts or ascites. As a result, venous return and preload decrease resulting in reduced cardiac output and hypotension.

f. *Dyspnea:* Pulmonary function may be compromised as enlarged ovaries and ascites restrict diaphragmatic movement. This may be due to pleural effusion, pulmonary edema, atelectasis, pulmonary embolism, acute respiratory distress syndrome (ARDS), and pericardial effusion.

g. *Hypercoagulable state:* This is likely due to hemoconcentration and hypovolemia resulting from third spacing and fluid shift. It is also related to increased estrogen levels. Patients have an increased risk of developing deep venous thromboses and pulmonary embolisms.

h. *Electrolyte imbalance:* This occurs due to the extravasation of fluid and resultant renal dysfunction resulting from decreased perfusion. Increased reabsorption of sodium and water occurs in the proximal tubule, leading to oliguria and low urinary sodium excretion.

The exchange of hydrogen and potassium for sodium in the distal tubule is reduced. As a result, hydrogen and potassium ions accumulate and cause hyperkalemia and acidosis.

i. *Acute renal failure:* Hypovolemia in OHSS leads to hemoconcentration and creates a hypercoagulable state. Microthrombi form in tubules, leading to decreased renal perfusion. Acute renal failure may result.

Etiology

The pathogenesis of ovarian hyperstimulation syndrome (OHSS) is unknown, but the process is related to increased vascular permeability in the region surrounding the ovaries and their vasculature. Beta human chorionic gonadotropin (hCG) as well as estradiol, prolactin, histamine, and prostaglandins, have been implicated in the past.

Currently, vasoactive substances such as interleukins, tumor necrosis factor (TNF)-alpha, endothelin-1, and VEGF secreted by the ovaries have been implicated in increasing vascular permeability.

hCG plays a critical role in enhancing ovarian angiogenesis and triggering the cascade of vascular permeability in ovarian vessels that leads to third spacing and OHSS. These changes in the ovarian vasculature are exaggerated responses to normal luteinizing hormone. The function of hCG is similar to that of LH. Moreover, hCG exerts a follicle stimulating hormone-like action in stimulating the ovaries. In addition, it has a prolonged half-life. All of these properties of hCG lead to ovarian stimulation and changes in periovarian vasculature even after ovulation.

Risk Factors

Age younger than 35 years, low body mass index (BMI), gonadotropin treatment, high estradiol concentrations, large number of follicles, history of polycystic ovarian syndrome, administration of exogenous hCG, and endogenous hCG from treatments resulting in pregnancy increase a patient's risk of developing OHSS.

If the pre-hCG estradiol amount is greater than 3000 pg/mL and/or if more than 15 follicles are present, the rate of severe OHSS approaches 80%.

The incidence of ovarian hyperstimulation syndrome (OHSS) depends on definitions, risk factors, stimulation protocols, and conception. Rates of occurrence have been estimated as follows:

- Mild—8–23%
- Moderate—1–7%
- Severe—0.25–5%

Only women of childbearing age are affected by ovarian hyperstimulation syndrome.

Ovarian hyperstimulation syndrome usually has two phases. The first phase (**early onset OHSS**) develops between the second and seventh day after ovulation, and the second phase (**late onset OHSS**) only occurs if the patient becomes pregnant. Ovarian hyperstimulation syndrome is self-limited, and the symptoms subside within 2–6 weeks.

Prevention

1. By coasting; not done nowadays where hCG trigger is delayed or dose is reduced to 2500 from 10000 IU.
2. Cancellation of cycles when follicles were big in size and >15 in numbers or E_2 level > 3000 pg/mL.
3. Cabergolin 0.25 mg daily to start before hCG injections till the pick up.

4. Use of GnRH antagonists in the subsequent cycles.
5. By use of preservation of oocytes and frozen embryo transfer in the next cycles.
6. Adminstering prophylactic albumin after hCG trigger.

Treatment

Patients with mild and moderate ovarian hyperstimulation syndrome are treated at home with bedrest and strict control of fluid intake and output. If a weight gain greater than 2 lb occurs, the patient should be evaluated to determine, if hospitalization is required.

Patients with severe ovarian hyperstimulation syndrome are often hospitalized and confined to bed, with strict control of fluid intake and output. Intravenous fluids (i.e. isotonic sodium chloride solution) must be administered until hemodilution is achieved. If the urinary output remains low, albumin 25% (50 mL/hr IV for 4 hrs) has been effective in promoting diuresis. Transvaginal or abdominal paracentesis should be performed, if the patient becomes uncomfortable. Thoracocentesis is rarely indicated in cases of pleural effusion. Because of the risk of thrombosis, heparin (5000 U SC every 12hr) is recommended. In severe cases, renal failure and DIC results which can be life-threatening.

Prognosis

The prognosis in mild or moderate cases of ovarian hyperstimulation syndrome (OHSS) is excellent. However, morbidity may be clinically significant in cases of severe OHSS, and fatalities do occur. However, the prognosis is optimistic in severe OHSS, if proper (or adequate) treatment is given.

Death from OHSS is largely due to hypovolemic shock and electrolyte imbalance, hemorrhage, and thromboemboli (hypercoagulability may endanger the patient). Estimated fatality rates are 1 per 400,000–500,000 stimulated cycles.

Treatment of Unexplained Infertility

Only 5–10% of these couples eventually achieve a pregnancy within 5 years. Empirical treatment with controlled ovarian hyperstimulation followed by intrauterine insemination has improved the pregnancy rate in those patients. If pregnancy does not occur during the first 4–6 intrauterine insemination cycles, other alternatives include IVF or any of the associated assisted reproductive technologies procedures.

Assisted Reproductive Technologies

The first successful human IVF attempt resulted in delivery of Louise Brown in England in 1978 and is considered the beginning of a new era for the treatment of infertility. Edward and Steptoe are considered the forefather of 1st IVF pregnancy born in their laboratory. Prof. Suhash Mukherjee, a Bengali Professor in physiology from Kolkata presented and reported earlier his concept of IVF pregnancy though not recognized by the then authority. But later his work was recognized and followed in our country.

In Vitro Fertilization

IVF consists of retrieving a preovulatory oocyte from the ovary and fertilizing it with sperm in the laboratory, with subsequent embryo transfer (replacement) within the endometrial cavity. The pioneering work of Edwards and Steptoe has been duplicated worldwide, and IVF is now recognized as an established treatment for infertility.

Indications

- Absence of the fallopian tubes and severe pelvic adhesions and bilateral tubal block.
- Endometriosis unsuccessfully treated medically or surgically with distorted anatomy.
- Husbands with severe oligospermia or a history of obstructive azoospermia.
- Patients with unexplained infertility.

Procedure

IVF consists of retrieving preovulatory oocytes from the ovary and fertilizing them with sperm in the laboratory, with subsequent embryo transfer (replacement) within the endometrial cavity. The following steps are required during an IVF cycle:

- Ovarian stimulation
- Follicular aspiration
- Oocyte classification
- Sperm preparation
- Oocyte insemination
- Embryo culture
- Embryo transfer

Ovarian Stimulation for IVF

Although the world's first IVF pregnancy, which occurred in England, followed the fertilization of a single oocyte obtained during a spontaneous menstrual cycle, IVF success is related to the patient's age and the number of embryos transferred into the endometrial cavity, among other factors. The number of embryos obtained in any given IVF cycle depends on the number of oocytes obtained after ovulation induction, follicular aspiration, and fertilization.

Several protocols are available for ovarian stimulation, and all are based on the principles of follicular recruitment, selection, and dominance.

Clomiphene Citrate

- Today, this is used infrequently in IVF. A clomiphene-only protocol consists of 5–7 days of treatment, with doses of 50–150 mg starting on the second menstrual cycle day. The ovarian response is monitored using pelvic ultrasonography and determinations of serum E_2 and LH levels. When the follicle diameter reaches 18 mm, LH must be measured every 3–4 hours to detect a premature LH surge that generally occurs when the follicle reaches 23–24 mm in diameter. Oocyte retrieval must be performed within 24–26 hours after the LH surge.
- The advantages of the CC protocol include low cost and an almost nonexistent risk of ovarian hyperstimulation syndrome.
- The major disadvantages include (1) low oocyte yield (1–2 per cycle), (2) frequent LH surges that lead to oocyte retrieval at any time of the day, (3) high cancellation rate (25–50%), and (4) low pregnancy rate.

Clomiphene Citrate and Human Menopausal Gonadotropins

- This combination has the advantage of increasing the number of recruited follicles. The doses of CC are similar, but HMG (150 IU daily) is administered for a period of 2–7 days after the CC. Frequent pelvic ultrasonography and daily determinations of E_2 levels are required, as are frequent determinations of LH once the follicular diameter reaches 15 mm. The follicle completes its development at 17–18 mm; therefore, hCG (10,000 IU IM) must be administered at this time to complete the oocyte maturation. Oocyte aspiration should be performed 35 hours after the hCG injection.
- The advantage of the CC/HMG protocol is an increase in the number of recruited follicles. The disadvantages of the protocol are premature luteinization, spontaneous LH surge (20–50%), and high cancellation rate (15–50%).

Human Menopausal Gonadotropins

- The use of HMG has evolved with the introduction of new technologies and the generation of pure FSH gonadotropins that can be used subcutaneously. Furthermore, recombinant FSH and LH gonadotropins are currently available.

- The doses of gonadotropins (based on FSH amounts) vary from 150–450 IU/day depending on the patient's age and history of previous ovulatory response. In general, patients are started on the second or third menstrual cycle day. The response is monitored using daily serum E_2 determination and later using pelvic ultrasonography.
- Once most of the follicles reach 17–18 mm in diameter, the gonadotropins are discontinued. hCG (10,000 IU) is administered and oocyte retrieval is performed 35 hours later. With the use of gonadotropins, ovulation induction appears to be more predictable. However, a spontaneous LH surge occurs in approximately 25% of cycles, which is one of the reasons for cancellation.

Regardless of the use of gonadotropins, a group of patients, known as **poor responders**, develops only 2–3 follicles, and their oocytes are of poor quality. The possibility of a successful pregnancy in this group of patients is seriously compromised. In general, these patient responses are related to poor ovarian reserve (POR). This is defined by an elevated baseline FSH level (>10 mIU/mL), a low E_2 level (< 20 pg/mL) associated with an absence of follicle development on sonograms, or elevated AMH level characterize poor ovarian reserve.

GnRH Agonists (GnRH-a)

Initially, GnRH agonists were used in IVF patients who had a history of premature luteinization, spontaneous LH surge, and an ovarian stimulation response that was less than ideal. The GnRH-a can be used in 3 protocols known as long protocol, short protocol, ultra short protocol.

The long protocol

- GnRH-a is given for two to three weeks. Down regulation of the pituitary gland is achieved as confirmed by the very low level of serum E_2.
- The GnRH is usually started in the mid-luteal phase or early in the early follicular phase.
- FSH or HMG therapy is started after down regulation.

Disadvantage of long protocol

- It is more expensive.
- Takes longer time.
- Larger dose of GnRH analogue.
- Larger number of ampoules of HMG.

GnRHa short protocol

- GnRH-a is started on day one or two of the cycle.
- Exogenous FSH administration, then is started on day 3 of the cycle to continue follicular stimulation, meanwhile complete pituitary desensitization occur.

Advantage of short protocol

1. Shortening the stimulation time.
2. Reducing the amount of GnRH used.
3. Reducing the amount of HMG used. Thus the total cost of the procedure will be lower.

The protocol has been criticized for being unphysiological, as it increases the LH levels in the early stages of the follicular phase, which is harmful to the growing follicles.

Ultrashort protocol

- GnRH-a is given for only three days with the flare up technique.
- LH could be suppressed till the mid-cycle.
- This protocol will help to retrieve more oocytes with a minimal risk of premature LH surge.

Potential risks and disadvantages with the use of GnRH-a include (1) increased requirements of gonadotropins, (2) increased costs due to additional days of therapy, (3) the risk of ovarian hyperstimulation syndrome due to excessively high E_2 levels, and (4) an increased rate of multiple pregnancies.

GnRH Antagonists

- The GnRH antagonists are the latest generation of GnRH that block LH secretion without a flare-up effect. The GnRH antagonists (e.g. cetrorelix, ganirelix) are administered (1) as a single dose on the eighth menstrual cycle day; (2) in small amounts over several days, starting on a given menstrual cycle day; (3) when the largest follicle reaches a diameter of 14 mm; or (5) when the LH levels in serum are greater than 10 mIU/mL.
- GnRH antagonists have the advantage of blocking the LH surge at the periovulatory period; therefore, premature luteinization or spontaneous LH surge does not occur. Because the pituitary gland is not downregulated at the beginning of the menstrual cycle, smaller amounts of gonadotropins are required to stimulate ovulation. Another advantage with this protocol is the prevention of ovarian hyper-stimulation syndrome, especially in patients with elevated E_2 levels (>3000 pg/mL) or more than 15 follicles during the stimulation. Because the half-life of the GnRH antagonist is short, it is possible to elicit the preovulatory LH surge by the administration of

leuprolide acetate and avoid the long-term effects of the hCG injection that are responsible for triggering the ovarian hyperstimulation.

Oocyte aspiration is undertaken 35–36 hours after hCG administration. This is followed by **sperm preparation** and **embryo culture.** Day 3 embryo is **transferred** into the uterine cavity.

Management of the Luteal Phase

Progesterone supplementation during the luteal phase is started 36–72 hours after oocyte retrieval. The exogenous progesterone is administered because of concerns that superovulation and the aspiration of granulosa cells at the time of oocyte retrieval may induce an abnormal endocrine milieu.

Normally, progesterone supplementation is continued for approximately 2 weeks. If the pregnancy test result is positive, progesterone is continued until the 12th week of gestation.

NICE Guidelines

Ovulation Induction

Classification of Ovulatory Disorders

Anovulation and oligo-ovulation are ovulatory disorders into three groups:
- *Group I:* Hypothalamic pituitary failure (hypothalamic amenorrhea or hypogonadotropic hypogonadism).
- *Group II:* Hypothalamic pituitary dysfunction (predominantly polycystic ovary syndrome).
- *Group III:* Ovarian failure

Antiestrogens

Women with PCOS should be offered treatment with clomiphene citrate or tamoxiphen as the first line of treatment for up to 12 months to induce ovulation.(A)
- Women with unexplained infertility should be informed that treatment with clomiphene citrate increases chance of pregnancy but that needs to be balanced by possible risk of treatment like multiple pregnancy.(A)
- Women undergoing treatment with clomiphene citrate should be offered ultrasound monitoring during at least the first cycle of treatment to ensure that they receive a dose that minimizes the risk of multiple pregnancy.

Metformin

- Metformin is not currently licensed for the treatment of ovulatory disorders in UK. Anovulatory women with PCOS who have not responded to clomiphene citrate and who have a BMI of >25 should be offered metformin combined with clomiphene citrate because this increases ovulation and pregnancy rates.(A)
- Women on metformin should be informed of the side effects associated with its use like nausea, vomiting and other GI disturbances.

Ovarian Drilling

Women with PCOS who have not responded to clomiphene citrate should be offered laparoscopic ovarian drilling because it is as effective as gonadotropin treatment and is not associated with increased risk of multiple pregnancy.(A)

Gonadotropin Use in Ovulation Induction Therapy for Ovulatory Disorders

- Women with WHO group-II ovulation disorders who do not ovulate with clomiphene citrate or tamoxifen can be offered treatment with gonadotropins. HMG, urinary FSH and recombinant FSH are equally effective in achieving pregnancy.(A)
- Women with WHO group-II ovulation disorders with PCOS who are ovulating with clomiphene citrate but do not get pregnancy after 6 months should be treated with clomiphene stimulated IUI.(A)

Gonadotropin use during IVF Treatment

HMG, urinary FSH and recombinant FSH are equally effective in achieving live birth when used following pituitary downregulation as a part of IVF treatment.(A)

GnRH Analogues in Ovulation Induction Therapy

Women with PCOS who are being treated with gonadotropins should not be offered treatment with GnRH agonists concomitantly because it does not improve pregnancy rates and it is associated with an increased risk of ovarian hyperstimulation.(A)

GnRH Analogues during IVF Treatment

For pituitary downregulation as part of IVF treatment using GnRH agonist in addition to gonadotropin stimulation facilitates cycle control and results in higher pregnancy rate than use of gonadotropin alone. The routine use of GnRH analogue long protocol in IVF cycles is strongly recommended.(A)

The use of GnRH antagonist is associated with less pregnancy rates and, therefore, except in some indicated cases, its routine use in IVF cycles is not recommended. (A)

Growth Hormone as an adjunct to Ovulation Induction Therapy

The use of adjuvant growth hormone treatment with GnRH agonist and/or HMG during ovulation induction in women with PCOS who do not respond to clomiphene citrate is not recommended because it does not improve pregnancy rates.(A)

Pulsatile Gonadotropin-releasing Hormone

Women with WHO group-I should be offered pulsatile administration of gonadotropin-releasing hormone or gonadotropins with luteinizing hormone activity because these are effective in inducing ovulation.(B)

Dopamin Agonists

Women with ovulatory disorders due to hyperprolactinemia should be offered treatment with dopamine agonists like bromocriptine. (A)

Monitoring Ovulation Induction during Gonadotropin Therapy

Ovarian ultrasound monitoring to measure follicular size and number should be an integral part of patient management during gonadotropin therapy to reduce the risk of multiple pregnancy and ovarian hyperstimulation. (C)

Other Risks and Side Effects Associated with Ovulation Inducing Agents

Women who are offered ovulation induction should be informed that a possible association between ovulation induction therapy and ovarian cancer remains uncertain. It should be used at the lowest effective dose with minimum duration of use.(C)

Tubal and Uterine Surgery

Tubal microsurgery and laparoscopic tubal surgery: For women with mild tubal disease tubal surgery may be more effective than no treatment.(D)

Tubal Catheterization or Cannulation

For women with proximal tubal obstruction selective salpingography plus tubal catheterization or hysteroscopic tubal cannulation may be treatment options because these treatments improve the chance of pregnancy.(B)

Uterine Surgery

Women with amenorrhea who are found to have intrauterine adhesions should be offered hysteroscopic adhesiolysis because this is likely to restore menstruation and improve the chance of pregnancy.(C)

Medical and Surgical Management of Endometriosis

Medical treatment of minimal and mild endometriosis by ovarian suppression does not enhance fertility in subfertile women and should not be offered.(A)

Surgical Ablation

* Women with minimal or mild endometriosis who undergo laparoscopy should be offered surgical ablation or resection of endometriosis plus laparoscopic adhesiolysis because this improves the chance of pregnancy. (A)
* Women with ovarian endometriosis >4 mL should be offered laparoscopic cystectomy because this improves the chance of pregnancy.(A)
* Women with moderate to severe endometriosis should be offered surgical treatment to restore the anatomy because that improves the chance of pregnancy. (A)
* Postoperative medical treatment does not improve pregnancy rate in women with moderate to severe endometriosis, therefore, is not recommended. (A)

Intrauterine Insemination

* Where IUI is used to manage male factor fertility problems ovarian stimulation should not be offered because it is no more clinically effective than unstimulated IUI and it carries risk of multiple pregnancy.(A)
* Where IUI is used to manage minimal or mild endometriosis couples should be informed that ovarian stimulation increases pregnancy rates compared with no treatment but that the efficacy of unstimulated IUI is uncertain.(A)
* Where intrauterine insemination is undertaken single rather double insemination should be offered.(A)
* Where intrauterine insemination is used to manage unexplained infertility fallopian sperm perfusion of 4 mL processed sperm is used for insemination because it improves pregnancy rates compared to standard technique.(A)

Surgery for Hydrosalpinges before IVF Treatment

Women with hydrosalpinges should be offered salpingectomy preferably by laparoscopy before IVF treatment because this improves chance of live birth.

Female Age

Women should be informed that chance of a live birth following IVF treatment varies with female age and the optimal female age range for IVF treatment is 23–39 years. Chance of live birth per treatment cycle are:

a. Greater than 20% for women aged 23–35 yrs
b. 15% for women aged 36–38 yrs
c. 10% for women aged 39 yrs
d. 6% for women aged 40 yrs and above

Number of Embryos to be Transferred to Avoid Multiple Pregnancy

Couples should be informed that chance of multiple pregnancy following IVF treatment depends on the number of embryos transferred per cycle of treatment. To balance the chance of a live birth and the risk of multiple pregnancy and its consequences, no more than two embryos should be transferred during any one cycle of IVF treatment.

12C. IN VITRO FERTILIZATION (IVF)

In vitro **fertilization (IVF)** is a process by which an egg is fertilized by sperm outside the body: *in vitro*. IVF is a major treatment for infertility when other methods of assisted reproductive technology have failed. The process involves monitoring and stimulating a woman's ovulatory process, removing ovum from the woman's ovaries and letting sperm fertilize them in a fluid medium in a laboratory. The fertilized egg (zygote) is cultured for 2–6 days in a growth medium and is then transferred to the mother's uterus with the intention of establishing a successful pregnancy.

The first successful birth of a "test tube baby", Louise Brown, occurred in 1978. Louise Brown was born as a result of natural cycle IVF where no stimulation was made. Robert G. Edwards, the physiologist who developed the treatment, was awarded the Nobel Prize in Physiology of Medicine in 2010.

Indications

1. Bilateral irreversible tubal disease or block.
2. Male subfertility with obstructive azoospermia or oligoasthenospermia where there is a defect in sperm quality; in such cases intracytoplasmic sperm injection (ICSI) may be used, where a sperm cell is injected directly into the egg cell. This is used when sperm have difficulty penetrating the egg, and in these cases the partner's or a donor's sperm may be used.
3. In unexplained infertility for women that have not conceived after 2 years of regular unprotected sexual intercourse.{NICE Guideline}
4. IVF also has an expanded indication when there is need of some artificial procedure that is usually not necessary for the IVF procedure itself, but is virtually impossible to perform without concomitantly performing IVF. These include *in vitro* fertilization with intracytoplasmic sperm injection (ICSI), assisted hatching (AHA), embryo cryopreservation, blastocyst culture, TESE and MESA for male factor, and embryo biopsy for pre-implantation genetic diagnosis.

Step-by-Step Descriptions of the IVF Procedures

Step 1: Control Ovarian Hyperstimulation (COH)

COH is done using different protocols. The most common one is a long GnRH-agonist protocol where the secretion of gonadotropin hormones is suppressed in order to prevent premature ovulation. Once optimal suppression is achieved, the next step is the recruitment of multiple follicles by daily injections of gonadotropins. Ultrasound imaging and hormone assessments are used to monitor follicular development. When the lead follicles have reached the appropriate size (18–20 mm and ET 8 mm), the final maturation of eggs is done by hCG administration. Egg retrieval is scheduled 34–36 hours after hCG injection.

Step 2: Egg Retrieval (Follicular Aspiration)

Egg retrieval is performed in an adjacent OT under intravenous sedation. Ovarian follicles are aspirated transvaginally using a needle guided by transvaginal ultrasonography (Fig. 12.31). The patient is placed in the dorsal lithotomy position for the transvaginal oocyte aspiration. The vaginal wall is washed with saline. A 5- to 9-MHz ultrasonographic probe with a sterile cover and attached needle guide is inserted in the vagina to localize the ovaries and the follicles. A 17-gauge needle is subsequently passed via the needle guide through the vaginal fornix into the ovaries. The fluid is delivered to the IVF laboratory, which, ideally, is located adjacent to the operating room. Follicular fluids are scanned by the embryologist to locate all available eggs. The eggs are placed in a special media and cultured in an incubator until insemination.

Oocyte classification: The classification of the oocyte is a crucial step for success with IVF. The oocytes are

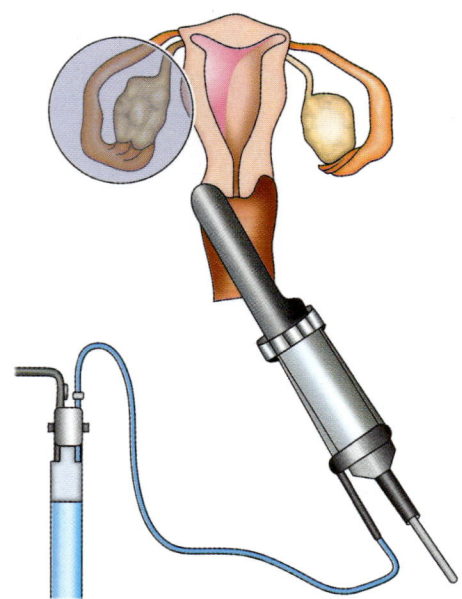

Fig. 12.31: Follicular aspiration through transvaginal route

graded according to the appearance of the corona-cumulus complex (Fig. 12.32). The presence of a polar body (metaphase II stage) and/or germinal vesicle (prophase stage) is a determining factor for the preincubation time prior to the insemination. Other oocytes are degenerated (atretic and fractured zona). The last category constitutes fewer than 15% of the total oocytes obtained.

Step 3: Fertilization and Embryo Culture

Sperm preparation and oocyte insemination—A semen sample is obtained after a 3- to 5-day period of sexual abstinence immediately prior to the oocyte retrieval. For IVF and intracytoplasmic sperm injection (ICSI) procedures, the removal of certain components of the ejaculate (i.e. seminal fluid, excess cellular debris, leukocytes, morphologically abnormal sperm) with the retention of the motile fraction of sperm is desirable.

For most specimens, the greatest recovery of the motile portion results from separation via centrifugation through a discontinuous density gradient system.

However, for certain very poor specimens with low original concentrations of motile sperm, the use of the gradient system results in such a negligible recovery. In that case, swim up method is preferred.

In this method, a washed pellet of sperm is layered with nutrient media allowing the motile fraction to swim up into the media before being separated. Finally, the supernatant containing the motile fraction of sperm is collected. Sperm concentration and motility are determined. A final number of 200,000 motile sperm in a small volume of media is added to the oocytes.

If sperm parameters are normal, approximately 50,000 to 100,000 motile sperm are transferred to the dish containing the eggs. This is called standard insemination.

Embryo culture: The inseminated oocytes are incubated in an atmosphere of 5% carbon dioxide in air with 98% humidity. Ideally, the presence of 2 pronuclei and the extrusion of a second polar body are the criteria required to ascertain fertilization, which should occur approximately 18 hours after insemination (Fig. 12.33).

The ICSI technique is utilized to fertilize mature eggs, if sperm parameters are abnormal. This procedure is performed under a high-powered microscope. The embryologist picks up a single spermatozoa using a fine glass micro-needle and injects it directly into the egg's cytoplasm (Fig. 12.34). ICSI increases the chance that fertilization will occur, if the semen sample has a low sperm count and/or motility, poor morphology or poor progression. If there are no sperm in the ejaculate, sperm may be obtained via a surgical procedure. ICSI is always used to achieve fertilization if the sperm is surgically retrieved.

Fertilization is assessed 16–18 hours after insemination or ICSI. The fertilized eggs are called

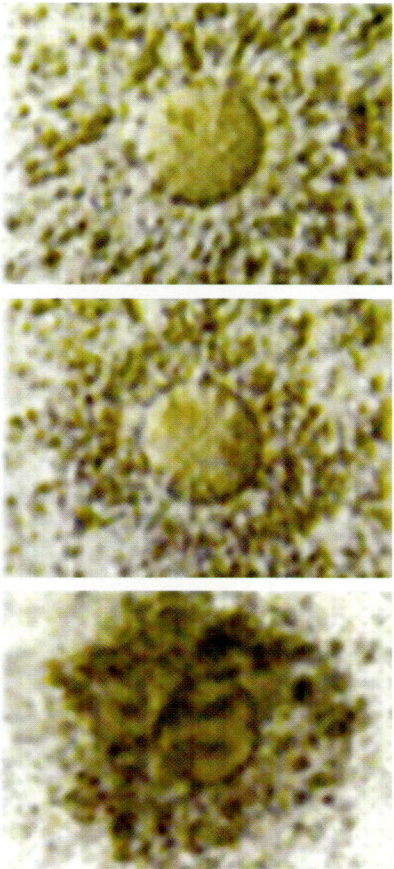

Fig. 12.32: Eggs surrounded by cumulus complex at retrieval

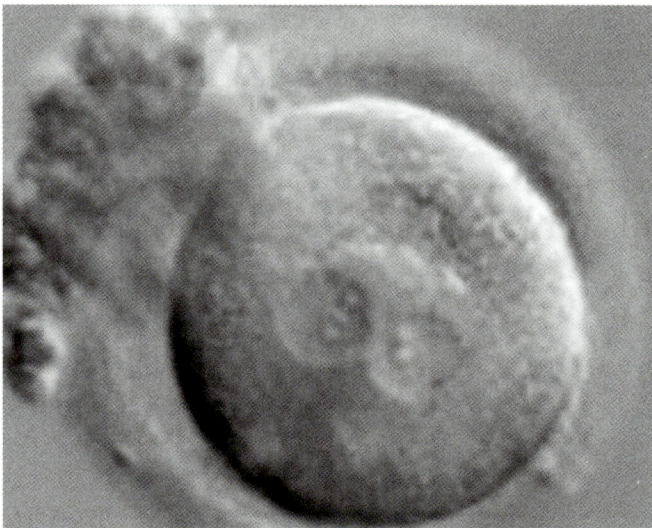

Fig. 12.33: A normally fertilized egg is called a zygote. Two pronuclei are seen in the center

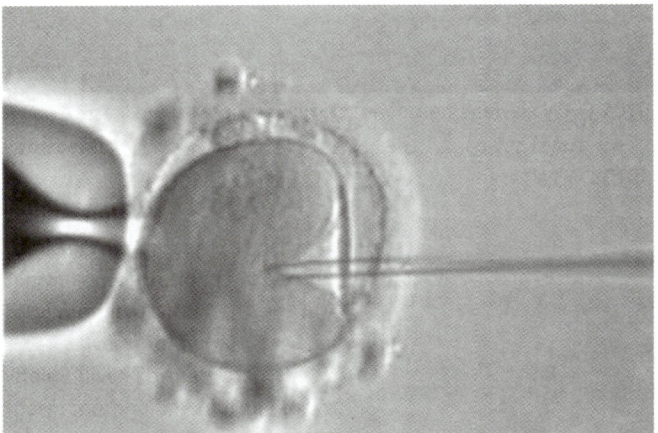

Fig. 12.34: Intracytoplasmic Sperm Injection (ICSI) procedure where a single spermatozoon, as shown by an arrow, is in the process of being injected into a mature egg's cytoplasm

zygotes and are cultured in a specially formulated culture medium that supports their growth. They will be assessed on the second and third day after retrieval. A 4- to 8-cell stage pre-embryo is observed approximately 36–48 hours after insemination (Fig. 12.35). A 10- to 16-cell embryo is observed after 48–72 hours. The morula or blastocyst stage is observed after 96–120 hours.

Blastocyst culture has several advantages. Embryos at this stage have a higher potential for implantation, therefore, fewer embryos can be transferred on day 5 to reduce the chance of multiple pregnancies. A day 3 embryo transfer is recommended for cycles with low numbers and/or poor quality.

Step 4: Embryo Quality

There are several criteria used to assess the quality of the embryo. This is especially important when trying to decide which embryos to choose for embryo transfer. Before transfer, the embryos are evaluated and photographed by the embryologist who along with the physician will select the best quality embryos based on the rate of development and its appearance. The number of embryos transferred is decided on basis of ASRM recommendation depending on the age.

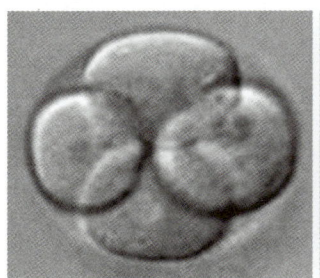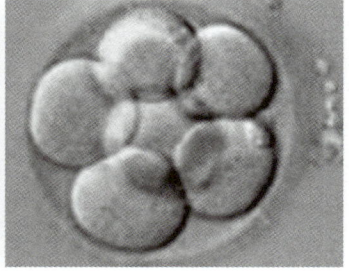

Fig.12.35: Embryos at the cleavage stage: A 4-cell embryo (left) and a 6-cell embryo (right)

Typically embryos are transferred at the cleavage stage (day 3 after oocyte retrieval) or at the blastocyst stage (day 5).

Day 3 transfers: Day three embryos are called cleavage stage embryos and have approximately 4–8 cells. These embryos are analysed to see how symmetrical they are and whether there is any fragmentation. Fragmentation occurs when the cells divide unevenly resulting in crowding of the embryo. No fragmentation is preferable. Embryos are classified into grades 1 through 4. Grade 4 represents the best quality embryos (Fig. 12.36A).

Day 5 transfers: Day 5 embryos are called blastocyst embryos. At this stage, the embryos are increased in size and are analysed to see how expanded these embryos are. The more expanded they are the better is the quality of the embryo. These embryos are also classified by a number scale, 1 through 6. Grade 6 represents the best quality blastocyst (Fig. 12.36B).

Step 5: Embryo Transfer

Embryos are transferred on day 3 when they are at the cleavage stage (6–8 cells) or on day 5 when they have reached the blastocyst stage. Embryo transfer is a simple procedure that does not require any anesthesia.

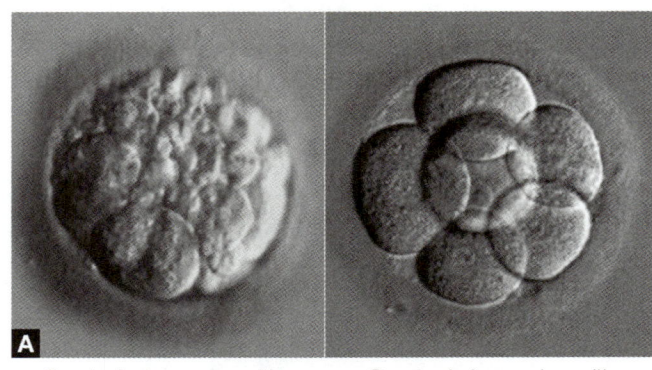

A

Grade 1: A poor quality cleavage embryo   Grade 4: A good quality cleavage embryo

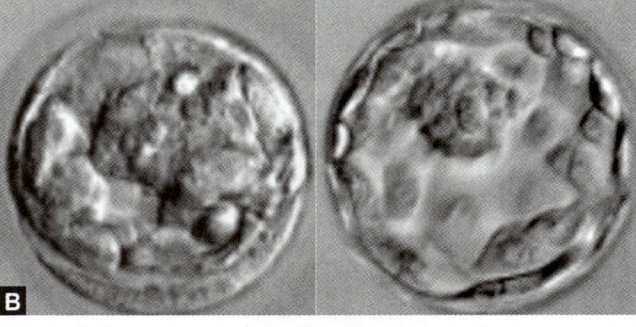

B

Grade 1: A poorly expanded blastocyst   Grade 6: A nicely expanded blastocyst

Fig. 12.36: Different quality blastocysts

Embryos are loaded in a soft catheter and are placed in the uterine cavity through the cervix.

Assisted Fertilization Techniques

Assisted fertilization techniques historically include partial zona dissection (PZD), subzonal sperm injection (SUZI), ICSI, and assisted hatching (AH). Currently, only ICSI and AH are used clinically.

PZD consists of creating a small opening at the zona pellucida level either mechanically or using low-pH solutions to digest a small portion of the zona. The intent is for the sperm to take advantage of this weak spot to make contact with the oocyte membrane so that fertilization will occur. The rate of fertilization per oocyte is approximately 20–25%, the incidence rate of polyspermia is elevated (50%), and the pregnancy rate is only 5% per cycle. To succeed with PZD requires the recovery of approximately 500,000 sperm after the sperm wash.

The SUZI procedure is indicated in patients for whom conventional IVF or PZD does not work. The procedure consists of suspending the oocyte in a sucrose medium. By osmosis, the oocyte is dehydrated; therefore, the perivitelline space is enlarged. Next, 3–5 spermatozoa are injected into the perivitelline space using a microneedle. Fertilization occurs in approximately 15–20% of the oocytes, the pregnancy rate is less than 3%, and the incidence of polyspermia is 50%.

PZD and SUZI are obsolete and have been replaced by the ICSI procedure. Palermo et al developed the ICSI procedure in Belgium. ICSI has revolutionized the treatment of severe male factor infertility because only a single live sperm is required per oocyte. The sperm can be obtained through masturbation, epididymal aspiration, testicular biopsy, or needle puncture of the testes. ICSI gives the opportunity to males with a history of obstructive azoospermia (perhaps due to congenital absence of the vas deferens) to have a biological child.

The sperm is paralyzed by stroking the distal portion of its tail. The oocyte is stripped from the cumulus using a solution of hyaluronidase. To inject the sperm, first the oocyte is stabilized with a micropipette, then the sperm is loaded, tail first, into a microneedle. The oocyte membrane is pierced with the microneedle, and the oolemma is entered. The spermatozoon is released inside the oolemma, and the microinjected oocyte is kept in the incubator.

The fertilization rate varies from 50–75% per oocyte. The current fertilization rate is 95% per patient, and the pregnancy rate is comparable to that of IVF. The risks involved with the procedure are few and include

oocyte rupture and damage and/or retention of the second polar body with the presence of 3 pronuclei. Currently, an increased risk of congenital malformation and chromosome abnormalities exists with ICSI. However, no significant difference exists between IVF and ICSI outcome.

Assisted embryo hatching (Fig. 12.37) is an obligatory step in the process of embryo implantation. This is needed when some of the IVF embryos demonstrate thick zona pellucida; this zona thickness may represent an obstacle for the normal embryo hatching, therefore, interfering with the implantation. The procedure is performed a couple of hours before the embryo transfer. AH can be performed mechanically, creating a microrent at the zona level by laser, or by chemical digestion of the zona using a Tyrode solution (low pH). Either of the procedures creates a weak spot within the zona, facilitating the break of the zona and the hatching of the embryo. AH is recommended for patients undergoing IVF who are older than 38 years, patients with multiple ART failures, and in all cryopreserved embryos.

Embryo Cryopreservation

The use of GnRHa-COH protocols to prevent the LH surge not only decrease the number of cancelled cycles but also increase the number of follicles and their synchronization; therefore, more embryos are available than the ideal number to be transferred. Embryo cryopreservation become an important part of ART to prevent multiple pregnancies, maternal and fetal complications, and to decrease the cost of ART because patients have the opportunity to achieve a pregnancy from the same IVF cycle.

Embryo cryopreservation can be performed at the 2-pronuclei stage, on cleaved embryos, and at the

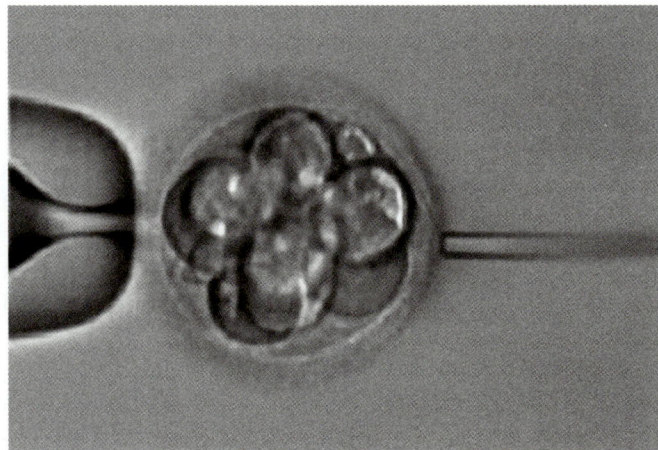

Fig. 12.37: An assisted hatching procedure where a part of the zona is thinned by expelling acidified medium by micropipette

blastocyst stage. The embryos are stored in liquid nitrogen for a period of 3–5 years, and their subsequent disposition should be outlined in the consent form, to include (1) embryo donation to another couple, (2) donating the embryos for research, or (3) disposition of the embryo after thawing.

Frozen Embryo Transfer

The transfer of cryopreserved embryos can be performed during a natural menstrual cycle or during an artificial endometrium-stimulated cycle. No differences in the pregnancy rate occur, provided that the endometrium, during a natural menstrual cycle, demonstrates a 10 mm thick triple-line pattern. The embryos are thawed 24, 48, or 96 hours after ovulation, depending on the stage at which cryopreservation was performed. The thawed embryos are incubated 24 hours before embryo transfer.

The artificially stimulated endometrium requires detection of ovulation during a previous menstrual cycle and downregulation of the pituitary gland with GnRHa starting on the 21st menstrual cycle day and is followed by increasing doses of estrogen starting with the onset of the menstrual bleeding. Estrogen is administered for 2 weeks. At that time, pelvic ultrasonography is performed to determine endometrial thickness. If the above-mentioned criteria are fulfilled, progesterone is added to the estrogen for 48 hours, then the embryos are thawed, cultured, and transferred. The administration of estrogen and progesterone is continued until the day of the pregnancy test. If the pregnancy test result is positive, the hormonal support must be continued until the 10th week of pregnancy.

IVF-Related Procedures

Though rarely performed, gamete and zygote intrafallopian transfer have been used as alternatives to IVF.

Gamete Intrafallopian Transfer

In 1985, Asch et al described the gamete intrafallopian transfer (GIFT) procedure. The procedure consists of ovarian stimulation, monitored follicular development, and oocyte aspiration similar to IVF. It differs in that the patient must have at least 1 normal-appearing and patent fallopian tube.

On the day of oocyte retrieval, the male provides a semen sample 2 hours before the procedure to perform the sperm wash and capacitation. Once the oocytes have been classified, a laparoscopy or a minilaparotomy is performed. The oocytes, along with 150,000 sperm, are loaded into a special catheter in the laboratory under a microscope. The loaded catheter passed through the fimbrial ostium and advanced up to the ampulla of the fallopian tube, where the gametes are released. Fertilization should occur inside the fallopian tube.

The major drawback of the GIFT procedure is that it does not allow for confirmation of fertilization and laparoscopy or minilaparotomy is required.

Zygote Intrafallopian Transfer

The zygote intrafallopian transfer (ZIFT) procedure is a combination of IVF and GIFT. Fertilization occurs in the IVF laboratory. However, the pre-embryo is transferred into the fallopian tube via laparoscopy at the 2-pronuclei stage or 24 hours after oocyte retrieval. One variant of the ZIFT procedure is the transfer of the cleaved pre-embryos at 48 hours (tubal embryo transfer). This procedure requires that the patient be taken to the operating room twice, which represents additional expense and doubles the risk for complications.

Indications of ART

The primary indications for ART are as follows:
- Tubal factor—9.0%
- Male factor—17.0%
- Endometriosis—5.0%
- Uterine—1.0%
- Ovulatory dysfunction—6.0%
- Diminished ovarian reserve—13.0%
- Unknown factor—11.0%

Success rates for fresh cycles were as follows:
- Overall pregnancy rate per initiated cycle—35.0%
- Live birth rate per initiated cycle—28.6%
- Live births per oocyte retrieval—31.9%
- Live births per embryo transfer—35.7%
- Live birth rate from frozen pre-embryos—28.9%.

The incidence of spontaneous miscarriage (15.0%), stillbirths (0.5%), congenital malformation, or chromosome abnormality is similar to that of the general population. Ectopic pregnancy occurs in approximately 0.7% of cases.

The pregnancy rate for fresh cycles by patient age is approximately 44.7% among women younger than 35 years and decline to approximately 17.7% in those older than 40 years.

The percentage of multiple births following ART are 30.8% (twins—28.8%; triplets or more—2.1%) whereas it is 3% in the general population.

Alternative Methods

Donor oocyte: Patients with poor ovarian reserve can go for either adoption or an oocyte donation. The source of the oocyte can be any healthy one or known (i.e. younger relative). Ideally, the donor should preferably be aged 21–30 years.

The donor undergoes ovulation induction according to the standard IVF protocol. Meanwhile, the recipient takes increasing doses of estrogens to synchronize her endometrium in preparation for a fresh embryo transfer.

Because oocyte cryopreservation is still in a preliminary stage of development, only fresh oocytes without quarantine are used. However, the donor must be screened for numerous transmissible diseases (e.g. HIV, syphilis, hepatitis, gonorrhea, chlamydia) according to FDA regulations, and a complete physical and gynecological evaluation is performed. The oocyte recipient and her partner are required to have the same kinds of screening tests as the oocyte donor. The legal aspects of the procedure and future offspring must be discussed. A thorough consent form must be signed by all parties involved.

The success of donor oocyte programs surpasses the success of conventional IVF. Since the risk of multiple pregnancy is very high, the conservative approach of transferring only two embryos is highly recommended to the recipient couple.

Donor sperm: Men who cannot produce sperm or women who do not have a partner and wish to become pregnant may opt for donor sperm. Many opt to use sperm banks, which require strict and rigorous infectious testing. After deposition, the samples are frozen and quarantined for at least 6 months. Once repeat infectious testing is confirmed to be negative, the sample is available for selection and intrauterine insemination or IVF is performed in synchronization with the patient's cycle.

Gestational Carriers

Patients who were unable to have a biological child because of absence of the uterus (congenital or acquired) or patients in whom a pregnancy is contraindicated are now able to have a biological child by the use of a gestational carrier or surrogate mother. A gestational carrier is a woman who is carrying a pregnancy resulting from embryos created by IVF, using the gametes of the intended parents. The gestational carrier program must be designed under the strictest policies because of the medicolegal implications.

The selection or approval of the gestational carrier or surrogate should be based on the premise that the pregnancy does not imply a risk for the carrier and that all the consent forms have been signed once the carrier and the genetic parents have completed the psychological evaluations and screening tests. The endometrium of the gestational carrier is artificially stimulated through the administration of estrogen and progesterone.

Microsurgical Epididymal Sperm Aspiration (MESA) or Testicular Sperm Extraction (TESE)

Some patient's semen samples contain no spermatozoa due to a congenital obstruction of the sperm ducts, vasectomy, failed vasectomy reversal or primary testicular failure. In these conditions, a urologist can obtain sperm surgically from the epididymis (MESA) or from the testis (TESE). This sperm can be frozen and used for fertilization by ICSI.

Preimplantation Genetic Diagnosis (PGD)

Preimplantation genetic diagnosis (PGD) is a procedure that is performed in conjunction with *in vitro* fertilization (IVF). It is designed to help detect genetic abnormalities in embryos before implantation, thereby avoiding the transfer of affected embryos.

Indications for PGD

PGD is indicated for the patients who have a history of recurrent miscarriages, advanced maternal age (>38 yrs), repeated IVF failures in spite of high grade embryos, unexplained infertility, severe male factor infertility or inherited genetic disorders, e.g. cystic fibrosis, Tay-Sachs disease, myotonic dystrophy, etc. Currently, there are more than 50 types of single gene mutations that can be diagnosed.

In order to perform genetic testing on an embryo, a single cell is removed from the embryo on the third day of development. Embryos must have 5 or more cells. This procedure is called embryo biopsy. It has been shown that removal of one or two cells from an 8-cell embryo does not impede its development (Fig. 12.38). This biopsied cell is lysed for fluorescence in situ hybridization (FISH) analysis to detect chromosomal anomalies or for polymerase chain reaction (PCR) analysis to detect single gene mutation. The embryos that are normal based on the genetic analysis results are transferred.

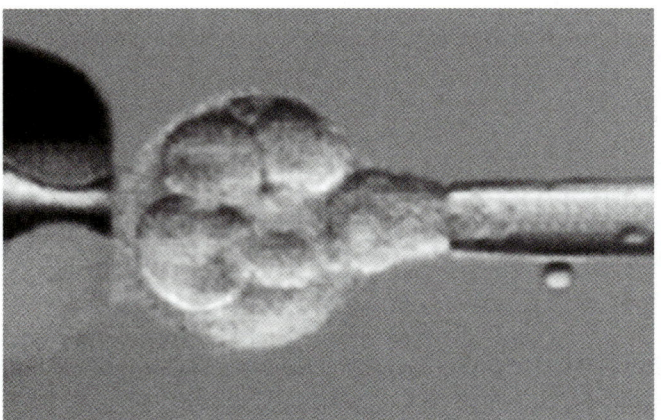

Fig. 12.38: **PGD producre:** An embryo biopsy procedure where one cell is removed from an 8-cell embryo

Benefits of PGD

Patients who are carriers of single gene mutations can avoid transmitting those disorders to their offspring by testing the embryos at the preimplantation stage and choosing not to transfer those which are affected. Patients who have had several miscarriages in the past can benefit from PGD for aneuploidy screening (PGD-AS) by avoiding the transfer of embryos that are aneuploid and will eventually fail to implant. The likelihood of having a trisomic pregnancy increases with advanced maternal age (>38 yrs). PGD allows selection of normal embryos at the pre-implantation stage and reduces the chance of detecting abnormal fetal development during an aminocentesis in the second trimester. Another group of patients who can benefit from PGD are those who carry translocations, which are detected by karyotyping.

Risks

There are certain risks associated with any micromanipulation procedure but these are minimal and are outweighed by the benefits. Occasionally nuclear material from the blastomeres is lost during processing. Due to poor hybridization of chromosome probes, sometimes results for all chromosomes are not able to be determined. This often happens when embryos are of poor quality on day 3 of development and exhibit extensive fragmentation. In single gene mutation analysis, if DNA material from the biopsied cells is degraded, amplification will be poor and sometimes no results can be obtained. A 10% misdiagnosis rate is not uncommon in aneuploidy screening due to mosaicism, a condition where one cell of a multicellular embryo is genetically different than another cell.

Biomarkers

Biomarkers that affect the pregnancy chances of IVF include:
- Antral follicle count, with higher count giving higher success rates.
- Anti-müllerian hormone levels, with higher levels indicating higher pregnancy chances.
- Level of DNA fragmentation as measured, e.g. by Comet assay, advanced maternal age and semen quality.
- Progesterone elevation (PE) on the day of induction of final maturation is associated with lower pregnancy rates in IVF cycles in women undergoing ovarian stimulation using GnRH analogues and gonadotropins.

Other Factors

- Tobacco smoking reduces the chances of IVF producing a live birth by 34% and increases the risk of an IVF pregnancy miscarrying by 30%.
- A body mass index (BMI) over 27 causes a 33% decrease in likelihood to have a live birth after the first cycle of IVF.
- Salpingectomy or laparoscopic tubal occlusion before IVF treatment increases chances for women with hydrosalpinges.
- The autoimmune diseases play a role in decreasing IVF success rates by interfering with proper implantation of the embryo after transfer. Aspirin is sometimes prescribed to women for the purpose of increasing the chances of conception by IVF, but there is insufficient evidence to show that it actually works.

Complications of IVF Procedure

Multiple Births

The major complication of IVF is the risk of multiple births. This is directly related to the practice of transferring multiple embryos at embryo transfer. Multiple births are related to increased risk of pregnancy loss, obstetrical complications, prematurity, and neonatal morbidity with the potential for long-term damage. Recent evidence also suggest that singleton offspring after IVF is at higher risk for lower birth weight for unknown reasons.

Other Risks to the Egg Provider/Retriever

A risk of ovarian stimulation is the development of ovarian hyperstimulation syndrome, particularly if hCG is used for inducing final oocyte maturation. This results in swollen, painful ovaries. It occurs in 30% of patients.

During egg retrieval, there is a small chance of bleeding, infection, and bowel and bladder injury(transvaginal ultrasound aspiration).

Ectopic pregnancy may also occur, if a fertilized egg develops in the fallopian tubes and requires immediate treatment.

Birth Defects

Babies resulting from IVF (with or without ICSI) have a relative risk of birth defects of 1.32 compared to naturally conceived infants. Certain birth defects conceived through IVF include septal heart defects, cleft lip with or without cleft palate, esophageal atresia, and anorectal atresia; the mechanism of causality is unclear.

Other Risks to the Offspring

Some concurrent medical disorders like gestational hypertension, impaired fasting glucose, thyroid disorder may be carried over.

An IVF-associated incidence of cerebral palsy and neurodevelopmental delay are believed to be related to the confounders of prematurity and low birth weight.

Overall, IVF does not cause an increased risk of childhood cancer though some studies have shown increased risk of certain cancers like retinoblastoma, hepatoblastoma and rhabdomyosarcoma.

Fertility Preservation in Cancer Patients

Introduction

Fertility preservation methods are still applied relatively infrequently in the cancer population because of limited knowledge about success and effects of different potential anticancer interventions to minimize risk of tumor recurrence and thereby neglecting therapeutic and psychological aspect of fertility preservation attempts. Cancer and cancer treatments vary in their likelihood of causing infertility. Individual factors such as disease, age, treatment type and dosages, and pretreatment fertility should be considered in counseling patients about the likelihood of infertility.

Patients who are interested in fertility preservation should consider their options as soon as possible to maximize the likelihood of success. Some treatments in females are dependent upon phase of the menstrual cycle and can be initiated only at monthly intervals.

The two methods of fertility preservation with the highest likelihood of success are sperm cryopreservation for males and embryo freezing for females. Conservative surgical approaches and transposition of ovaries or gonadal shielding prior to radiation therapy may also preserve fertility in selected cancers. There appears to be no detectable increased risk of disease recurrence associated with most fertility preservation methods and pregnancy, even in hormonally sensitive tumors. Aside from hereditary genetic syndromes and *in utero* exposure to chemotherapy, there is no evidence that a history of cancer, cancer therapy, or fertility interventions increases the risk of cancer or congenital abnormalities in the progeny.

Treatment-related infertility may be associated with psychosocial distress, and early referral for counseling may be beneficial in moderately distressed people.

Causes of Male Infertility in Cancer Patients

- The disease itself like Hodgkin's lymphoma
- Retrograde ejaculation or anejaculation
- 1° or 2° hormone insufficiency
- Damage or depletion of germinal stem cells

Anti-tumor agents that can cause prolonged azoospermia

Radiation (2.5 GY to testis)	Cisplatin (500 mg/m^2)
Chlorambucil (1.4 g/m^2)	Procarbazine (4 g/m^2)
Cyclophosphamide (19 g/m^2)	Melphalan (140 mg/m^2)

New agents like oxaliplatin, irinotecan, monoclonal antibodies, tyrosine kinase inhibitors and taxanes also affect sperm production but its mode of action is not known.

Current Options for Preservation of Fertility in Males (Table 12.3)

- Sperm cryopreservation
  - Antegrade ejaculate
  - Retrograde ejaculate
  - Testicular aspirate (outpatient surgery)
- Gonadal shielding during radiation
- Testicular suppression with GnRH analogs or antagonists—not effective

Use of Cryopreserved Sperm

- 10–30% of the men who banked sperm before cancer treatment return to use the sperm
- Storage fees are rarely the reason for specimen discard.

Table 12.3: Summary of fertility preservation options in males

Intervention	Definition
Sperm cryopreservation (S) after masturbation	Freezing sperm obtained through masturbation
Sperm cryopreservation (S) after alternative methods of sperm collection	Freezing sperm obtained through testicular aspiration or extraction, electroejaculation under sedation, or from a postmasturbation urine sample
Gonadal shielding during radiation therapy (S)	Use of shielding to reduce the dose of radiation delivered to the testicles
Testicular tissue cryopreservation; testis xenografting; spermato-gonial isolation (I)	Freezing testicular tissue or germ cells and reimplantation after cancer treatment or maturation in animals; not established in humans
Testicular suppression with GnRH analogs or antagonists (I)	Use of hormonal therapies to protect testicular tissue during chemotherapy or radiation therapy

Causes of Female Infertility

- DNA damage to oocytes
- Destruction of the primordial follicles
- Hormonal imbalances due to damage to the pituitary
- Damage to uterus, ovaries and tubes

Effect of Radiation on Female Fertility

- Direct and indirect damage to DNA of oocytes
- Small primordial and growing follicles damaged
- Damage to the pituitary

Table 12.4 grades risk of ovarian damage in different types of cancers as well as shows different options for fertility preservation in females.

Table 12.4: Risk of ovarian damage in following cancers

Low risk	Moderate risk	High risk
• Wilms'	• Stage IV breast	• Leukemia
• Lymphomas	• Adeno cervix	• Neuroblastoma
• Stage I-III breast CA (infiltrating and ductal)	• Colorectal	• Stage IV lobular breast
• Nongenital rhabdomyosarcoma		
• Osteogenic sarcoma		
• Squamous cell cervix Ewing sarcoma		

Options for fertility preservation

The now
- Embryo cryopreservation

Near future
- Oocyte cryopreservation
  - Still considered experimental

Long range planning
- Ovarian tissue cryopreservation
- Cytotoxic protectants

Embryo Cryopreservation

Embryo cryopreservation is considered an established fertility preservation method because it has routinely been used for storing surplus embryos after in vitro fertilization. Approximately 2 weeks of ovarian stimulation with daily injections of follicle-stimulating hormone is required and must be started within the first 3 days of the menstrual cycle.

Limitations of Embryo Cryopreservation

a. Time—need 2–6 weeks; may delay therapy for cancer
b. Relationship status—must have partner or donor sperm
c. Age—not acceptable for children
d. High cost/cycle plus storage fees
e. Risks—hyperstimulation syndrome
   - Exposure to higher level of estradiol

Cryopreservation of unfertilized oocytes. Cryopreservation of unfertilized oocytes is an option, particularly for patients without a partner or those with religious or ethical objections to embryo freezing. It is an option for pubertal girls. Ovarian stimulation is required. Oocyte cryopreservation should be performed only in centers with the necessary expertise according to institutional review board (IRB)—approved protocols.

Ovarian tissue cryopreservation. Ovarian tissue cryopreservation and transplantation procedures should be performed only in centers with the necessary expertise under IRB-approved protocols that include follow-up for recurrent cancer. Tissue is removed laparoscopically and cryopreserved. This contains primordial and primary follicles. They are reimplanted when ready to have children and oocytes are matured in the lab and fertilized. A concern with reimplanting ovarian tissue is the potential for reintroducing cancer cells, although in fewer than 20 procedures reported thus far, there are no reports of cancer recurrence.

Limitations of ovarian tissue cryopreservation:

a. Large follicular loss due to ischemia (about 25% of primordial follicles are lost)
b. Possibility of residual malignant cells

c. Oocytes arrested in prophase I must undergo *in vitro* maturation, if not reimplanted.

d. Expensive

Ovarian suppression. Currently, there is insufficient evidence regarding the safety and effectiveness of gonadotropin-releasing hormone analogs and other means of ovarian suppression on fertility preservation.

Ovarian transposition. Ovarian transposition (oophoropexy) can be offered when pelvic radiation is administered as cancer treatment. Because of the risk of remigration of the ovaries, this procedure should be performed as close to the radiation treatment as possible. This may be performed laparoscopically, if laparotomy is not needed for treatment. The success rate judged by short-term menstrual function is 50%. The failure is attributed to scatter radiation, alteration of the ovarian blood supply and total radiation dose. On many occasions, ovarian repositioning may or may not be required.

Conservative gynecologic surgery. It has been suggested that radical trachelectomy is restricted to stage IA2-IB cervical cancer disease with diameter less than 2 cm and invasion less than 10 mm. In the treatment of other gynecologic malignancies, interventions to spare fertility have generally centered on doing less-radical surgery and/or lower-dose chemotherapy with the intent of sparing the reproductive organs as much as possible.

Other considerations. Of special concern in breast and other gynecologic malignancies, there is possibility that fertility preservation interventions and/or subsequent pregnancy may increase the risk of cancer recurrence.

Use of Cytoprotective Agents

These are:

a. NRF2 activators—sulforaphane

b. Amifostine

c. Trental/vitamin E

d. Dexrazoxane

e. GnRh-analogue or antagonist (doubtful role); is claimed to have lower incidence of premature ovarian failure and infertility in prepubertal girls receiving alkylating agents.

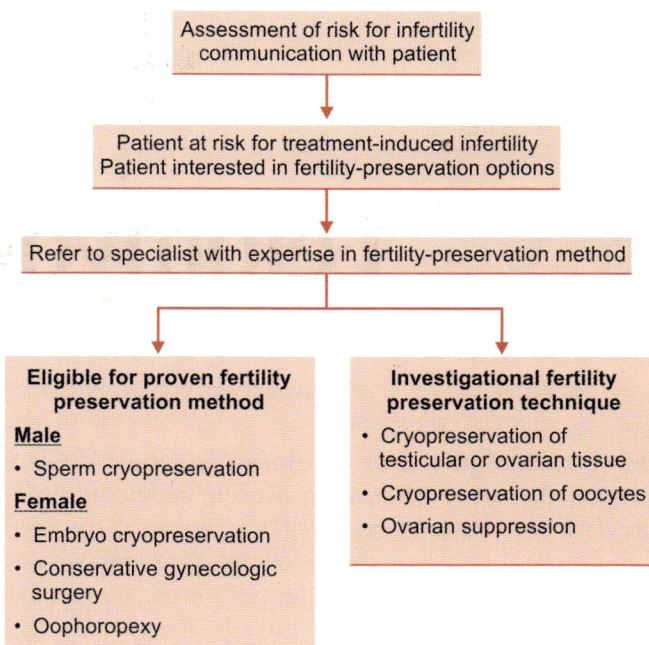

Fig. 12.39: Flowchart of fertility preservation protocol

Special Considerations: Fertility Preservation in Children

Use of established methods of fertility preservation (semen cryopreservation and embryo freezing) in postpubertal minor children requires patient assent and parental consent. The modalities available to prepubertal children to preserve their fertility are limited by the sexual immaturity of the children and are essentially experimental. Efforts to preserve fertility of children using experimental methods (e.g. gonadal tissue cryopreservation) should be attempted only under IRB-approved protocols (Fig. 12.39).

Conclusion

Oncologists should answer basic questions about whether fertility preservation options decrease the chance of successful cancer treatment, increase the risk of maternal or perinatal complications, or compromise the health of offspring. Patients should be encouraged to participate in registries and clinical studies as available to define further the safety of these interventions and strategies. Currently, women with a history of cancer and cancer treatment should be considered high risk for perinatal complications and would be prudent to seek specialized perinatal care.

13 | Leiomyoma Uterus

This is a benign tumor of uterus and pelvic tissue composed mainly of smooth muscle cells containing varying amount of connective tissue. The term 'Leiomyoma' is reasonably accurate as it emphasyses the origin of the tumor from smooth muscle cells. The tumor is well-circumscribed but not encapsulated. It produces compressed tissues in the surrounding to produce false or pseudocapsule. It is the most common tumor of the uterus and pelvis.

Incidence

The true incidence is very difficult to ascertain because many women with fibroids remain asymptomatic. It is responsible for one-third of all gynecology admission in hospitals. Incidence varies from 40–70% between age group of 35–50 years.

- The incidence is much higher in blacks than in whites. There is no explanation for this racial difference.
- Patients with uterine leiomyoma often have a positive family history suggesting presence of a gene encoding for its development. About 50% of leiomyomas show detectable chromosomal abnormality. Submucous myomas have fewer cytogenetic abnormality (12%) than subserous (29%) and interstitial myomas (35%).
- The lifetime risk of woman over 45 years of age developing fibroids is greater than 60%.

Epidemiology

- Age and parity: Fibroids are more common in elderly women more with low parity. Increasing parity decreases the incidence and number of fibroids.
- Fibroid growth is dependent on both estrogen and progesterone. Therefore, fibroids appear only after menarche and show reduction in size after menopause. Fibroids have increased local estrogen and estrogen receptor levels compared to normal myometrium. Progesterone receptor levels are also increased in fibroids relative to myometrium. The highest mitotic activity is seen in fibroids in secretory phase giving rise to prospect of use of mifepristone, antiprogesterone to decrease in tumor volume.

- Use of combined OCP and ERT in postmenopausal women with higher dose of estrogen shows some association in increase in size of fibroids in the initial months of use. But with current low dose of COC and ERT risk of growth of fibroid is minimum.
- Obesity, diabetes, PCOS and hypertension may likely be associated with increase in size of fibroids.

Pathophysiology

Fibroids are round- or oval-shaped tumors with a characteristic white whorled appearance on cut section. Fibroids may be single or multiple and of varying sizes and can arise at different sites. There can be many small seedling fibroids in association with large fibroids which may grow to big size over the years. Fibroids usually do not grow after menopause unless they undergo sarcomatous changes (0.5%).

Fibroid can undergo many other degenerative changes like: (a) Cystic degeneration, (b) hyaline degeneration, (c) fatty degeneration, (d) calcarious degeration, (e) red degeneration and (f) sarcomatous degeneration.

Growth Factors

There are many growth factors, polypeptides produced which are overexpressed in fibroids locally stimulate fibroid growth by increasing extracellular matrix. TGF-α, and bFGF (basic fibroblastic growth factor) increase DNA synthesis and EGF (epidermal growth factor), and PDGF (platelet-derived growth factor) stimulate synthesis of extracellular matrix and VEGF (vascular endothelial growth factor) promotes angiogenesis.

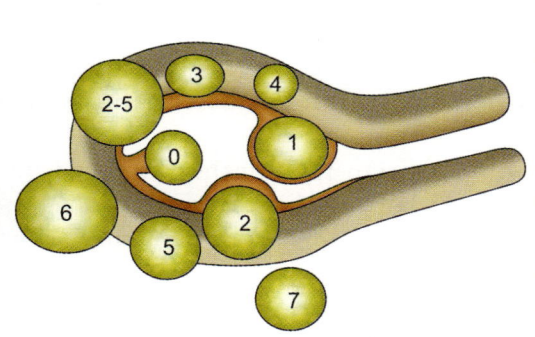

SM–Submucosal	0	Pedunculated intracavitary
	1	<50% intramural
	2	≥50% intramural
O–Other	3	Contacts endometrium; 100%
	4	Intramural
	5	Subserosal ≥50% intramural
	6	Subserosal <50% intramural
	7	Subserosal pedunculated
	8	Other (specify, e.g. cervical, parasitic)

Hybrid: Leiomyomas (impact both endometrium and serosa)

Two numbers are listed separated by a hyphen. By convention, the first refers to the relationship with the endometrium while the second refers to the relationship to the serosa. One example is below:

2–5	Submucosal and subserosal, each with less than half the diameter in the endometrial and peritoneal cavities, respectively.

Fig. 13.1: Leiomyoma subclassification system

Microscopic Appearance

Fibroids are mainly composed of smooth muscle cell bundles admixed with variable amount of connective tissue. The term 'Cellular leiomyoma' is used when density of smooth muscles is proportionately more without any abnormal mitotic features. There are fibroids which are composed of polygonal cells rather than spindle cells. They are termed as 'symplasmic' or 'atypical' leiomyomas. The malignant counterpart of leiomyoma is 'leiomyosarcoma' which shows high cellularity, nuclear metamorphosis, abnormal mitoses and areas of necrosis with infiltrating margins. Usually the number of cellular mitoses exceed 10 per 10 high power fields in contrast to always less than five in case of benign form of leiomyomas.

Risk Factors

- *Age:* Incidence of fibroids increase with age.
- *Endogenous hormonal factors:* Early menarche and late menopause increases greater exposure to endogenous estrogens and progesterone and increases the likelihood of uterine fibroids.
- *Family history:* First degree relatives of women with fibroids have 2.5 times increased risk of developing fibroids.
- *Ethnicity:* African American women have 2.9 times greater risk of having fibroids than white women.
- *Weight:* Risk of fibroid increase with increase in body weight and BMI.

Classification of Fibroids (Fig. 13.1)

FIGO fibroid classification system categorises submucous, intramural, subserosal and transmural fibroids.
- *Type 0:* Intracavitary, i.e. submucus fibroid entirely within the cavity.
- *Type 1:* Less than 50% of fibroid diameter within the myometrium.
- *Type 2:* 50% or more of fibroid diameter within the myometrium.
- *Type 3:* Interstitial fibroid abut the endometrium (in contact) without any intracavitary component.
- *Type 4:* Intramural entirely within the myometrium without any extension to either endometrial surface or serosa.
- *Type 5:* Subserosal with at least 50% intramural
- *Type 6:* Subserosal with less than 50% intramural
- *Type 7:* Subserosal attached to serosa by a stalk.
- *Type 8:* In other areas without any involvement of myometrium; that includes cervical, round or broad ligament and 'parasitic' fibroids.

Transmural fibroids are categorized by its relationship to both endometrial and serosal surface with endometrial relationship noted first, i.e. "type 2–5".

Clinical Features

Fifty percent of the women with fibroids may remain asymptomatic. Symptoms do not always correlate with size of fibroids.

Out of the women who become symptomatic, menstrual disorder is the commonest symptom.

1. Abnormal Uterine Bleeding (30%)

- Heavy/prolonged bleeding (menorrhagia) iron deficiency anemia. Bleeding is due to incrased endometrial surface area (up to 200 sqm insted of normal 15 sqm). It may be due to endometrial hyperplasia because of frequent anovular cycle with hyperestrogenic state.
- Submucous myoma causes pre- and post-menstrual spotting and metrorrhagia. Bleeding is due to interruption of blood supply to the endometrium, distortion and congestion of surrounding vessels or ulceration of the overlying endometrium.

2. Pain

It may be dysmenorrhea of congestive type or continuous not related to menstruation dates. This can be due to following reasons:

- Vascular occlusion producing necrosis, infection.
- Torsion of a pedunculated fibroid resulting in acute pain.
- Myometrial contractions to expel the myoma.
- Red degeneration.
- Heaviness or fullness in the pelvic area or feeling a mass.
- If the tumor gets impacted in the pelvis, it produces pressure on nerves producing back pain radiating to the lower extremities or bladder and rectal symptoms.
- Dysparunea, if it is polypoid protruding into vagina.

3. Pressure Effects

- Large fibroids may distort or obstruct organs like ureters, bladder or rectum producing urinary symptoms, hydroureter, constipation, pelvic venous congestion and edema.
- Rarely a posterior fundal tumor produces extreme retroflexion of the uterus distorting the bladder base causing urinary retention.
- Parasitic tumor may cause bowel obstruction. Cervical tumors result in serosanguinous vaginal discharge, bleeding, dyspareunia or infertility.

4. Infertility

- The relationship is uncertain. Fibroid per se does not cause infertility and its removal may not enhance fertility.
- 27–40% of women with multiple fibroids are infertile but other causes of infertility are present.

- Presence of submucous fibroid acts as a cause of implantation failure.
- Cornual fibroid can produce mechanical obstruction to ascent of sperms.
- Co-existing anovulation, salpingitis causing tubal block, associated endometriosis can cause subfertility.
- Increased tubo-ovarian relationship, delayed or defective ovum pickup, and increased macrophages induced altered peritoneal current may be responsible for subfertility.
- Various other theories have been advanced to explain the potential subfertility effect of fibroids:
  a. Dysfunctional uterine contractility
  b. Focal endometrial vascular disturbance
  c. Endometrial inflammation,
  d. Secretion of vasoactive substances,
  e. Enhanced endometrial androgen environment.

5. Spontaneous Abortions

Incidence of spontaneous abortion before myomectomy is 40% and after myomectomy 20%.

Examination

General: Look for anemia, edema, pulse and BP.

Abdominopelvic Examination

Presence of a suprapubic mass which has the following characters:

- Size corresponds to uterine shape (pyriform)
- Surface—smooth
- Consistency—firm
- Margin—well defined
- Mobility—from side-to-side present but not in above downwards

Pelvic Examination

- Uterus and the mass is continuous.
- No adnexal SOL and Hingarani groove is absent.
- Try to identify sites of the tumor.
- Cul-de-sac: Any mass in the POD.
- Presence of cervical/broad ligament/anterior/ posterior fibroid.
- Mass moves with the cervix.
- Cervix if dilated with a rim around a pedunculated fibroid polyp.
- External os is totally effaced in cervical fibroid; if os is anteriorly pushed behind symphysis, cervical fibroid is posterior and it is reversed when cervical fibroid is anterior.

Table 13.1: Clinical differential diagnosis with ovarian tumor

Serial no.	Topic	Fibroid	Ovarian tumor
1	Age	Mostly in reproductive age group	All ages
2	Parity	In low parity women	Not related
3.	Menstrual disorder	Commonest symptom	Not common
4.	GI symptoms	Absent	Very common
5.	Rate of growth	Slow	May be rapid
6.	Shape	Pyriform unless multinodular	Oval or spherical
7.	Number	Single mass	May be bilateral
8.	Surface	Smooth or nodular	Smooth
9.	Feel	Firm	Cystic or variegated
10.	Tenderness	Not tender	May be tender
11.	Mobility	Mobile from side-to-side but not above downwards	Mobile in all directions
12.	Ascites (shifting dullness)	Absent	Present in maligant mass
13	Vaginal exam	Mass moves with cervix	Mass separate from uterus
14	Rectovaginal exam	No mass in POD	Nodular metastasis in POD in malignant mass

- **Rectovaginal examination,** identify any retroperitoneal extension in case of retroperitoneal leiomyosarcoma.

Confirmation of Diagnosis

1. *Sonography (transabdominal/transvaginal)* is a reliable noninvasive technique to differentiate fibroids from other pelvic pathology. Fibroids on sonography appear symmetrical, well-defined, hypoechoic (cystic degeneration), heterogenous hyperechoic (calcification or hemorrhagic)mass.
2. *Saline infusion sonography, hysteroscopy* can identify cavity fibroids with a sensitivity and specificity of 90%
3. *MRI* allows evaluation of number, size, sites and infiltration of different types of fibroids and assess its proximity to bladder, rectum and endometrial cavity. This is required before any plan for myomectomy.

Differential Diagnosis

- Exclude pregnancy
- Ovarian SOL (Table 13.1)
- Tubo-ovarian abscess
- Endometriostic cysts
- Adenomyosis
- Koch's abdomen congenital anomalies with hematometra
- Endometrial or cervical cancer with hematometra

Treatment

It depends on (a) age, (b) parity, (c) pregnancy status, (d) desire for future pregnancy, (e) general health, (f) symptoms, (g) size, and (h) location.

a. Emergency Measures

- Blood transfusion/PRBC to correct anemia.
- Emergrncy surgery is indicated for (a) infected myoma, (b) acute torsion, and (c) intestinal/ureteric obstruction.
- In general, myomectomy is contraindicated during pregnancy.

b. General Principles of Management

- Most cases are asymptomatic and may not need treatment.
- Postmenopausal small fibroids need no treatment.
- Initial follow up every 6 months to determine the rate of growth of the myoma.
- The only indication for myomectomy in pregnancy is torsion of a pedunculated fibroid.
- Myomectomy is not recommended during cesarean section unless it is found pedunculated subserosal or in line of cesarean section. Presently, it is being practised in selected cases of elective cesarean section with blood in hand to spare the women from another surgery.
- Pregnant women with previous multiple myomectomy (especially if the cavity was entered) should be delivered by CS to reduce risk of scar rupture in labor.

c. Expectant Management

The mere presence of small asymptomatic fibroids <3 cm does not need any treatment. At least 50% of fibroids may remain asymptomatic. Spontaneous regression of fibroids may occur after menopause. But it is not suitable in case fibroid sustain its growth potential over a period of time.

d. Medical Management

This is expected to serve two important purpose: 1) Relief of symptoms; 2) reduction in size. Most of the drugs used do not help in shrinkage of the tumor to a substantial extent. Moreover, the shrinkage effect on fibroid disappears immediate after cessation of treatment.

- Non-steroidal anti-inflammatory agents, e.g. mefenamic acid, reduce menstrual blood loss and dysmenorrhea.
- Antifibrinolytic agents, e.g. tranexamic acid, 1–2 gm daily reduce menorrhagia.
- The combined oral contraceptive pill is also effective, if the patient requires contraception.
- Danazol in the dose of 200–400 mg/day for 3–6 months reduces menorrhagia, by suppressing gonadotropin secretion and abolishing cyclical ovarian function. It also reduces size of fibroids so long it is used.
- Gonadotropin-releasing hormone (GnRH) agonists:
  a. Produce reduction in the size of fibroids, in the region of 50% within three months but, once discontinued, fibroids regrow to their former size within two months; therefore, they are mainly useful preoperatively.
  b. GnRH agonists should be commenced in midluteal phase for rapid downregulation and after a few breakthrough bleeding, amenorrhea results. Uterine volume is reduced by 35% after 3 months and 60% after 6 months. The optimal duration of presurgical treatment with GnRH agonists is 3 months.
  c. The currently available GnRH agonists include: Goserelin 3.6 mg, leuproline 3.75 mg by monthly subcutaneous depot insertion and buserelin 900–1200 mg or nafarelin 800 μg intranasal spray in divided doses.
  d. They are associated with significant side effects, including amenorrhea, menopausal symptoms and bone loss which can lead to osteoporosis in long-term use.
  e. For this reason, low dose estrogen-progesterone combination, oral progesterone alone or tibolone

is used to ameliorate vasomotor symptoms and maintain bone mineral density.
- Antiprogesterone treatment with mifepristone is said to reduce uterine size and menstrual disorders, but there is risk of endometrial hyperplasia because of its anti-progesterone effect on endometrium.
- **Asoprisnil,** a selective progesterone receptor modulator (SPRM) with mixed agonist/antagonist effects, has been used to treat fibroids. It inhibits endometrial proliferation by its selective agonist effect on endometrium. It has been found that asoprisnil treatment for 3 months reduces fibroid-related symptoms and its size without hypoestrogenic symptoms and endometrial hyperplasia.

e. Surgical Measures

Myomectomy
- Open myomectomy
- Laparoscopic myomectomy
- Hysteroscopic myomectomy

Hysterectomy
- Vaginal hysterectomy
- Abdominal hysterectomy

Uterine artery embolization

I. Abdominal Myomectomy

- Although myomectomy allows preservation of the uterus, it carries higher risk of blood loss and greater operative time than with hysterectomy.
- There is a 15% recurrence rate for fibroids and 10% of women undergoing myomectomy will eventually require hysterectomy within 5 to 10 years.
- Women should be counselled about the risks of requiring hysterectomy at the time of planned myomectomy.
- Persistence of menorrhagia is observed in 5–10% cses even after myomectomy for some period.

Different Types of Myomectomy Incisions

- Midline anterior for anterior corporeal fibroid.
- Bonney's hood operation for fundal or upper posterior fibroid (Figs 13.2 and 13.3).
- Secondary tunneling incision for small interstitial fibroid.
- Transcavitary incision for posterior fibroids less than golfball in size (<6 cm).
- Direct posterior incision for big posterior fibroid.
- Rutherford Morison (bifurcation of uterus) incision for central cervical fibroid.
- Post box incision for broad ligament fibroid.

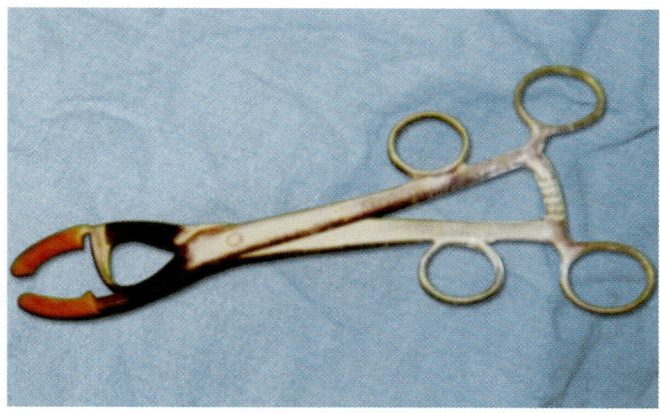

Fig. 13.2: Bonney's myomectomy clamp

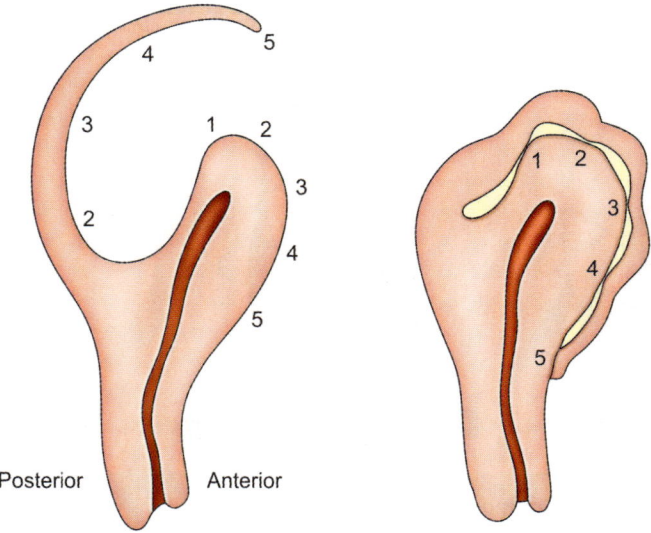

Posterior   Anterior

Fig. 13.3: Bonney's hood incision

Basic Principles of Abdominal Myomectomy

1. Type of myomectomy incisions will be decided after assessing the position and number of fibroids.
2. Incisions are planned in such a way that *maximum number of fibroids can be removed with minimum number of incisions.*
3. Incision preferably is placed in anterior wall to minimize adhesions sparing the attachment of fallopian tubes (Fig. 13.4).
4. To find out proper plane of incision.
5. Enucleation of fibroids through primary, and secondary tunneling and transcavitary incision.
6. Secure proper hemostasis by Tiers of circular mattress sutures with 1'0' vicryl starting from bottom.
7. Excision of redundant tissues to remove myohyperplasia.

8. Reconstruction of uterus. If cavity is opened, construct the cavity wall separate and a pediatric Foley catheter can be placed for a few days postoperative to maintain patency.
9. Some anti-adhesive measures, like immersion in heparinized Ringer lactated solution, omental patches, interceed patch over the repaired wound; can be taken, particularly if incision remains on posterior wall.

Techniques to Reduce Blood Loss

A variety of methods have been described that are aimed at minimizing blood loss. The two main approaches, medical and mechanical, diminish uterine blood flow to the myoma.

One step to decrease blood loss in myomectomy is use of 8-L-arginine vasopressin. Dilute solutions of vasoprassin (20 units in 200 mL distilled water) are injected directly into the myoma, raising a circumferential wheal and causing vasoconstriction. It blanches the tissue and provides better visualization of the tissue planes. However, its use is contraindicated in patients with epilepsy, migraine, asthma, heart failure, and nephritis. It may produce water intoxication, the early signs of which must be recognized. Headache, drowsiness, and listlessness always precede convulsions and coma, which can result from severe overdosage of this medication.

The most direct method to minimize blood loss during myomectomy is to use mechanical methods that decrease uterine blood flow. **Bonney** first described the use of an atraumatic clamp that compresses the uterine vessels and decreases uterine blood flow. The Bonney clamp is applied from the pubic end of the abdominal wound; it must contain the round ligament in its grip, or it slips below the uterine vessels. To stop uterine blood flow, blood flow from the infundibulopelvic ligament is compressed using a ring forceps.

Techniques to Prevent Adhesion Formation

Multiple strategies have been described for minimizing this potential complication. The vertical, anterior uterine incision can minimize blood loss and prevent the formation of adhesions that involve the tubes, ovaries, or bowel. This incision should be employed, if feasible. The intraperitoneal instillation of heparinized Ringer slution (5000 unit of heparin in 1000 mL infusion bottle) during and after surgery helps prevent adhesion. Other strategies include use of adhesion barriers such as Interceed, Gore-Tex and Seprafilm over the opearative sites.

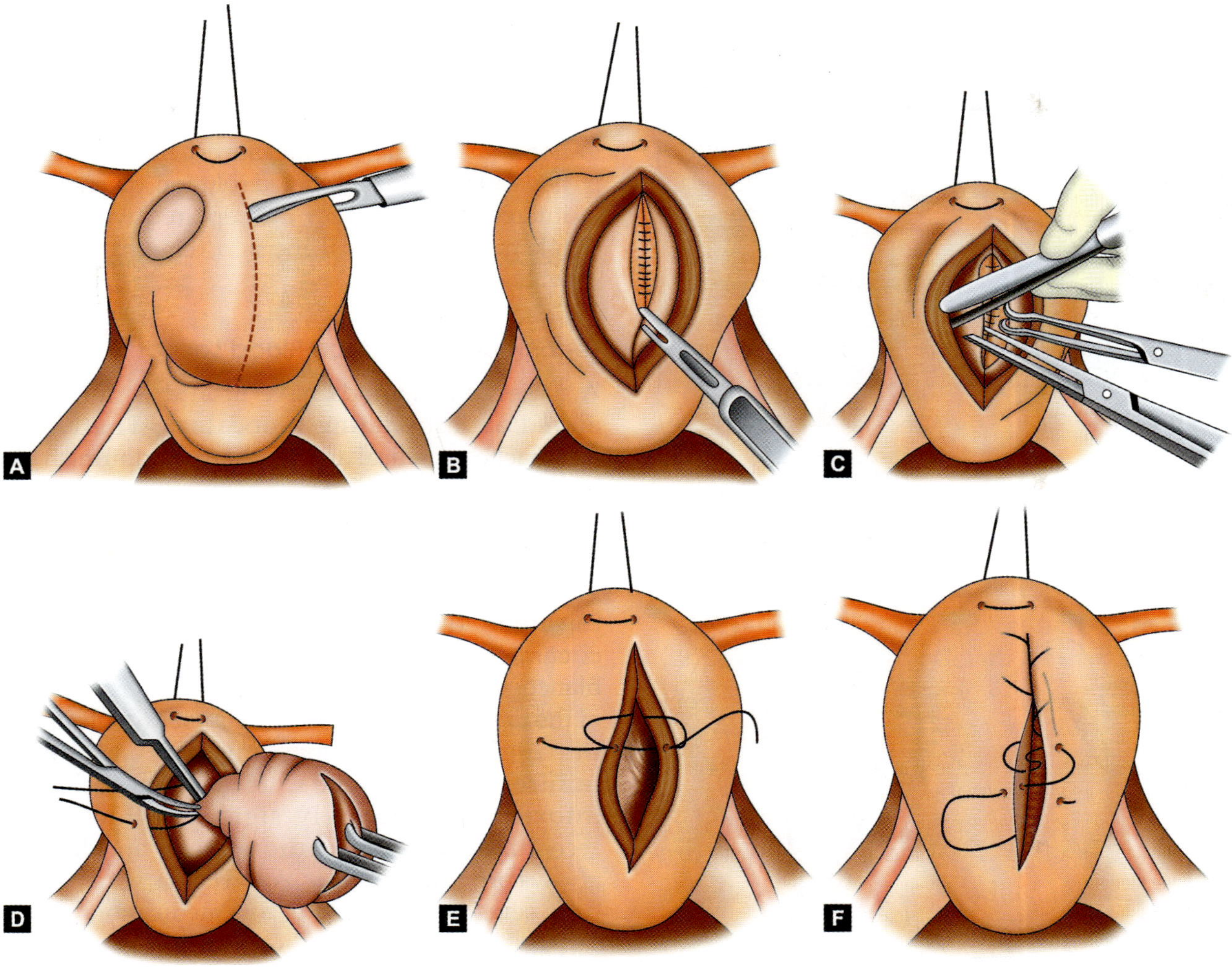

Fig. 13.4: Steps of myomectomy by midline anterior incision

II. Laparoscopic Myomectomy (Fig. 13.5)

- Myomas may be removed by laparoscopic approach.
- The challenges of this surgery rest with the surgeon's ability to remove the mass through 3–4 small abdominal incisions and to reconstruct the uterus.
- When compared to a laparotomy, the laparoscopic approach appears to take longer but is associated with a quicker recovery.
- Concerns have been raised regarding the ability to suture the uterus with an adequate multilayer closure laparoscopically.
- Uterine rupture during a subsequent pregnancy has been reported.
- The risk of recurrent myomas may be higher after a laparoscopic approach, with a 33% recurrence risk at 27 months.
- There are fewer postoperative adhesions in women who have undergone myomectomy laparoscopically but adhesion formation after laparoscopic myomectomy has still been reported to occur in 60% of cases.
- The choice of surgical approach is largely dependent on surgical expertise.

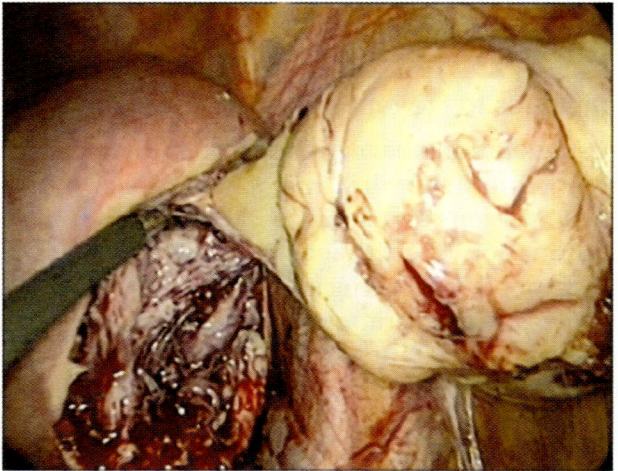

Fig. 13.5: Laparoscopic myomectomy

- Morcellators have permitted removal of larger myomas, but there is a danger of injury to surrounding organs.
- Current available recommendations for conventional abdominal myomectomy are indicated when:
  a. Fibroids exceeding 5 to 8 cm
  b. Multiple myomas, or
  c. When deep intramural leiomyomas are present.
- **Laparoscopic-assisted myomectomy** presents an opportunity to enucleate the myoma partially by laparoscopy, deliver the tumor through a small abdominal incision, then close the uterine defect through this laparotomy.

III. Hysteroscopic Myomectomy (Fig. 13.6)

- Intracavitary or submucous myomas are found in 30% of outpatient diagnostic hysteroscopies in women with abnormal uterine bleeding.
- Hysteroscopic myomectomy is considered in women with (a) symptomatic intracavitary, (b) submucous narrow-based intrauterine myomas, (c) infertility, and (d) repeated pregnancy losses.
- The pregnancy rate in women undergoing *in vitro* fertilization (IVF) may be reduced when myomas are submucosal or when they distort the uterine cavity.
- If fertility is not desired and abnormal uterine bleeding is the main symptom, concomitant endometrial ablation or resection may provide better resolution of abnormal/bleeding than myomectomy alone.
- Recently, electrosurgical loop electrodes using bipolar technology, as well as vaporizing electrodes using both monopolar and bipolar technology, have been described as new technologies to facilitate hysteroscopic myomectomy.
- Pretreatment with GnRH analogue for 3 months prior to myomectomy may increase the preoperative hemoglobin and hematocrit in women with anemia and result in shrinkage of the fibroid, decrease of uterine blood flow and endometrial cavity size, as well as thinning of the endometrium.
- Hysteroscopic myomectomy needs good endoscopic expertise. It has been associated with significant complications:
  a. Intraoperative bleeding may lead to an emergency hysterectomy.
  b. Electrical burns to the genital tract, and bowel have been reported.
  c. Hyponatremia, pulmonary edema, heart failure, cerebral edema, blindness, coma, and death from excessive irrigant fluid absorption have also been rarely reported.
- Prolonged surgical procedures require careful monitoring of irrigant fluid balance. Termination of procedure is recommended when fluid deficit exceeds 1000 mL or after introduction of 1500 mL of non-electrolyte solution and 2000 mL of an electrolyte solution.

Laparoscopic Myolysis

- Myolysis refers to the procedure of delivering energy to myomas in an attempt to desiccate them directly or disrupt their blood supply.
- Myomata deprived of their blood supply would presumably shrink or completely degenerate as they receive less nutrients, sex hormones, and growth factors.

The indications for myolysis include symptomatic myomas requiring surgical treatment for:

a. Abnormal uterine bleeding
b. Pelvic pain
c. Pressure to adjacent organs.

Women may be considered candidates for myolysis, if (a) they have fewer than four myomas of 5 cm or (b) their largest myoma measures less than 10 cm in diameter.

- Concomitant hysteroscopic endometrial ablation or resection is recommended to further assist in the management of menorrhagia and can be performed at the end of laparoscopic myolysis.
- Complications (<1% cases) consist of (a) pelvic infection, (b) bacteremia, and (c) bleeding.
- In general, 3 months of GnRH agonist pretreatment reduces the total uterine myoma volume by approximately 35 to 50%.

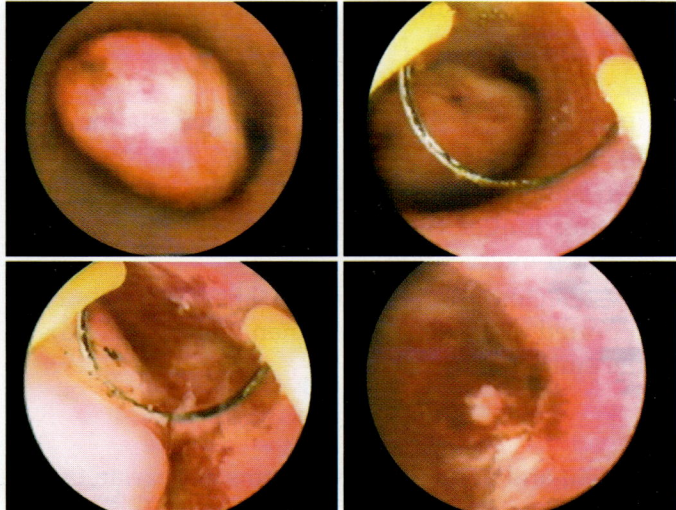

Fig. 13.6: Hysteroscopic myomectomy

- Following myoma coagulation, the total uterine myoma volume is reduced permanently by 80%.
- It is recommended that pregnancy should not be undertaken by women who have undergone myolysis although some women who underwent the procedure have conceived and have uneventfully been delivered by cesarean section.
- Three cases of uterine rupture during the third trimester of pregnancy have been reported. Thus, myolysis can be considered only after a woman expresses her desire not to conceive again.

Uterine Artery Embolization (Fig. 13.7)

- The most popular approach to uterine artery occlusion is selective uterine artery catheterization and embolization.
- Eligible women include those with symptomatic fibroids who wish to avoid surgical therapy.
- Before undergoing uterine artery embolization, all women should be counselled that this procedure is (a) less than 10 years old, and (b) its long-term effects and durability, including fertility and pregnancy outcomes, are not yet known.
- Preoperative evaluation should include: (a) A thorough history, (b) physical and pelvic examination, (c) complete blood count (CBC), (d) electrolytes, (e) renal function tests, and (f) coagulation profile.
- Routine cervical cytology and endometrial sampling should be performed.
- Uterine artery embolization is performed in a medical imaging suite by interventional radiologists using aseptic sterile techniques.

Perioperative risks and complications include:
(a) Infection, (b) bleeding, (c) hematomas at the femoral artery puncture site, (d) allergic or anaphylactic

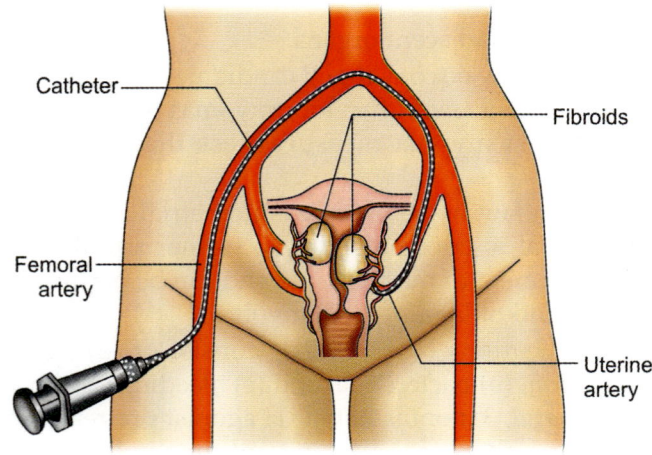

Catheter

Fibroids

Femoral artery

Uterine artery

Fig. 13.7: Uterine artery occlusion

reactions to the iodinated contrast dye, and (e) incomplete uterine artery occlusion, (f) misembolization of non-target organs. Such complications occur in approximately 1 to 2% of procedures.

Post–uterine Artery Occlusion— Side Effects and Complications

1. *Early or Acute Abdominal Pelvic Pain*

a. Virtually, all women experience some degree of acute pain, often requiring hospitalization.
b. The pain is thought to be due to nonspecific ischemia of the uterus and fibroids, and responds to opiates and nonsteroidal anti-inflammatory drugs (NSAIDs).

2. *Post-embolization Syndrome*

Up to 40% of women experience (a) diffuse abdominal pain, (b) generalized malaise, (c) anorexia, (d) nausea, vomiting, and (e) low-grade fever, and leukocytosis.

The syndrome is self-limiting and usually resolves within 48 hours to 2 weeks with conservative and supportive therapy, consisting of intravenous fluids and adequate pain control, including NSAIDs.

3. *Infection*

a. The incidence of febrile morbidity and sepsis following embolization has been reported to be between 1.0 and 1.8%.
b. The infections include pyometra with endomyometritis, bilateral chronic salpingitis, tuboovarian abscess, and infected myomas.
c. The most frequent pathogen isolated is *Escherichia coli*. Some women have responded to antibiotic therapy but others have required prolonged hospitalization, intensive therapy, and hysterectomy.

4. *Persistent or Chronic Pain*

a. In 5 to 10% of women, the pain persists for more than 2 weeks.
b. Persistent pain in the absence of infection or pain lasting longer than 2 to 3 months may require surgical intervention.
c. Hysterectomy for postembolization pain has been reported in up to 2% of women within 6 months of the embolization.

5. *Ovarian Dysfunction*

Transient and permanent symptoms of ovarian failure have been reported in 10% of women after uterine artery embolization.

6. Menstrual Dysfunction

- Improvement in menstrual bleeding in up to 90% of women following uterine artery embolization has been reported.
- Transient or permanent amenorrhea has been reported in 15% and 3% of women, respectively.
- Amenorrhea after embolotherapy is also highly age-dependent and is reported to be related to waning ovarian function.

7. Transcervical Myoma Expulsion

- Following artery embolization, spontaneous expulsion of myomas through the cervix has been reported to occur in approximately 5 to 10% of women.
- 60% of women with submucous myomas, confirmed by hysteroscopy, expel myomas vaginally, following uterine artery embolization.

8. Uterine Wall Integrity

- The physical characteristics, integrity, and the histopathologic features of the uterine wall after uterine artery embolization remain unknown.
- Uterine wall defects, uterine fistula, and diffuse uterine necrosis following uterine artery embolization have been reported.
- Although normal pregnancies and deliveries following uterine artery occlusion have been reported, there is insufficient long-term data regarding reproductive outcome following this procedure and it would be prudent to reserve embolization for women who will not wish pregnancy.

9. Hysterectomy

- The number of women who proceed to hysterectomy following uterine artery embolization has been used as an indicator for the measurement of treatment failure.

- The rate of hysterectomy within 6 months of embolization is 1 to 2%, and the indications are persistent bleeding, persistent pain, prolapse of fibroids, and uterine malignancies.

10. Mortality

The mortality is approximately 0.1 to 0.2 per 1000 procedures.

IV. Hysterectomy

- The only indications for hysterectomy in a woman with completely asymptomatic fibroids are: (a) Rapidly enlarging fibroids or (b) when enlarging fibroids raise concerns of leiomyosarcoma (specially after menopause).
- In women who have completed childbearing, hysterectomy is indicated as a permanent cure for leiomyomas causing substantial bleeding, pelvic pressure, or anemia.
- When considering hysterectomy for menorrhagia attributed to fibroids, other causes should be ruled out.
- Endometrial biopsy should be considered, to exclude endometrial malignancy.

Special Situations

I. Fibroids and Pregnancy

Prevalance of fibroids in pregnancy ranges from 0.09% to 3.9%.

- Less than two-thirds of women with fibroids and unexplained infertility conceive after myomectomy.
- Approxemately 90% of the fibroids exhibit no change in size during pregnancy. The mean increase in fibroid volume in pregnancy is 12%. Fibroid growth occurs most commonly in the first trimester, less in the second and third trimesters. Larger fibroids (>5 cm in diameter) are more likely to grow, whereas smaller fibroids remain stable in size.

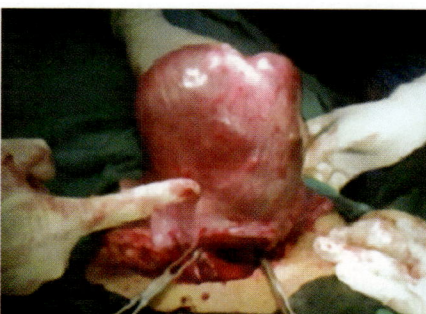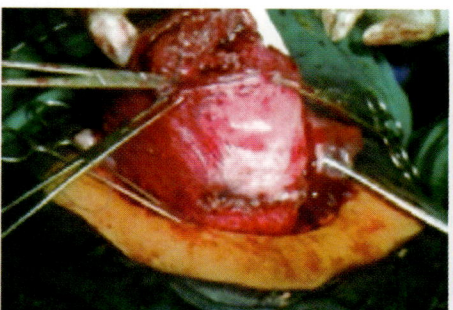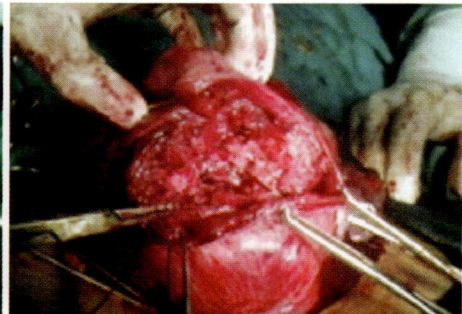

Fig. 13.8: Cesarean myomectomy done by author

Red Degeneration

In the 2nd or 3rd trimester of pregnancy, rapid increase in size results in vascular deprivation and degeneration. It causes pain and uterine tenderness. It may initiate preterm labor. It is managed conservatively with bedrest, narcotics and tocolytics, if indicated. After the acute phase subsides, pregnancy will continue to term.

Effect of Fibroids during Pregnancy

- If the placenta implants over or in close proximity to a myoma, there may be an increased risk of miscarriage, preterm labor, abruption, prelabor rupture of membranes, or intrauterine growth restriction.
- Fibroids located in the lower uterine segment increase the likelihood of fetal malpresentation, antepartum hemorrhage, and cesarean section.
- Large fibroids, defined as greater than 20 cm in diameter, can cause abruption and acute abdominal pain.

Effect of Fibroids during Labor

Fibroid produces:
- Uterine inertia
- Malpresentation
- Obstructed labor particularly in case of cervical or isthmic myoma which necessitates cesarean section.
- Retained placenta and PPH.
- Myomectomy should not be performed in pregnant women because of the increased risk of uncontrolled bleeding.
- The exception is (a) symptomatic subserous fibroids on a pedicle less than 5 cm thick, in which case the risk of hemorrhage may be reduced and (b) fibroid at the line of incision. The working advantage is in pregnancy tissue plane dissection is easy and all oxytocic drugs work very well for hemostasis on puerperal uterus, particularly, if myomectomy is done in upper segment.

II. Fibroids and Uterine Leiomyosarcomas
(Figs 13.9 and 13.10)

- Uterine sarcoma is a rare gynecologic malignancy, occurring in 1.7 per 100 000 women.
- Sarcomas represent 1.2 to 6% of all uterine malignancies, with leiomyosarcomas representing approximately 25% of these.
- The mean age at diagnosis for uterine leiomyosarcoma is between 44 and 57 years.
- 50% of the women experience abnormal bleeding pain, enlarging abdomen, or abnormal vaginal discharge.

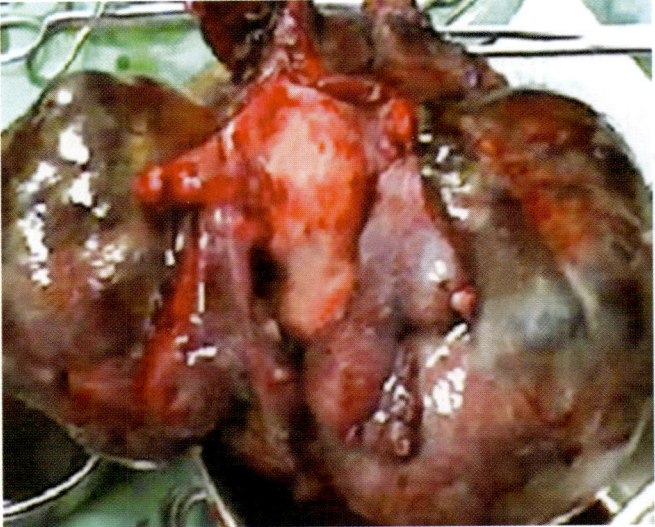

Fig. 13.9: Macroscopic appearance of leiomyosarcoma

- A uterine mass increasing in size in a postmenopausal woman suggests leiomyosarcoma rather than a benign leiomyoma.
- The masses tend to be softer due to tissue necrosis and internal cystic degeneration and hemorrhage.
- Leiomyosarcomas tend to be difficult to separate from the surrounding myometrium at attempted myomectomy because of their invasive nature.
- Fewer than 1 in 10 leiomyosarcomas arise within the cervix.
- Cervical cytology, endometrial sampling, and ultrasound (including color Doppler) have not been found to be reliable.
- There is insufficient evidence to support routine biopsy of uterine fibroids.
- Magnetic resonance imaging (MRI) is promising in distinguishing between benign and malignant smooth muscle tumors. An ill-defined margin of a uterine smooth muscle tumor on MRI is more in keeping with a malignant process.
- The clinical diagnosis of a rapidly growing leiomyoma prior to menopause has not been shown to predict uterine leiomyosarcoma in the absence of any other symptomatology, and thus should not be used as the sole indication for myomectomy or hysterectomy.
- Typically leiomyosarcomas is a large solid mass with a mean diameter of 10 cm. Approximately 25% of the tumor masses are <5 cm in size. About two-thirds of leiomyosarcomas are intramural, 1/5th submucosal, 1/10th subserosal and 5% arise in the cervix. The cut surface is typically bulging, fleshy, focally necrotic, and hemorrhagic.

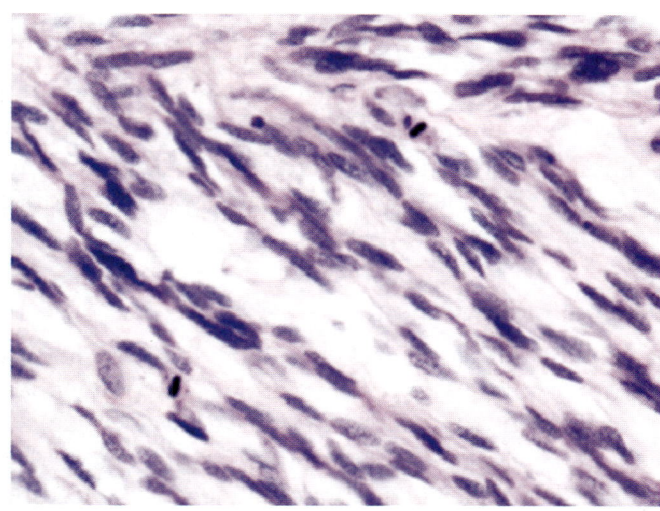

Fig. 13.10: Histological appearance of leiomyosarcoma

- Microscopically, it shows moderate hyper-cellularity, moderate to marked nuclear atypia usually of diffuse type, with high mitotic rate of 10 or more mitotic figures/10 HPF and 90% of them have >15 mitotic figures/10 HPF. It is characterized by tumor necrosis with an abrupt transition from viable cells to necrotic cells without an interposed zone of granulation tissue or fibrous tissue. Preserved nuclei with marked pleomorphism and hyperchromasia can still be seen within the necrotic area and often there is a perivascular growth of viable tumor cells.

SOGC Clinical Practice Recommendations

- Medical management should be tailored to the needs of the woman presenting with uterine fibroids and to alleviating the symptoms. Cost and side effects of medical therapies may limit their long-term use. (IIIC)
- In women who do not wish to preserve fertility, hysterectomy may be offered as the definitive treatment for symptomatic uterine fibroids and is associated with a high level of satisfaction. (IIA)
- Myomectomy is an option for women who wish to preserve their uterus, but women should be counseled regarding the risk of requiring further intervention. (IIB)
- It is important to monitor ongoing fluid balance carefully during hysteroscopic removal of fibroids. (IB)
- Laparoscopic myolysis may present an alternative to myomectomy or hysterectomy for selected women with symptomatic intramural or subserous fibroids who wish to preserve their uterus but do not desire future fertility. (IIB)

- Uterine artery occlusion may be offered as an alternative to selected women with symptomatic uterine fibroids who wish to preserve their uterus.(IC)
- Women choosing uterine artery occlusion for the treatment of fibroids should be counseled regarding possible and patient satisfaction are lacking. (IIIC)
- Removal of fibroids that distort the uterine cavity may be indicated in infertile women, where no other factors have been identified, and in women about to undergo *in vitro* fertilization treatment. (IIIC)
- Concern of possible complications related to fibroids in pregnancy is not an indication for myomectomy, except in women who have experienced a previous pregnancy with complications related to these fibroids. (IIIC)
- Women who have fibroids detected in pregnancy may require additional fetal surveillance when the placenta is implanted over or in close proximity to a fibroid. (IIIC)
- Hormone replacement therapy may cause myoma growth in postmenopausal women, but it does not appear to cause clinical symptoms. Postmenopausal bleeding and pain in women with fibroids should be investigated in the same way as in women without fibroids. (IIB)
- There is currently no evidence to substantiate performing hysterectomy for an asymptomatic leiomyoma for the purpose of alleviating the concern that it may be malignant. (IIIC)

An Evidence-based Guideline for the Management of Uterine Fibroids (*Working Party for the New Zealand Guidelines Group April 2000*)

Summary of the Recommendations

- Transvaginal ultrasound of the endometrium is accurate in excluding endometrial hyperplasia but is often unable to distinguish submucosal fibroids and polyps. (A)
- Transabdominal ultrasound may be required for uteri greater than 12 weeks' size as these will be beyond the reach of the transvaginal ultrasound. (D)
- Transvaginal ulrasound and transvaginal sonohysterogram are both more accurate in diagnosing the location of fibroids than hysteroscopy. (A)
- When recommending hysteroscopy the following should be considered: Normal saline should be used as it offers advantages (shorter and less discomfort) over carbon dioxide instillation. (A)

- There is insufficient evidence to recommend magnetic resonance imaging (MRI) and CT scanning as an initial diagnostic test for uterine pathology. (D)

Medical Treatments

- Progestogens should not be recommended in the treatment of uterine fibroids as there is insufficient evidence of benefit. (D)
- Oral contraceptives are not effective in shrinking uterine size but may reduce menstrual blood loss with a resultant improvement in haematiocrit. (C)
- Hormone replacement therapy (HRT) should not be used to treat fibroids as it is not effective in reducing uterine fibroid size. (A)
- Women who bleed while on continuous combined HRT in patients should have adjustments made to their HRT by either decreasing the estrogen dose or increasing the progesterone dose. (D)
- RU486 is effective in reducing uterine fibroid size without causing a reduction in bone mineral density. (D)
- Danazol should not be recommended as initial treatment for fibroids as it is not as effective as gonadotropin-releasing hormone analogues and has androgenic side effecs which limit its use. (C)
- Gestrionone is effective in reducing uterine and fibroid size but androgenic side effects may limit its use. (A)
- Nonsteroidal anti-inflammatory drugs (NSAIDs) are not effective as a treatment for women with fibroids in reducing heavy menstrual bleeding. (B)
- Gonadotropin-releasing hormone analogue (GnRHa) treatment effectively reduces uterine and fibroid size but unpleasant side effects and a reduction in bone mineral density limit its sole use beyond 6 months. (A)
- Gonadotropin-releasing hormone (GnRH) analogue treatment for 3 months followed by combined 'addback' therapy (estrogen plus progestin) results in fibroid shrinkage and is an alternative for women who have contraindications to surgey or who do not wish to undergo. But once therapy stops then the fibroids will return to pretherapy size. (B)
- There is insufficient evidence to recommend progestogen-releasing intrauterine systems to reduce uterine fibroid size. (C)

Surgical Management

- Administration of GnRH analogues for 2 to 4 months prior to surgery for uterine fibroids is recommended for women with a large uterine (>18 weeks size).
- Women who are diagnosed with submucous uterine fibroids and heavy or abnormal menstrual bleeding should be offered hysteroscopic ablation or resection as an alternative to hysterectomy. (C)
- Laparoscopic myomectomy should be undertaken in women who wish to conceive because of less adhesion risks.
- There is insufficient evidence to recommend the routine use of adhesion barriers. (B)
- There is insufficient evidence to recommend the routine use of vasopresin in reducing operative blood loss. (C)
- There is insufficient evidence to support the routine use of laser-induced interstitial thermotherapy, myolysis or cryomyolysis technique. (D)
- Embolization of uterine fibroids may be an effective alternative to myomectomy or hysterectomy but RCTs are awaited. (D)
- The low incidence of leiomyosarcoma discovered incidentally in asymptomatic women with uterine fibroids does not support operative management of fibroids as prevention of leiomyosarcoma. (D)
- The decision whether hysterectomy or myomectomy is undertaken is dependent on: the woman's preference, age and fertility profile of the woman and the position and number of the fibroids. (D)

14 Genitourinary Prolapse

Incidence

Almost 40% of females have some degree of prolapse. The incidence of uterine prolapse is 14–16% and rectocele is 20%. The incidence of posthysterectomy vault prolapse varies from 0.2 to 4.4%. Whether this is more following vaginal or abdominal hysterectomy is not clear. The vault prolapse following abdominal hysterectomy is due to failure to detect the already pre-existing element of vaginal descent which is ignored. The vault prolapsed following vaginal hysterectomy is mainly due to faulty repair in primary surgery.

Risk Factors

Multiparity, operative vaginal delivery, obesity, aging, chronic increased intra-abdominal pressure, connective tissue disorders are considered risk factors for genitourinary prolapse.

Definitions of Prolapse

A hernia of one or more pelvic organs (uterus, vaginal apex, bladder, rectum) and its associated vaginal segment from its normal location.

Anterior vaginal prolapse (cystocele/urethrocele): Pathologic descent of anterior vaginal wall and overlying bladder base.

Enterocele: Hernia in which peritoneum is in contact with vaginal mucosa. The normal intervening endopelvic fascia is absent, and small bowel fills the hernia sac.

Rectocele: Defect of posterior vaginal wall support. May be asymptomatic or associated with disorders of defecation.

Uterovaginal prolapse: Descent of uterus/apical vagina due to attenuation of uterosacral/cardinal ligament support complex.

Classification of Prolapse

Prolapse may be external or internal. Congenital nulliparous or general (acquired).

Two Systems of Classification

- Baden-Walker (1968) (Figs 14.1, 14.2 and Table 14.1) and Beecham (1980)
- Pelvic Organ Prolapse Quantification, 1996

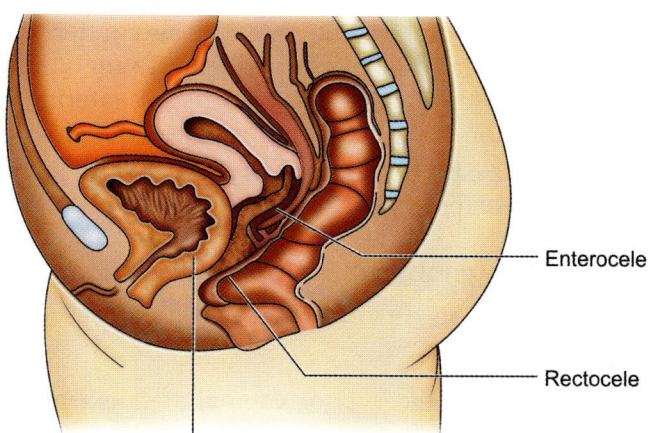

Fig. 14.1: Bayden-Walker grading of prolapse

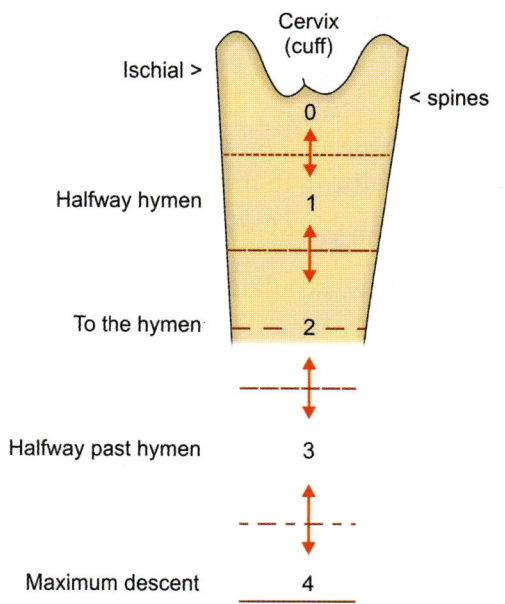

Fig. 14.2: Baden-Walker system for the evaluation of pelvic organ prolapse on physical examination

211

Table 14.1: Baden-Walker system for evaluation of pelvic organ prolapse on physical examination

Grade	Posterior urethral descent, lowest part of other sites
0	Nomal position for each respective site
1	Descent halfway to the hymen
2	Descent to the hymen
3	Descent halfway past the hymen
4	Maximum possible descent for each site

Cystocele

First degree: The anterior vaginal wall, from the urethral meatus to the anterior fornix, descends halfway to the hymen.

Second degree: The anterior vaginal wall and underlying bladder extend to the hymen.

Third degree: The anterior vaginal wall and underlying urethra and bladder are outside the hymen. This cystocele is often part of the third degree uterine or posthysterectomy vaginal vault prolapse.

Cystocele can be central or lateral and often dominant prolapse.

Uterine or Vaginal Vault Prolapse

First degree: The cervix or vaginal apex descends halfway to the hymen.

Second degree: The cervix or vaginal apex extends to the hymen or over the perineal body.

Third degree: The cervix and corpus uteri extend beyond the hymen or the vaginal vault is everted and protrudes beyond the hymen.

Rectocele

First degree: The saccular protrusion of the rectovaginal wall descends halfway to the hymen.

Second degree: The sacculation descends to the hymen.

Third degree: The sacculation protrudes or extends beyond the hymen.

Enterocele

The depth of the enterocele sac, relative to the hymen, should be described anatomically, with the patient in the supine and standing positions during Valsalva maneuver.

First degree: 2.5 cm below posterior fornix; 2nd degree: 5 cm below; 3rd degree: 7.5 cm below up to hymen; 4th degree: outside hymen.

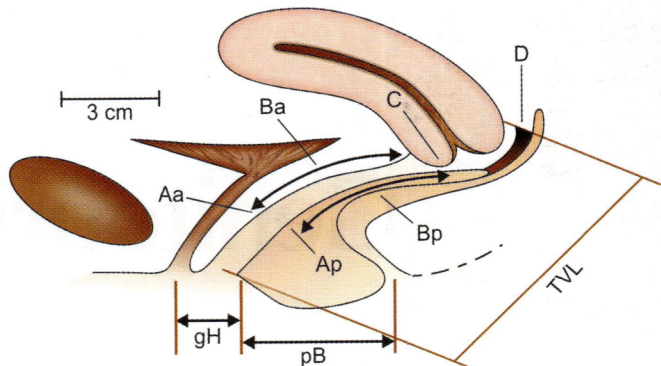

Fig. 14.3: Normal position.

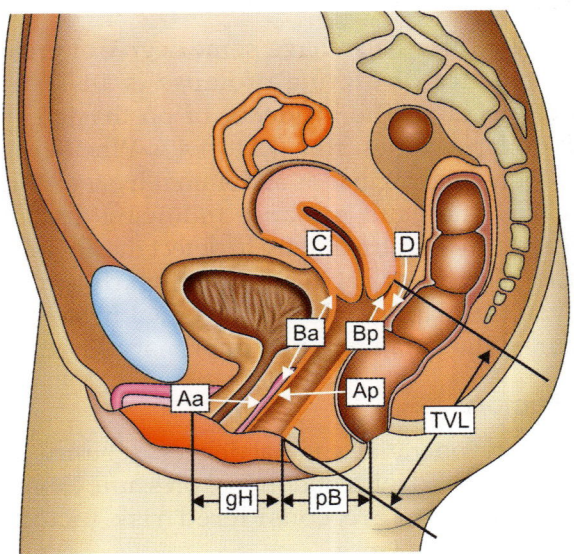

Fig. 14.4: Normal site specific points

*Six sites: Points Aa,Ba, C,D, Bp, and Ap, the genital hiatus (g H), perineal body (pB), and total vaginal length (TVL).
Hymen is fixed point of reference
Point Aa: Point in midline of anterior vaginal wall 3 cm proximal to external urethral meatus (approximately the bladder neck or urethral vesical junction). By definition it can only range from –3 cm (no prolapse) to +3 cm (complete prolapse)
Point Ba: The most distal point of the upper anterior vaginal wall. Point Ba is –3 when there is no prolapse and would have a positive value equal to Point C in a patient with total vaginal eversion.

POP Q

Approved by the International Continence Society, the American Urogynecologic Society for the description of female pelvic organ prolapse (Table 14.2).

Advantage of POP Q (Figs 14.3 to 14.6):
POP Q: Objective, site-specific system for describing, quantifying, and staging pelvic support in women.

POP Q: Provides standardized means for documenting, comparing, and communicating clinical findings with proven interobserver and intraobserver reliability.

Table 14.2: Staging of pelvic organ prolapse by POP-Q measurements

Stage	Description
0	No descensus of pelvic structures during straining.
I	The leading surface of the prolapse does not descend below 1 cm above the hymenal ring.
II	The leading edge of the prolapse extends from 1 cm above the hymen to 1 cm through the hymenal ring.
III	The prolapse extends more than 1 cm beyond the hymenal ring, but there is not complete vaginal eversion.
IV	The vagina is completely everted.

POP Q: Approved by the International Continence Society, the American Urogynecologic Society, and the Society of Gynecologic Surgeons for the description of female pelvic organ prolapse.

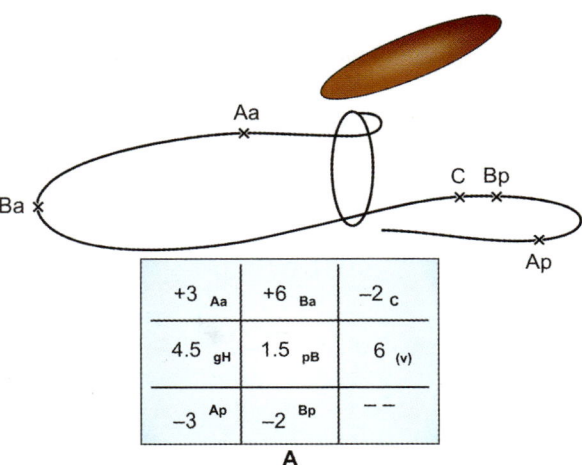

+3 Aa	+6 Ba	−2 c
4.5 gH	1.5 pB	6 (v)
−3 Ap	−2 Bp	− −

A

Fig. 14.5: Anterior wall prolapse.
A= anterior wall prolapse
Leading edge of pr olapse of upper anter ior vaginal wall represented by Point Ba at +6 cm
Point Aa is maximally distal at +3 cm.
The vaginal cuff is 2 cm above the hymen (Point C = −2)
The total vaginal length is 6 cm. This means that if the vaginal apex or cuff was in its normal position, Point C would be −6. Since point C representing the a pex or vaginal cuff is −2 cm, one can deduce that the apex or cuff has undergone 4 cm of descent.
In summary, this is an example of Stage III prolapse as the leading edge of the prolapse (Point Ba) is beyond the hymen at +6 cm.

Disadvantage

POP Q: Too many variations to allow grouping patients into comparable populations for study purposes

POP Q: Too complex for simple clinical communication.

Anatomical Considerations

The normal position, support and suspension of uterus, vagina, bladder and rectum is well supported by an interrelated system of bony, muscular and connective tissue elements.

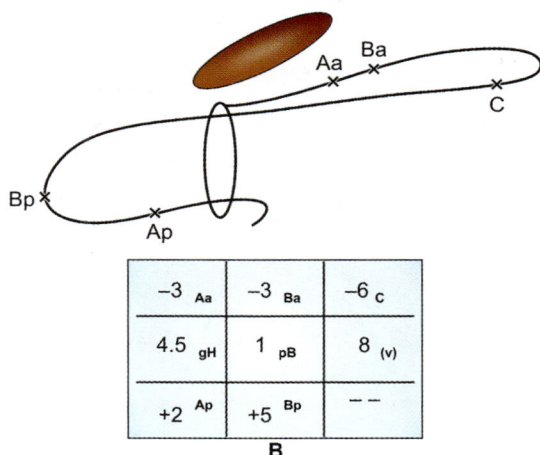

−3 Aa	−3 Ba	−6 c
4.5 gH	1 pB	8 (v)
+2 Ap	+5 Bp	− −

B

Fig. 14.6: Posterior wall prolapse.
B= posterior wall prolapse
Leading edge of pr olapse, if upper poster ior vaginal wall represented by Point Bp at +5 cm
Point Ap is 2 cm distal to the hymen so is +2
The vaginal cuff is 6 cm above the hymen (Point C = −6)
The total vaginal length is 8 cm. This means that if the vaginal apex or cuff was in its normal position, Point C would be −8. Since point C representing the a pex or vaginal cuff is −6 cm, one can deduce that the apex or cuff has undergone 2 cm of descent.
In summary, this is an example of Stage III prolapse as the leading edge of the prolapse (Point Bp) is beyone the hymen at +5 cm.

In a standing female, upper 2/3rd vagina remains almost horizontal to pelvic floor and lower 1/3rd of vagina is oblique vertical with an angle of 135° in between at the fornices. The posterior aspect of the pelvic inlet is approximately 60° above the anterior aspect. This partially vertical orientation of the pelvic inlet deflects force on to the superior symphysis pubis with no direct effect on pelvic outlet.

DeLancey has proposed a 3 Level pelvic support system (Fig. 14.7):

Level-I support (Table 14.3): This is contributed by strong condensed endopelvic fascial structures comprising of Mackenrodt-uterosacral-pubocervical complex.

Level-II support (Table 14.4): On each side of the pelvis, a dense layer of endopelvic fascia envelopes the uterus and cervix and attaches to pelvic sidewall. It also serves as neurovascular conduit and is composed of collagen, smooth muscle, blood vessels and nerves.

Level-III support: Support of pelvic organs is achieved through a complex interplay between pelvic ligaments, muscles, and endopelvic fascia which attach the pelvic organs to the bony pelvis to form a continuous support structure.

The **levator ani** group of muscles is the major structural component of pelvic floor. Laterally, the

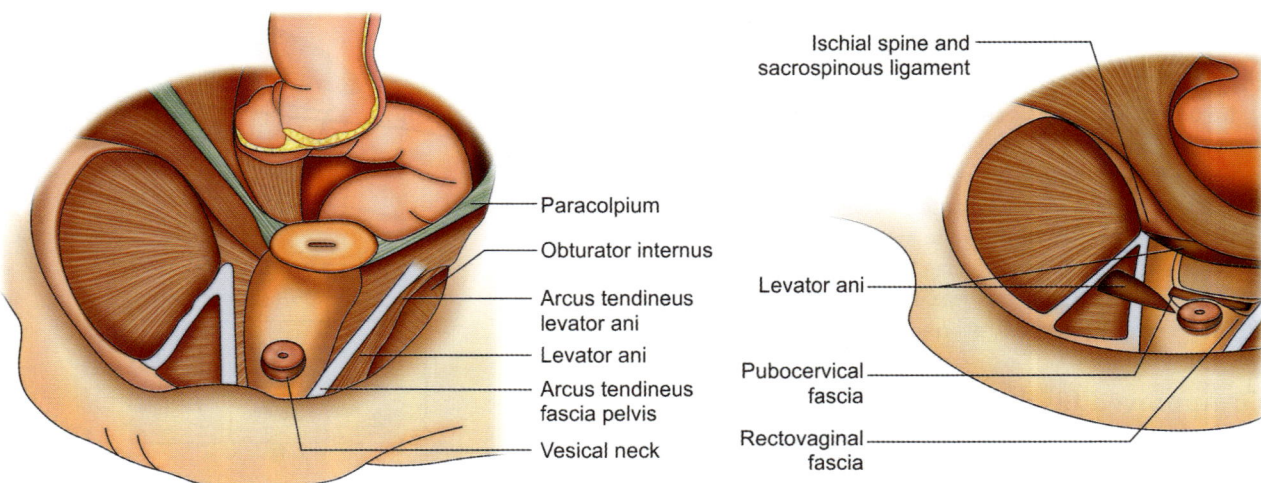

Fig. 14.7: DeLancey pelvic floor support

			Table 14.3: Anatomical distribution of Level-I pelvic support structre			
Deep endopelvic fascia component	*Origin*	*Insertion*	*Nerve supply*	*Vascular supply*	*Muscular component*	*Function*
1. Uterosacral	S2, S3, S4	On the posterior and lateral wall of pericervical ring of vagina at 5 & 7 o'clock position	Uterosacral plexus of autonomic nerves	Minimal	Rectouterine muscle	This hold the cervix behind the urogenital hiatus in the posterior pelvis at the level of ischial spines
2. Mackenrodt's ligament	Fibrous connection with lateral abdominal and pelvic walls	To lateral supravaginal cervix at 3 o'clock and 9 o'clock position with pericervical ring	Portion of uterosacral complex	Uterine artery and veins	Uterine artery muscle content	Provides lateral attachment of cervix at the level of ischial spines
3. Pubocervical ligaments	Inferior surface of the superior pubic ramus medially and arcus tendineus fascia pelvis laterally	To the anterior and lateral supravaginal cervix at 11 o'clock and 1 o'clock positions to form pericervical ring	Perivesicular nerve plexus	Vessels of bladder pillar Minimum smooth muscle		Provides a minimum degree of cervical stabilization anteriorly but provides support to bladder

levator mucle is composed of iliococcygeus, a thin muscle layer which originates from the arcus tendineus levator ani. These insertions are thickening of the pelvic sidewall parietal fascia that extend from the ischial spines posteriorly to pubic tubercles. Immediately inferior to the muscular arches are thickening of the parietal fascia of the ileococcygeus muscles called **arcus tendineus fascia pelvis** or white lines. These structures are the lateral attachment of pubocervical fascia and proximal rectovaginal septum. The white line is nearly horizontal in standing position and vertical in lithotomy position.

Another fascial thickening termed as **arcus tendineus rectovaginalis** runs posteriorly from the white line and serves as lateral support for the distal rectovaginal septum of the posterior vagina. The lateral supports of the anterior and posterior vaginal septa merge. The obturator internus muscle forms the lateral borders of the upper portion of the pelvic basin. Posterior to iliococcygeus, the pelvic floor is covered by the coccygeous muscle and sacrospinous ligament which pass between ischial spine and coccyx. The most posterior portion of pelvis is covered by piriformis muscle. The midline confluence of the levator muscles

Table 14.4: Anatomical distribution of Level-II pelvic support structure

Fascial component	Shape	Contents	Function	Boundaries				
				Distal	Lateral	Proximal	Superior	Inferior
Pubocervical septum	Trapezoid	Connective tissue and muscle	Anterior vaginal support	Pubic tubercles and pubic arch	Arcus tendineus fascia pelvis	Pericervical ring centrally and pubo-cervical and cardinal ligament laterally	Visceral fascia of bladder	Vaginal epithelium
Rectovaginal septum	Trapezoidal	Connective tissue and smooth muscle	Posterior vaginal support and suspension	Fusion with perineal body at the central tendon of perineum	Arcus tendineus fascia pelvis proximally and arcus tendineus fascia recto-vaginalis distally	Pericervical ring centrally and uterosacral ligament at periphery	Vaginal epithelium	Visceral fascia of rectum
Pericervical ring	Collar of connective tissue around the supravaginal cervix	Fibroelstic connective tissue	Cervical stabilization within the interspinous diameter	Located between base of bladder and anterior cervix connects with pubo-cervical ring at 11 o'clock and 1 o'clock positions	Connected with cardinal ligament at 3 and 9 o'clock positions	Located between rectum and posterior cervix; connects with uterosacral ligament at 5 and 7 o'clock positions and proximal RVS centrally		

forms a strong band of connective tissue between coccyx and anus known as levator plate or **anococcygeal raphe.** The plate is oriented horizontal in the standing patient. The vagina and the rectum are supported from below by the endopelvic fascia over levator plate. The nerve and muscle injury to the pubococcygeus and iliococcygeus muscles allows levator plate to sag and descend permanently. This causes the genital hiatus to remain open as it does during defecation. This increased opening changes the normal horizontal axis of the proximal vagina to a vertical orientation and predisposes the central pelvic organs to prolapse.

The pudendal nerve runs in the area posterior to ischial spine into Alcock's canal and is, therefore, subjected to significant stretch and pressure during descent through the pelvis during labor. The injury to pudendal nerve weaken the levator muscles which significantly contribute to development of pelvic organ prolapse.

The connective tissues of the pelvis are collectively known as *endopelvic fascia.* It supports and invests all the midline organs and structures of the pelvis except the tubes and ovaries. It may be divided into three parts: parietal fascia, visceral fascia and deep endopelvic connective tissue. When the septa and their supports are intact, vaginal and rectal axis have a posterior angle of approximately 130° at the anterior point of their suspension over levator plate. The apical or proximal 2/3rd of the vagina is nearly horizontal and is suspended over the levator plate. The normal vaginal axis is oriented posteriorly over a point just above the center of the fourth sacral vertebra.

The **pericervical ring** is the location where all the deep endopelvic fascial support structures converge. Tear of the structures attached to the ring can be a sequel to the obstetric injury to the neuromuscular bundle. Level III support is attributed to fusion to the urogenital diaphragm anteriorly and to the proximal perineum posteriorly. Damage at these sites results in urinary incontinence anteriorly and in perineal body defects posteriorly. Cystocele and rectocele are defects within the pubocervical and rectovaginal septa, respectively.

Confirmed Risk Factors

- Increasing age
- Vaginal delivery
- Increasing parity
- Obesity (BMI >30)
- Spina bifida and spina bifida occulta (congenital prolapse)

Relative Risk Factors

- Race
- Family history of prolapse
- Constipation
- Connective tissue disorders, e.g. Marfan's syndrome, Ehlers-Danlos syndrome
- Previous hysterectomy
- *Menopause:* Atrophy of support structures
- Occupations involving heavy lifting

Intrapartum Variables

- Fetal macrosomia
- Prolonged second stage of labor
- Episiotomy
- Anal sphincter injury
- Epidural anesthesia
- Use of forceps

Clinical Features

Vaginal/General Symptoms

- Sensation of pressure, fullness or heaviness.
- Sensation of a bulge/protrusion or something coming down.
- Seeing something coming out from vagina.
- Spotting (in the presence of ulceration of the prolapse).

Urinary Symptoms

- Incontinence
- Frequency
- Urgency
- Incomplete bladder emptying
- Weak or prolonged urinary stream
- The need to reduce the prolapse manually before voiding
- The need to change position to start or complete voiding

Bowel Symptoms

- Constipation/straining
- Urgency of stool
- Incontinence of flatus or stool
- Incomplete evacuation
- The need to apply digital pressure to the perineum or posterior vaginal wall to enable defecation (splinting)

Coital Defects

- Dyspareunia
- Loss of vaginal sensation
- Vaginal flatus

Examination

- Evaluate the patient in both the lithotomy and standing positions, during relaxation and maximal straining, in empty and full bladder.
- To perform the evaluation, place a standard double-bladed Sim's speculum in the vaginal vault to visually examine the vagina and cervix.
- The speculum is removed and keeping the posterior blade into the posterior vagina, the anterior wall is visualized.
- The speculum is then overturned into the anterior vagina to view the posterior wall.
- Note the point of maximal descent of the anterior, lateral, and apical walls in relation to the ischial spines and hymen.
- Next, place 2 fingers into the vagina such that each finger opposes the ipsilateral vaginal wall, and ask the patient to bear down.
- After evaluating the lateral vaginal support system, assess the apex (cervix and apical vagina).
- Repeat the examination with the patient standing and bearing down in order to note the maximum descent.
- Assess for 'dominant prolapse' (i.e. which portion is coming out first on straining—that indicates maximum damage of pelvic support)and also assess type of cystocele. Cystocele can be of two types—central and lateral or combined. The last is the most common variety.
- Next, grade the strength and quality of pelvic floor contraction, asking the patient to tighten the levators around the examining finger.
- Assess the external genitalia, noting estrogen status, diameter of the introitus, and length of perineal body.
- Perform a careful **bimanual examination** and note uterine size, mobility, and adenexa.
- Palpate pubococcygeal fibers of levator ani.
- Lastly, perform a **rectal examination,** assessing the external sphincter tone and checking for the presence

of rectocele or enterocele, tone of levator plate and feel the anococcygeal raphe.

Examination for Enterocele

- *Inspection:* Sims' speculum depresses posterior vagina with rectocele; posterior lip held with sponge forceps and pulled anterior, posterior vault seen for enterocele on coughing.
- *Rectovaginal examination:* Thumb and index finger guard rectocele and enterocele palpated for any descent coming from above on coughing. Three types of enterocele:
  a. Congenital—elongation of sac of POD.
  b. Acquired: (i) Traction type—associated with defect in vault support mechanism, (ii) Pulsion type—associated with increased intra-abdominal pressure.

Examination for Urinary Incontinence

When the patient has significant anterior vaginal wall prolapse (cystocele), look for stress incontinence both with prolapse remaining outside and after it has been reduced. It is important to exclude the development of postoperative potential incontinence (PI) prior to management of uterine prolapse.

Investigations

1. *Bladder function evaluation:* This includes clean catch urine sample to test for infection, a postvoid residual volume (PVR), and cystometry for assessment of bladder sensation.
2. *Bowel function evaluation:* By stool examination, proctoscopy, and anal sphincter tone assessment.
3. *Pelvic muscle function assessment:* Done by digital assessment of pubococcygeus and puborectalis muscle along the pelvic sidewalls within the vagina at 4 and 8 o'clock position. Many women have urethral hypermobility which is defined as resting urethral angle or maximal strain angle greater than 30° which can be measured by a genitometer. A swab is placed in the urethra at the urethrovesical junction and with this instrument the baseline urethral angle from the horizontal and maximal strain angle is measured.
4. *Imaging:* It is not routinely recommended but if indicated, USG of pelvis and KUB is done. MRI for suspected uterine and renal anomaly and defecography is indicated when rectal mucosal prolapse is suspected.

Considerations for Nonsurgical or Surgical Decision Making

- Medical condition and age
- Severity of symptoms
- Patient's choice
- Presence of other pelvic conditions requiring simultaneous treatment, including urinary or fecal incontinence.
- Presence or absence of urethral hypermobility.
- Presence or absence of pelvic floor neuropathy.
- History of previous pelvic surgery

Conservative Treatment

- Pelvic exercises and pessaries are the current mainstays of nonsurgical management of patients with uterine prolapse.
- Routine Kegel exercises can improve pelvic floor muscle tone and stress incontinence.
- Vaginal estrogen cream

Nonsurgical (conservative) management of pelvic organ prolapse is recommended by ACOG and should be attempted before surgery is contemplated.

Conservative management confers several advantages:
a. It is safe and inexpensive.
b. It is not usually associated with morbidity and mortality.
c. Most appropriate for comorbid medical disease producing unfit for surgery.
d. It can lead to a high patient satisfaction.
e. It may be used for patients awaiting surgery or patients who want to postpone.

Pelvic muscle exercises (PMEs) and vaginal support devices (pessaries—Fig. 14.8) are the main nonsurgical treatments for patients with pelvic organ prolapse.

Pelvic muscle exercises can improve pelvic floor muscle tone and stress urinary incontinence, but improvement of pelvic floor muscle tone does not lead to regression of pelvic organ prolapse.

Vaginal support devices (pessaries) are manufactured from medical-grade silicone and are safe, cost-effective, and minimally invasive options for treating patients with pelvic organ prolapse.

Pessary use has few contraindications:
a. Need to remain in follow-up and timely replacement
b. Vaginitis
c. Undiagnosed vaginal bleeding.

An important adjunct is application of topical estrogen prior to pessary use, particularly if signs of hypoestrogenism (atrophic vaginitis) exist. Once the

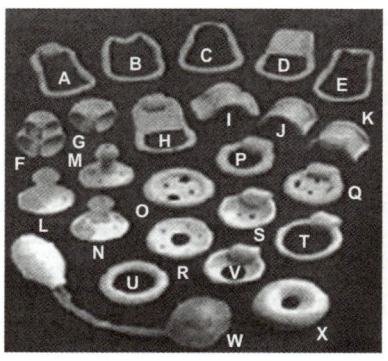

Different pessary available

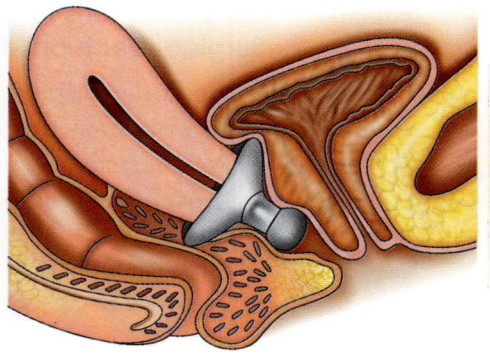

Gellhorn placement

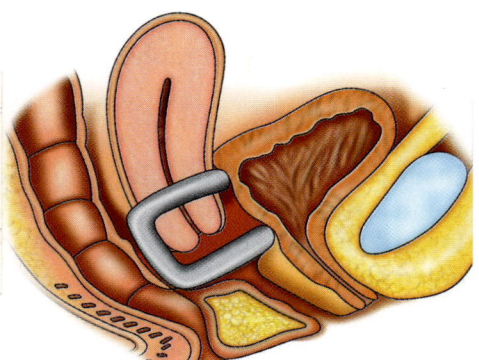

Gehrung pessary

Fig. 14.8: Different types of pessaries

pessary is in place, continued vaginal estrogen cream application (i.e. 1–2 times per week) or application of vaginal estrogen ring once every 3 months is indicated. Vaginal erosions are indications for temporary pessary removal and treatment with topical estrogen.

Many different types of pessaries (Fig. 14.8) can be used. Pessaries may be classified as supportive (e.g. ring), or space-occupying (e.g. doughnut, cube, Inflatoball). The most common pessaries in use today are the ring (with or without support), Gellhorn, doughnut, and cube. Other types are the Inflatoball, Hodge and Shaatz pessaries.

Types of Pessaries (Table 14.5)

- Two most common types, i.e. ring with support and space filling Donut pessary, depending on concomitant pelvic floor defects.
- The ring support pessary is recommended for stages I and II prolapse and space filling pessaries are used for stages III and IV prolapse.
- The Gellhorn is most often used for patients with significant uterine prolapse and a large introital diameter who have not obtained relief with other pessaries.

The Smith-Hodge pessaries facilitate retro-displacement of the uterus and should be used for patients with a well-defined pubic notch and adequate vaginal width.

Table 14.5: Indication of uses of different pessaries

Serial no	Pathology	Type of pessary
1	1st and 2nd degree uterine prolapse	Ring with support
2	3rd degree uterine prolapse	Shaatz, Donut, Gellhorns Inflatoball
3	Cystocele/rectocele	Gehrung
4.	Cystocele with SUI	Gehrung with knob

Surgery for Anterior Compartment Defect

  i. *Vaginal approach*
- Anterior colporrhaphy
- Vaginal paravaginal repair

  ii. *Abdominal approach*
- Anterior abdominal colporrhaphy
- Abdominal paravaginal repair
- Laparoscopic repair

A thorough history and physical examination should distinguish a central or a transverse vaginal defect from a paravaginal defect. However, most patients have a combination of these.

The purpose of anterior colporrhaphy, is to plicate the vaginal muscularis fascia overlying the bladder (pubocervical fascia) to diminish the bladder and anterior vaginal protrusion. Anterior colporrhaphy is indicated especially for patients with a central vaginal defect. The vaginal mucosa is incised in the midline, and then it is sharply dissected away from the pubocervical fascia laterally to the inferior pubic ramus. Several layers of interrupted delayed absorbable sutures are placed laterally on the pubocervical fascia in a mattress fashion. Excess vaginal mucosa is trimmed and the resulting vaginal mucosa is closed with running or interrupted sutures.

Paravaginal defect repair may be performed laparoscopically, abdominally, or vaginally. In this procedure, the retropubic space of Retzius is entered to reattach the anterolateral vaginal sulcus with its overlying endopelvic fascia to the obturator internus and pubococcygeus muscles and fascia at the level of the arcus tendineus fascia of the pelvis (ATFP) bilaterally, and thus restores the lateral vagina to its normal place of attachment (DeLancey's level II support).

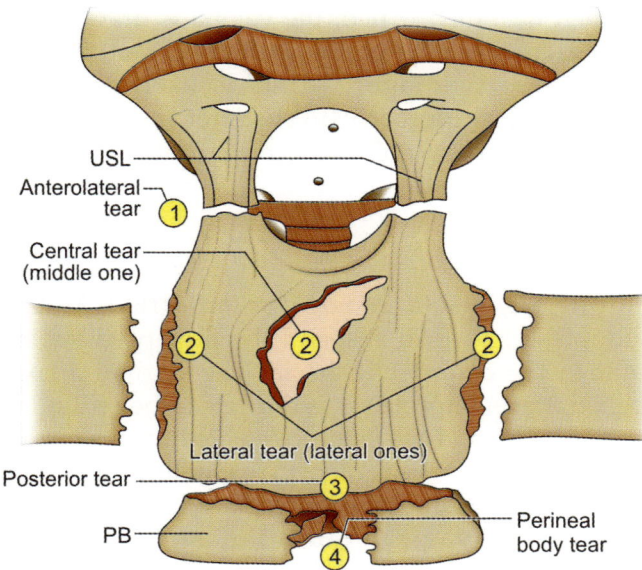

USL
Anterolateral tear ①
Central tear (middle one)
② ② ②
Lateral tear (lateral ones)
Posterior tear
PB
③
④
Perineal body tear

Fig. 14.9: Defect in rectovaginal septum

Surgery for Posterior Compartment Defect

i. *Vaginal*

a. Posterior colporrhaphy
b. Defect specific posterior colporrhaphy
c. Transanal rectocele repair

Posterior vaginal repair (posterior colporrhaphy) is performed to repair the posterior vaginal defect, usually a rectocele. Traditionally, posterior colporrhaphy has been performed via a transvaginal approach with levator ani muscle plication. In this surgery, posterior vagina is cut in midline and rectocele is opened. The torn rectovaginal fascia is plicated in the midline, thus eliminating the posterior vaginal protrusion, and the excess vaginal mucosa is excised and repaired with absorbable sutures (Fig. 14.9).

Defect-specific, or site-specific defect repair, was introduced by Richardson in 1972. It attempts to identify and repair specific areas of deficiency in the rectovaginal fascia. This type of repair does not attempt to plicate the levator ani fascia and, thus, may be associated with a lower incidence of postoperative morbidity.

Transanal repair is performed mainly by colorectal surgeons. This technique involves plication of the rectal muscularis fascia and its attachment to the bilateral levator ani muscles. Transvaginal posterior vaginal repair is generally recommended as better procedure than transanal repairs.

II. *Abdominal*

Mesh abdominal sacral colpoperineorrhaphy.

III. *Laparoscopic*

Laparoscopic mesh sacral colpoperineopexy.

Surgery for Apical Compartment Defects

I. *Vaginal*

• Enterocele repair
• Sacrospinous ligament suspension
• Iliococcygeal suspension
• Uterosacral ligament vaginal vault suspension
• Manchester-Fothergill procedure.

II. *Abdominal*

• Uterosacral ligament suspension
• Abdominal sacral colpopexy.

III. *Laparoscopic*

• Laparoscopic mesh sacral colpopexy
• Laparoscopic uterosacral ligament suspension.

IV. *Obliterative Procedures*

Preoperative Care

Surgery for pelvic organ prolapse repair is an elective procedure. Preoperatively, a thorough discussion with the patient should lead to patient acknowledgment of the possibility of incomplete resolution or recurrence of pelvic organ prolapse and complications of surgery (e.g. injury to bladder, urinary dysfunction, urinary retention, possible need for prolonged catheterization). The vaginal tissue wall may be optimized with vaginal estrogen for 1–2 months prior to the surgery. Women with pelvic organ prolapse and pelvic pain and sexual dysfunction need to be counseled that, while pelvic organ prolapse surgery repairs the anatomic vaginal defect, surgery does not necessarily lead to relief of pelvic pain or improvement of sexual function.

The choice of procedure depends largely on the surgeon's experience and preference, but other factors to consider are the patient's general health status, degree and type of pelvic organ prolapse, need for preservation or restoration of coital function, concomitant intrapelvic disease, and desire for preservation of menstrual and reproductive function. Patients who wish to retain their uterus may undergo a Manchester repair or a LeFort colpocleisis. A Papanicolaou test, ultrasonography, and endometrial biopsy should be performed prior to surgical repair to rule out any pathology.

I. Vaginal Approach

Vaginal surgery is preferred by many surgeons because the patient may have a shorter recovery time and it may take less intraoperative time compared with abdominal surgery. The most common vaginal procedures to suspend the prolapsed vaginal apex are sacrospinous ligament fixation, modified McCall culdoplasty, iliococcygeus suspension, and high uterosacral ligament suspension.

A. *Sacrospinous Ligament Fixation* (Fig. 14.10)

Sacrospinous ligament fixation is usually performed on the patient's right side to avoid rectum and sigmoid colon injury. The right perirectal space is dissected, and a window is made to expose the coccygeus muscle overlying the sacrospinous ligament on the right side with the help of Breisky-Navratil retractors. The ischial spine is palpated with the index finger and 2 pulley sutures of permanent or delayed absorbable material are placed through the sacrospinous ligament, 2 fingerbreadths medial to the ischial spine to avoid injury to the pudendal neurovascular bundle. The safe and nerve-free zone for placement of the sacrospinous ligament sutures is situated approximately in the middle of the sacrospinous ligament, more than 2.6 cm medial to the ischial spine. The passage of sutures through the sacrospinous ligament (SSL) may be facilitated by a series of instruments that include the long-handled Deschamps ligature carrier, Miya hook ligature carrier. The sacrospinous ligament pulley sutures are then attached to the vaginal vault and tied to pull up the vaginal cuff.

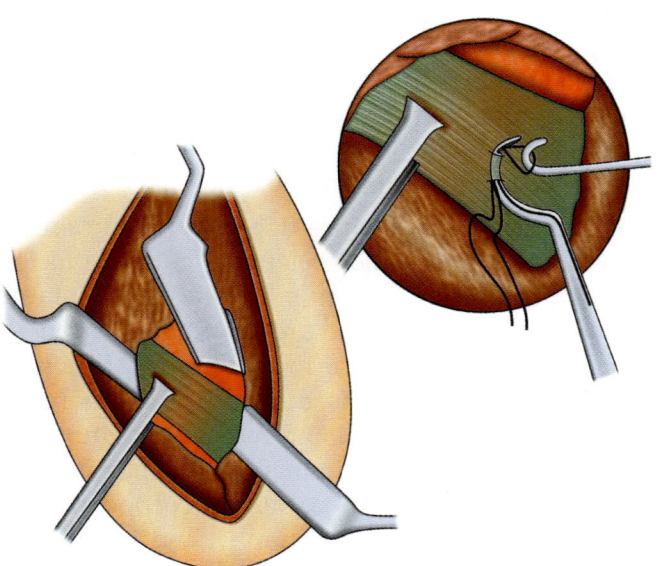

Fig. 14.10: Sacrospinous fixation

When the stitch is tied, the vagina is drawn up to the SSL at the level of the ischial spine.It has the following advantages: (a) It is a transvaginal extraperitoneal approach; (b) posterior vagina tied to a strong SSL ; (c) very quick procedure; (d) durable repair with rare recurrence.

B. *Endopelvic Fascia Repair*

Endopelvic fascia repair (or modified McCall culdoplasty) aims to suspend the prolapsed vaginal vault to the endopelvic fascia. The vaginal apex is opened, the enterocele sac is dissected, the redundant sac is excised, and the enterocele is reduced. Next, the bilateral uterosacral ligaments are identified and up to 3 modified McCall sutures are placed to incorporate the posterior vaginal vault, the peritoneum, the uterosacral ligaments, and the endopelvic fascia of the upper vagina and rectum. Sutures are then tied to secure the vaginal vault to the upper portion of the endopelvic fascia ensuring an adequate closure of the cul-de-sac peritoneum.

C. *Iliococcygeus Suspension*

Iliococcygeus suspension was described initially by Inmon in 1963 and has the purpose of suspending the vaginal vault to the fascia of the iliococcygeus muscle in patients with attenuated uterosacral ligaments. Iliococcygeus muscle is a component muscle of the levator ani; it originates from the arcus tendineus levator ani and inserts into the anococcygeus raphe and the coccyx. The securing suture is placed into the iliococcygeus fascia bilaterally 1–2 cm caudal and posterior to the ischial spine.

D. *High Uterosacral Ligament Suspension*

High uterosacral ligament suspension aims to suspend the prolapsed vaginal vault bilaterally to the uterosacral ligaments. Similarly to the modified McCall culdoplasty procedure, the enterocele sac is dissected, the redundant sac is excised, and the enterocele is reduced. The uterosacral ligaments are identified, and 2–3 delayed absorbable sutures are placed through the middle portion of the uterosacral ligaments (at approximately the level of the ischial spine) taking care to avoid ureteral injury.

The distal portions of the uterosacral ligaments are plicated across the midline with 1–3 permanent sutures to obliterate the cul-de-sac. Each uterosacral ligament suture is then passed through the full thickness of the posterior vaginal wall. The vaginal vault is then closed medial to uterosacral sutures. Tying the vault suspension sutures will suspend the vagina deep into the pelvis, up to the level of the ischial spine. Cystoscopy should be performed at the end of each procedure to rule out ureteral injury.

E. Manchester-Fothergill Procedure

Manchester procedure for pelvic organ prolapse is indicated for patients with anterior vaginal defects, an elongated cervix, no evidence of uterine descent, and those who wish to retain their uterus. This procedure was developed by Arachibald Donald and later modified by his pupil Fothergill. It consists of (a) preliminary D&C, (b) anterior colporrhaphy, (c) amputation of the cervix, (d) tightening of Neocervix by placation of Mackenrodt's ligament, and (e) posterior colporrhaphy.

F. Vaginal Hysterectomy with Pelvic Floor Repair

Hysterectomy is performed in the elderly patient though it is not the pathological organ to remove. This is done because:

1. Uterus is in the midline.
2. It is a potential malignant organ—pre- or post-menopausal.
3. Due to attenuated structural support available for repair it is difficult with uterus kept *in situ*.
4. Presence of uterus can act as midline pivot for future recurrence of prolapse.

Principal steps

1. Remove uterus vaginally with or without salpingo-oophorectomy.
2. To remove ovaries vaginal route, after uterus is removed, superior pedicle is caught hold with Ovarian clamps and lateral clamp is placed in infundibulopelvic ligament lateral to ovaries.
3. Peritoneal closure is followed by internal and external McCull culdoplasty tightening the Mackenrodt's and uterosacral ligaments in the midline.
4. This is followed by anterior and posterior colporrhaphy.

Other Procedures

Vaginal obliterative procedures, partial (LeFort) colpocleisis and total colpocleisis are indicated for patients who are medically unfit for prolonged anesthesia or long surgical procedures, and who are not contemplating sexual activity. These procedures may be performed under regional or local anesthesia with intravenous sedation. Since the uterus is retained with partial colpocleisis, preoperative uterine evaluation is indicated prior to surgery.

With the LeFort colpocleisis, a rectangular portion of anterior and posterior vaginal mucosa is removed. The anterior pubocervical septum is sutured to the posterior rectovaginal septum using Lambert inverting sutures and as the approximation is continued progressively on each side, the most dependent portion of the prolapse is gradually inverted. A perineorrhaphy is usually performed to support the inverted vagina and help prevent pelvic organ prolapse recurrence.

Total colpocleisis procedures are performed for patients with posthysterectomy vaginal vault prolapse. These procedures do not intend to correct enterocele since they are both extraperitoneal procedures. Also, these procedures carry risk of postoperative de novo stress urinary incontinence, and thus a concomitant anti-incontinence procedure may be performed in at-risk patients prior to closing the vagina.

II. Abdominal Approach

A. Repair of Anterior Compartment Defect

The main abdominal operations performed for apical vaginal prolapse and uterine prolapse are abdominal sacral colpopexy and total abdominal hysterectomy with high uterosacral ligament suspension. These operations allow fixation of the upper vagina or the uterus to the sacrum, with the help of grafts and sutures through the anterior sacral ligament (presacral fascia) at the level of the sacral promontory or at S1–S2. The strongest presacral fascia is found at the sacral promontory. The abdominal approach allows a higher vaginal fixation in the pelvis and provides durable repairs with an adequate vaginal length.

1. *Anterior abdominal colporrhaphy* (Fig. 14.11): A high **central defect** can be corrected by dissecting

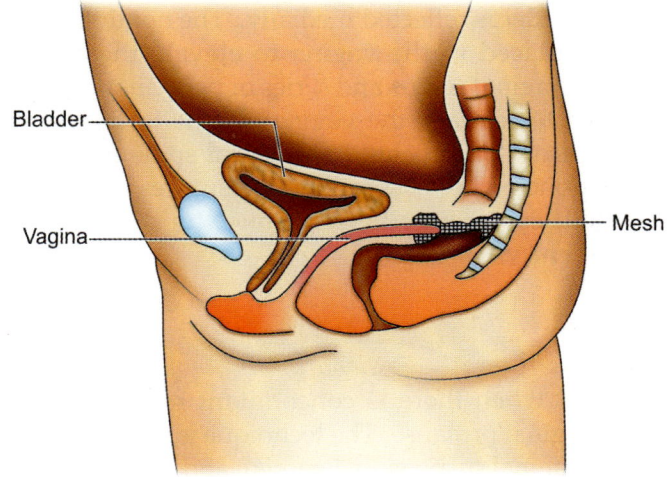

Fig. 14.11: Abdominal approach

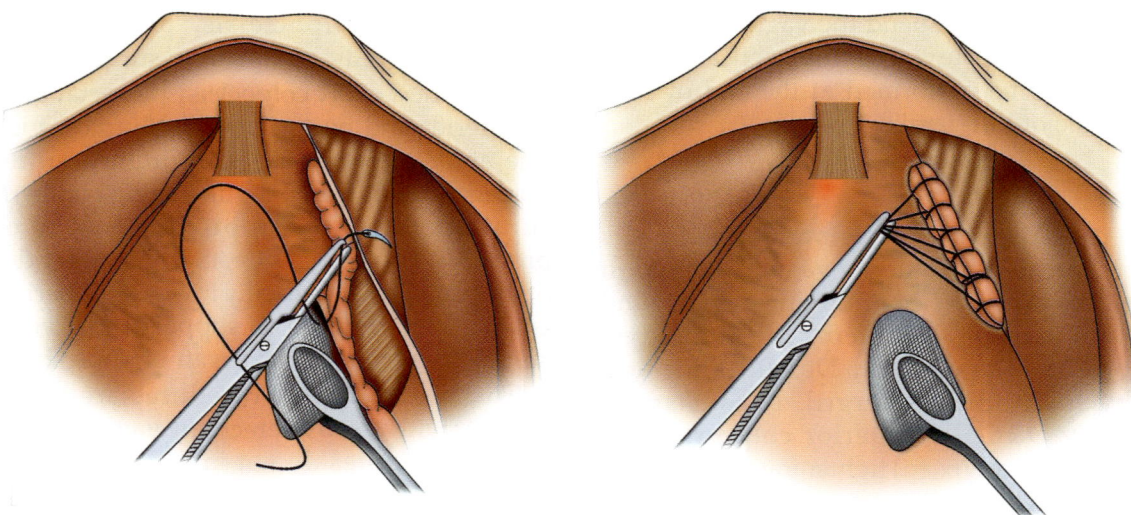

Fig. 14.12: Mesh paravaginal repair

between the base of the blader and the upper one-third of the anterior vaginal wall. The defective tissue is may then be wedged out and the defect is closed with interrupted sutures.

2. *Paravaginal repair* (Fig. 14.12): The paravaginal or lateral defect repair involves reattachment of the anterior lateral vaginal sulcus to the obturator internus fascia and muscle at the level of arcus tendineus fascia pelvis (ATFP). It is usually performed as bilateral procedure. It has been found that most patients with anterolateral detachments always has separation of the upper vaginal fornices from the arcus tendineus adjacent to the ischial spine. After entering into the retropubic space, careful blunt dissection is performed to mobilize the bladder, urethra and paravaginal tissue. A Foley catheter is placed to delineate urethrovesical junction.

The ATFP is identified along the obturator internus muscle from the inferior pubic ramus to the ischial spine as the bladder is reflected medially. The nondominant hand is placed in the vagina to elevate the lateral superior vaginal sulcus and series of permanent suture are used to reattach the vaginal sulcus to the ATFP starting from 1 cm behind the ischial spine medially. This is done on both sides. After all sutures are placed and tied, cystoscopy is performed to identify any bladder entry.

B. *Repair of Posterior Compartment Defect*

Mesh abdominal sacral colpoperineopexy: This is indicated when there is concomitant rectocele with apical vaginal prolapse. The technique is to replace the normal vaginal suspensory ligament and replace it with graft material that runs from the sacrum to the perineal body. Its purpose is to correct the posterior compartment defects and suspend the perineal body thus preventing descent and opening of genital hiatus. It can be performed transabdominally or as a combined abdominovaginal procedure with Mersilene mesh. Mesh erosion recur frequently (16–40%).

C. *Sacrocolpopexy Repair for Apical Vaginal Prolapse* (Figs 14.13 and 14.14)

This procedure may be performed by an open laparotomy or laparoscopic approaches. The graft is sutured to the posterior and anterior vaginal wall after the peritoneum covering the vagina is dissected from the vaginal wall. The peritoneum covering the sacral promontory is incised and the vascular structures are avoided (particularly the common iliac and the middle sacral vessels) by performing careful blunt and sharp dissection. The graft is sutured over the anterior sacral

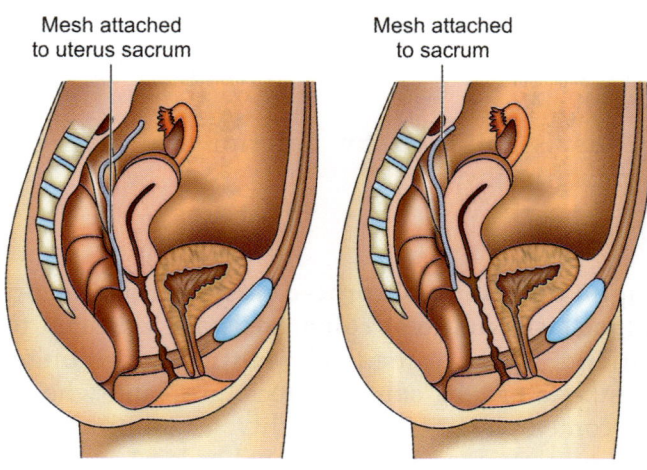

Mesh attached to uterus sacrum

Mesh attached to sacrum

Fig. 14.13: Mesh sacrocolpopexy

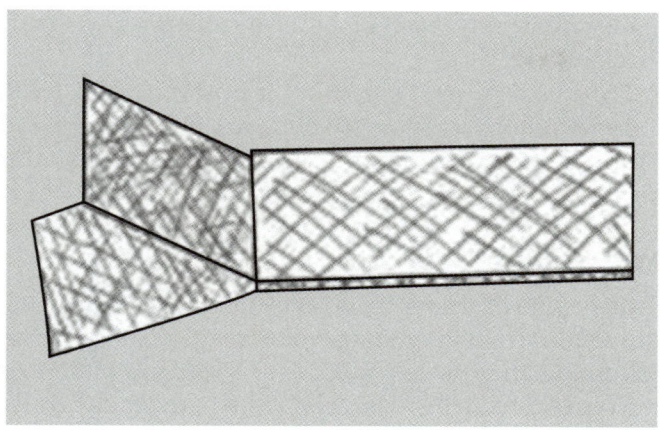

Fig. 14.14: Y-shaped mesh

longitudinal ligament over the S2–S3 vertebrae or preferentially over the sacral promontory, thus correcting the apical vaginal prolapse. The peritoneum over the presacral space is closed and the graft is peritonealized to prevent mesh erosions.

A variety of grafts have been used for sacropexy procedures (e.g. harvested fascia lata abdominal fascia, cadaveric fascia lata, Marlex, Prolene, Mersilene with variable success rates. The ideal biocompatible material used should be chemically and physically inert, durable, noncarcinogenic, noninflammatory, readily available, and inexpensive.

The synthetic polypropylene mesh has been shown to be superior to autologous fascia lata. Multifilament mesh (i.e. Mersilene) has been associated with chronic inflammation that can be detrimental compared to monofilaments. Moreover, mesh with large pore size (>75 micrometers) allows ingrowth of fibroblast, collagen and blood vessels, and allows for macrophage and leukocyte infiltration and passage, thus decreasing the chance of mesh infection and mesh erosion.

Grafts are placed from the vaginal cuff, or the amputated cervical stump to the presacral fascia with permanent suture in a tension-free fashion. The graft is peritonealized and some surgeons obliterate the rectovaginal pouch (pouch of Douglas) to prevent future enterocele.

The most important complications in sacrocolpopexy include bleeding and graft erosion. The peroperative hemorrhage is difficult to control as sacral veins retract into the sacrum. The use of hemosatic sutures, pressure and bone wax or applying sterile thumbtacks into the bone to taponade the veins are found to stop the bleeding. Otherwise, a small 1 cm piece of rectus abdominis muscle is iced over the bleeding veins and then electrocautery is applied.

Mesh erosion is treated by transvaginal excision of the exposed mesh or sometimes excision of entire grafts with severe infection. The risk of erosion ranges from 3.5 to 12%.

The other complications include postoperative ileus, intestinal obstruction and intra-abdominal adhesion.

The **Marion-Moschcowitz** abdominal procedure entails a spiral suture placed around the rectovaginal pouch to close it circumferentially.

The **Halban procedure** involves placement of several sutures in the sagittal plane that close the anterior and posterior leaves of the pouch of Douglas. Whether performing a total hysterectomy at the time of sacrocolpopexy increases the chance of vaginal exposure or erosions is debatable.

Laparoscopic Approach

Procedures used are:

a. *Laparoscopic paravaginal defect repair for anterior compartment defect*

The space of Retzius is exposed from the anterior pubovesical attachments adjacent to the pubic symphysis to the posterlateral ischial spine and the extent of defect is assessed. Using the vaginal finger to elevate the vaginal wall at the defect site, interrupted sutures are placed from the ATFP to vaginal layer medially. Approximately 4–5 interrupted 2–0 permanent sutures are placed on each side. Once the sutures are placed, Burch retropubic urethropexy can also be placed laparoscopically, if there is associated stress incontinence.

b. *Laparoscopic mesh sacral colpoperineopexy for posterior repair*

In this method, laparoscopically placed sacral colposcopy mesh is attached to perineal body by opening the posterior vagina. The mesh affixed to the perineal body is retrieved via laparoscopy to attach to the sacrum.

c. *Laparoscopic repair for apical compartment defect*

1. *Laparoscopic mesh sacral colpopexy:* Space is created in the rectovaginal space by placing EEA sizers in vagina and in rectum. The posterior peritoneum over a vascular plane over sacral promontory to expose the anterior longitudinal ligament. The vascular structures to be in danger of injury are: (a) left iliac vein not protected by artery as it is on the right side, (b) middle sacral vessels, and (c) presacral venous plexus. One limb of the polypropylene mesh is attached to posterior vagina as low as possible to the RVS and one arm is attached to anterior vagina. At least 6 permanent monofilament of 2-0 polypropylene sutures are placed to fix the

mesh in the vagina. Both the leaves of the mesh are brought back to sacral promontory and appropriate tension is adjusted by finding a suitable location of the area on the mesh where it can be sutured over the anterior longitudinal ligament by two permanent 2-0 sutures.

2. *Laparoscopic uterosacral ligament suspension:* The uterosacral ligaments are identified with its attachment to the upper vagina and cervix back to lateral sacrum at S2-3 level. The suspension suture of 2-0 size polypropylene is placed in the middle segment of the ligament and then into the ipsilateral vaginal cuff. Another suture is placed in the sacral portion of the ligament to the medial ipsilateral cuff. Care is taken to identify the ipsilateral ureter and rectum before placing suture. The contralateral suture is placed in a similar fashion. Once the sutures are tied, cystourethroscopy should be performed to assure normal bladder integrity and ureteral patency.

IV. Obliterative Procedures

a. *Total colpectomy with colpocleisis:* This is an option for patients who have posthysterectomy vaginal vault prolapse where all of the vaginal skin is removed from the hymen posteriorly to within 0.5 to 2 cm of the external urethral meatus anteriorly.

b. Partial colpocleisis where some portion of the vaginal epithelium is left to provide drainage tracts for cervical or upper genital discharge.

These techniques also include high perineorrhaphy and plication of puborectalis muscle to reinforce the posterior support and to reduce the genital hiatus and recurrent prolapse. Success rate is claimed to be as high as 100%. These procedures can be performed quickly and with relatively low morbidity though it can produce some troublsome voiding dysfunction and coloractal dysfunction.

Complications of Abdominal Approach

- Bleeding is the most serious complication of sacral colpopexy. Injuring the presacral venous plexus or the middle sacral artery while operating in the presacral space is possible.
- Other complications include ureteral injury, graft erosion, and suture pullout causing recurrence of the prolapse.
- Erosion of synthetic grafts through the vagina has been reported as 3%.

Complications of Vaginal Approach

- Pelvic infection, hemorrhage, and injury to the ureters, bladder, urethra with fistula formation,

bowel injury, sacral osteomyelitis, and graft rejection.
- The two most serious complications from sacrospinous ligament fixation are hemorrhage and nerve injury from the pudendal neurovascular bundle.

Postoperative Care

Patients must avoid strenuous exercise or heavy lifting and refrain from intercourse for 6 weeks postoperative. Following the 6-week follow-up visit, the patient is instructed to progressively return to usual daily activities.

Patients must avoid increased intra-abdominal pressure, such as constipation, weight lifting for at least 3 months. This will facilitate adequate healing and may prevent pelvic organ prolapse recurrence.

For postmenopausal patients, vaginal estrogen therapy is continued (unless it is contraindicated) to maintain the integrity of pelvic tissues.

When grafts are used for pelvic floor reconstruction, a postoperative follow-up visit must check for any graft erosions.

NULLIPAROUS PROLAPSE

Incidence: In India nulliparous prolapse cases constitute 1.5–2% cases of genital prolapse.

Etiology

1. Connective tissue disorders—Ehlers-Danlos syndrome
2. Congenital defect of pelvic floor muscles
3. Congenital spine defect—spina bifida occulta, split pelvis

Surgical Procedures

- Shirodkar's posterior sling
- Purandare's anterior cervicopexy
- Khanna's sling
- Virkud's composite sling
- Joshi's sling
- Soonawala's sling

Shirodkar's Sling (Fig. 14.15)

Dr VN Shirodkar used fascia lata femoris to strengthen the uterosacral ligaments fixing it to sacral promontory retroperitoneally. It is now replaced by Mersilene tape. Mersilene tape has definite advantage over fascia lata as it is inert material, nonabsorbable, non-irritant with predictable tensile strength. Tape is fixed to the

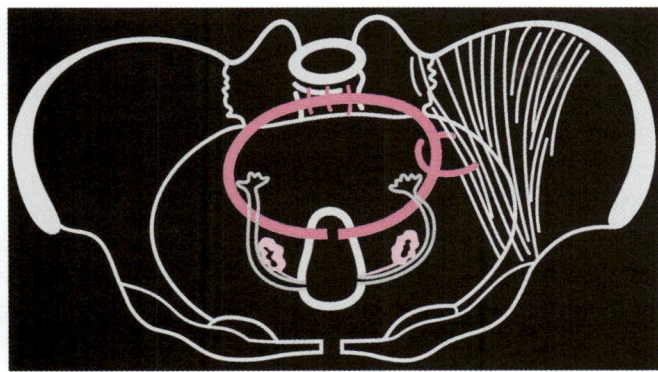

Fig. 14.15: Shirodkar's sling

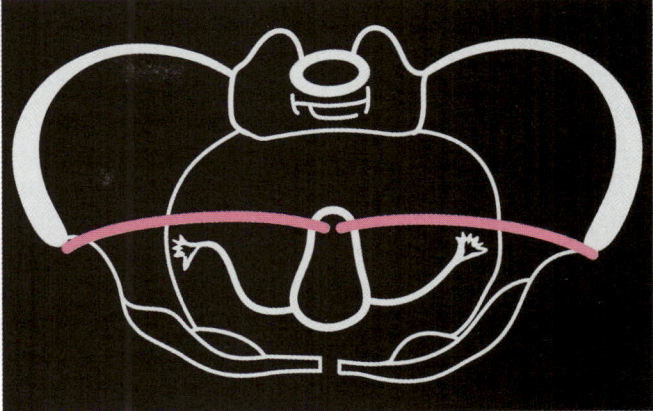

Fig. 14.17: Khanna's sling

posterior aspect of isthmus and sacral promontary. It is anatomically correct but difficult to perform.

Purandare's Cervicopexy (Fig. 14.16)

Here, rectus sheath fascial strips are anchored to the anterior aspect of isthmus of uterus with the lateral ends remain attached to its original sites.

Advantage: Easy to perform, dynamic support, Minimal blood loss.

Disadvantage: Alters pelvic anatomy by obliterating uterovesical fold, vagina is being pulled forward to increase risk of enterocele formation.

Khanna's Sling Operation (Fig. 14.17)

Tape is anchored to anterior aspect of isthmus and anterior superior iliac spine. It is easier to perform and safer.

Joshi's Sling

Anterior surface of uterus at the level of internal os is suspended to the pectineal ligament on both sides with Mersilene tape.

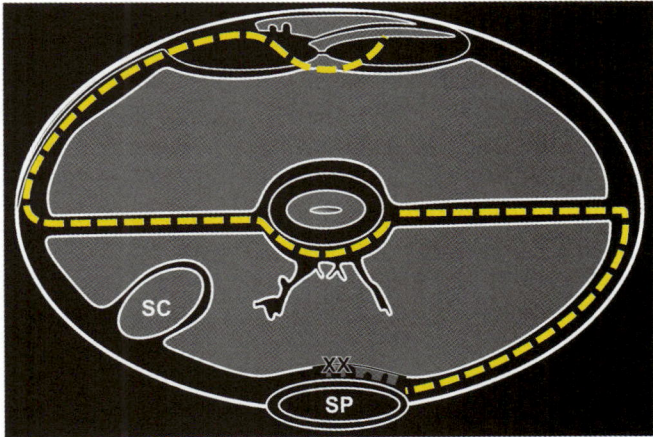

Fig. 14.18: Virkud's sling

Virkud's Sling (Fig. 14.18)

One end of Marsilene tape is attached to sacral promontory. Subperitoneally, it is extended on right pelvic wall, then to broad ligament and fixed to posterior surface of isthmus. Then it is passed between left broad ligament through left internal inguinal ring. It is then turned medially and sutured to rectus sheath.

Soonawala's Sling

It is attached to anterior longitudinal ligament on S1 vertebra and then it is carried along right uterosacral ligament of isthmus of uterus and then ratracted extraperitoneally to S1 vertebra.

Vaginal Vault Prolapse

Introduction

Vaginal vault prolapse has been defined by the International Continence Society as descent of the vaginal cuff below a point that is 2 cm less than the

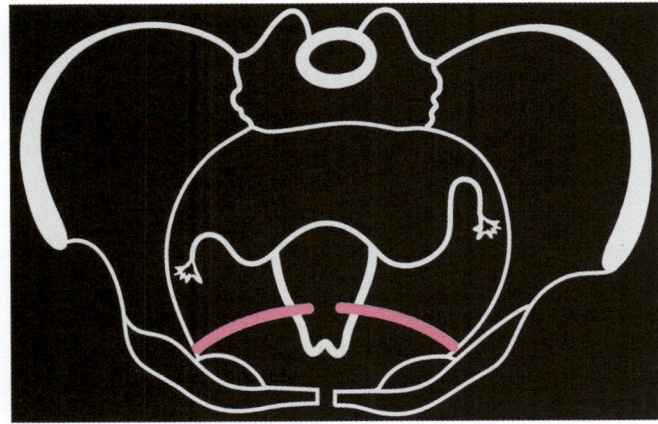

Fig. 14.16: Purandare's cervicopexy

total vaginal length above the plane of the hymen. It occurs when the upper vagina bulges into or outside the vagina. Coexistent pelvic floor defects like cystocoele, rectocoele or enterocoele are present in 72% of patients with vault prolapse.

The surgical options for the correction of vault prolapse lie between the vaginal and the abdominal approach. The choice of procedure should be based on the patient's age, comorbidity, previous surgery and the level of physical and sexual activity . Of course, the experience of the surgeon influences the choice of operation. Importantly, greater awareness of the pelvic anatomy and the technique at the time of the original hysterectomy will significantly reduce the incidence of subsequent vault prolapse.

Incidence

The incidence of prolapse, which require surgical correction following hysterectomy, is 3.6 per 1000 per years of risk. The cumulative risk rises from 1% three years after a hysterectomy to 5% at 15 years after hysterectomy. Also the risk of prolapse following hysterectomy is 5.5 times in women whose initial hysterectomy was for genital prolapse as opposed to other reasons.

Evaluation and Description of Vault Prolapse

Most vaginal cuff prolapses include apical enterocele where the pubocervical and rectovaginal fascia have separated. The peritoneum becomes stretched and comes in direct contact with the vaginal epithelium creating a true hernia. The vaginal epithelium is stretched and becomes very smooth without rugae. There is always some degree of high cystocele formation and high rectocele formation associated with the vaginal vault prolapse.

Vaginal prolapse is distressing and disabling condition to women. The symptom of feeling "something coming down", "feeling pressure in the vagina" is always a common complaint. Urinary symptoms, such as poor stream, hesitancy, straining to void, incomplete emptying, recurrent urinary tract infections, and the need to reduce the bulge digitally to void or defecate may also present especially when associated with anterior and posterior compartment prolapse.

Non-surgical Management

Conservative management will include pelvic floor exercise and pessaries, commonly ring and shelf pessaries. Their role in vault prolapse management is unclear and there is no evidence to suggest that pelvic floor exercise is helpful. However, pessaries may have a limited role in the very frail and elderly in whom surgery is not an option.

Surgical Management (Vaginal Approach)

For the patient with good pelvic floor muscle strength as assessed by clinical examination and reasonably substantive endopelvic fascia, a vaginal approach using native tissues may be appropriate. The vagina is anchored to existing stable structures like the sacrospinous ligament, iliococcygeous muscle and endopelvic fascia. Women with attenuated fascia, poor pelvic floor muscle strength, repeat repair or severe ongoing physical stress are better served by a technique of vault suspension that provides compensatory repair either through vaginal or abdominal approach using the mesh.

Prevention of Vault Prolapse (McCall Culdoplasty)

It was described by McCall in 1957 as a technique to correct enterocoele and involves the suspension of the vault into the origins of the uterosacral ligaments and obliteration of the cul-de-sac. More recently Elkins described a high McCall culdoplasty. The technique was described to repair the prolapsed vagina at hysterectomy. After the uterine fundus was delivered through an anterior colpotomy incision, the uterosacral ligaments are systematically plicated from the posterior cervix back into the pelvic cavity, until two fingerbreadths remain between the rectum and the plicated ligaments. The main problem with this technique is the risk of ureteric injury. However, this can be eliminated by the use of routine cystoscopy with or without methylene blue to identify ureteric efflux following the procedure.

Sacrospinous Fixation

It was originally described as a bilateral procedure but subsequently being done as a unilateral procedure. The later results in less tension, though the bilateral technique is more anatomical and maintain a wide vaginal vault.

The technique comprises dissection into the paravaginal space and the ischial spine is identified. Using a Deschamps ligature carrier, two nonabsorbable sutures are placed through the sacrospinous ligament, one and a half to two fingerbreadths medial to the ischial spine. One end of each suture is attached to the under surface of the posterior vaginal wall at the apical area. When the posterior colporrhaphy reaches the mid-portion of the vagina, the sacrospinous sutures are tied, firmly attaching the vaginal apex to the surface of the coccygeal-sacrospinous ligament complex with no intervening bridge of suture material.

Although infrequent, haemorrhage is the most common complication but it is rarely of a life threatening nature. It may be a result of injuring the pudendal artery or vein, or the hypogastric venous plexus.

Other complications include injury to the bladder or rectum. Transient and self-limiting gluteal pain could result from injuring the small nerve that runs through the coccygeal-sacrospinous ligament complex. Immediate and severe postoperative gluteal pain radiating to the posterior surface of the leg, and often associated with perineal parathesia, indicates posterior cutaneous, pudendal, or sciatic nerve trauma. The recommended treatment for the latter is immediate reoperation and releasing the offending suture and repositioning it to a more medial position.

Iliococcygeal Fixation

The technique comprises the fixation of the everted vaginal apex to the ilioccygeal fascia just below the ischial spine. It is usually done as a bilateral procedure as it imposes less tension on the vaginal wall than sacrospinous fixation. The iliococcygeal muscle can be approached through either an anterior or posterior vaginal wall incision. It is relatively easier than sacrospinous fixation and can be done in conjunction with vaginal hysterectomy or as a separate procedure for correction of vault prolapse. There has been reports of reduced risk of lower rate of postoperative cystocele, bleeding and pain, injury to the pudendal nerves and vessels, and less chance of vaginal shortening, but certainly iliococcygeal fixation offers no additional benefit over sacrospinous fixation (RCOG).

Uterosacral Suspension

This has been described as a bilateral procedure carried out vaginally. It can also be carried out via an abdominal or laparoscopic approach. The aim is to place sutures through the uterosacrals at the level of the ischial spine, with one arm brought out through the lateral aspect of the rectovaginal fascia and the other through the pubocervical fascia on each side. These are tied anchoring the vaginal cuff to the uterosacrals. The biggest risk is injury to the ureters (up to 10.9%) due to its proximity to the anterior border of the uterosacrals, especially at the level of the cervix. Most gynecologist believe the concept that the uterosacral ligaments are compromised in the first place, for prolapse to occur,

and for this reason will prefer sacrospinous fixation, while some suggest that the uterosacral ligaments are not weakened, but instead break at specific points resulting in enterocoele and vault prolapse. The later school of thought believe that the uterosacral can be used, even in severe prolapse by identifying the distal portion of breakage and anchoring the vagina high above this point to the uterosacral ligament using an intraperitoneal approach

Abdominal Approach
Abdominal Sacrocolpopexy

The abdominal sacral colpopexy employs the interposition of a synthetic mesh or tissue graft between the vagina and sacrum. The point of sacral attachment does not affect the vaginal axis and attachment to the sacral promontory allows effective restoration of vaginal support, while maintaining both vaginal capacity and coital function. It involves a double attachment of the mesh to the anterior and posterior vaginal surfaces with reported good results. Consistent cure rate of more than 90% has been reported.

This procedure has added advantage over the traditional procedures because it maintains the normal axis of the vagina, with preservation of maximal vaginal length which is desirable for optimal sexual function. It also provides a source of strength in patients with weak tissue or recurrent prolapse. It is further associated with a lower rate of recurrent prolapse and dyspareunia which makes it popular choice amongst surgeons especially in fit patients. Its main drawback includes that it is performed via laparotomy with all the associated risk of internal organ injury, longer operation time and hospital stay, so these need to be balanced against the benefits. In the very elderly with coexisting medical pathology, the risk of laparotomy coupled with the extra risk of general anesthesia will make this procedure unsuitable.

Laparoscopic Approach
I. Laparoscopic Sacral Colpopexy

In theory, laparoscopic approach to the repair of the vault prolapse should follow the same principle as in the open technique, with laparoscopy only being the mode of surgical access. However, a highly skilled and experienced laparoscopic surgeon is needed. This approach has a steep learning curve and takes many years of practise to acquire the necessary skills.

II. Laparoscopic Uterosacral Ligament Vault Suspension

The technique begins with the identification of the vaginal vault apex, and the rectovaginal and pubocervical fascia facilitated by the use of a vaginal probe. Traction is placed on the vaginal probe forward to stretch the uterosacral ligaments so they can be identified and traced backwards. At this stage, both ureters are identified. The peritoneum overlying the vaginal apex is incised to expose the pubocervical fascia anteriorly and the rectovaginal fascia posteriorly. The uterosacral ligament on each side is attached using nonabsorbable sutures to the ipsilateral side of the vaginal vault. Intra- or extracorporeal knots can be used depending on the surgeon's preference.

There is a high risk of ureteric injury, so cystoscopy is advised after suture placement. Success rate of up to 90% over a 2-year period has been reported.

Laparoscopic surgery has a steep learning curve and not all surgeons will have the necessary skill to excel especially considering the technical difficulty and longer operation time. The main advantage is good exposure of the operation field enabling the surgeon to fully evaluate and treat other components of the prolapse effectively. Most recently new innovations like robotics, though in its infancy is helping to address some of the limitations of laparoscopy by providing better technical features such as 3D vision and more precise robotic instrument manoeuvrability.

Colpocleisis

This is a procedure that may gain in popularity in the coming years and as life expectancy rises in an aging population.

Colpocleisis involves surgical obliteration of the lumen of the vagina. Basically, the vaginal epithelium is mobilized anteriorly and posteriorly leaving about 2 cm from the vault above and also from the urethral meatus below. The prolapse is reduced by placing progressive sutures anteroposteriorly, till the prolapsed tissues are above the level of the levator plate. It can also be carried out as a partial or total procedure. The partial procedure is usually reserved for women with an intact prolapsed uterus with the aim of giving access to any discharge or bleeding from the uterus via a small opening.

It is suitable for the frail elderly woman who is not sexually active and for whom conservative methods like the pessary is not ideal. It has the advantage that it can also be carried out under local anesthesia and involves a shorter operation time. The complications of urinary stress incontinence of up to 27% in previously continent women has been reported though no intraoperative complication has been reported in the literature. Success rate of 97% and above have also been reported.

Prevention of Genitourinary Prolapse

- Good intrapartum care, including avoiding unnecessary instrumental trauma and prolonged labor.
- The role of hormone replacement therapy in preventing prolapse is uncertain.
- Pelvic floor exercises may prevent prolapse occurring secondary to pelvic floor laxity and are strongly advised after childbirth.
- Smoking cessation will reduce chronic cough.
- Weight loss, if overweight or obese.
- Avoidance of heavy lifting occupations.
- Treatment of constipation throughout life.

RCOG Guidelines for Vault Prolapse

1. *Can vaginal vault prolapse be prevented at the time of hysterectomy?*
   a. McCall culdoplasty at the time of vaginal hysterectomy is a recommended measure to prevent enterocele formation.
   b. Suturing the cardinal and uterosacral ligaments to the vaginal cuff at the time of hysterectomy is a recommended measure to avoid vault prolapse.
   c. Sacrospinous fixation at the time of vaginal hysterectomy is recommended when the vault descends to the introitus during closure.
   d. Does subtotal hysterectomy have a place in the prevention of PHVP?
      Subtotal hysterectomy is not recommended for the prevention of PHVP. [*New 2015*]
   e. Are there preferred suture materials for vault support at the time of hysterectomy?
      There is inadequate and conflicting evidence over the use of permanent sutures in the short term and no evidence of benefit in the long term; they can be associated with high suture exposure rates. [*New 2015*]
2a. *Is there a role for conservative management?*
    The role of conservative measures for post-hysterectomy vaginal vault prolapse is unclear.
   b. *Is pelvic floor therapy of value in the management of PHVP?*
      Pelvic floor muscle training (PFMT) is an effective treatment option for women with stages I–II vaginal prolapse, including PHVP. [*New 2015*]

c. *What is the place of vaginal devices?*

Vaginal pessaries are an alternative treatment option for women with stages II–IV PHVP. [*New 2015*]

3. *How can post-hysterectomy vaginal vault prolapse be repaired surgically?*

Anterior and posterior repairs along with obliteration of the enterocele sac are inadequate for post-hysterectomy vaginal vault prolapse.

Abdominal sacrocolpopexy and sacrospinous fixation should be considered in terms of their relative benefits and risks. Abdominal sacrocolpopexy is an effective operation for post-hysterectomy vaginal vault prolapse. In comparison, sacrospinous fixation may have a higher failure rate but has lower postoperative morbidity.

4. *What criteria can be used to determine which procedure to use?*

The following criteria should be considered when helping women choose between the two procedures.

a. For a choice to be made, it is important that the surgeon is experienced in both procedures and able to choose between them before surgery.

b. Vaginal sacrospinous fixation requires adequate vaginal length and vault width to enable reaching the sacrospinous ligament.

c. Abdominal sacrocolpopexy can be carried out, if women require laparotomy for other indication.

d. Vaginal sacrospinous fixation is more suitable for physically frail women, because of the morbidity associated with abdominal surgery.

e. Abdominal sacrocolpopexy is more suitable for sexually active women, as sacrospinous fixation is associated with exaggerated retroversion of the vagina, leading to a less physiological axis than following sacrocolpopexy.

f. Vaginal length is also well maintained after sacrocolpopexy whereas sacrospinous fixation can cause vaginal narrowing and/or shortening, especially when carried out alongside repair of anterior and/or posterior vaginal wall defects, leading to dyspareunia.

g. ASC is associated with significantly lower rates of recurrent vault prolapse, dyspareunia and postoperative stress urinary incontinence (SUI) when compared with SSF. However, this is not reflected in significantly lower reoperation rates or higher patient satisfaction.

5a. *Should prophylactic continence surgery be performed at the time of sacrocolpopexy?*

It is not clear whether prophylactic continence surgery is beneficial in women who are urodynamically continent and it should not be routinely recommended.

b. *Is there an indication for concomitant surgery for occult SUI?*

Colposuspension performed at the time of sacrocolpopexy is an effective measure to reduce postoperative symptomatic SUI in previously continent women. [*New 2015*]

c. *Is there an indication for concomitant surgery for PHVP and overt SUI?*

Colposuspension at the time of ASC does not appear to be effective treatment for SUI. [*New 2015*] Concomitant mid-urethral sling surgery may be considered when vaginal surgical approaches are used for the treatment of PHVP. [*New 2015*]

6. *What is the role of unilateral or bilateral sacrospinous fixation?*

There is no evidence to recommend bilateral or unilateral sacrospinous fixation as prophylactic continent surgery.

7. *What is the role of iliococcygeus fixation?*

Iliococcygeus fixation does not reduce the incidence of anterior vaginal wall prolapse associated with vaginal sacrospinous fixation and should not be routinely recommended.

8. *Is vaginal uterosacral ligament suspension recommended for post-hysterectomy vaginal vault prolapse?*

Caution is advised with vaginal uterosacral ligament suspension, although it is effective for posthysterectomy vaginal vault prolapse, there is a risk of ureteric injury.

9. *Are laparoscopic procedures recommended?*

a. Clinicians should be aware that laparoscopic procedures involve a high level of expertise and longer operation times. Laparoscopic sacrocolpopexy appears to be as effective as open sacrocolpopexy.

b. The ureters are particularly at risk during laparoscopic uterosacral ligament suspension. There is insufficient evidence to judge the value of other laparoscopic techniques.

c. Laparoscopic techniques used to treat this condition are sacrocolpopexy, uterosacral ligament suspension and sacrospinous fixation.

d. *Laparoscopic and robotic sacrocolpopexy (LSC and RSC):* LSC can include mesh extension or be combined with other vaginal procedures to correct other compartment prolapse.

There is limited evidence on the effectiveness of RSC; therefore, it should only be performed in the context of research or prospective audit following local governance procedures. [*New 2015*]

10. *When should colpocleisis be used?*

    Colpocleisis is a safe and effective procedure that can be considered for those women who do not wish to retain sexual function.

11. *Sling procedures*

    Sling procedures should not be used without adequate patient counselling and special provisions for audit and research.

12. *Is there a role for total mesh reconstruction?*

    There is insufficient evidence to judge the safety and effectiveness of total mesh reconstruction.

    Under what circumstances would transvaginal mesh (TVM) kits/grafts be considered?

    a. The limited evidence on TVM kits does not support their use as first-line treatment of PHVP.

    b. If TVM is considered, women should be fully informed of the permanent nature of the mesh and potential mesh complications, some of which are serious and have long-term effects that can be difficult to treat. [*New 2015*]

    c. If TVM is considered, women should be fully informed of alternative surgical and nonsurgical options and referral to other surgeons/units arranged as appropriate. [*New 2015*]

13. *Vault suspension to the anterior abdominal wall.*

    Vault suspension to the anterior abdominal wall can be a simple measure. However, there are not enough studies assessing this technique to judge its value.

14. *When should colpocleisis be used?*

    Colpocleisis is a safe and effective procedure that can be considered for frail women and/or women who do not wish to retain sexual function.

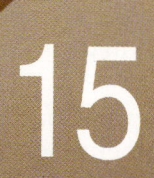

15 | Endometriosis

Introduction

Endometriosis is one of the commonly encountered problems in gynecology. Its pathogenesis is still poorly understood and remains controversial. The first histological description of a lesion consistent with endometriosis was given by Von Rokitansky (1860) and Cullen (1896) who suggested endometriomas, or adenomyomas, resemble mucous membrane of the uterus.

Definition

This is defined as a disease characterized by the presence of tissue that is morphologically and biologically similar to normal endometrium and contains functional endometrial glands and stroma in ectopic locations outside the uterine cavity. This ectopic endometrial tissue undergoes cyclical changes of growth and shedding in response to rise and fall of gonadal hormones. Cyclical bleeding from the endometriotic deposit induces a local inflammatory reaction, fibrous adhesion and firm implants in the peritoneum including the pelvic organs outside the uterus.

Prevalence

Endometriosis is primarily a disease of the reproductive years and is only rarely described in adolescence in case of outflow tract obstruction or in postmenopausal state with estrogen replacement therapy.

Prevalence of endometriosis in various clinical settings	
Unexplained infertility	70–80%
Infertile women	15–20%
Diagnosed on laparoscopy	0–53%
Women undergoing sterilization	2%
In women with affected 1st degree relative	7%

Etiopathogenesis

Among the theories concerning the pathogenesis of endometriosis, three main concepts can be discerned (Box 15.1). The oldest concept that of **in situ development**, is that endometriosis develops on the spot where it is found. Development may occur from the remnants of the Wolffian ducts or the müllerian ducts, or alternatively from metaplasia of the peritoneal or ovarian tissue.

> **Box 15.1:** Etiopathogenesis of endometriosis
> i. **In situ development from:**
>   a. Germinal epithelium of the ovary
>   b. Embryonic cell rests
>   Mesonephric (Wolffian knob, Wolffian duct)
>   Paramesonephric (müllerian ducts)
>   c. Coelomic metaplasia
>   d. Metaplasia by inflammation
>   e. Metaplasia by hormonal stimulation
>   f. Metaplasia by induction
> ii. **Transplantation**
>   a. Implantation, retrograde menstruation
>   b. Implantation, mechanical transplantation
>   c. Benign lymphogenous metastasis
> iii. **Combination of in situ development and endometrial transplantation and implantation**

A second concept, **the induction theory,** is based on the assumption that endometriosis results from differentation of mesenchymal cells, activated or induced by substances released by degenerating endometrium that arrives in the abdominal cavity.

A third concept, the **transplantation or implantation theory**, is based on the transplantation and subsequent implantation of endometrial tissue. This would include transportation of viable endometrial cells during menstruation via the Fallopian tubes into the abdominal cavity, implantation of these cells on to the peritoneum and the development of these cells into endometriosis.

In situ Development

Von Recklinghausen offered several arguments in support of endometriosis originating from the Wolffian duct.

He noted a great similarity in the structure of 'adenomyomas' and the mesonephros and emphasized that mesonephros develops close to the uterus, the tubes and the ovaries. In particular, Meyer (1923) disputed the theories of von Recklinghausen. He opined that endometriosis is supposed to develop where peritoneum was found. According to this theory, the histogenesis of endometriosis is explained by metaplasia of the original coelomic membrane. These metaplastic changes could occur secondary to inflammatory processes or hormonal influences.

The Implantation Theory (Fig. 15.1)

The conditions that have to be met for the implantation theory are threefold: Firstly, retrograde menstruation has to occur; secondly, retrograde menstruation should contain viable endometrial cells; and thirdly, adhesion to the peritoneum has to occur with subsequent implantation and proliferation. Retrograde menstruation and peritoneal adhesion of endometrial tissue is an essential element in the pathogenesis of endometriosis according to Sampson's theory.

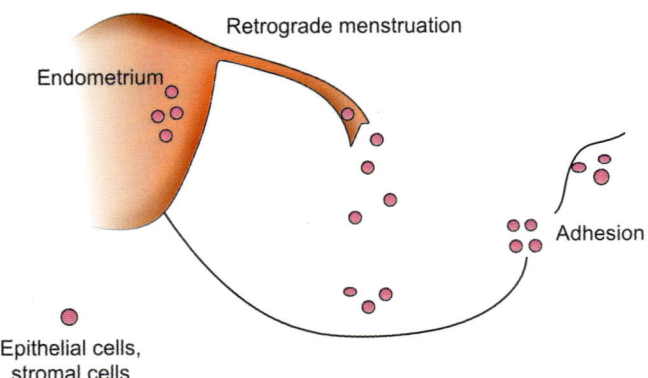

Fig. 15.1: Implantation theory

The Induction Theory

Levander and Normann (1955) introduced the induction theory. This theory is based on the assumption that specific substances which are released by degenerating endometrium induce the development of endometriosis from omnipotent blastema, present in connective tissue.

Causes of Persistence and Growth of Endometriosis

- **Impaired immune system.** Women with endometriosis have fewer natural killer (NK) cells. In their absence, the immune system is weakened and may allow endometrial tissue to invade and implant.

- **Growth factors and angiogenesis.** Macrophages and endometriotic implants produce growth factors like VEGF, which are of particular interest because they play important roles in angiogenesis, a natural process by which new blood vessels form to promote implantation outside.

- *Other growth factors are:* Transforming growth factors-beta (TGF-β), platelet-derived endothelial growth factor (PD-ECGF), and tumor necrosis growth factors.

In conclusion, the transplantation theory (suggesting the implantation and subsequent growth of retrogradely-shed viable endometrial cells) still remains the most widely-accepted theory to explain the pathogenesis of endometriosis, although the development of endometriosis is probably a multifactorial event. A plausible alternative could well be the induction theory (transformation of mesothelium to endometrium-like tissue under the influence of products of regurgitated endometrium). Both theories require retrograde menstruation and adhesion of shed endometrial cells to the peritoneal lining.

Anatomic Spread (Fig. 15.2)

- The ovary is the most common site for endometriosis. Spread to the ovary is believed to be lymphatic, although superficial implants may be due to retrograde menstrual flow because the ovaries are in a dependent part of the pelvis. Lesions can vary in size from spots to large endometriomas. The classic lesion is chocolate cyst of the ovary that contains old blood which has undergone hemolysis. Once intracystic pressure rises, the cyst perforates, spilling its contents within the peritoneal cavity. This can cause severe abdominal pain. The inflammatory response causes adhesions that further increase the morbidity of the disease.

- Uterine serosa can be affected. Vesicular lesions may provoke an inflammatory response and scarring that cause the bladder to adhere anteriorly. Posteriorly, the disease may cause obliteration of the cul-de-sac and form dense adhesions between the posterior vaginal wall or cervix and the anterior rectum. Severe dyspareunia, dyschezia, and alteration of bowel habits are the clinical sequelae of this common spread.

- Deep peritoneal disease is caused by infiltration of the uterosacral ligaments and rectovaginal septum by endometriotic nodules. Tethering of the uterus can lead to fixed retroversion. Dyspareunia is an important feature.

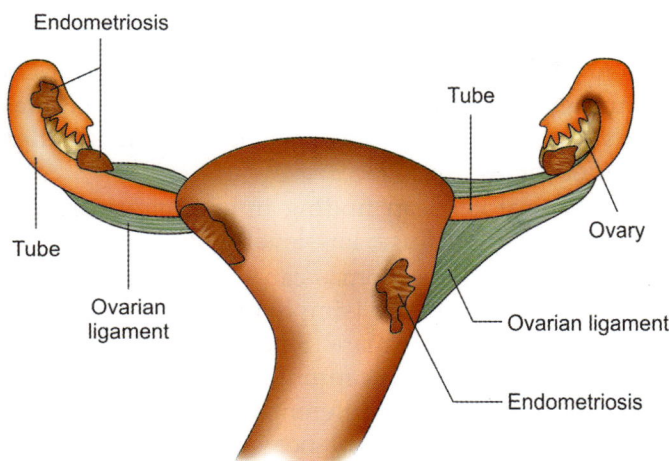

Fig. 15.2: Common sites of endometriosis in pelvis

- Through contiguous spreading, endometriosis may invade the rectovaginal septum and the anterior rectal wall. It may also involve the upper rectum and sigmoid colon, infiltrating the muscularis. Cyclical rectal bleeding (hematochezia) is pathognomonic of endometriosis. However, transmural bowel involvement by endometriosis remains a rarity. The ileum, appendix, and cecum may also be involved, leading to intestinal obstruction.

- Although uncommon, interference in the genitourinary tract by endometriosis can affect the bladder, ureters, and kidneys by invasion, compression, or scarring. Medical therapy has less than satisfactory results, and surgical intervention is often required.

- Uncommon sites include incisional scars, the umbilicus, and the thoracic cavity. Catamenial or cyclic pneumothorax can cause hemoptysis.

- Ectopic endometrial tissue rarely can undergo malignant transformation—all endometriotic lesions, therefore, should be biopsied.

- Postmenopausal endometriosis may be encountered in women who are on estrogen replacement therapy (ERT). Occasionally, if ERT is administered after total abdominal hysterectomy, endometriosis can be stimulated in an ovarian remnant. Extrapelvic endometriosis is believed to be hormone-resistant when it occurs after surgical castration. Transplantation of endometrial implants during the original surgery is believed to explain this occurrence. Another possible explanation is coelomic metaplasia.

Symptoms—outlined in Table 15.1.

Table 15.1: Diagnosis—frequency of symptoms in endometriosis	
Symptoms	*Frequency (%)*
Dysmenorrhea	60–80
Pelvic pain	30–50
Infertility	30–40
Dyspareunia	25–40
Menstrual irregularity	10–20
Cyclical dysuria/hematuria	1–2
Dyschezia	1–2
Rectal bleeding (cyclic)	<1

Clinical Signs

- *Abdominal examination:*
  - Bilateral/unilateral ovarian cysts—soft cystic with restricted mobility
  - Umbilical scar endometriosis
- *Pelvic examination:*
  - Fixed retroverted tender bulky uterus owing to adhesion and adenomyosis.
  - Endometrioma of ovary
  - Nodularity of the uterosacral ligaments and the cul-de-sac.
  - Cervical endometriosis.
  - Occasionally, a bluish nodule may be seen in the vagina due to infiltration from the posterior vaginal wall.
  - Perineal scar endometriosis

Causes of Dyspareunia

- Deep dyspareunia due to scarring of the uterosacral ligaments, nodularity of the rectovaginal septum, cul-de-sac obliteration, and/or uterine retroversion. All of these may also lead to chronic backache.
- These symptoms are exaggerated during menses.
- Women with deep infiltration of the uterosacral ligaments have the most severe impairment of sexual function.

Causes of Infertility

I. *In mild disease*

- *Ovarian function:* Anovulation, luteolysis by PGF$_{2\alpha}$, altered prolactin release
- *Tubal function:* Defective ovum pickup, altered tubo-ovarian relation, altered tubal and ciliary motility
- *Sperm function:* Phagocytosis by macrophages
- *Endometrium:* Interference by endometrial antibodies, defective implantation by adenomyomatous changes
- *Coital function:* Dyspareunia and, therefore, reduced coital frequency

II. *In moderate-to-severe disease*

Anatomical obstruction due to tubal block, formation of peritoneal inflammation and dense pelvic adhesions.

Diagnosis

I. *Laparoscopy* (Figs 15.3 to 15.9)

Laparoscopy is the gold standard in diagnosis of endometriosis.

For a definitive diagnosis of endometriosis, visual inspection of the pelvis at laparoscopy is the best form of diagnostic tool, unless disease is visible in the posterior vaginal fornix or elsewhere.

II. *USG* (Fig. 15.10)

Patients with suspected endometriosis referred for US scanning evaluation should receive a transvaginal study, because this is more sensitive for smaller endometriomas.

The typical US scan finding in endometriosis is a cystic mass with diffuse, low-level echoes.

However, endometriomas can vary in appearance. They may appear cystic (simple or complex), or they may resemble a solid mass. Small implants typically are not seen with US scanning. Doppler waveform analysis is not helpful in differentiating endometriomas from other masses. Low-resistance waveforms resembling malignancy are encountered in endometriomas.

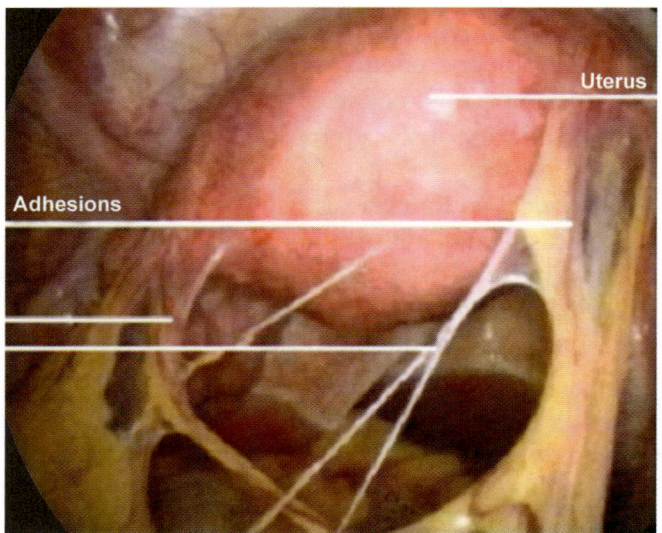

Fig. 15.3: Dense adhesions in endometriosis

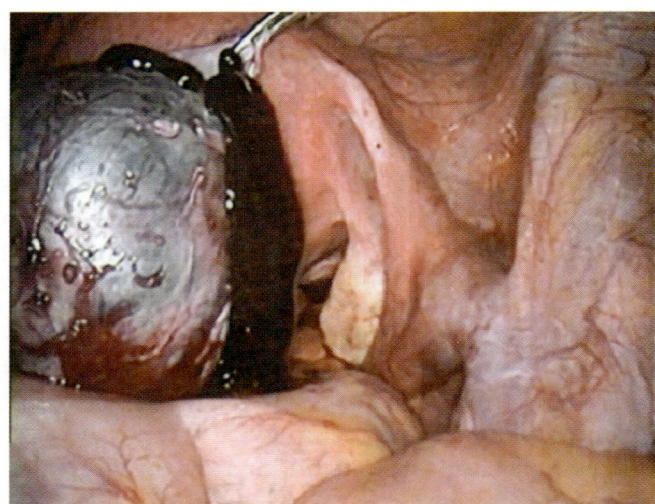

Fig. 15.5: Rare site on appendix

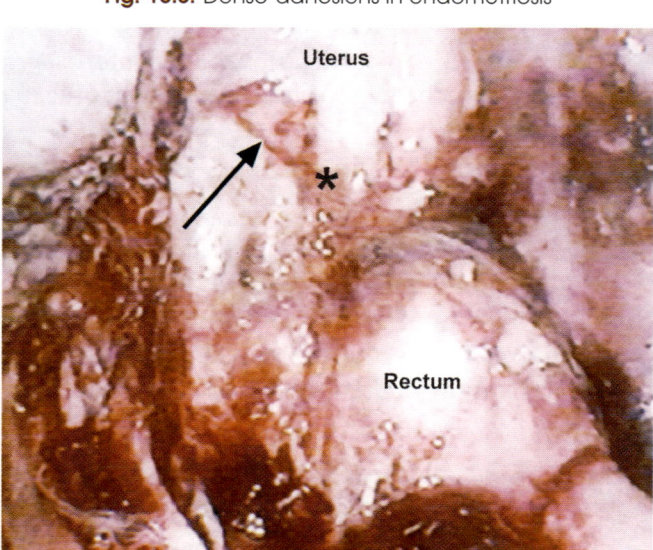

Fig. 15.4: Chocolate cyst of ovarian endometrioma

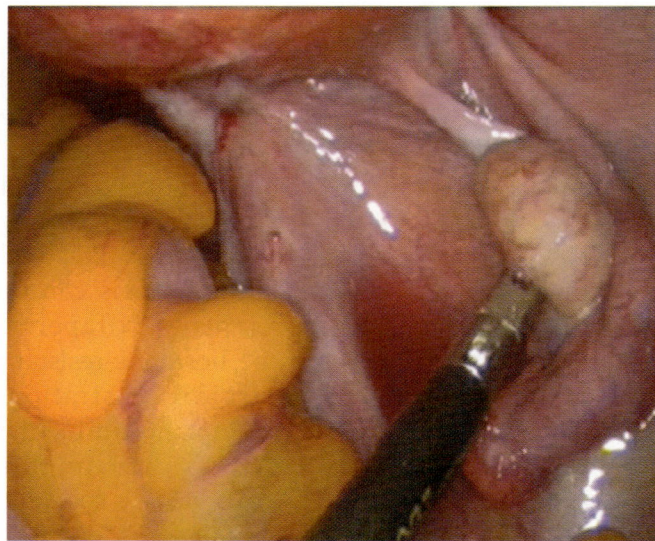

Fig. 15.6: Rectovaginal endometriosis

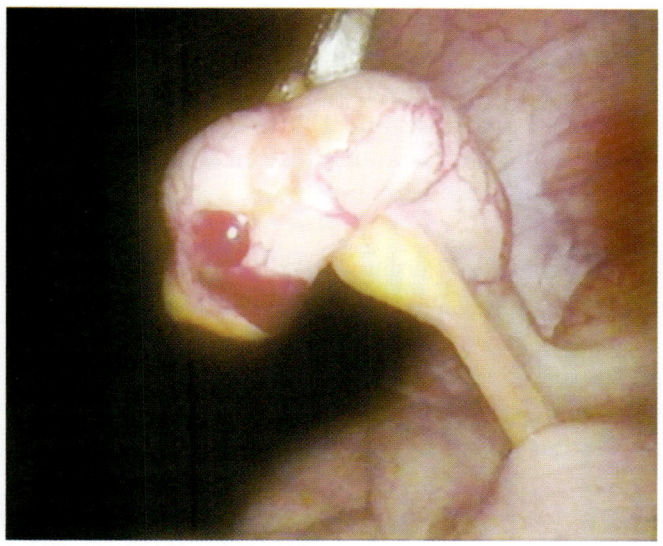

Fig. 15.7: Endometriosis obstruction of right ureter

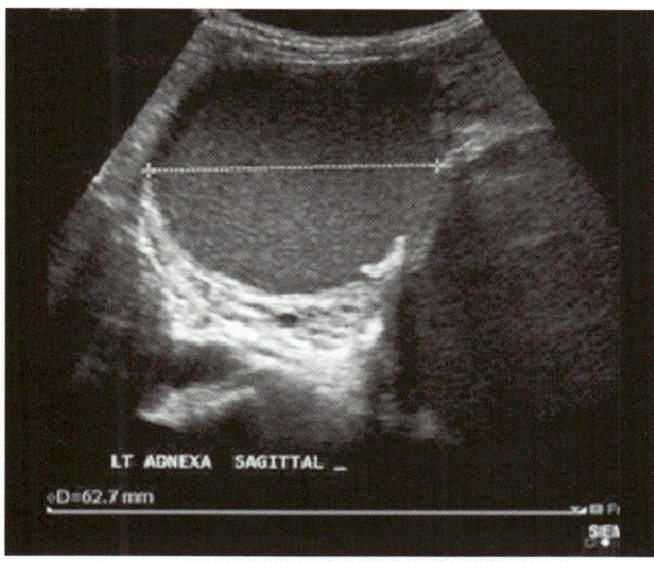

Fig. 15.10: USG of ovaries

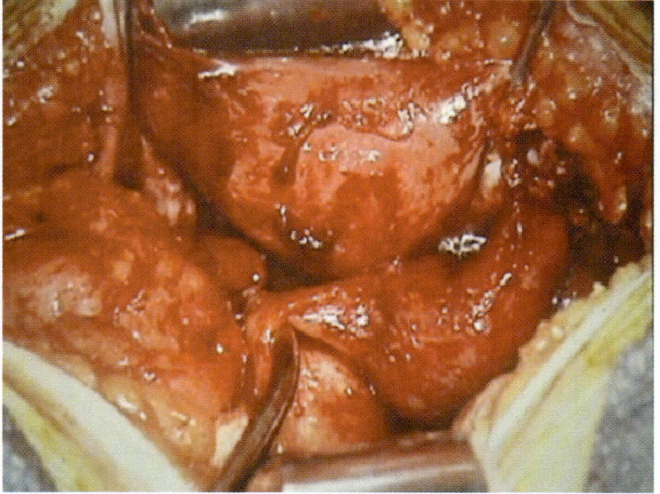

Fig. 15.8: Severe endometriosis

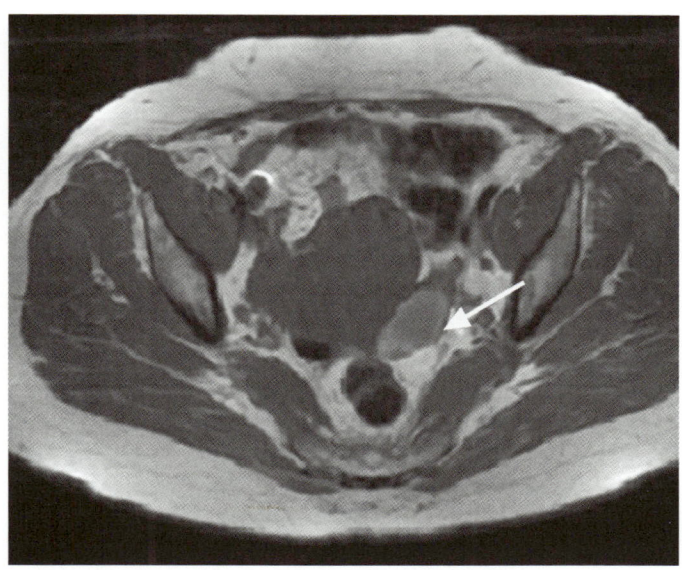

Fig. 15.11: MRI of ovaries

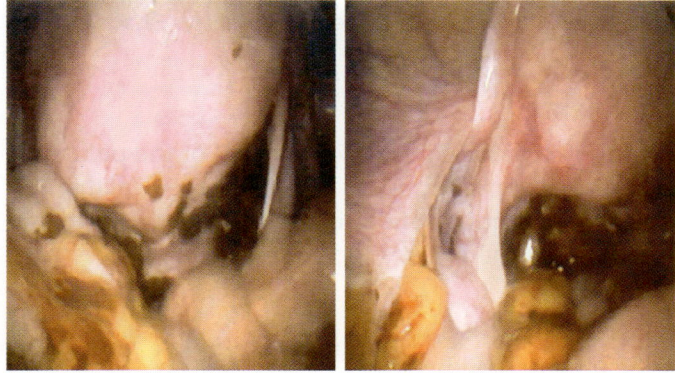

Fig. 15.9: Endometriosis over bowel

III. *MRI* (Figs 15.11 and 15.12)

US scanning is not as specific as MRI in the evaluation of endometriosis. The appearance of a cystic mass with homogeneous, diffuse, low-level echoes is highly suggestive of an endometrioma.

MR images include sagittal and axial fast spin-echo T2-weighted images and gradient echo T1-weighted images with and without fat suppression, before and after injection of gadolinium.

The appearance of endometriomas on MRIs is variable and depends on the concentration of iron and protein in the fluid, products of blood degradation. Most endometriomas have the gross appearance of chocolate cysts, representing highly concentrated blood products. MRI demonstrates these endometriomas as cystic masses with very high signal intensity on T1-

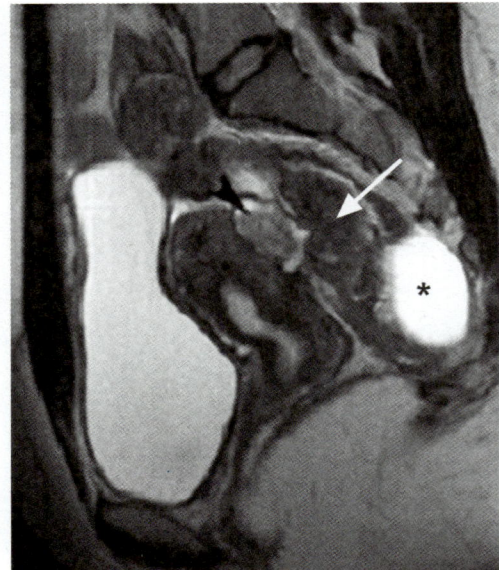

Fig. 15.12: MRI on endometriosis of rectosigmoid colon

weighted images and very low signal intensity on T2-weighted images.

IV. *Histological Confirmation*

- Positive histology confirms the diagnosis of endometriosis.
- Negative histology does not exclude it.
- Visual inspection is usually adequate but histological confirmation of at least one lesion is ideal.
- In cases of ovarian endometrioma (greater than 3 cm in diameter) and in deeply infiltrating disease, histology should be obtained to identify endometriosis and to exclude rare instances of malignancy.

Table 15.2: Correlation of histological lesion with laparoscopic lesion	
Nature of	*Histological correlation*
Black	94%
White	80%
Red	75%
Glandular	66%
Subovarian adhesions	39%
Patches	22%
Yellow brown pockets	39%

A fertility score (EFI) has been developed that predicts probability of pregnancy of an infertility endometriosis patient with endometriosis with standard non-IVF treatment after surgical staging. It is expected that male and female gamets are sufficiently functrional to enable attempts at non-IVF conception. One factor that is not included in the EFI is uterine

abnormality because it is quite uncommon in infertile endometriotic patients (Fig. 15.13).

The EFI score ranges from 0–10, with 0 representing the poorest prognosis and 10 the best prognosis. Half of the point comes from the historical factors and half from the surgical factors.

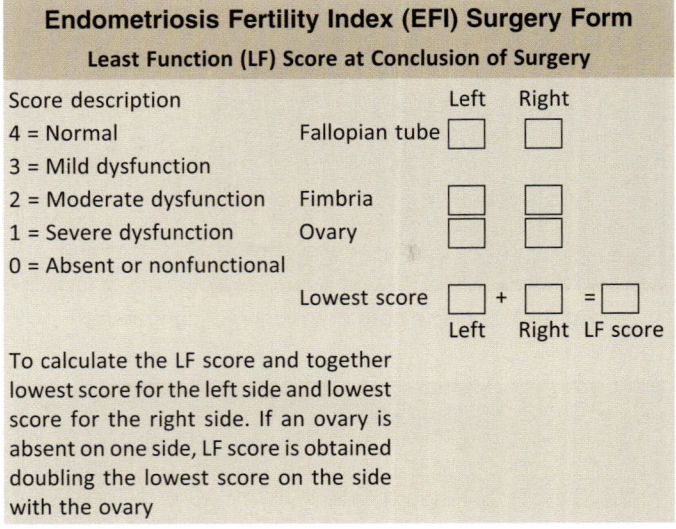

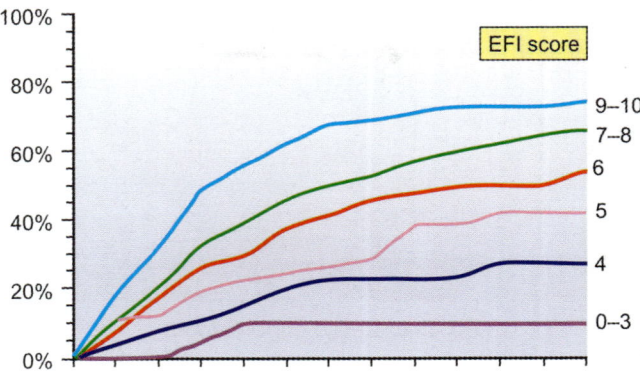

Fig. 15.13: Estimated percent pregnant by EFI score

Treatment

This is directed according to the need of the patient. If the pain is the predominant symptom, medical therapy is the treatment of option. If infertility is the problem, surgical treatment gives the better result.

Medical Therapy

- Oral contraceptives
- Progesterone
- Danazol
- GnRH agonists
- Progesterone depot
- LNG-IUD

Endometriosis Fertility Index (EFI)			
Historical factors		**Surgical factors**	
Factor description	Points	Factor description	Points
Age		LF Score	
If age is ≤35 yrs.	2	If LF score = 7 to 8	3
If age is 36 to 39 yrs.	1	If LF score = 4 to 6	2
If age is ≥40 yrs.	0	If LF score = 1 to 3	0
Years infertile		AFS endometriosis score	
If years infertile is >3	2	If AFS endometriosis lesion score is <16	1
If years infertile is <3	0	If AFS endometriosis lesion score ≥16	0
Prior pregnancy		AFS total score	
If there is a history of a prior pregnancy	2	If AFS total score <71	1
If there is no history of prior pregnancy	0	If AFS total score ≥71	0
Total historical factors	☐	**Total surgical factors**	☐
EFI = Total historical factors + Total surgical factors		☐ + ☐ = ☐ Historical Surgical EFI score	

- RU-486 (misoprostol)
- Centchroman

Combined oral contraceptive pills (COCPs), danazol, progestational agents, and GnRH analogs form the mainstay of medical therapy. All these therapies have similar clinical efficacy in terms of reduction in pain-related symptoms and duration of relief.

- COCPs act by ovarian suppression and continuous progestin administration causes atrophy of endometriotic tissue.
- Initially, continuous or cyclic COCPs are administered for 3 months. If pain is relieved, this treatment is continued for 6–12 months. Subsequent pregnancy rates upon discontinuation of the pill are 40–50%.
- Continuous noncyclical administration of COCPs for 3–4 months produce amenorrhea and relieve pain.
- Women with endometriosis are at increased risk of epithelial ovarian cancer, and COCPs are believed to protect against this.
- All progestational agents act by decidualization and atrophy of the endometrium.
- Medroxyprogesterone acetate is effective in pain suppression in both the oral and injectable depot preparations. Oral doses of 10–20 mg/day can be administered continuously. The time to resumption of ovulation is longer and variable with depot preparations. Adverse effects include weight gain, fluid retention, depression, and breakthrough bleeding.

- Megestrol acetate, another progesterone preparation is also effective in doses of 40 mg/day with similarly good results.
- The levonorgestrel intrauterine system (LNG-IUS) has been shown to reduce endometriosis-associated pain. When inserted at the time of laparoscopic surgery, it has been found to reduce the recurrence by 35%.
- Danazol acts by inhibiting the midcycle FSH and LH surges and prevents steroidogenesis in the corpus luteum.
- Its androgenic property produces side effects which include oily skin, acne, weight gain, deepening of the voice, and facial hirsutism.
- The recommended dose is 400–800 mg/day.
- Because of the possibility of virilizing changes in a female fetus, **additional barrier contraception must be used while on danazol therapy.**
- GnRH analogs produce a hypogonadotropic-hypogonadic state by downregulation of the pituitary gland. Currently, goserelin and leuprolide acetate are the commonly used agonists.
- Once again, efficacy is limited to pain suppression and fertility rates may show no improvement. GnRH therapy may lead to improvement in pain associated with endometriosis in 85–100% of women. Pain relief is believed to persist for 6–12 months after cessation of treatment.
- Treatment is usually restricted to monthly injections for 6 months.
- Loss of trabecular bone density caused by GnRH is restored by 2 years after cessation of therapy. Other prominent adverse effects include hot flashes and vaginal dryness.
- Much interest has been shown in whether add-back therapy should be instituted to prevent osteoporosis and hypoestrogenic symptoms. Hormone replacement therapy preparations, progestins, tibolone maleate, and bisphosphonates have all been shown to be effective. Add-back therapy is used to prevent loss in bone density and relieve vasomotor symptoms without reducing the efficacy of GnRH regimens. GnRH agonists can be used for 12 months with low dose estrogen and norethindrone add-back therapy with good results.

Aromatase inhibitors

- Aromatase is a protein in the body that is responsible for producing estrogen. Normally, it is found in the ovaries, and to a much lesser extent in the skin and fat.
- Aromatase is also found in high levels in the ectopic endometrial tissue of women with endometriosis.

Revised American Society for Reproductive Medicine Classification of Endometriosis 1985

Patient's Name _____   Date _____

Stage I   (Minimal)   1–5   Laparoscopy _____   Laparotomy _____   Photography _____

Stage II   (Mild)   6–15   Recommended treatment _____

Stage III (Moderate)   18–40   _____

Stage IV   (Severe)   >40

Total _____   Prognosis _____

	ENDOMETRIOSIS	< 1cm	1–3 cm	> 3 cm
Peritoneum	Superficial	1	2	4
	Deep	2	4	6
	R Superficial	1	2	4
Ovary	Deep	4	16	20
	L Suprficial	1	2	4
	Deep	4	16	20
	Posterior cul-de-sac Obliteration	Partial 4	Complete 40	
	Adhesions	<1/3 Enclosure	1/3–2/3 Enclosure	>2/3 Enclosure
	R Filmy	1	2	4
Ovary	Dense	4	8	16
	L Filmy	1	2	4
	Dense	4	8	16
	R Filmy	1	2	4
Tube	Dense	4	8	16
	L Filmy	1	2	4
	Dense	4	8	16

- Aromatase inhibitor suppresses the growth of endometriosis and reduces the associated inflammation by decreasing aromatase expression in endometriotic tissue and thereby rereducing estrogen synthesis.
- Aromatase inhibitors combined with progestins, oral contraceptive pills or GnRh analogues reduces pain and lesion size.
- Even after total abdominal hysterectomy with bilateral salpingo-oophorectomy, endometriosis persists or recurs in some patients because of extraovarian estrogen production. Use of aromatase inhibitors such as letrozole or anastrozole–reduces circulating estrogen dramatically and gives relief of symptoms of endometriosis.

LNG-IUS (Fig. 15.14)

Insertion of an LNG-IUS after laparoscopic surgery for symptomatic endometriosis significantly reduces the risk of recurrence of moderate or severe dysmenorrhea. There is only limited evidence of this beneficial role for endometriosis.(*Cochrane review*)

Mifepristone

- It appears to be effective in improving the symptoms and causing regression of endometriosis in the absence of significant side effects.
- Subcutaneous implantation of mifepristone-loaded capsules is an effective means for long-term treatment of endometriosis.
- Treatment with mifepristone, 50 to 100 mg daily, results in amenorrhea, anovulation, and symptomatic improvement in women with endometriosis.

GnRH analogue in endometriosis with infertility

- GnRHa is commonly used in severe endometriosis.
- Moderate to severe endometriosis needs reconstruction procedure aimed to restore the

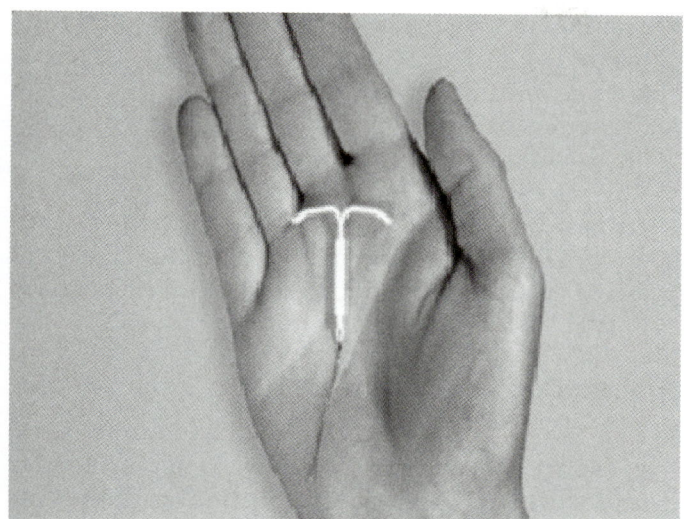

Fig. 15.14: LNG-IUS

anatomy. GnRHa usually is given before and after surgery.

- GnRHa makes operative procedure simpler, reduce the diameter of the cyst, makes detachment easier.
- The success in cure rate of pelvic pain and dysmenorrhea is 80–90%, whereas pregnancy rate is 52%.

Preoperative GnRHa

Advantages

- Decreases vascularity: Decreases operative blood loss.
- Decreases size and extent of surgical excision.
- Higher pregnancy rate is achieved.

Disadvantages

- Smaller lesions may not be visible during surgery leaving uncorrected and that lead to recurrence.
- Planes appear not clear during surgery.
- Expensive

Postoperative GnRHa

This eradicates microscopic lesions which could not be removed during surgery. However, it delays the chance of conception which is maximum within 2 years of surgery. Three-step approach of treatment:

- Straightway surgery
- 6 month treatment with GnRHa before surgery.
- 2nd look laparoscopy with removal of residues.
- **Sandwich therapy**—GnRHa–Surgery–GnRHa

Surgical Care

Surgical care can be broadly classified as **conservative** when reproductive potential is retained, **semiconservative** when reproductive ability is eliminated but ovarian function is retained, and **radical** when the uterus and ovaries are removed. Age, desire for future childbearing, and deterioration of quality of life are the main considerations when deciding on the extent of surgery.

1. Conservative Surgery

- With conservative surgery, the aim is to destroy visible endometriotic implants and lyse peritubal and periovarian adhesions that are a source of pain and may interfere with ovum transport. The laparoscopic approach is the method of choice for treating endometriosis conservatively. Ablation can be performed with laser or electrodiathermy. Overall, the recurrence rate is 19% and is similar for all techniques. Laparoscopic ablative surgery with bipolar diathermy or laser for endometriomas is effective for relieving pelvic pain in 87% of patients. Ovarian endometriomas can be treated by drainage or cystectomy. Laparoscopic cystectomy yields better pain relief and pregnancy rates than drainage. Medical therapy with GnRH agonists reduces the size of the cyst but does not reduce pain relief.
- The absolute benefit for women undergoing surgical ablation of endometriosis is 30–40% over women having only diagnostic laparoscopy. In cases of rectovaginal endometriosis, significant short-term pain relief is reported 80%, but at 1-year follow-up, 50% again require analgesics or hormones for pain relief. During postoperative treatment, GnRH analogs result in significantly reduced pain scores in women who have received treatment for 6 months.
- Tubal flushing with oil-soluble media improve pregnancy rates in women with endometriosis-associated infertility.
- Presacral neurectomy is used to relieve severe dysmenorrhea. The nerve bundles are transected at the level of the third sacral vertebra, and the distal ends are ligated. Vascular injury to the middle sacral artery and vein is a potential complication. Also, constipation is a long-term adverse effect (94%) of this procedure and should be considered while deciding whetheror not to perform this procedure.
- Nodularity of the uterosacral ligaments may contribute to dyspareunia and low back pain. The transmission of neural pathways is via the Lee-Frankenhäuser plexus. Laparoscopic uterine nerve ablation (LUNA) is performed to interrupt the pain fibers. Potential complications of this procedure include uterine prolapse and pelvic denervation. When combined with laparoscopic ablation, LUNA significantly reduce pain attributed to endometriosis.

In patients with subfertility, tissue ablation significantly increase the cumulative pregnancy rate. *A recent Cochrane review, however, fail to show any benefit from either LUNA or presacral neurectomy.*

- For patients with mild disease, postoperative adjunctive hormonal treatment is effective in reducing pain but has no impact on fertility. GnRH analogs, danazol, and medroxyprogesterone have all been found to be useful for this indication. However, for severe endometriosis, the efficacy of preoperative or postoperative hormonal treatment has not yet been established.

2. Semiconservative Surgery

- The indication for this type of surgery is mainly in women who have completed their childbearing, are too young to undergo surgical menopause, and are debilitated by the symptoms. Such surgery involves hysterectomy and cytoreduction of pelvic endometriosis. Ovarian endometriosis can be removed surgically because one tenth of functioning ovarian tissue is all that is needed for hormone production. Patients who undergo hysterectomy with ovarian conservation have a 6-fold higher rate of recurrence compared to women who undergo oophorectomy.
- Medical therapy in women who have completed childbearing is equally efficacious for symptom suppression.

3. Radical Surgery

- This involves total hysterectomy with bilateral oophorectomy and cytoreduction of visible endometriosis. Adhesiolysis is performed to restore mobility and normal intrapelvic organ relationships.
- Ureteric obstruction may warrant surgical release or excision of a damaged segment. Bowel obstruction may require a resection anastomosis or a wedge resection if the obstruction is confined to the anterior rectosigmoid.
- Endometriosis may recur in 15% of women after extirpative surgery, irrespective of whether ERT is given postoperatively. ERT can be instituted safely immediately after surgery, especially in younger women who face the prospect of accelerated bone loss and vasomotor symptoms.

IVF-ART for Treatment of Infertility

- VF is appropriate treatment, especially if tubal function is compromised, if there is also male factor infertility, and/or other treatments have failed.

- Treatment with a GnRH agonist for 3–6 months before IVF in women with endometriosis increases the rate of clinical pregnancy.
- Presence of adenomyoma is detrimental for implantation in embryo transfer.
- Role of estrogen, aspirin, progesterone, IGF are claimed to be useful in helping implantation. Assay of AMH, Doppler flow in endometrium is used to assess endometrium preparedness for implantation in IVF.

Specific Causes of Failure of ART in Endometriosis

- *Poor endometrial receptivity:* In endometrium, presence of various abnormal cell adhesion molecules, lack of favorable matrix metalloproteinase, growth factor enzymes and steroid hormone receptors–reduce endometrial receptivity.
- *Bad quality oocytes:* Presence of abnormal immune cells like cytokines, interlukins, lack of growth factor in the follicular fluid–poor oocyte quality receptivity.
- *Poor ovarian reserve* due to repeated surgical trauma or ovarian destruction.

Figure 15.15 underlines systemetic approach in management of endometriosis.

RCOG Guidelines

1. *Which symptoms are typically associated with endometriosis?*

Based on clinical and patient experience, endometriosis can cause the following symptoms:

- Severe dysmenorrhea
- Deep dyspareunia
- Chronic pelvic pain
- Ovulation pain
- Cyclical or perimenstrual symptoms, such as bowel or bladder, with or without abnormal bleeding or pain
- Infertility
- Chronic fatigue
- Dyschezia (pain on defecation).

2. *When in the menstrual cycle is clinical examination most reliable for diagnostic purposes?*

Deeply infiltrating nodules are most reliably detected when clinical examination is performed during menstruation.

3. *What is the 'gold standard' diagnostic test?*

For a definitive diagnosis of endometriosis, visual inspection of the pelvis at laparoscopy is the gold standard investigation, unless disease is visible in the posterior vaginal fornix or elsewhere.

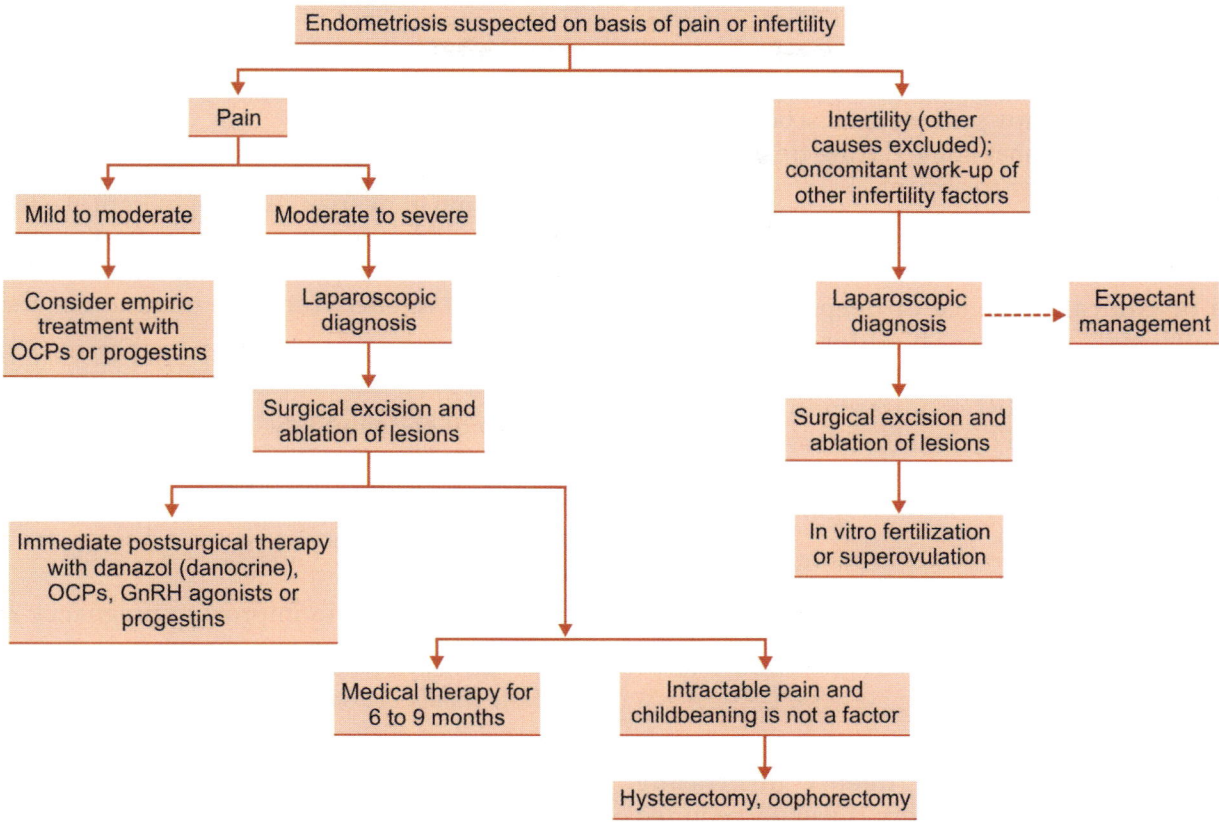

Fig. 15.15: Schematic approach of endometriosis management

Good surgical practice is to use an instrument such as a grasper, via a secondary port, to mobilize the pelvic organs and to palpate lesions, which can help determine their nodularity. It is also important to document in detail the type, location and extent of all lesions and adhesions in the operative notes.

4. *Is histological confirmation necessary?*

Positive histology confirms the diagnosis of endometriosis; negative histology does not exclude it. Whether histology should be obtained, if peritoneal disease alone is present is controversial. Visual inspection is usually adequate but histological confirmation of at least one lesion is ideal. In cases of ovarian endometrioma (greater than 3 cm in diameter) and in deeply infiltrating disease, histology should be obtained to identify endometriosis and to exclude rare instances of malignancy.

5. *How reliable is imaging for diagnostic purposes?*

Compared with laparoscopy, transvaginal ultrasound (TVS) has limited value in diagnosing peritoneal endometriosis but it is a useful tool both to make and to exclude the diagnosis of an ovarian endometrioma.

6. *How reliable is serum CA125 measurement for diagnostic purposes?*

Serum CA125 levels may be elevated in endometriosis. However, compared with laparoscopy, measuring serum CA125 levels has no value as a diagnostic tool.

7. *What is the empirical treatment of pain symptoms without a definitive diagnosis*

If a woman wants pain symptoms suggestive of endometriosis to be treated without a definitive diagnosis, a therapeutic trial of a hormonal drug to reduce menstrual flow is appropriate.

8. *How effectively do nonsteroidal anti-inflammatory drugs (NSAIDs) treat endometriosis-associated pain?*

There is inconclusive evidence to show whether NSAIDs are effective in managing pain caused by endometriosis.

9. *How effectively do hormonal drugs treat endometriosis-associated pain?*

Suppression of ovarian function for 6 months reduces endometriosis-associated pain. Symptom recurrence is common following medical treatment of endometriosis.

10. *Is there a role for the levonorgestrel intrauterine system (LNG-IUS)?*

LNG-IUS appears to reduce endometriosis-associated pain.

11. *Can bone mineral density loss while taking a GnRH agonist be prevented using 'add-back' therapy?*
The use of a GnRH agonist with 'add-back' (estrogen and progestogen) therapy protects against bone mineral density loss at the lumbar spine during treatment and for up to 6 months after treatment.

12. *What investigations are recommended to assess disease extent?*
In case of clinical evidence of deeply infiltrating endometriosis, ureteric, bladder and bowel involvement should be assessed. Consideration should be given to perform MRI or ultrasound (transrectal and/or transvaginal and/or renal), with or without IVP and barium enema studies, to map the extent of disease as it may be multifocal.

13. *How should suspected endometriomas be managed?*
A guideline for the management of suspected ovarian malignancy should be followed in cases of ovarian endometrioma.

14. *How should suspected severe/deeply infiltrating disease be managed?*
The management of severe/deeply infiltrating endometriosis is complex. Surgery is usually required and multiple organs are sometimes involved. Therefore, if disease of such severity is suspected or diagnosed, referral to a center with the necessary expertise to offer all available treatments in a multidisciplinary context, including advanced laparoscopic surgery and laparotomy, is strongly recommended.

15. *When should surgical treatment be considered?*
Ideal practice is to diagnose and remove endometriosis surgically.

16. *Does surgical treatment relieve pain?*
Ablation of endometriotic lesions reduces endometriosis-associated pain compared with diagnostic laparoscopy.

17. *Does nerve ablation provide pain relief?*
Laparoscopic uterine nerve ablation by itself does not reduce endometriosis-associated pain.

18. *What is the role of more radical surgery?*
Endometriosis associated pain can be reduced by removing the entire lesions in severe and deeply infiltrating disease.

19. *Is there a role for hormonal treatment before or after surgery?*

There is insufficient evidence of benefit to justify the use of preoperative or postoperative hormonal treatment.

20. *Is there a role for hormonal treatment in endometriosis-associated infertility?*
Suppression of ovarian function to improve fertility in minimal–mild endometriosis is not effective and should not be offered for this indication alone. There is no evidence of its effectiveness in more severe disease.

21. *Does surgery for minimal–mild disease improve pregnancy rates?*
Ablation of endometriotic lesions plus adhesiolysis to improve fertility in minimal–mild endometriosis is effective compared with diagnostic laparoscopy alone.

22. *Does surgery for moderate–severe disease improve pregnancy rates?*
The role of surgery in improving pregnancy rates for moderate–severe disease is uncertain.

23. *How should ovarian endometriomas be managed?*
Laparoscopic cystectomy for ovarian endometriomas is better than drainage and coagulation.

24. *Is there a role for hormonal treatment after surgery?*
Postoperative hormonal treatment has no beneficial effect on pregnancy rates after surgery.

25. *Is there a role for flushing the fallopian tubes?*
Tubal flushing appears to improve pregnancy rates in women with endometriosis-associated infertility.

26. *Does intrauterine insemination (IUI) improve pregnancy rates?*
Treatment with IUI improves fertility in minimal to mild endometriosis.

27. *Is in vitro fertilization (IVF) indicated?*
IVF is appropriate treatment, especially if tubal function is compromised, if there is also male factor infertility, and/or other treatments have failed.

28. *Is there a role for surgical treatment of endometriomas before IVF?*
Laparoscopic ovarian cystectomy is recommended for endometriomas >4 cm in diameter

29. *Is there a role for hormonal treatment before IVF?*
Treatment with a GnRH agonist for 3–6 months before IVF in women with endometriosis increases the rate of clinical pregnancy.

16 Menopause and Hormone Therapy (HT)

Menopause is defined as amenorrhea for at least one year due to permanent cessation of follicular development.

Many women experience a variety of symptoms as a result of the hormonal changes associated with the transition through menopause.

Premature Menopause

The average age of women at the time of menopause is **51 years**. The most common age range at which women experience menopause is 48–55 years. If menopause occurs in a woman younger than 40 years, it is considered to be premature. About 1% of women experience premature menopause. Menopause is considered **late,** if it occurs in a woman older than 55 years. Menopause is more likely to occur at a slightly earlier age in women who smoke, have never been pregnant, or live at high altitudes.

Perimenopause/Perimenopausal Transition

The hormonal changes associated with menopause actually begin prior to the last menstrual period during three to five years period called the perimenopause. During this transition, women may begin to experience menopausal symptoms and may lose bone density, even though they are still menstruating. This is characterized by elevated FSH levels associated with variable cycle lengths and missed menses.

Surgical Menopause

Surgical menopause is menopause induced by the removal of the ovaries and uterus. Women who have had surgical menopause often have a sudden and severe onset of the symptoms of menopause.

Physiology

Although menopause is associated with changes in hypothalamic and pituitary hormones that regulate the menstrual cycle, menopause is not a central event but rather an outcome of primary ovarian failure.

At the level of ovary, there is a gradual depletion of ovarian follicles due to apoptysis or programmed cell death. The ovary, therefore, is no longer responsive to the pituitary hormones LH, FSH. As a result, estrogen and progesterone production ceases. The pituitary FSH and later LH rises due to intact functioning HPO axis and negative feedback from ovary which is a cardinal sign of menopause.

Androgen production from ovary continues beyond the menopausal transition because of sparing of the stromal compartment but androgen concentration is lower in menopausal age than in women of reproductive age. Menopausal women continue to have low level of circulating estrogen (20–30 pg/mL) principally derived from peripheral aromatization of ovarian and adrenal androgens.

Causes for Menopause

Menopause occurs due to a complex series of hormonal changes. The important change associated with menopause is a decline in the number of functioning eggs within the ovaries. At the time of birth, most females have about 1 to 3 million eggs, which are gradually lost throughout a woman's life. By the time of first menstrual period, she has an average of about 400,000 eggs. By the time of menopause, a woman may have fewer than 10,000 eggs. About 400 eggs are lost through normal ovulation every month. Most eggs die off through a process called atresia.

- Normally, FSH is responsible for the growth of ovarian follicles during the first half of menstrual cycle. As menopause approaches, the remaining eggs become more resistant to FSH, and the ovaries dramatically reduce their production of estrogen.
- Estrogen affects many parts of the body, including the blood vessels, heart, bone, breasts, uterus, urinary system, skin, and brain. Loss of estrogen is believed

to be the cause of many of the symptoms associated with menopause. At the time of menopause, the ovaries also decrease their production of testosterone—a hormone involved in the libido, or sexual drive.

Menopause Symptoms

I. Immediate Effects of Estrogen Deficiency

Vasomotor symptoms	Psychological problems	Urogenital symptoms
Hot flushes	Loss of libido	Vaginal dryness
Night sweats	Loss of confidence	Dyspareunia
Palpitation	Ansomnia	Frequency
Headache	Depressed mood	Urgency
	Irritability	Dysuria
	Forgetfulness	

Hot Flushes

Hot flushes are the most common symptom of menopause. It may occur in as many as 75% of perimenopausal women. Hot flush symptoms vary among women. Commonly, the hot flush is a feeling of warmth that spreads over the body, lasting from around 30 seconds to a few minutes. Flushed (reddened) skin, palpitations and sweating often accompany hot flashes. Hot flushes often increase skin temperature and pulse, and they can cause insomnia, or sleeplessness. Hot flushes usually last 2 to 3 years, but many women can experience them for up to 5 years. The physiologic mechanism underlying the cause of hot flushes are ill-understood. This may be due to:

a. Central event—probably initiated in hypothalamus, produces an increased core body temperature, metabolic rate and skin temperature; this results in peripheral vasodilatation and sweating in some women. This central event may be triggered by noradrenergic, serotonergic and dopaminergic activation.

b. LH surge which often accompany hot flushes is not directly responsible for this as it often is present even in pituitary destruction.

c. Acute estrogen deficiency can alter the vascular permeability and the thermoregulatory center.

Various factors seem to be related to hot flush frequency. Warm temperatures increase a women's core body temperature and makes her more likely to reach the sweating threshold. Cooler air temperatures are associated with a lower incidence of hot flushes.

In perimenopausal women, a high BMI (>30 kg/m^2) is associated with an increased risk of hot flushes as compared to women with low BMI (<24.9 kg/m^2). But in postmenopausal women, this association is not found.

Strenuous exercise may trigger hot flushes, however daily exercise is associated with an overall decreased incidence. Women who have less physical activity have an increased risk of hot flushes.

Cigarette smoking (past and current) is associated with an increased risk of hot flushes. There is no significant association between alcohol intake and rate of hot flushes. There is no evidence supporting relationship of hot flushes with emotional stress and consumption of caffeine, hot or spicy food.

Treatment

Before starting treatment, a detailed history of woman regarding frequency and severity of hot flushes and their effect on the woman's daily activities should be enquired into.

- No treatment is required unless hot flushes are bothersome to the patient and disrupt her day-to-day activities.
- Therapy should be tailored to each woman's needs. The decision to start treatment should be based on the severity of symptoms, individual woman's attitude towards menopause and medication and assessment of risks related to treatment.
- There is a tendency of natural regression of symptoms over time in most women. In majority of women, treatment for hot flushes can be discontinued within a year.
- Since obesity and sedentary lifestyle are related to hot flushes, patient should be advised to maintain a healthy weight and to do regular exercise.
  1. For mild vasomotor symptoms, the first strategy should be lifestyle changes like regular exercise, keeping the core body temperature cool with paced respiration.
  2. When the desired relief from hot flushes is not achieved, addition of non-prescription remedies may be considered, as these are comparatively free of side effects. Vitamin E, 800 iu/day is nontoxic at this doses, inexpensive and can be tried for relief of hot flushes.
  3. Soy may have some estrogen agonist activity. A healthy diet incorporating soy protein seems reasonable.

When to start hormone therapy?

Systemic estrogen therapy has been approved by FDA for treatment of vasomotor symptoms. For patients with persistent and severe hot flushes, HT is the most effective intervention. **HT should be used for the**

shortest duration of time necessary to control symptoms at the lowest dose.

The short-term use (5 years or less) of estrogen and progestin does not seem to be associated with significant risk.

Estradiol is the first-line estrogen (orally or transdermally). In a cyclic regimen-progestational agent should be added for 10–14 days in women with intact uterus.

Treatment should be periodically evaluated to determine, if it is still necessary, as in almost all women, menopause-related vasomotor symptoms will abate over time without any intervention.

Urogenital Atrophy

Atrophic changes in the urogenital region is a frequent occurrence of postmenopausal women essentially due to estrogen deficiency. The vulva loses most of its collagen and adipose tissue thus becoming flat and thin. Lubrication through transudation from blood vessels and glandular secretions diminish. The vaginal surface becomes thinner, less elastic and more friable. These changes result in symptoms of vaginal dryness, itching, discomfort and painful intercourse.

In Indian women, urogenital symptoms have an incidence of more than 40% after menopause. A thorough history of symptom frequency and precipitating factors is important.

Women with urinary symptoms, such as frequency, urgency and nocturia, should be investigated by doing a urine culture and blood glucose estimation. If these investigations are normal for menopausal women vaginal estrogen therapy should be offered along with lifestyle modification, bladder drill and anti-muscarinic therapy are recommended for the treatment of urge urinary incontinence.

Treatment

Estrogen therapy (ET), if not contraindicated, is the treatment of choice for postmenopausal women with features of urogenital atrophy.

Local vaginal estrogen therapy is preferable and is probably also more efficacious for vaginal problems.

Women experiencing vaginal atrophy can be offered any of the following effective vaginal estrogen replacement therapies: conjugated equine estrogen (CEE) cream, estriol or estradiol cream, a low-dose estradiol tablet or a sustained-release intravaginal estradiol ring.

Vaginal estrogen creams are usually prescribed daily at bedtime for a week followed by twice weekly for a maximum of three months.

25 µg 17 β-estradiol vaginal tablet has been approved by the FDA for atrophic vaginitis at a dosage of one tablet every day for 2 weeks. This is followed by one tablet twice every week. These tablets are equal in efficacy and sometimes preferred over creams by women as they are less messy. However, the creams provide lubrication, which may provide additional benefit for women with dyspareunia.

Vaginal rings are a new FDA approved estrogen-delivery system, not available in India at present. These flexible 2 mg silicone rings deliver estradiol at a continuous rate of 6.5–15 µg/24 hours at a sustained rate for up to 12 weeks.

Estradiol vaginal rings should be pressed into an oval and then inserted into the upper third of the vaginal vault. The woman with clean, dry hands or health care provider with gloved hands can insert the ring with the woman standing with one leg up, squatting, or lying down in knees-up position. It is removed by hooking a finger into it and pulling it out. It is replaced every 3 months.

Although systemic absorption of estrogen can occur with local preparations, there is insufficient data to recommend annual endometrial surveillance or progesterone addition in asymptomatic women using local estrogens.

Adverse Effects

Overall, intravaginal products are tolerated well, with few reports of spotting or discharge, headache, and genital pruritus. If the discharge is foul smelling or is associated with vaginal itching or other signs of vaginal infection, further evaluation is warranted.

Alternative Treatment

Tibolone 2.5 mg/day for 6 months in postmenopausal women with vaginal atrophy has significantly shown to improve vaginal dryness, dyspareunia, and signs of atrophic vaginitis without causing endometrial proliferation.

Non-hormonal Treatment

Lubricants: Regular sexual activity generally maintains vaginal health. Lubricants are generally considered a temporary measure to relieve vaginal dryness during intercourse.

Moisturizers: Vaginal moisturizers (containing polycarbophil gel) applied on a regular basis have an efficacy equivalent to local hormone replacement for the treatment of local urogenital symptoms such as vaginal itching, irritation, and dyspareunia, and should be offered to women wishing to avoid use of hormone therapy. The polymer attaches to mucin and epithelial cells on the vaginal wall through anionic binding. Polycarbophil carries up to 60 times its weight in water and holds water in place against the vaginal epithelial surface until it is sloughed off, typically after 24 hours or more. Due to this prolonged contact with the vaginal surface, moisturizers require only two to three applications a week and reapplication before sexual intercourse is not essential.

Recommendations

Urogenital Problems

1. Conjugated estrogen cream, an intravaginal sustained release estradiol ring, or estradiol vaginal tablets are recommended as effective treatment for vaginal atrophy. (IA)

2. Routine progestine cotherapy is not required for endometrial protection in women receiving vaginal estrogen therapy in appropriate dose. (IIIC)

3. Vaginal lubricants may be recommended for subjective symptom improvement of dyspareunia. (IIIC)

4. Health care providers can offer polycarbophil gel (a vaginal moisturizer) as an effective treatment for symptoms of vaginal atrophy including dryness and dyspareunia. (IA)

5. As part of the management of stress incontinence, women should be encouraged to try nonsurgical options such as weight loss in obese women, pelvic floor physiotherapy with or without biofeedback weighted vaginal cones, functional electric stimulation and/or intravaginal pessaries. (II-IB)

6. Lifestyle modifications, bladder drill (II-IB), antimuscarinic therapy (IA) are recommended for urge urinary incontinence.

7. Estrogen therapy should not be recommended for the treatment of postmenopausal urge or stress urinary incontinence but may be recommended before corrective surgery. (IA)

8. Vaginal estrogen therapy can be recommended for the prevention of recurrent urinary tract infections in postmenopausal women. (IA)

9. Following treatment of adenocarcinoma of the endometrium (Stage 1), estrogen therapy may be offered to women distressed by moderate to severe menopausal symptoms. (IB)

10. Routine evaluation of sex hormone levels in postmenopausal problems with loss of libido is not recommended. (IIIA)

II. Long-term Effect of Estrogen Deficiency

Cardiovascular disease is the collecting term for angina, myocardial infarction, stroke and peripheral vascular disease. Despite an overall reduction in mortality from CVD, this is still the leading avoidable cause of deaths in the globe. CVD is also age dependent and is underdiagnosed in females. The prevalence of CVD increases after menopause. Women with premature menopause and surgical oophorectomy are more at risk of CHD.

Table 16.1: Death rate in critical disease in menopause	
Cause of CVD in women	*Death rate per 100,000*
Ischemic heart disease	23
Respiratory disease	21
Cerebrovascular disease	21
Cancer of rectum and colon	13

CVD and HRT

Contrary to the initial advice when WHI (Women's Health Initiative) was published in 2002 which raised questions about safety of HT, recent studies clearly show that HT is clearly safe in younger women (age between 50 and 59 years). There may be some beneficial effect, if HT is used within 10 years of menopause perhaps due to relatively healthier state of the underlying vasculature and lower baseline CVD risk. Most of the studies have shown HT as cardiac neutral and, therefore, is not used to promote HT as cardioprotective in younger women. Therefore, prior to use of HT, every women should have a health assessment to identify CVD risk factors like hypertension, diabetes mellitus, smoking, dyslipidemia, obesity and metabolic syndrome. Where risk factors are identified lifestyle changes and pharmacological intervention should be introduced early in premenopause. If dyslipidemia is identified, starting HT has a protective effect on lipid profile where HDL cholesterol increases and LDL cholesterol decreases. Estrogen in comparison to estrogen-progesterone combination has most favorable effect and oral administration is more favorable than transdermal on lipid metabolism except in hypertriglyceridemia (WHI, 2002).

There is evidence that types of HRT have an effect on CVD risk. Currently there is no evidence that estrogen only preparation carry a risk on CVD; but E+P combination will definitely carry an absolute risk on CVD specially, if started late age (>60 yrs) or used for a prolonged time. A history of myocardial infarction, stroke, pulmonary embolism is contraindication to start HT (IMS, 2008).

Key Points

1. All perimenopausal women should have an individual CVD risk assessment. Where risk factors are identified women should receive lifestyle advice like stop smoking, weight reduction, healthy diet, increased regular exercise.
2. HT can be given to women around the age of natural menopause without increasing the risk of coronary heart disease.
3. HT is not contraindicated in presence of hypertension and in some cases treatment may even reduce the blood pressure.
4. In women with POF, HT is strongly recommended till the age of natural menopause.
5. Health care providers should not initiate or continue HT for the sole purpose of preventing CVD (CAD or stroke). IA
6. Health care providers should not prescribe HT in those at high risk for venous thromboembolism. (IA)
7. Health care providers should initiate other evidence-based therapy or interventions to effectively reduce risk of CVD events in women of high risk for vascular disease. (IA)
8. Risk factors for stroke (obesity, hypertension, smoking) should be addressed to all post-menopausal women. (IA)
9. In prescribing HT to elderly postmenopausal women, low or ultralow dose estrogen is preferred. (IB)
10. HT may be prescribed to diabetic women for relief of menopausal symptoms. (IA)

Bone Loss (Osteoporosis)

Rapid bone loss is common during the perimenopausal years. Most women reach their peak bone density at 25 to 30 years. After that, bone loss averages 0.13% per year. During perimenopause, bone loss accelerates to about 3% loss per year. Later, it drops off to about 2% loss per year. However, bone loss can cause osteoporosis, a condition that increases the risk of bone fractures.

Osteoporosis is the thinning of bone tissue and loss of bone density over time. In osteoporosis, the bone mineral density (BMD) is reduced, bone micro-architecture is deteriorating, and the amount and variety of proteins in bone is altered. Osteoporosis occurs when there is an imbalance between new bone formation and old bone resorption. Two essential minerals for normal bone formation are calcium and phosphate. Bone is a living dynamic tissue where remodeling is constantly taking place. In children, osteoblasts work faster and increase density and strength of bone mass which reaches its peak in late 20s. The balance between breakdown and formation remains stable till the age of 35 years. After menopause sets in, oestrogen levels fall, and bone turnover increases and reformation does not keep up with its breakdown and this leads to osteoporosis. Decreased dietary intake of calcium, lack of weight-bearing exercise also contribute to the setting-in of osteoporosis (Table 16.2).

Symptoms of Osteoporosis

Osteoporosis is a silent disease. It may not cause any symptoms till there are minute fractures called fragility fractures, which commonly occur in vertebra, rib, wrist, and hip. Multiple vertebral fractures lead to a stooped posture, loss of height, and chronic pain with resultant reduction in mobility in the elderly.

How can one Prevent Osteoporosis?

Doing weight-bearing exercises for about half an hour per day after the age of 35 is a good way of keeping osteoporosis away. Taking calcium-rich food like milk

Table 16.2: Risk factors for osteoporosis	
Major risk factors	*Minor risk factors*
Age >65 years	Rheumatoid arthritis
Vertebral compression fractures	H/O clinical hyperthyroidism
Family history of osteoporotic fracture	Long-term anticonvulsant therapy
Systemic glucocorticoid therapy for >3 months	Low dietary calcium therapy
Malabsorption syndrome	Smoking
Primary hyperparathyroidism	Excessive alcohol intake
Hypogonadism	Excessive caffeine intake
Early menopause	Weight <57 kg
	Weight loss of 10% of weight at age of 25 years
	Long-term heparin therapy
	Low BMI <19 g/m^2

or milk products, green leafy vegetables, and legumes, can also prevent osteoporosis. Calcium excretion is enhanced with intake of tea or coffee and one should cut down on their consumption.

Testing for Osteoporosis

Periodic testing of the bone mineral density is done by special tests like DEXA (dual energy X-ray absorptiometry) scan usually of the hip and spine. A fracture risk assessment tool has been developed by WHO and is increasingly used to identify the women who are at risk of osteoporosis.

Treatment of Osteoporosis

The main aim of treatment is to prevent fragility fractures. The specific treatments include as per NICE, 2008 are:

1. Biphosphonates
2. Selective estrogen receptor modulators (SERMs)
3. Calcium and vitamin D
4. Parathyroid hormone
5. Strontium ranelate
6. Calcitriol
7. Calcitonin

For all women at risk of osteoporosis, they must consume adequate (700 mg/day) calcium and vitamin D along with sufficient exposure to sunlight.

HT and Osteoporosis

Women who are already on HT for menopausal symptoms will continue to get benefit from prevention of osteoporosis while on treatment. **Although HT is a not a 1st line drug of choice in osteoporosis prevention,** it is specifically indicated in:

1. Women with premature menopause
2. Postmenopausal women with increased risk of fracture
3. Early physiological and surgical menopause

Recommendations

1. The goals of osteoporosis management include assessment of fracture risk and prevention of fracture and height loss. (1B)
2. A stable or increasing BMD reflects a response to therapy in the absence of trauma, fracture or height loss. Progressive decreases in BMD indicate a lack of response to current therapy. (1A)
3. Physicians should identify the absolute fracture risk in postmenopausal women by integrating the key risk factors for fracture; namely, age, BMD, prior fracture, and glucocorticoid use. (1B)

Calcium and Vitamin D

Adequate calcium and vitamin D supplementation is key to ensuring prevention of progressive bone loss. For postmenopausal women a total intake of 1500 mg of elemental calcium and supplementation with 800 IU/ day of vitamin D are recommended. (1B)

Hormone Therapy

1. Usual-dosage HT should be prescribed for symptomatic postmenopausal women for relief of menopausal symptom (1A) and a reasonable choice for the prevention of bone loss and fracture. (1A)
2. Physicians may recommend low- and ultralow-dose estrogen therapy to symptomatic women for relief of menopausal symptoms (1A) but should inform their patients that despite the fact that such therapy has demonstrated a beneficial effect in osteoporosis prevention (1A), no data are yet available on reduction of fracture risk.

Bisphosphonates

1. Treatment with alendronate, risedronate, or zoledronic acid should be considered to decrease the risk of vertebral, nonvertebral, and hip fractures. (1A)
2. Etidronate is a weak antiresorptive agent and may be effective in decreasing the risk of vertebral fracture in those at high risk. (1B)

Selective Estrogen Receptor Modulators

Treatment with raloxifene should be considered to decrease the risk of vertebral fractures. (1A)

Calcitonin

Treatment with calcitonin is considered to decrease the risk of vertebral fractures and to reduce pain associated with acute vertebral fractures. (1B)

Parathyroid Hormone

Treatment with teriparatide should be considered to decrease the risk of vertebral and nonvertebral fractures in postmenopausal women with severe osteoporosis. (1A)

Menopausal Hormone Therapy (MHT)

Menopause Population in India

India has 71 million people over 60 years of age and the number of menopausal women is about 43 million. Projected population in India by 2026 will be 1.4 billion, people over 60 years will be 173 million, and the menopausal population will be 103 million. Average age of menopause is 47.5 years in Indian women with an average life expectancy of 71 years. Menopausal symptoms are different in rural and urban areas. Urogenital symptoms, fatigue and weakness, body aches, and pains are the predominant symptoms in both rural and urban menopausal women. Hot flushes, psychological symptoms, mood swings, and sexual dysfunctions are seen more in urban women. Not all women require routine hormone therapy as well as HT does not suit everyone. Each woman needs to be aware of the benefits and potential risks of HT so that she can make an informed decision. **HT should be given at the lowest effective dose for the shortest length of time necessary to achieve the desired clinical effect.** HT is the best available treatment for relieving hot flushes and night sweats. HT reduces the risk of osteoporotic fracture. HT can effectively relieve vaginal and urinary symptoms of the menopause.

I. Risks and Benefits of Hormone Use after Menopause

The most comprehensive evidence about the risks and benefits of taking hormones after menopause to prevent disease comes from the Women's Health Initiative (WHI). The WHI Hormone Program involved two studies—the use of estrogen plus progestin for women with a uterus (the Estrogen-plus-Progestin Study), and the use of estrogen alone for women without a uterus (the Estrogen-Alone Study). The WHI Estrogen-plus-Progestin Study was stopped in July 2002, when investigators reported that the overall risks of estrogen-plus-progestin outweighed the benefits. The researchers found that use of this estrogen-plus-progestin pill increased the risk of breast cancer, heart disease, stroke, blood clots, and urinary incontinence. However, the risk of colorectal cancer and hip fractures was lower among women using estrogen-plus-progestin than among those taking the placebo. In addition, the WHI Memory Study showed that estrogen-plus-progestin doubled the risk for developing dementia in postmenopausal women age 65 and older. The risk increased for all types of dementia, including Alzheimer's disease.

The WHI Estrogen-Alone Study, which used estrogen alone was stopped in February 2004, when the researchers concluded that estrogen alone increased the risk of stroke and blood clots. In contrast with the WHI Estrogen-plus-Progestin Study, the risk of breast cancer was decreased in women using estrogen alone compared with those taking the placebo. Use of estrogen alone did not increase or decrease the risk of colorectal cancer. Similar to the results seen in the Estrogen-plus-Progestin Study, women using estrogen alone had an increased risk of urinary incontinence and a decreased risk of hip fractures.

II. Effect of Menopausal Hormone Use on Breast Cancer Risk and Survival

The WHI Estrogen-plus-Progestin Study concluded that estrogen-plus-progestin increases the risk of invasive breast cancer. After 5 years of follow-up, women taking these hormones had a 24% increase in breast cancer risk compared with women taking the placebo. The increase amounted to an additional 8 cases of breast cancer for every 10,000 women taking estrogen-plus-progestin for 1 year compared with 10,000 women taking the placebo.

The WHI Estrogen-Alone Study concluded that taking estrogen did not increase the risk of breast cancer in women with a prior hysterectomy, at least for the 7 years of follow-up in the study. Further analysis of data from the study indicated a 20% decrease in risk of breast cancer in women taking estrogen alone, although this decrease was seen mainly in the occurrence of early-stage breast cancer and ductal breast cancer, but this lower incidence was not statistically significant. The Estrogen-Alone Study also showed a substantial increase in the frequency of abnormal mammograms.

III. Effects of Hormone Use on the Risk of Endometrial Cancer

Studies have shown that long-term exposure of the uterus to estrogen alone increases a woman's risk of endometrial cancer. The risk associated with estrogen-plus-progestin appears to be much less. The long-term effects of estrogen-plus-progestin on endometrial cancer risk remain uncertain.

The Million Women Study confirmed a lower risk of endometrial cancer in women taking estrogen-plus-progestin in comparison with those taking estrogen only or tibolone.

IV. Effect of Menopausal Hormone Use on the Risk of Ovarian Cancer

Several observational studies have found that the use of estrogen alone is associated with a slightly increased risk of ovarian cancer for women who used this hormone for 10 or more years. The results from the Million Women Study showed that women currently using menopausal hormones had an increased risk of developing ovarian cancer and a 20% likelihood of dying from the disease compared with nonusers. However, the increased risk disappeared after hormone use stopped.

Data from the WHI Estrogen-plus-Progestin Study indicate that there may be an increased risk of ovarian cancer with use of estrogen-plus-progestin. After 5.6 years of follow-up, a 58% increased risk of ovarian cancer was reported in women using estrogen-plus-progestin compared with nonusers, but the increased risk was not statistically significant. More research is needed to clarify the relationship between menopausal hormone use, particularly for estrogen-plus-progestin, and the risk of ovarian cancer.

V. Effect of Menopausal Hormone Use on the Risk of Colorectal Cancer

After 5 years of follow-up of women taking estrogen plus progestin, the WHI Estrogen-plus-Progestin Study reported a 37% reduction in colorectal cancer cases compared with women taking the placebo. The WHI Estrogen-Alone Study concluded that estrogen alone had no significant effect on colorectal cancer risk.

VI. Does the Way in which Hormones are Administered Make a Difference?

Most of the data on the long-term health effects of hormones come from studies in which hormones (estrogen-alone or estrogen-plus-progestin) are administered orally in the form of pills. Hormones in the form of transdermal patches or gels are also used to treat menopause-related symptoms. Estrogen-containing vaginal creams and rings can be used specifically for vaginal dryness. Progesterone is also available as a pill or gel. The amount of estrogen that enters the bloodstream from estrogen-containing vaginal creams and rings depends on the types of hormones and the dose. Generally, vaginal administration of hormones results in lower levels of circulating hormones compared with an equivalent oral dose. Because the vaginal epithelium responds to very small doses of estrogen, low-dose estrogen-containing creams or gels can be used.

VII. Principles of Taking Menopausal Hormones

Although menopausal hormones have short-term benefits such as relief from hot flushes and vaginal dryness, several health concerns are associated with their use. Women should discuss with their health care provider whether to take menopausal hormones and what alternatives may be appropriate for them. **The US Food and Drug Administration (FDA) currently advises women to use menopausal hormones for the shortest time and at the lowest dose possible to control symptoms.**

VIII. What are the alternatives for women who choose not to take menopausal hormones?

To decrease the risk of chronic disease, women can adopt a healthy lifestyle by exercising regularly, eating a healthy diet, limiting the consumption of alcohol, and not starting to smoke or, for smokers, trying to quit. Eating foods rich in calcium and vitamin D or taking dietary supplements containing these nutrients can help prevent osteoporosis. Results from the WHI showed that taking calcium and vitamin D supplements provided some benefit in preserving bone mass and preventing hip fractures, particularly in women age 60 and older. Although generally well tolerated, these supplements are associated with an increased risk of kidney stones. Other drugs, such as alendronate, raloxifene and risedronate, have been shown to prevent bone loss. In addition, parathyroid hormone is approved by the FDA for treatment of osteoporosis .

Estrogens in HT

I. Oral

- *Conjugated equine estrogen (CEE):* 0.625 mg (estrone sulfate + equilin sulfate +17 dihydroequilin)
- Estradiol valerate (1, 2, 4 mg).

II. Transdermal (estradiol)

- *Patches:* 25 µg, 50 µg/24 hour twice weekly.
- *Gel :* 75 µg/24 hours daily.

III. Subcutaneous implant (estradiol)

- 25/50/100 mg 6 monthly.

IV. Vaginal: Cream.

Progestins in HT

I. Oral route

- Norgestrel: 150 mg/day.
- Micronized progesterone: 200 mg/day.
- Dydrogesterone: 20 mg/day.
- Medroxyprogesterone acetate: 10 mg/day.
- Norethisterone acetate: 0.7–2.5 mg/ day.

II. Hormone-releasing intrauterine system.

- Levonorgestrel: 20 µg / day.
- Progestasert: 65 µg/day.

III. Vaginal—natural progesterone gel/pessary.

IV. Transdermal—sequential/continuous patch.

Low Dose HT

- Low-dose estrogen is defined as less than 0.625 mg (0.3 mg), conventional-dose or standard estrogen is defined as 0.625 mg, and high-dose estrogen is defined as more than 0.625 mg.

- Transdermal estrogens may have a less adverse effect in terms of cardiovascular risk, both arterial and venous.

HOPE Study (Women's Health, Osteoporosis, Progestin, Estrogen Study)

- Overall, lower doses of HRT provided benefits comparable to commonly prescribed regimens with significantly fewer side effects, such as leg cramps, breast pain and bleeding.
- Patients in the lower dose HRT groups experience more cycles without bleeding than those in the group using the most commonly prescribed doses.
- This study evaluated conjugated equine estrogen CEE (0.3 or 0.45 mg/day) combined with medroxy-progesterone acetate MPA (1.5 or 2.5 mg/day).
- Low-dose HRT—0.45 mg of conjugated estrogens and 1.5 mg of MPA significantly decreased the number and severity of hot flushes in postmenopausal women, compared to placebo. Improvement was seen within the first week of therapy.
- Lower doses of HRT provided significant improvement in lipid or cholesterol levels—HDL-cholesterol ("good" cholesterol) increased by approximately 10%; LDL-cholesterol ("bad" cholesterol) decreased by approximately 7% by the end of one year.

Standard Dose of HRT

- CCE: 0.625 mg
- Micronized E: 1–2 mg
- Estradiol valerate: 1–2 mg

Reduced dose of HRT

- CEE: 0.3 to/0.45 mg
- 0.45 CEE + 1.5 mg MPA
- 0.3 CEE + 1.5 mg MPA

Tibolone

Tibolone is a steroid with oestrogenic, progestogenic and androgenic properties. It is single dose, oral postmenopausal therapy, with a moderately effective action on menopausal and urogenital symptoms, libido and bone. Its potential lack of breast stimulation makes it a good option for the treatment of menopausal symptoms.

Tibolone is structurally related to 19-nortestosterone progestins. Its activity depends on its metabolism. Tibolone is metabolized to three biologically active metabolites, the 3α-hydroxy metabolite and 3β-hydroxy metabolite with estrogen agonist property and Δ4-ketoisomer with progestogenic and androgenic activity. The Δ-4 isomer is primarily concentrated within the endometrium, binds to progesterone receptor and protects the endometrium from the other two estrogenic metabolites. The Δ-4 isomer of tibolone has also direct androgenic effect with decrease in sex-hormone binding globulin and rise in circulatory free testosterone which has good influence on sexual activity.

Specific binding affinity of tibolone and its primary metabolites

Tibolone and its metabolites	Estrogen receptor	Progesterone receptor	Androgen receptor
3-α-OH tibolone	+	+	+
3-β-OH tibolone	+	−	−
Δ-4 tibolone	−	+	+

Effect of Tibolone on Breast

Breast tissue contains all the enzymes necessary for formation of estrogens (sulfatase, aromatase, and 17β-OH steroid dehydrogenase) and conversion of estrogens into their sulfates (sulfotransferase). Tibolone and its metabolites inhibit estrone sulfatase and 17β-OH steroid dehydrogenase in breast normal and abnormal cells and thereby inhibit conversion of estrone sulfate to estradiol. On the contrary, its 3-hydroxy metabolites increase conversion of estrone back to estrone sulfate by increasing the activity of sulfotransferase. Therefore, tibolone-induced enzyme changes lower the active estrogen concentration in breast tissue.

Tibolone effect on breast enzymes

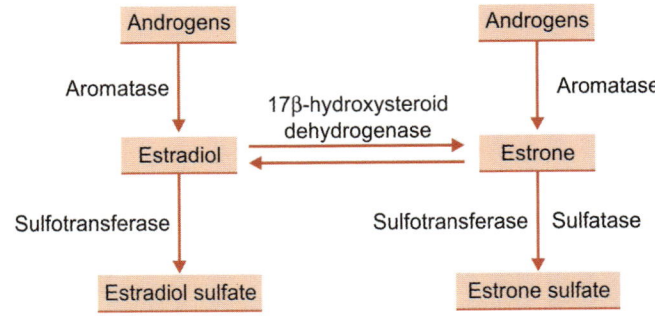

Low Dose Tibolone

- 1.25 mg instead of 2.5 mg/day does not have major loss of efficacy.
- Tibolone has different effects on different tissues.

- Treats hot flushes, vaginal dryness as CEE and improves libido. Endometrial safety and prevention of bone loss are equal to CEE/MPA.
- Less breakthrough bleeds.

LIFT (Long-term Intervention on Fractures with Tibolone) Study

- Multicentric RCT with 1.25 mg tibolone is used for 3 years.
- Reduced vertebral fractures by 45% and non-vertebral fractures by 25%.
- Risk of stroke is 2-fold more in patients >70 yrs.
- Avoid tibolone in elderly women at risk of stroke.

Tibolone comes closest to being the ideal product for long-term HRT because of the specific actions (Fig. 16.1).

- *Brain:* Enhances mood, libido.
- *Heart:* Beneficial effects on CVS.
- *Breast:* Lower incidence of breast tenderness and no effect on mammography.
- *Endometrium:* No proliferation.
- *Urogenital symptoms:* Improve.
- *Bone:* Prevents bone loss.
- It induces amenorrhea.

Thus it is a menstruation free HRT, which is most welcome to most women, with an intact uterus.

Specific Indications of Tibolone

- Breast cancer risk
- Breast cancer treated
- Family history
- Low parity/nulliparity
- Racial factor
- Endometrial cancer risk
- Past history of endometriosis/fibroid
- Patients with NIDDM
- Patients with hypertriglyceridemia and history of thromboembolic phenomena.

Low Dose Transdermal Patch

Transdermal patches are considered low dose, if they contain 50 μg or less estrogen; patches containing more than 50 μg estrogen are considered high-dose patches.

Indicated for those:

a. Women at high risk for VTE.
b. Women with spontaneous or estrogen-induced hypertriglyceridemia.
c. Obese women with metabolic syndrome.
d. In smokers, hypertension with impaired sexuality

These types of formulation comprise of transdermal estradiol 50 μg/24 hrs (2 × wkly) + Trandsermal norethisterone 170 μg/24 hrs for 14 days/28 though they are not available in India.

Low-dose, transdermal hormone therapy (HT) does not appear to increase the risk for stroke compared with no HRT use.

Patchless Transdermal E2

- More recently, 'patchless' formulations of transdermal estrogen have been developed that share the advantages of transdermal therapy.

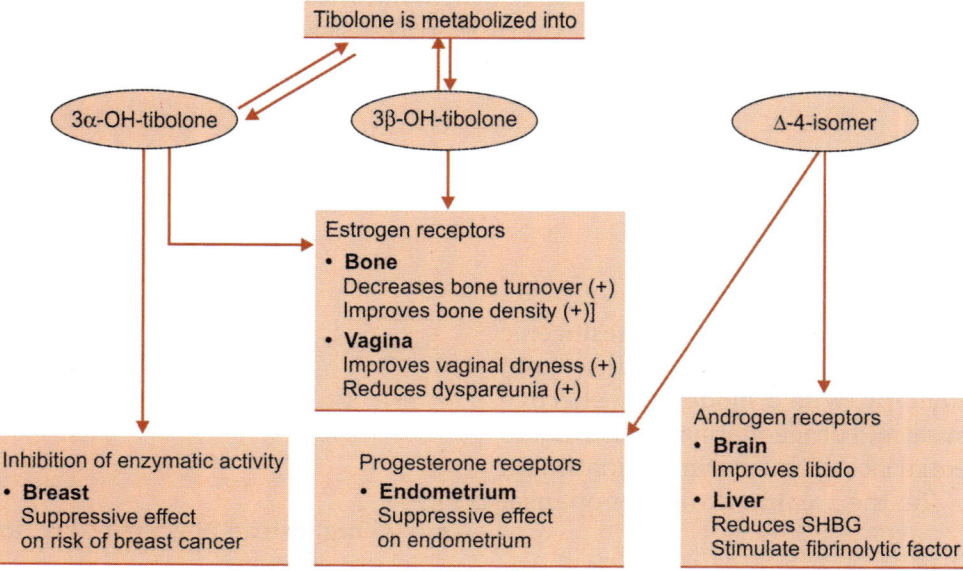

Fig. 16.1: Tissue specific effects of tibolone metabolites

- Avoid application-site reactions and obviate cosmetic concerns about patch visibility.
- FDA has approved three new low-dose patchless transdermal estrogen preparations for the US market. This is not available in India.

Patchless E2

- Estradiol gel received FDA approval in December 2006. It contains 0.06% estradiol in a hydroalcoholic gel base that is supplied in a non-aerosol, metered-dose pump, and is applied once-daily. Each depression of the pump delivers a unit dose of 0.87 g gel, which contains 0.52 mg of estradiol.
- Two daily doses (0.87 and 1.7 g, containing 0.52 and 1.04 mg estradiol, respectively) have been approved for the treatment of moderate to severe vasomotor symptoms associated with menopause.
- Estradiol transdermal spray approved by FDA in 2007 is a homogeneous liquid solution of 1.7% estradiol in alcohol.
- Each spray delivers 90 µL solution containing 1.53 mg estradiol to an area on the inner surface of the arm between the elbow and wrist.
- One, two, or three sprays are applied daily to non-overlapping areas of the inner arm for the treatment of moderate to severe vasomotor symptoms associated with menopause.
- The most frequently reported adverse events during short-term treatment with estradiol gel or spray are breast tenderness and metrorrhagia.
- There are no reports of adverse changes in hematology, blood chemistry, urinalysis, lipid, coagulation, and carbohydrate values following 12 weeks of treatment with any of the low dose transdermal estradiol preparations.
- These 'patchless' estradiol preparations combine the advantages of low doses and transdermal delivery with the practical conveniences of once-daily application and minimal application site reactivity.

LNG-IUS

In women on ERT, this can be used in combination with oral or transdermal estrogen preparations without progestogens.

Use of SERMs in Menopause

Apart from the uterus and breasts—the main reproductive organs, estrogen also acts on other tissues of the liver, brain, heart and bones. It acts on target tissues by binding to the estrogen receptors which are located in the cell nucleus.

Hormone therapy (HT) offered to postmenopausal women for relief from menopausal symptoms and protection from long-term consequences bring with it some undesirable complications in the form of Ca breast and Ca endometrium. The need for an ideal drug which proves beneficial in some organs and avoids the undesirable effects on other organs has resulted in the development of selective estrogen receptor modulators (SERMs) that can confer all the benefits of estrogen without any of its risks. These compounds exhibit selective agonistic or stimulatory effects (i.e. estrogenic) on one organ system and neutral or antagonistic (i.e. antiestrogenic) effects on other organ systems.

Types of SERMs

Synthetic and natural SERMs are available.
1. *Synthetic SERMs:* Belong to 5 chemical groups: Triphenylethylenes, benzothiophenes, tetrahydron-aphtylenes, indoles and benzopyrans.
2. *Natural SERMs:* These are phytoestrogens, plant-derived substances that are structurally and functionally similar to estrogens and are found in many foods. They exhibit estrogenic activity in the body by acting on estrogen receptors. They too have both weak estrogenic and antiestrogenic activity.

SERMs widely used are:
1. Clomiphene—which is used for ovulation.
2. Tamoxifen—used for the treatment of ER-positive. Breast cancer and chemoprotection for women at risk of breast cancer.
3. Toremifene—a tamoxifen derivative, indicated for the treatment of ER-positive breast cancer.
4. Raloxifene—used for the prevention and treatment of osteoporosis.

SERMs in Menopause Management

As the risk of osteoporosis increases once women reach menopause, prevention as well as treatment is necessary for them. Raloxifene is a drug for prevention and treatment of postmenopausal osteoporosis.

Those women found to be at risk should be evaluated by performing bone densitometry by dual-energy X-ray absorptiometry (DEXA). Prophylaxis needs to be planned for women with BMD T-scores below –2.0 SD in the absence of risk factors and in women with T-scores below –1.5 SD, if other risk factors are present.

Treatment with Raloxifene

Raloxifene has been approved for the prevention of postmenopausal osteoporosis in 1997 and the treatment of postmenopausal osteoporosis in 1999.

The Multiple Outcomes of Raloxifene Evaluation (MORE) trial found that treatment with raloxifene 60 and 120 mg/day for 3 years significantly reduced vertebral fracture risk by 30% and 50% compared with placebo respectively, in postmenopausal women with osteoporosis. Raloxifene does not stimulate endometrial proliferation which is beneficial for women with a uterus.

a. *Action on breast tissue:* In the MORE Study of 5,129 postmenopausal women with osteoporosis treated with raloxifene, a 76% overall reduction of breast cancer and a 90% reduction in estrogen receptor-positive breast cancer were noted in comparison with placebo.

 A head-to-head comparative **Study of Tamoxifen and Raloxifene (STAR)** showed that the drug raloxifene, currently used to prevent and treat osteoporosis in postmenopausal women, works as well as tamoxifen in reducing breast cancer risk for postmenopausal women at increased risk of the disease.

b. *Action on lipids and cardiovascular system:* In an analysis of MORE data, raloxifene decreased total cholesterol (8.5%) and LDL cholesterol (15%) without significant changes in HDL and triglycerides. Homocysteine and lipoprotein levels were also found to decrease significantly.

 The Raloxifene Use and the Heart (RUTH) study was designed to investigate possible cardioprotective effects of raloxifene in elderly women with CAD or at risk for CAD. Results demonstrated a neutral effect on CAD risk during 5.6 years of follow-up.

c. *Action on brain:* Its beneficial effects on the brain, such as the cognitive benefits associated with estrogen use are yet unknown, although raloxifene does not appear to impair cognition or affect mood in postmenopausal women.

Adverse effects

- Raloxifene may induce hot flushes and leg cramps.
- It is not beneficial for vaginal atrophy.
- Raloxifene increases the risk of deep vein thrombosis (DVT) by 1% similar to that observed with estrogen.

Contraindications

- Premenopausal women.
- Post-menopausal women with vasomotor symptoms.
- Women who have had thrombophlebitis/DVT.
- Hepatic and renal impairment

Dose: A single oral dose of 60 mg/day. It can be taken with or without food. Use should be commenced at least one year after the menopause. Efficacy and safety have been determined for up to 40 months.

Contraindication of Use of HRT

- Active or past breast cancer
- Recurrent or active endometrial cancer
- Abnormal vaginal bleeding
- Recurrent or active blood clots
- History of stroke
- Liver disease
- Known or suspected pregnancy

Side Effects of HT

Most common side effects are:
- Monthly bleeding
- Irregular spotting
- Breast tenderness

Less common side effects of HRT include:
- Blood clots and stroke (rare, but the most serious risk)
- Fluid retention
- Headaches (including migraine)
- Dizziness
- Skin discoloration (brown or black patches)
- Increased breast density

Key Recommendations for Prescription of HT

- Individualization of HT, i.e. the dose, type, route, is adjusted according to the need of the individual woman.
- Use unopposed estrogen only for women who have undergone hysterectomy.
- Progesterone needs to be added, if prescribed for women with an intact uterus.
- The art of prescribing HT is to use the minimum effective dose judiciously on indication, after appropriate counseling.
- A specific indication for starting HT must be present, and it must be documented.
- Symptoms which definitely require HT are vasomotor symptoms and symptoms as a result of urogenital atrophy.
- The main rule for giving HT is to use the "lowest possible dose for shortest possible duration."
- For prevention and treatment of osteoporosis, other modalities (bisphosphonates) should be preferred over estrogens.
- Assessment of risk factors prior to starting HT is an essential prerequisite.

- Lifestyle modification is an integral component of managing postmenopausal women.

Choice of Preparation

- *Hypertension:* Non-oral estrogens are of choice.
- *Thromboembolism:* Transdermal route is preferable.
- *Gallbladder disease:* Non-oral route.
- *Side effects:* Change to non-oral.
- *Poor response:* May be due to inadequate absorption from intestine/transdermal site—implant is beneficial.
- *Lactose intolerance:* Lactose present in oral preparation, so non-oral route is of choice.

Benefits of HRT

- *Vasomotor symptoms:* Hot flushes and night sweats resulting from hyperactivity of midbrain–hypothalamic–pituitary axis and characteristic of climacteric are relieved by HRT.
- *Atrophy of genital tract:* This leads to vaginal dryness and postmenopausal bleeding from atrophic vaginitis/atrophic endometrium respond to estrogen therapy.
- *Dyspareunia* due to vaginal dryness is not a problem in menopause, but it is a problem during climacteric.
- *Loss of libido* also responds to estrogen replacement. Some also get benefit from testosterone.

Urinary Symptoms

- Incontinence—urethral abnormality, detrussor instability, overflow incontinence.
- Frequency, urgency, dysuria.
- Difficulty in voiding.
- Estrogen may produce considerable improvement in these symptoms by increasing.
  - Epithelial thickness, vascularity, closing pressure of urethra.
  - Adrenergic receptor in bladder urethral muscle.
  - Collagen content of connective tissue

Sleep Disturbances

Early morning awakening and inability to get back to sleep is a frequent complaint in postmenopausal women. Estrogen receptors are present in reticular activation system, preoptic area, and hypothalamus. Estrogen replacement improves sleep by acting at these sites.

Mood and Psychological Changes

Estrogen replacement appears to have a direct mental tonic effect on the cognitive functions even in the absence of vasomotor symptoms. It overcomes anxiety, over sensitivity, tearfulness, irritability, aggression. However, if progesterone is also given, it may reduce the beneficial effects of estrogen on libido and mood.

Bone and Skeleton

- Post-menopausal women, due to increased bone resorption, exceeding the rate of new bone formation loose 30% of their total bone mass. It leads to osteoporosis, and fracture may occur with minimal/trivial trauma.
- Estrogens cause stimulation of C cells of thyroid resulting in increased level of calcitonin, which causes inhibition of osteoclastic bone resorption.
- Progesterone has synergistic action, as it binds competitively with glucocorticoid receptors in bone, thus inhibiting the resorbing effect of cortisone.

Cardiovascular System

- In menopause, as there is increased level of plasma total cholesterol and LDL and decreased level of HDL, leading to atherosclerosis, there is increase in cardiovascular diseases.
- Estrogen causes decreases in the incidence and mortality of IHD, due to its beneficial effect on the lipid metabolism.

Skin, Hair, Body Fat

In postmenopausal women, there is decrease in content of collagen in skin. So the skin becomes wrinkled. Estrogen increases the collagen content. It also prevents varicose ulceration.

Neuroprotection

- It reduces the risk of Alzheimer's disease by reducing β amyloid protein and cholinergic dysfunction in brain.
- It enhances the proliferation of neuronal cell population within the hippocampus.
- It regulates the synaptic neurotransmission and increases nerve growth factor. Thus it enhances neuroplasticity, memory, and cognition.
- It delays the onset of Parkinson's disease by its action on dopaminergic system in midbrain.

Other Effects

- Estrogen prevents tooth loss and periodontal disease.
- There is substantial decrease in the risk of fatal colon cancer.
- There is reduction in age-related macular degeneration, cataract and severe nuclear sclerosis.

- Less risk of osteoarthritis.
- Alleviates the worsening symptoms of multiple sclerosis.

Recommended Follow-up when on HT

After commencement or change of HT, women should be reviewed after 3 months to:

1. Assess effect of therapy
2. Enquire about side effects and bleeding pattern
3. Assess any rise in blood pressure and weight gain.
   Thereafter, a review should be arranged at least annually to:

- Check effectiveness of therapy and presence of side effects.
- Review best type of therapy for patient, i.e. consider changing from sequential to continuous combined therapy when known to be postmenopausal.
- Discuss pros and cons of continuing long-term HT particularly in respect of increased risk of breast cancer which should be weighed against benefits.
- Check blood pressure.
- Encourage breast awareness.
- Cervical smear three or five yearly depending on local recommendation.
- Pelvic examination, if required
  Overall despite highly publicized and overestimated risk of HRT, the benefits of HRT outweighed its risks in many women provided it is used appropriately for its licensed indication.

IMPORTANT STUDIES ON HRT

WHI Study, 2005

- This randomized controlled trial examined the risks and benefits of long-term combined HT use in 16,608 asymptomatic postmenopausal women compared to the placebo group. The trial has been halted prematurely, after 5 years of an 8-year study, due to an increased risk of invasive breast cancer.
- This randomized controlled trial examined the risks and benefits of long-term combined HT use in 16,608 asymptomatic postmenopausal women compared to the placebo group.
- The trial has been halted prematurely, after 5 years of an 8-year study, due to an increased risk of invasive breast cancer.
  The another WHI trial on estrogen use alone was published in the July, 2002.
  The key findings after five years 10,000 women treated per year:
- Breast cancer increased from 30 to 38 cases (did not appear in the first four years of use).

- Coronary heart disease increased from 30 to 37 cases (appeared in first year of use)
- Stroke increased from 21 to 29 cases (were greatest during the first 2 years).
- Blood clots: Increased from 16 to 34 cases

The benefits were:
- A reduction in colorectal cancer from 16 to 10 cases after 3 years.
- Hip fracture (reduced from 15 to 10)

Drawback of the study:
1. This study caters to old group of late menopause patients.
2. The study group had many women who were already affected with comorbid conditions.

MWS (Million Women's Study), 2005

The Million Women Study is a multicenter, population-based prospective cohort study of women aged 50 and over invited to routine breast cancer screening in the UK.

Aims

The Million Women Study was set up with the aim of recruiting 1,000,000 women in the UK into a cohort study, to provide the following correlation with HT:

I. HRT and Breast Cancer

Follow-up of over 1 million women in the Million Women Study confirmed that women currently using HRT are more likely to develop breast cancer than those who are not using HRT. Past users are not at increased risk. The study was able to show that this effect is substantially greater for combined (estrogen-progestogen) HRT than for estrogen-only HRT; and that the effects were similar for oral, transdermal and implanted HRT. Current users of estrogen-progestogen HRT are at 2-fold increased risk of developing breast cancer, and current users of estrogen-only HRT are at 1.3-fold risk.

II. HRT and Endometrial Cancer

It is well known that post-menopausal women who have not had a hysterectomy are at increased risk of cancer of the endometrium, if they take estrogen-only HRT. Follow up of over 700,000 women in the Million Women Study confirmed this and showed that the risk of endometrial cancer is also increased in women who take tibolone; but is reduced, in women taking combined estrogen-progestogen HRT.

III. *HRT and Ovarian Cancer*

Results of the study show a small increase in risk of ovarian cancer in women taking HRT. The risk in current users was increased about 1.2-fold; for every 1000 women using HRT, 2.6 developed ovarian cancer over 5 years, compared with 2.2 in those not taking HRT. The risk was the same for estrogen-only, combined estrogen-progestogen and tibolone.

HERS Study, 2002 (Heart and Estrogen/ Progestin Replacement Study)

This study was designed to look at the effect of hormone replacement therapy on the rate of recurrent heart problems in women who already had heart disease. The HERS trial found that taking estrogen plus progestin for up to 4 years did not prevent further heart attacks or death from previous heart disease in post-menopausal women who already had a previous heart attack or known heart disease.

For the entire four-year HERS trial period, there were no significant differences in heart problems between the active hormone and the placebo groups. In the first year of HERS, the active hormone group had more heart problems than the placebo group, but after 2 or more years the active hormone group had somewhat fewer heart problems.

Conclusion

The latest data on HT do not warrant the fear and ultra-conservative approach issued in 2002. However, there are potential side effects and risks involved in taking HT that may be reduced by tailoring the therapy to individual patients. Emerging data suggest that side effects are reduced by:

- Using lower HRT doses;
- Minimising or eliminating systemic progestogens by use of intrauterine progestogen delivery systems;
- Using non-oral routes in some women;
- Initiating HRT in symptomatic women from near menopause.

HT can be offered to informed women for as long as they have debilitating symptoms, but the data are not yet strong enough to advocate it for chronic disease prevention, except perhaps for osteoporosis prevention near menopause, with the option of other effective fracture prevention treatments at a later age.

Systematic reviews of HT show that the main side effects are irregular uterine bleeding and breast tenderness when excessive estrogen is used.

Long-term therapy is appropriate for women with prolonged symptoms who are aware of the potential risks.

When HT is initiated near menopause for symptom control and subsequent improved quality of life, there are likely to be additional benefits (reduced fracture and cardiovascular risk, and possibly cognitive benefits) that outweigh the risks (which are not significantly raised in women under age 60 years).

Beyond this age, women can try stopping HT to see, if their quality of life is maintained without therapy. However, some women have continuing symptoms into their seventh decade, and they should not be denied HT, if their therapy and risks are assessed on an individual basis, and each patient is aware of the risks.

IMS and FOGSI Guidelines for Hormone Therapy in Menopause

Both Indian Menopause Society and FOGSI have set guidelines for HT which are similar in many respects.

Issues to be Dealt with Before Commencing HT

- Specific indication for starting HT must be present and it must be documented.
- Symptoms which definitely require HT are vasomotor and symptoms of urogenital atrophy.
- Main rule for HT—lowest possible dose for shortest possible duration.
- Assessment of risk factors prior to starting HT is essential.
- Lifestyle modification is an integral component of managing postmenopausal women.

Tests before Initiation of Therapy (IMS recommendation)

- Minimum investigations required are lipid profile and endometrial thickness on transvaginal ultrasound.
- Any pre-existing breast cancer is to be ruled out by mammography and/or sonography.

FOGSI Recommendation

- Routine screening tests—CBC, urine test, Pap test, serum TSH, blood sugar, lipid profile, TVS and mammogram.
- Tests to be done on indication—TSH, estradiol, endometrial sampling, BMD, tests for thrombosis.

Counseling before Starting HT

Counseling for HT must include explanation of the associated risks. HT, particularly estrogen and medroxyprogesterone acetate, leads to a small increase in breast cancer incidence, which increases with duration of therapy and age. The relative and absolute risks of pulmonary embolism, stroke and breast cancer should be explained. The documented additional risks for these are eight cases of each of these/10,000 women per year i.e. <1/1000 women/year. Women who are taking only estrogen therapy without the progesterone need not be concerned about breast cancer as these are not relevant to them. In fact the estrogen only arm has been found to be advantageous with regards to breast cancer.

Hormone Therapy (IMS and FOGSI)

- Type, dose, regimen and route of HT to be based on patient preference, efficacy in individual patient, side effects and costs.

- Lower than standard doses of EPT should be considered such as 0.3 mg of oral conjugated estrogen or 0.25 to 0.5 mg of micronized estradiol, but these have not been tested in long-term trials.

- Local estrogens should be preferred wherever possible since less rigorous follow-up and monitoring are required particularly for genitorurinary complaints.

- Unopposed estrogen for women with hysterectomy, progestin be added to the estrogen for women with uterus.

- Use of HT is recommended long term to patients with premature menopause uptil the expected age of menopause, i.e. 50 years as a form of replacement therapy.

- HT is recommended to patients with surgical menopause till 50 years of age. This may be started in the immediate postoperative phase. HT should be weaned off gradually.

- For prophylaxis, the role of HT, if any, is only in women at high risk for developing osteoporosis and in these it should be started after 6–12 months of amenorrhea when diagnosis of menopause is certain.

Duration of therapy: It depends on the indication of use and therapeutic response. Hormones should be gradually weaned off or symptoms may recur with abrupt withdrawal. Women should be counseled that risk is small when HT duration is less than 5 years.

Follow-up on HT: Follow-up for all women on HT is mandatory. This should initially be after 1 and 3 months to confirm adequacy of treatment and thereafter annually.

Recommendations for Symptomatic Treatment Osteoprotection (FOGSI Recommendations)

- Overall, HT is effective in the prevention of all osteoporosis-related fractures, even in patients at low risk of fracture. [A]

- Although no head-to-head studies have compared HT to bisphosphonates in terms of fracture reduction, there is no evidence to suggest that bisphosphonates or any other antiresorptive therapy is superior to HT.

- It is, therefore, suggested that, in 50–59 years old postmenopausal women, HT is a cost-effective firstline treatment in the prevention of osteoporotic fractures.

- Even lower than standard-dose preparations maintain a positive influence on bone indices such as bone mineral density. [A]

- HT has a positive effect on osteoarthritis and the integrity of intervertebral disks.

- Duration of therapy should be for a minimum of 5 years for benefit to be apparent.

- Bone mineral density declines after discontinuation of estrogen and approaches that of non-users. Another osteoprotective agent should be initiated prior to cessation of HT. (IMS guideline)

HT-Coronary Heart Disease, Stroke and Thromboembolism (FOGSI Recommendations)

- HT in women aged 50–59 years does not increase CHD risk in healthy women and may even decrease the risk in this age group. [A]

- Estrogen-alone therapy in the age group 50–59 is associated with significantly less coronary calcification. [A]

- Early harm (more coronary events during the first 2 years of HT) is not observed in the early post-menopausal period.[A]

- It is unclear at present whether there is a statistical increase in ischemic stroke with standard HT in healthy women aged 50–59. The WHI data showed no statistically significant increase in risk; nevertheless, even if statistically increased, as found in Nurses' Health Study, the lower prevalence of this occurrence in this age group makes the attributable risk extremely small. [A]

- The risk of venous thrombosis is approximately two fold higher with standard doses of oral HT, but it is extremely low in a healthy woman under 60 years of age. [A]

- The risk of venous thrombosis is possibly less with transdermal, compared with oral estrogen therapy. [B]

HT-Breast

- After 5 years' use of combined estrogen and progesterone, there is a small increase in risk of breast cancer in North American women of about eight extra cases per 10,000 women per year. However, no significant increase was seen in women without prior use of HT in the WHI study. [A]

- Estrogen-only use does not cause an increase in breast cancer for up to 7 years. In observational studies, a small increase in the risk with estrogen-alone therapy appears with long-term use. [B]

- Combined estrogen and progesterone therapy may cause increased breast density in up to 50% of postmenopausal women, dependent on the regime (dose, type of progesterone). The effect of estrogen alone is a smaller. [A]

- The effect on breast density is dose-related. Ultra-low-dose regimes do not cause any perceptible change in density. [A]

- The average increase in breast density under standard dose HT is only about 5–10%. [A]

- Increased baseline breast density is a risk factor for breast cancer. There are no data to support a direct association between HT-induced breast density changes and the risk of developing breast cancer.

HT-Neuroprotection (FOGSI Recommendation)

- At present, there is no evidence of substantial cognitive decline across the menopausal transition. However, many women experience cognitive difficulties in association with vasomotor symptoms, sleep disturbances and mood changes. [A]

- Cognitive benefits from estrogen replacement therapy appear to depend on age of initiation.

- Observational studies show a decreased risk of Alzheimer's disease in hormone users and typically involve women who initiated estrogen therapy early in the menopausal transition.

- Limited data exist on the effect of progesterone added to estrogen in the early postmenopause period. Clinical trials data suggest no cognitive benefit with MPA early in the menopause. [A]

No consensus: There is no consensus whether cessation of hormone therapy should be abrupt or tapered.

Evidence-based prescription of HT is to start early, use minimum effective dose judiciously on indication, after appropriate counseling.

Postmenopausal Bleeding

Definition

Postmenopausal bleeding (PMB) is defined as vaginal bleeding occurring after 12 months of amenorrhea of natural menopause, However, it can apply to younger women following premature ovarian failure or premature menopause.

Epidemiology

Postmenopausal bleeding is a common problem representing 5% of all gynecology outpatient attendances.

Etiology

- *Vaginal atrophy:* The most common cause of PMB (65%)
- Use of *HRT* (10–15%).
- *Endometrial hyperplasia;* simple, complex, and atypical (10%).
- *Endometrial cancer:* The probability of a woman presenting with PMB having endometrial cancer is 10%. However, 90% of women with endometrial cancer present with PMB.
- Endometrial polyps or cervical polyps (12%).
- Cervical cancer.
- Uterine sarcoma (rare).
- *Ovarian cancer,* especially oestrogen-secreting (theca cell) ovarian tumors.
- *Vaginal cancer* (very uncommon).
- *Vulval cancer* may bleed, but the lesion should be obvious.
- Non-gynaecological causes including trauma or a *bleeding disorder.*

Clinical Investigation of Women with Postmenopausal Bleeding

Physical Examination

Pelvic examination should be performed searching for visual evidence of lesions or bleeding from gynecologic (e.g. vulva, vagina, exocervix) and non-gynecologic (e.g. perineum, periurethral, perianal) sources.

Investigations

Evaluation of the Endometrium

Transvaginal ultrasound scan (TVUS) is an appropriate first-line procedure to identify which women with PMB are at higher risk of endometrial cancer. The mean endometrial thickness in postmenopausal women is much thinner than in premenopausal women.

Thickening of the endometrium may indicate the presence of pathology. In general, the thicker the endometrium, the higher is the likelihood of endometrial cancer. The threshold of endometrial thickness is 4 mm; a thickness of >4 mm gives 7.3% likelihood of endometrial cancer. In a woman with PMB, if endometrial thickness is less than 4 mm uniformly, the probability of carcinoma is less than 1%. But still some pathology may be missed and therefore it is recommended that hysteroscopy and, biopsy, should be performed if clinical suspicion is high.

Compared with premenopausal women, the measured thickness of the endometrium (by convention a double layer in the midsagittal view; Fig. 16.2) should be thinner in postmenopausal women not receiving HRT (Fig. 16.3). This double-thickness layer is called the EEC. If there is uniformly sonolucent fluid—generally a nonconcerning finding—the thickness of the fluid echo is subtracted from the measurement from baseline to baseline to obtain the EEC (Fig. 16.4). The morphologic features should be uniform and, if there are irregularities, or if the EEC cannot be adequately

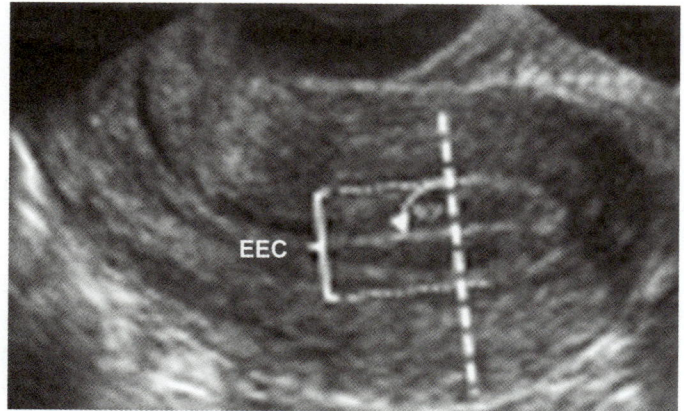

Fig. 16.2: Endometrial echo complex (EEC) measurement in the sagittal plane

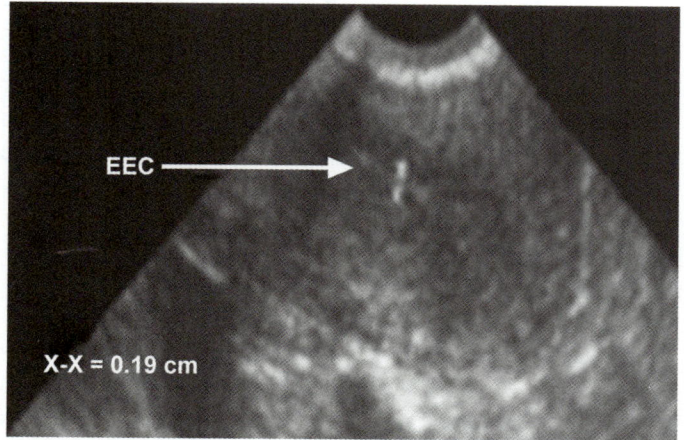

Fig. 16.3: Typical measurement of normal postmenopausal endometrial echo complex (EEC) (< 4 mm) (arrowhead)

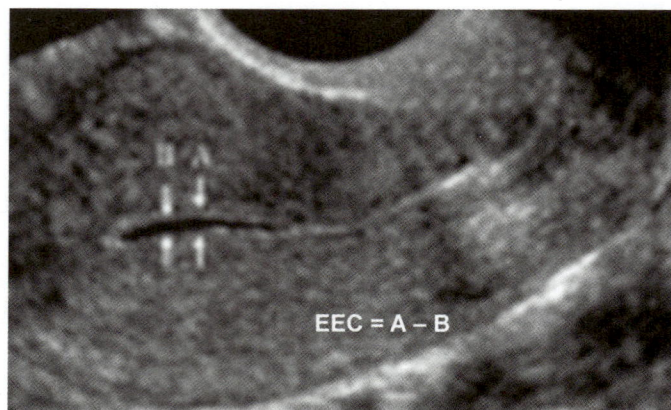

Fig. 16.4: Measurement of endometrial echo complex (EEC) when there is fluid in the cavity

evaluated, other investigations are warranted, such as contrast sonography, hysteroscopy, and/or endometrial sampling.

In general, thicker EECs are associated with a greater likelihood of endometrial or intracavitary pathology, including endometrial polyps, hyperplasia, and cancer. On the other hand, the reliability of TVUS allows the clinician to identify a group of women with postmenopausal bleeding who have a thin endometrium and thus a very low likelihood of hyperplasia or neoplasia. Unless there is a recurrence of bleeding, this group of women with postmenopausal bleeding and a thin EEC generally require no more investigation.

There is some evidence that TVUS may be less sensitive for the detection of early endometrial carcinomas regardless of the EEC threshold and it has been demonstrated that 17% of patients with postmenopausal bleeding and early endometrial cancer had an EEC of less than 4 mm.

Endometrial Biopsy

A definitive diagnosis in PMB is made by histology. Historically, endometrial samples have been obtained by dilatation and curettage. Nowadays, it is more usual to obtain a sample by endometrial biopsy, which can be undertaken using samplers like vibra aspirator as outpatient procedure.

Dilatation and Curettage

Dilatation and curettage (D&C) should no longer be the first method of sampling the endometrium in most cases. Comparison of office-based endometrial sampling with the Pipelle device with combined curettage and hysteroscopy reveals that each blind procedure is an acceptable screening tool but does miss usually benign lesions such as endometrial polyps. However, it is not completely clear that D&C is equivalent to endometrial sampling with a suction catheter.

Procedure and Tissue Yield Failure Rates of Office-based Endometrial Sampling

When inadequate tissue is obtained to allow histologic assessment, the specimen is typically called "nondiagnostic." Evidence suggests that such patients may have underlying intrauterine lesions, including malignancy, especially if results of transvaginal ultrasonography (TVUS) are nondiagnostic or in excess of an acceptable threshold value such as 5 mm. Office-based sampling of the endometrium is associated with a procedure failure rate of approximately 10% and a tissue yield failure rate of 10%.

Hysteroscopy

Hysteroscopy and biopsy are the preferred diagnostic technique to detect polyps and other benign lesions. Hysteroscopy may be performed as an outpatient procedure, although some women may require general anesthesia.

Saline-infused Sonogram

Saline is placed in the uterus through the cervix with a small, thin tube. The doctor looks by ultrasound to see if there are any masses within the uterine lining. It is often done along with an endometrial biopsy.

Cautions

Most women with PMB will not have significant pathology. But
- PMB in women on HRT still needs investigation.
- An obvious lesion like atrophic vaginitis does not exclude another lesion.
- Many women are unable to distinguish between vaginal and urinary or rectal in women presenting with PMB, the prevalence of bladder tumors and rectal cancers may be was 1.07% and of bladder cancer was 0.7%.

Risk of Endometrial Cancer

Endometrial cancer is one of the most commonly diagnosed reproductive tract malignancy in postmenopausal women. Although endometrial cancer accounts for 6% of all female cancers, a number of intrinsic clinical features, like early diagnosis (because of investigation of abnormal or postmenopausal bleeding) relatively slow spread of majorityof endometrial cancerous growth and prompt use of effective therapy, causes only about 3% cancer-related deaths.

There are 2 distinct types of endometrial cancer; most are Type 1, which develops secondary to unopposed estrogen-induced endometrial hyperplasia with an endometrioid appearance on histopathologic evaluation. Type 2 lesions comprise the minority, are of serous or clear cell origin, are not related to estrogen exposure, and are associated with a relatively poor prognosis. Recent data reveal that approximately 90% are Type 1 and about 10% are Type 2 lesions.

For women with postmenopausal bleeding who do not use HRT, the incidence of endometrial cancer ranges from 4.9 to 11.5%. There appears to be a greater risk of endometrial cancer in women who present with postmenopausal bleeding 10 or more years following menopause.

Incidence of Postmenopausal Bleeding on HRT

There are no reliable data regarding the incidence of endometrial carcinoma in women using estrogen and progestin-containing HRT regimens. However, the estimated proportions range from 0.02 to 0.05% per annum. For women receiving tamoxifen, the risk of endometrial cancer is likely above 10% depending in part on the dose and in part on the duration of therapy.

Investigation of Postmenopausal Bleeding on HRT

Evaluation of women with postmenopausal bleeding while using HRT is affected by a number of factors, including the type of regimen, the dose of estrogen, and, if used, the scheduling of progestin administration (cyclic or continuous). These and other factors have an effect on the nature and timing of anticipated and unscheduled bleeding and may have a role in the timing and interpretation of ultrasound findings.

Causes of Abnormal Uterine Bleeding using HRT

- Poor compliance
- Poor gastrointestinal absorption (particularly for oral preparations)
- Drug interactions
- Coagulation defects
- Liver disease
- Gynecologic disorders apart from, endometrial cancer, endometrial polyps, and cervical or vaginal lesions
- Nonreproductive tract origins (e.g., urinary tract, gastrointestinal tract lesions).

History of Patients on Hormone Therapy

The clinician should determine if the bleeding pattern is within acceptable limits. In addition, the provider should ascertain if there are any other factors or symptoms that may place the patient at increased risk of endometrial cancer. Pertinent questions to ask include the following:

When does the bleeding occur with respect to progestin administration?
Women receiving cyclical progestin therapy should have bleeding near the end of or shortly after discontinuation of the progestin component of the regimen.

How long does the bleeding last? How heavy is it?
Heavy bleeding, even when experienced in the context of a cyclically administered progestin, may suggest the presence of intrauterine pathology.

Was there a period of amenorrhea after HRT was started?
For continuous combined regimens, breakthrough bleeding is common, especially in the first six months, but should a period of amenorrhea be established initially, bleeding, even within the first six months, suggests intrauterine abnormalities.

Is there a reason to suspect poor gastrointestinal absorption?
A history of nausea, vomiting, or diarrhea is a potential explanation for incomplete absorption and resultant bleeding.

Is there any evidence of hepatocellular disease?
The liver is responsible for metabolizing estrogen. Should there be active or chronic hepatocellular disease, the circulating levels of estrogen may be higher than normal and abnormal bleeding may occur secondary to endometrial stimulation.

Is the patient receiving any other drugs?
The intentional or inadvertent use of other gonadal steroids (estrogens with or without progestins) may explain unexpected bleeding.

Tamoxifen

Women with breast cancer who take tamoxifen on a long-term basis are at increased risk of endometrial cancer. Tamoxifen can cause variable changes to the endometrium, and ultrasound may be more difficult to interpret. All women with PMB on tamoxifen would normally have hysteroscopy and biopsy in addition to ultrasonography.

Tamoxifen-related Bleeding

Postmenopausal patients receiving tamoxifen experience an increased risk of endometrial neoplasia which is highest after four years of exposure. Whereas there is no evidence to support the use of routine biopsy of such patients, any who present with bleeding while receiving tamoxifen should undergo office-based endometrial sampling if possible. If not feasible, such patients should undergo hysteroscopy and curettage.

Investigation of Postmenopausal Uterine Bleeding in Women Receiving Tamoxifen

The tamoxifen-induced impact on the endometrium frequently, creates a thickened EEC, often with diffuse subendometrial cystic change that is in no way indicative of endometrial hyperplasia or malignancy. As a result, TVUS for evaluation of EEC thickness is not useful in the evaluation of tamoxifen-related postmenopausal bleeding.

Many patients with tamoxifen-related bleeding have endometrial polyps. Consequently, if bleeding persists, evaluation of the endometrial cavity is indicated, generally with hysteroscopy, with hysteroscopically guided excision of any identified polyps and curettage for reassessment of the endometrium. Contrast sonography may also be useful in this regard; however, there is evidence that saline infusion sonography is inferior to hysteroscopy in detecting focal lesions in these patients.

For patients who are receiving tamoxifen, who have persistent episodes of postmenopausal bleeding without any evidence of focal lesions, and for whom both the cervical canal and endometrial cavity have been adequately evaluated with imaging and adequate endometrial sampling showing benign tissue, annual repeated sampling is indicated.

Treatment of PMB

1. Endometrial atrophy—oral estrogen (CEE 0.625 mg daily for 3 months) or Premarin ointment to apply inside vagina for 6 weeks stops bleeding

2. Endometrial hyperplasia and polyp—may be treated with hysteroscopic polypectomy and endometrial ablation or hysterectomy

3. Endometral cancer—surgery followed by chemo-radiotherapy

4. Bleeding from ERT—should be controlled by progesterone or by stopping hormone therapy before endometrium is properly evaluated.

5. Surgical treatment is done for cancer cervix, granulosa theca cell tumor producing PMB.

17

Contraception and Family Planning

Family planning services are defined as "educational, comprehensive medical or social activities which enable individuals, including minors, to determine freely the number and spacing of their children and to select the means by which this may be achieved.

The world population is expected to be around 8 billion in 2025 with a fertility rate of 2.1 per children per women. Approximately 96% of the population growth now occurs in developing countries.

In India, during the 1965–2009 period, contraceptive usage has more than tripled (from 13% of married women in 1970 to 48% in 2009) and the fertility rate has more than halved (from 5.7 in 1966 to 2.6 in 2009), but the national fertility rate is still high enough to cause long-term population growth. India adds up to 10 lakh (10,00,000) people to its population every 15 days.

India's Population 2016	
Current population of India in 2016	1,33,2743,359 (1.33 billion)
Total male population in India	628,800,000 (628.8 million)
Total female population in India	591,400,000 (591.4 million)
Sex ratio	940 females per 1,000 males
Age structure	
0 to 25 years	50% of India's current population
Currently, there are about 51 births in India in a minute	
India's population in 2011	1.21 billion
India's population in 2001	1.02 billion
Population of India in 1947	350 million

Throughout the world, 45% of married women of reproductive age practice contraception. About 71 million living in developing countries are at risk of unplanned pregnancy. Fewer than 15% of women in reproductive age are using oral contraceptives. Demographic Health Survey data for India (2005–06) reveals that 52% of illiterate women do not use any contraceptive method.

Unmet demand for (modern) contraceptives refers to women who want to avoid pregnancy but are not using a modern contraceptive method. Illiterate women in India have risen to 272.95 million in 2011. Not infrequently, opposition from the male partner has been found to thwart aspirations of the female to use family planning methods. Such opposition may arise because of the apprehension that allowing women freedom to make reproductive decisions will:
a. Erode the authority of the male partner within the family
b. Encourage the wife to be unfaithful, or
c. Loose face within the community.

Contraception

Efficacy of Contraception

It is generally assessed by measuring the number of unplanned pregnancies that occur during a specified period of exposure and use of a contraceptive method. The two methods used to measure the contraceptive efficacy are the Pearl Index and Life- Table Analysis.

Pearl Index

This index created by Raymond Pearl in 1933 is defined as the number of failures per 100 woman years of exposure. The denominator is the total months or cycles of exposure from the onset of a method until completion of the study. The quotient is multiplied by 1200, if the denominator consists of months and by 1300 if the denominator consists of cycles.

Calculation and usage

$$\text{Pearl index} = \frac{\text{Number of pregnancies} \times 12}{\text{Number of women} \times \text{Number of months}} \times 100$$

$$\text{Pearl index} = \frac{\text{Number of pregnancies} \times 1200}{\text{Number of women users} \times \text{Number of months of exposure}}$$

There are two calculation methods for determining the Pearl index:

The Pearl Index is sometimes used as a statistical estimation of the number of *unintended pregnancies* in 100 woman-years of exposure (e.g. 100 women over one year of use, or 10 women over 10 years). It is also sometimes used to compare birth control methods, a lower Pearl index representing a lower chance of getting unintentionally pregnant.

Usually, two Pearl indices are published from studies of birth control methods:

- **Actual use** Pearl Index, which includes all pregnancies in a study and all months (or cycles) of exposure.
- **Perfect use** or **method** Pearl Index, which includes only pregnancies that resulted from correct and consistent use of the method, and only includes months or cycles in which the method was correctly and consistently used.

Life–Table Analysis

This calculates a failure rate for each month of use. A cumulative failure rate can then compare methods for any specific length of exposure.

Medical Eligibility Criteria for Contraception (Table 17.1)

This is WHO recommendation, 2008 assigned all present methods of contraception to any of four categories of suitability. The categories are (Table 17.1):

1. A condition for which there is no restriction for the use of the contraceptive method.
2. A condition where the advantages of using the method generally outweigh the theoretical or proven risks.
3. A condition where the theoretical or proven risks usually outweigh the advantages of using the method.
4. A condition which represents an unacceptable health risk, if the contraceptive method is used.

Where resources for clinical judgement are limited, such as in community-based services, the four-category classification framework can be simplified into two categories. With this simplification, a classification of category 3 indicates that a woman is not medically eligible to use the method.

Types of Birth Control

- Reversible methods of birth control
  - Fertility awareness-based methods
  - Barrier methods
  - Intrauterine contraception (IUD, IUS)
  - Hormonal methods
- Permanent methods of birth control
  - Female sterilization
- Male sterilization (non-scalpel vasectomy)

Periodic Abstinence

Coitus Interruptus

Coitus interruptus involves withdrawal of the entire penis from the vagina before ejaculation. Fertilization is prevented by lack of contact between spermatozoa and the ovum. This method of contraception remains a significant means of fertility control in the developing world.

Efficacy

Effectiveness depends largely on the man's capability to withdraw prior to ejaculation. The failure rate is estimated to be approximately 4% in the first year of perfect use. In typical use, the rate is approximately 19% during the first year of use.

Table 17.1: Categories of suitability according to medical eligibility, WHO		
Category	*With clinical judgement*	*With limited clinical judgement*
1	Use method in any circumstances	
2	Generally use the method	Yes (use the method)
3	Use of method not usually recommended unless other more appropriate methods are not available or not acceptable	
4	Method not to be used	No (do not use the method)

Advantages

Advantages include immediate availability, no devices, no cost, no chemical involvement, and a theoretical reduced risk of transmission of sexually transmitted diseases (STDs).

Disadvantages

The probability of *pregnancy* is high with incorrect or inconsistent use.

Lactational Amenorrhea

Elevated prolactin levels and a reduction of gonadotropin-releasing hormone from the hypothalamus during lactation suppress ovulation. This leads to a reduction in luteinizing hormone (LH) release and inhibition of follicular maturation. The duration of this suppression varies and is influenced by the frequency and duration of breastfeeding and the length of time since birth. Mothers only need to use breastfeeding to be successful; however, as soon as the first menses occurs, she must begin to use another method of birth control to avoid pregnancy.

Efficacy

The perfect-use failure rate within the first 6 months is 0.5%. The typical-use failure rate within the first 6 months is 2%.

Advantages

Involution of the uterus occurs more rapidly. Menses are suppressed. This method can be used immediately after childbirth. This method facilitates postpartum weight loss.

Disadvantages

Return to fertility is uncertain. Frequent breastfeeding may be inconvenient. This method should not be used, if the mother has human immunodeficiency virus (HIV) infection.

Natural Family Planning

Natural family planning is one of the most widely used methods of fertility regulation, particularly for those whose religious or cultural beliefs do not permit devices or drugs for contraception. This method involves periodic abstinence, with couples attempting to avoid intercourse during a woman's fertile period, which is around the time of ovulation. Techniques to determine the fertile period include the calendar method, cervical mucus method, or the symptothermal method.

The calendar method is based on 3 assumptions as follows: (1) A human ovum is capable of fertilization only for approximately 24 hours after ovulation, (2) spermatozoa can retain their fertilizing ability for only 48 hours after coitus, and (3) ovulation usually occurs 12–16 days before the onset of the subsequent menses. The menses is recorded for 6 cycles to approximate the fertile period. The earliest day of the fertile period is determined by the number of days in the shortest menstrual cycle subtracted by 18. The latest day of the fertile period is calculated by the number of days in the longest cycle subtracted by 11.

With the cervical mucus method, the woman attempts to predict her fertile period by quantifying the cervical mucus with her fingers. Under the influence of estrogen, the mucus increases in quantity and becomes progressively more elastic and copious until a peak day is reached. This is followed by scant and dry mucus, secondary to the influence of progesterone, which remains until the onset of the next menses. Intercourse is allowed 4 days after the maximal cervical mucus until menstruation.

The symptothermal method predicts the first day of abstinence by using either the calendar method or the first day mucus is detected, whichever is noted first. The end of the fertile period is predicted by measuring basal body temperature. The basal body temperature of a woman is relatively low during the follicular phase and rises in the luteal phase of the menstrual cycle in response to the thermogenic effect of progesterone. The rise in temperature can vary from 0.2–0.5°C. The elevated temperatures begin 1–2 days after ovulation and correspond to the rising level of progesterone. Intercourse can resume 3 days after the temperature rise.

Efficacy

The failure rate in typical use is estimated to be approximately 25%.

Advantages

No adverse effects from hormones occur. This may be the only method acceptable to couples for cultural or religious reasons. Immediate return of fertility occurs with cessation of use.

Disadvantages

This is most suitable for women with regular and predictable cycles. Complete abstinence is necessary during the fertile period unless backup contraception is used. The failure rate is relatively high. This method does not protect against STDs.

Barrier Methods

Male Condom

The condom consists of a thin sheath placed over the glans and the shaft of the penis that is applied before any vaginal insertion. It is one of the most popular mechanical barriers. Among all of the barrier methods, the condom provides the most effective protection of the genital tract from STDs. Its usage has increased from 13.2–18.9% among all women of reproductive age because of the concern regarding the acquisition of HIV and STDs. It prevents pregnancy by acting as a barrier to the passage of semen into the vagina.

Efficacy

The failure rate of condoms in couples that use them consistently and correctly during the first year of use is estimated to be approximately 3%. However, the true failure rate is estimated to be approximately 14% during the first year of typical use. Common errors with condoms usage include failure to use condoms with every act of intercourse and throughout intercourse, improper lubricant use with latex condoms (e.g. oil-based lubricants), incorrect placement of the condom on the penis, and poor withdrawal technique.

Advantages

Condoms are readily available and are usually inexpensive. This method involves the male partner in the contraceptive choice. Condoms are effective against both pregnancy and STDs.

Disadvantages

Condoms possibly decrease enjoyment of sex. Some users may have a latex allergy. Condom breakage and slippage decrease effectiveness. Oil-based lubricants may damage the condom.

Female Condom

The female condom (Fig. 17.1) is a polyurethane sheath intended for one-time use, similar to the male condom. It contains 2 flexible rings and measures 7.8 cm in diameter and 17 cm long. The ring at the closed end of the sheath serves as an insertion mechanism and internal anchor that is placed inside the vaginal canal. The other ring forms the external patent edge of the device and remains outside of the canal after insertion.

The female condom prevents pregnancy by acting as a barrier to the passage of semen into the vagina. **Simultaneous use of both the female and male condom is not recommended** because they may adhere

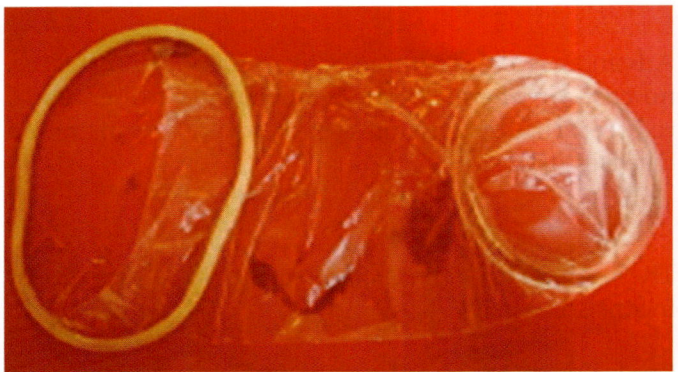

Fig. 17.1: Female condom

to each other, leading to slippage or displacement of either device.

Efficacy

Efficacy trials are limited. Initial trials have demonstrated pregnancy rate of 15% in 6 months. Less than 1% of women in the United States use this method of contraception. It is not available in India.

Advantages

The female condom provides some protection to the labia and the base of the penis during intercourse. The sheath is coated on the inside with a silicone-based lubricant. It does not deteriorate with oil-based lubricants. It can be inserted as long as 8 hours before intercourse.

Disadvantages

The lubricant does not contain spermicide. The device is difficult to place in the vagina. The inner ring may cause discomfort. Some users consider the female condom cumbersome. The female condom may cause a urinary tract infection, if left in vagina for a prolonged period.

Diaphragm

The diaphragm is a shallow latex cup with a spring mechanism in its rim to hold it in place in the vagina (Fig. 17.2). Diaphragms are manufactured in various diameters. A pelvic examination and measurement of the diagonal length of the vaginal canal determines the correct diaphragm size. It is inserted before intercourse so that the posterior rim fits into the posterior fornix and the anterior rim is placed behind the pubic bone. Spermicidal cream or jelly is applied to the inside of the dome, which then covers the cervix.

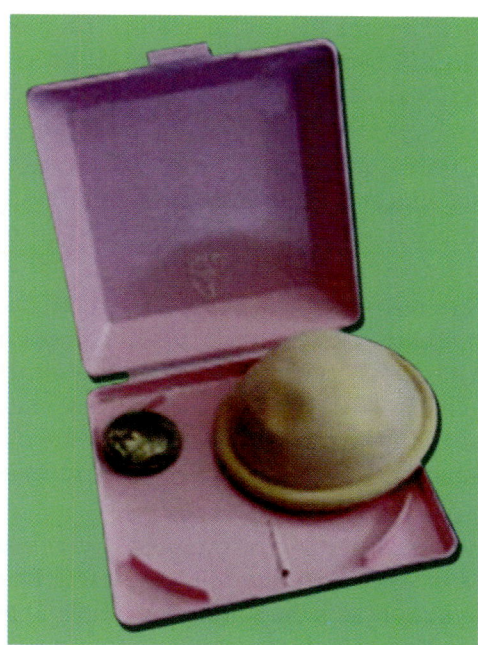

Fig. 17.2: Contraceptive diaphragm

Contraceptive Action

It prevents pregnancy by acting as a barrier to the passage of semen into the cervix. Once in position, the diaphragm provides effective contraception for 6 hours. If a longer interval has elapsed without removal of the diaphragm, fresh spermicide is added with an applicator. After intercourse, the diaphragm must be left in place for at least 6 hours.

Efficacy

Effectiveness of the diaphragm depends on the age of the user, experience with its use, continuity of use, and the use of spermicide. The typical-use failure rate within the first year is estimated to be 20%.

Advantages

The diaphragm does not entail hormonal usage. Contraception is controlled by the woman. The diaphragm may be placed by the woman in anticipation of intercourse.

Disadvantages

Prolonged use during multiple acts of intercourse may increase the risk of urinary tract infections. Usage for longer than 24 hours is not recommended due to the possible risk of *toxic shock syndrome (TSS)*. The diaphragm requires perfect fitting. Poorly fitted diaphragms may cause vaginal erosions. Diaphragms have a high failure rate. The diaphragm may develop an odor, if not properly cleansed.

Cervical Cap

The cervical cap is a cup-shaped latex device that fits over the base of the cervix. A groove along the inner circumference of the rim improves the seal between the inner rim of the cap and the base of the cervix. The cap must be filled one-third full with spermicide prior to insertion. It is inserted as long as 8 hours before coitus and can be left in place for as long as 48 hours.

A cervical cap acts as both a mechanical barrier to sperm migration into the cervical canal and as a chemical agent with the use of spermicide.

Efficacy

Effectiveness depends on the parity of women due to the shape of the cervical os. With perfect use in the first year, the failure rate for nulliparous women is 9%, as opposed to 20% in parous women. With typical use within the first year, the failure rate is 20% in nulliparous women and 40% in parous women.

Advantages

It provides continuous contraceptive protection for its duration of use regardless of the number of intercourse acts. Unlike with the diaphragm, additional spermicide is not necessary for repeated intercourse. The cervical cap does not involve ongoing use of hormones.

Disadvantages

Cervical erosion may lead to vaginal spotting. The cervical cap is associated with a theoretical risk of TSS, if it is left in place longer than the prescribed period. The cervical cap requires professional fitting and training for use. Severe obesity may make placement difficult. It has a relatively high failure rate. Women must have history of normal results on Papanicolaou (Pap) tests.

Spermicidal Agents

Vaginal spermicides consist of a base combined with either nonoxynol-9 or octoxynol. The actual spermicidal agent consists of a surfactant that destroys the sperm cell membrane. Bases include vaginal foams, suppositories, jellies, films, foaming tablets, and creams. These must be inserted into the vagina prior to each coital act. Use of spermicidal agents also reduces the risk of infection by both viral and bacterial organisms that cause STDs; however, clinical data on their efficacy for preventing the transmission of HIV are limited. Nonoxynol-9 is toxic to the lactobacilli that are part of the normal vaginal flora. Adverse effects include increased vaginal colonization with the bacteria

Escherichia coli, which may predispose to bacteriuria after intercourse.

Spermicides prevent sperm from entering the cervical os by attacking the sperm's flagella and body, reducing their mobility, and disrupting their fructolytic activity, thereby inhibiting their nourishment.

Efficacy

The perfect-use failure rate within the first year is 6%. The typical-use failure rate within the first year is 26%.

Advantages

The lubrication provided by spermicides may heighten satisfaction in both partners. Another advantage is the ease of application. It is easily accessible, available over the counter, and inexpensive. It requires minimal patient education. It augments contraceptive efficacy of the cervical cap and diaphragm. Spermicides produce no adverse systemic effects.

Disadvantages

Spermicides provide minimal protection from STDs. Insertion may be uncomfortable for some couples. Vaginal irritation is possible, and spermicides may cause an allergic reaction.

Hormonal Contraceptives

Combination Oral Contraceptives
(Tables 17.2 and 17.3)

Dr. Gregory Goodwin Pincus, Dr. M. C. Chang and Dr. John Rock are three "fathers" of the birth-control pill since they developed a relatively safe and simple oral contraceptive that has revolutionized family planning. In 1957, the pill was released as a treatment for gynecological disorders. Finally, in 1960, it became FDA approved as contraceptive and by 1963, 1.2 million women started using it all over the globe. Prior to 1992, the estrogenic component of oral contraceptives consisted of either ethinyl estradiol or mestranol. Today, ethinyl estradiol is used in all preparations containing 35 µg or less (up to 15 µg) of estrogen.

The progestin component consists of norethindrone, levonorgestrel, norgestrel, norethindrone acetate, ethynodiol diacetate, norgestimate, and desogestrel. The most recent addition to the progestin group is the addition of drospirenone in birth control pills.

The other major development is the reduction in the dosage of ethinyl estradiol to 20 µg. The major impetus for this change is to improve the safety and reduce adverse effects. These lower doses are associated with a decrease in the incidence of estrogen-related adverse effects, such as weight gain, breast tenderness, and nausea.

Another recent development is the release of a combined oral contraceptive pill to raise folate serum levels. Beyaz contains the same progestin and estrogen contents as Yaz (drospirenone 3 mg/ethinyl estradiol 20 µg) plus 0.451 mg levomefolate calcium (folic acid metabolite).

Monophasic oral contraceptives have a constant dose of both estrogen and progestin in each of the hormonally active pills. Phasic combinations can alter either or both hormonal components. Use should be initiated either on the first day of the menses or the first Sunday after menses has begun. Most of the formulations have 21 hormonally active pills followed by 7 placebo pills. This facilitates consistent daily pill intake.

If a woman misses 1 or 2 pills, she should take 1 tablet as soon as she remembers. She then takes 1 tablet twice daily until coverage of the missed pills is achieved. Women who have missed more than 2 consecutive pills should be advised to use a backup method of contraception simultaneous to finish up the packet of pills until their next menses.

Prevention of ovulation is considered the dominant mechanism of action. Either estrogen or progesterone

	Estrogen				**Progestogen**	
Mechanism	Suppresses FSH release from anterior pituitary	Increases concentration of progesterone receptors	Enhances progestin effect	Suppresses LH release from anterior pituitary	Cervical mucus thickening	Decidualized endometrial bed with exhausted and atrophied glands
Result	Inhibits follicular development	Endometrial stabilization	Enabled progestogen dose reduction	Inhibits ovulation	Impervious to sperm penetration	Not receptive to embryo implantation

Table 17.2: Mechanism of action of COC components

alone is capable of inhibiting both FSH and LH sufficiently to prevent ovulation. The combination of the 2 steroids creates a synergistic effect that greatly increases their antigonadotropic and ovulation-inhibitory effects. They also alter the consistency of cervical mucus, affect the endometrial lining, and alter tubal transport.

Efficacy

Failure rates are correlated to individual compliance. Rates range from 0.1% with perfect use to 5% with typical use.

Table 17.3: Types of oral contraceptive pills

Low dose oral contraceptive	Products containing less than 50 µg EE
1st generation oral contraceptive	Products containing less than 50 µg EE
2nd generation oral contraceptive	Products containing 20, 30, or 35 µg EE and norethindrone progesterone family of either levonorgestrel, norgestimate
3rd generation oral contraceptive	Products containing desogestrel or gestodene with 20, 25 or 30 µg EE

All contraceptive progestogens have a similar 4-ring steroid skeleton and can be classified according to the time of introduction (first, second, third generation and other) (Table 17.4).

Estranes correspond to first-generation progestogens, such as norethisterone (NE), norethindrone (NE), ethynodiol diacetate, lynestrenol (LYN) and norethynodrel as well as dienogest (DNG).

Gonane progestogens correspond to second-generation, e.g. levonorgestrel (LNG) and norgestrel (NG) and third-generation progestogens, e.g. desogestrel (DSG), gestodene (GSD) and norgestimate (NGM). Examples of pregnanes in COCs are cyproterone acetate, chlormadinone acetate and nomesgestrol.

Second-generation progestogens were introduced into the market in the 1970s. During the 1980s, three new third-generation progestogens (DSG, GSD and NGM) were developed. Both desogestrel (acting as 3-keto desogestrel) and norgestimate (acting mainly through levonorgestrel) are prodrugs. DRSP is progestogen derived from 17-α spironolactone and possesses anti-mineralocorticoid and mild anti-androgenic activity.

Advantages

Oral contraceptives are used as treatment for menstrual irregularity because menses is more regular and predictable.

a. In the prevention of ovulation, oral contraceptives can reduce and sometimes eliminate mittelschmerz.

b. Women with anemia secondary to menorrhagia increase their iron stores. Women can manipulate the cycle to avoid menses during certain events, such as vacations or weekends, by extending the number intake days of hormonally active pills or by skipping the placebo pill week.

c. Oral contraceptives prevent benign conditions, such as benign breast disease, pelvic inflammatory disease (PID), and functional cysts. Functional cysts are reduced by the suppression of stimulation of the ovaries by FSH and LH. Ectopic pregnancies are prevented by the cessation of ovulation.

d. Oral contraceptives are noted to prevent epithelial ovarian and endometrial carcinoma. Studies have noted an approximate 40% reduced risk of malignant and borderline ovarian epithelial cancer. Use of oral contraceptives is associated with a 50% reduction of risk of endometrial adenocarcinoma. Protection appears to persist for at least 15 years following discontinuation of use.

Disadvantages

Adverse effects include nausea, breast tenderness, breakthrough bleeding, amenorrhea, and headaches.

Table 17.4: Evolution of progestins in available COCs

Pregnanes	Estranes	Gonanes 1st generation	Gonanes 2nd generation	Other/unclassified 3rd generation
Medroxyprogesterone acetate	Norethindrone acetate	Dinorgestrel	Desogestrel (DSG)	Drospirenone (DRSP)
Cyproterone acetate	Ethynodiol diacetate	Levonorgestrel	Gestodene	Cyproterone acetate
Chlormadinone acetate	Lynestrenol		Norgestimate (NGM)	
Nomegestrol, Nestorone	Norethynodrel			

Oral contraceptives do not provide protection from STDs. Daily administration is necessary, and inconsistent use may increase the failure rate. A few months of delay of normal ovulatory cycles may occur after discontinuation of oral contraceptives. Women who continue to have amenorrhea after a discontinuation period of 6 months require a full evaluation.

Metabolic Effects and Safety

Venous Thrombosis

- Venous thromboembolism, including pulmonary embolism and deep venous thrombosis, is the most common serious cardiovascular event among women who use oral contraceptive pills. Despite a low absolute risk (15 cases per 100,000 cardiovascular events per year), women who are taking oral contraceptive pills have a three to six times greater risk of venous thromboembolism than women who do not use this contraceptive method.

  The absolute risk of venous thromboembolism associated with oral contraceptive pills increases with age, obesity, recent surgery and some forms of thrombophilia. This risk is highest during the first year of use and is not related to the estrogen component of currently available pill formulations. The dose and type of progestin may influence the effect of an oral contraceptive on lipid metabolism as well as coagulation and fibrinolytic markers. But the association between third-generation progestins and risk of venous thromboembolism is not strong enough to recommend discontinuation.

- The blood of women with an inherited antithrombin III defect or factor V leiden mutation has abnormally increased coagulability. Women with these conditions who take oral contraceptive pills are at increased risk for venous thromboembolism. Progestin-only pills should be considered for use in these patients. Ideally, some experts believe that all first-time oral contraceptive pill users should be screened for factor V Leiden.

- The estrogen component of oral contraceptives has the capability of activating the blood clotting mechanism. Use of low-estrogen oral contraceptives is associated with a lower risk of thromboembolism than use of oral contraceptives with higher levels of estrogen. Although use of oral contraceptives is not associated with a detectable hypercoagulable state for most women, users at a greater risk for thromboembolism include women who smoke heavily, women with high or abnormal blood lipids, women with severe diabetes with damage to the arteries, women with consistently elevated blood pressures, and women who are obese.

- *Hypertension:* Oral contraceptives have a dose-related effect on blood pressure. With the older, high-dose pills, as many as 5% of patients can expect to have blood pressure elevations of 140/90 mm Hg or higher. This elevation is believed to be secondary to estrogen-induced increase in renin substrate in susceptible individuals. Although today's low-dose pills have minimal blood pressure effects, maintaining a surveillance of blood pressure is advisable.

- *Atherogenesis and stroke:* Limited preliminary data have demonstrated that oral contraceptive use does not lead to coronary atherosclerosis. The risk of myocardial infarction, ischemic stroke and hemorrhagic stroke does not become higher with increasing duration of oral contraceptive pill use or because of past use. The risk of mortality from cardiovascular disease attributable to oral contraceptive pill use is up to 10 times higher in women 40 to 44 years of age than in women 20 to 24 years of age. Despite the increased cardiovascular risk in older women, the risk of pregnancy is still greater in women who use no other form of contraception.

- *Hepatocellular adenoma:* These benign liver tumors have been associated with the use of oral contraceptives. Although these tumors are histologically benign, their danger lies in the risk of rupture of the capsule of the liver, leading to extensive bleeding and, possibly, death. With the current low-dose oral contraceptive combination, the risk for liver tumors is much lower.

- *Cancer:* The association of oral contraceptive use and breast cancer in young women is controversial. The Collaborative Group on Hormonal Factors in Breast Cancer demonstrated that current oral contraceptive users, and those who had used oral contraceptives within the past 1–4 years, had a slightly increased risk of breast cancer. Thus, although the consensus states that oral contraceptives can lead to breast cancer, the risk is small and the resulting tumors spread less aggressively than usual. Further, the risk becomes equal 10 years after stopping OC pill to normal age related risk without OCP.

- The relationship between oral contraceptive use and cervical cancer is also quite controversial. A weak association may exist between oral contraceptive use and squamous cell cancer of the cervix. Important risk factors include early sexual intercourse and exposure to the human papillomavirus. The overall consensus is that oral contraceptive use increases the risk of cervical neoplasia though it is a minimal risk. Thus, women who use oral contraceptives should have annual Pap tests.

Contraindications

- Cerebrovascular disease or coronary artery disease
- A history of deep vein thrombosis
- Pulmonary embolism, or congestive heart failure, untreated hypertension
- Diabetes with vascular complications
- Estrogen-dependent neoplasia; breast cancer
- Undiagnosed abnormal vaginal bleeding
- Known or suspected pregnancy
- Active liver disease
- Age older than 35 years and cigarette smoking.

Finally, drospirenone has antimineralocorticoid properties. It is contraindicated in patients with kidney or adrenal gland insufficiency or liver problems. Potassium levels should be checked during the first month of use, especially if drospirenone is taken daily with drugs that can increase potassium levels (e.g. nonsteroidal anti-inflammatory drugs, ACE inhibitors).

91-Day Combination Oral Contraceptives

Seasonale is a 91-day oral contraceptive regimen in which tablets containing the active hormones are taken for 12 weeks (84 days), followed by 1 week (7 day) of placebo tablets. With the Seasonale dosing regimen, the expected menstrual periods are reduced from once a month to approximately once every 3 months.

Although Seasonale users have fewer scheduled menstrual cycles, clinical trials show that many women, especially in the first few cycles of use, has more unplanned bleeding and spotting between the expected menstrual periods than women taking a conventional 28-day cycle of oral contraceptive.

To counteract the unplanned bleeding, a newer version of Seasonale (**Seasonique**) was developed. This new brand completely eliminates the hormone-free interval. Seasonique also has 84 active pills (30 μg of ethinyl estradiol and 150 μg of levonorgestrel) but is followed by 7 more active pills (10 μg ethinyl estradiol) instead of the traditional placebo. Therefore, no hormone-free weeks occur.

The two main advantages to replacing the placebo week with a week of low-dose estrogen are a diminished amount of unplanned bleeding and spotting and fewer or no symptoms (e.g. cramping, bloating, headaches) for women who are sensitive to the placebo-week hormone fluctuations (in particular, low estrogen). The risks of using **Seasonale** are similar to the risks of other conventional combination oral contraceptives and include an increased risk of blood clots, heart attack, and stroke.

Lybrel is the first FDA-approved oral contraceptive with 365-day combination dosing. It contains a low combined daily dose of the hormones levonorgestrel and ethinyl estradiol (90 μg and 20 μg, respectively). It provides women with more hormonal exposure on a yearly basis (13 additional weeks of hormone intake per year) than conventional cyclic oral contraceptives that contain the same strength of synthetic estrogens and similar strength of progestins.

The incidence of pill failure that results in pregnancy is approximately 1–2% per year (1–2 pregnancies per 100 women per year of use) if taken every day as directed. The average failure rate is approximately 5% per year (5 pregnancies per 100 women per year of use), including women who do not always take the pill exactly as directed without missing any pills.

Checklist for Oral Contraceptive Pill Use in Women 35 Years of Age

1. Check for any reason (**WHO criteria; Table 17.5**) that the patient should not take oral contraceptive pills.
2. Ask the patient about a history of headaches, hypertension and diabetes; ask about a family history of premature cardiovascular disease.
3. Measure the patient's blood pressure; in addition, measure the patient's fasting blood sugar, total cholesterol, high-density lipoprotein cholesterol, low-density lipoprotein cholesterol and triglyceride cholesterol levels.
4. Record the patient's height and weight; perform a breast examination, and consider mammography is age >35 years.
5. Ask the patient about smoking habits.

Missing pills: Figure 17.3 shows the recommendation to be followed.

Advantages and Disadvantages

Advantages of the pill include:

- It does not interrupt sex.
- It usually makes bleeds regular, lighter and less painful.
- It reduces risk of cancer of the ovaries, uterus and colon.
- It can reduce symptoms of premenstrual syndrome.
- It can sometimes reduce acne.
- It may protect against pelvic inflammatory disease.

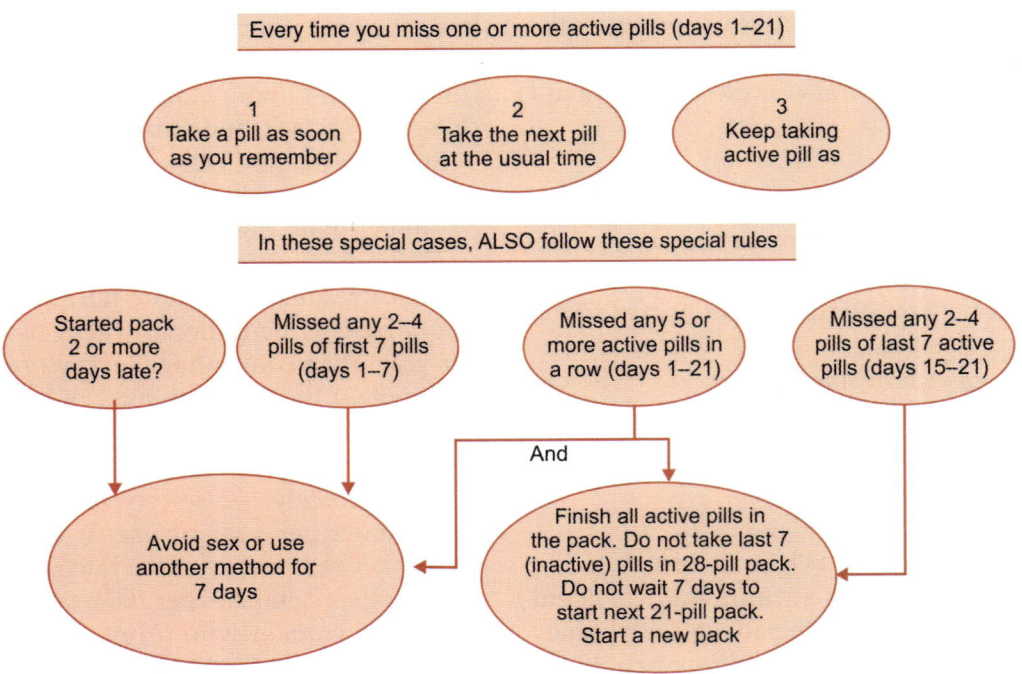

Fig. 17.3: Recommendations to be followed for missing pills

The World Health Organization (WHO) now promote a graded scheme of "precautions," rather than "contraindications," in considering which patients should not use oral contraception

Table 17.5: World Health Organization precautions for the use of oral contraceptive pills

Category 4 (refrain from use)	Category 3 (exercise caution)	Category 2 (advantages outweigh risks)	Category 1 (no restrictions)
Venous thromboembolism	Postpartum <21 days	Severe headaches after initiation of oral contraceptive pills	Postpartum ≥21 days
Cerebrovascular or coronary artery disease	Lactation (6 weeks to 6 months)		Postabortion, with abortion performed in first or second trimester
Structural heart disease	Undiagnosed vaginal or uterine bleeding	Diabetes mellitus	History of gestational diabetes
Diabetes with complications	Age >35 years and smoke fewer than 20 cigarettes per day	Major surgery without prolonged immobilization	Varicose veins
Breast cancer		Sickle-cell disease or sickle-cell- hemoglobin C disease	Mild headaches
Pregnancy		Blood pressure of 140/100 to 159/109 mm Hg	Irregular vaginal bleeding patterns without anemia
Lactation (<6 weeks postpartum)	History of breast cancer but no recurrence in past 5 years		Past history of PID
Liver disease	Interacting drugs	Undiagnosed breast mass	Current or recent history of PID
Headaches with focal neurologic symptoms	Gallbladder disease		Current or recent history of STD
			Vaginitis without purulent cervicitis
Major surgery with prolonged immobilization		Cervical cancer	Increased risk of STD
			HIV-positive or at high risk for HIV infection or AIDS
Age >35 years and smoke 20 cigarettes or more per day		Age >50 years	Benign breast disease
Hypertension (blood pressure of >160/100 mm Hg or with concomitant vascular disease)		Family history of lipid disorders	Family history of breast cancer or endometrial or ovarian cancer
			Cervical ectropion
		Family history of premature myocardial infarction	Viral hepatitis carrier
			Uterine fibroids
			Past ectopic pregnancy
			Obesity
			Thyroid conditions.

A careful personal and family medical history (with particular attention to cardiovascular risk factors) and an accurate **blood pressure** measurement are recommended before the initiation of oral contraceptive pills. A **physical examination including breast and Papanicolaou smear** (with screening genital cultures as indicated) are usually performed at the time oral contraceptive pills are initially prescribed.

- It may reduce the risk of fibroids, ovarian cysts and non-cancerous breast disease.

Disadvantages of the pill include:
- It can cause temporary side effects initially such as headaches, nausea, breast tenderness and mood.
- It can increase *blood pressure with prolonged use.*
- It does not protect against *sexually transmitted infections.*
- Breakthrough bleeding and spotting is common in the first few months of using the pill.
- It has been linked to an increased risk of some serious health conditions such as thrombosis (blood clots) and breast cancer.

In Special Situations

Age

>40 years: The risk of cardiovascular disease increases with age and may also increase with combined hormonal contraceptive use. In the absence of other adverse clinical conditions, combined low dose hormonal contraceptives can be used until menopause.

Postpartum

<21 days: There is some theoretical concern regarding the association between combined hormonal contraceptive use up to three weeks postpartum and risk of thrombosis in the mother. Blood coagulation and fibrinolysis are essentially normalized by three weeks postpartum.

Past Ectopic Pregnancy

The risk of future ectopic pregnancy is increased among women who have had an ectopic pregnancy in the past. Combined hormonal contraceptives provide protection against pregnancy including ectopic gestation.

Deep Vein Thrombosis/Pulmonary Embolism

Family history of DVT/PE (first-degree relatives): some conditions which increase the risk of DT/PE are heritable.

Superficial Venous Thrombosis

Varicose veins are not risk factors for DVT/PE.

Valvular Heart Disease

Among women with valvular heart disease, combined hormonal contraceptive use may further increase the risk of arterial thrombosis; women with complicated valvular heart disease are at greatest risk.

Headaches

Aura is a specific focal neurologic symptom. Migraine is a relative condraindication.

Vaginal Bleeding Patterns

Irregular menstrual bleeding patterns are common among healthy women.

Unexplained Vaginal Bleeding

There are no conditions that cause vaginal bleeding which will be worsened in the short term by use of combined hormonal contraceptives.

Cervical Ectropion

Cervical ectropion is not a risk factor for cervical cancer, and there is no need for restriction of combined hormonal contraceptive use.

Cervical Cancer

There is some theoretical concern that combined hormonal contraceptive use may affect prognosis of the existing disease. While awaiting treatment, women may use combined hormonal contraceptives. In general, treatment of this condition renders a woman sterile.

Breast Disease

Breast cancer: Breast cancer is a hormonally sensitive tumor, and the prognosis of women with current or recent breast cancer may worsen with combined hormonal contraceptive use.

Endometrial Cancer

COC use reduces the risk of developing endometrial cancer. While awaiting treatment, women may use COCs, CICs, patch or ring. In general, treatment of this condition renders a woman sterile.

Ovarian Cancer

COC use reduces the risk of developing ovarian cancer. While awaiting treatment, women may use COCs, CICs, patch or ring. In general, treatment of this condition is hysterectomy along with bilateral ovariotomy and does not need contraception further.

Uterine Fibroids

COCs do not appear to cause growth of uterine fibroids, as well as CICs, patch and ring.

Table 17.6: Factors to consider in starting or switching oral contraceptive pills	
Objective	*Action*
To minimize high risk of thrombosis	Select a product with a lower dosage of estrogen
To minimize nausea, breast tenderness or vascular headaches	Select a product with a lower dosage of estrogen
To minimize spotting or breakthrough bleeding	Select a product with a higher dosage of estrogen or a progestin with greater potency
To minimize androgenic effects	Select a product containing a third-generation progestin, low-dose nore-thindrone or ethynodiol diacetate.
To avoid dyslipidemia	Select a product containing a third-generation progestin, low-dose nore-thindrone or ethynodiol diacetate.

Pelvic Inflammatory Disease (PID)

COCs may reduce the risk of PID among women with STIs, but do not protect against HIV or lower genital tract STIs. Whether CICs, patch or ring reduce the risk of PID among women with STIs is unknown but they do not protect against HIV or lower genital tract STIs. Table 17.6 considers selection of different pill formulations according to patients medical profile.

Gallbladder Disease

COCs, CICs, patch or ring may cause a small increased risk of gallbladder disease. There is also concern that COCs, CICs, patch or ring may worsen existing gall-bladder disease. However, unlike COCs, CICs have been shown to have minimal effect on liver function in healthy women, and have no first-pass effect on the liver.

History of Cholestasis

a. *Pregnancy related:* History of pregnancy-related cholestasis may predict an increased risk of developing COC-related cholestasis.
b. *History of cholestasis:* Past history of COC related cholestasis predicts an increased risk with subsequent COC use.

Liver Tumors

There is no evidence regarding hormonal contraceptive use among women with hepatocellular adenoma. COC use in healthy women is associated with development and growth of hepatocellular adenoma.

Thalassemia

There is anecdotal evidence from countries where thalassemia is prevalent that COC use does not worsen the condition.

Iron-deficiency Anemia

Combined hormonal contraceptive use may decrease menstrual blood loss.

Potential Interactions between Oral Contraceptive Pills and Selected Drugs

Drug decreases effectiveness of oral contraceptive pills	
• Amoxicillin	• Ampicillin
• Carbamazepine	• Ethosuximide
• Metronidazole	• Phenobarbital
• Phenytoin	• Primidone
• Rifampin	• Tetracycline
• Troglitazone	
Oral contraceptive pills decrease effectiveness of drug	
• Clofibrate	• Lorazepam
• Oxazepam	• Salicylates
• Temazepam	
Oral contraceptive pills potentiate effect of drug	
• Benzodiazepines	• Beta blockers
• Caffeine	• Corticosteroids
• Theophylline	

Summary of Key Recommendations (Faculty of Sexual and Reproductive Health Care Clinical Guidance, 2012)

I. What should be discussed with women when prescribing drugs to women using hormonal contraception?

Health professionals supplying hormonal contraception should ask women about their current and previous drug use including prescription, over the counter, herbal, recreational drugs and dietary supplements.

II. Advice for women using drugs that may reduce contraceptive efficacy (Fig. 17.4)

- All women starting enzyme-inducing drugs should be advised to use a reliable contraceptive method unaffected by enzyme inducers [e.g. progestogen-only injectable, copper-bearing intrauterine devices (Cu-IUDs) or the levonorgestrel containing intrauterine system (LNG-IUS)].
- With the exception of the very potent enzyme inducers rifampicin and rifabutin, women who are

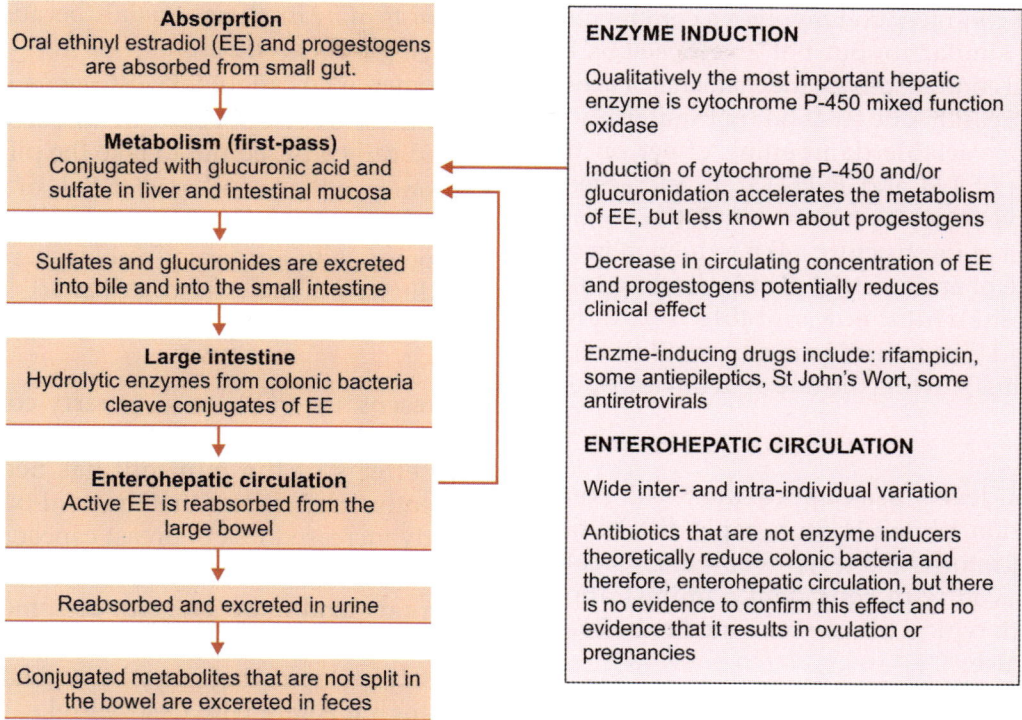

Fig. 17.4: Drug interaction with hormonal contraceptive and pharmacokinetics of hormonal contraceptives

on an enzyme-inducing drug and who do not wish to change from COC may increase the dose of COC to at least 50 µg EE (maximum 70 µg) and use an extended or tricyclic regimen with a pill-free interval of 4 days.

- Women who do not wish to change from the progestogen-only pill (POP) or implant while on short-term treatment with an enzyme-inducing drug or within 28 days of stopping treatment may opt to continue the method together with additional contraceptive precautions (e.g. condoms).
- Women using enzyme-inducing drugs who require emergency contraception (EC) should be advised of the potential interactions with oral methods and offered a Cu IUD.
- Women who request oral EC while using enzyme-inducing drugs or within 28 days of stopping them, should be advised to take a total of 3 mg LNG (two 1.5 mg tablets) as a single dose as soon as possible and within 120 hours of unprotected sexual intercourse though use of LNG >72 hours after intercourse and double dose are off label use.
- **Ulipristal acetate (UPA)** is not advised in women using enzyme-inducing drugs or who have taken them within the last 28 days. Women should be advised that UPA has the potential to reduce the efficacy of hormonal contraception. Additional precautions are advised for 14 days after taking UPA.

- Women using drugs that have effect on gastric pH (e.g. antacids, H_2 antagonists and proton pump inhibitors) and who require EC should be offered a CuIUD or LNG as the efficacy of UPA may be reduced.

What advice should be given to women using hormonal contraception and antibacterial drugs that are not enzyme inducers?

Additional contraceptive precautions are not required during or after courses of antibiotics that do not induce enzymes. Women should be advised about the importance of correct contraceptive practice during periods of illness.

Effect of contraceptive hormones on drug metabolism: Women on **lamotrigine monotherapy** should be advised that due to the risk of reduced seizure control whilst on combined hormonal contraception (CHC), and the potential for toxicity in the CHC-free week, the risks of using CHC may outweigh the benefits.

Progestin-only Oral Contraceptives

Progestin-only oral contraceptives, also known as minipills, are not used widely. Less than 1% of users of oral contraceptives use them as their sole method of contraception. Candidates for use include women who are breastfeeding and women with contraindications to estrogen use.

Prevention of contraception involves a combination of mechanisms similar to, but not as efficacious as, combination oral contraceptives. Mechanisms of action include (1) suppression of ovulation (not uniformly in all cycles), (2) a variable dampening effect on the midcycle peaks of LH and FSH, (3) an increase in cervical mucus viscosity by a reduction in its volume and an alteration of its structure, (4) a reduction in the number and size of endometrial glands, leading to an atrophic endometrium not suitable for ovum implantation, and (5) a reduction in cilia motility in the fallopian tube, thus slowing the rate of ovum transport.

Efficacy

Serum progestin levels peak approximately 2 hours after administration. Within 24 hours, rapid distribution and elimination returns the level to baseline. Greater efficacy is achieved with consistent administration. Failure rates with typical use are estimated to be 7% in the first year of use.

Advantages

Due to the lack of estrogen, evidence of serious complications to which estrogen can contribute (i.e. thromboembolism) is minimal. Noncontraceptive benefits include decreased dysmenorrhea, decreased menstrual blood loss, and decreased premenstrual symptoms. Unlike DMPA, fertility is immediately reestablished after the cessation of progestin-only oral contraceptives.

Disadvantages

The most significant disadvantage is the continuous need for compliance with usage. Users need to be counseled on the need for a backup method of contraception, if a pill is missed or taken late. A pill is considered late, if ingestion occurs 3 hours after the established time of administration. If a pill is missed, it should be taken as soon as possible; the next pill should be taken at the scheduled time. Backup contraception should be used for the next 48 hours. Unscheduled bleeding and spotting are common even with correct use. Other adverse effects include nausea, breast tenderness, headache, and amenorrhea.

What special categories of women take the mini-pill?

Although nearly all women can use the mini-pill, if they want to, in practice it is commonly taken by people who would have difficulties with the ordinary pill. These include:

- *Breastfeeding* mothers—mainly because the pill tends to stop milk production.
- Women who cannot take estrogens
- Women over 35 years of age who have been medically advised not to take the pill.
- Women who are at special risk of *heart disease* or strokes.
- Women who are heavy smokers—*smoking* and the ordinary pill may cause *heart attacks* or clots

What are the side effects of the mini-pill?

At present, the POP seems to carry considerably less risk than the ordinary pill though research into long-term effects of the mini-pill has been rather less. Currently, it is believed that the mini-pill might carry a slightly increased risk of breast cancer.

The chief known side effects are:
- Periods tend to be irregular or sometimes produce amenorrhea.
- Risk of ectopic pregnancy in POP failed pregnancy though it is rare with desogestrel.
- Acne and skin pigmentation
- Breast tenderness
- Small risk of cysts in the ovaries–indeed, it is best not to use the POP in woman with ovarian cyst
- Nausea, headache, dizziness, depression and weight change.

Who shouldn't take the mini-pill?

This should not be taken by women with:
- Undiagnosed vaginal bleeding
- Severe artery disease
- Liver tumors
- Acute intermittent porphyria
- History of breast cancer
- Should only be used 'with caution' by certain women with history of previous ectopic pregnancy.

What are the various kinds of mini-pill?

The brands are:
Group 1 : Contains norethisterone.
Group 2: Contains ethynediol diacetate.
Group 3: Contains levonorgestrel.
Group 4 :.Contains desogestrel.

In 2009, the Royal College of Obstetricians' and Gynaecologists' Faculty of Sexual and Reproductive Health Care issued new guidelines about the mini-pill. The essence of them is as follows:

1. The mini-pill should not be used by women who currently have breast cancer.

2. A proper clinical history is taken from the woman to make sure it is safe for her.

3. If taken properly, the mini-pill is over 99 per cent effective.

4. At present, there is no evidence that one mini-pill is better than another.

5. If a woman vomits within two hours of taking a mini-pill, then another one should be taken as soon as possible.

6. Women who are using drugs called 'liver enzyme-inducers' must be told that the effectiveness of the mini-pill may be reduced by them.

7. After stopping the mini-pill, there is no delay in return of fertility.

8. The mini-pill commonly causes changes in menstrual patterns, and that 20% of females will have no bleeding.

9. There is no scientific evidence that the mini-pill causes weight gain, depression, or headache.

10. The mini-pill can be used up to age of 55. If a woman wants to use it after that age, she should have her blood levels of hormone checked to see, if it is still necessary.

Desogestrel-only Pill

This new progestogen-only pill (POP) is licenced in 2002. Each tablet contains 75 µg of desogestrel, which is metabolized to etonorgestrel. Etonorgestrel is a selective progestogen with high affinity for progesterone receptors and low affinity for androgen receptors.

How does the desogestrel-only pill work?

It inhibits ovulation in 97% of cycles. Thick cervical mucus changes in women using desogestrel daily are evident (by Insler score for hostility to sperm) but this is likely to be less important contraceptive action.

How should the desogestrel-only pill be taken?

Recent recommendations from the World Health Organization (WHO), however, have suggested that POPs can be started up to day 5 without the need for barrier methods, as the risk of ovulation is acceptably low. Steady-state levels of hormone are achieved within 4–5 days and maximal cervical mucus effects occur in about 2 days. Barrier contraception should be advised for 48 hours following pill starts after day 5 or following missed pills. The half-life of desogestrel is about 30 hours and pills should be taken every day without omission. A delay of more than 3 hours (27 hours since the last dose) should be treated as a missed pill and barrier contraception used until two consecutive pills have been taken. Although ovulation inhibition appears to be the primary mode of action, it is advised to take tablets daily within 3 hours of the same time every day.

How effective is the desogestrel-only pill?

The overall failure rate of desogestrel (including those women who are breastfeeding and poor compliers) is 0.41 per 100 women-years and for levonorgestrel 1.55 per 100 woman-years. Pearl index calculated in non-breastfed women is 0.17 for desogestrel and 1.41 for levonorgestrel.

What are the contraindications for use of the desogestrel-only pill?

WHO Medical Eligibility Criteria for all POPs suggest few absolute contraindications for use. A WHO Classification 3 (theoretical risks outweigh benefits) is given for current deep vein thrombosis or pulmonary embolism; past history of breast cancer; severe active liver disease; malignant hepatoma and liver enzyme inducing drugs (due to reduced efficacy). This is true for desogestrel-only pills also.

What are the side effects of the desogestrel-only pill?

1. *Irregular bleeding pattern:* Discontinuation rates due to abnormal bleeding, however, is similar: 22.5% for desogestrel and 18% for levonorgestrel.

2. Headache, acne, breast pain, nausea, vaginitis and dysmenorrhea.

3. In more than 1% women suffer from mood changes and decreased libido

4. About 0.1% women may have vomiting, alopecia, fatigue, rash urticaria, erythema nodosum and problems with contact lenses.

5. *Ectopic risk:* No ectopic pregnancies are reported with its use.

What does this new desogestrel-only pill add to current contraceptive choice for women?

POPs are used by only 5% of women. POPs may be the method of choice for (a) older women, (b) Postpartum women who are breastfeeding. This new desogestrel-only pill has been shown to reliably inhibit ovulation in 97% of cycles with Pearl index of 0.41. In contrast, levonorgestrel-only POP inhibit ovulation in 71% of cycles with Pearl index of 1.55.

Combination Patch Contraceptive

The contraceptive transdermal patch releases estrogen and progesterone directly into the skin. Each patch contains a 1-week supply of hormones of both norelgestromin and ethinyl estradiol. It releases a sustained low daily dose of steroids equivalent to the lowest-dose oral contraceptive. The failure rate for the patch is 1 pregnancy per 100 women per year, similar to that of other combination methods. Advantages include greater compliance and decreased adverse effects, such as nausea and vomiting, due to the avoidance of the first-pass effect. However, the patch may cause skin irritation, and, if it is removed unnoticed, this may compromise efficacy. Disadvantages and contraindications are similar to those of combination oral contraceptives. It may be less effective in obese women.

Contraceptive Vaginal Ring

The actual design of vaginal rings as a mode of contraception was first developed in the 1970s. The vaginal rings can deliver progesterone or progesterone-estrogen combinations. Today, the combination contraceptive vaginal ring is a new form of contraception that is approved by FDA in 2001.

NuvaRing (Fig. 17.5), a vaginal contraceptive ring, is a nonbiodegradable, flexible, colorless ring made up of a polymer of ethylene vinyl acetate and magnesium stearate. The outer diameter of the ring is 54 mm and the cross-sectional diameter is 4 mm. The ring contains 11.7 mg of etonogestrel and 2.7 mg of ethinyl estradiol.

It releases 120 µg of etonogestrel and 15 µg of ethinyl estradiol each day. The hormones are released slowly and are absorbed directly from vagina.

The ring is used in the same schedule as oral contraceptives, with 3 weeks of ring usage (ring is left in place for 3 wk) and 1 week without to produce a withdrawal bleed. The ring can be inserted any time during the first 5 days of the menstrual cycle. The ring should be placed in the vagina, even if the woman has not finished bleeding, and she should use a backup contraceptive method for 7 days. A new ring should be inserted each month. If the ring comes out during the first 3 weeks of use, it should be washed with lukewarm water and replaced. If the ring-free interval is more than 3 hours, a backup contraceptive method should be used for 7 days. The ring should never be left in the vagina for more than 4 weeks. If left in for more than 4 weeks, pregnancy should be excluded before inserting a new ring and a backup contraceptive method should be used for 7 days after inserting a new ring.

Advantages

NuvaRing is highly effective because it results in complete suppression of ovulation. The steady release of hormone provides exceptional cycle control. The ring is a very effective reversible method of birth control. With typical use, the ring is presumed to be more effective than combination oral contraceptives. With typical usage, 8 of 100 pill users become pregnant; with perfect use of the NuvaRing, fewer than 1 of 100 women becomes pregnant.

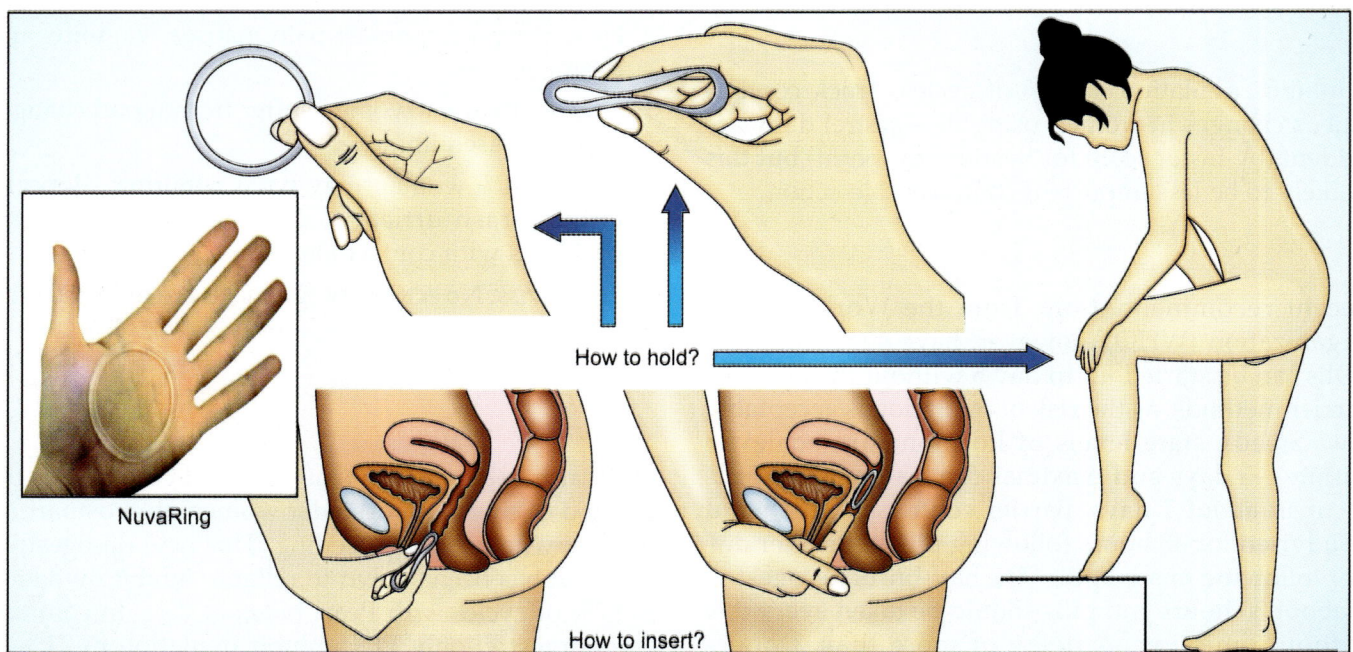

NuvaRing

How to hold?

How to insert?

Fig. 17.5: Insertion of NuvaRing

Since daily intake is not needed in NuvaRing contraception, can be easily inserted and removed by the woman herself, and because return of fertility is rapid upon discontinuation, NuvaRing is a highly acceptable method for women and their partners. Because the hormones are absorbed directly into the blood through the vaginal mucosa, the hepatic first-pass metabolism of progestin is prevented. The ring delivers the lowest dose of ethinyl estradiol compared with other combined hormonal contraceptives. Unlike combined oral contraceptives, the adverse effects of nausea and vomiting are avoided with ring use. It is assumed that the noncontraceptive advantages associated with the NuvaRing will be similar to those known to be associated with the combination oral contraceptives.

Disadvantages

Adverse effects include headaches and vaginal irritation or discharge. The ring may accidentally slip out during intercourse and either the user or the partner may feel the ring during sexual intercourse. Contraindications are similar to those of combined oral contraceptives.

Implants

FDA approved levonorgestrel implant (Norplant) as contraceptive in 1990. This method consists of 6 silicone rubber rods, each measuring 34 mm long and 2.4 mm in diameter and each containing 36 mg of levonorgestrel. The implant releases approximately 80 µg of levonorgestrel per 24 hours during the first year of use, achieving effective serum concentrations of 0.4–0.5 ng/mL within the first 24 hours. The rate of release decreases to an average of 30 µg/day in later years of use. Release of the progestational agent by diffusion provides effective contraception for 5 years. Contraceptive protection begins within 24 hours of insertion, if inserted during the first week of the menstrual cycle. The rods are inserted subcutaneously, usually in the woman's upper arm, where they are visible under the skin and can be easily palpated.

The mechanism of action is a combination of suppression of the LH surge, suppression of ovulation, development of viscous and scant cervical mucus to deter sperm penetration, and prevention of endometrial growth and development.

Efficacy

The contraceptive efficacy of the method is similar to that of surgical sterilization. Overall, pregnancy rates increase from 0.2% in the first year to 1.1% by the fifth year.

Advantages

The long-term effectiveness is an advantage. It is not related to its use in regard to coitus. Exogenous estrogen is absent. Prompt return to the previous state of fertility occurs upon removal. No adverse effect on breast milk production occurs.

Disadvantages

A minor surgical procedure is necessary for incision. Difficulty in removal is a disadvantage. Menstrual irregularities are common along with other adverse effects, including headaches, mood changes, hirsutism, galactorrhea, and acne.

Absolute contraindications include active thrombophlebitis or thromboembolic disease, undiagnosed genital bleeding, acute liver disease, benign or malignant liver tumors, known or suspected breast cancer, and history of idiopathic intracranial hypertension. Relative contraindications include heavy cigarette smoking, history of ectopic pregnancy, diabetes mellitus, hypercholesterolemia, severe acne, hypertension, and history of cardiovascular disease, severe vascular or migraine headaches, and severe depression.

Appropriate candidates are women who are postpartum or breastfeeding, women who have less contraceptive compliance, women in whom pregnancy is contraindicated due to a medical condition, and patients with contraindications to the use of estrogen.

Another FDA-approved implant is the 2-rod levonorgestrel system, termed Norplant II. Each rod is 4.4 cm long and contains a homogenous mixture of the drug and a polydimethylsiloxane elastomer covered by silicone tubing. Norplant II is approved for 3 years of use but has been shown to be effective for as long as 5 years.

Implanon is a single-rod implant that is 4 cm long and 2 mm in diameter. It consists of 68 mg of etonogestrel in an ethylene vinyl acetate copolymer core. **Etonogestrel** is a biologically active metabolite of desogestrel. Desogestrel is significantly more potent than levonorgestrel; a serum concentration of 0.09 ng/mL can inhibit ovulation in most women. Serum concentrations are adequate for contraception coverage for approximately 3 years. However, etonogestrel implant may be less effective in women who are overweight.

Compared with the Norplant system, Implanon is associated with a higher frequency of amenorrhea and oligomenorrhea, a decrease in the prevalence of frequent and prolonged bleeding, and a decrease in the frequency of adverse effects such as weight gain, headache, and acne. When the rod is removed, the return to fertility is rapid, with the return of ovulation within 3 weeks. However, Implanon is not associated with loss of bone mineral density (BMD).

Injectable Depot Medroxyprogesterone Acetate (DMPA)

DMPA is a suspension of a synthetic progestin that is injected intramuscularly. Pharmacologically active levels are achieved within 24 hours after injection, and serum concentrations of 1 ng/mL are maintained for 3 months. During the fifth or sixth month after injection, the levels decrease to 0.2 ng/mL, and they become undetectable by 7–9 months after injection.

DMPA acts by the inhibition of ovulation with the suppression of FSH and LH levels and eliminates the LH surge. This results in a relative hypoestrogenic state. Single doses of 150 mg suppress ovulation in most women for as long as 14 weeks. The contraceptive regimen consists of 1 dose every 3 months.

Efficacy

DMPA is an extremely effective contraceptive option. Neither varying weight nor use of concurrent medications has been noted to alter efficacy. Within the first year of use, the failure rate is 0.3%.

Advantages

- DMPA does not produce the serious adverse effects of estrogen, such as thromboembolism.
- Anemia improves because of reduced blood loss.
- Dysmenorrhea improves.
- The risks of endometrial and ovarian cancer are decreased.
- It is safe for breastfeeding mothers.

Disadvantages

- Disruption of the menstrual cycle to eventual amenorrhea occurs in 50% of women within the first year. Persistent irregular bleeding can be treated by administering the subsequent dose earlier or by prescribing temporary low-dose estrogen therapy.
- Because DMPA persists in the body for several months in women it can delay the return to fertility. Approximately 70% of users desiring pregnancy conceive within 12 months, and 90% of users conceive within 24 months of stopping the drug.
- Adverse effects, such as weight gain, depression, and menstrual irregularities, may continue for as long as 1 year after the last injection.

- Bone loss may not be completely reversible even after stopping inj. DMPA (FDA, 2004). Therefore, women are advised not to use Depo-Provera for long. But recent studies have contradicted the FDA warning. Women who have stopped using DMPA experience an average bone gain of 1.34% at the hip versus a loss of 0.19% for women who have never taken the drug. Spine density has increased 2.86% for women who have stopped using the drug, compared with an increase of 1.32% for nonusers.
- A subcutaneous version of the drug is now available (depo-subQ provera 104) that delivers a lower dose of medroxyprogesterone acetate (MPA) than does the intramuscular formulation (104 mg vs 150 mg). The subcutaneous route opens the possibility for home self-injections, and the lower dose can decrease suppression of pituitary function and ovarian estradiol production effectively for a month.
- Subcutaneous DMPA is also associated with lower decreases in bone mineral density as compared with the intramuscular route and possess the same reversible effect.

The clinician making an assessment of women using hormonal contraception with unscheduled bleeding should:

- Take a detailed clinical history
- Exclude sexually transmitted infections (STIs)
- Check the cervical screening history
- Do a urine pregnancy test.
  1. A clinical history should be taken from women using hormonal contraception with unscheduled bleeding to identify the possibility of an underlying cause. (Grade C)
  2. Hormonal contraceptive users with unscheduled bleeding who are at risk of STIs (i.e. those aged <25 years old, or who have a new sexual partner, or more than one partner in the last year) should be tested for *C. trachomatis* as a minimum. Testing for *N. gonorrhoeae* will depend on sexual risk and local prevalence.(Good Practice Point—GPP)
  3. Women using hormonal contraception who have unscheduled bleeding should have a cervical screen. (GPP)
  4. A pregnancy test is indicated for women using hormonal contraception with unscheduled bleeding, if the clinical history identifies the possibility of incorrect method use, drug interactions or illness, which may lead to malabsorption of oral hormones. (GPP)

When examination may NOT be required?

Unscheduled bleeding in the first 3 months after starting a new hormonal contraceptive method is common.

Genital examination is not required, if after taking a clinical history there are no risk factors for STIs, no concurrent symptoms suggestive of underlying causes, and the woman is participating in a national cervical screening program. Some women may be happy to continue with the method after this initial assessment but follow-up should be planned as bleeding may persist.

When is examination required?

Provided, there has been consistent and correct use of hormonal contraception, pelvic examination is warranted to visualize the cervix by speculum examination:

- For persistent bleeding beyond the first 3 months use
- For new symptoms or a change in bleeding after at least 3 months use of a method
- If the woman has not participated in a National Cervical Screening Programme
- If requested by the woman
- After a failed trial of the limited medical management available
- If there are other symptoms such as pain, dyspareunia or postcoital bleeding when these symptoms would also warrant bimanual examination).

Provided there has been consistent and correct use of hormonal contraception, a speculum examination and a bimanual examination should be performed for women using hormonal contraception with unscheduled bleeding if they have: persistent bleeding or a change in bleeding after at least 3 months use; failed medical treatment; if they have not participated in a National Cervical Screening Programme or if they have other symptoms (such as pain, dyspareunia or heavy bleeding (Good Practice Point).

How to manage unscheduled bleeding in women on OC pills?

Figures 17.6 and 17.7 show the management of unscheduled bleeding in women on OC pills.

When is further investigation (endometrial biopsy, ultrasound scan or hysteroscopy) required?

- In general, an endometrial biopsy should be considered in women aged >45 years (or in women aged <45 years with risk factors for endometrial cancer (e.g. obesity or polycystic ovarian syndrome) who have persistent unscheduled bleeding after the first 3 months of starting a method or who present with a change in bleeding pattern. (GPP)
- Nevertheless, for all women using hormonal contraception with unscheduled bleeding, if such a structural abnormality is suspected a transvaginal ultrasound scan and/or hysteroscopy may be indicated. (GPP)
- It is not generally recommended that a combined oral contraceptive pill is changed within the first 3 months of use as bleeding disturbances often settle in this time. (GPP)
- For women using a combined oral contraceptive, pill the lowest dose of ethinyl estradiol (EE) to provide good cycle control should be used. However, the dose of EE can be increased to a maximum of 35 µg to provide good cycle control. (GPP)
- Bleeding is common in the initial months of progestogen-only method use and may settle without treatment. If treatment may encourage women to continue with the method, it may be considered. (GPP)
- For women with unscheduled bleeding using a progestogen-only injectable, implant or IUS who wish to continue with the method and are medically eligible, a COC may be used for up to 3 months in the usual cyclic manner or continuously without a pill-free interval. (GPP)
- For women using a progestogen-only injectable contraceptive with unscheduled bleeding, mefenamic acid 500 mg twice or thrice daily for 5 days can reduce the length of a bleeding episode but has little effect on bleeding in the longer term. (Grade B)

Very recently, 50 mg mifepristone every 2 weeks increases endometrial estrogen receptors and reduces breakthrough bleeding in new users of both DMPA and LNG implant. Treatment with doxycycline inhibits matrix metalloproteinase which plays a regulatory role in the breakdown of endometrium to produce normal menstruation.

Alternatively, a regime of mifepristone 25 mg twice a day for one day followed by EE 20 µg twice a day for 5 days reduces bleeding days by about 50%.

Intrauterine Devices

Description

Although intrauterine device (IUD) is a highly effective method of contraception, it is used by less than 2% of women of reproductive age. The reason for such a small

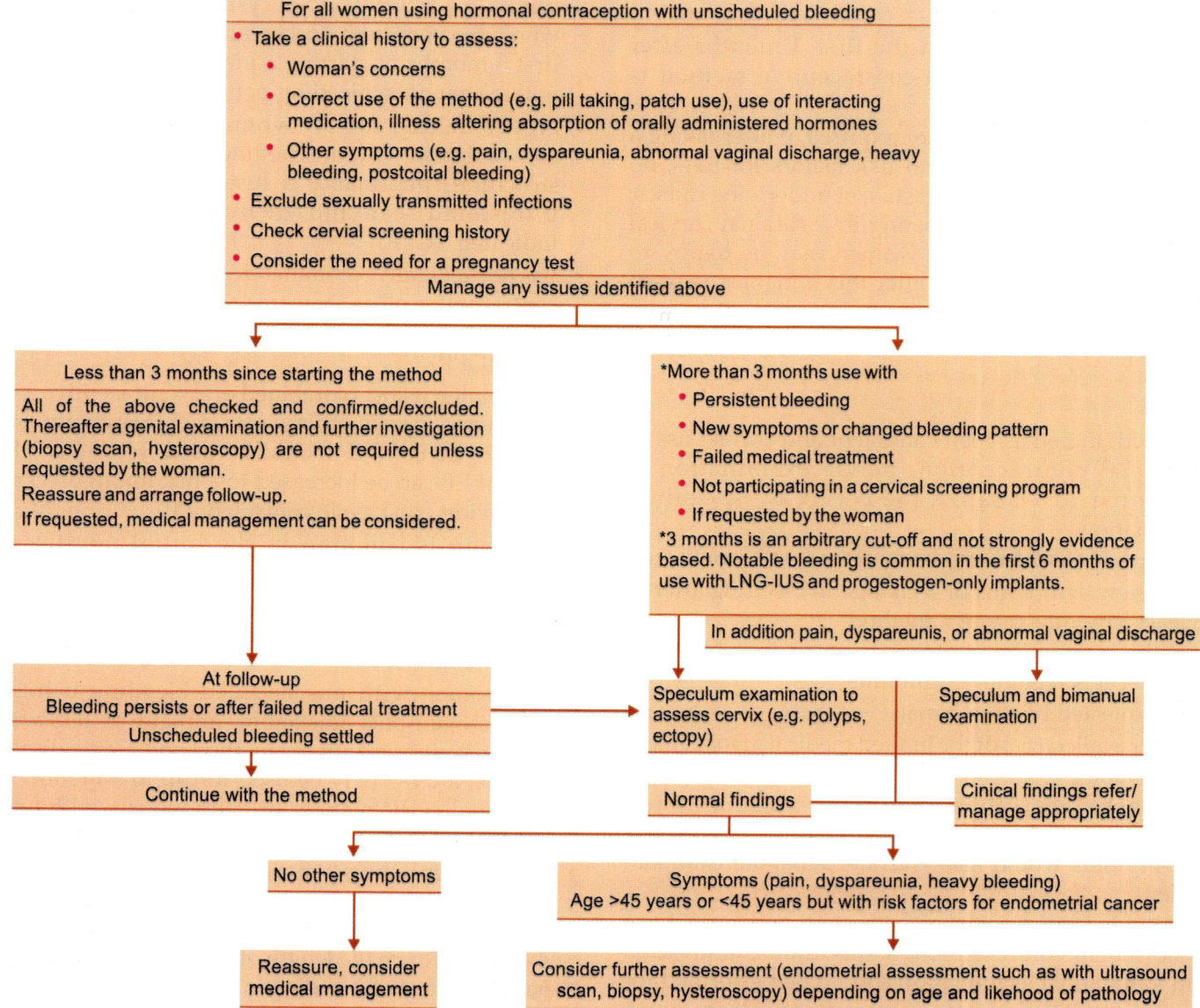

For all women using hormonal contraception with unscheduled bleeding
- Take a clinical history to assess:
  - Woman's concerns
  - Correct use of the method (e.g. pill taking, patch use), use of interacting medication, illness altering absorption of orally administered hormones
  - Other symptoms (e.g. pain, dyspareunia, abnormal vaginal discharge, heavy bleeding, postcoital bleeding)
- Exclude sexually transmitted infections
- Check cervial screening history
- Consider the need for a pregnancy test

Manage any issues identified above

Less than 3 months since starting the method
All of the above checked and confirmed/excluded. Thereafter a genital examination and further investigation (biopsy scan, hysteroscopy) are not required unless requested by the woman.
Reassure and arrange follow-up.
If requested, medical management can be considered.

*More than 3 months use with
- Persistent bleeding
- New symptoms or changed bleeding pattern
- Failed medical treatment
- Not participating in a cervical screening program
- If requested by the woman
*3 months is an arbitrary cut-off and not strongly evidence based. Notable bleeding is common in the first 6 months of use with LNG-IUS and progestogen-only implants.

In addition pain, dyspareunis, or abnormal vaginal discharge

At follow-up
Bleeding persists or after failed medical treatment
Unscheduled bleeding settled

Speculum examination to assess cervix (e.g. polyps, ectopy)

Speculum and bimanual examination

Continue with the method

Normal findings

Cinical findings refer/manage appropriately

No other symptoms

Symptoms (pain, dyspareunia, heavy bleeding)
Age >45 years or <45 years but with risk factors for endometrial cancer

Reassure, consider medical management

Consider further assessment (endometrial assessment such as with ultrasound scan, biopsy, hysteroscopy) depending on age and likelihood of pathology

Fig. 17.6: Management of unscheduled bleeding in women on OC pills

percentage stems from the fear of bleeding, sepsis and uterine perforation.

Currently, only 2 IUDs are available; one is Copper T380A and levonorgestrel intrauterine system marked as Mirena. Figure 17.8 shows early IUDs which were not available now.

The T-shaped progesterone-releasing IUD Progestasert, which is placed into the uterine cavity, is made of ethylene vinyl acetate copolymer. It contains 38 mg of progesterone and minimal amounts of barium sulfate for greater visibility on X-ray films. The vertical limbs are 36 mm long, and the horizontal arms are 32 mm wide. It has a pair of dark-blue double-strings that hang from the lower limb. Approximately 65 µg/day of progesterone is released from the progesterone form

from a reservoir in its stem. This is a sufficient amount of hormone to last for 400 days; therefore, this IUD must be replaced yearly.

The Copper T380 was introduced in 1988. The T-shaped IUD is made of polyethylene with fine copper wire wrapped around the vertical stem. The string is clear or white and hangs from the lower limb of the IUD. This device consists of 308 mg of copper covering portions of its stem and arms. Contraceptive effectiveness continues for 10 years, after which time it must be replaced.

Mirena is similar in shape to the Copper T380 in that it also consists of a small T-shaped frame with a reservoir that contains levonorgestrel, a progesterone. This intrauterine system releases 20 µg of levonorgestrel

Medical therapy options for women using hormonal contraception with unscheduled bleeding
(Based on expert clinical judgment of the multidisciplinary group developing this Guidance)

Combined hormonal contraceptive users	Progestogen-only pill users	Progestogen-only implants, injectable or intrauterine system
In general, continue with the same pill for at least 3 months as bleeding may settle in this time.	May try a different POP although there is no evidence that changing the progestogen type or increasing the dose improves bleeding.	A first-line COC (30–35 mg EE with levonorgestrel or norethisterone) may be considered for up to 3 months continuously or in the usual cyclical regimen (unlicensed).
Use a COC with a dose of EE to provide the best cycle control.		No evidence reducing injection interval for DMPA improves bleeding, however, the injection can be given up to 2 weeks early.
May consider increasing the EE dose up to a maximum of 35 mg.	No evidence that desogestrel-only pills have better bleeding patterns than traditional POPs.	
May try a different COC but no evidence that one better than other in terms of cycle control.	No evidence to support the use of two POPs per day to improve bleeding.	Mefenamic acid 500 mg thrice daily for 5 days for women with bleeding on DMPA to reduce the duration of the bleeding interval, no long-term benefit.
No evidence changing progrestogen dose or type improves cycle control but may help on an individual basis.		
There are no data on managing bleeding associated with the patch. Continue for at least 3 months as bleeding may settle in this time.		

Fig. 17.7: Treatment options for women using hormonal contraceptive with unscheduled bleeding

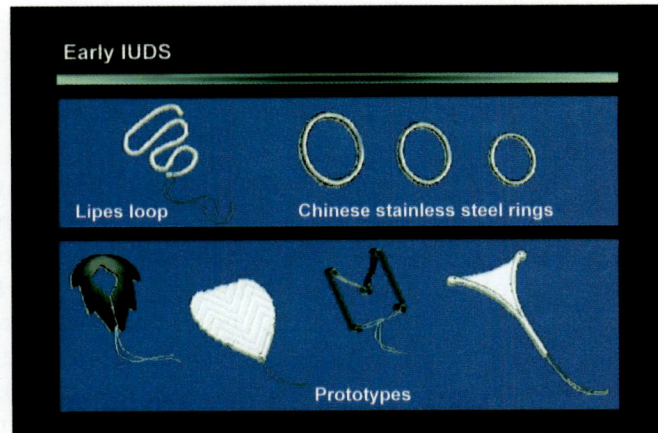

Fig. 17.8: Early days' IUD

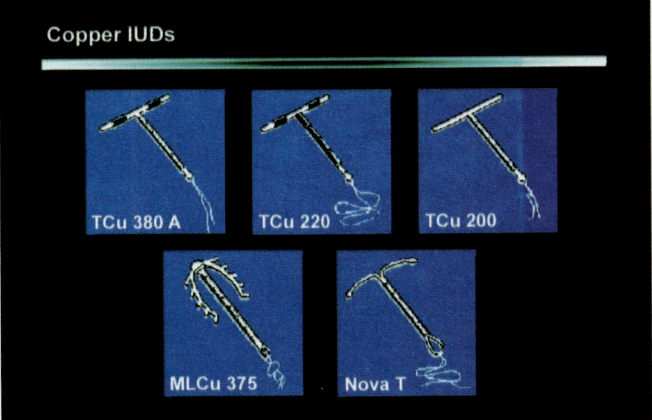

Fig. 17.9: Different types of copper IUD

per day into the uterine cavity for as long as 5 years. It consists of a polyethylene frame with a cylinder containing a polydimethylsiloxane-levonorgestrel mixture enveloping the vertical arm. The cylinder is coated with a membrane that regulates the release of the hormone. This model is also visible on X-ray films. The Mirena is now FDA approved for treating menorrhagia as well (Fig. 17.9).

Efficacy

The failure rate is 0.6% with the Copper T380, and of 0.1% with Mirena, respectively.

Advantages

- IUDs produce no adverse systemic effects.
- Ectopic pregnancies are reduced overall; however, the ratio of extrauterine to intrauterine pregnancy is increased, if conception does occur.
- Menstrual blood loss and dysmenorrhea are decreased with Progestasert. Twenty percent of women experience amenorrhea with Mirena.

Disadvantages

- IUDs are associated with a risk of uterine perforation at the time of insertion.

- Increased dysmenorrhea occurs with the Copper T380.
- Increased menstrual blood loss occurs in the first a few cycles with use of the Copper T380 and Mirena IUDs.
- Whether IUDs increase the risk of PID is controversial. IUDs have none of the potential non-contraceptive benefits of hormonal contraceptives.
- IUDs may be expelled unnoticed, and they do not protect against STDs.
- Ectopic pregnancies are half as likely in IUD users as they are in women using no birth control. Ectopic pregnancies are more likely in women who use Progestasert than the Copper T380; however, the overall risk still remains less than for women who do not use birth control. Of those using Progestasert who become pregnant, approximately half of the pregnancies are ectopic. The overall risk of ectopic pregnancy when using the IUD is very low, at about 1 in 1000 in 5 years. If a woman becomes pregnant with the IUD *in situ*, the risk of ectopic pregnancy is about 1 in 20, and she should seek advice to exclude ectopic pregnancy.

Contraindications

- History of previous PID in the past year or active PID
- Abnormal or distorted uterine cavity
- Undiagnosed genital bleeding
- Uterine or cervical malignancy
- History of ectopic pregnancy
- Increased susceptibility to infection (e.g. those with leukemia, diabetes, valvular heart disease, or AIDS)
- Wilson disease
- Known or suspected pregnancy
- History of genital actinomyces, and active cervical or endometrial infections.
- History of previous PID in the past year or active PID
- Abnormal or distorted uterine cavity
- Undiagnosed genital bleeding
- Uterine or cervical malignancy
- History of ectopic pregnancy
- Increased susceptibility to infection (e.g., those with leukemia, diabetes, valvular heart disease, or AIDS)
- Wilson disease
- Known or suspected pregnancy
- History of genital actinomyces, and active cervical or endometrial infections.

Guidance for Health Care Providers to Address Common Misconceptions

Intrauterine Devices

1. *Intrauterine devices are safe to use among adolescents:* Current evidence demonstrates the safety of modern IUDs. Good evidence suggests that the relative risk of pelvic inflammatory disease (PID) is increased only in the first 20 days after IUD insertion and then returns to baseline, while the absolute risk remains small. Bacterial contamination associated with the insertion process is the likely cause of infection, not the IUD itself. The risk of PID with IUD placement is 0–2% when no cervical infection is present and 0–5% when insertion occurs with an undetected infection. Women with positive chlamydia cultures after IUD insertion are unlikely to develop PID, even with retention of the IUD, if the infection is promptly treated. The levonorgestrel intrauterine system may lower the risk of PID by thickening cervical mucus and thinning the endometrium.

2. *Intrauterine devices do not increase an adolescent's risk of infertility:* Infertility is not more likely after discontinuation of IUD use than after discontinuation of other reversible methods of contraception. Baseline fecundity returns rapidly after IUD removal.

3. *Intrauterine devices may be inserted without technical difficulty in most adolescents and nulliparous women:* Little evidence suggests that IUD insertion is technically more difficult in adolescents compared with older women. More than one-half of young nulliparous women report discomfort with IUD insertion. The treatment of pain during IUD insertion may include supportive care, nonsteroidal anti-inflammatory drugs (NSAIDs), narcotics or paracervical blocks. Use of buccal or vaginal misoprostol 2–3 hours before IUD insertion to soften a nulliparous cervix does not appear to reduce insertion pain.

4. *Adolescents should be routinely screened for STIs (e.g. gonorrhea and chlamydia) at the time of IUD insertion:* Women aged 15–19 years have the second highest rates of chlamydia and the highest rates of gonorrhea of any age group. It is reasonable to screen for STIs and place the IUD on the same day and administer treatment, if the test results are positive. If an STI is diagnosed after the IUD is in place, it may be treated without removing the IUD. Routine antibiotic prophylaxis is not recommended before IUD insertion.

5. *Intrauterine device expulsion is uncommon in adolescents:* Intrauterine device expulsion rates

range from 3 to 5% for all IUD users and from 5 to 22% in adolescents. Young age, previous IUD expulsion, and nulliparity may slightly increase the risk of expulsion. Prior expulsion should not be considered a contraindication for another IUD provided that appropriate counseling is given.

6. *Intrauterine devices cause changes in bleeding patterns:* Adolescents using either copper IUDs or the levonorgestrel intrauterine system can expect changes in their menstrual bleeding especially in the first months of use. The copper IUD may cause heavier menses that can be treated with NSAIDs. Women using the levonorgestrel intrauterine system will have a decrease in bleeding over time that will lead to light bleeding, spotting, or amenorrhea. Health care providers should counsel adolescents so they understand that these changes are expected.

Postpartum and Postabortal Long-acting Reversible Contraception (LARC) Initiation

1. *Postpartum long-acting reversible contraception:* Adolescent mothers are at high risk of rapid repeat pregnancy; 20% give birth again within 2 years. Insertion of an IUD or implant immediately postpartum ensures reliable contraception for adolescents when they are highly motivated to prevent pregnancy and are already in the health care system.

2. *Postabortal long-acting reversible contraception:* Inserting an IUD or implant immediately after abortion significantly reduces the risk of repeat abortion. As is the case with older women, the benefits of providing LARC to adolescents after a spontaneous or induced abortion outweigh the risks. The implant is safe to place after any abortion, including second-trimester or septic abortion. Intrauterine devices are safe to place after a first-trimester or second-trimester abortion; however, the adolescent should be counseled about the possibility of IUD expulsion (Table 17.7).

Healthcare professionals should be aware that:
- IUD use is not contraindicated in nulliparous women of any age.

Table 17.7: Expulsion rate in postpartum insertions

Timing of insertion	Expulsion rate
Interval (>4 weeks after delivery)	Low (3% in skilled inserter)
Immediate postpartum (within 10 min)	Slightly higher (up to 9.5%)
Early postpartum (between 10 min and 48 hrs)	Moderately higher (up to 37%)

Table 17.8: Comparison of copper IUDs

	1st yr failure per 100 women	Recommended lifespan
CuT 380A	0.3	12 years
Multiload Cu250	1.2	3 yrs
Multiload Cu 375	1.4	5yrs
CuT200	2.3	3yrs
Nova T	3.3	5 yrs

- Women of all ages may use IUDs.
- IUDs can safely be used by women who are breastfeeding.
- IUD use is not contraindicated in women with diabetes.
- IUD use is a safe and effective method of contraception for women who are HIV-positive or have AIDS (safer sex using condoms should be encouraged in this group).

Practical Details of Fitting IUDs

- The most effective IUDs contain at least 380 mm sq of copper and have banded copper on the arms.
- Provided that it is reasonably certain that the woman is not pregnant, IUDs may be inserted (a) at any time during the menstrual cycle, (b) immediately after first- or second-trimester abortion, or at any time thereafter, (c) from 4 weeks postpartum, irrespective of the mode of delivery.
- Emergency drugs including antiepileptic medication should be available at the time of IUD insertion in a woman with epilepsy because there may be an increased risk of a seizure at the time of cervical dilation.
- IUD may be used as **emergency contraceptive** when inserted within 5 days of intercourse.

Advice for Women at Time of Fitting

- Women should be informed about symptoms of uterine perforation or infection that would warrant an early review of IUD use.
- That insertion of an IUD may cause pain and discomfort for a few hours and light bleeding for a few days, and they should be informed about appropriate pain relief.
- About how to check for the presence of IUD threads and encouraged to do this regularly with the aim of recognising expulsion.

Insertion of Copper 380A (Fig. 17.10)
Preparation
- Non-steroidal anti-inflammatory analgesia 1 hour previously.

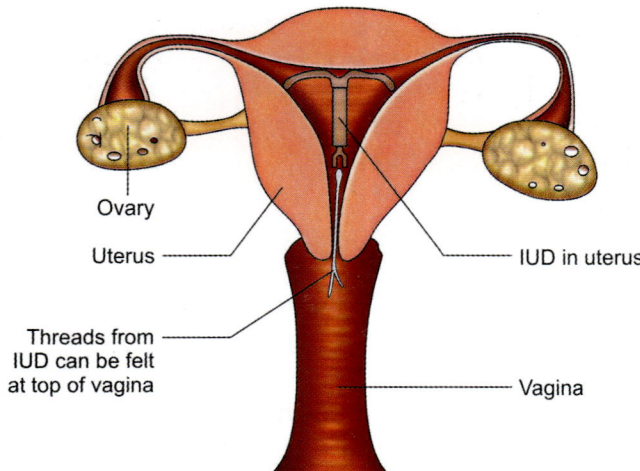

Fig. 17.10: Copper T insertion

- Cervical cleansing with antiseptic solution.
- 'No-touch' sterile technique.
- Assessment of uterine length/distance by sound measure.
- Allis tissue forceps are used to stabilize the cervix during insertion and reduce perforation.

Copper-releasing Devices

- The blue flange must be aligned with the IUCD arms at the uterine distance.
- Insert the white inserter rod into the insertion tube at the opposite end to the arms of the IUCD.
- Insert the IUCD into the uterus until the flange reaches the back of the cervix.
- Pull back the inserter tube to allow the inserter rod arms to adopt the T position (2 cm approximately).
- Slowly advance the insertion tube to ensure correct positioning before removing the insertion rod.
- Cut the threads to a length of 3 cm approximately and keep a portion for her feel in the vagina.

Follow-up Visits for Managing Problems

- A follow-up visit should be recommended after the first menses or 3–6 weeks after insertion to exclude infection, perforation or expulsion.
- Heavier and/or prolonged bleeding associated with IUD use can be treated with nonsteroidal anti-inflammatory drugs and tranexamic acid.
- Women who find heavy bleeding associated with IUD use unacceptable may consider changing to a levonorgestrel intrauterine system (LNG-IUS).
- The presence of Actinomyces-like organisms on a cervical smear in a woman with a current IUD requires ion and treatment with doxycycline. Routine removal is not indicated in women without signs of pelvic infection.
- Women who have an intrauterine pregnancy with an IUD *in situ* should be advised to have the IUD removed before 12 weeks' completed gestation, whether or not they intend to continue the pregnancy.

Missing Threads

Steps

1. Ask about pain abdomen
2. Amenorrhea or her LMP
3. Fever/GI symptoms
4. Duration of use
5. Time of use—postpartum, postabortal, etc.

Examination

1. General signs of sepsis like tachycardia, abdominal tenderness, rise in temperature
2. P/S examination:
   a. Look for the threads
   b. See for the displaced vertical stem
   c. Coiling of threads in vaginal vault
3. PV examination:
   a. Uterine size—rule out pregnancy, bulkiness may be due to fibroids
   b. Tenderness of uterus, fornices
   c. Any evidence of cervical infection

Investigations

1. USG is to find out the location of Copper T.
2. Straight X-ray can identify the missed Copper T but cannot definitively say about its location.
3. HSG is not currently used with or without dilators or lateral view.
4. Hysteroscopy to identify and extract the copper T, if it remains within the uterus.

Causes

1. Torn threads
2. Thread coiled inside
3. Pregnancy
4. Spontaneous expulsion unnoticed
5. Intrauterine displacement
6. Perforation

Management

1. *Suspected perforation:* Laparotomy or laparoscopic removal. It is removed always as it is susceptible to sepsis, intra-abdominal adhesion.

2. *Intrauterine displacement:* Removal by hysteroscopy or dilatation and curettage or hook.
3. *Pregnancy:*
   a. Counsel for termination, if she agrees.
   b. If want to continue pregnancy, remove the thread, if it can be removed easily. If not, counsel them regarding the small risk of congenital anomaly or remove it at 3rd stage after delivery.

PPIUCD Programme

Timing of PPIUCD Insertion

1. *Postplacental insertion:* Immediate following placental removal after vaginal delivery by AMTSL, IUD is inserted with a long forceps or manually in the uterine fundus.
2. *Intracesarean:* Immediately following removal of placenta during cesarean section, IUD is inserted manually in the uterine fundus before closure of uterine incision.
3. *Early pospartum:* IUD is inserted within 48 hours after vaginal delivery, preferably within the first 24 hours manually or by long ring forceps.

There should not be any interaction between AMTSL and PPIUCD. All three steps of AMTSL(IM oxytocis, controlled cord traction, massaging uterus) are done before PPIUCD insertion.

IUD should not be inserted between after 48 hours to within next 4 weeks of delivery because of risk of infection and expulsion. Beyond 4 weeks, it is called *interval insertion.*

Immediate and early postpartum changes in uterus and vagina favors easy insertion of IUD.

1. Uterus is approximately 20 weeks in size, 1 kg in weight and 30 cm in length. The anterior and posterior walls are close together and each wall is 4–5 cm in thickness and hence not easily perforable.
2. The lower uterine segment is stretched thin and extremely floppy which adds to the marked mobility and forward tilting of the body of the uterus.
3. This disparity in weight and consistency between upper and lower segments of the uterus creates a sharp angle between the vagina and the uterus.
4. The cervical opening is large, its outer margin is ragged and extremely soft. Therefore, in the first 10 minutes after delivery, the cervix can be easily stretchable to admit one small closed hand or an instrument easily to insert copper T. Beyond 10 minutes and till 48 hours after delivery, the cervix is closed for manual insertion but easily dilatable for instrument introduction.

Technique of PPIUCD Insertion

1. Elevate the uterus by special maneuver to straighten the lower uterine segment.
2. Negotiation of the uterovaginal angle with the hand or the instrument so that IUD can be reached at the fundus not in the midcavity.
3. **Kelly placental long forceps** holding the copper T or hand is used to position the IUD in the fundus; not the inserter tube. The forceps is long enough to reach the fundus and rigid enough to overcome the uterovaginal angle.
4. Careful confirmation of the fundal placement is made by feel of the forceps touching the fundus and even by feel through abdominal palpation and the hand holding the forceps reaching up to the perineum. No part of IUD including the strings should be seen after the fundal insertion.

Frequently Asked Questions with Answers

Q.1. Aren't the expulsion rates for immediate postpartum IUCDs unacceptably high?

Ans. In general, the expulsion rate is thought to be between 10 and 14%. While this is higher than the expulsion rate when the IUCD is inserted in the interval period, it is still an acceptable expulsion rate because it can provide 86–90% of users with an effective, continuing method of family planning.

Q.2. What is the best way to ensure a low expulsion rate?

Ans. High fundal placement of the IUCD by an experienced provider is the best current approach to ensure a low expulsion rate. Immediate PPIUCD placement with a Kelly placental forceps is associated with a lower expulsion rate.

Q.3. Is there a difference between manual and instrumental insertion?

Ans. Studies comparing manual and instrumental insertion technique have failed to show a difference in expulsion rates. Manual insertion should only be attempted in the postplacental period, i.e. <10 minutes after expulsion of the placenta when the cervix is maximally dilated and can accommodate a hand without excessive force. If the cervical canal is too tight to accommodate the provider's hand, instrumental insertion is recommended. All other immediate PPIUCD insertions beyond 10 minutes and at <48 hours postpartum should be performed with a long Kelly placental forceps.

Q.4. Which kinds of patients can get the postpartum IUCD?

Ans. Almost all women regardless of age, marital status or parity are candidates for IUCD placement at <48 hours postpartum. Studies have shown that even women with the following characteristics and conditions are excellent candidates for the immediate PPIUCD:

- Under 20 years of age
- HIV-infected and clinically well
- AIDS and on antiretroviral therapy (ARV) and clinically well
- History of ectopic pregnancy
- History of PID (assuming not at current high individual risk for STIs)

Q.5. Which kinds of patients should not get the IUCD in the immediate postpartum period?

Ans. IUCDs should never be offered to women with the following conditions, most of which occur rarely in the general population:

- Current PID, gonorrhea or chlamydia
- Purulent (pus-like) vaginal/cervical discharge
- Immediately after a septic abortion
- Suspected puerperal sepsis
- A distorted uterine cavity
- Malignant trophoblastic disease
- Pelvic tuberculosis
- Genital tract cancers (cervical or endometrial)

Although WHO MEC do not address these issues specifically, immediate PPIUCD placement is not recommended for women with unresolved postpartum hemorrhage, ruptured membranes for more than 18 hours or suspected chorioamnionitis because of concerns regarding increased expulsion and infection rates. Because of documented increase in perforation rates, immediate PPIUCDs are generally not offered to women between 48 hours and 4 weeks postpartum unless other methods are not available or acceptable (WHO Category 3).

Q.6. If the IUCD is placed immediate postpartum or intracesarean, how should the strings be managed?

Ans. Regardless of whether placement occurs within 48 hours after vaginal delivery or intracesarean, strings should not be cut at the time of insertion. During cesarean section, IUCD strings should never be passed through the cervix into the upper vagina but should be left in the lower uterine segment. Strings generally descend during involution and will be found curled in the posterior vaginal fornix at the follow-up visit. Strings can be cut at a follow-up visit, but only if the woman complains or if they protrude from the introitus.

Q.7. Can women who have anemia get the IUCD immediate postpartum?

Ans. Yes. Monthly menstrual bleeding increases slightly with the IUCD, especially in the first 3 months after insertion. Blood loss which results in anemia is rare and it is safe to provide an already anemic woman with an IUCD. Standard treatment with iron and folate should be continued.

Q.8. What kind of follow-up is necessary for women who get an IUCD immediate postpartum?

Ans. A follow-up visit at 4 to 6 weeks postpartum is generally recommended. If possible, a pelvic examination and a string check can be conducted at that visit. If IUCD strings are neither visible nor palpable on pelvic examination, proper IUCD positioning can also be confirmed by ultrasound or X-ray examination.

Q.9. What special precautions should be taken for patients who have heart disease?

Ans. No special intervention is required for women with uncomplicated valvular heart disease such as mitral valve prolapse. Prophylactic antibiotics as per national guidelines are advised before providing the immediate PPIUCD to women with complicated valvular heart disease such as pulmonary hypertension, atrial fibrillation, or a history of subacute bacterial endocarditis.

Preinsertion Tasks

1. If insertion is performed by the same provider that assisted the delivery, put on new pair of sterile gloves.
2. Ensure that active management of third stage of labor has been performed.
3. Arrange IUCD insertion instruments and supplies on sterile tray or draped area. Keep IUCD in sterile package to the side of sterile draped area.
4. Inspect perineum, labia and vaginal walls for lacerations. If lacerations are not bleeding heavily, insert the IUCD and repair the lacerations, if needed.

Insertion of IUCD

1. Gently visualize cervix by depressing the posterior wall of the vagina.

2. Clean cervix and vagina with antiseptic solution 2 times using 2 swabs and wait for 2 minutes.

3. Gently grasp the anterior lip of the cervix with the ring forceps (speculum may be removed at this time, if necessary, leave forceps at the side gently).

4. Open sterile package of IUCD from bottom by pulling back plastic cover approximately 1/3 upwards.

5. Hold IUCD package, stabilize IUCD in package and remove pluger rod, inserter tube and card from the package.

6. Grasp IUCD with Kelly placental forceps in the sterile package using no-touch technique.

7. Gently lift anterior lip of cervix using ring forceps and apply gentle traction to steady the cervix.

8. Insert placental forceps holding IUCD into lower uterine cavity up to the point of feeling slight resistance against back wall of the uterus. Avoid touching walls of the vagina. Gently remove ring forceps from the cervix and leave it on the sterile towel.

9. Move hand to the lower part of abdomen (base of hand on lower part of uterus and fingers towards fundus) and gently push uterus upward in the abdomen to reduce the angle and curvature between the uterus and vagina.

10. Gently move the placental forceps holding the IUCD upward towards the uterine fundus. Lower right hand (hand holding the placental forceps) down to enable forceps to easily pass vaginal-uterine angle and follow the curve of the uterine cavity. Keep placental forceps closed while moving up so IUCD does not become displaced. Take care not to perforate the uterus.

11. Continue advancing the forceps until uterine fundus is reached. Confirm that the end of the forceps has reached the fundus.

12. Open the forceps, tilt it slighty towards midline, and release IUCD at the fundus.

13. Continue to stabilize the uterus with the hand on the abdomen.

14. Sweep placental forceps to side wall of uterus.

15. Slowly remove forceps from uterine cavity, sliding instrument along the side wall of the uterus and keeping it slightly open. Take particular care not to dislodge the IUCD or catch IUCD strings as forceps are removed.

16. Stablize the uterus until the forceps are completely out of the uterus. Place forceps on sterile towel or tray.

17. Examine cervix to see if any portion of IUCD or strings are visible protruding from the cervix. If IUCD or strings are seen protruding from cervix, remove IUCD, reload in sterile package and reinsert. Ensure that there is no bleeding from cervix.

18. Remove all instruments used and place them in 0.5% chlorine solution in open position and ensure that they are totally sub-merged.

19. Allow the woman to rest for few minutes. Support the initiation of routine postpartum care, including immediate breasfeeding.

WHO MEC Category 1

There is no restriction of use of Copper T.

Women with conditions that fall into this category include the following:

1. *Reproductive:*
   - Women with history of etopic pregnancy.
   - Women with immediate after 1st trimester induced or spontaneous abortion without any evidence of sepsis.
   - Women who are 4 weeks or more postpartum.
   - Women with benign ovarian tumor or fibroids which do not distort uterine cavity.

2. *STI or genital infections:*
   - Women with vaginitis like candidiasis, bacterial vaginosis without evidence of STI.
   - Women with history of past PID with subsequent pregnancy.
   - Women who have breast disease or cancer.
   - Women who have viral hepatic disease or malaria.
   - Women who have diabetes, hypertension or uncomplicated valvular disease. Women who smoke or obese.

Category 2

Where women can generally use Copper T with benefits outweighing the risks but need to be monitored. The women with disease with category 2 are as follows:

1. *Reproductive*
   - Women who are 20 years or less and nulliparous or are simply nulliparous irrespective of age with a greater risk of expulsion due to small size of the uterus.
   - Women with heavy menstrual flow, dysmenorrhea, endometriosis where other methods are contraindicated.
   - Women who are immediately following 2nd trimester abortion where there is no evidence of infection.
   - Women who are less than 48 hours postpartum with no evidence of infection.

- Women with uterine anomaly which do not distort the uterine cavity.
2. *STI* (IUD do not protect against STI; those at risk should take protection by condoms).
   - Women with STI other than gonorrhea, syphilis like herpes, syphilis.
   - Women who are at risk of STI like herpes, HIV, syphilis, hepatitis.
   - Women with a history of PID without a subsequent pregnancy assuming there are no current risk factors for STI
3. *HIV/AIDS*
   - Women who are HIV infected but clinically well.
   - Women with AIDS and on ARV therapy but clinically well.
4. *General*
   - Women with complicated heart disease like rheumatic heart disese, artificial shunts although prophylactic antibiotics are advised during IUD insertion to prevent endocarditis.
   - Women with iron deficiency anemia, sickle cell disease, thalassemia though there are concern for increase blood loss on IUD.

Category 3

For the following women, IUD is not recommended since the risks outweigh the benefits. It is advised only when no other suitable alternative is available. These are:

1. *Reproductive:*
   - Women who are 48 hrs to 4 weeks postpartum.
   - Women with benign trophoblastic disease.
   - Women who have ovarian cancer should not insert Copper T although they are category 2 for continuation.
2. *STI:* Women who have high individual risk for gonorrhea and Chlamydia should not get IUD inserted but they are category 2 for continuation.
3. *HIV/AIDS:* Women who have AIDS but not on ARV therapy should not get IUD inserted but are category 2 for continuation.

Category 4

These are the following conditions where IUD is never recommended.

1. *Reproductive*
   - Women who are pregnant.
   - Women who have malignant trophoblastic disease.
   - Women with cervical or endometrial cancer should not get IUD inserted though they are in

category 2 for continuation while following evaluation.
   - Women with uterine abnormality or fibroid that distort the uterine cavity that may interfere with IUD insertion.
   - Women with pelvic tuberculosis.
   - Women with unexplained vaginal bleeding should not have IUD inserted but in category 2 for continuation while awaiting evaluation.
2. *STI:* Women who have current PID, purulent cervicitis, Chlamydia or gonorrhea should not have an IUD inserted but in category 2 while awaiting evaluation or undergoing treatment.

Intrauterine System (IUS)

LNG (hormonal)-IUD

Mirena (Fig. 17.11A, B) was approved by the FDA for use in 2000 for intrauterine contraception and in 2009 to treat heavy periods for women who choose intrauterine contraception. The cylinder reservoir contains 52 mg of levonorgestrel (LNG) in a 1:1 mixture with polydimethylsiloxane. The system releases the active ingredient, LNG, over an extended period of up to 5 years at a virtually constant rate. The initial release rate of the LNG is 20 µg every 24 hours. It has a shelf-life of 3 years.

Mode of Action of Mirena IUS (Fig. 17.12)

- Downregulate endometrial estrogen and progesterone receptors.
- Glands of the endometrium become atrophic.
- Stroma becomes swollen and decidual.

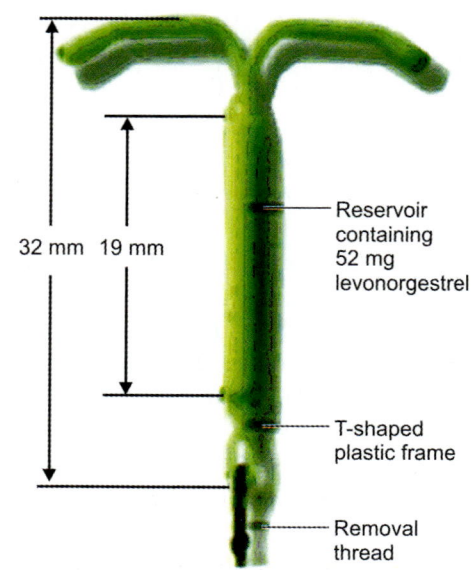

32 mm　19 mm

Reservoir containing 52 mg levonorgestrel

T-shaped plastic frame

Removal thread

Fig. 17.11A: Mirena

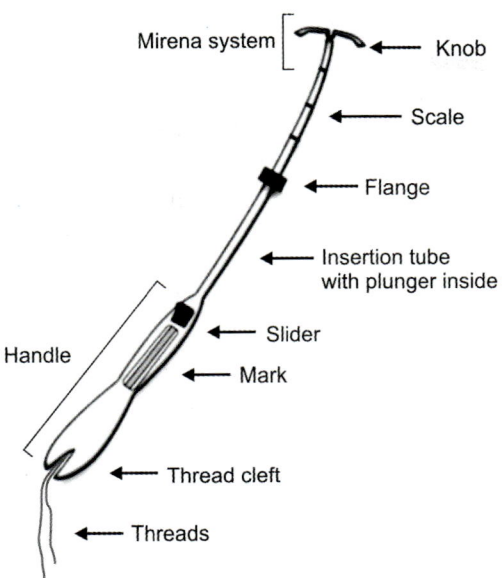

Fig. 17.11B: Parts of mirena

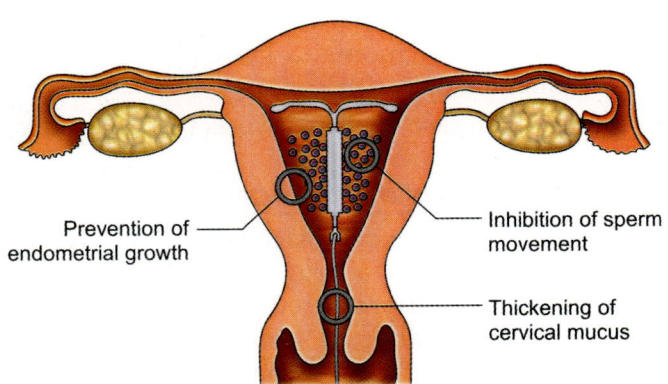

Fig. 17.12: Mirena provides contraception through a combination of three actions

- Mucosa thins and the epithelium becomes inactive and monostratified.

When to Insert Mirena?

- It is recommended that postpartum insertion of the levonorgestrel-releasing intrauterine system be delayed until uterine involution is complete (approximately six weeks after delivery).
- The device can be inserted immediately after termination of a first-trimester pregnancy.

Contraceptive Efficacy

The IUS may act predominantly by preventing implantation and sometimes by preventing fertilization. The pregnancy rate associated with the use of the IUS is very low (fewer than 10 in 1000 over 5 years). The licensed duration of use for IUS is 5 years for contraception. There is no evidence of delay in the return of fertility following removal or expulsion of the IUS.

Effects on Periods

- Irregular bleeding and spotting are common during the first 6 months following IUS insertion.
- Oligomenorrhea or amenorrhea is likely by the end of the first year of IUS use.

Risks and Possible Side Effects

- Up to 60% of women stop using the IUS within 5 years. The most common reasons are unacceptable vaginal bleeding and pain. There is no evidence that IUS use causes weight gain.
- There may be an increased likelihood of developing acne as a result of absorption of progestogen, but few women discontinue IUS use for this reason.
- The risk of uterine perforation at the time of IUS insertion is very low (less than 1 in 1000).
- The risk of developing pelvic inflammatory disease following IUS insertion is very low (less than 1 in 100) in women who are at low risk of STIs.
- The IUS may be expelled, but this occurs in fewer than 1 in 20 women in 5 years.
- The overall risk of ectopic pregnancy when using the IUS is very low, at about 1 in 1000 in 5 years.
- If a woman becomes pregnant with the IUS in situ, the risk of ectopic pregnancy is about 1 in 20, and she should seek advice to exclude ectopic pregnancy.

Other Issues to Consider before Fitting an IUS

- Women who are aged 45 years or older at the time of IUS insertion and who are amenorrheic may retain the device until they no longer require contraception.
- Fertility rapidly returns to normal after removal of Mirena.
- All pregnancies are normal after Mirena.
- Conception rate is 96/100 after 12 months of removal of LNG-IUS.

Testing for the following infections should be undertaken before IUS insertion:
- *Chlamydia trachomatis* in women at risk of STIs.
- *Neisseria gonorrhoeae* in women from areas where the disease is prevalent and who are at risk of STIs.
- If testing for STIs is not possible, or has not been completed, prophylactic antibiotics should be given before IUS insertion in women at increased risks of STIs.

Summary of Recommendations

- There is no evidence that the effectiveness of the IUS is reduced when taking any other medication.
- IUS use is not contraindicated in women with diabetes.
- IUS is a safe and effective method of contraception for women who are HIV positive or have AIDS (safer sex using condoms should be encouraged in this group).
- IUS, may be used by women who have migraine with or without aura.
- Women with a history of venous thromboembolism may use the IUS.
- IUS is medically safe for women to use, if estrogen is contraindicated.

Practical Details of Fitting the IUS

Provided that it is reasonably certain that the woman is not pregnant, the IUS may be inserted:

- At any time during the menstrual cycle (but if the woman is amenorrheic or it has been more than 5 days since menstrual bleeding started, additional barrier contraception should be used for the first 7 days after insertion).
- Immediately after first- or second-trimester abortion, or at any time thereafter from 4 weeks postpartum, irrespective of the mode of delivery.
- Emergency drugs including antiepileptic medication should be available at the time of IUS insertion in a woman with epilepsy because there may be an increased risk of a seizure at the time of cervical dilatation.

Advice for Women at Time of Fitting

Women should be informed:

- About symptoms of uterine perforation or infection that would warrant an early review of IUS use.
- That insertion of an IUS may cause pain and discomfort for a few hours and light bleeding for a few days.
- About how to check for the presence of IUS threads.

Follow-up and Managing Problems

A follow-up visit should be recommended after the first menses, or 3–6 weeks after insertion, to exclude infection, perforation or expulsion. Thereafter, a woman should be strongly encouraged to return at any time to discuss problems, if she wants to change her method of contraception, or if it is time to have the IUS removed.

The presence of Actinomyces-like organisms on a cervical smear in a woman with a current IUS requires an assessment to exclude pelvic infection. Routine removal is not indicated in women without signs of pelvic infection.

Women with an intrauterine pregnancy with an IUS in situ should be advised to have the IUS removed before 12 completed weeks of gestation whether or not they intend to continue the pregnancy.

Extended Gynecological Use of LNG-IUS

- LNG-IUS is licensed for use in menorrhagia and to provide endometrial protection to perimenopausal and postmenopausal women on estrogen replacement therapy.
- There is limited evidence to suggest that LNG-IUS may also be beneficial in women with endometriosis, adenomyosis, fibroids, endometrial hyperplasia and early stage endometrial cancer (where the patient is deemed unfit for primary surgical therapy) or as adjuvant therapy with tamoxifen to prevent endometrial carcinoma, a known side effect of tamoxifen therapy.
- Before IVF in case of adenomyosis with infertility

Emergency Postcoital Contraception

Description: Emergency postcoital contraception is defined as the use of a drug or device to prevent pregnancy after unprotected sexual intercourse. Unwanted pregnancy is common; worldwide, approximately 50 million pregnancies are terminated each year. The widespread use of emergency contraception may have prevented more than 1 million abortions and 2 million pregnancies every year.

1. Emergency Contraceptive Pills and the Minipill Emergency Contraception Method

The ECP consists of 2 pills, which each contain 0.5 mg of levonorgestrel and 50 µg of ethinyl estradiol, ingested 12 hours apart for a total of 4 pills. The first dose should be taken within the first 72 hours after unprotected intercourse.

Only the progestin levonorgestrel has been studied for the use in MECM. It is marketed as Plan B. Its treatment schedule comprises 1 dose of 750 µg levonorgestrel taken as soon as possible and no later than 48 hours after unprotected intercourse and a second dose taken 12 hours later.

Ulipristal is a selective progesterone receptor modulator with antagonistic and partial agonistic effects. When taken immediately before ovulation, ulipristal postpones follicular rupture. It is thought that the primary mechanism of action for emergency contraception is inhibition or delay of ovulation; however, alterations to the endometrium that may affect implantation may also occur. The treatment regimen is 1 tablet of 30 mg orally as soon as possible within 120 hours (5 days) after unprotected intercourse or a known/suspected contraceptive failure. If vomiting occurs within 3 hours after the dose, consider repeating the regimen.

The **mechanism of action** of either the ECP or MECM is not clearly established. If administered before ovulation, both methods may inhibit follicular development and maturation, resulting in anovulation and deficient luteal function. Treatment following ovulation may affect the endometrium, thus inhibiting implantation. They also may affect tubal transport of the sperm or ova. However, menses and fertility return with the next cycle.

WHO recommends levonorgestrel for emergency contraceptive pill use. Ideally, this progestogen-only method should be taken as a single dose (1.5 mg) within five days (120 hours) of unprotected intercourse. Alternatively, a woman can take the levonorgestrel in two doses (0.75 mg each; 12 hours apart).

Efficacy

Most studies cite an effectiveness rate of 55–94%, with the true effectiveness rate likely to be approximately 75%. Despite this significant reduction in the rate of pregnancy, patients must understand that this method of contraception should be used only in emergencies and that they should be encouraged to use other more consistent forms of contraception.

Several factors complicate the calculation of a failure rate. Factors include dependence on the patient's history of their last menstrual period and day of exposure, effect of regular and irregular menstrual cycles on the calculation of the estimated time of ovulation, the possibility of the patient being pregnant, and the possibility that more than one unprotected coitus has occurred during that period.

Disadvantages

Adverse effects include nausea and emesis, minor changes in menses, breast tenderness, fatigue, headache, abdominal pain, and dizziness. Ectopic pregnancy is possible, if treatment fails.

The date of the patient's last menses, her contraceptive history and the dates of unprotected intercourse should be determined. The patient's likely risk of pregnancy should be discussed, as well as decision to continue the pregnancy in the event that emergency treatment is not effective.

Indications for Pelvic Examination before Use of Emergency Contraception

- Suspected pregnancy
- Assessment for sexually transmitted disease
- Consideration of insertion of intrauterine device
- Overdue Papanicolaou smear

The patient should be advised that 98% of women will bleed within 21 days of use of emergency contraception. If bleeding does not occur within four weeks of emergency contraception, a pregnancy test should be performed.

Most importantly, patients should be counseled to consistently use a precoital method of birth control. The failure rates of emergency postcoital contraception accumulate over time, and this method is not as effective as precoital birth control. Physicians should take this opportunity to educate women about more effective options.

Key Facts

- Emergency contraception can prevent most pregnancies when taken after intercourse.
- Emergency contraception can be used following unprotected intercourse, contraceptive failure, incorrect use of contraceptives, or in cases of sexual assault.
- There are two methods of emergency contraception: Emergency contraceptive pills (ECPs) and copper-bearing intrauterine devices (IUDs) (Table 17.9).
- When inserted within five days of unprotected intercourse, a copper-bearing IUD is the most effective form of emergency contraception available.
- The emergency contraceptive pill regimen recommended by WHO is one dose of levonorgestrel 1.5 mg, taken within five days (120 hours) of unprotected intercourse.

Emergency contraception is effective only in the first few days following intercourse before the ovum is released from the ovary and before the sperm fertilizes the ovum. Emergency contraceptive pills cannot interrupt an established pregnancy or harm a developing embryo.

In What Situations should Emergency Contraception be Used?

Emergency contraception can be used in a number of situations following sexual intercourse.

Table 17.9: Different regime of emergency contraceptives

Regimen	Timing of first dose after intercourse	Reported efficacy
Estrogen and progestin (100 μg of ethinyl estradiol and 0.5 mg of levonorgestrel given twice, with 12 hours between doses)	0 to 72 hours	About 75% of pregnancies prevented
Levonorgestrel (0.75 mg given twice, with 12 hours between doses)	0 to 72 hours	75 to 85% of pregnancies prevented
High-dose estrogen (e.g. 50 μg of ethinyl estradiol daily for 5 days)	0 to 72 hours	Equivalent to estrogen-progestin 85 to 100%
Mifepristone (a single dose of 10, 50 or 600 μg)	0 to 120 hours	85 to 100% effective
Copper intrauterine device	0 to 120 hours after the earliest estimated day of ovulation	Failure rate <1%

- When no contraceptive has been used.
- When there is a contraceptive failure or incorrect use.
- Condom breakage, slippage, or incorrect use.
- Three or more consecutively missed combined oral contraceptive pills;
- The progestogen-only pill (minipill) taken more than three hours late (or more than 12 hours late if taking a 0.75 mg desogestrel-containing pill).
- Norethisterone enanthate (NET-EN) progestogen-only injection taken more than two weeks late.
- Depot-medroxyprogesterone acetate (DMPA) progestogen-only injection taken more than four weeks late.
- Failed withdrawal (e.g. ejaculation in the vagina or on external genitalia).
- Miscalculation of the periodic abstinence method, or failure to abstain or use a barrier method on the fertile days of the cycle.
- Expulsion of an intrauterine contraceptive device (IUD) or hormonal contraceptive implant.
- In cases of sexual assault when the woman was not protected by an effective contraceptive method.

Safety

Levonorgestrel-alone emergency contraception pills are very safe and do not cause abortion or harm future fertility. Side effects are uncommon and generally mild.

Medical Eligibility Criteria and Contraindications

- Emergency contraceptive pills prevent pregnancy. They should not be given to a woman who already has a confirmed pregnancy. However, if a woman inadvertently takes the pills after she becomes pregnant, the available evidence suggests that the pills will not harm either the mother or her fetus.
- Emergency contraceptive pills are for emergency use only and are not appropriate for regular use as an ongoing contraceptive method because of the higher

possibility of failure compared with non-emergency contraceptives.

- In addition, frequent use of emergency contraception can result in side effects such as menstrual irregularities, although their repeated use poses no known health risks.
- There are no medical contraindications to the use of levonorgestrel emergency contraception pills.

2. Copper-bearing Intrauterine Devices (IUDs)

WHO recommends that a copper-bearing IUD, as an emergency contraceptive, be inserted within five days of unprotected intercourse. This may be an ideal emergency contraceptive for a woman who is hoping for an ongoing, highly effective contraceptive method. Insertion of the IUD is significantly more effective than either the ECP or MECP regimen, reducing the risk of pregnancy following unprotected intercourse by more than 99%.

Mode of Action

As emergency contraception, the copper-bearing IUD primarily prevents fertilization by causing a chemical change that damages sperm and egg before they can meet.

Effectiveness

When inserted within five days of unprotected intercourse, a copper-bearing IUD is over 99% effective in preventing pregnancy. This is the most effective form of emergency contraception available. Once inserted, the woman can continue to use the IUD as an ongoing method of contraception, and she may choose to change to another contraceptive method in the future.

Safety

A copper-bearing IUD is a very safe form of emergency contraception. The risks of infection, expulsion or perforation are low.

Medical Eligibility Criteria and Contraindications

The only situation in which a copper-bearing IUD should never be used as emergency contraception is if a woman is already pregnant.

3. Mifepristone

Mifepristone inhibits ovulation and blocks implantation by causing a delay in maturation of the endometrium. It causes actual regression of the corpus luteum in 50% of women when given in the middle or late luteal phase.

Sterilization

Description

Sterilization is considered an elective permanent method of contraception. Although both female and male sterilization procedures can be reversed surgically, the surgery is technically more difficult than the original procedure and may not be successful. In regard to reversal of sterilization, success is greater with tubal reanastomosis than with reanastomosis of the vas deferens.

1. Female Sterilization

India

India is a country where overpopulation is a main problem. Poor families do not have access to birth control and medical advances in the past 50 years have lowered the death rate, resulting in large population density and overcrowding. In 1959, the Second Five-Year Plan offered monetary compensation to low income men who underwent vasectomy. These incentives partially served as a way to educate men that sterilization was the most effective way of contraception and that vasectomies did not affect sexual performance. However, mass sterilization efforts resulted in lack of cleanliness and poor technique, potentially resulting in botched surgeries and major complications. In 1976, compulsory sterilization policies were put in place. However, these, along with "sterilization camps" (where large amounts of sterilizations were performed quickly and often unsafely), backfired and discouraged people to participate in sterilization. The compulsory laws were removed. The focus of population policies has changed in the 21st century. The government is more concerned with empowering women, protecting them from violence, and providing basic necessities to families. Sterilization efforts are still in existence and still target poor families.

History of the Procedure

- In 1823, Blundell first suggested tubal ligation for sterilization before the Medical Society of London.
- In 1895, Dührssen used a double ligature and was the first to perform tubal ligation via colpotomy.
- In 1919, Madlener crushed and ligated the tubes with nonabsorbable suture.
- In 1924, Irving published his method in which the proximal portion of the severed tube is buried in a small myometrial tunnel on the anterior uterine surface.
- In 1930, Pomeroy technique was posthumously published in the *New York State Journal of Medicine.*
- In 1940, Hajime Uchida developed his technique, which can be performed as an interval or puerperal procedure.
- In 1960, the era of laparoscopy began with unipolar electrocoagulation of the fallopian tube.
- In 1973, Jaroslav Hulka devised a spring clip that could be applied laparoscopically.
- In 1981, Filshie introduced a titanium and silicone clip that was widely used in Europe.
- In 2002, the Essure hysteroscopic sterilization procedure was approved for use in the United States. Sterilization can be performed surgically in the postpartum period with a small transverse infraumbilical incision or during the interval period. Sterilization during the interval period can be performed with laparoscopy, laparotomy, or colpotomy. The methods of fallopian tube sterilization include occlusion with Falope rings, clips, or bands; segmental destruction with electrocoagulation; or suture ligation with partial salpingectomy.

Preoperative Details

Informed Consent and Preoperative Counseling

- Inform the patient that a sterilization procedure is intended to be permanent and irreversible. Furthermore, this consent cannot be obtained, if the patient is younger than 21 years, in labor, under the influence of drugs or alcohol, mentally incompetent, or having an abortion. In India a sterilization form is available which is to be signed by the acceptor, husband/guardian and surgeon. The Govt. of India give incentive of 250/- to acceptor, 75/- to surgeon and spent total of 545/- per patient.
- As with any form of contraception, 0.5–1% chance of failure exists.
- The relative likelihood of an ectopic pregnancy is increased when sterilization failure occurs in all

procedures involving occlusion or excision of the isthmic or ampullary segments of the tube, but ectopic pregnancy has not been demonstrated in the hysteroscopic approach.

- Inform the patient that complications exist, although the incidence of major complications is low.
- For minilaparotomy and laparoscopic techniques, complications may include injuries to the gastrointestinal and genitourinary tracts, infection, hemorrhage, and complications of anesthesia.
- For the hysteroscopic approach, the same complications associated with diagnostic hysteroscopy apply—uterine perforation, bleeding, excessive absorption of distention media, and infection.

Laboratory Studies

- Urinalysis and hemogram; critical level of Hb is 8 gm/dL.
- Medical and psychiatric counseling is to be done and necessary investigations are done accordingly including CDC, KFT, PPBS, chest X-ray, ECG.
- Gonorrhea and chlamydia screening: Sterilization using any technique is contraindicated in the presence of active pelvic infection.
- Papanicolaou test: A Papanicolaou test should be performed within 6 months of the procedure.

Surgical Therapy

Surgical approaches for female sterilization include laparoscopy, hysteroscopy, microlaparoscopy, laparotomy (concurrent with cesarean delivery), minilaparotomy, and vaginal approaches. Although minilaparotomy is the most common approach worldwide, laparoscopy is used most commonly for interval procedures. Vaginal colpotomy approaches are rarely used because they are associated with a higher incidence of infection and can no longer be recommended.

Puerperal Tubal Sterilization

In comparison with interval sterilization, infra-umbilical minilaparotomy following delivery in the early puerperium is convenient, simple, and cost-effective. However, if maternal or infant complications exist, sterilization should be delayed.

Bilateral tube ligation (BTL) may be performed after closure of the uterine incision during cesarean delivery or following completion of a vaginal delivery within 72 hours. Postpartum BTL is technically simple because the uterine fundus is at the level of the umbilicus,

making the fallopian tubes readily accessible through a small periumbilical abdominal incision.

Minilaparotomy

Minilaparotomy is defined as a laparotomy with an incision size smaller than 5 cm. The operation can be performed through a suprapubic incision in the interval after pregnancy and through a subumbilical incision within the first 48 hours after delivery.

A 2- to 5-cm periumbilical semilunar incision is made with the skin tented with Allis clamps. Dissection is carried down to the fascia, which is grasped with hemostats or Allis clamps and opened transversely, exposing the peritoneum, which can then be entered sharply. With uterine manipulation and retraction, the tubes can be visualized and grasped with a Babcock clamp (Fig. 17.13). Often, the oviducts can be palpated at their uterotubal junction and the uterus may then be rotated to position the isthmus of the tube under the incision anteriorly with the aid of Army-Navy retractors. The fallopian tube is "walked" with Babcock clamps until the fimbriated end is identified. A major cause of failure of sterilization is the inadvertent ligation of the round ligament mistakenly identified as the fallopian tube.

After the BTL, the minilaparotomy incision is closed in layers. Closure of the peritoneum is optional. The fascia is closed with running 2-0 or 0 delayed absorbable suture. Subcutaneous closure is optional, and the skin is closed with 3-0 or 4-0 absorbable suture in a subcuticular manner or with acrylic glue.

Pomeroy Technique (Fig. 17.14)

This technique is the simplest and most commonly performed puerperal tubal sterilization.

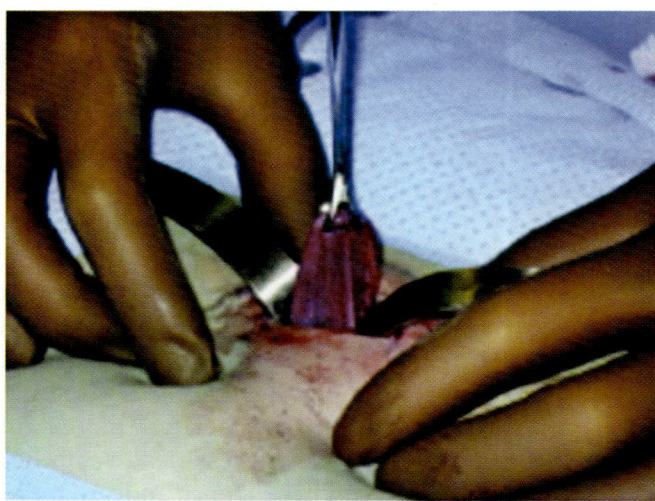

Fig. 17.13: Elevation of the fallopian tube through the incision

The mid-portion of the oviduct is grasped with a Babcock clamp, creating a loop, which is tied with 2-0 or 0 plain catgut suture, and each limb of the tubal knuckle is cut separately. Specimens are submitted to pathology. The ligation sutures are held while the tube is cut to prevent retraction of the tubal stumps into the peritoneal cavity before they can be adequately examined for hemostasis.

The original description consists of forming a loop of the ampullary segment of the fallopian tube and ligating the base of the loop with a double strand of 1-0 chromic catgut, followed by resection of the top of the ligated loop. The rationale for this technique is based on prompt absorption of the suture ligature with subsequent separation of the cut ends of the tube, which then become sealed by spontaneous reperitonealization and fibrosis. A resultant natural gap of 2–3 cm should occur between the severed proximal and distal segments of the tube (Fig. 17.15A).

Many modifications of the Pomeroy technique have been described; the most common involves doubly ligating each loop.

Failure rates are reported to be 1 case in 300–500 patients.

Parkland Technique (Fig. 17.15C)

The Parkland technique is a midsegmental resection similar to the Pomeroy technique, except each leg of the loop is tied separately. The Parkland technique was designed to avoid the intimate approximation of the tubal cut ends, as occurs with the Pomeroy technique,

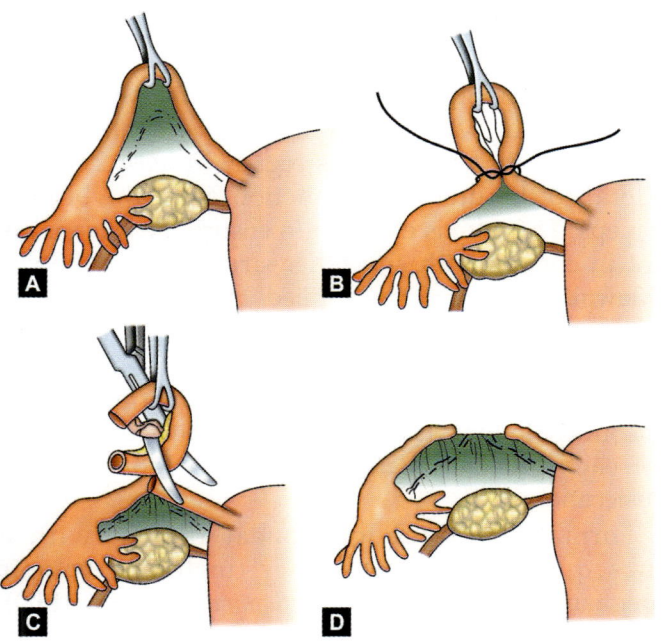

Fig. 17.14: Pomeroy method

thereby theoretically reducing the risk of subsequent recanalization.

An avascular area in the mesosalpinx directly under the tube is perforated with a hemostat, and the jaws are opened to spread the mesosalpinx, thereby freeing approximately 2.5 cm of tube. The tube is then ligated proximally and distally with a 0 or 00 plain or chromic suture, and a 1- to 2-cm tubal segment is excised and submitted for pathologic confirmation.

Failure rates are reported to be 1 in 400 patients.

Uchida Technique

The mid-portion of the oviduct is raised with 2 Babcock clamps. The tubal serosa is hydrodissected from the muscularis by subserosal injection of a dilute (1:100,000) saline solution of epinephrine or isotonic sodium chloride solution. A linear incision is made parallel to the axis of the tube in the ballooning serosa on the antimesosalpingeal aspect with a scalpel. The serosal peritoneum is grasped on either side of the tubal incision with hemostats, and a third hemostat is used to bluntly dissect and reflect the serosa and the surrounding areolar tissue from the tubal muscularis. With the tubal muscularis exposed, a relatively long (5 cm) segment of tubal muscularis is ligated proximally and distally with a 0 or 0-0 plain catgut suture and resected. The serosal edges are then reapproximated, burying the proximal exposed tubal end within the leaves of the broad ligament, leaving the distal end exposed.

During the puerperium, Uchida modified the sterilization procedure by including fimbriectomy. Clearly, the excision of such a large segment of tube, combined with a fimbriectomy, accounts for the low rate of failure for this technique.

Irving Technique (Fig. 17.15B)

The Irving technique is designed to be used in conjunction with cesarean delivery. A mesosalpingeal window is created beneath the tube approximately 4 cm from the uterotubal junction. The tube is doubly ligated with 0 or 00 absorbable suture and severed, with the sutures on the proximal end left long. The proximal tubal stump may require mobilization by dissecting it free from the mesosalpinx. A small nick is made into the serosa on the posterior (or anterior) uterine wall near the uterotubal junction. A hemostat is used to deepen the incision, creating a pocket in the myometrium approximately 1–2 cm deep. The 2 free ends of the proximal stump ligature are then individually threaded onto a curved needle and brought deep into the myometrium tunnel and out

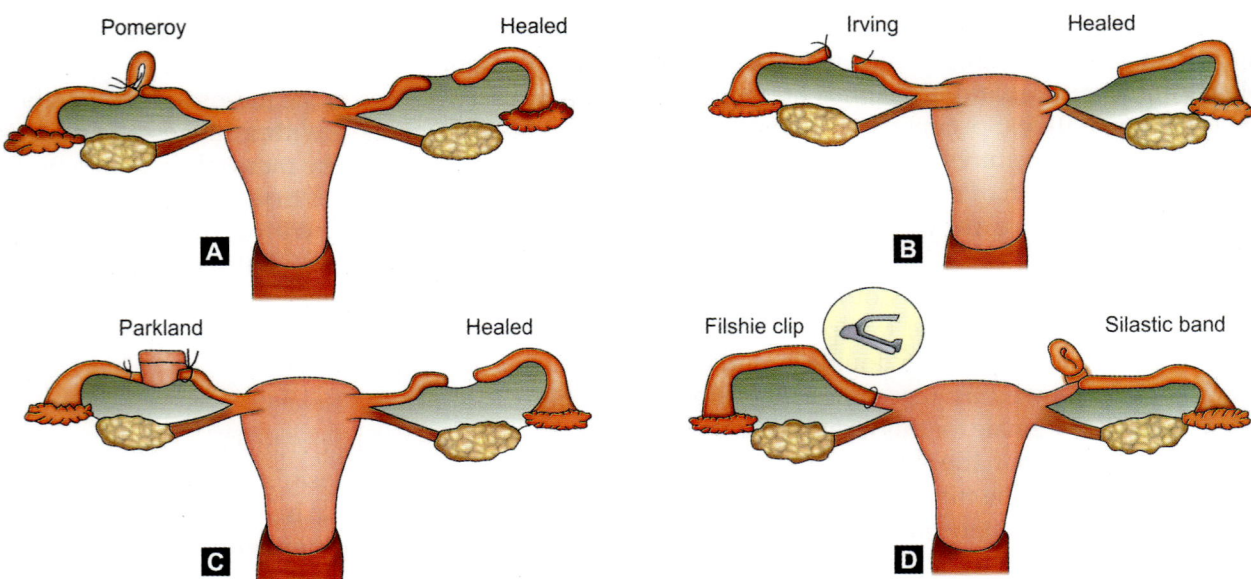

Fig. 17.15: Different methods of tubectomy

through the uterine serosa. Traction on the sutures draws the proximal tubal stump deep into the myometrial tunnel, and the sutures are tied. The serosal opening of the tunnel is then closed around the tube with fine absorbable suture. An additional option is to bury the distal end of the tube between the leaves of the broad ligament as originally described by Irving. Failure rates are less than 1 in 1000 patients.

Laparoscopic Techniques

Laparoscopy

Advantages include small incisions, full access to the oviducts, rapid recovery, and the ability to inspect the pelvis and upper abdomen.

Disadvantages include the need for general anesthesia, the risks of vessel/viscera injury with needle insufflation/trocar entry, and difficulty associated with laparoscopy in patients who are obese or in the presence of abdominal and/or pelvic adhesions. Entry accounts for 30–50% of all laparoscopic sterilization complications.

The failure rate of the laparoscopic approach ranges from 7.5 per 1000 procedures for unipolar coagulation to as high as 36.5 per 1000 for the spring clip. The failure rate of Filshie clip is between 1 and 2%.

Microlaparoscopy

Microlaparoscopy involves use of 1.2- to 2-mm microendoscopes with 5- to 7-mm suprapubic ports for bipolar coagulation or mechanical occlusive devices. This surgery is possible because of improved technology in light transmission and fiberoptic bundles.

Electrodesiccation Technique

The use of electrosurgery is preferable when the fallopian tube is edematous, thickened, or cannot be mobilized easily for mechanical device placement. This technique should always be readily available during laparoscopic BTL, both as a backup method of sterilization and for control of unexpected bleeding. However, the technique causes greater tubal damage, making tubal reversal more difficult, if the patient regrets her decision.

I. Bipolar Current

Bipolar current is theoretically safer than unipolar current because tissue destruction is essentially confined to the area between and immediately adjacent to the bipolar paddles. The oviduct is identified and grasped at the mid-isthmus region, at least 2.5–3 cm lateral to the uterotubal junction, with the bipolar forceps. The tube is elevated to ensure the forceps are not in contact with any other structure (e.g. bowel, sidewall), and current is applied. High voltage results in excessive heat and tissue charring, sometimes causing sticking of the electrodes. Extensive damage to the tissue may facilitate future fistula formation and encourage failure. The procedure is repeated 2–3 times for each tube to create a 3 cm contiguous area of desiccation.

Formation of tuboperitoneal fistula, with a subsequent risk of pregnancy (including ectopic pregnancy) or possible *pelvic inflammatory disease* (PID), is minimized by maintaining the most proximal burn no closer than 2 cm to the uterine cornu. Leaving a 2-

to 3-cm pedicle allows enough space for absorption of intrauterine fluid under pressure, such as during menstruation, and minimizes the risk of fistula formation.

II. Monopolar Current

In surgery, using monopolar energy, the current passes through the entire patient to complete the circuit between the electrode and the electrosurgical generator. The initial popularity of unipolar current occurred during the early years of laparoscopic sterilization when it was often the only instrumentation available. Its use has diminished following many documented bowel injuries. For this reason, unipolar current has largely been replaced with bipolar electrodesiccation.

III. Mechanical Methods

a. *Falope (Yoon) ring technique:* A nonreactive silicone rubber band measuring 3.6 mm in outer diameter and incorporating 5% barium sulfate for radiographic identification is used. The applicator consists of inner grasping prongs and an outer double-barreled sheath. The Falope ring is stretched around the base of the applicator sheath. Some devices allow for double-loading of the rings so that the applicator needs to be inserted into the abdominal cavity only once.

The isthmic portion of the fallopian tube is identified. The forceps of the applicator are extended and a segment at least 3 cm from the uterine cornu is grasped, taking care to avoid the proximity of any vessels in the mesosalpinx. Approximately 2.5 cm of tube is gently pulled into the barrel using a slow "milking" technique. This may be difficult with edematous tubes, or in the presence of chronic pelvic adhesions. The larger-diameter outer barrel then pushes the Falope ring over the knuckle of tube, and the ring then returns to its former state, with an inner diameter of 1 mm.

The loop of tube should clearly contain 2 complete lumens of tube. Slowly advancing the entire applicator toward the tube while gradually retracting the tongs and tube into the applicator and avoiding excessive traction on the tube are important.

Failure to do this can result in mesosalpingeal hemorrhage and tubal laceration, which occur in approximately 1–5% of cases. This can be treated with bipolar coagulation, or a Falope ring may be placed on each transected end.

Falope ring application has traditionally been considered more painful postoperatively secondary to ischemia. The failure rate is reported to be 3.3 cases per 1000 patients.

b. *Hulka-Clemens clip technique:* The clip is designed to be applied at a right angle to the isthmic portion of the tube 2.5–3 cm from the uterotubal junction. When properly applied, only 4 mm of tube and virtually none of the blood supply is destroyed.

The clip consists of 2 toothed jaws of Lexan plastic joined by a stainless steel hinge pin. The lower jaw has a distal hook. A gold-plated spring maintains the clip in an open position. When completely advanced, the spring closes and locks the jaw.

The applicator is withdrawn from the abdomen and reloaded, and the contralateral tube is treated in the same fashion.

Failure of the Hulka clip should not exceed 2–3 cases per 1000 patients.

c. *Filshie clip technique* (Fig. 17.15D): This technique involves a 12.7 mm long clip of titanium with a silicone rubber lining. The clip is applied laparoscopically with an applicator, much like the Hulka spring clip, at right angles to the isthmus approximately 2–2.5 cm from the uterotubal junction. Initially, the clip occludes the tubal lumen by pressure. As tubal necrosis occurs, the rubber expands to maintain blockage of the lumen. The tube eventually divides, and the stumps heal closed. The Filshie clip usually remains attached and is eventually covered by peritoneum.

Rare reports of migration of the Filshie clip into the bladder, vagina, peritoneal cavity, and appendix and its expulsion from the vagina, urethra, and rectum are reported.

Filshie clip application has a reported failure rate of 7 cases per 1000 patients.

Hysteroscopic Techniques

Hysteroscopy

Essure has been shown to be 99.80% effective in preventing pregnancy after 4 years of follow-up (Fig. 17.16).

The Essure microinserts device consists of polyethylene terephthalate (PET) fibers wrapped around a stainless steel core, surrounded by 24 coils of nickel-titanium alloy, a substance widely used for coronary artery stents and cardiovascular devices. The microinserts are dynamic, spring-like devices that are inserted into each fallopian tube. Once deployed, the effectiveness of the Essure microinserts is believed to be due to a combination of the space filling design of the device and a local occlusive, benign tissue response to the PET fibers. This process takes approximately 3 months to form complete occlusion. Hysteroscopy

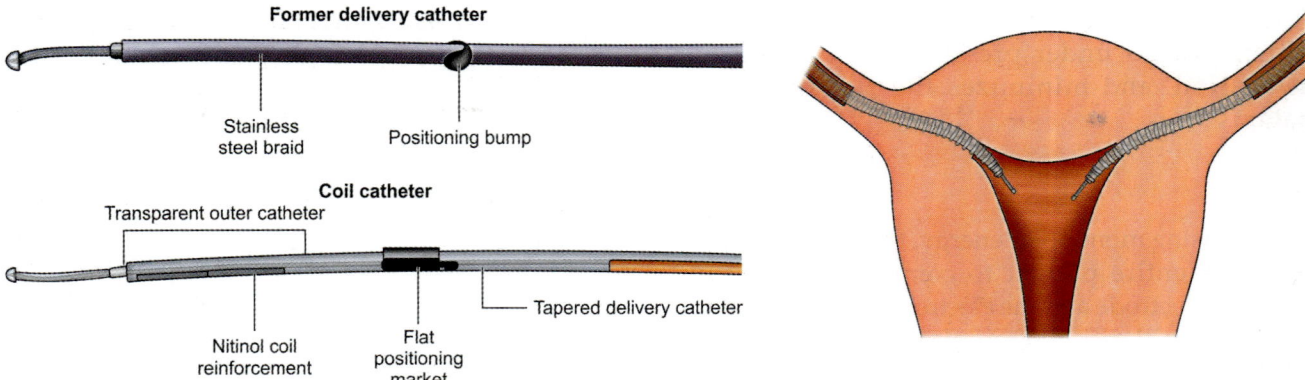

Fig. 17.16: Transcervical sterilization by Essure

may be performed in the office setting under local anesthesia, which is preferred, although regional or *general anesthesia* may be selected according to patient or surgeon preference. Successful bilateral placement rates vary from 94.6–99%.

A 5 mm operative hysteroscope with a 5-French operating channel is inserted under direct vision through the cervical os, and the uterine cavity is entered. Normal saline is used for the distension medium, which minimizes the risk of fluid overload and virtually eliminates the risk of electrolyte imbalance inherent in the use of isotonic solutions (glycine and sorbitol).

Both tubal ostia are identified. The device is passed through the operating channel and guided into the tubal ostium through the hysteroscope to the depth of the black indicator on the outer cannula. With the applicator steadied against the hysteroscope, the wheel on the handle is rotated, which causes the outer sheath to retract, exposing the wound-down coils of nickel-titanium. The device is then deployed by pressing a release button and turning the wheel again. The device is then retracted from the operating channel and the procedure is repeated on the contralateral side. Out of the 24 coils, 3–8 coils must be visible trailing in the uterine cavity to confirm proper placement of the device. Since the Essure microinserts are clearly visible via HSG, this provides physicians and patients reassurance regarding proper placement and tubal occlusion.

Another hysteroscopic device was recently approved and is commercially available. **Adiana** uses radiofrequency energy from a separate electrosurgical generator to desiccate a small segment of the interstitial portion of the fallopian tube, after which a small silicone plug is inserted. This method, using monopolar electrosurgery, requires glycine as the distension medium. It therefore carries the risk of electrolyte imbalance inherent in the use of nonionic solutions as well as the potential risk of thermal injury should the electrode perforate into the abdominal cavity. Since the silicone plug is not radiopaque, its final location cannot be confirmed on HSG to aide in confirmation of occlusion. Twelve-month data for Adiana report a 1.07% failure rate.

Follow-up

The follow-up visit for open or laparoscopic approaches is 1–2 weeks postoperatively. This is to notify if she develops fever (38°C or 100.4°F), increasing or persistent abdominal pain, or bleeding or purulent discharge from the incision.

Patients who have undergone hysteroscopic sterilization must be counseled to use an alternate form of contraception for 3 months at which time a low-pressure hysterosalpingogram must be obtained to confirm placement and bilateral tubal occlusion. The importance of the 3-month hysterosalpingogram needs to be communicated to patients at the time of microinsert placement; subsequent office follow-up may be required to ensure patients comply with confirmation test.

Complications

1. *Mortality:* The risk of death from tubal sterilization is 1–2 cases per 100,000 procedures; most of these are complications of *general anesthesia.* The most common cause of death during laparoscopic BTL appears to be hypoventilation related to anesthesia. **Cardiopulmonary arrest** and hypoventilation are reported as the leading cause of death in most cases. **Sepsis** as a cause of death from laparoscopic sterilization is directly related to bowel perforations or electrical bowel burns. No deaths have been reported from the hysteroscopic approach.

2. *Unintended laparotomy:* Unintended laparotomy occurs with 1–2% of laparoscopic procedures; most of these conversions are attributable to technical inability to complete the laparoscopic procedure rather than to complications of the procedure.

3. *Bowel injury:* Bowel injury can occur during insertion of the insufflation needle or trocar or during electrocoagulation. Small injuries from the needle or trocar with no bleeding or leakage of enteric contents can usually be managed expectantly; otherwise, prompt laparotomy is indicated.

4. *Vascular injury:* Vascular injury can occur during insufflation needle or trocar insertion. Injury to a large vessel is a life-threatening emergency. Perform an immediate laparotomy with direct pressure over the injury to control bleeding until repair can be performed.

5. *Method failure (pregnancy or ectopic pregnancy):* Although sterilization is highly effective and considered the definitive form of pregnancy prevention, it has a failure rate during the first year of 0.1–0.8%. At least one-third of these are ectopic pregnancies.

BTL failures can be grouped into the following categories:

- Luteal phase pregnancy is defined as a pregnancy in which conception occurs before the BTL, but pregnancy is diagnosed after an interval tubal sterilization.

- Misidentification of the oviduct because of poor visualization from inadequate exposure, adhesions, adnexal pathology, or poor lighting may result in mistakenly ligating the round ligament, ovarian ligament, infundibular ligament, or dilated broad ligament blood vessels instead of the oviduct. Therefore, initially identifying the fimbriated tubal ends and then tracing the tube medially to the isthmic region is imperative. In postpartum minilaparotomy BTL, Babcock clamps should be placed sequentially along the oviduct until the fimbria is visualized.

- Incomplete occlusion of the oviduct occurs because of poorly placed mechanical clips or the use of mechanical devices on edematous or dilated tubes. With correct clip application, the mesosalpinx on the surface of the tube is pulled upward to resemble the flat triangular shape of an envelope flap (**Kleppinger envelope sign**). When silastic rings are used, the tubal serosa, but not the tubal lumen, may be pulled into the ring, with absence of the vertical crease formed when the entire loop of tube is included in the ring.

- Incomplete tubal occlusion with electrocoagulation is generally associated with too brief an application of current or with the use of coagulation current instead of cutting current.

- Improper technique occurs with the use of the wrong sutures or failure to preserve a 2 cm proximal tubal segment. If a short proximal stump is left, the fluid pressure from uterine contractions could either prevent complete closure of the tubal lumen during healing or cause a fistula to form to relieve pressure after healing is complete.

6. *Pain:* After laparoscopy, patients may experience some degree of chest and shoulder pain due to trapped gas and mechanical blocking devices are believed to cause ischemic pain.

7. *Infection/hemorrhage:* Wound infections and hematoma have been associated with minilaparotomy. Hemorrhage is a rare complication that usually occurs following major vessel injury during laparoscopic entry and occasionally occurs following mesosalpingeal vessel injury during the occlusion procedure.

8. *Visceral (bowel, bladder, uterus) injuries:* Organ injuries can occur from sharp trauma (e.g. insufflation needle, trocar, scalpel), blunt trauma (e.g. from adhesiolysis), or electrical-thermal trauma. Injuries can also occur during inadvertent application of the occlusion device to the incorrect structure. If recognized at the time of occurrence, injuries to the bowel and bladder (which are more common in the presence of adhesions) are relatively easy to manage and will not result in long-term adverse sequelae. Injuries to the uterus, most often caused by uterine manipulators, do not usually lead to adverse sequelae unless bowel or bladder has been perforated simultaneously.

9. *Patient regret:* Sterilization is intended to be permanent, but patient regret is not rare. Poststerilization regret is a complex condition often caused by unpredictable life events.

10. The proportion of women who actually undergo microsurgical tubal reanastomosis is only 0.2% in the first 5 years after BTL. The most important factor in determining the success of reversal by tubal anastomosis is the length of healthy tube remaining after sterilization. Isthmic-to-isthmic anastomoses are most likely to be successful. Sterilization reversal using a sutureless laparoscopic approach yielded a 59% ongoing pregnancy rate with a 3.9% ectopic rate.

Noncontraceptive benefits are as follows:

1. *Ovarian cancer:* Several studies report a protective effect of sterilization against ovarian cancer, with a relative risk ranging from 0.2–0.8. Protection is hypothesized to result from reduced exposure of the ovaries to potential environmental carcinogens as well as oncogenic viruses.

2. *Pelvic inflammatory disease:* Although BTL does not protect against the acquisition of sexually transmitted disease, sterilization has been demonstrated to reduce the spread of organisms from the lower genital tract to the peritoneal cavity and thus protect against PID. However, in cases of infection occurring within weeks of surgery, manipulation of the cervix, uterus, or oviducts is postulated to exacerbate a chronic infection or facilitate bacterial ascent from the lower genital tract at the time of surgery (e.g. chlamydial or gonococcal cervicitis).

Post-tubal Ligation Syndrome

Proposed in 1951, this syndrome is a controversial constellation of symptoms, including pelvic discomfort, ovarian cystic changes, and menorrhagia, which are suggested to occur as a result of disruption of the uteroovarian blood supply, with resultant disturbances of ovulatory function after BTL.

However, the CREST (Collaborative Review of Sterilisation) study indicates that, women who are sterilized are more likely to have reduced bleeding, menstrual pain, with increased cycle irregularity.

Efficacy

The cumulative 10-year failure rate with each method of tubal ligation is as follows: spring clip method, 3.7%; bipolar coagulation, 2.5%; interval partial salpingectomy, 2%; silicone rubber bands, 2%; and postpartum salpingectomy, 0.8%. Essure system is 99.8% effective in preventing pregnancy after 2 years of follow-up.

Advantages

Female sterilization does not involve hormones. It is a permanent form of contraception. There is no change in libido, menstrual cycle, or in lactation. Female sterilization is usually a same-day procedure.

Disadvantages

- Female sterilization is a procedure that involves general or regional anesthesia.
- Patients who undergo the Essure system procedure require a backup method of contraception for the first 3 months.

- It is permanent contraception, and patients may regret the decision later, especially women younger than 30 years. Some studies have reported "regret" in 26% of women, and less than 10% undergo the reversal procedure.
- Sterilization does not protect the patient from STDs.
- Sterilization causes short-term discomfort, and it involves all the risks of surgery.

2. Male Sterilization—Vasectomy

The incidence of vasectomy procedure account for 5.6% of all contraceptive use (WHO). While female sterilization is far more common than male sterilization, as a procedure vasectomy is safer, simpler, about half the cost of female sterilization, and probably more effective.

Vasectomy involves incision of the scrotal sac, transection of the vas deferens, and occlusion of both severed ends by suture ligation or fulguration. The procedure is usually performed with the patient under local anesthesia in an outpatient setting. Complications include hematoma formation and sperm granulomas. Spontaneous resolution is rare. After sterilization, remnant sperm remains in the ejaculatory ducts. The man is not considered sterile until he has produced sperm-free ejaculates as documented by semen analysis. This usually requires 15–20 ejaculations. Vasectomy prevents the passage of sperm into seminal fluid by blocking the vas deferens.

Efficacy

The failure rate is approximately 0.1%.

There are different ways for men to be sterilized. One type does not require an incision—a cut. The other types of vasectomy require an incision. Incision methods take about 20 minutes. The no-incision method takes less time.

Incision Methods

Usually, a local anesthetic is injected into the pelvic area. Then, the doctor makes an incision on each side of the scrotum to reach each vas deferens—the tubes that carry sperm. Sometimes a single incision is made in the center. Each tube is blocked. In most procedures, a small section of each tube is removed. Tubes may be tied off or blocked with surgical clips. Or, they may be closed using an instrument with an electrical current.

No-Incision Method

With the no-incision ("no-scalpel") method, the skin of the scrotum is not cut. One tiny puncture is made to reach both vasa. The vasa are then tied off, cauterized, or blocked. The tiny puncture heals quickly. No stitches are needed, and no scarring takes place.

The no-scalpel method reduces bleeding and decreases the possibility of infection, bruising, and other complications.

Vasectomy is safe and, because it lasts for life, it is simple and convenient.

Vasectomy does not change hormones or masculinity. It will not produce impotence. It also will not affect sex organs, sexuality, and sexual pleasure. No glands or organs are removed or altered. Ejaculate will be about the same amount as before.

Vasectomy is appropriate when:

- Other methods are unacceptable.
- Couple has fear to pass on a hereditary illness or disability.
- Partner's health likely to be threatened by a future pregnancy.
- Husband want to spare wife of tubal sterilization due to health risk.

No Scalpel Vasectomy

No-scalpel vasectomy was developed in China by Dr. Li Shunqiang with the aim of reducing men's fear related to the incision and increasing vasectomy use in China. Since 1974, over 10 million Chinese men have undergone vasectomy by the no-scalpel technique.

No-scalpel vasectomy is less invasive than the incision approach because tissue trauma or blood vessel injury caused by sharp or blind dissection is avoided. It is a breakthrough advance in vasectomy practice with the main clinical advantage being a low surgical complication rate, especially haematoma and infection.

The Indian Government launched a national no-scalpel vasectomy project in 1998 in collaboration with the United Nations Population Fund (UNFPA) to promote male participation in contraception and arrest the declining trend in male sterilization. The prevalence of vasectomy increased from 0.7% in 1997 to about 3% in 2003. Today India is one of the leading nations in the world with regard to the use of no-scalpel vasectomy. The main steps are shown in Figs 17.17 to 17.27.

Possible Risks of Vasectomy

Major complications with vasectomy are rare and are usually caused by infection.

Complication rates for vasectomy are generally lower for the no-incision method than for methods that include cutting the skin.

- Signs of infection: (a) a fever over 100°F, (b) blood or pus oozing from the site of the incision, (c) excessive pain or swelling
- Bruising, which usually clears up on its own.
- Hematomas—they usually clear up by themselves, or with bed rest or ice packs. In rare cases, they need to be drained.
- Hydrocele—swellings that contain fluid and tenderness near the testicles. They usually clear up in about a week. Applying heat and wearing an athletic supporter can help.
- Granuloma—sperm that leaks from the tubes and causes a small lump under the skin near the site of the surgery. This usually clears up by itself. Surgical treatment is sometimes required.
- Pain or discomfort in the testicles. This is usually temporary, but in about 2 out of 100 cases the pain may be chronic and severe.
- Very rarely, the cut ends of a tube grow back together. This most often happens within four months of the operation and may allow pregnancy to happen.
- Decreased sexual desire or impotency occurs in 4 out of 1,000 cases. The most likely cause is emotional — there is no physical cause for sexual dysfunction associated with vasectomy.

Future Methods of Contraception

Many new contraceptive designs are under investigation to provide more contraceptive options that have fewer adverse effects, are safer, and are more efficacious. A few of the newer methods and forms of contraception are discussed below.

1. One of the more exciting new developments is a hormonal contraceptive method for men. The male birth control pill manipulates steroid hormones to decrease spermatogenesis and testosterone secretion.
2. Uniplant is a single-rod implant system that consists of 55 mg of nomegestrol acetate in a capsule that is 3.5 cm long and 2.4 mm in diameter. Uniplant has been shown to be highly effective for as long as 1 year, with a frequency and degree of menstrual irregularities similar to those of Norplant.
3. Clinical studies are in progress for a biodegradable implant, **Capnor**, to eliminate the necessity of implant removal. This is a single 40 mm rod that contains levonorgestrel and maintains contraceptive protection for 1 year.
4. Biodegradable pellet implants containing norethindrone and cholesterol are currently undergoing investigation. They dissolve within

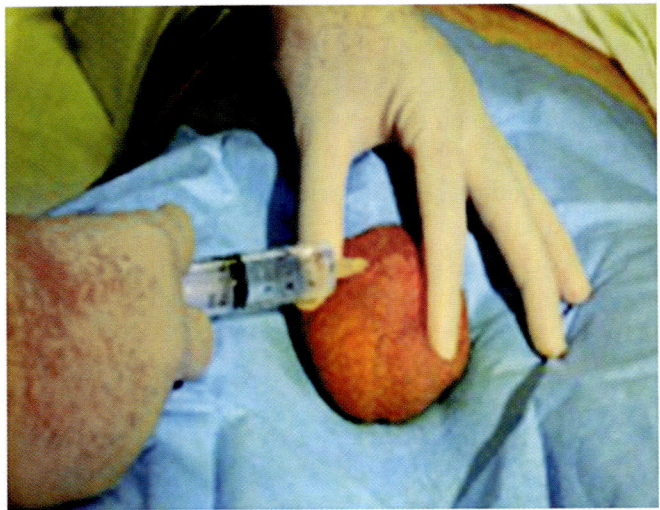

Fig.17.17: Step1: Injection of local anesthetics to 'numb' the skin area superficial

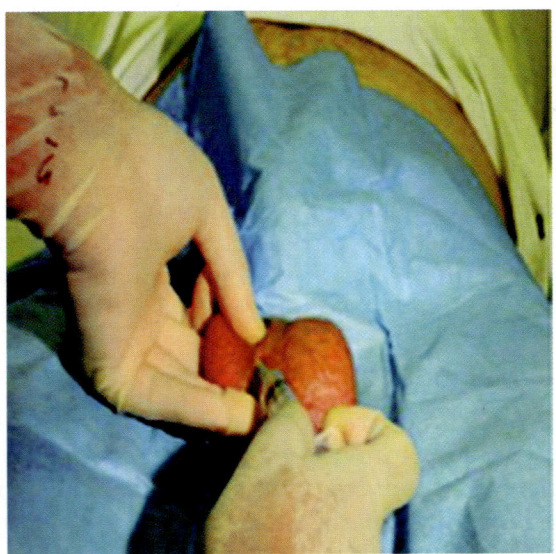

Fig.17.18: Step 2: A slightly deeper injection ar ound the vas. The needle does not penetrate any structure and is not very painful

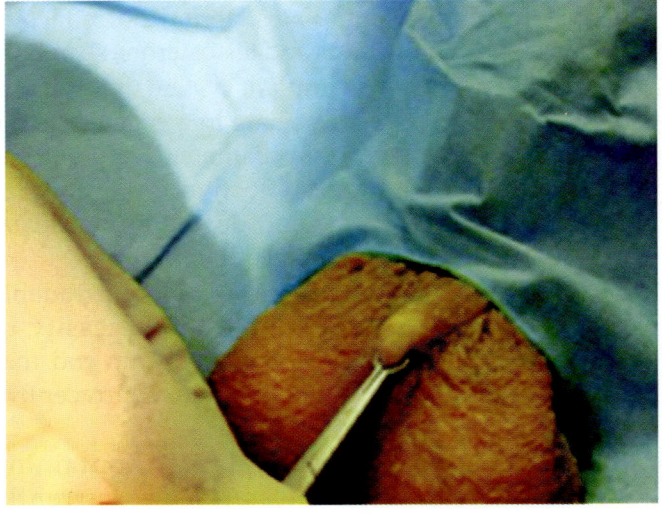

Fig.17.19: Step 3: Vas is lifted up by a vasectomy 'Ring'

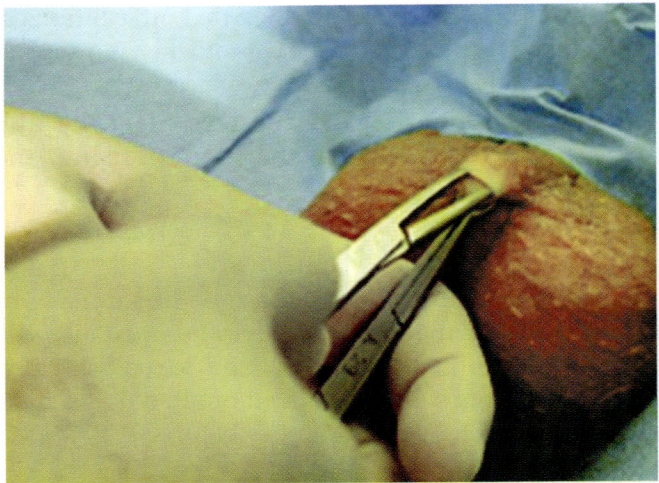

Fig.17.20: Step 4: Small opening made in the skin

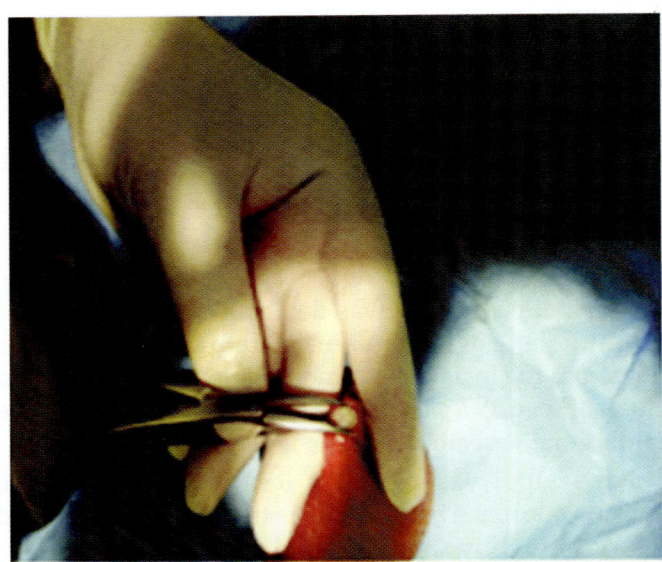

Fig.17.21: Step 5: Vas showing through the skin aperture

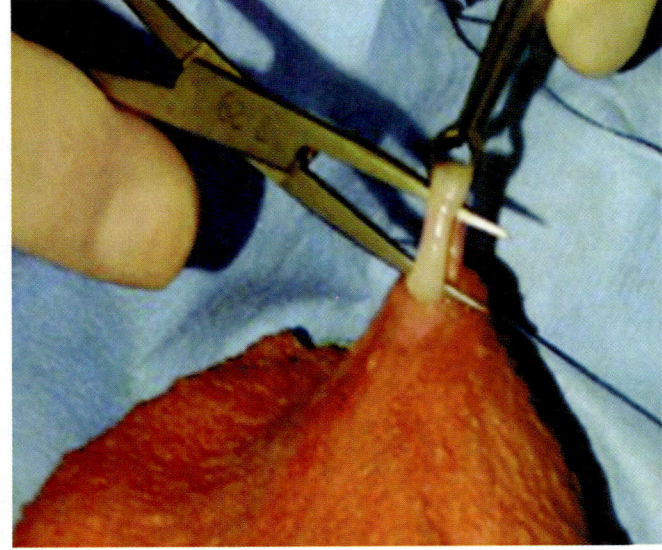

Fig.17.22: Step 6: Vas lifted out of the scrotum

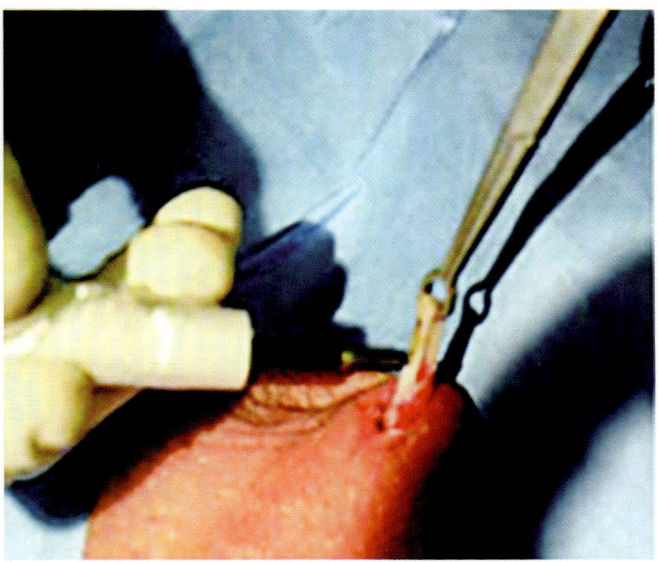

Fig.17.23: Step 7: The exposed loop of vas being cauterized

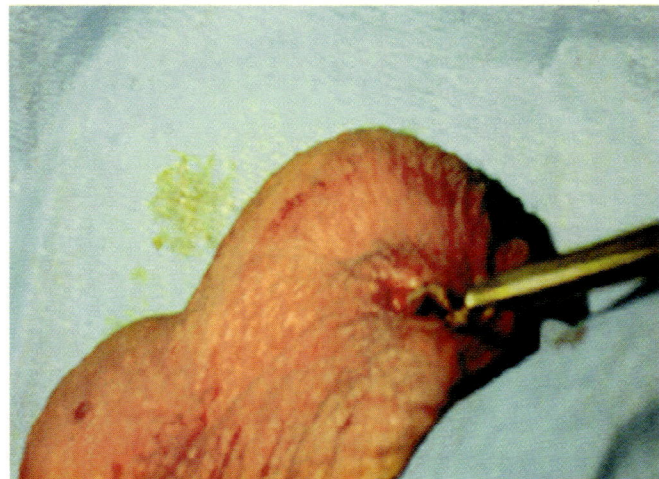

Fig.17.25: Step 9: Cauterized loop is cut and returned to scrotum. The procedure repeated for other side of v as through same skin opening

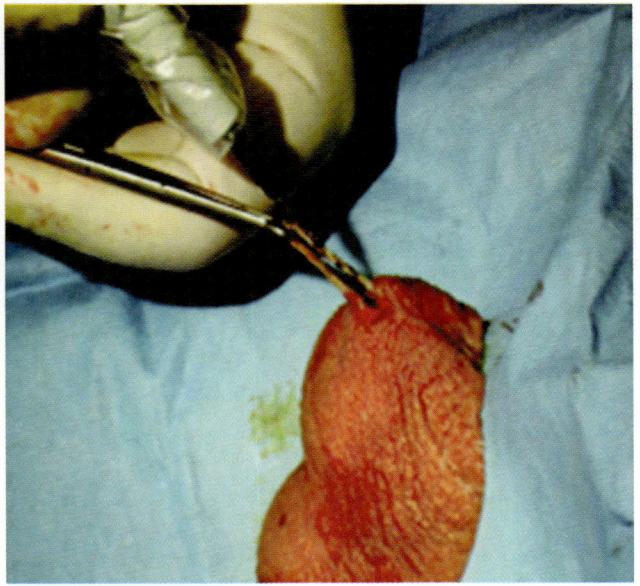

Fig.17.24: Step 8: Cauterizing extended further to a larger portion of vas

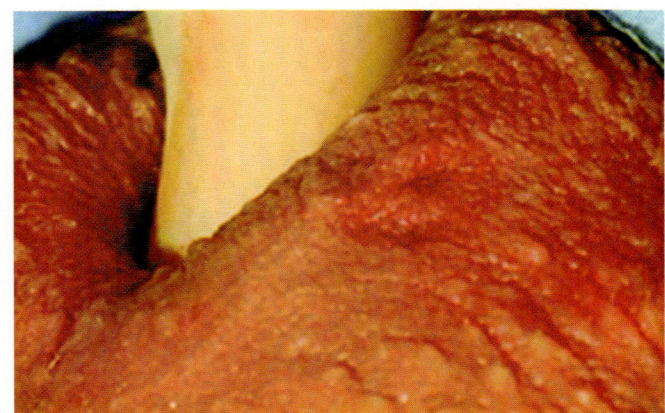

Fig.17.26: Step 10: After both vasa are completed and retur ned to scrotum, only a small skin wound is left which does not require any suture

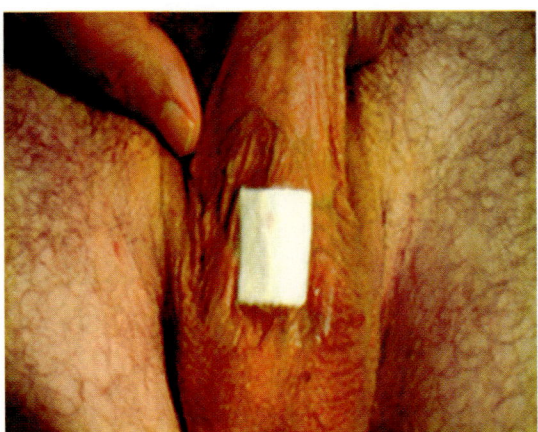

Fig.17.27: Step 11: Wound covered by a small dressing which may be removed after 48 hrs

Table 17.10: Summary of changes from the fourth edition to the fifth edition of the MEC (changes are highlighted in bold)

Condition	COC/P/CVR	CIC	POP	DMPA NET-EN	LNG/ETG	Cu-IUD		LNG-IUD	
Breastfeeding									
a. <6 weeks postpartum	4	**4**	**2**	**3**	**2**				
b. ≥6 weeks to <6 months (primarily breastfeeding)	3	**3**	1	**1**	1				
c. ≥6 months postpartum	2	**2**	1	**1**	1				
Postpartum (non-breastfeeding women)									
a. <21 days			1	**1**	1				
(i) without other risk factors for VTE	3	3							
(ii) with other risk factors for VTE	**4**	**4**							
b. ≥21 days to 42 days			1	**1**	1				
(i) without other risk for VTE	2	2							
(ii) with other risk factors for VTE	**3**	**3**							
c. >42 days	1	1	1	**1**	1				
Postpartum (breastfeeding or non-breastfeeding women, including after cesarean section)									
a. <48 hours including insertion immediately after delivery of the placenta						1		not BF = 1; BF = 2	
b. ≥48 hours to <4 weeks						3		3	
c. ≥4 weeks						1		1	
d. Puerperal sepsis						4		4	
Superficial venous disorders									
a. Varicose veins	1	1	1	1	1	1		1	
b. Superficial venous thrombosis	2	2	1	1	1	1		1	
Know dyslipidemias without other know cardiovascular risk factors	**2**	**2**	2	2	2	1		2	
STIs						*I*	*C*	*I*	*C*
a. Current purulent cervicitis or chlamydial infection or gonorrhea	1	**1**	1	1	1	4	2	4	2
b. Other STIs (excluding HIV and hepatitis)	1	**1**	1	1	1	2	2	2	2
c. Vaginitis (including *Trichomonas vaginalis* and bacterial vaginosis)	1	**1**	1	1	1	2	2	2	2
d. Increased risk of STIs	1	**1**	1	1	1	2/3	2	2/3	2
HIV/AIDS									
High risk of HIV	1	**1**	1	1	1	2	2	2	2
Asymptomatic or mild HIV clinical disease (WHO stage 1 or 2)	1	**1**	1	1	1	2	2	2	2
Severe or advanced HIV clinical disease (WHO stage 3 or 4)	1	**1**	1	1	1	3	2	3	2
Antiretroviral therapy						*I*	*C*	*I*	*C*
a. Nucleoside reverse transcriptase inhibitors (NRTIs)									
Abacavir (ABC)	1	1	1	1	1	2/3	2	2/3	2
Tenofovir (TDF)	1	1	1	1	1	2/3	2	2/3	2
Zidovudine (AZT)	1	1	1	1	1	2/3	2	2/3	2
Lamivudine (3TC)	1	1	1	1	1	2/3	2	2/3	2
Didanosine (DDI)	1	1	1	1	1	2/3	2	2/3	2
Emtricitabine (FTC)	1	1	1	1	1	2/3	2	2/3	2
Stavudine (D4T)	1	1	1	1	1	2/3	2	2/3	2

(Contd.)

Table 17.10: Summary of changes from the fourth edition to the fifth edition of the MEC (changes are highlighted in bold) *(Contd.)*

Condition	COC/P/CVR	CIC	POP	DMPA NET-EN	LNG/ETG	Cu-IUD	LNG-IUD
b. Non-nucleoside reverse transcriptase							
inhibitiors (NNRTIs)	2	2	2	1= DMPA	2	2/3 2	2/3 2
				2 = NET-EN			
Efavirenz (EFV)	1	1	1	1	1	2/3 2	2/3 2
Nevirapine (ETR)	2	2	2	1 = DMPA	2	2/3 2	2/3 2
				2 = NET-EN			
Rilpivirine (RPV)	1	1	1	1	1	2/3 2	2/3 2
c. Protease inhibitors (PIs)							
Ritonavir-boosted atazanavir (ATV/r)	2	2	2	1 = DMPA	2	2/3 2	2/3 2
				2 = MET-EN			
Ritonavir-boosted lopinavir (LPV/r)	2	2	2	1 = DMPA	2	2/3 2	2/3 2
				2 = NET-EN			
Ritonavir-boosted darunavir (DRV/r)	2	2	2	1 = DMPA	2	**2/3 2**	**2/3 2**
Ritonavir (RTV)	2	2	2	1 = DMPA	2	**2/3 2**	**2/3 2**
				2 = NET-EN			
d. Integrase inhibitors							
Raltegravir (ral)	1	1	1	1	1	**2/3 2**	**2/3 2**

Progesterone-releasing vaginal ring (PVR) (changes are highlighted in bold)	
Condition	Category
Pregnancy	**NA**
Breastfeeding and ≥ 4 weeks postpartum	**1**

Emergency contraceptive pills (ECPs) (changes are highlighted in bold)			
Condition	COC	LNG	UPA
Pregnancy	NA	NA	NA
Breastfeeding and ≥4 weeks postpartum	1	1	2
Past ectopic pregnancy	1	1	**1**
Obesity	1	1	**1**
History of severe cardiovascular disease (ischemic heart disease, cerebrovascular attack, or other thromboembolic conditions)	2	2	**2**
Migraine	2	2	**2**
Severe liver disease (including jaundice)	2	2	**2**
CYP3A4 inducers (e.g. rifampicin, phenytoin, phenobarbital, carbamazepine, primidone, rifabutin, St John's wort/hypericum perforatum)	1	1	**1**
Repeated ECP use	1	1	**1**
Rape	1	1	**1**

2 years and release the norethindrone for 12–18 months. Insertion of the pellets has been demonstrated to be simple; however, if the patient desires removal several months later, removal has been noted to be difficult.

5. The vaginal sponge is made of soft disposable polyurethane foam that contains the spermicide nonoxynol-9. It offers an immediate and continuous presence of spermicide throughout a 24-hour period. The polyurethane foam is designed to trap and absorb semen before the entry of sperm into the cervix. Unlike a diaphragm, the sponge does not have to be fitted and, it had overall equal efficacy in multiparous as nulliparous women. The main advantage of the sponge over a diaphragm is its ready availability. The greatest risk with its use is the possibility of toxic shock syndrome (TSS). TSS is a rare, life-threatening bacterial infection that may occur, if the sponge is left in place for more than 30 hours or if it is used while a woman is menstruating.

6. **Lea's shield** is a one-size-fits-all diaphragm like device. This device consists of a 1-way valve that allows air to escape during placement, thus creating a suction effect against the cervix. The unilateral

direction of the valve permits uterine and cervical fluids to be released into the vaginal canal but prevents sperm from entering.

7. Chemical scarring of the fallopian tubes by instilling phenol quinacrine that ultimately leads to blockage of the tubes.

8. Another nonsurgical form of tubal sterilization is by introduction of **methyl cyanoacrylate** into the fallopian tubes to produce a reversible chemical plug to block the tubes which can be removed later. Chemical scarring and plugs are also under investigation as potential methods of vasectomy.

9. A pregnancy vaccine is one of the most controversial and exciting forms of contraception under development. The pregnancy vaccine, unlike anti-infective vaccines, stimulates an immune response against one or more host-specific antigens like sperm antigens, zona pellucida antigens or chorionic gonadotropin.

Currently, the major research focus is on the development of a vaccine that works by producing antibodies against human chorionic gonadotropin (hCG). In pregnant women, hCG is formed on about the 23rd day following midcycle conception. The hCG sends a signal to prevent menstruation. The presence of vaccine-induced anti-hCG antibodies can inhibit this signaling process and allow menstruation to proceed.

Medical Eligibility Criteria Wheel for Contraceptive Use 2015 (Table 17.10)

Introduction

This document is part of the process for improving the quality of care in family planning. *Medical eligibility criteria for contraceptive use* (MEC), the first edition of which was published in 1996, presents current World Health Organization (WHO) guidance on the safety of various contraceptive methods for use in the context of specific health conditions and characteristics. This is the fifth edition of the MEC—the latest in the series of periodic updates. In comparison to the fourth edition

of the MEC, summaries given in Table 17.10 highlight changes that appear in the fifth edition of the guideline.

In the MEC, the safety of each contraceptive method is determined by several considerations in the context of the medical condition or medically relevant characteristics; primarily, whether the contraceptive method worsens the medical condition or creates additional health risks, and secondarily, whether the medical circumstance makes the, contraceptive method less effective. The safety of the method is weighed along with the benefits of preventing unintended pregnancy.

This document covers the following family planning methods: low-dose ($\leq$35 μg ethinyl estradiol) combined oral contraceptives (COCs), combined patch (P), combined vaginal ring (CVR), combined injectable contraceptives (CICs), progestogen-only pills (POPs), depot medroxyprogesterone acetate (DMPA), norethisterone enanthate (NET-EN), levonorgestrel (LNG) and etonogestrel (ETG) implants, emergency contraceptive pills (ECPs), copper-bearing intrauterine devices (Cu-IUDs), levonorgestrel-releasing IUDs (LNG-IUDs), copper-IUD for emergency contraception (E-IUD), progesterone-releasing vaginal ring (PVR), barrier methods (BARR), fertility awareness-based methods (FAB), lactational amenorrhea method (LAM), coitus interruptus (CI), and female and male sterilization (STER).

For each medical condition, contraceptive methods are placed into one of four numbered categories. Depending upon the individual, more than one condition may need to be considered together to determine contraceptive eligibility. These conditions and characteristics include: age, weeks/months postpartum, breastfeeding status, venous thromboembolism, superficial venous disorders, dyslipidemias, puerperal sepsis, past ectopic-pregnancy, history of severe cardiovascular disease, migraines, severe liver disease, use of CYP3A4 inducer, repeat use of ECPs, rape, obesity, increased risk of sexually transmitted infections, high risk of HIV infection, living with HIV, use of antiretroviral therapy.

Urinary Flow Disorders

18A. PHYSIOLOGY OF URINARY FLOW AND CONTINENCE

The main organs involved in urination are the urinary bladder and the urethra. The smooth muscle of the bladder, known as the detrusor, is innervated by sympathetic nervous system fibers from the lumbar spinal cord and parasympathetic fibers from the sacral spinal cord. Fibers in the pelvic nerves constitute the main afferent limb of the voiding reflex; the parasympathetic fibers to the bladder that constitute the excitatory efferent limb also travel in these nerves. Part of the urethra is surrounded by the external urethral sphincter, which is innervated by the somatic pudendal nerve originating in the cord, in an area termed Onuf's nucleus.

Smooth muscle bundles pass on either side of the urethra, and these fibers are sometimes called the internal urethral sphincter, although they do not encircle the urethra. Further along the urethra is a sphincter of skeletal muscle, the sphincter of the membranous urethra (external urethral sphincter). The bladder's epithelium is termed transitional epithelium which contains a superficial layer of dome-like cells and multiple layers of stratified cuboidal cells underneath when remains empty. When the bladder is fully distended the superficial cells become squamous (flat) and the stratification of the cuboidal cells is reduced in order to provide lateral stretching.

Physiology

The physiology of micturition and the physiologic basis of its disorders are sometimes difficult to assess especially at the supraspinal level. Micturition is fundamentally a spinobulbospinal reflex facilitated and inhibited by higher brain centers such as the pontine micturition center subject to voluntary facilitation and inhibition.

In healthy individuals, the lower urinary tract has two discrete phases of activity:
a. The storage (or guarding) phase, when urine is stored in the bladder;
b. The voiding phase, when urine is released through the urethra.

The state of the reflex system is dependent on both a conscious signal from the brain and the firing rate of sensory fibers from the bladder and urethra. At low bladder volumes, afferent firing is low, resulting in excitation of the outlet (the sphincter and urethra), and relaxation of the bladder. At high bladder volumes, afferent firing increases, causing a conscious sensation of urinary urge. When the individual is ready to urinate, she consciously initiates voiding, causing the bladder to contract and the outlet to relax. Voiding continues until the bladder empties completely, at which point the bladder relaxes and the outlet contracts to re-initiate storage. The muscles controlling micturition are controlled by the autonomic and somatic nervous systems. During the storage phase, the internal urethral sphincter remains tense and the detrusor muscle relaxed by sympathetic stimulation. During micturition, parasympathetic stimulation causes the detrusor muscle to contract and the internal urethral sphincter to relax. The external urethral sphincter (sphincter urethrae) is under somatic control and is consciously relaxed during micturition.

In the adult, the volume of urine in the bladder that normally initiates a reflex contraction is about 300–400 mL.

Storage Phase

During storage, bladder pressure stays low, because the bladder is highly compliant in nature and shows a very slight rise as the bladder is filled. This phenomenon is a manifestation of the law of Laplace. In the case of the bladder, the tension increases as the organ fills, but so does the radius. Therefore, the pressure increase is slight until the organ is relatively full.

Action potentials carried by sensory neurons from stretch receptors in the urinary bladder wall travel to the sacral segments of the spinal cord through the pelvic nerves. Since bladder wall stretch is low during the storage phase, these afferent neurons fire at low frequencies. Low-frequency afferent signals cause relaxation of the bladder by inhibiting sacral parasympathetic preganglionic neurons and exciting lumbar sympathetic preganglionic neurons. Conversely, afferent input causes contraction of the sphincter through excitation of Onuf's nucleus, and contraction of the bladder neck and urethra through excitation of the sympathetic preganglionic neurons.

Voiding Phase

Voiding begins when a voluntary signal is sent from the brain to begin urination, and continues until the bladder is empty.

Bladder afferent signals ascend the spinal cord to the periaqueductal gray, where they project both to the pontine micturition center and to the cerebrum. At a certain level of afferent activity, the conscious urge to void becomes difficult to ignore. Once the voluntary signal to begin voiding has been issued, neurons in pontine micturition center fire maximally, causing excitation of sacral preganglionic neurons. The firing of these neurons causes the wall of the bladder to contract; as a result, a sudden, sharp rise in intravesical pressure occurs. The pontine micturition center also causes inhibition of Onuf's nucleus, resulting in relaxation of the external urinary sphincter. When the external urinary sphincter is relaxed urine is released from the urinary bladder since the pressure in the bladder is great enough to force urine to flow out of the urethra. The micturition reflex normally produces a series of contractions of the urinary bladder. The flow of urine through the urethra has an overall excitatory role in micturition, which helps sustain voiding until the bladder is empty.

Voluntary Control

The mechanism by which voluntary urination is initiated remains unsettled. One possibility is that the voluntary relaxation of the muscles of the pelvic floor causes a sufficient downward tug on the detrusor muscle to initiate its contraction. Another possibility is the excitation or disinhibition of neurons in the pontine micturition center, which causes concurrent contraction of the bladder and relaxation of the sphincter.

The bladder can be made to contract by voluntary facilitation of the spinal voiding reflex when it contains only a few milliliters of urine. Voluntary contraction of the abdominal muscles aids the expulsion of urine by increasing the pressure applied to the urinary bladder wall, but voiding can be initiated without straining even when the bladder is nearly empty.

Voiding can also be consciously interrupted once it has begun, through a contraction of the perineal muscles. The external sphincter can be contracted voluntarily, which will prevent urine from passing down the urethra.

The Urethral Support System (Fig. 18.1)

The urethral support system consists of all the structures extrinsic to the urethra that provide a supportive layer upon which the urethra rests. The major components of this supportive structure include the anterior vagina, the endopelvic fascia, the arcus tendineus fasciae pelvis, and the levator ani muscles.

The *endopelvic fascia* is a dense fibrous connective tissue layer, which surrounds the vagina and attaches it to the arcus tendineus fasciae pelvis laterally. The *arcus tendineus fasciae pelvis* in turn is attached to the pubic bone ventrally and to the ischial spine dorsally. The arcus tendineus fasciae pelvis is a tensile structure located bilaterally on either side of the urethra and vagina. It provides the support needed to suspend the urethra on the anterior vaginal wall. Although well-defined near its origin as a fibrous band at the pubic bone, the arcus tendineus fasciae pelvis becomes a broad aponeurotic structure as it passes dorsally to the ischial spine.

The *levator ani muscle* consists of three parts—the pubococcygeus, the puborectalis, and the iliococcygeus muscles. The pubococcygeus and the puborectalis muscles form a U-shape as they originate from the pubic bone on either side of the midline and pass behind the rectum to form a sling. This sling of muscle is composed of predominantly Type I striated muscle fibers and, therefore, is suited to maintaining constant tone. It is this constant tone that normally keeps the urogenital hiatus closed.

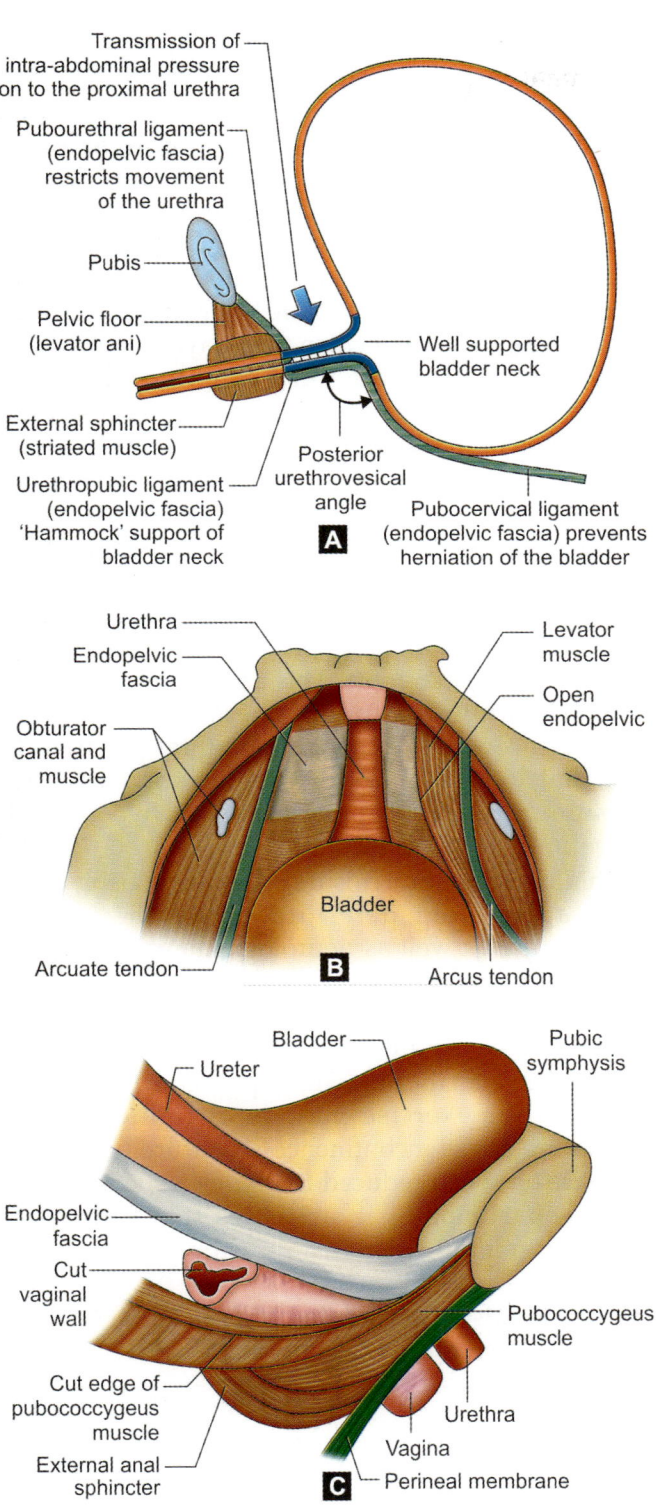

Fig. 18.1: Anatomy of female pelvis

displacement of about 10 mm. This displacement is due to a simultaneous contraction of the diaphragm and abdominal wall muscles. This downward momentum must then be arrested by stretch resistance of the pelvic floor structures which compresses the proximal intra-abdominal portion of the urethra against the underlying supportive layer, which is composed of the endopelvic fasciae, the vagina, and the levator ani muscles.

Additionally, the constant tone maintained by the pelvic muscles relieves the tension placed upon the endopelvic fascia. If the nerves to the levator ani muscle are damaged during childbirth, the denervated muscles would undergo atrophy thereby leaving pelvic organ support upon the endopelvic fascia alone. Elderly striated muscle takes 35% longer to develop the same force as in the young adult. These changes are not due to alterations in neural recruitment, but due to age-related changes in striated muscle contractility. This decrease in muscle strength, in turn, will be associated with a loss of pelvic muscle stiffness or resistance to stretch.

If the muscle is normally innervated and is sufficiently attached to the endopelvic fascia, then many women can simply learn to use a voluntary muscle contraction during a cough to help prevent urine loss.

The Sphincteric Closure System (Figs 18.2 and 18.3)

The sphincteric closure of the urethra is normally provided by the urethral striated muscles, the urethral smooth muscle, and the vascular elements within the submucosa. Each is thought to contribute equally to the resting urethral closure pressure.

Anatomically, the urethra can be divided into percentiles with the internal urethral meatus representing point 0 and the external meatus representing the 100th percentile mark. The urethra passes through the wall of the bladder at the level of the vesical neck where the detrusor muscle fibers extend below the internal urethral meatus to as far as the 15th percentile. The striated urethral sphincter muscle begins at the termination of the detrusor fibers and extends to the 64th percentile. It is circularly oriented and completely surrounds the smooth muscle of the urethral wall. Starting at the 54th percentile the striated muscles of the urogenital diaphragm, the compressor urethrae and the urethrovaginal sphincter can be seen. They are continuous with the striated urethral sphincter and extend to the 76th percentile. Their fiber direction is no longer circular. The compressor urethrae passes over the urethra to insert into the urogenital diaphragm near the pubic ramus. The urethrovaginal sphincter surrounds both the urethra and the vagina. The distal

Functionally, the levator ani muscle and the endopelvic fascia serve an interactive role in maintaining continence and pelvic support. In a hard cough, intraabdominal pressure can increase suddenly by about 150 cm H_2O and this causes the proximal urethra to undergo a mid-sagittal caudodorsal

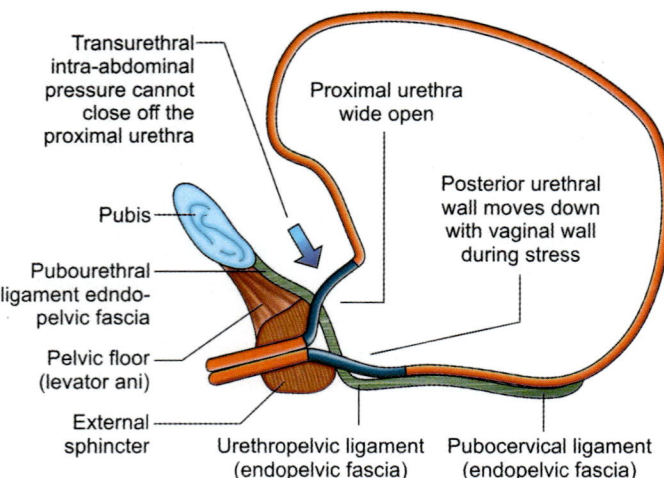

Fig. 18.2: Anatomy of the urethra shown in longitudinal section

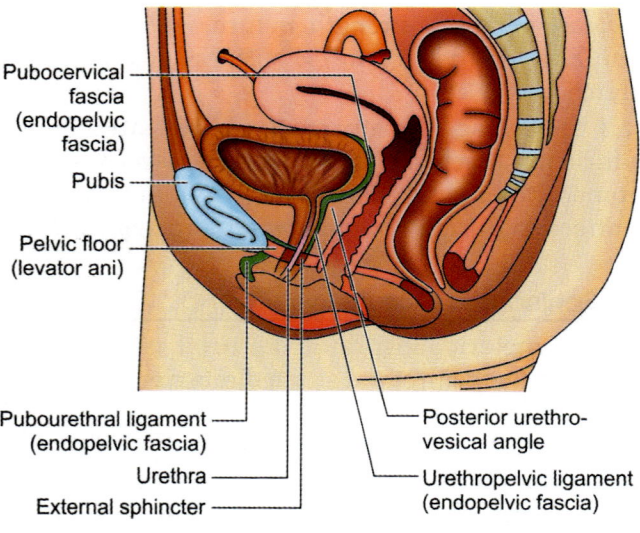

Fig. 18.3: Urethral support mechanism

thought to contribute to continence by forming a watertight seal via coaptation of the mucosal surfaces. Surrounding this plexus is the inner longitudinal smooth muscle layer, which is in turn surrounded by a circular layer that itself lies inside the outer layer of striated muscle. The smooth muscle layers are present throughout the upper four-fifths of the urethra. The circular configuration of the circular smooth muscle layer and outer striated muscle layer suggests a role in constricting the lumen when these layers contract. The mechanical role of the inner longitudinal smooth muscle layer is presently unresolved. It is possible that contraction of this longitudinal layer may help to open the lumen to initiate micturition, rather than constrict the lumen.

There are several important clinical correlates of urethral muscular anatomy. Perhaps the most important of these is that stress incontinence is caused by disorder of the urethral sphincter mechanism as well as with urethral support. This appears because of the fact that urethral support operations cure stress incontinence without changing urethral function. The fact that urethral support operations cure stress incontinence does not implicate urethral hypermobility as the cause of stress incontinence.

This loss of urethral closure pressure probably results from age-related deterioration of the urethral musculature as well as neurologic injury. Substantial decreases in closure pressure are seen with age . Pelvic floor exercise increases urethral resting closure pressure by about 30% only after an intensive 8–12 weeks which is much less than the intravesical pressure during a hard cough. Thus exercise may be of limited help in alleviating stress incontinence when urethral resting pressure has been reduced too much, especially if the woman participates in activities that cause large increases in intra-abdominal pressure.

Factors Involved in Maintaining Urethral Closure and Continence

Intrinsic Urethral Mechanism (Fig. 18.4)

The urethra consists largely of a rich vascular "sponge", lined by a moist mucosal layer and surrounded by a coat of smooth muscle, fibroelastic tissue and striated muscle. The mucosa provides coaptation. The vascular submucosa creates the "washer effect" for the continence mechanism. Functionally, the surrounding smooth muscle coat contains this mechanism by directing submucosal expansile pressures inward towards the mucosa. Muscle tone is mediated by alpha-adrenoceptors in the sympathetic nervous system. All three layers are under estrogen control.

terminus of the urethra runs adjacent to, but does not connect with the bulbocavernosus muscles.

Functionally, the urethral muscles maintain continence in various ways. The U-shaped loop of the detrusor smooth muscle surrounds the proximal urethra favoring its closure by constricting the lumen. The striated urethral sphincter is composed mainly of Type I (slow twitch) fibers, which are well-suited to maintain constant tone as well as allow voluntary increases in tone to provide additional continence protection. Distally, the recruitment of the striated muscle of the urethrovaginal sphincter and the compressor urethrae compress the lumen.

The smooth muscle of the urethra may also play a role in determining stress continence. The lumen is surrounded by a prominent vascular plexus that is

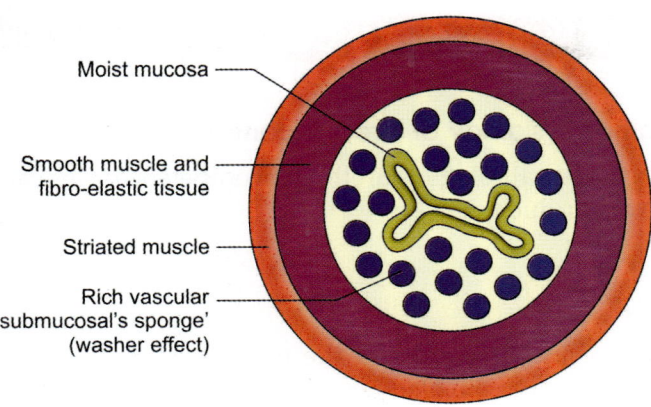

Moist mucosa

Smooth muscle and
fibro-elastic tissue

Striated muscle

Rich vascular
submucosal's sponge'
(washer effect)

Fig. 18.4: Integrity of urethral resistance

Extrinsic Factors

1. Levator ani muscles (pelvic diaphragm) support all of the pelvic organs and the pubourethralis portion form the "external sphincter".
2. The endopelvic fascia condenses to form three distinct ligaments:
   a. Pubourethral ligament—stabilizes the urethra
   b. Urethropelvic ligament—supports the bladder neck and the urethra.
   c. Pubocervical fascia—supports the bladder.
   Their attachments to the side wall of the urethra and pelvic wall (arcuate tendons) form a "hammock"

behind the urethra. When intra-abdominal pressure increases, (e.g. when coughing, sneezing and during exercise), the urethra is forced closed against the posterior "hammock".

3. Urogenital diaphragm (perineal muscles and fascia).
4. *Uterus and cervix*—The cardinal ligaments laterally, and the uterosacral ligaments posteriorly provide direct and indirect support of the bladder as the endopelvic fascia (pubocervical fascia), is fixed to the cervix.

Integration of the Stress Continence Control System

The levator ani muscles, endopelvic fascia, and muscular structures of the urethra comprise a system. These muscles are recruited during a cough to help prevent urine loss during stress. The coordinated action of these elements depends upon the central nervous system.

Recent evidence has shown that nerve dysfunction accompanies stress incontinence. This is supported by the observation that many women, simply by learning to time a pelvic muscle contraction to occur during a cough, are able to eliminate stress incontinence during that cough.

18B. URETHRAL SPHINCTER INCONTINENCE (GENUINE STRESS INCONTINENCE)

Introduction

The International Continence Society (ICS) defines SUI as the complaint of involuntary leakage on effort or exertion, or on coughing or sneezing.

Normally, at rest the intraurethral pressure is greater than the intravesical pressure. The pressure difference between the bladder and the urethra is known as the urethral closure pressure. If intra-abdominal pressure increases as it does with a cough, sneeze, or strain, and if this pressure is not equally transmitted to the urethra, then continence is not maintained and leakage of urine occurs (Fig. 18.5).

Urinary incontinence is an underdiagnosed and underreported problem that increases with age—affecting 50–84% of the elderly and is more than 2 times more common in females than in males.

Incidence of Subtypes of Urinary Incontinence in Women

1. Stress incontinence—50%
2. Urge incontinence—20%
3. Mixed—30%

Genuine Stress Incontinence

Definition

The involuntary loss of urine when the intravesical pressure, as a result of an increase of intra-abdominal pressure, exceeds the resistance produced by the urethral closure mechanisms, in the absence of bladder activity (unassociated with the desire to void).

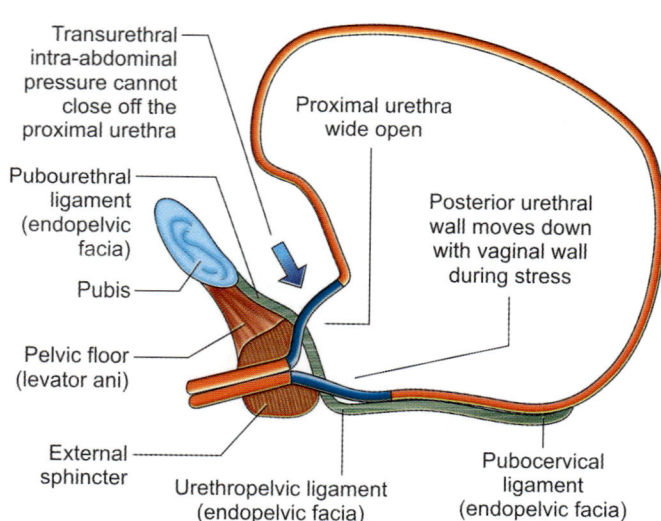

Transurethral intra-abdominal pressure cannot close off the proximal urethra

Proximal urethra wide open

Pubourethral ligament (endopelvic facia)

Pubis

Posterior urethral wall moves down with vaginal wall during stress

Pelvic floor (levator ani)

External sphincter

Urethropelvic ligament (endopelvic facia)

Pubocervical ligament (endopelvic facia)

Fig. 18.5: Normal urethral support

Pathophysiology of Stress Incontinence

The basic pathology is urethral incompetence. This can be either due to:

A. *Urethral Hypermobility (80–90% of patients)*

This results from loss of the normal pelvic support mechanism of the bladder and urethra due to:
- Trauma and stretching of vaginal delivery
- Hysterectomy
- Hormonal changes in menopause
- Pelvic denervation
- Congenital weakness

As the bladder neck support is weakened, the increase in intra-abdominal pressure is no longer transmitted equally to the bladder outlet, and, therefore, instantaneous leakage occurs.

B. *Intrinsic Sphincter Dysfunction (10–20% of patients)*

This results from damage to the sphincter due to:
- Multiple prior operations
- Trauma
- Radiation
- Neurogenic disorders including diabetes mellitus
- *Atrophic changes:* Lack of estrogen.

Evaluation of Urinary Incontinence

History

1. Type of incontinence (urge or stress): Immediate leak after coughing or standing up is stress incontinence. Leaking after a few seconds is a detrusor contraction.
2. Straining to void/incomplete emptying (?overflow)
3. Medications (alpha-blockers)
4. Frequency (>7–8 diurnal voids)
5. Pattern (diurnal, nocturnal, after taking medications)
6. Associated symptoms (dysuria, hematuria, suprapubic or perineal discomfort)—bladder carcinoma, bladder stone or infection.
7. Alteration in bowel habits/sexual function
8. Other diseases (cancer, diabetes, neurologic disease)

Voiding Record

A diary kept over a 24- or 48-hour period which records the times and volumes that the patient voids will give an idea of the largest single voided volume but also of

Voiding Record					
Date	Time	Volume voided	Wet or dry	Volume of incontinence	Comments cough, sneeze, running water, on way to toilet, teat coffee, alcohol, etc.

frequency and polyuria and severity of incontinence problems.

Physical Examination

1. *Abdominal examination*—distended bladder, abdominal mass.
2. *Pelvic examination*—atrophic vaginitis/urethritis, pelvic muscle laxity, bladder neck descent, cystocele, rectocele, uterine/vault prolapse, pelvic mass.
3. *Stress test*—leakage with a full bladder after coughing—immediate (stress incontinence) or delayed (detrusor contraction). Bilateral elevation of the vaginal wall, lateral to the bladder neck, will stop leakage in patients with hypermobility of the urethra, but not in patients with intrinsic sphincter dysfunction (Bonney–Marshall urethral elevation test).
4. *Rectal examination*—skin irritation, anal sphincter control, fecal impaction
5. *Neurologic examination*—mental status, sacral reflexes, perineal sensation (S2,3,4)
6. *Other medical conditions*—congestive heart failure, peripheral edema

Laboratory Investigation

1. Creatinine and electrolytes
2. Fasting glucose and calcium
3. Renal ultrasound in patients with incomplete emptying
4. Urine culture.

Urodynamic Evaluation of Urinary Incontinence

In approximately 10–15% of women with symptoms of stress incontinence, this is actually due to detrusor instability. Urodynamic testing reveals that approximately 20% of women with symptoms of urge, frequency, and overactive urge incontinence actually have underlying genuine stress incontinence, rather than detrusor overactivity.

1. *Post-void residual urine:* This test is essential in all incontinent women and distinguishes between true incontinence (residual urine <50 mL) and overflow incontinence (residual urine >100 mL).
2. *Voiding record:* A diary kept over a 24- or 48-hour period which records the times and volumes that the patient voids will give an idea of the largest single voided volume but also of frequency and polyuria and severity of incontinence problems.
3. *Uroflow:* A poor flow can be an indication of urethral obstruction and should be treated during surgery to prevent postoperative retention or difficulty to void (Fig. 18.6).
4. *Pressure flow study:* A small catheter in the bladder measures the pressure during voiding while her flow is also measured. This helps to differentiate true urethral obstruction from underactivity of the detrusor. Obstruction = detrusor pressure more than 50 cm H_2O and flow <15 mL/s.
5. *Cystometrogram:* The pressure in the bladder and rectum is measured during bladder filling. Intra-abdominal pressure is subtracted from bladder pressure to give a real indication of detrusor function (Fig. 18.7).
6. *Abdominal leak-point pressure (ALPP):* This is the measurement of the total bladder pressure during coughing or Valsalva maneuver to determine the pressure in the bladder required to induce leakage. In hypermobility of the urethra, the ALPP will be more than 60 cm H_2O, but with intrinsic sphincter dysfunction, the ALPP is less than 60 cm H_2O and often less than 20 cm H_2O (Fig. 18.8).
7. *Cystoscopy:* Cystourethroscopy allows an anatomical assessment of the bladder and the urethra. The precise role of cystourethroscopy in the evaluation of female urinary incontinence is controversial. Fewer than 2% of bladder tumors have been identified by routinely performing cystoscopy in incontinent women.

On the other hand, cystoscopy helps detect bladder lesions, such as a foreign body (e.g. suture, mesh material from prior surgery for prolapse or incontinence), bladder cancer, and bladder stones, which would otherwise remain undiagnosed, if only urodynamic findings are assessed. A visual inspection of the urethra helps establish the presence of urethral stricture or gross evidence of poor urethral closure.

Cystoscopy is indicated for patients with persistent irritative voiding symptoms or hematuria, persistent postoperative incontinence, voiding dysfunction, and findings suggestive of a diverticulum or fistula. Obvious causes of bladder overactivity, such as cystitis, stone, and tumor, can be easily diagnosed.

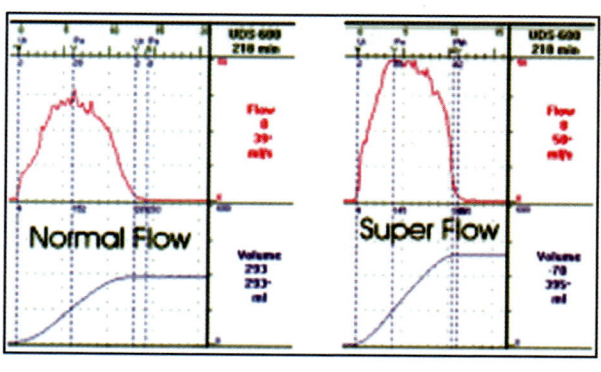

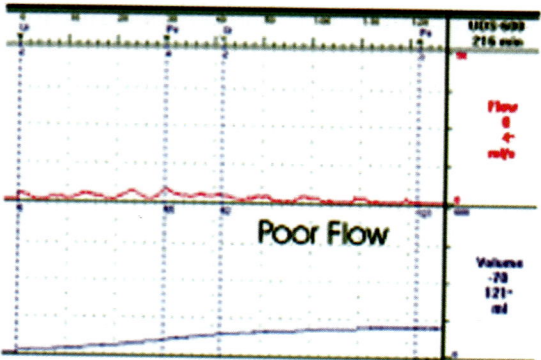

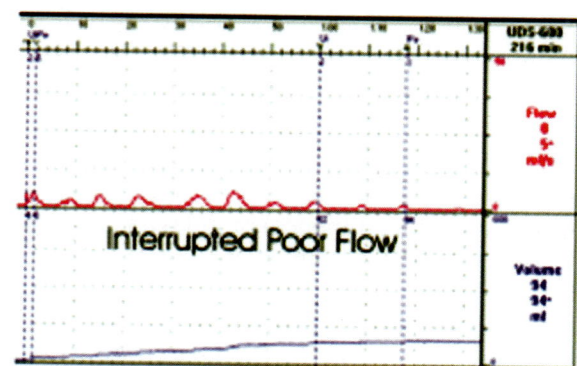

Fig. 18.6: Uroflowmetry

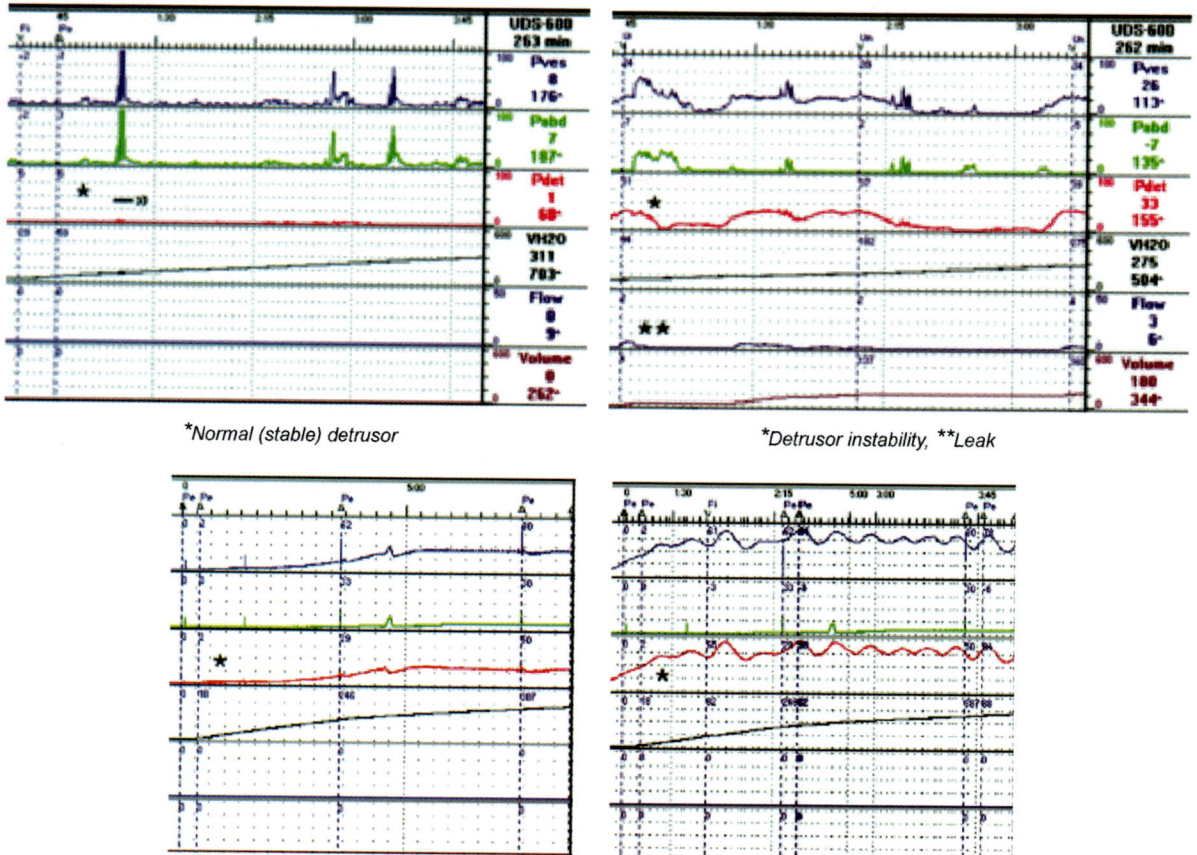

*Normal (stable) detrusor   *Detrusor instability, **Leak*

*Small volume bladder with poor compliance   *Detrusor hyperreflexia (neurogenic bladder)*

Fig. 18.7: Cystometrogram

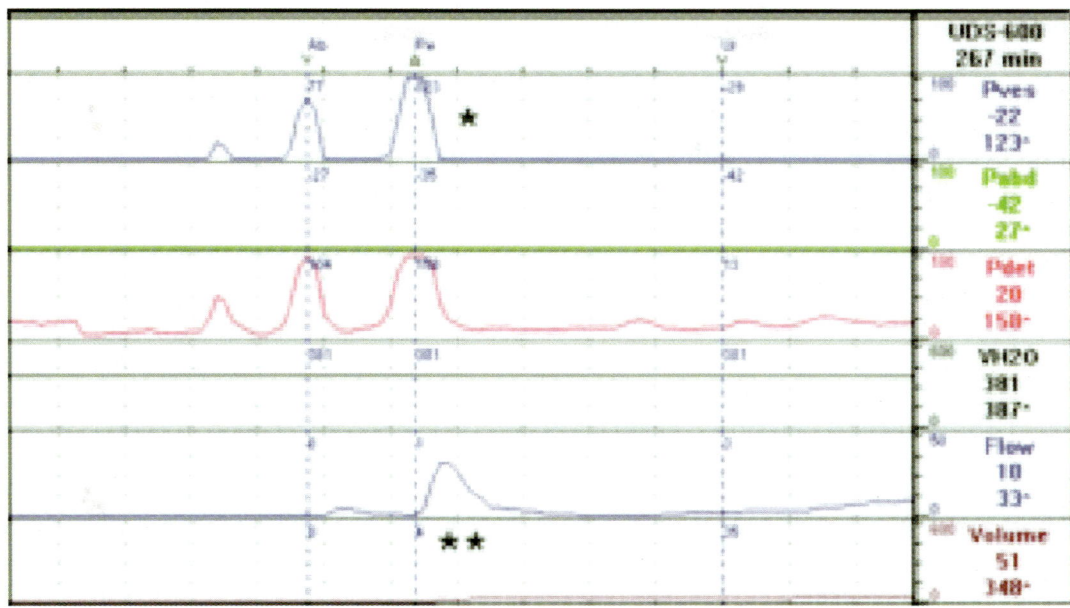

* Leak point pressure
** Leak

Fig. 18.8: ALPP

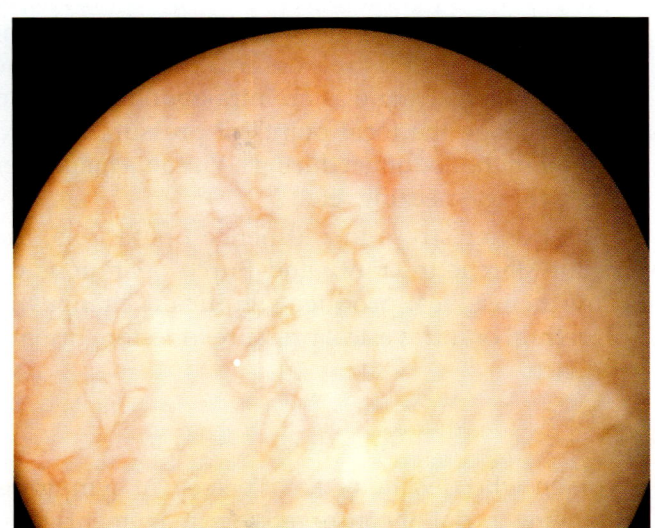

Fig. 18.9: Pale white detrusor bands are obser ved against a vascular mucosal background evidence of detrusor instability (DI)

A fixed, rigid, nonfunctioning urethra can be a finding in severe cases of intrinsic sphincter deficiency. Rounding of the urethra or the presence of bladder trabeculations (thick, band-like cords of detrusor muscle) during bladder filling may point to the diagnosis of detrusor overactivity (Fig. 18.9).

Treatment of Stress Urinary Incontinence

Nonsurgical Measures

For most patients with SUI, the simplest, least invasive, and least costly interventions is considered.

1. Dietary modification, weight restriction, reduction in consumption of caffeinated beverages and alcoholic drinks should be encouraged. Timed voiding to prevent filling the bladder to a capacity that causes urine loss should be undertaken with the use of a urine diary.

2. *Pelvic floor muscle exercises* or Kegel exercises have been found to be extremely helpful in patients with mild to moderate forms of incontinence. Focused repetitive voluntary contractions of the levator ani muscles (pubococcygeus, coccygeus, and iliococcygeus) created by having the patient contract or "squeeze" the muscle as if to prevent the passage of rectal gas is an effective therapy. The contractions exert a closing force on the urethra and increase muscle support to the pelvic organs. The patient should be provided written and verbal instructions on performing the exercises. Repetitions, with each contraction held for 3–5 seconds alternated with periods of relaxation, should be begun at 45–100 repetitions daily. In settings in which the patient is motivated and thorough follow-up and support, results for cure or improvement of bladder control (reduction in urine loss) can be up to 75%.

3. *Biofeedback:* Biofeedback is an adjunct to pelvic floor exercises that is used to facilitate the patient's comprehension of the proper muscles to contract. By using a pressure catheter and myographic monitoring, a visual or auditory signal of the physiologic response that can be provided to the

patient to help refine exercise skills. Using surface electromyography on the perineum to measure levator contraction and a pressure monitor in the vagina or rectum to indicate abdominal pressure, the patient can be instructed to preferentially contract the pelvic floor without concomitant abdominal contraction. Studies using a variety of techniques demonstrate a 54–95% cure rate or improvement in SUI. The efficacy of this modality is highly dependent on patient motivation and compliance.

4. *Electrical stimulation:* As an alternative to active patient contraction of the levator muscles, electrical stimulation of the muscles via small electrical currents can be used to help both SUI and mixed incontinence. Using intravaginal or transrectal electrodes with stimulators, the pelvic muscles automatically contract and are thereby artificially "trained." When used long term, weakened muscles are strengthened and innervations become re-established during activation.

5. *Pessaries:* Intravaginal devices or pessaries to correct the anatomic deficits associated with *stress incontinence* have long been used. Pessaries, traditionally used for treatment of genital prolapse, have also been shown to have a potential role in supporting the bladder neck and urethra and preventing *stress incontinence.* Continence can often be achieved because many devices adequately obstruct the bladder neck and urethra. As with all intravaginal devices, it is essential to avoid urinary obstruction and vaginal erosion, if the pessary is kept too long.

Surgery for Hypermobility of the Urethra

Surgical treatment of SUI
• Retropubic urethropexy
– Burch
– Marshall-Marchetti-Krantz (MMK)
• Needle urethropexy
• Suburethral sling
• Midurethral sling
– Retropubic (TVT, uretex, SPARC)
– Transobturator
• Urethral bulking agents

The pathology in these patients is malposition of a normal sphincteric unit and, therefore, the goal of surgery is repositioning of the bladder neck and urethra to a high retropubic position (bladder neck suspension). At present, the primary forms of surgical management of stress urinary incontinence are retropubic urethropexy and midurethral sling procedures. The three most common abdominal procedures are the Marshall-Marchetti-Krantz (MMK) procedure, the Burch procedure, and the paravaginal fascial repair.

  i. *Kelly, cystourethropexy (vaginal approach):* This is a very common operation done through the vaginal route along with genital prolapsed. A midline incision is made in the anterior vaginal wall and the vaginal mucosa is accurately separated from the pubocervical fascia. Urethropexy is performed placing two no.1 chromic catgut sutures. The first suture is placed about 2 cm proximal to the urethral meatus into the pubocervical fascia on the left and on the right of the forming a capital 'U'. The second suture is placed and tied in the same way underneath the first one to re-establish the posterior urethrovesical angle. This operation is not favored nowadays because of its high failure rate.

  ii. *Retropubic urethropexy: Marshall-Marchetti-Krantz and Burch operations:* The Marshall-Marchetti-Krantz (MMK) and Burch colposuspension operations for stress incontinence of urine are two of the retropubic urethropexy "pin-up" operations that essentially return the urethrovesical angle as an intra-abdominal organ and change the focal points of pressure applied through the abdomen during a Valsalva maneuver (coughing, sneezing, etc.)

Unlike other stress incontinence operations, the Marshall-Marchetti-Krantz and Burch operations do not, by themselves, produce significant changes in intraurethral or intravesical pressure to restore urinary continence.

Indications

1. Women who decline or have persistent symptoms following a trial of conservative management.
2. Women who have mixed urinary incontinence and able to control symptoms of urge incontinence.
3. The patient requiring concomitant abdominal surgery that cannot be performed vaginally is a candidate for an open Burch colposuspension.

Recommendation: The procedure is performed only if the patient has adequate vaginal mobility and capacity to allow elevation and approximation of the lateral vaginal fornices to Cooper's ligament on either side.

Contraindications

1. Patients with type III stress urinary incontinence (a fixed, nonfunctioning proximal urethra) are not candidates for a Burch procedure as no

hypermobility exists to correct. These patients are better served by a mid-urethral *sling procedure*.

2. The Burch procedure does not allow for correction of central defect *cystocele*, *rectocele*, or introital deficiency, and, thus, consideration of an alternative treatment is indicated.

Physiologic changes. The Marshall-Marchetti-Krantz and Burch operations rarely change the relationship between intraurethral pressure and intravesical pressure. They make the proximal urethra and bladder neck as intra-abdominal organ and equalize intra-abdominal pressures on the bladder wall that are precipitated by a Valsalva maneuver.

Points of caution. To ensure the integrity of the bladder and ureters, cystoscopy should be performed.

When operating in the space of Retzius, bleeding from the plexus of Santorini can be sometimes difficult to control. However, total hemostasis is essential before these operations are completed.

Technique

For the Marshall-Marchetti-Krantz and Burch operations, the patient is placed in the supine lithotomy position, i.e. the ski position. There are two acceptable incisions, the lower midline incision and the transverse incision. The supine lithotomy position (ski) with a transverse incision (Fig 18.10A) is preferred unless the patient is undergoing surgery for a gynecologic oncologic problem. The patient is prepped and draped, and a Foley catheter with a 30 mL bag is inserted.

The incision is made in the rectus fascia. The fascia is excised. The space of Retzius is entered. The bladder and the urethrovaginal angle are identified with the aid of the Foley catheter (Fig. 18.10B and C).

In **Fig. 18.11A** (MMK), the periurethral tissue with the adjacent pubovesical cervical *(PVC)* fascia sling is sutured to the periosteum of the symphysis pubis. The bladder *(B)* and proximal urethra have been brought back into the abdomen where intraurethral and intravesical pressures can be stabilized (Figs 18.12A to 18.17A).

In **Fig. 18.11B** (Burch), the urethra has been suspended by the pubovesical cervical fascia sling sutured to Cooper's ligament (Figs 18.12B to 18.17B).

In reality, the pubovesical cervical fascia in both operations has been made into a sling to bring the proximal one-third of the urethra and the neck of the bladder back into the abdomen. This new position allows even disposition of external pressures on all surfaces of the bladder and proximal urethra.

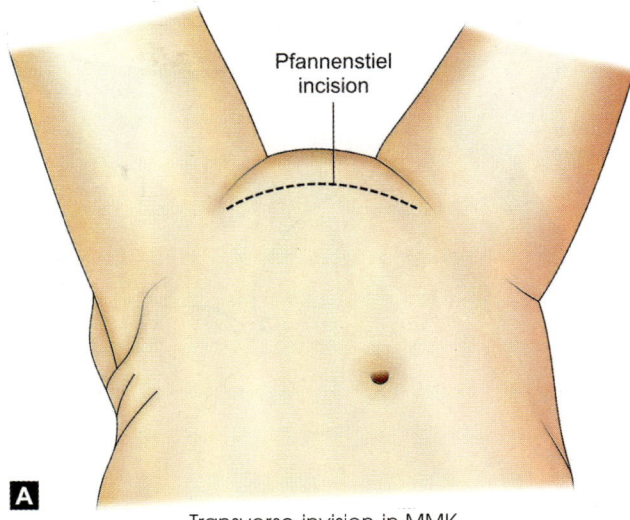

A Transverse invision in MMK

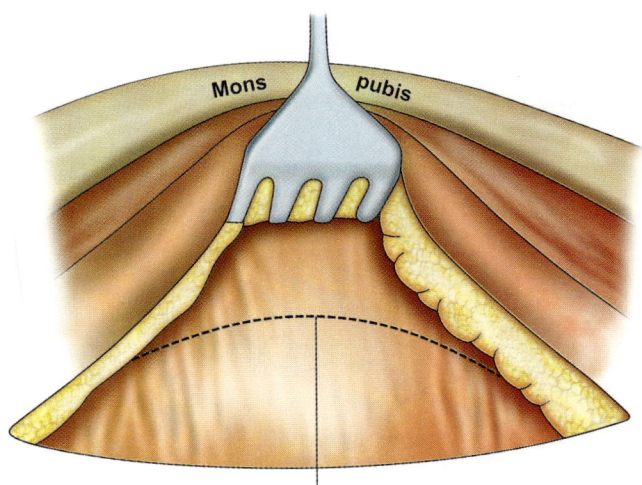

B Incision in conjoined fascia of the rectus m.

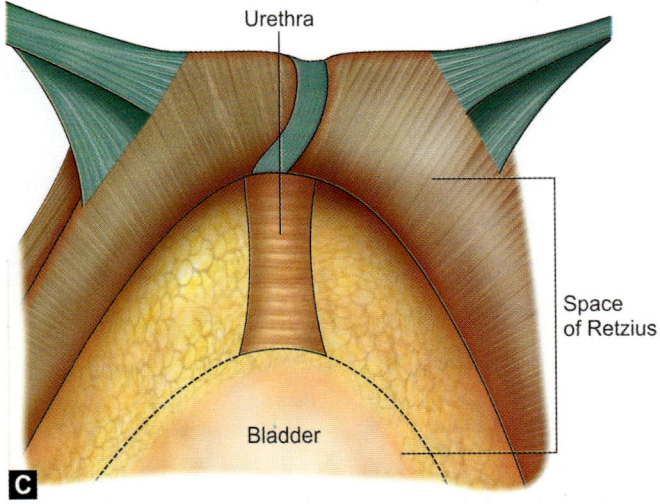

C

Fig. 18.10: Morbid anatomy of retropubic space

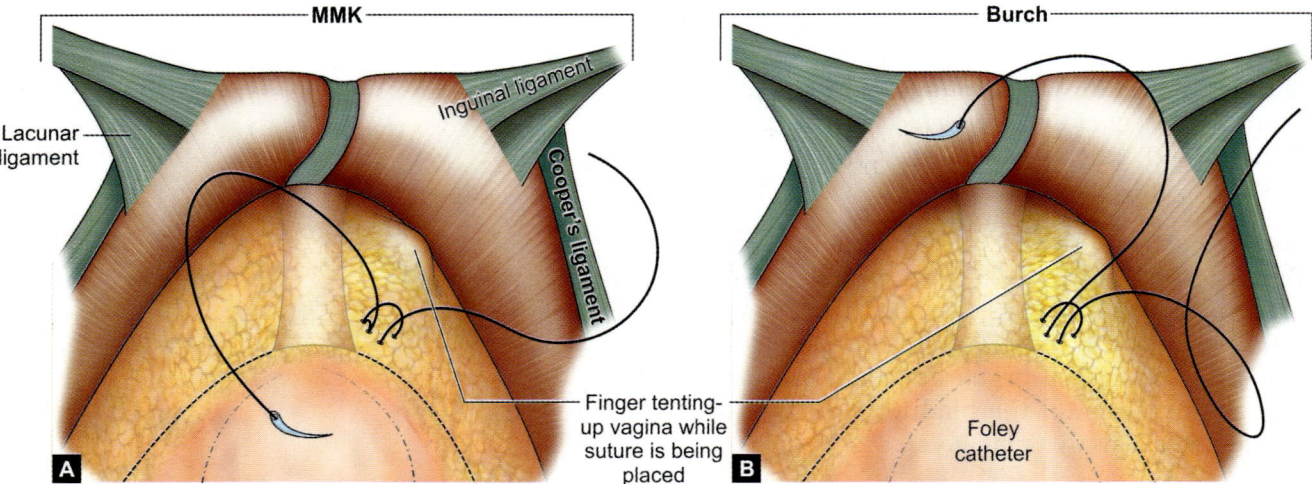

Fig. 18.11: A finger is inserted in the vagina to identify the perivaginal and periurethral areas for placement of 0 Prolene suture. Monofilament suture is preferred. A small, curved Mayo needle is used, and the position of the suture is confirmed by palpating the bladder and inserting a finger in the vagina before making each suture. The blood vessels should be avoided in placing the sutures in the periurethral tissue.

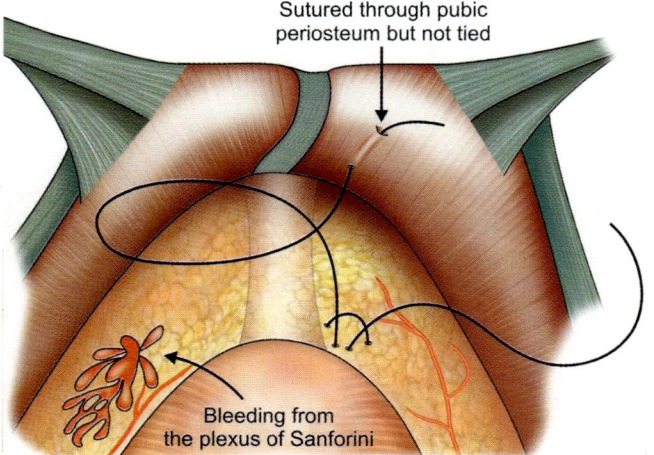

Fig. 18.12A: Showing the MMK operation, the suture placed in the periurethral tissue is tied to the periosteum of the pubic symphysis. Bleeding may occur from the vessels in the plexus of Santorini

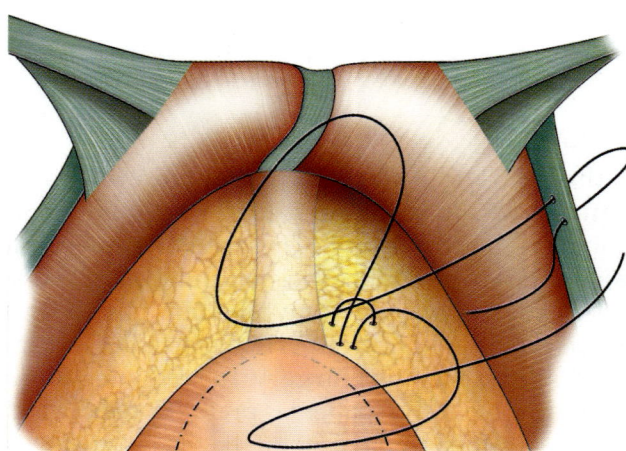

Fig. 18.12B: Showing the Burch operation, the suture placed in the periurethral tissue is brought through the conjoined tendon or Cooper's ligament

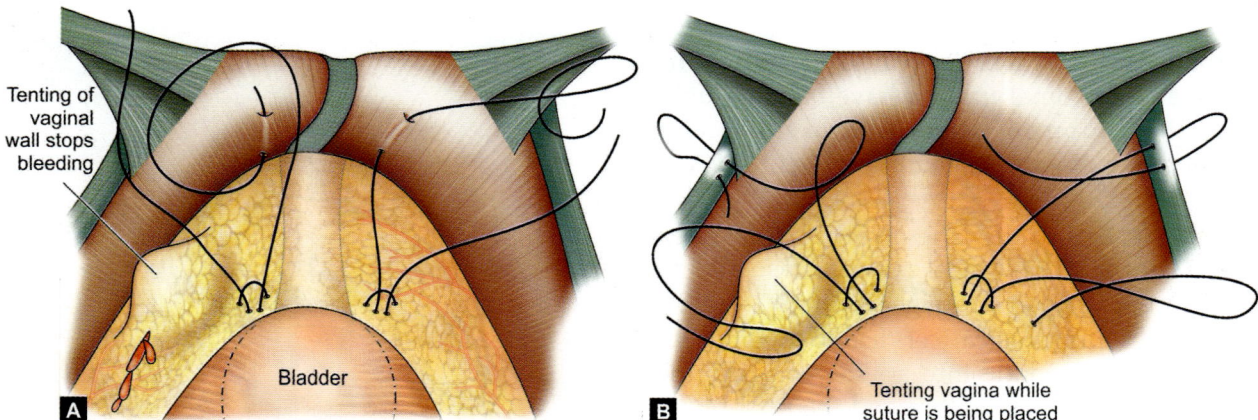

Fig. 18.13: The bleeding produced from the plexus of Santorini can be easily stopped by elevating the finger in the vagina. This allows for fulgurating or grasping and tying each of the bleeders specifically. The suture placed in the periurethral tissue is tied, respectively, to either the periosteum (MMK) (**A**) or Cooper's ligament (Burch) (**B**)

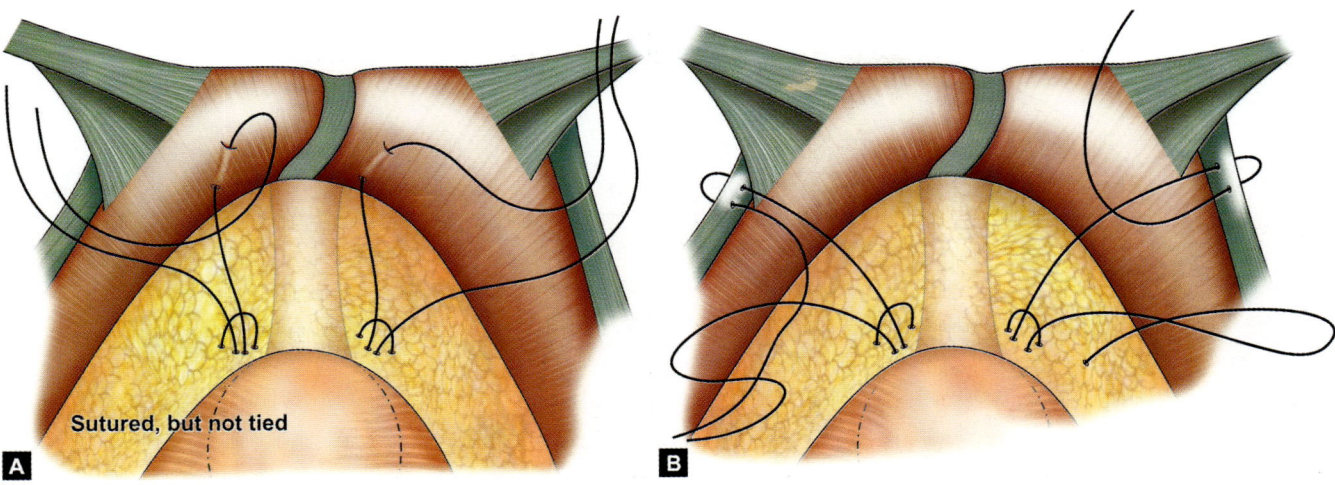

Fig. 18.14: The sutures have been completely placed but not tied

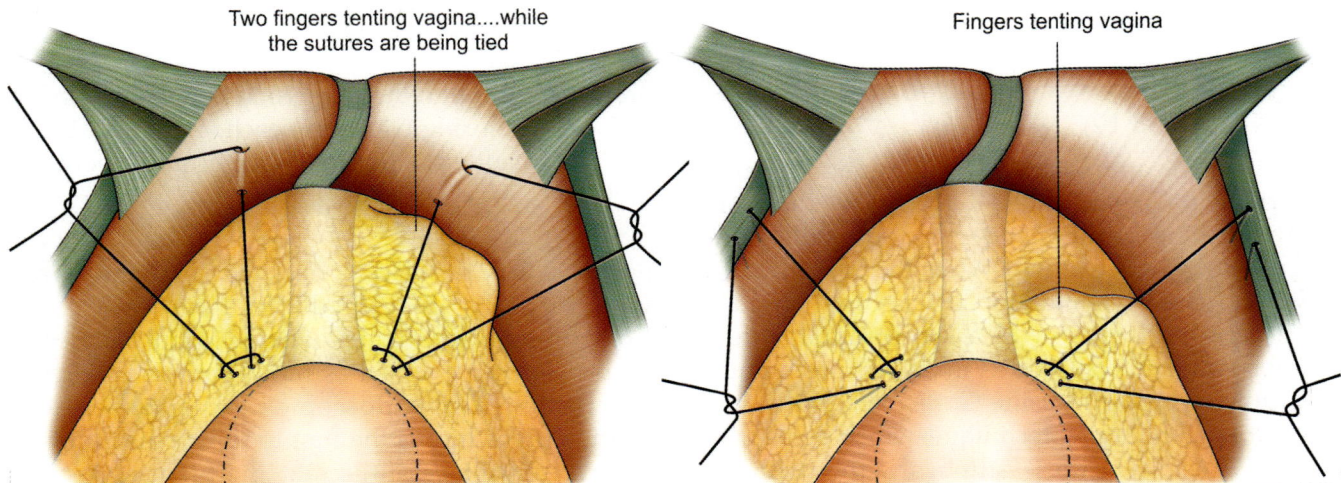

Fig. 18.15A: In **A** MMK, two vaginal fingers are used to tent up the anterior wall of the vagina while the sutures are being tied

Fig. 18.15B: The same is done in Burch, as the sutures are tied to Cooper's ligament

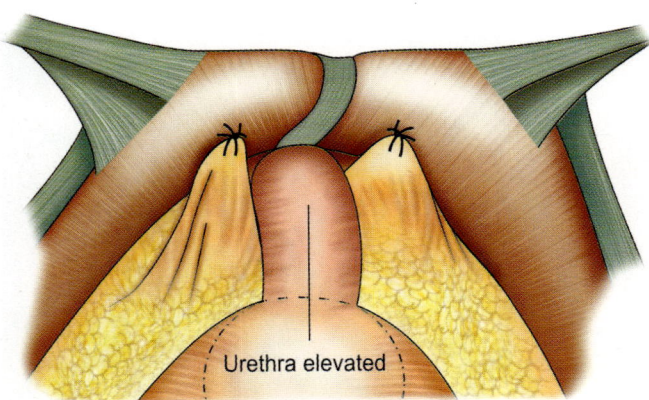

Fig. 18.16A: In MMK, the sutures are completely tied to the periosteum of the symphysis pubis. An additional one or two sutures can be placed if desired

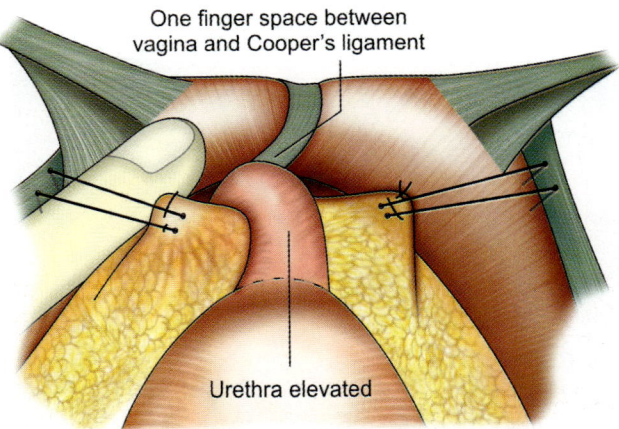

Fig. 18.16B: In Burch, a finger is inserted between the conjoined tendon or Cooper's ligament and the suture in the periurethral tissue. A 2 cm space (1 fingerbreadth) is desirable to prevent total occlusion of the urethra and postoperative urinary retention

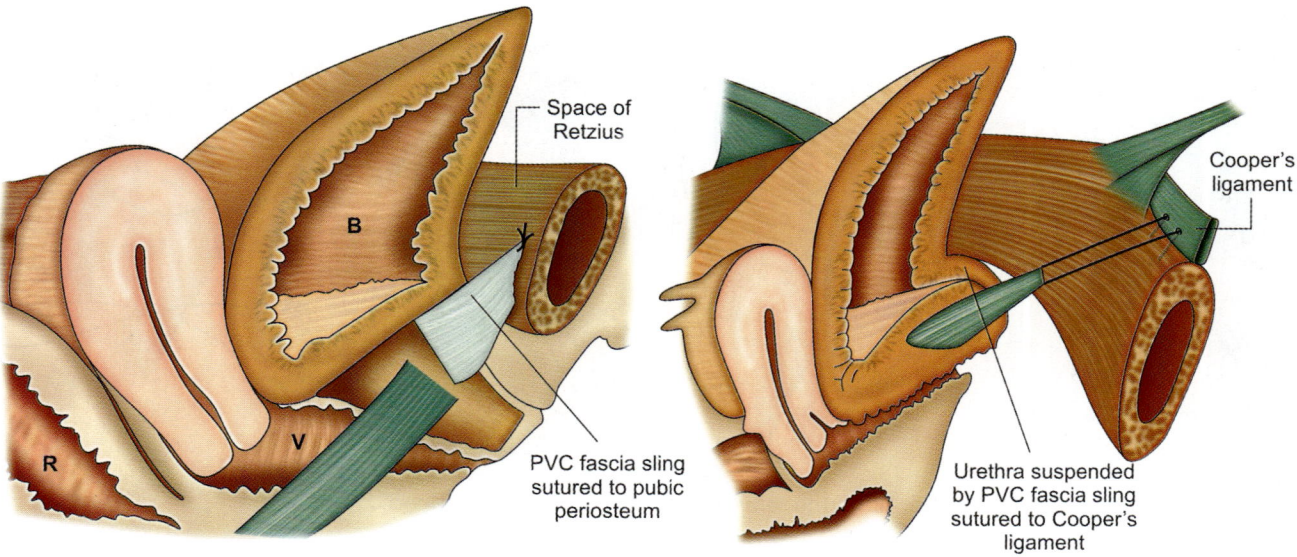

Fig. 18.17A: MMK operation   **Fig. 18.17B:** Burch operation

Laparoscopic Burch Colposuspension
(Figs 18.18 and 18.19)

The laparoscopic approach can be intra-abdominal or extraperitoneal. To gain access to the space of Retzius, retrograde filling of the bladder is done with saline (infused with indigo carmine). When the borders of the bladder are delineated, monopolar scissors are used to open up the peritoneum in a semilunar fashion. Dissection can then continue as in an open technique. The authors recommend using Gore-Tex sutures with extracorporeal knot tying technique, which helps with ease of laying down these stitches without undue tension.

Needle Suspension

Several needle suspension procedures have been developed, like Stamey, Raz, Gittes. Essentially, sutures are placed through the pubic skin or a vaginal incision into the anchoring tissues on each side of the bladder neck and tied to the fibrous tissue or pubic bone.

Stamey Bladder Neck Suspension

Suspension of the bladder neck via a vaginal approach was initially described by Peyrera in 1959. Contemporary techniques of transvaginal bladder neck suspension have arisen as modifications of Peyrera's description. The endoscopic needle suspension of Stamey procedure is the first to utilize the cystoscope to precisely place sutures at the bladder neck and visualize closure of the bladder neck with elevation of the suspension sutures. In addition, the procedure incorporates a knitted dacron graft as a bolster to buttress either side of the urethra and aid in the prevention of suture pull-out.

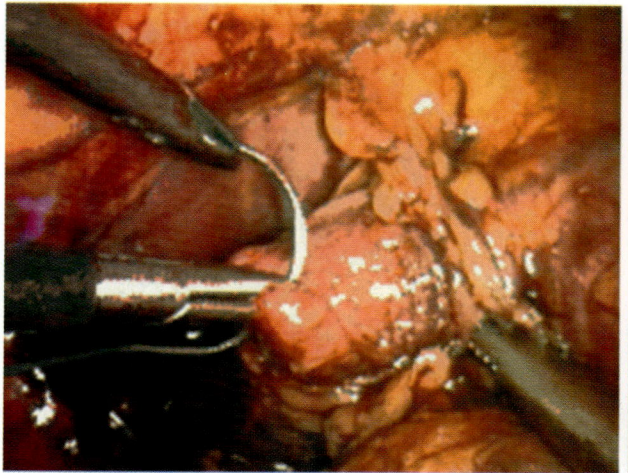

Fig. 18.18: Suture through the left urethropelvic ligament

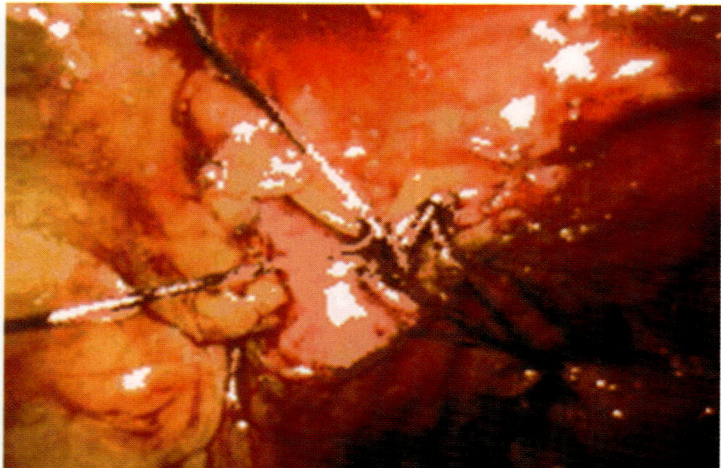

Fig. 18.19: Elevating suture fixed to Cooper's ligament (left side)

Indications for Surgery

The technique described by Stamey is indicated for correction of stress incontinence in the absence of a significant cystocele. Currently vaginal wall slings are preferred for patients with stress incontinence and no significant cystocele. The choice between these techniques depends on the surgeon's training and experience with the different procedures.

Surgical Technique

A T-shaped incision is made in the anterior vaginal wall. The dissection is carried down to the glistening periurethral fascia and continues laterally until the surgeon is able to palpate the balloon of the catheter. This identifies the bladder neck and allows adequate exposure for later placements of the dacron pledgets.

Needle Passage

Two suprapubic stab wound incisions are made on each side of the lower abdomen, and the anterior rectus fascia is exposed. The single-pronged Stamey needle is then inserted into the medial edge of one of the suprapubic wounds and advanced, under fingertip control, into the vaginal incision. The needle passes through the rectus fascia, adjacent to the periosteum, alongside the bladder neck, and through the periurethral fascia as it traverses from the abdomen to the vagina. The Foley catheter is removed, and cystoscopy is performed to confirm correct positioning of the needle. An appropriately positioned needle, when moved medially, will indent the ipsilateral bladder neck. If the needle penetrates the bladder, it should be removed and repassed. Cure rates that range from 53 to 80%.

Treatment of Intrinsic Sphincter Deficiency

A. Urethral Slings

In this condition, there is damage or paralysis of the sphincteric unit. The goal of surgery for intrinsic dysfunction is coaptation, support, and compression of the damaged sphincteric unit. Simple suspension of the bladder neck is unlikely to correct the problem. Urethral sling procedures are the best to achieve the goal.

A sling is put around the mid-urethra. There are different suburethral slings which include Sparc sling, TVT and IVS.

Tension-free Transvaginal Tape (TVT)

The tension-free transvaginal tape (TVT) sling procedure treats urinary stress incontinence by positioning a polypropylene mesh tape underneath the urethra. The procedure involves two miniature incisions in the suprapubic region and inserting a synthetic tape through the vagina in order to sit like a hammock under the urethra and prevent it moving down when the intra-abdominal pressure increases such as when coughing, and has an 86–95% cure rate. Complications, such as bladder perforation, can occur in the retropubic space, if the procedure is not done correctly. This minimally invasive procedure is a common treatment for stress urinary incontinence.

Transobturator Tape (TOT) (Fig. 18.20A–C)

The transobturator tape (TOT) sling procedure aims to eliminate stress urinary incontinence by providing support under the urethra. This minimally-invasive procedure eliminates retropubic needle passage and involves inserting a mesh tape under the urethra through three small incisions in the groin area. While the procedure has shown risks during its infancy, recent developments have increased the cure rate to 90%.

The operation can be performed under spinal or general anesthetic.

Special needles are used. The exit point for these needles is the groins (Fig. 18.21).

There will, therefore, be a small incision in each groin 5 cm lateral to the clitoris at the crural fold and another point in line with the external urethral meatus 2 cm below the previous point. This point is the entry or exit point of the needle.

Another small vertical incision is made below the urethral meatus in the anterior vagina. The lateral portion of the incision is extended by blind dissection till the space is created till the inferior ischiopubic ramus. Then the specially designed needle is passed from the point on the groin and rotated downward under the guidance of the finger through the created space into the vaginal opening and similar steps are done in the opposite side. This can be other way round also; one can start from the vaginal side through a guide and needle come out through the groin point. The needle and the covering plastic is removed and the mesh is placed snugly below the mid-urethra and the rest is cut flush with the skin in the groin points (Figs 18.22 and 18.23).

Specific Risks of TOT and TVT

Failure: 10% of women do not gain benefit from the operation. The operation, however, can be repeated.

Voiding difficulty: Approximately 10% of women will have retention or difficulty in emptying their bladder.

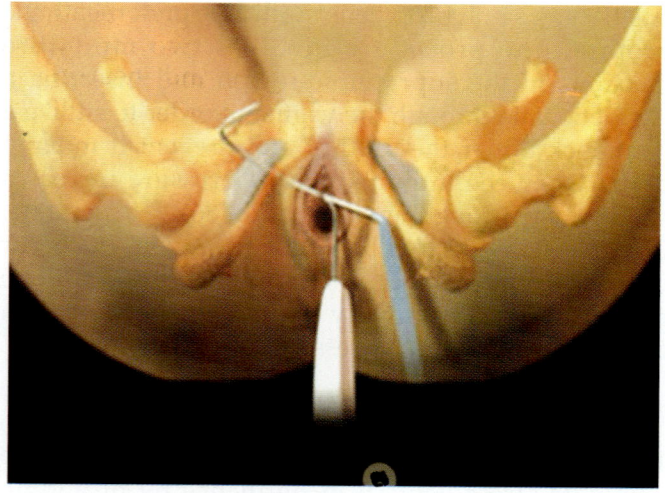

Fig. 18.20A: Inside out approach (TOT)

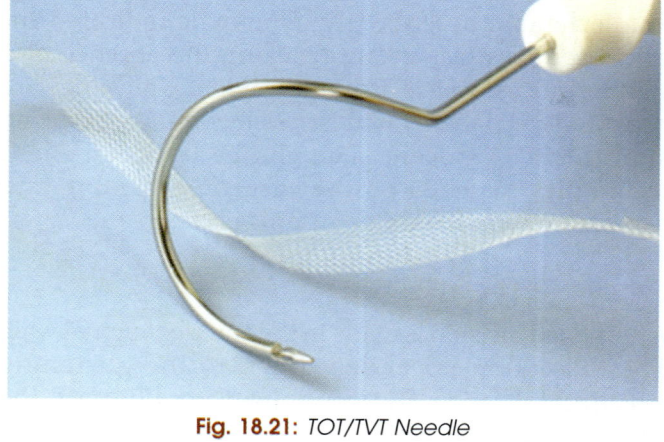

Fig. 18.21: *TOT/TVT Needle*

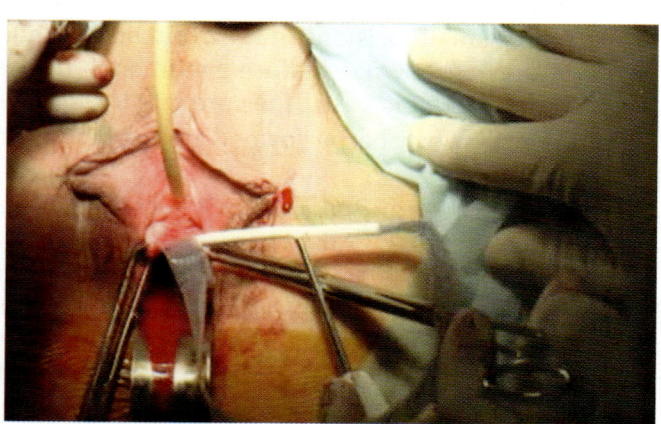

Fig. 18.20B: Needle being passed (TOT)

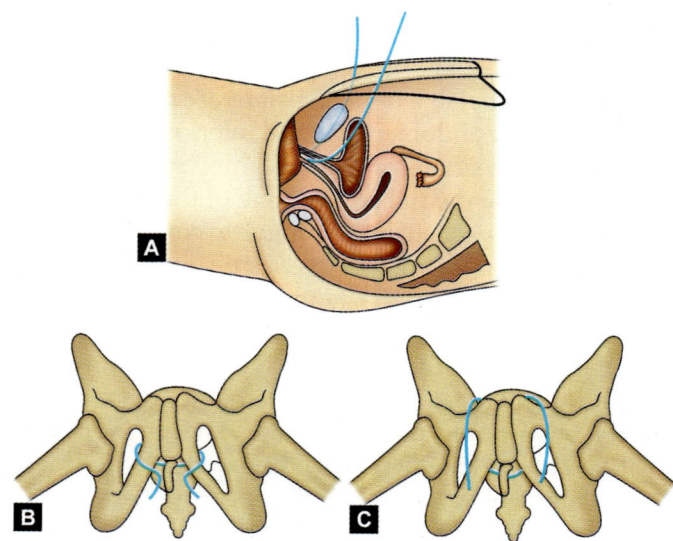

Fig. 18.22: (A) Placement of midurethral sling in the sagittal view; (B) Retropubic passage of midurethral sling; (C) Transobturator passage of midurethral sling

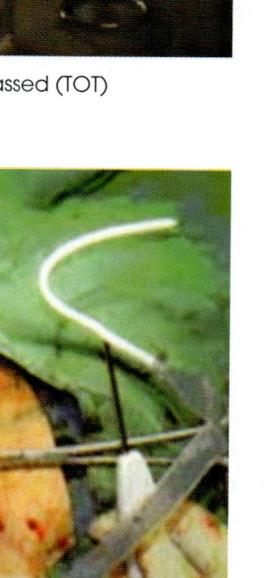

Fig. 18.20C: Mesh being placed (TOT)

overactive leading to symptoms such as urgency (needing to rush to the toilet) and frequency (needing to visit the toilet more often than normal).

Tape exposure and extrusion (10%): The vaginal area over the tape may not heal properly or get infected and therefore, part of the tape may need excising. Very rarely the tape might erode into the urethra or the bladder which would require removal by repeat surgery. The risk of exposure is increased by smoking and with certain diseases.

Pain on intercourse: This may arise from scar tissue in the vagina as a result of the incision.

Visceral trauma: During the suburethral sling operations, the needle used may injure the bladder, or

Bladder overactivity: Any operation around the bladder has the potential for making the bladder

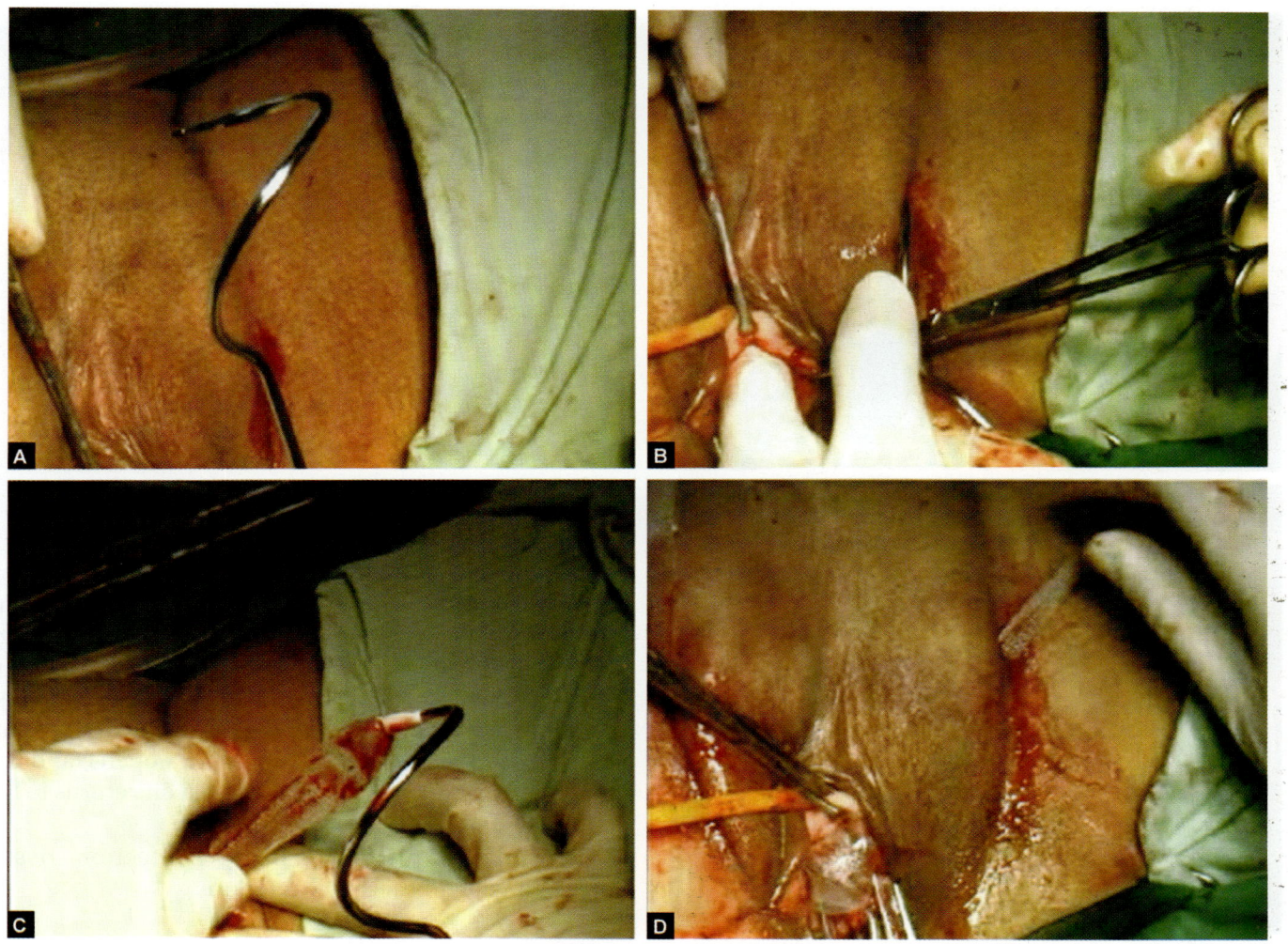

Fig. 18.23: Outside-in approach

urethra and need immediate repair. Therefore, routine cystoscopy is a must after sling operation.

Leg or groin pain: Occasionally, some patients describe pain in the groin or down the legs.

B. Periurethral and Transurethral Injections (Fig. 18.24A and B)

In patients with good support of the bladder neck, but with intrinsic sphincter deficiency, injections of substances, such as macroplastique and collagen, can cause coaptation of the urethral mucosa.

Periurethral or transurethral injection of a bulking agent into the submucosal space of the bladder neck causes narrowing or coaptation of the proximal urethra and bladder neck opening. This increases urethral resistance to involuntary urine loss without changing resting urethral closure pressure. Currently glutaraldehyde cross-linked bovine collagen is the most commonly used material. This procedure is generally reserved for genuine SUI caused by intrinsic sphincteric deficiency. The injections can be performed with the patient under sedation with local anesthetic in an outpatient or office setting. The bovine collagen degrades over 9–19 months, and repeat "booster" injections are often required. Pyrolytic carbon beads (Durasphere) is a permanent and hypoallergenic bulking agent that may obviate the need for repeat injections, but long-term cure rates are equally disappointing.

C. Artificial Sphincter (Figs 18.25 and 18.26)

The artificial urethral sphincter is an effective option for patients with incontinence not amenable to standard surgical treatment because of urethral scarring or atony. The artificial urinary sphincter is best used in patients with incontinence due to poor urethral sphincter function. The sphincter obstructs the urethra by compressing the bladder neck via a pressure-regulated balloon and releases the compression when the patient desires to void. Reported success rates are up to 91%,

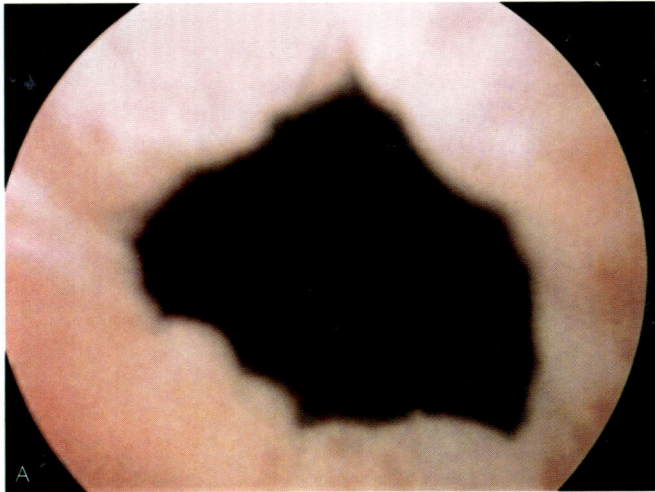

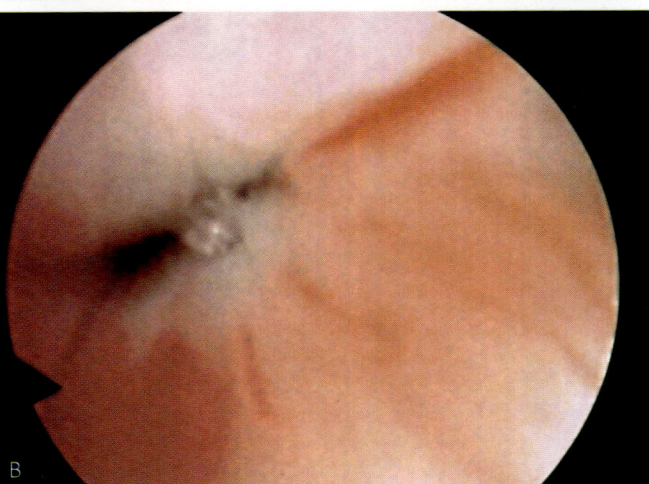

Fig. 18.24: (A) Bladder neck incompetence; (B) Bladder neck after macroplastique injection

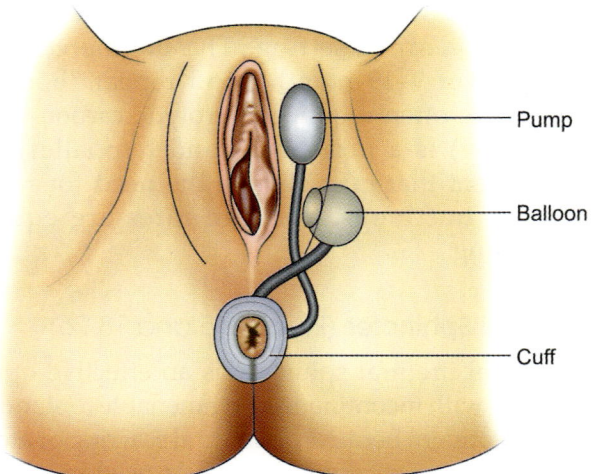

Fig. 18.25: Artificial sphincter device in place

but complication rates are high, with 21% of patients requiring surgical replacement of parts or the entire sphincter.

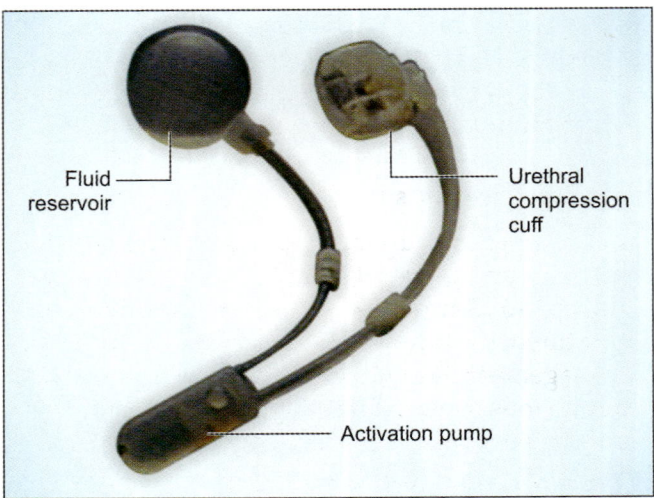

Fig. 18.26: Part of artificial sphincter

The device has three components: a pump, a balloon reservoir, and a cuff that encircles and closes the urethra. All three components are filled with fluid (e.g., saline). The cuff is connected to the pump, which is surgically implanted in the labia. The pump is activated by squeezing or pressing a button. The fluid in the cuff empties into the reservoir, the urethra opens, and the bladder empties. Fluid from the reservoir returns to the cuff, which again closes the urethra.

Possible **complications** include infection, tissue breakdown, and mechanical failure.

NICE Guidelines on UI

Urodynamic Testing

1. The use of multichannel cysometry, ambulatory urodynamics, or videourodynamics is not recommended before starting conservative treatment.
2. Multichannel filling and voiding cystometry is recommended in women before surgery for IUI, if:
   - There is clinical suspicion of detrusor overactivity, or
   - There has been previous surgery for stress incontinence or anterior compartment prolapse.
   - There are symptoms suggestive of voiding dysfunction.

Other Tests of Urethral Competence

1. The Q-tip, Bonney-Marshall and Fluid-Bridge tests are not recommended in the assessment of women with UI.

Cystoscopy is not recommended in the initial assessment of UI alone.

Imaging: MRI, computated tomography, X-ray are not recommended for the routine assessment of women with UI. USG is not recommended other than for the assessment of residual urine volume.

Procedures for Stress UI

- Retropubic mid-urethral tape procedures using a 'bottom-up' approach with macroporous (type 1) polypropylene meshes are recommended as treatment options for stress UI, if conservative management has failed. Open colposuspension and autologous rectus fascial sling are the recommended alternatives when clinically appropriate.

- Synthetic slings, using a retropubic 'top-down' or a transobturator foramen approach, are recommended as alternative treatment options for stress UI, if conservative management has failed.

- Synthetic slings, using materials other than polypropylene that are not of macroporous (type 1) construction, are not recommended for the treatment of stress UI.

- Intramural bulking agents (glutaraldehyde cross-linked antigen, silicone, hyaluronic acids/dextran copolymer) should be considered for the management of stress UI. If conservative management fails, women should be made aware that:
  - Repeat injections may be required to achieve efficacy
  - Efficacy diminishes with time
  - Efficacy is inferior to that of retropubic suspension or sling

- In view of associated morbidity, the use of artificial urinary sphincter should be considered for the stress UI in women, only if pressure surgery has failed. Life-long follow-up is recommended.

- Laparoscopic colposuspension is not recommended as a routine procedure for the treatment of stress UI in women. The procedure should be performed only by experienced surgeon with expertise in the assessment and treatment of UI.

- Anterior colporrhaphy, needle suspensions, paravaginal defect repair and Marshall-Marchetti-Krantz procedure are not recommended for the treatment of stess UI.

- Autologous fat and polytetrafluoroethylene used as intramural bulkings agents are not recommended for the treatment of stress UI.

18C. OVERACTIVE BLADDER

Overactive bladder (OAB) is a syndrome, defined by the International Continence Society (ICS), as consisting of the following symptoms: Urinary urgency, with or without urgency, urinary incontinence, usually with frequency and nocturia, in the absence of causative infection or pathologic conditions and suggestive of underlying detrusor overactivity. Other terms used include detrusor overactivity, detrusor instability, detrusor hyperreflexia, and involuntary bladder contractions.

Urgency is defined as the sudden compelling desire to urinate, a sensation that is difficult to defer. **Urgency urinary incontinence** (UUI) is urinary leakage associated with urgency. UUI is one of the most common types of urinary incontinence. Some women may have both stress urinary incontinence and UUI and this is called **mixed urinary incontinence**. Urinary frequency is defined as voiding 8 or more times in a 24-hour period. Nocturia is defined as the need to wake 1 or more times per night to void.

Anatomy

A normal bladder functions through a complex coordination of musculoskeletal, neurologic, and psychological functions that allow filling and emptying of the bladder contents. The prime effector of continence is the synergic relaxation of detrusor muscles and contraction of bladder neck and pelvic floor muscles.

Various efferent and afferent neural pathways and neurotransmitters are involved. Central neuro-transmitters (e.g. glutamate, serotonin, and dopamine) have a role in urination. Glutamate is an excitatory neurotransmitter in pathways that control the lower urinary tract. Serotonergic pathways facilitate urine storage. Dopaminergic pathways have both inhibitory and excitatory effects on urination. Dopamine D_1 receptors have a role in suppressing bladder activity, whereas dopamine D_2 receptors facilitate voiding.

In bladder filling, sympathetic nerve fibers that originate from T11 to L2 segments of the spinal cord, which innervate smooth-muscle fibers around the bladder neck and proximal urethra, cause these fibers to contract, allowing the bladder to fill. As the bladder fills, sensory stretch receptors in the bladder wall trigger a central nervous system (CNS) response. During bladder filling, the intravesical pressure remains low as a result of the viscoelastic properties of the bladder and antagonism of the parasympathetic nervous system.

The parasympathetic nervous system (PNS) causes contraction of the detrusor, while the muscles of the pelvic floor and external sphincter relax. The PNS fibers, as well as those responsible for somatic (voluntary) control of micturition, originate from the S2 to S4 segments of the spinal cord in the sacral plexus. The somatic fibers innervate the external sphincter and are responsible for the voluntary control of continence in the face of a pressing desire to void.

The normal adult bladder accommodates 300–600 mL of urine; a CNS response is usually triggered when the volume reaches 400 mL. However, urination can be prevented by cortical suppression of the PNS or by voluntary contraction of the external sphincter.

Pathophysiology

OAB appears to be multifactorial in both etiology and pathophysiology. Symptoms of OAB are suggestive of underlying detrusor overactivity. Overactivity of the detrusor muscle—neurogenic, myogenic, or idiopathic in origin—may result in urinary urgency and urgency incontinence.

The role of the M_2 receptor in the human bladder is not well established. It may have a role in detrusor overactivity related to obstruction and spinal cord injury.

Binding of acetylcholine to the M_3 receptor activates phospholipase C via coupling with G proteins. This action causes the release of calcium from the sarcoplasmic reticulum and contraction of the bladder smooth muscle. Increased sensitivity to stimulation by muscarinic receptors may lead to OAB. Leakage of acetylcholine from the parasympathetic nerve terminal may lead to micromotion of the detrusor, which may activate sensory afferent fibers, leading to the sensation of urgency.

Sensory afferent nerves may play a role in OAB. Activation of normally quiescent C sensory fibers produce symptoms of OAB in individuals with neurologic and other disorders. Several types of receptors identified on sensory nerves involved in OAB symptoms include vanilloid, purinergic, neurokinin A, and nerve growth factor receptors. Substances such as nitric oxide, calcitonin gene-related protein, and brain-derived neurotropic factor have a role in modulating sensory afferent fibers in the human bladder.

The urothelium communicates directly with suburothelial afferents acting as luminal sensors. Low pH, high potassium concentration, and increased osmolality in the urine can influence sensory nerves. Activation of suburothelial afferent fibers without changes in the smooth muscle may lead to urgency. Activation of the suburothelial afferents in the presence of enhanced smooth-muscle coupling may lead to urgency and unstable detrusor contractions.

Etiology

OAB is primarily a neuromuscular problem in which the detrusor muscle contracts inappropriately during bladder filling. OAB is a storage phase problem. These contractions often occur regardless of the amount of urine in the bladder. OAB may result from a number of different causes, both neurogenic and non-neurogenic.

Neurologic injuries that may cause OAB include the following:

- Spinal cord injury
- Stroke

Neurologic diseases that may cause OAB include the following:

- Multiple sclerosis
- Dementia
- Parkinson disease
- Medullary lesions
- Diabetic neuropathy

Detrusor overactivity can also occur in the absence of a neurogenic etiology. Contractions can be spontaneous or induced by rapid filling of the bladder, postural changes, or even walking or coughing. Idiopathic OAB is OAB in the absence of any underlying neurologic, metabolic, or other causes like urinary tract infection, bladder cancer, bladder stones, bladder inflammation, or bladder outlet obstruction.

Certain medications may lead to symptoms of OAB. Diuretics can cause symptoms of urge incontinence because of increased bladder filling, stimulating the detrusor. Bethanechol can also cause urge incontinence through its stimulation of bladder smooth-muscle contraction.

Risk Factors

Several risk factors are associated with OAB. Persons older than 75 years, those with increased BMI, persons with insulin-dependent diabetes and individuals with depression are 3 times as likely to develop OAB.

The physiological changes associated with aging, such as decreased bladder capacity and changes in muscle tone, favor the development of OAB when precipitating factors intervene. In postmenopausal women, many of these changes are related to estrogen deficiency. Perhaps the most important age-related change in bladder function that leads to incontinence is the increased number of involuntary bladder contractions (detrusor instability).

Any disruption in the integration of musculoskeletal and neurologic responses can lead to loss of control of normal bladder function and to urge incontinence.

Epidemiology

Incidence

According to *The National Overactive Bladder Evaluation (NOBLE) study,* incidence is around 16.5%; Of these, 6.1% suffer from OAB with urgency incontinence and 10.4% with OAB without urgency incontinence. Among individuals with OAB with urgency incontinence, 45% may have mixed incontinence symptoms (urgency incontinence plus stress incontinence).

Age-related Differences in Incidence

The prevalence of OAB increases with age. Twenty percent of the population aged 70 years or older report symptoms of OAB. Men tend to develop OAB slightly later in life than women do.

Impact on Quality of Life

OAB significantly impairs quality of life. It increases depression scores, and reduces quality of sleep. Individuals with OAB develop coping strategies to manage or hide their problems by modifying fluid intake, toilet mapping, reduced physical or social activity.

Worries and concerns regarding odor, uncleanliness and leakage during sexual activity may lead individuals to refrain from intimacy. Frequent urination and the need to interrupt activities may affect the person's work and ability to travel.

History

The patient's history should include information about the following:

- Onset, nature, duration and severity of lower urinary tract symptoms.
- Medical and surgical history.
- Obstetric and gynecologic history.
- Prescription of medications like anticholinergics or antimuscarinics, antidepressants, antipsychotics, sedatives or hypnotics, diuretics, alpha-adrenergic blockers, beta-adrenergic agonists, and calcium channel blockers.

- Bladder diary: This is used to record the times of micturitions and voided volumes, incontinence episodes, pad usage, and other information (e.g. fluid intake, degree of urgency, degree of incontinence); a 3-day diary is ideal.

Key screening questions should be asked, focusing on urgency, nocturia (>3 times per night), frequency (>8 times per day), and urinary incontinence. If the patient answers affirmatively to the screening questions, a bladder diary should be given to the patient to complete and review during a subsequent visit.

Physical Examination

A comprehensive physical examination can help to determine the nature, severity, and impact of the symptoms in patients with overactive bladder (OAB).

- Pulmonary and cardiovascular evaluation may be indicated to assess control of cough or the need for medications such as diuretics.
- Abdominal examination is performed to rule out diastasis recti, masses, ascites, and organomegaly, which can influence intra-abdominal pressure and urinary tract function. A palpable bladder may imply overflow incontinence or an obstructive problem.
- Pelvic examination is used to evaluate for inflammation, infection, atrophy, and pelvic organ prolapse. Such conditions can increase afferent sensation, leading to urinary urgency, frequency, dysuria, and OAB. Because the urethra and trigone are estrogen-dependent tissues, estrogen deficiency can contribute to urinary incontinence and urinary dysfunction. The most common signs of inadequate estrogen levels include thinning and paleness of the vaginal epithelium, loss of rugae, disappearance of the labia minora, and presence of a urethral caruncle.
- In females, the levator ani muscle function can be evaluated by asking the patient to tighten her vaginal muscles and to hold the contraction as long as possible. Normally, woman can hold such a contraction for 5–10 seconds. Voluntary levator ani muscle contractions that are very weak or absent are an indication that biofeedback training sessions with a pelvic floor physical therapist may be necessary.
- The bimanual examination should also include a rectal examination to check anal sphincter tone and, for fecal impaction, the presence of occult blood or rectal lesions.
- A neurologic examination is important. This involves assessment of the lumbosacral nerve roots and should include evaluation of the deep-tendon reflexes, lower extremity strength, sharp/dull sensation, and the bulbocavernosus and clitoral sacral reflexes. Abnormal findings (e.g. deep tendon hyperreflexia or an absent bulbocavernosus reflex) should alert the physician to possible underlying neurologic lesions contributing to urinary incontinence.

Comorbidity

Individuals with OAB and urinary incontinence may have other medical comorbidities. Urinary tract infections, skin infections, falls and fractures are more likely in persons with OAB and urinary incontinence.

In addition, depression is more common in individuals with OAB. However, it is unclear whether the depression is due to OAB or whether the two conditions share similar underlying neurologic etiologies.

Differential Diagnosis

The term overactive bladder (OAB) refers to a symptom complex. Therefore, the first part of the evaluation of OAB is to review the patient's lower urinary tract symptoms to ensure that the symptoms are consistent with OAB.

A diagnosis of OAB depends on the presence of urgency, which differs from a simple urge to void. A typical urge to void is a normal sensation that progressively strengthens when deferred. In contrast, urgency is an abnormal condition that is characterized by sudden onset of urgency and difficulty in deferring urination.

Nocturia is often confused with lower urinary tract symptoms (LUTS) and assumed to be a symptom of OAB. Most patients with nocturia do not have OAB and most patients with OAB do have nocturia.

Other causes of urinary frequency, urgency, and urinary incontinence must be excluded. Incontinence has several subtypes: Stress incontinence, mixed urinary incontinence, overflow incontinence, and transient incontinence.

Transient incontinence may be related to any of a number of conditions, easily recalled by means of the mnemonic: **DIAPPERS: D**elirium, **I**nfection, **A**trophy, **P**harmaceuticals, **P**sychological factors, **E**xcess urine output, **R**estricted mobility, and **S**tool impaction. Other conditions to consider include the following:

- Urinary stone disease
- Gastrointestinal (GI) or colonic pathology
- Gynecologic pathology

Guidelines for diagnosis of OAB by the American Urological Association (AUA) include the following:

- A thorough history, physical examination, and urinalysis should be done initially.

- If necessary, a urine culture, or postvoid residual assessment, or both can be done, along with use of bladder diaries or symptom questionnaires.
- Urodynamic study, cystoscopy, and diagnostic renal and bladder ultrasonography are not necessary in the initial workup of uncomplicated cases and should be reserved for refractory or otherwise complicated cases.
- Urine cytology is not recommended in the absence of hematuria when the patient responds to therapy.

Urine Study

Urinalysis is used to exclude microhematuria, pyuria, urinary tract infection, and glucosuria. In those individuals with microhematuria, further evaluation including a urine cytology is recommended.

Postvoid residual testing is not indicated in all patients. It is helpful in women who have undergone prior pelvic surgery (e.g. prior incontinence surgery), and those with significant pelvic organ prolapse. Postvoid residual volume is assessed by means of urethral catheterization or ultrasonography. There is no definitive upper level of normal for postvoid residual, but many would argue that postvoid residuals greater than 150–200 mL are indicative of incomplete bladder emptying and may warrant further evaluation.

Cystometry

Cystometry is a simple method for testing the bladder's storage function and provides information on bladder capacity, the extent of compliance, the ability to sense bladder filling, and temperature; it can also help assess for detrusor overactivity during bladder filling.

Urodynamic Study

Urodynamic study is not indicated as part of the first-line evaluation of patients with OAB unless a neurologic etiology is suspected. It is most commonly performed in individuals in whom first-line therapies for OAB fail and/or in whom a neurogenic etiology is suspected.

There are multiple components to a urodynamic study: **Cystometrography (CMG)** assesses the storage phase of bladder function—looking at bladder capacity, compliance, detrusor overactivity, sensation of filling, the voiding phase, and **uroflow/electromyelography** assesses detrusor pressure during voiding, relaxation of the pelvic floor muscles during voiding, the nature of the flow pattern (i.e. bell-shaped curve, staccato), and whether or not there is Valsalva voiding.

Intravesical pressure is a combination of intra-abdominal pressure and detrusor pressure. To determine the detrusor pressure, the intra-abdominal pressure is measured with a rectal catheter; this pressure is subtracted from the total intravesical pressure (measured with the bladder catheter).

Approach Considerations

Once diagnosed, overactive bladder (OAB) can be managed with several different methods. If a specific cause of OAB symptoms is identified, it should be treated appropriately; for example, urinary tract infection (UTI) should be treated with antibiotics; similarly, atrophic urethritis can be treated with topical application of estrogen vaginal cream.

Guidelines for the treatment of OAB by the American Urological Association (AUA) include the following:

- *First-line therapy:* Behavioral therapies and education should be offered first; starting antimuscarinic therapies along with behavioral therapies may prove clinically beneficial.
- *Second-line therapy:* Antimuscarinics; extended-release preparations should be used instead of immediate-release preparations when possible; transdermal **oxybutynin** can also be used.
- *Third-line therapy:* Surgery is rarely used to treat OAB and is reserved for patients in whom pharmacologic and behavioral therapy fail. Various surgical options are available, including sacral nerve neuromodulation and, rarely, bladder augmentation. Percutaneous tibial nerve stimulation **(PTNS)** is a minimally invasive option for patients in whom pharmacologic therapy fails or is contraindicated. Intradetrusor injection of **onabotulinumtoxin A** is another option.

The choice of a particular treatment depends on the severity of the symptoms and the extent that the symptoms interfere with the patient's lifestyle. The three main approaches to treatment include pharmacotherapy, behavioral therapy, and surgery.

Pharmacologic Therapy

Anticholinergics

Anticholinergic agents are currently the first-line therapy for OAB. These agents exhibit their primary action by inhibiting involuntary detrusor muscle contractions (at the level of the efferent pathway), but identification of muscarinic receptors in the urothelium/suburothelium suggests that they may also affect the afferent sensory pathway. The goals of therapy with anticholinergic agents are to prevent inappropriate detrusor contractions and to maintain normal bladder function.

Oxybutynin and tolterodine are the more commonly used anticholinergics in OAB treatment. Oxybutynin is among the first anticholinergic agents to be used to treat detrusor overactivity.

Tolterodine is the first major drug to address the problems of treatment tolerability. Unlike oxybutynin, tolterodine has a greater inhibitory effect on bladder contraction than on salivation.

Other anticholinergic agents used to treat OAB include trospium chloride, propiverine hydrochloride, solifenacin, darifenacin and oxybutynin patch. More recently, fesoterodine was approved by the FDA.

Darifenacin has the most selective M_3 activity and is safe with no effect on cognitive function, which make it useful in elderly patients.

Trospium is a large-molecule quaternary amine with minimal central nervous system (CNS) penetration. It has a unique liver metabolic pathway, making it the most suitable for patients receiving multiple drugs with cytochrome P-450 utilization.

Fesoterodine is the newest anticholinergic available for OAB. It shares the same active metabolite as tolterodine, 5-HMT; however, fesoterodine is efficiently and extensively metabolized to 5-HMT via ubiquitous esterases and is found superior in efficacy than tolterodine in the reduction of UUI episodes.

Anticholinergic agents cause frequent side effects such as dry mouth, constipation, blurred vision, and drowsiness. These effects are dose-related and can severely limit tolerability, especially in elderly patients. Anticholinergics may also produce confusion, especially in elderly patients with pre-existing dementia.

Anticholinergics are contraindicated in patients with urinary retention and untreated narrow-angle glaucoma. They should be used with caution in patients with clinically significant bladder outlet obstruction, decreased gastrointestinal motility, treated narrow angle glaucoma, and myasthenia gravis. More recently, cases of angioedema of the face, lips, tongue and/or pharynx have been reported with several of these agents, and patients should be counseled, if they experience swelling to seek care immediately.

Beta-3 Receptor Agonists

FDA approved the first beta-3 receptor agonist, mirabegron, for symptoms of urge urinary incontinence, urgency, and urinary frequency associated with OAB. Beta-3 receptor agonists act directly to inhibit afferent nerve firing independent of the relaxing effects on the bladder smooth muscle.

Botulinum Toxins

Detrusor injections of botulinum toxin A are approved by the FDA for the treatment of adults with OAB who cannot use, or do not adequately respond to anticholinergic medication. Most of the effects of botulinum toxin are the result of inhibition of the release of acetylcholine from the presynaptic nerve terminal, which prevents stimulation of the detrusor muscle.

It is also used for treatment of urinary incontinence due to detrusor overactivity associated with neurologic condition (e.g. spinal cord injury, multiple sclerosis) in adults.

Tricyclic Antidepressants

Tricyclic antidepressants, such as **imipramine and doxepin,** have also been used to treat OAB. These block the reuptake of noradrenaline and serotonin. However, whether this mechanism mediates its beneficial effects on bladder hyperactivity is unclear. These agents have been associated with cardiac dysrhythmias and mental status changes and thus should be used with caution in elderly patients. Tricyclic antidepressants are not recognized as first-line therapy for the treatment of overactive bladder.

Hormones

Hormones are used to treat OAB in association with atrophic urethritis and are not recommended as first-line therapies for OAB.

Estrogen (Premarin)

Detrusor overactivity can be associated with atrophic urethritis; topical application of estrogen vaginal cream should be considered in women with symptomatic atrophic urethritis/vaginits.

Behavioral Therapy

Behavioral therapy, also called behavioral modification, is a treatment approach that aims to alter an individual's actions or environment to improve bladder control. Components of behavioral therapy include (1) education, (2) dietary and lifestyle modification (see Dietary Measures), (3) bladder training, (4) pelvic floor muscle therapy (PFMT), and (5) self-monitoring with bladder or voiding diaries.

Bladder Training

Bladder training involves a program of patient education and a scheduled voiding regimen, which is progressively increased. The goals of bladder training are to normalize urinary frequency, to improve control over bladder urgency, to increase bladder capacity, to decrease incontinence episodes, to prolong voiding intervals and to improve the patient's confidence in bladder control

The mechanism by which bladder training works is not fully identified; however, theories include:

a. Improved cortical inhibition over detrusor contractions.

b. Improved cortical facilitation of urethral closure during bladder filling

c. Improved central modulation of sensory afferent impulses.

d. Changes in behavior due to improved awareness of lower urinary tract function.

e. Increased reserve capacity of the lower urinary tract.

Bladder retraining alone is successful in 75% of patients treated for urge incontinence.

Bladder retraining involves developing a schedule of when the patient should try to urinate; the patient should then try to consciously delay urination beteen these times. One method is to urinate at definite intervals (e.g. 30 min); then, as the patient becomes skilled at waiting, the time intervals are gradually increased by one-half hour until the individual is urinating every 3–4 hours.

Pelvic Floor Muscle Therapy (PFMT)

PFMT involves exercises designed to improve the function of the pelvic floor muscles. The rationale for use of PFMT in urgency urinary incontinence and OAB is that contraction of the muscles can reflexively or voluntarily inhibit contraction of the detrusor muscle. PFMT is defined as any program of repeated voluntary pelvic floor muscle contractions (VPFMC) taught by a healthcare professional.

Regular daily exercising of pelvic muscles can improve, and even prevent, urinary incontinence. This is particularly helpful in younger women. PFM exercises should be performed 30–80 times daily for at least 8 weeks. The principle behind PFM exercises is to strengthen the muscles of the pelvic floor, thereby improving function of the urethral sphincter.

Another approach is to use vaginal cones to strengthen the muscles of the pelvic floor. A vaginal cone is a weighted device that is inserted into the vagina. The woman contracts the pelvic floor muscles in an effort to hold the device in place. The contraction should be held for up to 15 minutes and should be performed twice daily. Within 4–6 weeks, symptoms improve in about 70% of women who try this method.

Biofeedback-assisted Therapy

Biofeedback is a method of positive reinforcement in which electrodes are placed on patient's abdomen and the anal area. Biofeedback-assisted behavioral therapy uses biofeedback to teach patients how to control normal physiologic responses of the bladder and pelvic floor muscles that mediate incontinence. Used in conjunction with PFM exercises, biofeedback helps patients gain awareness and control of the pelvic muscles.

Some therapists place a sensor in the vagina in women to assess contraction of the pelvic floor muscles. A monitor displays a graph that shows which muscles are contracting and which are at rest. The therapist can help the patient identify the correct muscles for performing Kegel exercises. About 75% of people who use biofeedback to enhance performance of Kegel exercises report symptom improvement, with 15% considered cured.

Pelvic Floor Electrical Stimulation

Pelvic floor electrical stimulation involves the use of mild electrical pulses to elicit contractions in a specific group of muscles. The current may be delivered using an anal or vaginal probe. Pelvic floor electrical stimulation should be performed in conjunction with PFM exercises. A treatment session usually last 20 minutes and may be performed every 1–4 days.

Success Rates

Behavioral therapy yield a mean 80.7% reduction in incontinence episodes. However, biofeedback is not necessary for everyone.

The International Continence Society (ICS) recommends that PFMT be offered as a first-line therapy to all women with stress, urge, or mixed urinary incontinence. Patients seem to benefit most from a PFMT program that provides intensive supervision.

Surgical Therapy

Augmentation cystoplasty is rarely necessary in idiopathic OAB. However, it may be used in individuals with refractory neurogenic OAB, particularly in those with poor compliance. In this reconstructive procedure, a segment of the bowel is removed and used to replace a portion of the bladder.

Neuromodulation (sacral nerve or tibial nerve stimulation): This is a new technique FDA approved for the management of OAB and UUI. It requires the surgical implantation of a small device at the level of the S3. Typically, an external stimulator is placed and if the patient experiences a 50% or greater reduction in symptoms, a permanent internalized stimulator is placed. Typically, twelve 30-minute sessions are performed, followed by a maintenance regimen.

Other Therapies under Investigation

Neurokinin receptor antagonists, alpha-adrenoceptor antagonists, nerve growth factor inhibitors, gene therapy, and stem cell-based therapies appear promising as future development of new modalities in OAB treatment.

Dietary Measures

Eliminate dietary caffeine in those with urge incontinence and encourage adequate dietary fiber. Some have suggested that the avoidance of certain foods and beverages (e.g. alcohol, spicy foods, nuts, chocolate, high-potassium foods, carbonated and caffeinated beverages) may improve the symptoms of OAB in some cases. Adequate fluid intake is important because many persons with OAB restrict fluids in hopes of voiding less; however, concentrated urine may act as a bladder irritant.

Management of Chronic Incontinence

Although management approaches, such as medical therapy, pelvic muscle exercises, and bladder training, improve continence in most patients, some never achieve complete dryness. Treatment failures are sometimes due to concurrent use of necessary medications such as diuretics or dementia or other physical impairments that keep them from being able to perform pelvic muscle exercises or to retrain their bladders.

The following recommendations can help keep persons with chronic incontinence improve symptoms and reduce their cost of care:

- Scheduled toileting: Take the patient to the toilet every 2–4 hours or according to his or her toilet habits.
- Prompted voiding: Check for dryness and encourage use of the toilet.
- Improved access to toilets.
- Managing fluids and diet—by eliminating dietary caffeine for those with urge incontinence and to encourage adequate fiber in the diet.
- Disposable absorbent pads or garments—use these to keep patients dry.

Prognosis

Behavioral therapy combined with pharmacologic therapy offer good results in OAB patients, with up to 80% of cases improve with excellent long-term results.

18D. GENITOURINARY FISTULA

Introduction

Any fistula is defined as an abnormal communication between two or more epithelial surfaces. Female urogenital fistula concerns primarily with fistula between the genital tract (vagina, cervix, uterus or perineum) and the urinary tract (bladder, urethra or ureter) (Fig. 18.27).

Incidence and Epidemiology

The majority of GUFs in developed countries are a consequence of gynecological surgery. The incidence rate of VVF after total abdominal hysterectomy is 0.5–2%, and of ureteric fistula is 0.05%. The estimated prevalence in the developing world is 1–2 per 1000 deliveries.

Classification of Female GUF (Fig. 18.28)

a. Vesicocervical
b. Juxtacervical
c. Midvaginal vesicovaginal
d. Suburethral vesicovaginal
e. Urethrovaginal

History

James Marion Sims published his famous discourse on the treatment of VVF in 1852. Using leaden or silver wire, Sims achieved success on his 30th surgical attempt on a slave named Anarcha. Sims emphasized the importance of good exposure, adequate resection of the fistula and scarred vaginal edges, and the critical

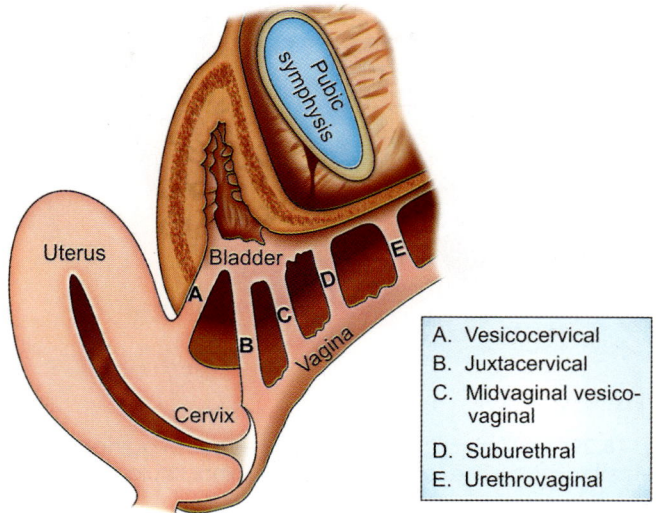

A. Vesicocervical
B. Juxtacervical
C. Midvaginal vesico-vaginal
D. Suburethral
E. Urethrovaginal

Fig. 18.28: Communication sites in GUF

importance of continuous postoperative bladder drainage.

Dr. Kelly also described both a vaginal repair of VVF in 1896, and a suprapubic closure in 1906. Dr Kelly also advocated the use of preoperative ureteral catheters to minimize the risk of ureteral injury. During the early 20th century, several additional techniques were used to improve outcome for the repair of VVF. In 1942, Latzko published his partial colpocleisis technique for repair of posthysterectomy VVF, in which he used the resection of scarred vaginal mucosa and a layered horizontal closure.

Classification according to Types of Fistula (Fig. 18.29)

- Vesicovaginal
- Vesicouterine
- Vesicocervical
- Vesicouterocervicovaginal
- Ureterovaginal

Anatomic Classification

Type I: Not involving the closing mechanism
Type II: Involving the closing mechanism
A. Not involving total urethra:
  a. Without circumferential defect
  b. With circumferential defect
B. Involving total urethra
  a. Without circumferential defect
  b. With circumferential defect
Type III: Miscellaneous, e.g. ureteric fistula.

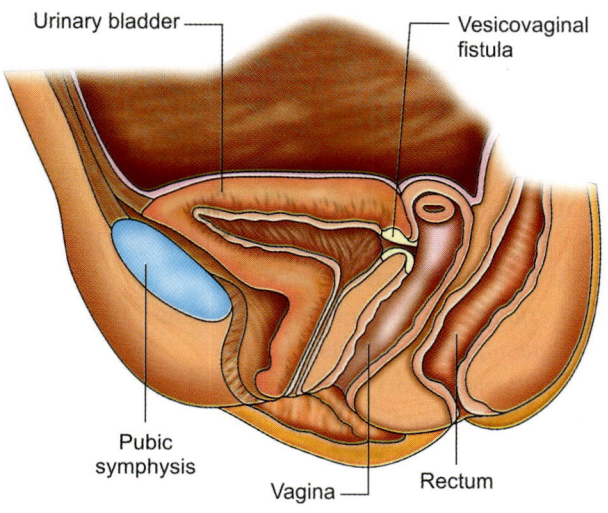

Fig. 18.27: Anatomic relations

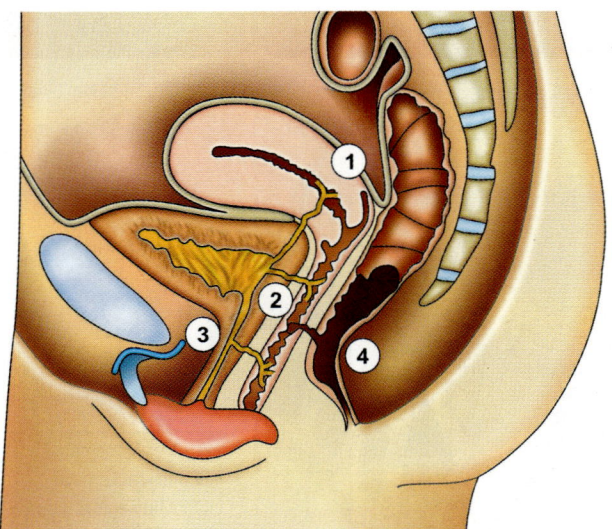

Fig. 18.29: 1—Vesicouterine fistula; 2—vesicovaginal fistula; 3—urethrovaginal fistula; and 4—rectovaginal fistula

Classification according to Size

- Small—<2 cm
- Medium—2–3 cm
- Large—4–5 cm
- Extensive— >5 cm

Classification according to the Site of Injury

- Juxtaurethral fistula
- Mid-vaginal fistula
- Juxta-cervical fistula
- Very large fistula
- Vault fistula
- Combined fistula
- Circumferential fistula
- Residual fistula

Etiology

Developing countries: Numerous factors are responsible for VVF in developing countries. These are:

a. Marriage and conception at a young age, often before full pelvic growth has been achieved.

b. Chronic malnutrition further limits pelvic dimensions, increasing the risk of CPD and malpresentation.

c. Few women are attended by qualified health care professionals or have access to medical facilities during childbirth; their obstructed labor may be protracted for days or weeks.

d. Effect of prolonged impaction of the fetal presenting part in the pelvis-tissue edema, hypoxia, necrosis, and sloughing resulting from prolonged pressure on the soft tissues of the vagina, bladder base, and urethra.

Typically, the urogenital fistula (UGF) is large and involves the bladder, urethra, bladder trigone, and the anterior cervix. Complex neuropathic bladder dysfunction and urethral sphincteric incompetency often result, even if the fistula can be repaired successfully.

Etiopathology

Vesicovaginal fistula can be congenital or acquired.

In most third world countries, >90% of fistulae are of obstetric etiology.

1. *Prolonged obstructed labor:* Commonest cause of VVF in developing countries; It accounts for >80% of the cases.

2. *Cesarean section:* Incision involving the posterior bladder wall.
   - During reflection of the bladder.
   - Accidental passage of suture through the posterior bladder wall during repair of the incision.

3. *Uterine rupture:*
   - Rupture of a previous cesarean section scar.
   - Rupture of the unscarred uterus from obstetric manipulations.
   - The bladder may be caught in the sutures during repair

4. *Direct trauma during operative vaginal delivery:* Forceps delivery, craniotomy, symphysiotomy, repair of vaginal or cervical lacerations

5. *Gynecological operations*
   - Pelvic floor repair, vaginal hysterectomy,
   - Abdominal hysterectomy, colporrhaphy.
   Commonest cause of VVF in developed countries, where it accounts for 75.3% of total.

6. Radiation necrosis.

7. *Malignancies:* Ca cervix, vagina, rectum and bladder.

8. *Traditional practices*: Gishiri cut, circumcision, caustic soda.
   - Gishiri cut accounts for 10–13% of all cases of VVF in the northern Nigeria.

9. *Infections:* Lymphogranuloma venereum, schistosomiasis, tuberculosis.

10. *Social factors:* Early marriage and early delivery.
    - 50% of cases are below 20 yrs.
    - 50% are in their first pregnancy.

11. *Others*: Coital injuries, excision of a urethral diverticulum

Risk Factors for Postoperative Fistulae

- Anemia—nutritional deficiency
- Radiotherapy—ionizing radiation
- Impaired vascularity, infections—endometriosis
- LSCS, vaginal hysterectomy, colporrhaphy
- Inflammation in pelvic surgery, malignancy
- Abnormal tissue adhesions
- Fibroids, ovarian mass producing anatomical distortion

Clinical Presentation

- Uncontrolled leakage of urine into the vagina is the hallmark symptom of patients soon after a prolonged obstructed labor, operative vaginal delivery, or cesarean section.
- In direct surgical injury to the bladder, the leakage of urine may occur from day one.
- In most surgical and obstetric fistulae symptoms develop between 5 and 14 days.
- History of previous surgeries or prolonged obstructed labor.
- Secondary amenorrhea.
- Secondary infertility

Traumatic Fistula

- History of previous pelvic or abdominal surgery
- Symptoms develop early, may be day 1
- Postoperative urinary leakage, oliguria
- Abdominal distension, pyrexia or loin pain
- Present earlier for repair than obstetric cases
- History of previous unsuccessful attempt at repair.
  Radiation-induced UGFs are associated with slowly progressive devascularization necrosis and may present 30 days to 3 months later. Patients with radiation-induced VVFs initially present with symptoms of radiation cystitis, hematuria, and bladder contracture.

Findings on Clinical Examination

- Ill-looking, malnourished, pale with evidence of intercurrent infections.
- Abdomen—kidneys may be enlarged and tender.
- Pelvic examination—vulva and thigh excoriations (ammoniacal dermatitis).
- Vaginal examination—best performed in Sims' lateral position, may also be done in dorsal position.
- Insert Sims' speculum of appropriate size, visualize anterior vaginal wall and then posterior vaginal wall.
- *Inspect:* Wherefrom the leaking is collected.
  Assess size, position, number, margins tissue—healthy, unhealthy/amount of scarring/vascularity/

any malignancy/proximity to lateral pelvic wall/urethra/cervix.

- Palpate the fistulous area during vaginal examination to confirm the inspection findings along with the mobility and amount of scar tissues around the fistulous margin and proximity to urethra, vault, bony walls.
- Do digital rectal examination to rule out RVF or any associated complete perineal tear.

Examination Under Anesthesia + Dye Tests

Digital vaginal examination and examination with a Sims' speculum may not confirm or exclude a fistula, thus necessitating EUA + DYE TESTS
  A malleable probe is passed through openings in the vaginal wall.

- For VVF and UVF, a metallic click against a catheter may be felt or seen via cystoscope.
- For RVF, the probe may be felt digitally in the rectum or seen via a proctoscope.
  - Enables assessment of available access.
  - Mobility of tissues for vaginal repair.
  - The decision to repair vaginally or an abdominal approach.
  - A full vaginal inspection is essential and should include assessment of tissue mobility; accessibility of the fistula to vaginal repair; determination of the degree of tissue inflammation, edema, and infection; and possible association of a rectovaginal fistula.
  - Urine should be collected for culture and sensitivity, and patients with positive results should be treated prior to surgery.

Specific Investigations—Dyes Studies

- Patient in lithotomy position.
- Examination best done under direct vision.
  'Three swab test' has limitations because of lack of adequate distension of the urinary bladder.
- If clear fluid leaks after instillation of dye, ureteric fistula is likely.
- Differentiate by "two dye test" .
- Phenazopyridine to stain renal urine
- Methylene blue to stain the bladder urine.

Other Specific Investigations

General Investigations

- FBC + Blood film + Malaria parasite
- Urine for urinalysis and culture sensitivity
- Stool for parasitic infestations
- Chest X-ray

Table 18.1: Differentiate between vesicovaginal fistula and ureterovaginal fistula

Points	Vesicovaginal fistula	Ureterovaginal fistula
Symptoms—continuous involuntary leakage of urine	True Incontinence	True incontinence
Presence of bladder filling sensation (filling of urge)	Absent	Present
Etiological factors	Both following obstetric and gynecologic assault	Mainly following gynecologic assault like LSCS/abdominal or vaginal hysterectomy
Time of onset	Delayed in obstetric fistula (uncommon nowadays); immediate in traumatic type	Usually immediate or within 1st 7 days of surgery
Site of fistula	High/mid or low vaginal	Always high fistula
Dye test	Positive with transurethral passage of methylene blue	Negative with transurethral passage of dye but positive with IV Indigo carmine
Cystoscopy	Fistulous opening seen in relation to trigone	Absence of urine spurt in one of the ureteric orifice
IVU	Bladder fistula with vaginal wall detected with dye filling in vagina	No filling of dye in lower part of affected ureter; often unilateral hydroureter/hydronephrosis/dye in vagina
Treatment	Surgical-approach mainly vaginal, abdominal in high fistula or failed cases	Alwalys urosugeon's job—abdominal approach with ureteroneocystostomy/ureteroureteral anastomosis/urinary diversion

- Serum urea/creatinine
- Intravenous urography

Table 18.1 differentiates between vesicovaginal and ureterovaginal fistula.

Preoperative Treatment

Timing of definitive repair—either immediate, if diagnosed within 24 hrs or at least three months after assault.

a. Improve patient's general health; high protein diet, antihelmintics, hematinics and treatment of intercurrent infections/diseases, vulval dermatitis with zinc oxide cream.
b. Bowel preparation, prophylactic antibiotics/urinary antiseptics.

Repair of VVF

- Route of repair; vaginal or abdominal
- Position of patient; lithotomy or reverse lithotomy (knee-elbow position)
- Type of suture materials; absorbable—vicryl 2/0 to 4/0
- Types of repair;(1) Dissection and repair in layers; (2) Saucerization

Patient Positioning

Lawson position: This position is ideal for proximal urethral and bladder neck fistulas. The patient is placed in a prone position with the knees spread and ankles raised in the air and supported by stirrups. Combining it with reverse Trendelenburg positioning enhances visualization with this technique.

Jackknife position: This is ideal for proximal urethral and bladder neck fistulas. The patient is placed in a prone position with the hips abducted and flexed and the table jackknifed.

Dorsal lithotomy position: Dorsal lithotomy position with standard Trendelenburg positioning provides excellent access for repair of a high VVF.

Excellent success rates for both the vaginal and abdominal approaches, if the following general surgical principles are followed:

1. Complete preoperative diagnosis
2. Adequate exposure
3. Secure hemostasis
4. Adequate mobilization of tissue
5. Tissue closure under no tension
6. Watertight closure of bladder during cystotomy repair
7. Proper timing to avoid infection and inflammation of tissue
8. Facilitate adequate blood supply at area of repair
9. 2–3 weeks continuous catheter drainage postoperatively for proper healing.

To Excise or not to Excise: The Fistula Tract Excision Debate

Routine excision of the fistula tract is not mandatory. This increase the risks of increasing the size of the fistula tract. Additionally, the fibrous ring of the fistula may add to the strength of the repair and prevent postoperative bladder spasms. Therefore, a small fistula may be resected as this ensures closure of all layers with viable tissues, but large tracts in bigger fistula should only be freshened by electrocoagulation or sharp knife dissection. There are also further risks of intracystic bleeding and blood clot formation from the mucosal edge of the bladder with fistula resection. Subsequent blockage of the catheter postoperatively would then increase the risk of failure of the VVF repair.

A. Vaginal Approach

This has the following advantages:

a. Minimal blood loss

b. Low postoperative morbidity

c. Shorter operative time

d. Shorter postoperative recovery time. The absolute contraindications for vaginal repair of VVF are the concomitant presence of fistulas with other abdominopelvic organs, such as ureters and small and large bowel, and multiple VVFs.

Exposure

- Suturing of the labial folds to the ipsilateral thigh provides improved visibility of the vaginal vault.
- Procedures used to facilitate exposure in the vagina include Dührssen and Schuchardt incisions.
- The **Dührssen incision** is a deep vagino-perineal incision or extended episiotomy for easy access to fistulaous opening in vagina. Its application to fistula surgery was recommended by Mackenrodt in 1894.
- **Schuchardt's parasacral incision** is an extension of a Dührssen incision, whereby a deep vaginoperineal incision is carried cephalad to the vault apex and then posteriorly toward the tip of the coccyx. Schuchardt's paravaginal incision is performed by incising the posterior vaginal wall in a direction angled toward the ischial tuberosity, going through the levator ani and the coccygeus muscle, to ultimately gain access into the ischiorectal fossa.

Catheterization of the fistula tract: Exposure and access to a VVF can be facilitated by catheterization of the fistula with a bulb catheter, such as a Foley's catheter. An uninflated catheter may thread the fistula where the bulb is inflated, then traction is placed on the catheter to draw the VVF into the field. A small VVF may be probed first with a lacrimal duct probe and dilated with cervical dilators to permit placement of a pediatric catheter/ureteral bulb catheter.

Low-tension Closure

- The critical issue of closure of suture lines without any tension is the key to successful surgical repair of VVF. In an attempt to reduce strain at the site of anterior vaginal wall closures, surgeons employ several strategies, including extensive vaginal wall dissection and mobilization from the underlying vesicovaginal endopelvic fascia. Alternatively, lateral radial or circumferential relaxing incisions can be created.
- To increase vascularization of the vaginal tissue, vascularized flaps or grafts at the site of fistula repair such as a Martius bulbocavernosus fibromuscular pedicle with or without intact skin patches applied. Such grafts are essential in the repair of large fistulas and radiotherapy-related fistulae, where large areas of devascularized and scarred vaginal walls commonly are observed.

Surgical Procedures for the Vaginal Approach

a. *Flap-splitting techniques* (Fig. 18.30)

In this technique, the vaginal wall is incised circumferentially around the fistula and widely dissected from the underlying endopelvic fascia in a standard anterior colporrhaphy technique. Leaving the tract unresected, the bladder is closed, tension-free, in two layers. The initial suture layer consists of 4-0 delayed absorbable suture placed in an extramucosal fashion and extending beyond the opening by 3–4 millimeters. Secondary imbricating suture is placed in a similar fashion into the bladder muscularis. The closure is tested for watertightness. Peritoneum may be available to interpose between the bladder and vagina. The vagina is then sutured closed over the bladder defect.

- Some surgeons prefer asymmetric J incision in the anterior vaginal wall whereby the lower curve of the J loops around the fistula site. This modification enables the surgeon to advance one flap over the fistula repair and prevent overlapping suture lines.
- Martius graft is added in cases where fistulal site appears poorly vascular and tissue defect is more.

Vaginal cuff excision

- *Technique:* The patient is placed in dorsal lithotomy position. Cystoscopy is performed. Traction on the fistula site is obtained by placing a Foley catheter into the fistula tract from a vaginal approach, inflating the balloon, and placing traction sutures at 1 cm distance from the fistula. The vaginal mucosa is denuded circumferentially for a radius of 3–5 mm from the vaginal cuff, including the fistula. This

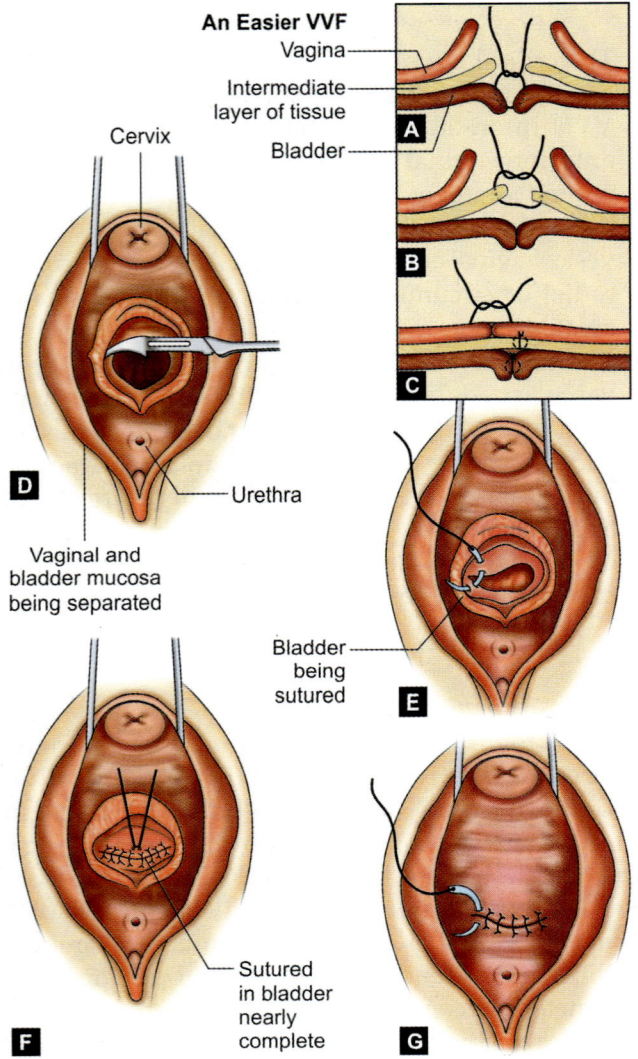

An Easier VVF

Vagina
Intermediate layer of tissue
Cervix
Bladder

A
B
C

D

Urethra

Vaginal and bladder mucosa being separated

Bladder being sutured

E

Sutured in bladder nearly complete

F

G

Fig. 18.30: Flap splitting procedures

fistula opening. The fistula at the bladder mucosa is not disturbed. A double row of sagittally oriented sutures is placed in the raw surfaces on either side of the fistula, with the second row imbricating the first. Suturing of the vaginal wall is then performed, providing a third layer of closure. The vaginal wall in contact with the bladder becomes the posterior vesical wall and eventually is reepithelialized with transitional epithelium.

- Numerous authors hold this time-honored procedure, with success rates of 93–100%, to be the standard for repair of simple posthysterectomy VVFs.
- Advantages of the Latzko procedure include simplicity of technique, high success rate, low morbidity, no impairment in bladder capacity, and no compromise of ureteral orifices, even with fistulas lying close to the orifices.

B. Abdominal Approach

The abdominal approach may be required:

a. For complex fistula involving the ureters, bowel, or other intra-abdominal structure.
b. The multiple operated fistula with significant scarring.
c. Fistula in the irradiated patient.
d. The inability to adequately expose the fistula vaginally.
e. When the position of the ureters to the fistula is very close.
f. When there is need for concomitant abdominal surgery, such as augmentation cystoplasty and ureteral reimplantation.

Exposure

As with the transvaginal approach, exposure with the transabdominal approach can be augmented with the use of traction sutures and with catheterization of the fistula with a Foley catheter. In this technique, superior bladder wall is bivalved up to the level of the fistula. The fistula tract is excised and the vagina and bladder are closed separately in layers. Stents may be placed following the incision cystotomy and removed during closure of the bladder . Peritoneum or omentum may be interposed between the vagina and bladder. Removal of the scarred fistula tract proceeds harvesting of the graft. The posterior bladder wall is sutured over the graft. Following abdominal fistula repair, a suprapubic catheter is inserted and retained for 10 to 14 days.

- The classic positioning of the patient for abdominal procedures is supine, with Trendelenburg

incision is then extended obliquely to the bladder wall so as to resect the fistula tract and vaginal cuff scar in a funnel-shaped specimen.

- The defect is closed in 4 layers. First, the bladder is closed with interrupted 4-0 sutures; the subvaginal pubocervicovaginal fascia then is closed in 2 layers with interrupted 3-0 sutures. This is followed by a vaginal wall closure. In each of the 4 layers, polyglycolic acid suture material is used.
- Intravenous Indigo carmine and cystoscopy is used to ensure bladder and ureteral integrity. A suprapubic catheter is the preferred method of bladder drainage and is maintained for approximately 3 weeks postoperatively.

b. *Latzko partial colpocleises procedure*

Latzko technique: Vaginal mucosa is sharply denuded in a circular fashion at a distance of 1.5 cm from the

orientation. However, modifying this by flexing the patient's hips and abducting and supporting her legs in stirrups is wise. Simultaneous access and examination of the vaginal vault may assist with laparotomy procedures.

- The choice of incision may include suprapubic V, Pfannenstiel, or midline vertical. The Turner-Warwick suprapubic V incision provides superior access to the lower abdomen and pelvis. The longitudinal suprapubic incision allows the surgeon to obtain omental graft easily.

Transvesical Extraperitoneal Technique

In 1885, Trendelenburg introduced the first transvesical extraperitoneal method of vesicovaginal repair. With the patient placed in a steep Trendelenburg position, a transvesical incision is performed to visualize the fistula. The bladder mucosa adjacent to the fistula is circumscribed and removed. The bladder is dissected off the vagina and the vaginal defects are closed first followed by the bladder defects separately.

Transperitoneal Technique

The transperitoneal technique was developed by von Dittel in 1803 for the repair of VVFs. In this procedure, a laparotomy is performed. The bladder is dissected from underlying gynecologic organs involved. The defects in the bladder and vagina or cervix are closed separately.

Transvesical Transperitoneal Suprapubic Technique

In this method, the peritoneal cavity is accessed by laparotomy and a sagittal incision is made in the bladder. This cystotomy incision is extended to the fistula. The bladder is mobilized off the vagina, and the bladder and vaginal defects are closed separately. This is suitable for patients with complex and difficult repairs, such as radiation-associated cases. Commonly, peritoneal or interposition grafts are added. A suprapubic catheter is brought out laterally to the sagittal closure. A transurethral catheter may be placed and discontinued on postoperative day 4 or 5; the suprapubic catheter is removed on postoperative day 14.

Different Methods of Closure of the Fistula

1. Vesical autoplasty where bladder flap is prepared to cover the bladder wall defect.
2. Electrocautery can be done to fulgarise the margins of very small fisula.

3. Fibrin glue: Occlusion therapy using fibrin glue is considered useful and safe for intractable fistulae. Fibrin glue facilitates healing by recruiting macrophages and providing a semisolid support structure rich in growth and angiogenic factors.
4. Laser welding can be used to fulgarise the fistula margins instead of cauterization.

C. Laparoscopic Approach

1. This method is applicable for those patients with clear indications for abdominal approach surgical treatment. The technique involves cystoscopy, catheterization of the fistula tract, dissection of the bladder from the vagina, laparoscopic cystotomy, excision of the tract, adequate dissection of the bladder from the vaginal wall, cystotomy, and colpotomy closure with interposition of a flap of healthy tissue.
2. *Transurethral suture cystorrhaphy (TUSC):* This technique involves suprapubic visualization with a shorter scope such as an arthroscope, large-caliber sheaths used transurethrally to allow passage of relatively large curved needles, self-righting needle driver, and adequate fulguration of the fistula tract and the surrounding bladder mucosa.

Interposition of Martius Labial Fat Pad Graft (Fig. 18.31)

a. The fat pad graft is mobilized by incising the labia majora. Care is taken to preserve the blood supply entering posteriorly.

b. The graft is rotated through the labial tunnel into the vaginal vault, covering the fistulous tract.

c. A Penrose drain is placed at the bed of the graft and brought out at a lateral site, if any persistent bleeding is noted. This drain is then removed on the third to fifth postoperative day.

d. In modified Martius flap, only the fibroadipose tissue in the labium majus is isolated. It is composed of fibrous septa, round ligament, and a superficial fibrous layer; it does not contain bulbocavernosus muscle. The risk of hemorrhage is more with the classic Martius graft technique because it requires a deep plane of dissection to isolate the bulbocavernosus muscle. The fibroadipose tissue isolated in their dissection possess sufficient blood supply and strength for success. Additionally, dual blood supply to this tissue and the bulbocavernosus muscle (dorsally via internal pudendal artery and ventrally via external pudendal artery) enables the surgeon the choice of using a flap with a superior or inferior base. Mild dyspareunia over the graft site is a

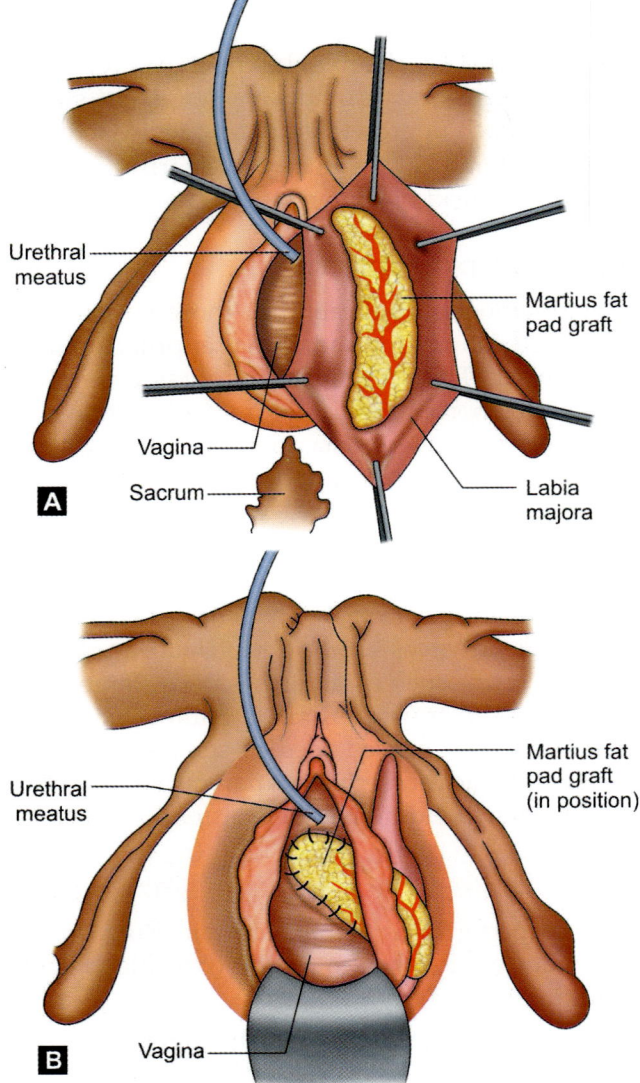

Urethral meatus

Martius fat pad graft

Vagina

Sacrum

Labia majora

A

Urethral meatus

Martius fat pad graft (in position)

Vagina

B

Fig. 18.31: Intrerposition of Martius graft

potential complication, which may be difficult to avoid and rectify.

I. *Vaginal Approach Interposition Grafts or Flaps*

a. *Martius flap*

b. *Gracilis muscle flap:* The predominant application for this flap is in total vaginal reconstruction following pelvic exenteration.

c. *Peritoneal flap:* The uterovesical peritoneal flap is approached through dissection between the vaginal wall and bladder in cephalad direction. Continuing dissection just beyond the posterior wall of the bladder exposes the peritoneum at the anterior cul-de-sac. It is mobilized carefully from the posterior bladder wall and brought down to reach beyond the fistula site and be secured over the fistula repair suture line with 2-0 polyglycolic sutures.

II. *Abdominal Approach Interposition Grafts or Flaps*

a. *Omental J flap:* Omentum, with its rich lymphatic and vascular supply, is ideal as an interposition graft. It has sufficient length to extend to the pelvis without tension. It can be mobilized from the transverse colon with right or left gastroepiploic artery to form a pedicle of sufficient length. The right is preferred because it has a better blood supply.

b. *Peritoneal flap*

c. *Rectus abdominis muscle flap*

d. *Autologous bladder mucosa interposition graft:* A site is selected at the bladder dome for harvesting of the donor mucosal graft. The graft is dissected from the muscularis and interposed between the bladder and vaginal walls so that the mucosal surface faces the vagina.

e. *Human dura mater interposition graft*

f. *Broad ligament flaps*

Postoperative Management

- To maintain adequate fluid balance with intake of 3–4 litres per day and output at 120–150 mL/hr.
- Continuous bladder drainage; check drainage and urine output hourly.
- Duration of drainage; 10–14 days on the average.
- Administer postoperative antibiotics.
- Prevention of deep vein thrombosis.
- Care of the perineum with vulva pads.
- Retraining of urinary bladder before discharge.
- Avoid pelvic and speculum vaginal examinations during the first 4–6 weeks postoperatively because the tissue is delicate.
- Pelvic rest: Prohibit coitus and tampon use for a minimum of 4–6 weeks. Other authors advocate strict pelvic rest for 3 months.

Complications

- Risks of infection
- Hemorrhage
- Injury to other organs, particularly the ureters
- Surgical failure of fistula repair; possible new fistula formation
- Thromboembolism and death
- Sexual dysfunction
- New-onset incontinence, and the progression of pre-existing urge and/or stress incontinence.
- Abdominal approach procedures carry risks of abdominal and pelvic adhesions.
- Vaginal approach procedures carry increased risks of dyspareunia, tenderness at the site of the donor Martius graft, and diminished vaginal length and caliber.

Instructions on Discharge

- Repeat EUA and dye test on day 21 before discharge.
- Refrain from sexual intercourse for 3 months.
- Counsel for antenatal care and hospital delivery in all subsequent pregnancies.
- Elective cesarean section in next pregnancy.
- Attempt for vaginal delivery is possible when: (a) fistula arise from nonrecurrent cases; (b) presence of interposition graft utilized in repair surgery; (c) labour is conducted in tertiary hospital.

Ureterovaginal Fistula

Normal Ureteric Anatomy

- Length of pelvic ureter: 15 cm (total length 25 cm).
- At pelvic brim:
  - It enters the pelvis retroperitoneally by crossing the bifurcation of common iliac artery near sacro-iliac joint.
  - It is related anteriorly to ovarian vessels as they cross the infundibulopelvic ligament. Ureter is adherent to medial flap of infundibulopelvic ligament (Fig. 18.32).
  - The ureter descends downward and medially along and anterior lower part of internal iliac artery.
  - The ureter forms the posterior boundery of ovarian fossa.
- The ureter cross over:
  - Common and internal iliac artery.
  - Obturator artery, vein, and nerve.
  - Obliterated hypogastric artery.
- At the level of ischial spine:
  - It curves forwards and medially below base of broad ligament.
- Then passes through upper part of cardinal ligament:
  - Below and at right angle to uterine artery.
  - 1.5 cm above and lateral to lateral vaginal fornix.
  - It enters the posterosuperior angle of the bladder and run in the bladder wall for 2 cm before opening in the trigone.

Blood Supply of Ureter

- Ureter has poor blood supply since it has segmental blood supply from the following vessels:
  - Abdominal aorta
  - Vesical artery
  - Renal artery
  - Internal iliac artery
  - Common iliac artery
  - Ovarian artery

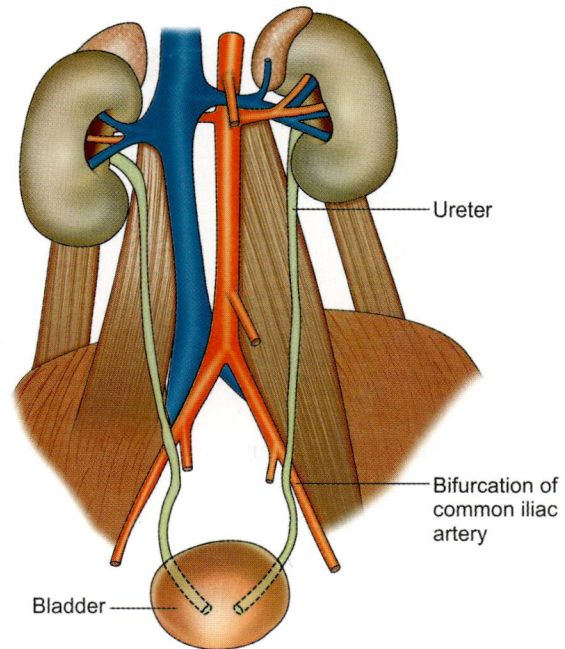

Fig. 18.32: Course of ureter

Incidence of Ureteric Injuries

- The incidence of ureteric injury varies between 0.1 and 30%, depending on the type of surgery.
- Obstetric and gynecological surgeries account for approximately 50% of ureteric injuries.
- Ureteric injuries are less common during vaginal (1%) than abdominal hysterectomies (1%).
- Prevalence of ureteric injury is higher following gynecological cancer surgery though benign gynecological surgery accounts for most cases.
- The incidence of all major complications associated with laparoscopy have declined but ureteric injuries still remains at approximately 1%.
- 38% occur during the treatment of endometriosis.

Risk Factors for Ureteric Injuries

a. *Anatomical risk factors:* The ureter is more prone to injury because of:
  - Its close attachment to the peritoneum.
  - Close relation to female genital tract.
  - Its variable course.
  - Not easily seen or palpable
b. *Pathological risk factors*
  - Congenital anomalies of ureter or kidney.
  - *Ureteric displacement produced by:*
    - Uterine size >12 weeks
    - Prolapse
    - Pelvic tumors like lateral fibroids, ovarian neoplasms.
    - Cervical or broad ligament swellings.

- *Adhesions:*
  - Previous pelvic surgery.
  - Endometriosis.
  - PID
- Distorted pelvic anatomy.

c. *Technical risk factors*

I. *Intraoperative*
- Crushing from misapplication of a clamp.
- Ligation with a suture.
- Transection (partial or complete).
- Angulation of the ureter with secondary obstruction.
- Ischemia from ureteral stripping, LASER, or electrocoagulation.
- Resection of a segment of ureter.

II. *Postoperative*
1. Avascular necrosis.
2. Kinking.
3. Subsequent obstruction over:
   - Hematoma, or
   - Lymphocele

Procedures associated with Increased Risk of Ureteric Injury

- Obstetrical procedures
- Gynecological procedures
- Urogynecology procedures
- Laparoscopic procedures

Sites of Ureteric Injuries

Common sites of ureteral injury are (Fig. 18.33):
- Lateral to the uterine vessels (commonest).
- The area of the ureterovesical junction close to the cardinal ligaments.
- The base of the infundibulopelvic ligament as the ureters cross the pelvic brim at the ovarian fossa.
- At the level of the uterosacral ligament.
- Bladder junction with ureter: During vaginal cuff closure, or anterior uterovesical pouch entry from the vagina.
- During laparoscopy, the ureter is injured most frequently adjacent to the uterosacral ligaments.

According to the organ injury scoring system developed by the committee of the American association for the surgery of trauma, ureteric injuries are classified as follows:

Sites of ureteric injuries			
Uretreic site	Lower third	Upper third	Middle third
Incidence of injury	51%	31%	19%

- *Grade I* *laceration:* Contusion or hematoma without devascularization.
- *Grade II* *laceration:* <50% transection.
- *Grade III* *laceration:* >50% transection.
- *Grade IV* *laceration:* Complete transection with < 2 cm of devascularization.
- *Grade V* *laceration:* Avulsion with >2 cm of devascularization.

Management Strategies of Ureteric Injuries

1. Anticipate the potential for specific injuries, based on the patient's known risk factors.
2. Prevent: The likelihood of injury.
3. Recognize: Take measures to identify any injuries as soon as they occur or soon thereafter.
4. Evaluate each injury to ascertain its full extent and plan its repair.
5. Repair the injury.
6. Test the integrity of the repair.
7. Follow up postoperatively to verify that the repair remains intact.

Preventive Strategies to Reduce the Risk of Ureteric Injuries

I. General preventive strategies
II. Specific preventive strategies

I. *Genereal Preventive Strategies*

A. *Preoperative measures*
1. Intravenous urogram (IVU).
2. Ultrasound scan.
   Both can identify ureteric dilatation and disclose anatomical variations.

B. *Intraoperative measures*
1. Appropriate operative approach.
2. Adequate exposure.
3. Avoid blind clamping of blood vessels.
4. Ureteric dissection and direct visualization.
5. Mobilize bladder away from operative site.
6. Short diathermy applications.

II. *Specific Preventive Strategies*

A. *During abdominal hysterectomy:*
- Clamp (cardinal, uterosacral) ligaments close to the uterus.
- Clamp, divide and ligate uterine vessels close to the uterus.
- Clamp infundibulopelvic ligament near to the ovary after dissection and palpation.

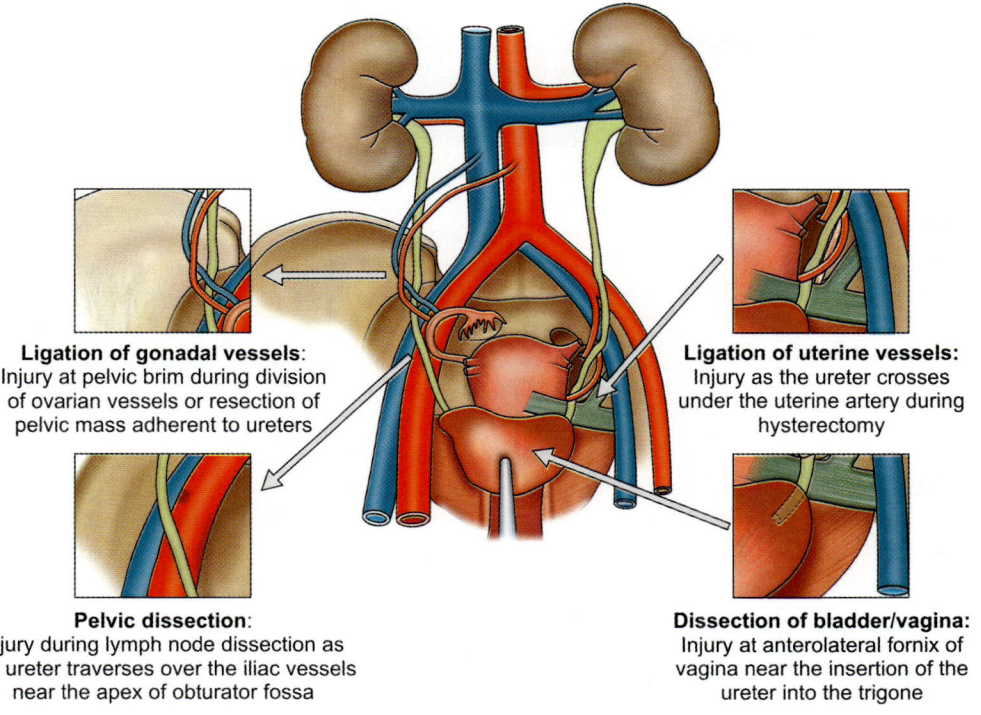

Ligation of gonadal vessels: Injury at pelvic brim during division of ovarian vessels or resection of pelvic mass adherent to ureters

Pelvic dissection: Injury during lymph node dissection as the ureter traverses over the iliac vessels near the apex of obturator fossa

Ligation of uterine vessels: Injury as the ureter crosses under the uterine artery during hysterectomy

Dissection of bladder/vagina: Injury at anterolateral fornix of vagina near the insertion of the ureter into the trigone

Fig. 18.33: Sites of ureteric injury

- Never to open vagina unless urinary bladder is dissected downward and laterally.
- Use of intrafacial technique.

B. *During vaginal surgery:*
1. Prevention of ureteric injuries can be achieved by adequate development of vesicouterine space, by:
   - Downward traction on the cervix.
   - Countertraction upward by Sims' speculum below the bladder.
2. All clamps:
   - Small bites.
   - Close to the uterus.
3. Avoid double clamping of uterosacral ligaments.
4. Vaginal oophorectomy should be avoided or done cautiously.
5. During anterior colporrhaphy:
   - Avoid too lateral dissection.
   - Avoid deep sutures: As the distance between needle and ureter in upper vagina $\geq$ 0.9 cm.

C. *During laparoscopy, safety of ureter can be achieved by:*
1. Moving the fallopian tubes away from pelvic side walls before coagulation.
2. The bleeding points at uterosacral ligaments should be secured with sutures or clips instead of electrocoagulation.
3. In LAVH place stapler or suture across uterine vessels and cardinal ligaments instead of electrocoagulation.

Identification of the Ureter

- The peritoneal reflection anterior to the uterus is incised and the bladder is reflected inferiorly with sharp dissection.
- The ureter is identified on the medial aspect of the broad ligament during the development of the perivesical and perirectal spaces, as is the superior vesical artery.

Management of Ureteric Injuries

Intraoperative Management (Table 18.2)

Aim is for quick repair which will reduce morbidity and decrease legal risks. Diagnose clinically:
- See cut ends of the ureter.
- Urine flow in the operative field.

Investigation

1. Intravenous administration of methylthioninium chloride or Indigo carmine—ureteric injury is suspected by extravasation of the dye.
2. Intraoperative transurethral cystoscopy or telescopy (through cystotomy) using an abdominal approach may be required to visualize ejaculation of dye stained urine from both ureteric orifices.
3. Ureteric catheter inserted:
   - From above: Ureterotomy.
   - From below: Through bladder.

Table 18.2: Intraoperative management of ureteric injury

Injury	Management
Needle Injury	No action unless bleeding or leakage
Crushed ureter	Ureteric catheter for 10–14 days
Ligated ureter	Remove ligature and ureteric catheter for 10–14 days
Small hole	Suture or ureteric catheter for 10–14 days
Partial transection	Stent placement
Complete transection (length) <5 cm from ureterovesical juntion	1. Ureteroneocystostomy (ureterovesical anastomosis) without no loss of tension—submucosal tunnel to avoid urine reflux when urinary bladder is distended with urine

Complete transaction >5 cm from ureterovesical junction (no loss of lenth)	2. Ureteroureterostomy (ureteroureteric anastomosis)
	    – End to end→Stricture
	    – End to side→Best
	    – Invaginate upper end into lower end.

Complete transaction (loss of length)	1. Ureteroneocystostomy:
	    a. Psoas hitch: mobilize bladder towards ureter (Fig. 18.34)
	    b. Boari flap with a psoas hitch: bladder flap prepared like tube
	2. Transureteroureterostomy
	3. Ureteroilecocystostomy
	4. Ureterocalycostomy
	5. Renal autotransplantation

Postoperative Management of Ureteric Injuries

- 70% of ureteric injuries are diagnosed postoperatively.
- Postoperative management of ureteric injuries:

a. Immediate postoperative.
b. Late postoperative, i.e. when ureteric fistula is already established.

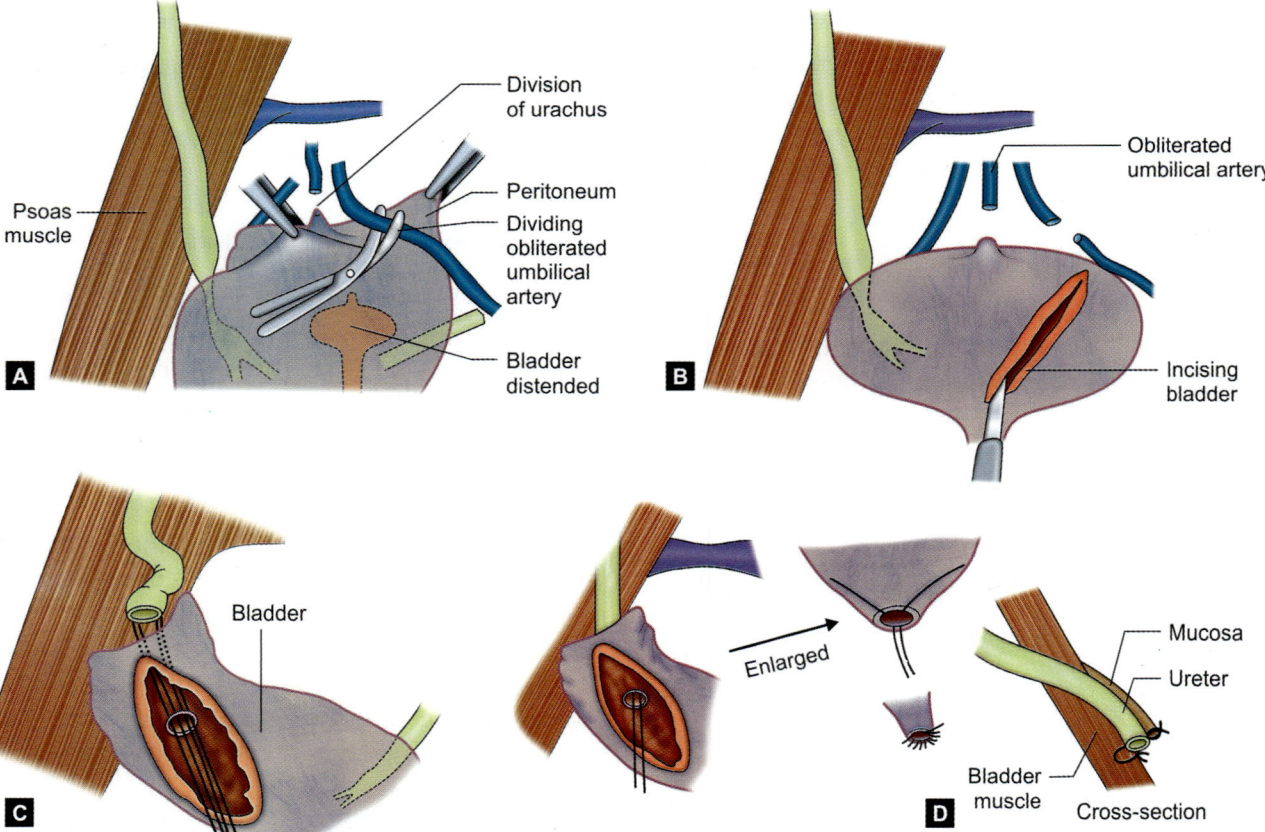

Fig. 18.34: Psoas hitch procedure

A. Immediate Postoperative Diagnosis

Clinically

1. Asymptomatic + Atrophy of the kidney.
2. Unexplained postoperative:
   - Stormy fever.
   - Abdominal distension.
   - Flank pain.
   - Urinoma as ascites
3. Hematuria—absent in 30%
4. Urinary leakage (vaginally or via abdominal wound).
5. Complications:
   - Postoperative anuria (due to ligation of one or both ureters or reflex spasm)
   - Abscess formation/sepsis
   - Peritonitis/ileus
   - Retroperitoneal urinoma
   - Secondary hypertension

Investigations

i. *Investigations are needed to establish renal function:*
   - Renal function tests.
   - A full blood count and an electrolyte profile.
ii. *Investigations to rule out hydronephrosis and to evaluate continuity of the ureter:*
   1. Intravenous urogram
   2. Abdominal and pelvic computerized tomography scan with intravenous contrast
   3. Retrograde ureterogram.
   4. Renal ultrasound.
   5. Cystoscopy.
   6. Contrast-dye tests.
   7. Analysis of fluid aspirated from the abdomen.

Immediate postoperative treatment: When recognition of ureteric injury has been delayed, repair should not be delayed.

Exceptions include

i. *Complications:* Sepsis, extensive hematoma or abscess formation at the site of injury.
ii. Woman is hemodynamically unstable

In these situations, it is preferable to perform (Fig. 18.35):
1. Percutaneous nephrostomy drainage of the renal pelvis or
2. A retrograde ureteric stent placement and delay surgery until the complication is resolved (Figs 18.35 and 18.36).

General Principles of Ureteric Repair (Fig. 18.37)

1. Meticulous ureteric dissection preserving adventitial sheath and its blood supply.

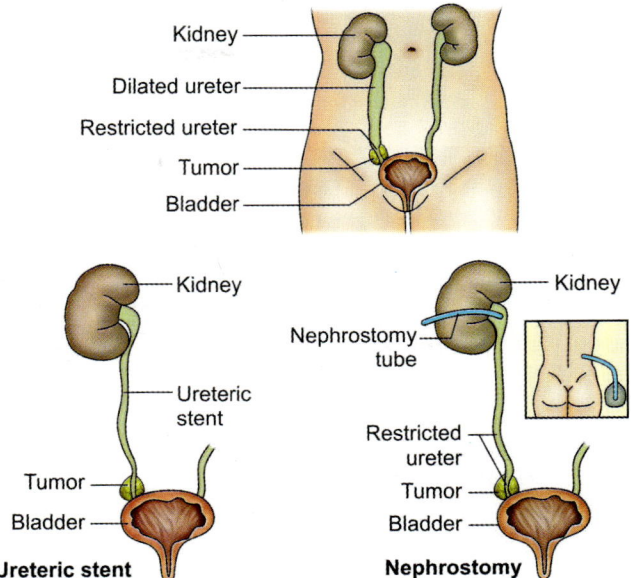

Fig. 18.35: Stenting and nephrostomy

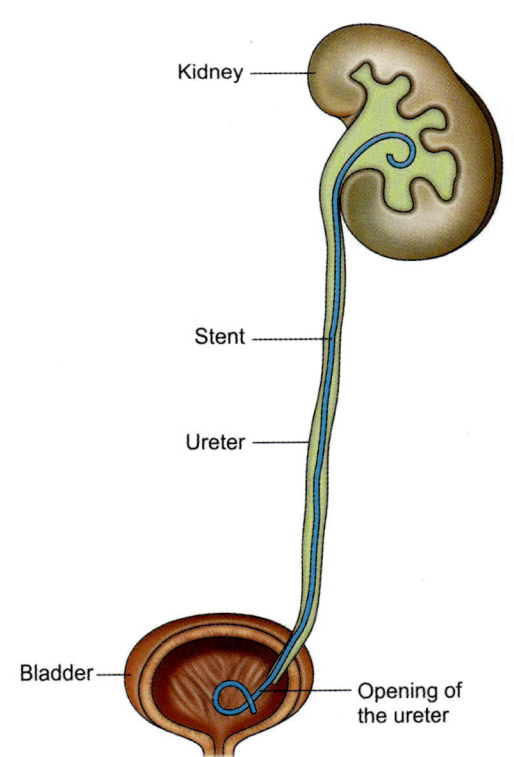

Fig. 18.36: Ureteric stent placement

2. Tension-free anastomosis by ureteric mobilization.
3. Repair over stent with a ureteric catheter.
4. Minimal use of fine absorbable suture to attain watertight closure.
5. Use of peritoneum or omentum to surround the anastomosis.

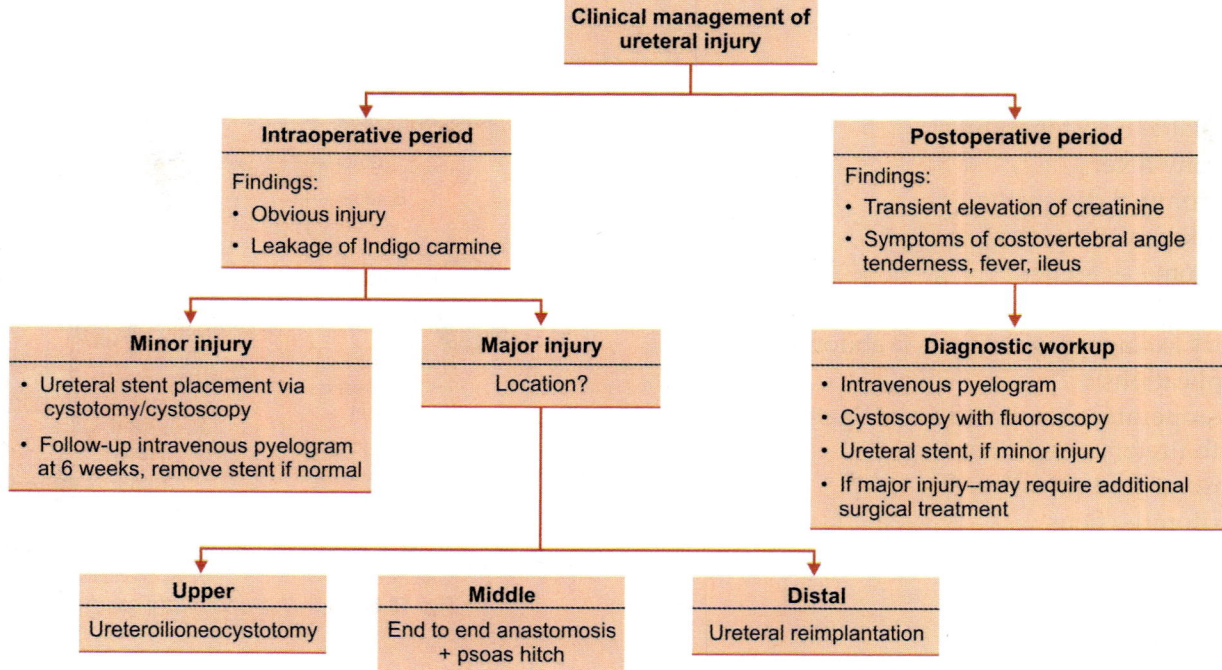

Fig. 18.37: Brief schematic chart of management of ureteric injury

6. Drain the anastomotic site with a passive (closed) drain to limit urinoma formation.
7. Consider a proximal diversion.

Complications following Surgery for Ureteric Injury

- Stricture
- Excessive drainage
- Stent and nephrostomy related problems
- Urinary tract infection
- Ureteric obstruction or reflux
- Boari flap complications
- Hematoma
- Wound infection

19

Cervical Lesion

The cervix is located at the base of the uterus and is normally characterized as having a stratified squamous epithelium. In cervical intraepithelial neoplasia (CIN), the cells of the cervix undergo changes that reflect a loss of controlled growth.

Cervical intraepithelial neoplasia (CIN), also known as **cervical dysplasia** and **cervical interstitial neoplasia**, is the potentially premalignant transformation and abnormal growth (dysplasia) of squamous cells on the surface of the cervix. CIN is not cancer, and is usually curable. Most cases of CIN remain stable, or are eliminated by the host's immune system without intervention. However, a small percentage of cases progress to become cervical cancer, usually cervical squamous cell carcinoma (SCC), if left untreated. The major cause of CIN is chronic infection of the cervix with the sexually transmitted human papillomavirus (HPV), especially the high-risk HPV types 16 or 18. Over 100 types of HPV have been identified. About a dozen of these types appear to cause cervical dysplasia and may lead to the development of cervical cancer.

The earliest microscopic change corresponding to CIN is dysplasia of the epithelial or surface lining of the cervix. Cellular changes associated with HPV infection, such as koilocytes, are also commonly seen in CIN. CIN is usually detected by a screening test, the Papanicolau or "Pap" smear. The purpose of this test is to detect potentially precancerous changes. Pap smear result is currently reported using the Bethesda system. An abnormal Pap smear result may lead to a recommendation for colposcopy of the cervix, during which the cervix is examined under magnification. A biopsy is taken of any abnormal appearing areas to diagnose cervical dysplasia.

Risk Factors

Risk factors that have been found to be important in developing CIN are:

- Women who become infected by a "high risk" type of HPV, such as 16, 18, 31, or 45
- Women who are immunodeficient
- Women who give birth before age 17

Besides, there are other risk factors which have been shown to increase a woman's likelihood of developing CIN, include poor diet, multiple sexual partners, lack of condom use and cigarette smoking.

Classification (Table 19.1)

Depending on several factors such as the type of HPV and the location of the infection, CIN can start in any of the three stages, and can either progress, or regress. CIN is classified in grades:

Symptoms and Signs

There are usually no symptoms. Usually pelvic examination is usually normal.

CIN 1: The essential feature is that the cells throughout the full thickness of the epithelium undergo cytoplasmic differentiation. But the cells in the lower

Table 19.1: Classification of CIN

Histology Grade	Corresponding Cytology	Description	Image
—	—	Normal cervical epithelium	
CIN 1 (Grade I)	LSIL	The least risky type, represents only mild dysplasia, or abnormal cell growth. It is confined to the basal 1/3 of the epithelium. This corresponds to infection with HPV, and typically will be cleared by immune response in a year or so, though can take several years to clear.	
CIN 2/3	HSIL	Formerly subdivided into CIN2 and CIN3	
CIN 2 (Grade II)		Moderate dysplasia confined to the basal 2/3 of the epithelium	
CIN 3 (Grade III)		Severe dysplasia that spans more than 2/3 of the epithelium, and may involve the full thickness. This lesion may sometimes also be referred to as cervical carcinoma *in situ*.	

third of the epithelium show no evidence of cytoplasmic differentiation or orderly stratification, lack clearly defined boundaries and have a high nucleocytoplasmic ratio with nuclear crowding while those in the middle and upper thirds of the epithelium show evidence of stratification and cytoplasmic maturation with decreasing nucleocytoplasmic ratio.

CIN 2: Here the undifferentiated nonstratified cells with pleomorphic nucleoli and a high nucleocytoplasmic ratio extend into the middle third from the lower third of the epithelium. But the cells in the upper third of the epithelium maintain a variable degree of stratification and of cytoplasmic differentiation.

CIN 3: In this condition, undifferentiated, nonstratified basaloid cells with nuclear crowding and nuclear pleomorphism with abnormal mitotic figures are commonly present in the upper third of the epithelium and move upwards from the lower third of the layers. This type of lesion is commonly seen in the proximal part of the transformation zone which may be within the endocervical canal and, therefore, not always visible on colposcopy.

NICE GUIDELINE ON CERVICAL SCREENING

Screening Program

All women between the ages of 25 and 64 years are eligible for cervical screening

- *Age 25 years:* First invitation.
- *Age 25–49 years:* Screening every 3 years.
- *Age 50–64 years:* Screening every 5 years.

Women 65 years of age or older should be screened, if:

- They have not had a cervical screening test since 50 years of age.
- A recent cervical cytology sample is abnormal.
- Before recall ceases because of age, a woman who has had mild dyskaryosis or borderline change

should have had at least three negative cytology results.

Taking an LBC (Liquid Based Cytology) Sample

- *Unless the woman will not re-attend, a cervical sample is not taken in the following circumstances:*
  - During menstruation.
  - If the woman is less than 12 weeks post-natally.
  - If there is discharge or infection. Treat the infection and take the sample on another occasion.
  - If the woman is pregnant and she is up-to-date with routine cytology.

To take the sample:

- Fully visualize the cervix by using a speculum.
- Insert the central bristles of the Cervex-Brush into the endocervical canal so that the shorter outer bristles contact the ectocervix fully.
- Rotate the brush 360° five times in a clockwise direction using pencil pressure (the brush is designed to collect cells in clockwise direction only).
- Ayres spatula can also be used for ectocervix sampling.
- Samples should be fixed immediately.

An endocervical brush should be used in the following circumstances in conjunction with a Cervex-Brush:

- If it is difficult to insert the Cervex-Brush into the os.
- If the os is narrow or stenosed.
- If the woman is being followed up for previous borderline changes in endocervical cells or for a previously treated endocervical glandular abnormality.
- A previous sample was inadequate because of the absence of endocervical cells.

If using an endocervical brush:

- Take the EndoCervex-Brush sample after the Cervex-Brush sample.
- Insert the EndoCervex-Brush gently into the os, with the lower bristles remaining visible, and rotate clockwise through one whole turn.
- Fix both samples in the same vial.
- **Fix the sample immediately** before withdrawing the speculum.

I. *Thin preparation*

- Using a vigorous swirling motion, rinse the brush into the fixative vial.
- Push the brush into the bottom of the vial at least 10 times, forcing the bristles apart. It is important to use firm pressure to prevent the cells clinging to the brush.

- Inspect the brush for any residual material and remove any remaining by passing the brush over the edge of the fixative vial.
- If there is any material on the edge of the vial, give it a shake.
- Label the vial.

II. *SurePath*

- Alternately, remove the head of the brush from the stem and place into the vial of fixative.
- Screw the lid on and label the vial.

HPV testing

- Since high-risk HPV has been implicated in more than 90% of cervical cancers, testing for the virus has been proposed as a screening modality either alone or combined with Papanicolaou tests. Digene Hybrid Capture 2 High-Risk HPV DNA Test, which is used to identify the presence of 14 high-risk HPV types found in cervical samples. It helps to triage cytologic abnormalities with HPV infection and indicate need for closer follow-up.
- HPV testing increase the sensitivity of cytology screening; however, it has lower specificity and, consequently, a lower positive predictive value when used as a primary screening test. HPV does improve specificity in women older than age 30 years when it is used as part of triaging Papanicolaou test results of atypical squamous cells of undetermined significance (ASC-US).

CYTOLOGIC ABNORMALITIES

ASC-US and ASC-H Cells

- Atypical squamous cells (ASC), including those designated as being ASC-US or in the category "cannot exclude high grade" (ASC-H), are an epithelial abnormality diagnosed when the degree of nuclear atypia is not sufficient for the cells to be defined as a squamous intraepithelial lesion (SIL), either low grade or high grade. ASC-H includes atypia that is suggestive of high-grade changes.
- Three follow-up strategies have been deemed appropriate when a diagnosis of ASC-US is made. These include repeat cytology at 6 and 12 months, colposcopy, and HPV testing. ASC-US lesions regress at 24 months in almost 70% of cases, with less than 10% progressing to high-grade squamous intraepithelial lesions (HSILs) and less than 1% progressing to invasive cancer. However, lesions that show high-risk HPV positivity have a shorter time frame to progression and take longer to regress than those who do not demonstrate HPV positivity.

Because of these findings, reflex HPV testing in these patients is appropriate as part of triaging for additional follow-up care. ASC-H lesions should prompt immediate colposcopic examination.

Low-grade Squamous Intraepithelial Lesions

- Low-grade squamous intraepithelial lesions (LSILs), as defined by the Bethesda system, are suggestive of mild dysplasia or expected CIN-1 on histology. Approximately 50% of these lesions will regress in 24 months, 20% will progress to HSILs, and about 0.2% will progress to cancer in the same time period.
- Progression and regression of LSILs are also affected by HPV positivity. However, it has been shown that 70–80% of LSILs are associated with high-risk HPV types, so reflex HPV testing does not help with triaging these patients to colposcopic examination.

High-grade Squamous Intraepithelial Lesions (HSILs)

HSILs are lesions consistent with moderate and severe dysplasia, corresponding with CIN-2, CIN-3, and carcinoma in situ on histology. These lesions have a lower likelihood of regression within 24 months, with only 35% regressing, 23.4% persisting, and 1.4% progressing to invasive cancer. Although HPV positivity does affect the time to regression, 90% or more of these lesions will be positive for high-risk HPV, so there is little use in testing for HPV as part of advocating for follow-up care.

Atypical Glandular Cells

Atypical glandular cells (AGC) seen on cytologic specimens can be associated with squamous cell and glandular abnormalities, including adenocarcinoma of the cervix or the endometrium. According to the Bethesda classification, these abnormalities can be subdivided into lesions associated with cervical, endocervical, or endometrial atypia. For all of these subcategories, except endometrial cells, the ASCCP guidelines recommend colposcopy with endocervical sampling and HPV testing for all women, and endometrial testing, if the patient is 35 years or older or at risk for endometrial neoplasia.

Immunohistochemistry

- Use of p16 immunohistochemistry can serve as a surrogate for the differentiation of benign lesions from precancerous ones. A cyclin-dependent kinase-4 inhibitor, p16 is identified as a biomarker for HPV transforming infections.

- It has been found that the proportion of p16-positive smears rise with the increasing severity of cytologic and histologic abnormality.
- Because of the lack of standardization, no current clinical guidelines exist for the use of p16 in primary cervical cancer screening or in the triage of low-grade Papanicolaou smears.

Frequency of Screening (NHS Cancer Screening Program)

Screening Intervals

The age and frequency of screening are as follows:

Age group (year)	Frequency of screening
25	First invitation
25–49	Three yearly
50–64	Five yearly
65+	Only screen those who have not been screened since age 50 or who have had recent abnormal tests

Age at Starting Screening

Recently published research and experience from the cervical screening program have shown that screening women under the age of 25 may do more harm than good. Cervical cancer is very rare in women under 25.

Age at Finishing Screening

Routine screening ends at the age of 65 years. Although it may possibly be safe to withdraw well screened women with three consecutive negative cervical samples from the screening programme at age 50 years, there is at present insufficient robust evidence to warrant this.

Unscheduled Cervical Screening

Additional cervical screening is not justified in any of the following situations, provided the woman is in the age group to be screened and has undergone screening within the previous three to five years:

- On an oral contraceptive
- With an IUCD in situ
- On hormone replacement therapy (HRT)
- In pregnancy—either antenatal or postnatal, or after termination unless a previous screening test was abnormal
- In women with genital warts
- In women with vaginal discharge
- In women with pelvic infection
- In women who have had multiple sexual partners
- In women who are heavy cigarette smokers.

Colposcopy (Fig. 19.1)

Colposcopy was pioneered in Germany by Dr. Hinselmann in 1920. He proved that microscopic examination of the cervix will detect cervical cancer in preinvasive stage. His work identified several atypical appearances which is still used today like: (a) leukoplakia, (b) punctation, (c) mosaicism, etc. The colposcopic examination serves to:

1. Identify normal landmarks
2. Identify abnormal areas in relation to these landmarks
3. Facilitate directed biopsy of abnormal areas for histologic diagnosis
4. Rule out invasive cancer

SQUAMOUS METAPLASIA

This is physiological replacement of the columnar epithelium with squamous epithelium. The region where this occurs is known as the Transormation zone (Fig. 19.2). This is important because almost all cervical cancers occur in this zone. Figure 19.3 depicts the schemetic diagramme of normal colposcopy (Fig. 19.4).

Indications of Colposcopy

- Suspicious visible lesion or palpable lesion of the cervix, vagina, vulva, perineum or perianal area.

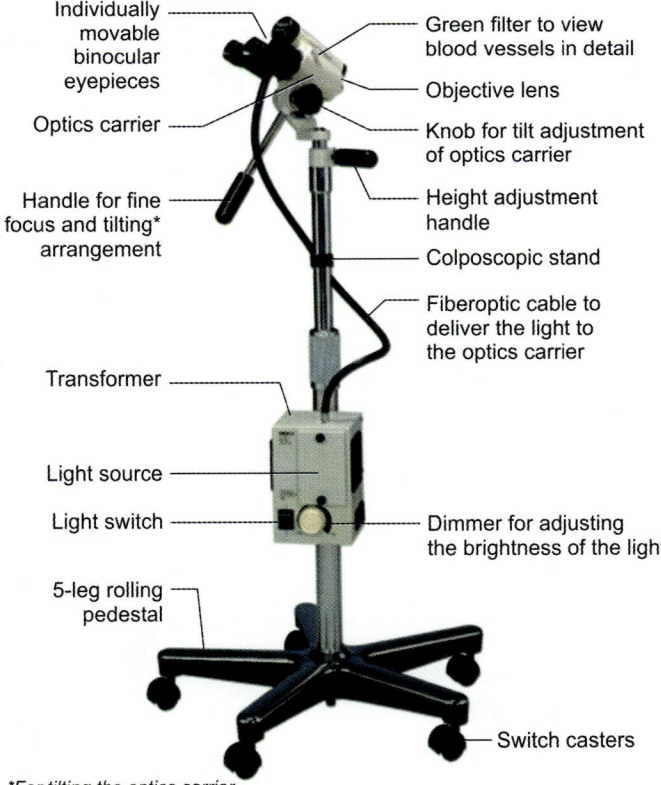

*For tilting the optics carrier

Fig. 19.1: Colposcope instrument

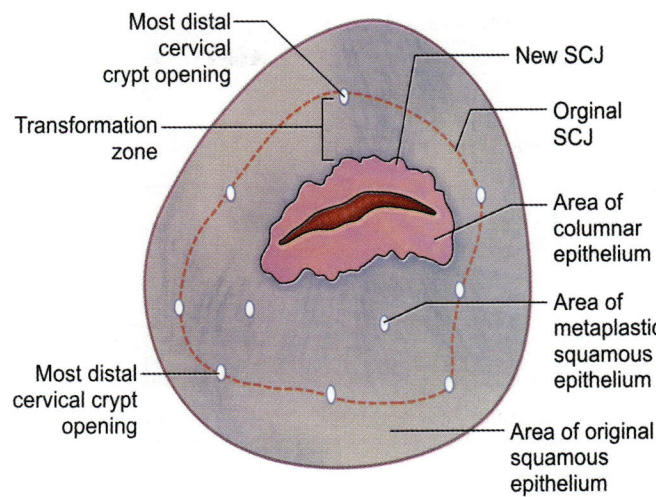

Fig. 19.2: A method of identifying outer and inner borders of the transformation zone (SCJ: Squamocolumnar junction)

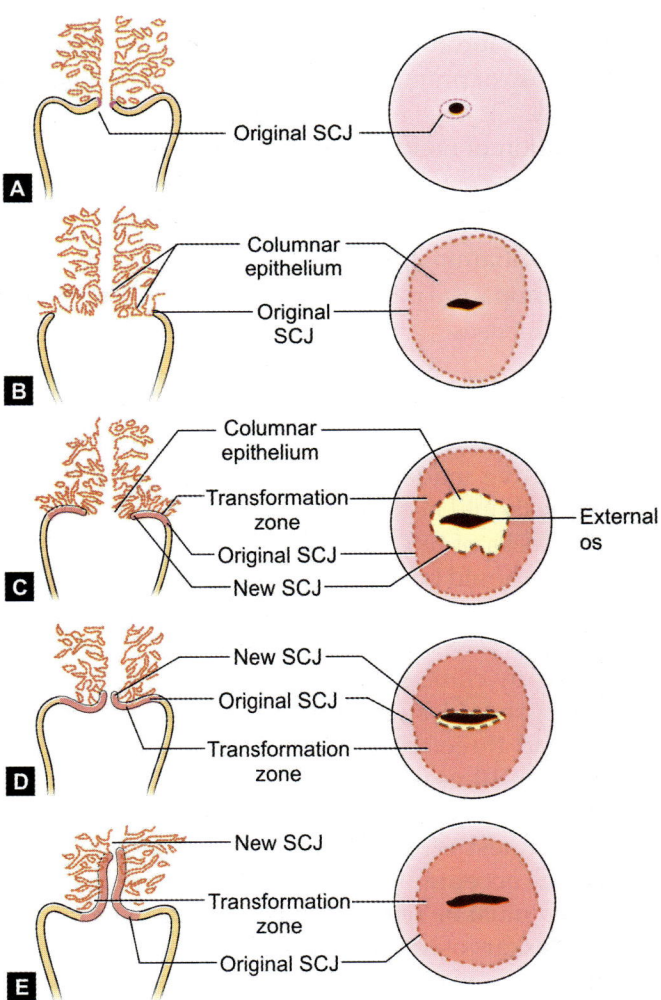

Fig. 19.3: Location of the squamocolumnar junction (SCJ) and transformation zone: (A) before menarche; (B) after puberty and at early reproductive age; (C) in a woman in her 30s; (D) in a perimenopausal woman; (E) in a postmenopausal woman

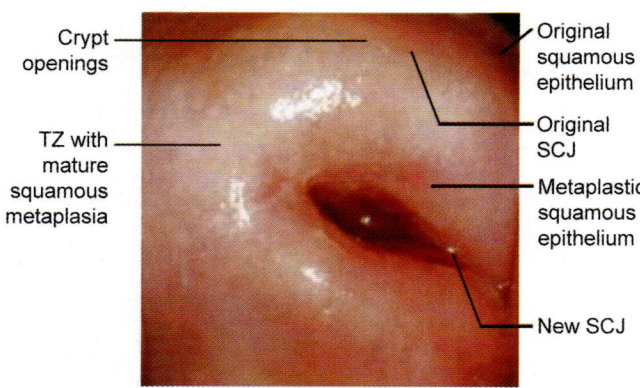

Fig. 19.4: The entire new squamocolumnar junction (SCJ) visible and hence the colposcopic examination is satisfactory; the transformation zone (TZ) is fully visualized. The metaplastic squamous epithelium is pinkish white compared to the pink original squamous epithelium

- Pap smear consistent with dysplasia or cancer.
- Pap smear with evidence of HPV infection (high-risk types).
- History of intrauterine DES exposure.
- Follow-up of previously treated patients or high-risk patients.
- Evaluation of child abuse or rape cases.

Contraindications

- Active, inflammatory cervicitis
- Postmenopausal patient who is not estrogen-primed
- Heavy menses

Guidelines for Colposcopy Referral

1. Women should be referred for colposcopy after three consecutive inadequate samples. At least 90% of women should be seen in a colposcopy clinic within eight weeks of referral.
2. Women should be referred for colposcopy after three tests reported as borderline nuclear change in squamous cells or endocervical cells to be seen in a colposcopy clinic within eight weeks of referral.
3. Women should be referred for colposcopy, if they have had three tests reported as abnormal at any grade in a 10-year period
4. Ideally, women should be referred for colposcopy after one test reported as mild dyskaryosis, but it remains acceptable to recommend a repeat test. Women must be referred after two tests reported as mild dyskaryosis to be seen by colposcopy within eight weeks of referral.
5. Women must be referred for colposcopy after one test reported as moderate and severe dyskaryosis (100%). They should be seen within four weeks of referral (90%).

6. Women must be referred for colposcopy after one test reported as possible invasion or glandular neoplasia (100%). They should be seen urgently within two weeks of referral (90%).

Steps in Colposcopy Examination

- Explain the procedure and obtain informed consent
- Obtain a relevant medical history
- Exclude pregnancy
- Perform bimanual examination, if not already done
- Examine vulva
- Insert sterile speculum
- Examine cervix using low power (inflammation, infection, leukoplakia, punctation, mosaicism, abnormal vessels)
- Obtain KOH/WP, (wet prepared), cultures and/or pap, if needed
- Use green filter and normal saline
- Apply 5% acetic acid. Wait for two minutes.
- Scan entire cervix with white light. Start with low power and move to higher magnification to document abnormal vascular patterns.
- Use endocervical speculum, if needed to view entire transformation zone (Fig. 19.5).
- The *entire TZ, including SCJ*, and borders of all lesions must be visualized in order for colposcopy to be satisfactory (Fig. 19.6).
- Apply Lugol's iodine solution to aid in delineating potential biopsy site (Fig. 19.7).

Perform endocervical curettage, if indicated (Figs 19.8 and 19.9)
- Glandular lesion
- Unsatisfactory colposcopy
- Normal colpoposcopy of ectocervix, yet abnormal cytology
- Contraindicated in pregnancy or active cervicitis

Assess abnormal areas when lesion is:
- Mild acetowhite or intensely acetowhite
- Irregular blood vessel pattern or punctation or mosaicism

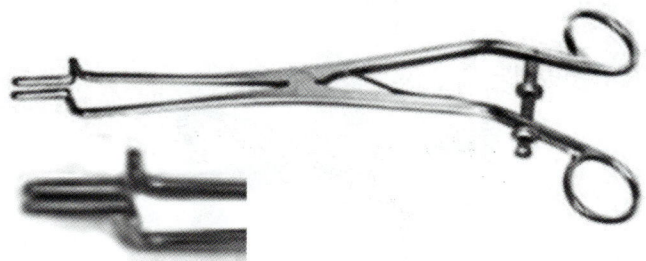

Fig. 19.5: Endocervical speculum

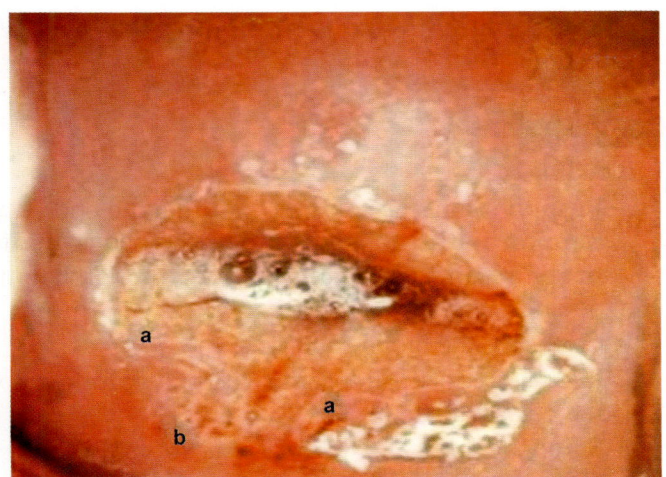

Fig. 19.6: The prominent white line corresponds to the ne w squamocolumnar junction and tongues of imm ature squamous metaplasia (a) with crypt opening at 4–8 o' clock positions (b) (after application of 5% acetic acid)

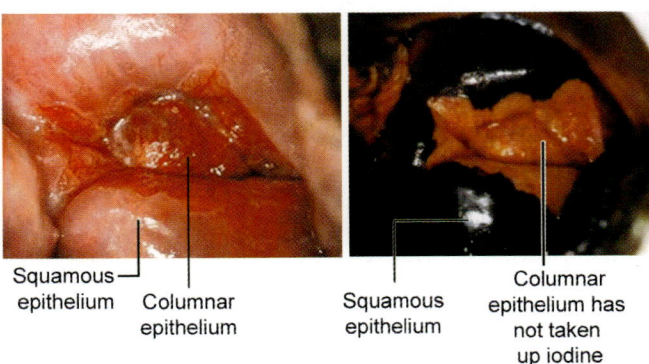

Squamous epithelium   Columnar epithelium   Squamous epithelium   Columnar epithelium has not taken up iodine

Fig. 19.7: Color changes after application of Lugol's iodine

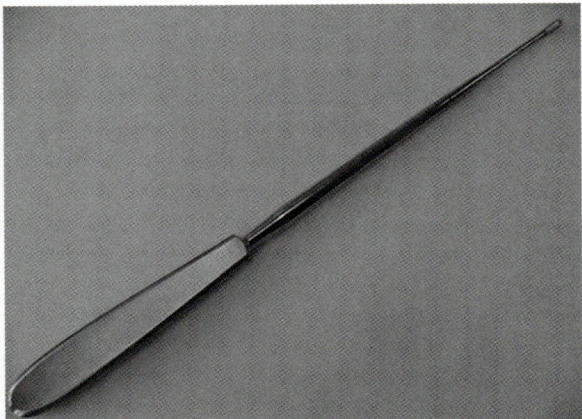

Fig. 19.8: Endocervical curette

- Diffuse vague borders or sharply demarcated borders
- Follows normal contours of the cervix or "humped up"

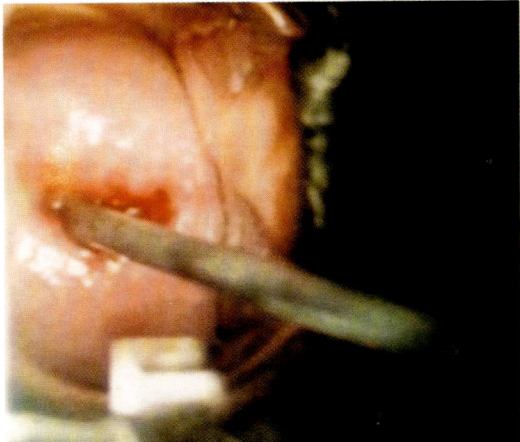

Fig. 19.9: Endocervical curettage used

- With leukoplakia
- Showing atypical vessels
- Normal iodine reaction (dark) or iodine-negative epithelium (yellow)

Perform cervical biopsies, if required (Figs 19.10 and 19.11)

- Biopsy posterior areas first.
- A depth of 3 mm is adequate.
- Biopsy area of the lesion with worst features and closest to SCJ, including the area with atypical vessels
- Apply pressure and Monsel's paste to bleeding sites after biopsy.
- Remove speculum and inspect vaginal walls, vulva, perineum, and perianal areas.

Post-procedure Instructions

- No douching, intercourse, or tampons until spotting subsides.
- Return for foul odor or discharge, pelvic pain, profuse bleeding or fever.

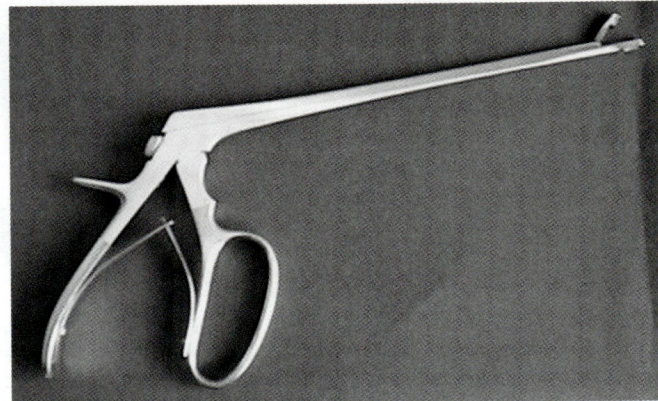

Fig. 19.10: Cervical punch biopsy forceps with sharp, cutting edges

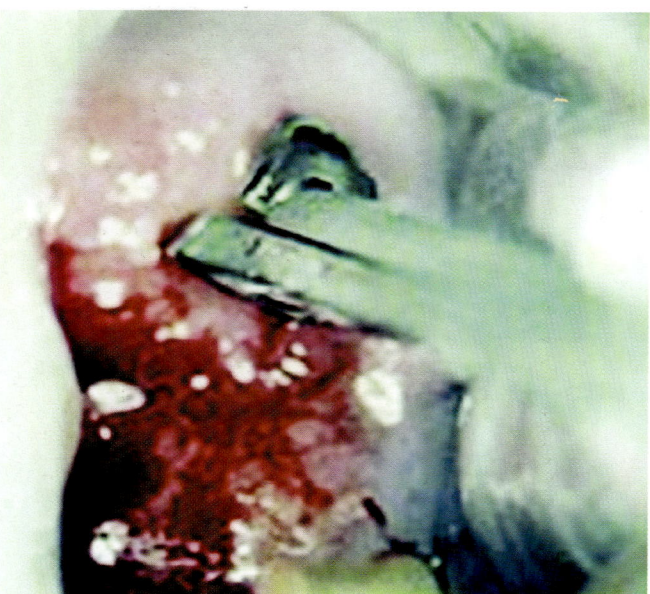

Fig. 19.11: Biopsy procedure

- Follow-up is usually 1–3 weeks to discuss histology results and definitive therapy.
- Encourage contraception once definitive therapy completed.
- Re-emphasize the relationship of cervical dysplasia with STDs, smoking, and non-monogamous sexual practices.

- Counsel patients about life-long risks of HPV infection.

Complications

- Bleeding
  - Reapply Monsel's solution. Saturate the end of a tampon with Monsel's and insert to provide pressure and astringent action for persistent oozing.
  - Cauterize the biopsy site.
  - Inject 1–2 cc of 2% lidocaine with epinephrine into the bleeding site.
  - Rarely, a cervical stitch of 4-0 absorbable suture across a deep biopsy site.
- Infection is rare but typically occurs on the 3rd or 4th day after biopsy.
- Avoid biopsy with active cervicitis.

Normal colposcopic findings will show the following (Fig. 19.12):
1. Original squamous epithelium
2. Columnar epithelium
3. Squamocolumnar junction
4. Squamous metaplasia
5. Transformation zone

Table 19.2 shows correlation of abnormal colposcopy findings with cervical dysplasia.

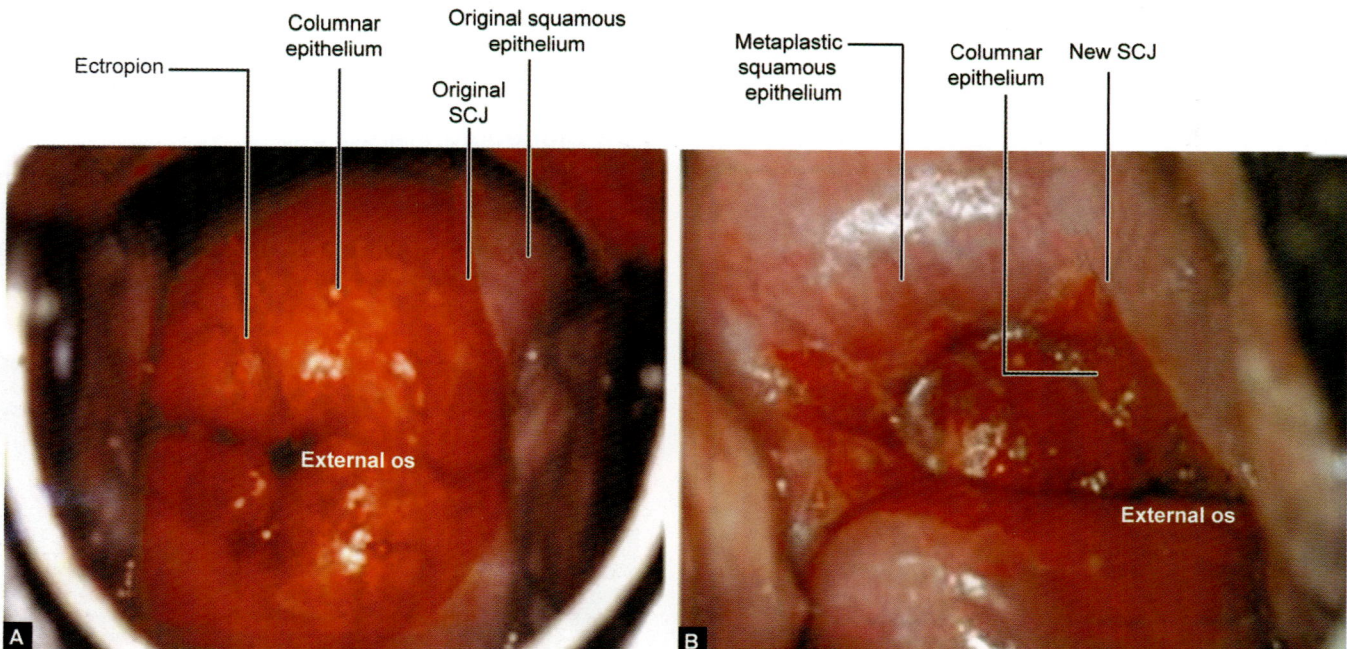

Fig. 19.12A and B: Normal colposcopic pictures: (A) Original squamocolumnar junction (SCJ) early reproductive age group. The SCJ is located far away from the external os. Note the presence of everted columnar epithelium occupying a large portion of the ectocervix producing ectropion. (B) The new SCJ has moved much closer to the external os in a woman in her 30s. The SCJ is visible as a distinct white line after the application of 5% acetic acid, due to the presence of immature squamous metaplastic epithelium adjacent to the new SCJ

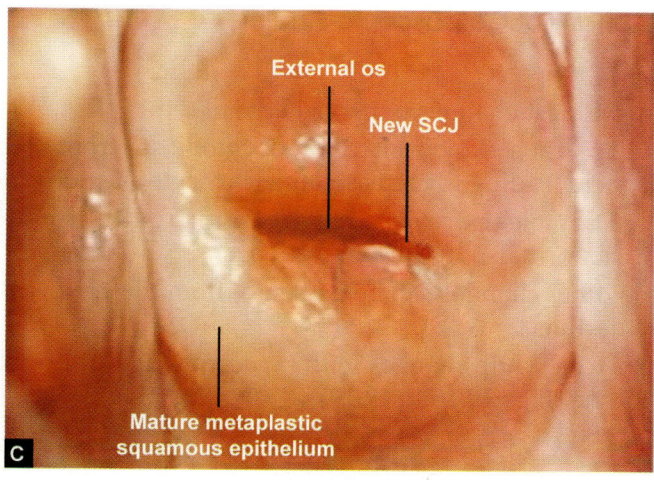

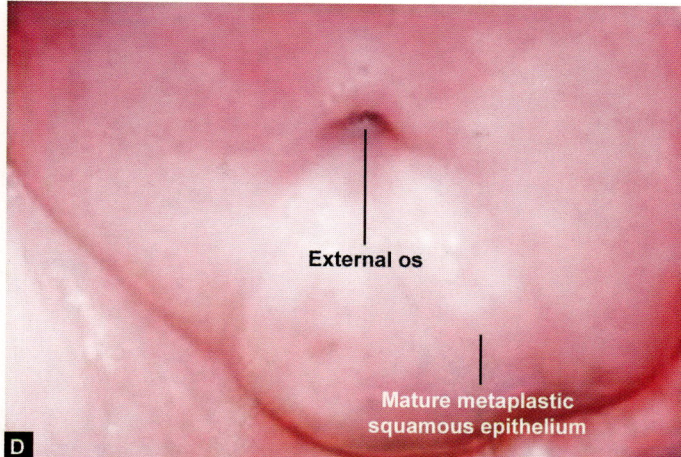

Fig. 19.12C and D: Location of squamocolumnar junction (SCJ). (C) The new SCJ is at the external os in a perimenopausal woman. (D) The new SCJ is not visible and has receded into the endocervix in a postmenopausal woman. Mature metaplastic squamous epithelium occupies most of the ectocervix

Table 19.2: Colposcopic correlation with dysplasia	
Mild dysplasia	*Severe dysplasia*
Acetowhite changes	Dull pearly grey epithelium
Bright white; clear demarcation between normal and abnormal epithelium	Indistinct demarcation between abnormal and normal epithelium
Fine punctation	Coarse punctations
	Mosaicism
	Abnormal vessels

Visual Inspection with Acetic Acid (VIA)

In the naked eye examination after 3% acetic acid is applied in the cervix, it works as a desiccant and the cellular cytoplasm is reduced enhancing a prominent nucleus which is enlarged secondary to HPV replication. This nuclear enlargement is seen as acetowhite changes (Fig. 19.13A to D).

VILI

The cervix is stained with Lugol's iodine solution which works by staining glycogen. The dysplastic tissue has an increased metabolic rate thereby lowering cellular glycogen. Normal tissue stains black/brown while dysplastic tissue appears highlighted or yellow (Fig. 19.14).

Adequacy of Colposcopy

1. Must evaluate the entrety of the lesion—upper border into the endocervix.
2. Must evaluate the entirety of the SCJ.

Normal Colposcopy

Figures 19.15A to D show normal colposcopy.

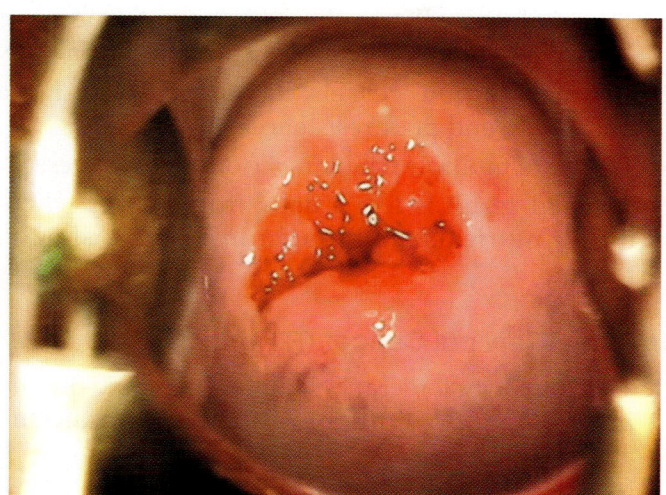

Fig. 19.13A: Before acetic acid

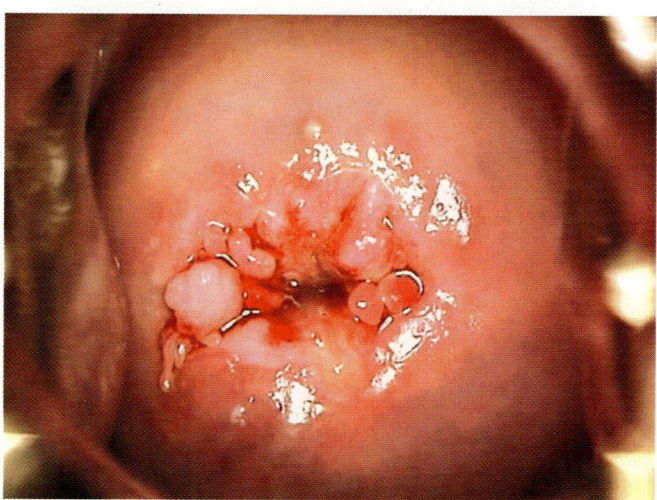

Fig. 19.13B: After 30 seconds of acetic acid

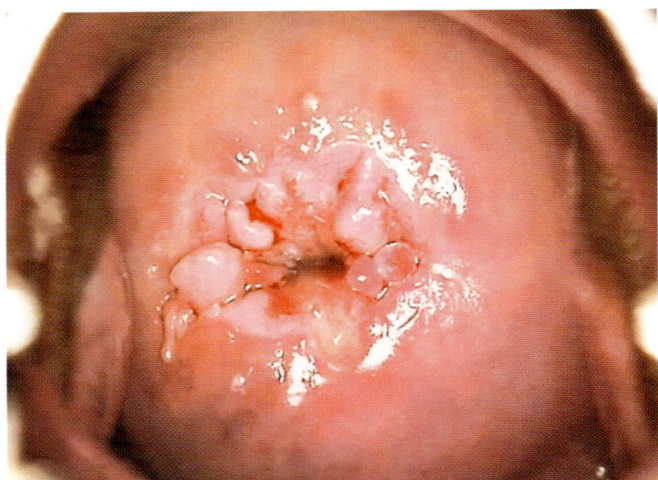

Fig. 19.13C: At 1 min of acetic acid

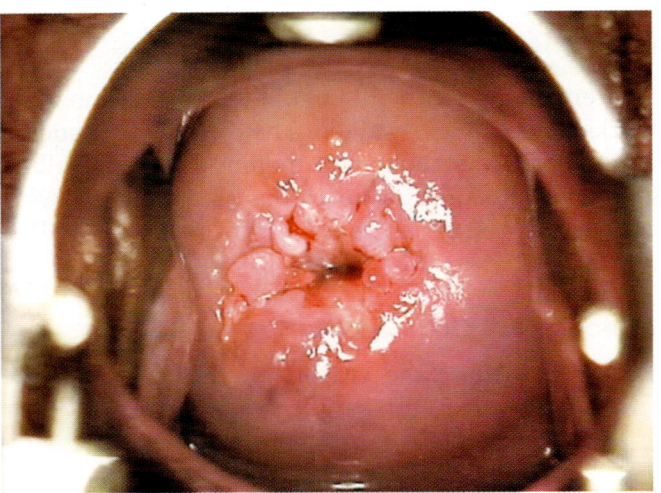

Fig. 19.13D: At 2 min of acetic acid

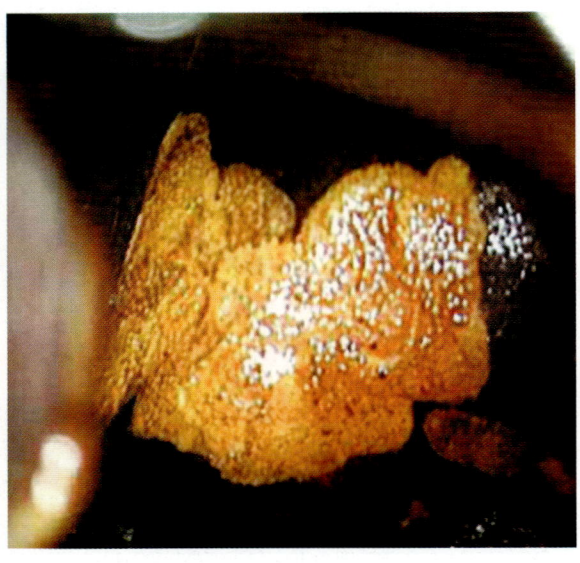

Fig. 19.14: Stain with Lugol's iodine in normal cervix

Abnormal Colposcopic Finding

I. *Acetowhite Changes*

a. Mildest changes of cervical dysplasia.

b. It is caused by desiccation of cytoplasm from acetic acid leading to increased nuclear/cytoplasmic ratio.

c. Very clear area of demarcation from normal to abnormal.

d. Other changes can be present within the acetowhite lesions.

   Acetowhite changes with (a) acetic acid, (b) Lugol's iodine (Figs 19.16 to 19.19).

II. *Punctations* (Fig. 19.20)

1. These are vessels that run perpendicular to the portion of the cervix.

2. They are seen end-to-end to the colposcopist.

3. The green filter removes red light, thus vessels are darkened.

4. Punctation can be small vessels (fine punctation) or large vessels (coarse punctation).

III. *Mosaicism* (Fig. 19.21)

1. A mosaic is a large image pieced together by smaller colorful tiles.

2. The lesion is made of small heaped epithelial islands and tiny vessels.

3. These islands look like a cobblestone road.

4. Islands are separated by vessels running parallel to the portio.

Abnormal Vessels (Fig. 19.22)

1. Angiogenesis is one key change that occur in progression of lesion to invasive cervical cancer.

2. The evolving cells in the cancerous tissue need oxygen and nutrients to grow at an exponential rate.

3. The new blood vessels have low flow, little pulsativity and poor resistance.

4. There are multiple tributaries from any one vessel.

5. The end result is like a delta from a river where lots of nutrients are brought in blood is slow to return.

Invasive Cervical Cancer (Fig. 19.23)

1. There are conglomeration of all colposcopic finding including acetowhite, punctuations, mosaicism, abnormal vessels.

2. Necrotic tissue resulting in anaerobic odors.

3. Lesion bleeding to touch.

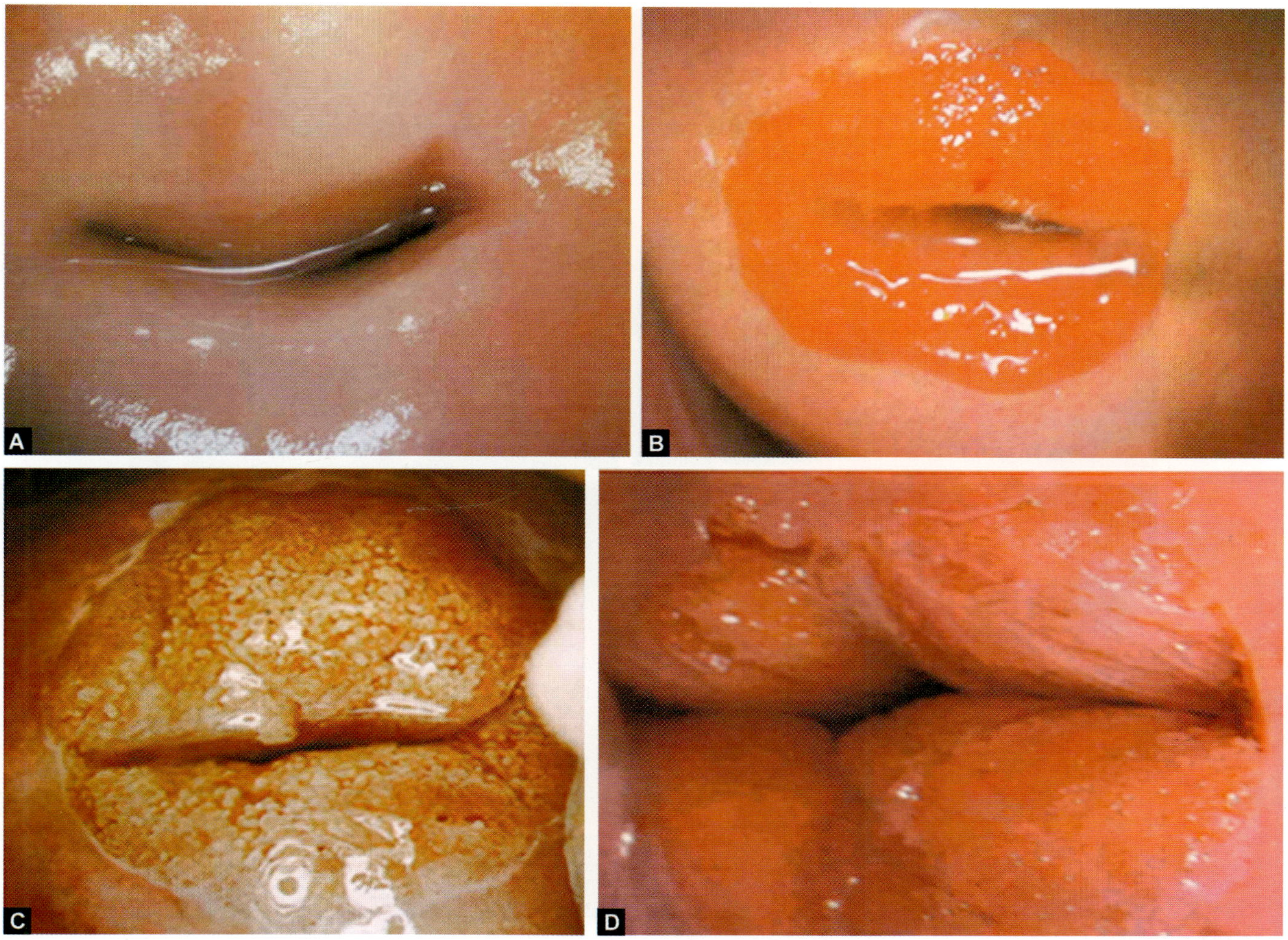

Fig. 19.15: Normal colposcopy

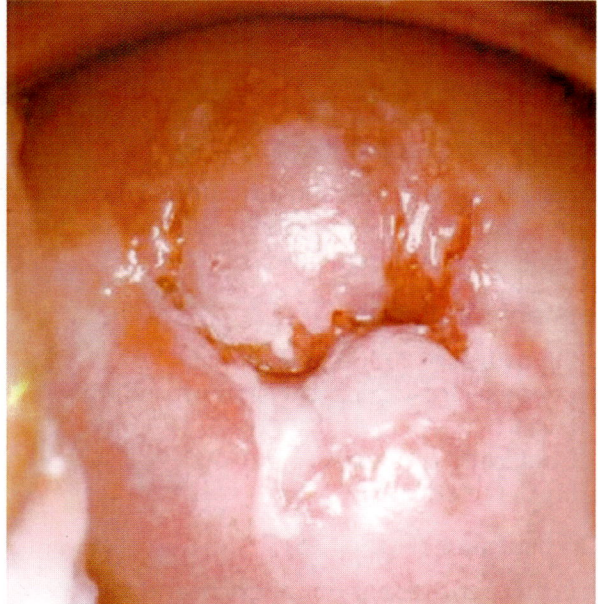

Fig. 19.16: Moderately dense acetowhite lesions with irregular margins in the anterior and posterior lips (CIN 1)

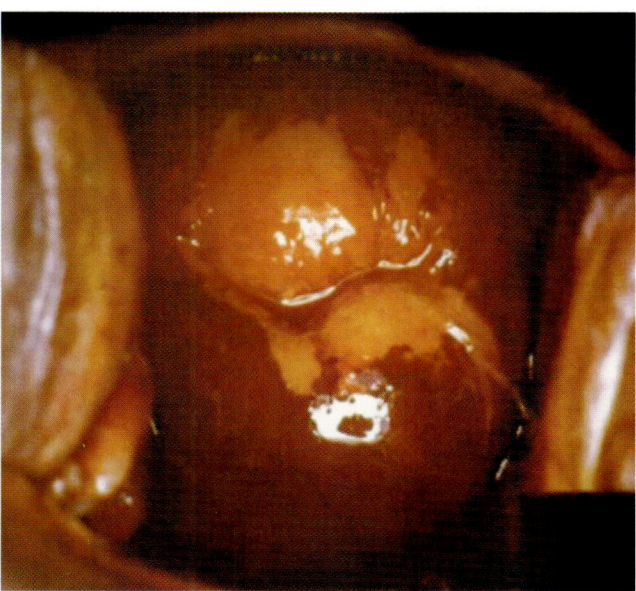

Fig. 19.17: A CIN 1 lesion with a mustard yellow iodine-nagative area with irregular margins (see the appearance after acetic acid application in Fig. 19.16)

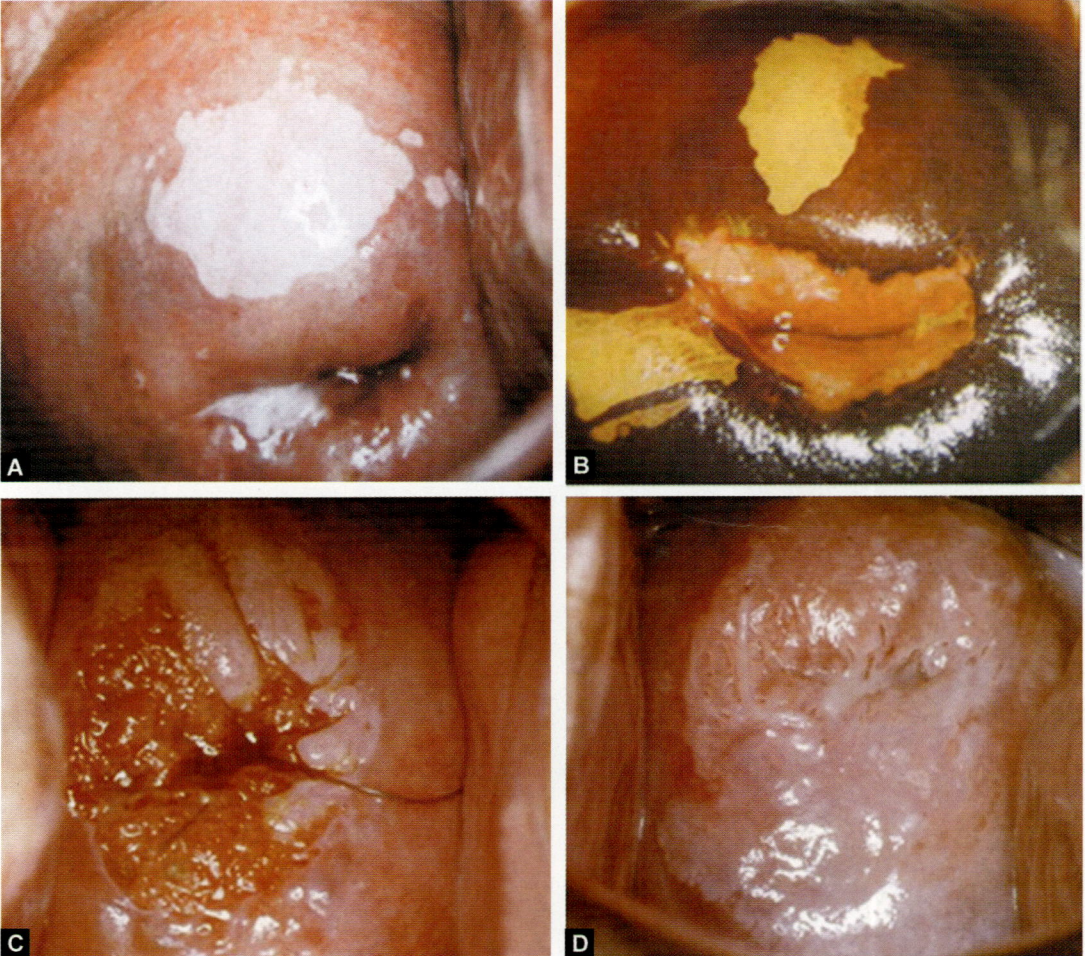

Fig. 19.18A to D: (A) Moderately dense acetowhite lesion in anterior lip; (B) Acetowhite lesion—iodine negative area; (C) Moderately dense acetowhite lesions with well-defined margins and coarse punctations in the anterior lip and in 3 o'clock position (CIN 2 lesion); (D) Note the intensely dense, complex, acetowhite lesion (CIN 3 lesion) with raised and rolled out margins, obliterating the external os

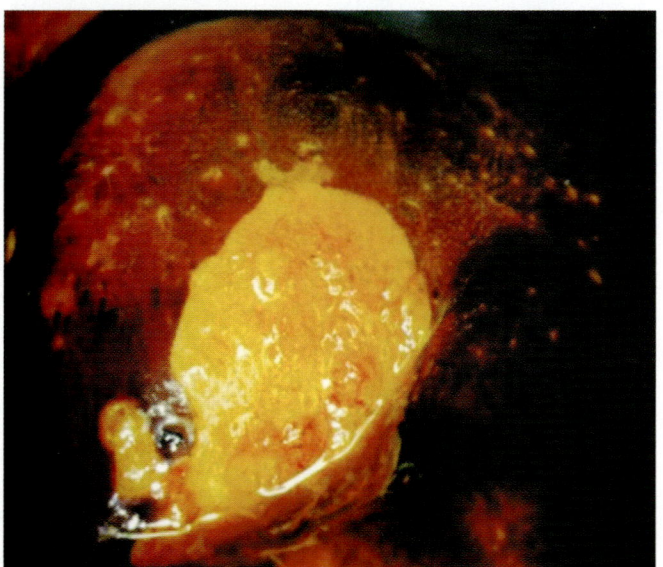

Fig. 19.19: A dense mustard yellow iodine-negative area in the upper lip suggestive of CIN 3 lesion

Glandular Lesions (Adenocarcinoma in Situ/Adenocarcinoma)

Figures 19.24A and B are showing gandular lesions.

Unusual Colposcopic Finging

Figures 19.25A to C are showing unusual colposcopic findings. Table 19.3 shows Reid colposcopic index to identify CIN of different grades.

Treatment Modality

   i. Cryosurgery
  ii. Loop electrosurgical excision procedure
 iii. Laser
 iv. Cold knife conization
  v. Hysterectomy

I. Cryosurgery (Fig. 19.26)

1. It is inexpensive, easy to perform and tolerated well by patients.
2. Cells are destroyed by cold thermal damage.

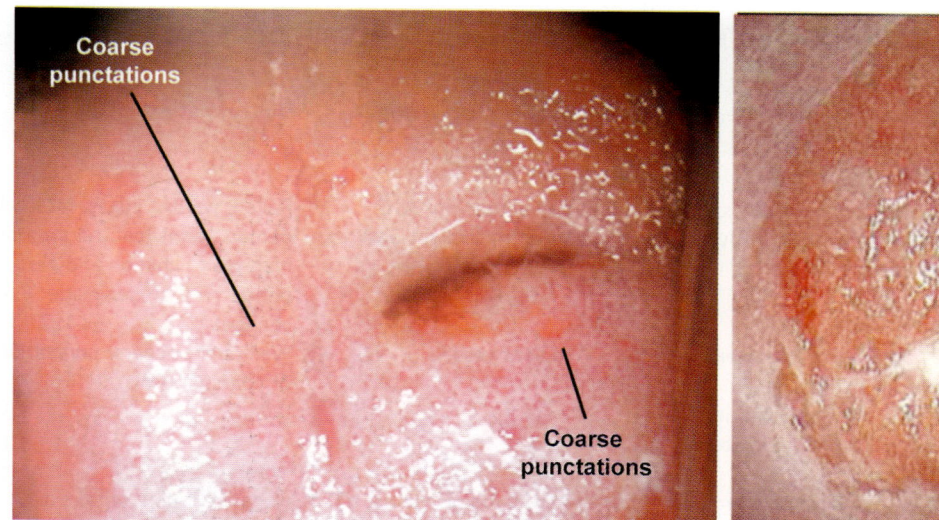
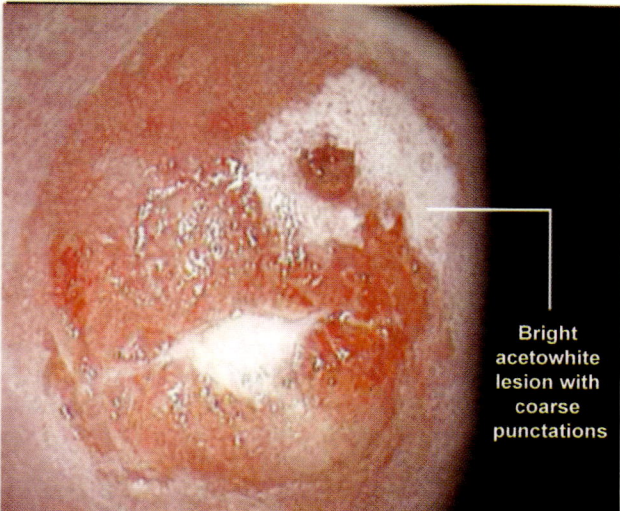

Fig. 19.20: Punctations

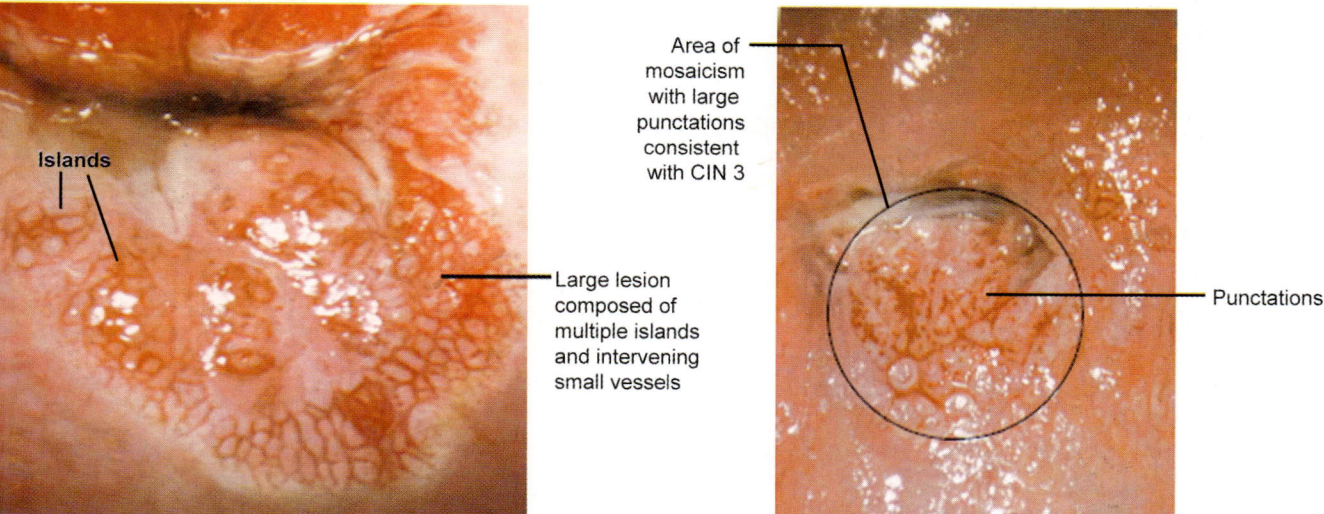

Fig. 19.21: Mosaicism

3. Freeze is done for 3 minutes followed by 1 minute thaw and again 3 minute freeze.
4. It may cause malodorus discharge for 2–3 weeks.
5. It hinders repeat colposcopy and often obscure SCJ.

Advantages of Cryosurgical Treatment

Cryosurgery is a recognised treatment procedure using low temperatures to destroy lesions. This allows freezing of tissue on a measured area and depth.

Properly carried out freezing is painless, and leaves no scars after healing. A procedure including two time freezing lasts about 15 minutes. After a few weeks of healing, there are no signs of lesions.

- Cryosurgical procedures are smokeless, in contrast to photocoagulation, electrocoagulation and laser vaporization. Extremely high temperatures produce smoke containing biological material, and unpleasant odor. It leads to contamination of the treatment field area. The smoke often contains virus genomes, e.g. HPV, which create danger of iatrogenous infection of air passages of people staying nearby. Cryosurgery procedures do not cause contamination of the room with vaporized tissue and smoke, so there is no risk of HPV infection.

- Contrary to other methods, the zone of tissue necrosis does not increase on the second day after the treatment. It is exactly as intended, and consistent with the borders of the frozen area. In case of coagulation methods, burn tissue demarcates deeper than can be seen during the procedure (Laser, LOOP).

Table 19.3: Modified Reid colposcopic index

Feature	0 points	1 points	2 points
Color of acetowhite (AW) area	Low-intensity acetowhitening; snow-white, shiny AW; indistinct AW; transparent AW; AW beyond the transformation zone	Grey-white AW with shiny surface	Dull, oyster-wihite; grey
AW lesion margin and surface configuration	Feathered margins; angular, jagged lesions; flat lesions with indistinct margins; microcondylom-atous or micropapillary surface	Regular lesions with smooth, straight outlines	Rolled, peeling edges; internal demarcations (central area of high-grade change and peri-pheral area of low-grade change)
Vessels	Fine/uniform vessels; poorly formed patterns of fine punctations and/or fine mosaic; vessels beyond the margin of transformation zone; fine vessels within microcondylomatous or micropapillary lesions	Absent vessels	Well-defined coarse punctation or coarse mosaic
Iodine staining	Positive iodine uptake giving mahogany brown color; negative uptake of lesions scoring 3 points or less on above three categories	Partial iodine uptake by a lesion scoring 4 or more points on above three categories—variegated, speckled appearance	Negative iodine uptake a lesion scoring 4 or more points on the above three criteria

Scoring: A score of 0 to 2 points = Likely to be CIN 1; 3–4 points = Overlapping lesion: likely to be CIN 1–2; 5 to 8 points = Likely to be CIN 2–3 lesions

Example of Normal Vessels

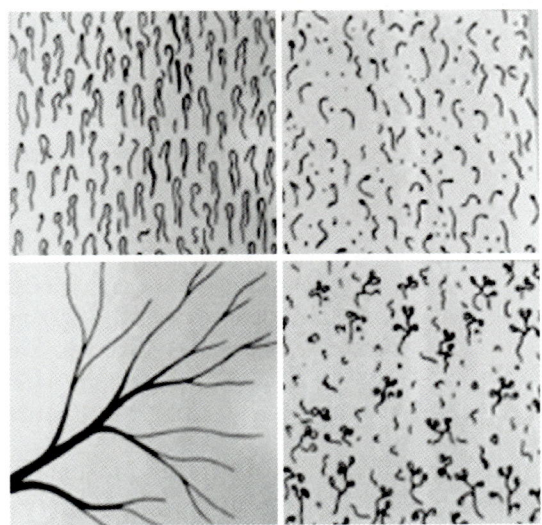

Fig. 19.22A: Fine vessels regular pattern

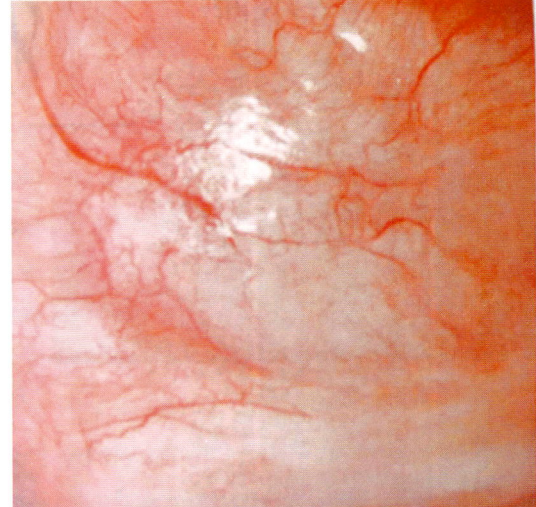

Fig. 19.22B: Normal branching

Abnormal vessels

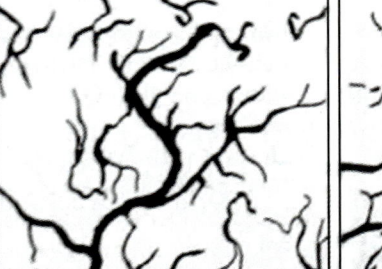

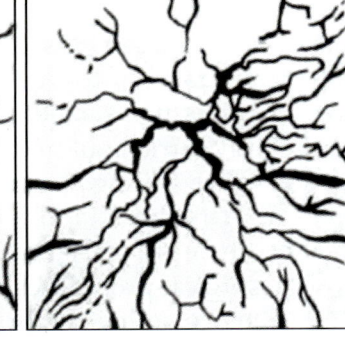

Fig. 19.22C: Prominent vessels   **Fig. 19.22D:** Coarse branching

- Cryosugical treatment of cervix pathologies is not associated with the risk of endometriosis. The frozen area remains covered with epithelium, which plays the role of a biological dressing.
- Treatment procedures are clean. The cryoprobes are autoclavable. A wide variety of cryoprobes allows for treatments of any section of genital ducts, e.g. in the cervix, which is very difficult, if not impossible with the use of photocoagulation or laser.
- Cryosurgical treatment is inexpensive and effective.

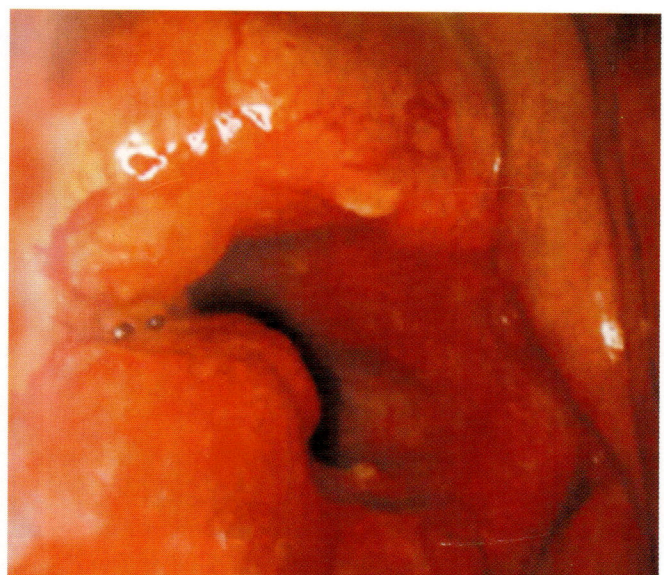

Fig. 19.22E: Coarse vessels

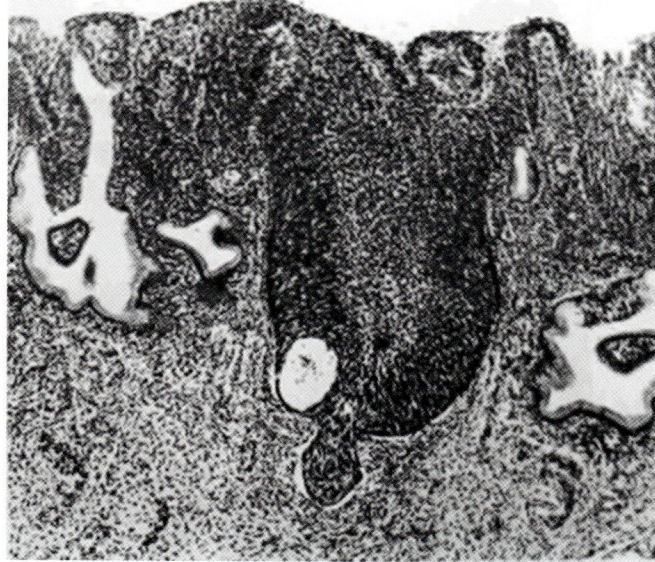

Fig. 19.23B: Invasive cells invading deep

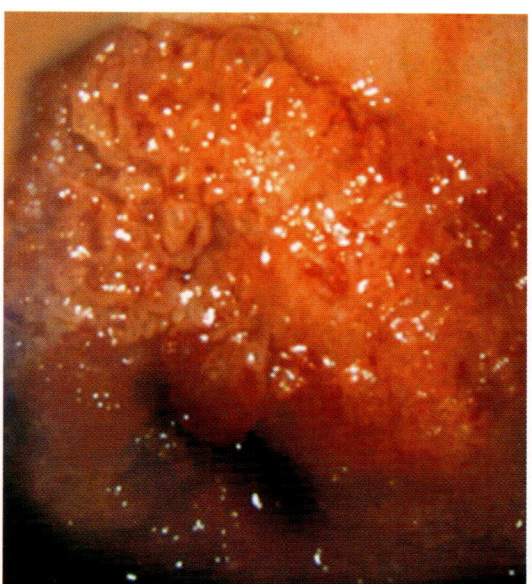

Fig. 19.23A: Coarse pattern of lesions

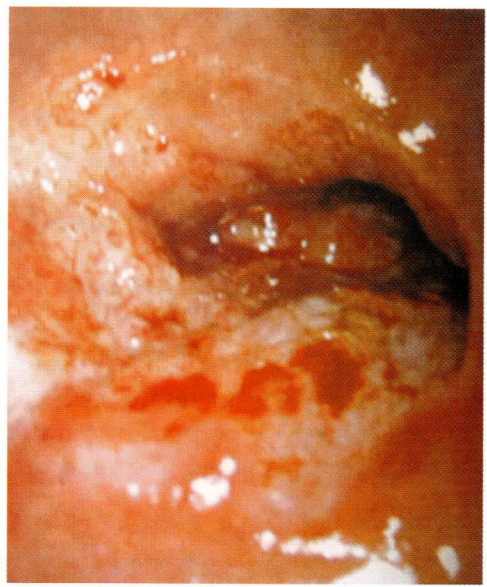

Fig. 19.23C: Prominent growth bleeding to touch

Procedure

Select the appropriate type of probe suitable to the shape and location of the lesion. Touch the affected place with probe, and activate the device pressing the pedal. The probe adheres to the tissue lowering its temperature. During about 2 minutes, a margin of frozen tissue is created. It is advisable to achieve freezing depth of 3–4 millimeters. Upon releasing the footswitch, the probe warms up in just 5 seconds. Gently remove the probe from the frozen area. Wait for self-thawing of tissue, and then repeat the procedure. Double freezing gives better therapeutic results. The entire procedure lasts up to 15 minutes.

Healing (Fig. 19.27)

Healing takes a few weeks. The site of freezing remains covered with dead epithelium, which plays the role of natural dressing, and then peels off. After the treatment, patient experiences metrorrhea-effusion from among frozen epithelium cells. However, it is advisable to maintain high personal hygiene. Sexual intercourse during the healing period is inadmissible.

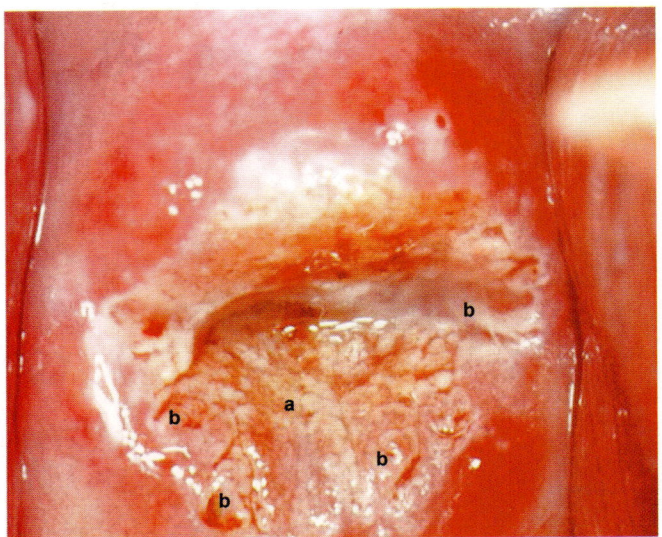

Fig. 19.24A: Adenocarcionoma in situ: Note the elevated lesions with an irregular acetowhite surface, enlarged and hypertrophied villi, papillary patterns (a), and atypical vessels (b), overlying the columnar epithelium

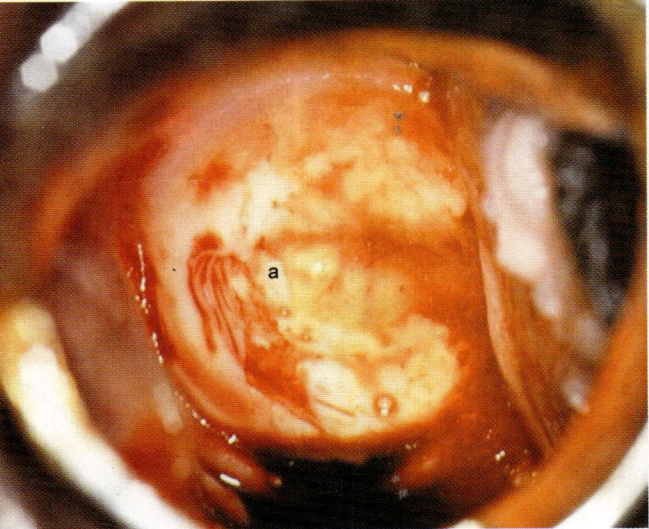

Fig. 19.24B: Adenocarcinoma: Note the greyish white dense acetowhite lesion with character writing-like atypical blood vessels (a)

Outcome

The final result is fully satisfactory. The physiological regeneration of tissue does not leave scars. The sore place becomes healthy, fully elastic. For this reason cryosurgery is permitted in nulligravida.

II. Conization of the Cervix by the Loop Electrical Excision Procedure (LEEP)

The indications for conization of the cervix are:

1. When the limits of the lesion in the cervix cannot be completely defined by colposcopy and directed biopsy, or the lesion is noted to extend up into the cervical canal and, therefore, is inaccessible to histologic examination by direct biopsy.

2. When there is severe cervical intraepithelial neoplasia (CIN) or carcinoma in situ in a young patient for whom a hysterectomy is contraindicated because of age and desire for fertility; and

3. When there is a failure of agreement between cytology, colposcopy, and histology. The purpose of conization of the cervix by the LEEP is to remove a cone-shaped piece of cervical tissue that will encompass the squamocolumnar junction. The procedure can be diagnostic as well as therapeutic.

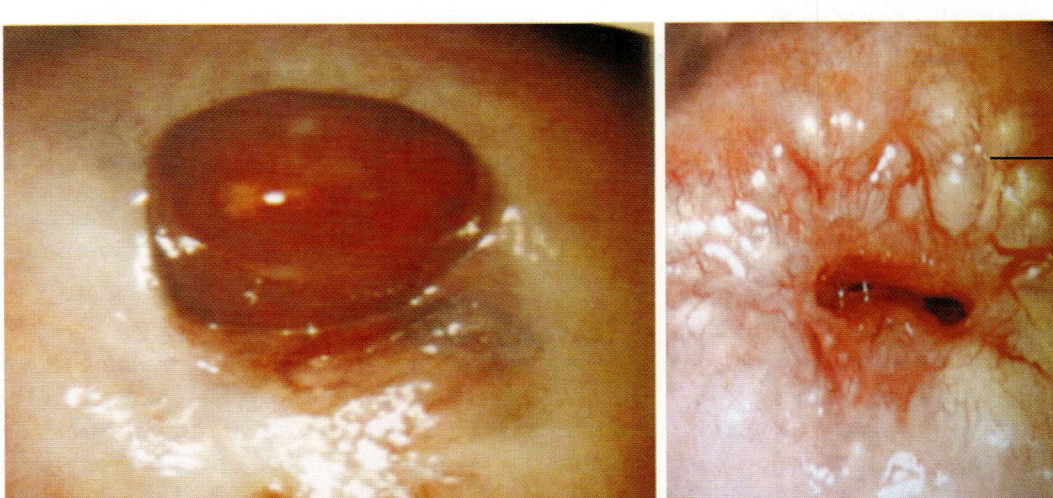

Prominent vessels of normal caliber surrounding multiple nabothian cysts

Fig. 19.25: (A) Polpy; (B) Nabothian cysts

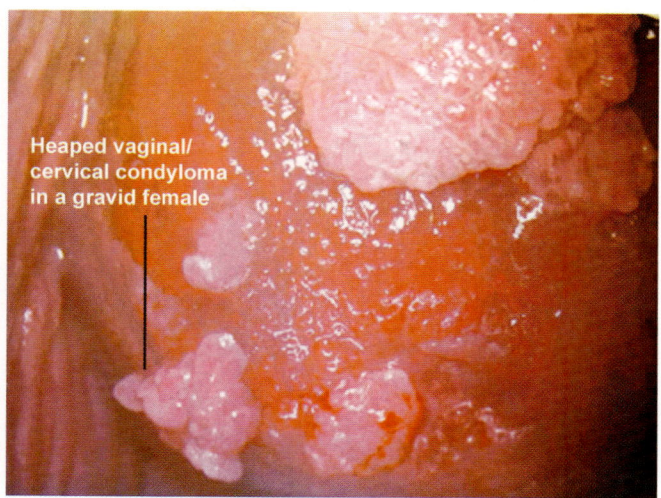

Heaped vaginal/
cervical condyloma
in a gravid female

Fig. 19.25C: Condyloma

Physiologic Changes

This operation removes the endocervical glands and in some patients has been associated with infertility because it reduces the production of cervical mucus. In addition, it may weaken the internal os of the cervix and, therefore, can be associated with second-trimester abortion.

Points of Caution

The surgical specimen should be adequate to provide an accurate diagnosis and remove the entire lesion. Hemostasis after conization is essential. These patients should be informed that there may be a small incidence of persistent cervical intraepithelial neoplasia following conization by the LEEP. Therefore, follow-up cytology and colposcopy are essential to this form of therapy.

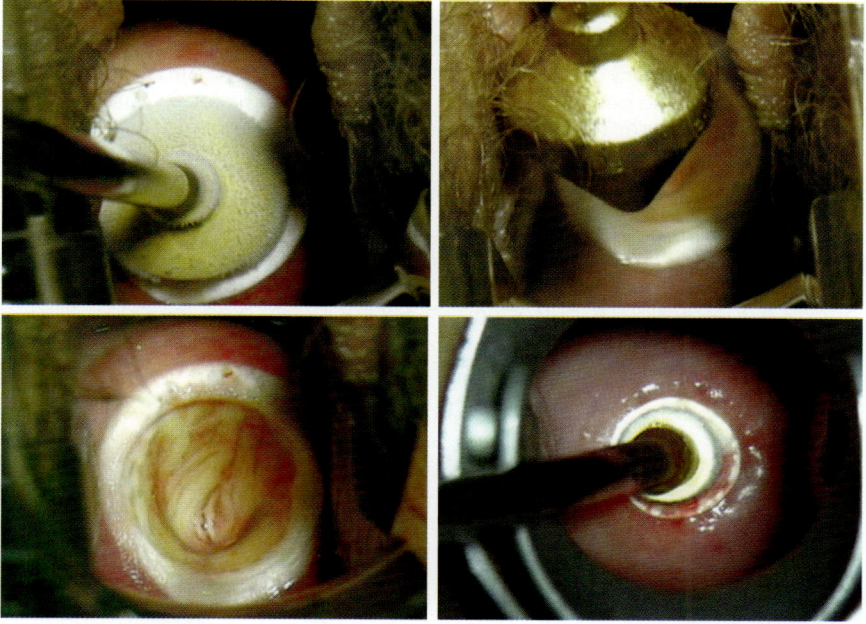

Fig. 19.26: Cryo probe used

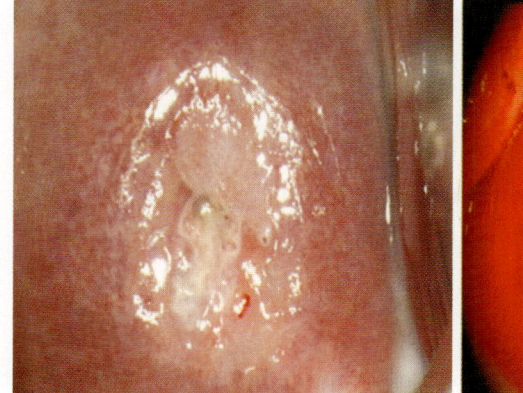

Pretreatment

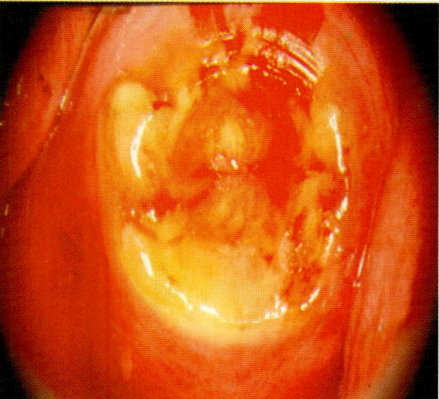

After double freezing treatment

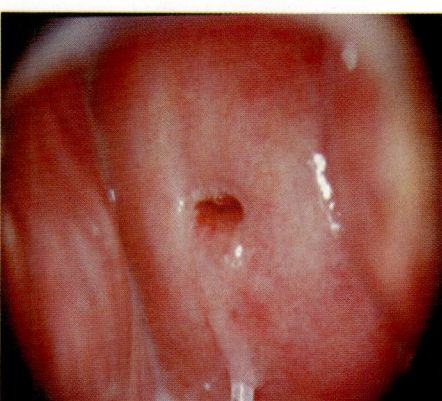

After 3 weeks

Fig. 19.27: Healing

Conization Procedure—Technique (Fig. 19.28A to N)

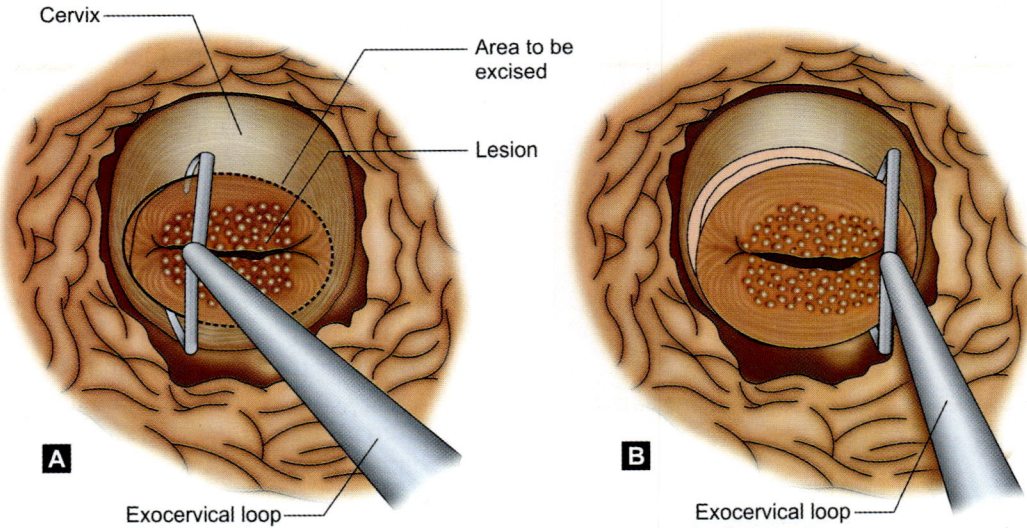

The patient may be anesthetized with general or local anesthesia. Local anesthesia consists of paracervical injections of 1% lidocaine at the 3, 5, 7, and 9 o'clock positions around the cervix. The cervix is stained with an iodine solution such as Schiller's solution to demarcate zones of glycogen depletion and thus neoplasia.   If the patient is under gener al anesthesia, a solution of Pitressin diluted with 10 inter national units to 30 mL of nor mal saline is injected around the entire surf ace of the cer vix. Vascular constricture and blanching of the cer vix will be noted. The injection of vasopressin solution is contraindicated in patients with cardiovascular disease and/or h ypertension. A pursestring vascular cerclage to control the bleeding is r arely indicated.

With the lesion adequately stained with Schiller's solution, the loop device with suction attached to the r od removes the smoke or fume. The loop is placed outside the lesion in the area of nor mal cervix. The electrocoagulator is adjusted to a blend between the cutting and the electr ocoagulation current. The loop de vice is inserted through the cervical tissue to the depth of the available loop and is slowly moved from one side of the portio of the cervix to the other side. By inserting the loop to the full depth of the cervix, the cone should contain the entire lesion.   When the surgeon has reached the opposite limits of the lesion as noted by Schiller's white area, the loop is lifted forward, and the specimen is removed.

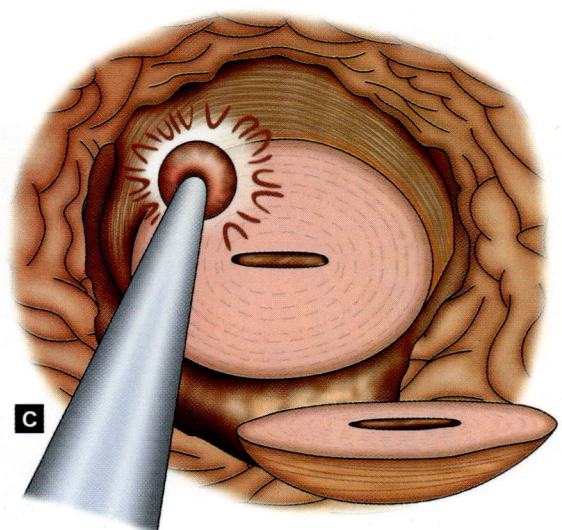

Electrocoagulation of any bleeding surfaces with the ball cautery is performed.

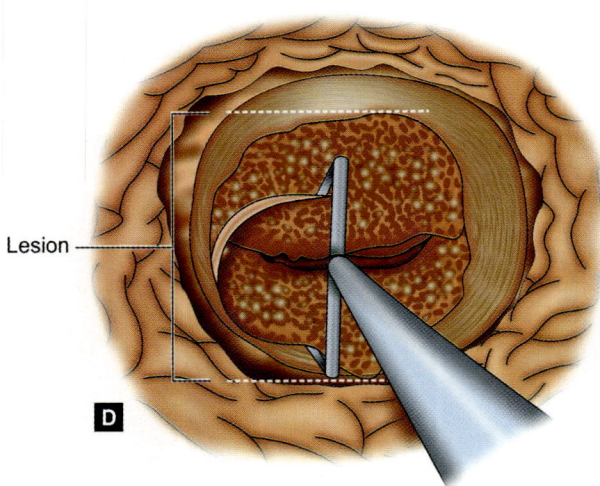

The lesion is larger than (extends outside the limits of) the available steel loops and m ust be re moved in sections (Fig. 19.28E to H). The electric wire of the loop is inseted and swept across the cervix in a routine fashion as shown in Figure 19.28A to C.

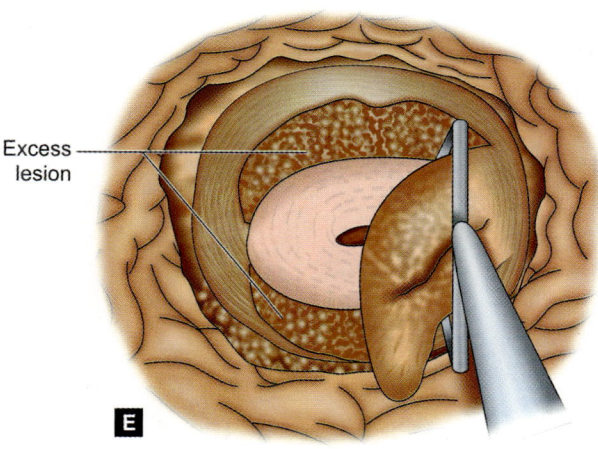

E

Excessive lesion remains outside that removed by the LEEP.

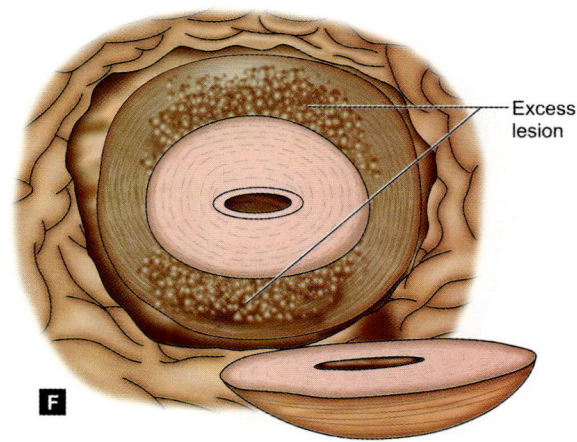

F

The cone is removed, but excessive lesion can still be seen outside the excised area.

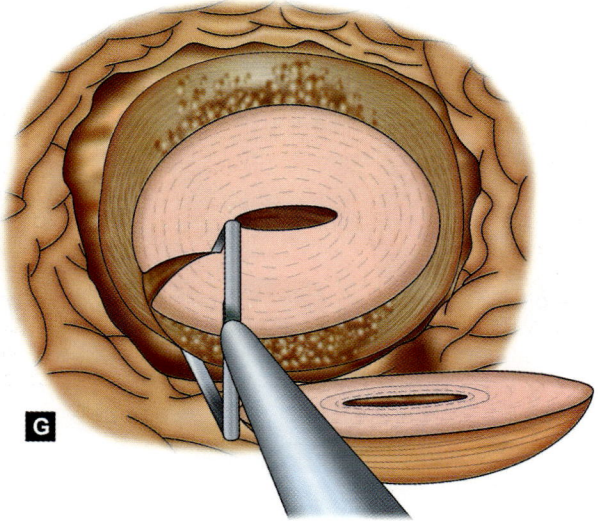

G

The remaining lesion can be removed by repeating the standard procedure, moving the electrical loop from one side to the other. The lesion that was outside the original cone has been removed.

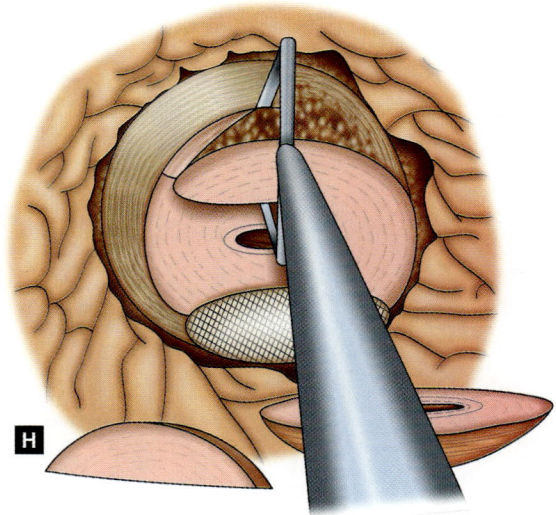

H

The lesion on the anterior lip of the cervix is removed in a similar manner.

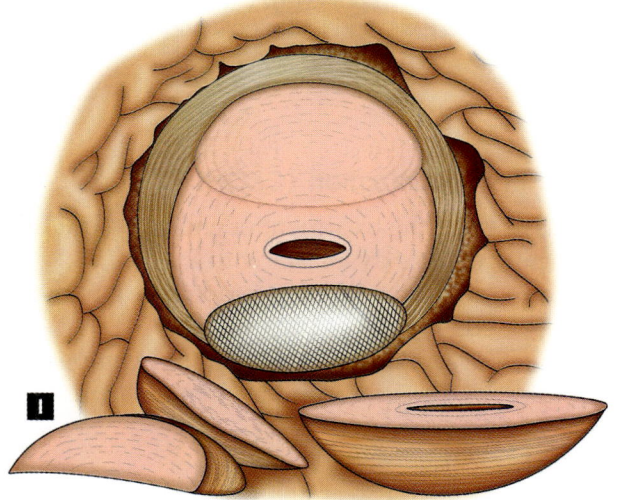

I

The three cone specimens of the cervix are removed by LEEP are (1) the original cone, (2) the posterior portion, and (3) the anterior portion.

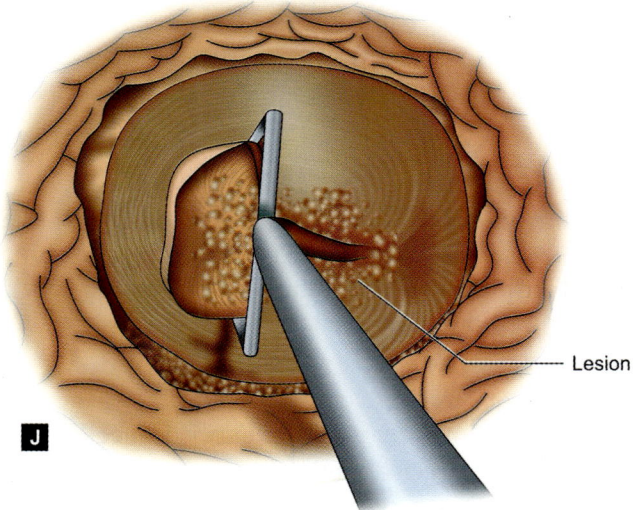

J

When the original lesion extends high into the endocervical canal, the cone specimen of the cervix is removed. Conization by the LEEP is moved from the patient's right to the left in the same technique as previously shown.

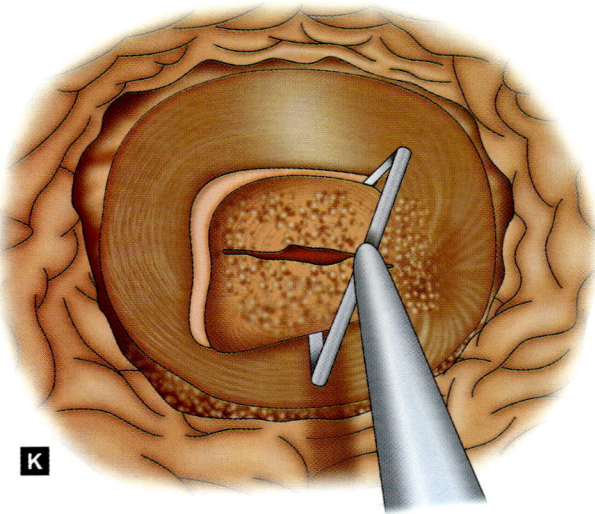

K

Most of the lesion has been removed by the LEEP.

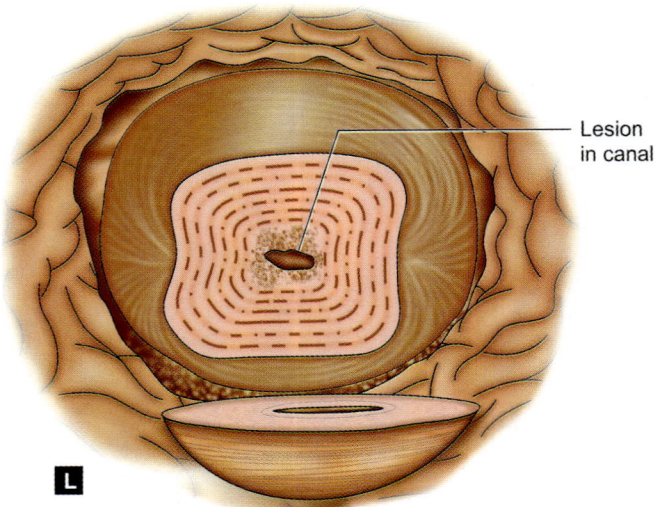

Lesion in canal

L

The exterior lesion on the portion is completely removed, but neoplasia remains in the cervical canal.

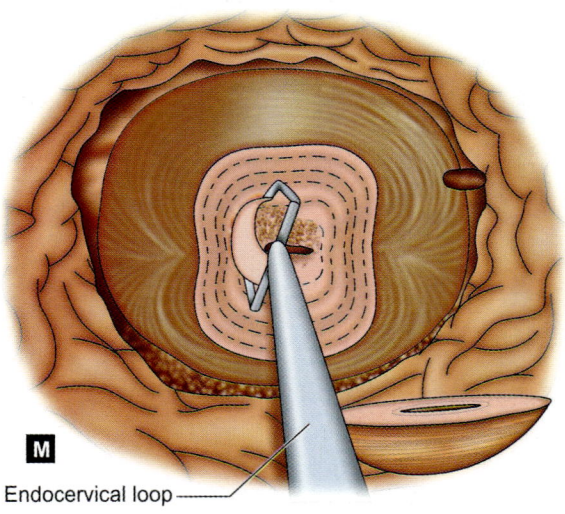

M

Endocervical loop

A smaller loop is placed up the canal. The remaining portion of the endocervical canal is removed by LEEP.

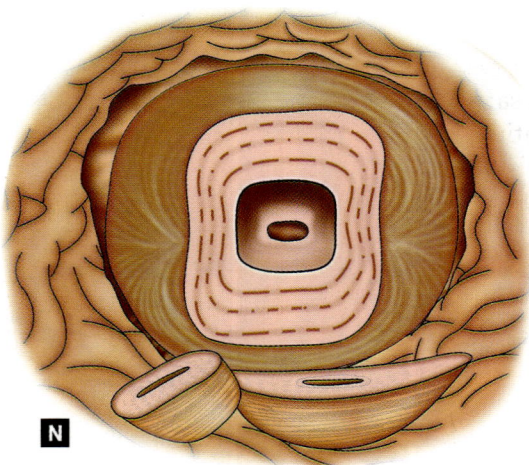

N

The two pathologic specimens, the cylinder and the cone, are shown here. Hemostasis can be achieved by the ball cautery. The specimens are sent to pathology clearly marked as upper cervical canal and lower squamous columnar junction of the cervix.

Fig. 19.28A to N: Conization procedure

It is advantageous to dip a tampon in a ferrous sulfate solution such as Monsel's. The tampon with the tip soaked in Monsel's solution is placed in the cervical cone for additional hemostasis.

III. Laser

1. CO_2 laser works by vaporizing cervical cells.
2. It is a very precise method; only need 5–7 mm of vaporization for treatment.
3. It heals great and spares cervical excisions.
4. Cost is a major problem.
5. It does not provide any specimen for tissue diagnosis.

IV. Cold Knife Conization (CKC) (Fig. 19.29)

1. It is used to be the treatment of choice before LEEP.
2. Surgically excises dysplasia with knife.
3. Indications are mainly when endocervical pathology is suspected.
4. Incompetent cervix is the postoperative complication.
5. It sometimes causes secondary hemorrhage.

V. Hysterectomy

1. It is the final definitive treatment for cervical dysplasia.
2. 10–20% of patients will continue to have abnormal PAP test due to vaginal dysplaia.

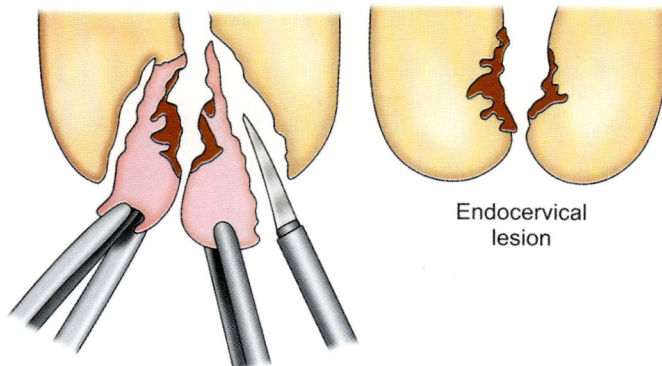

Fig. 19.29: Cold knife cone

3. Recovery time is prolonged, almost 6 weeks.
4. It can invite many complications like hemorrhage, bladder and bowel injury.

Management of Biopsy—Confirmed CIN 1 with Satisfactory Colposcopy

1. Treatment of women with biopsy-confirmed CIN 1 and satisfactory colposcopy includes individualized ablative or excisional modalities (AI recommendation).
2. Endocervical sampling is recommended before ablation of CIN (AII recommendation). Excisional modalities are preferred in women who have undergone previous ablative therapy and have recurrent biopsy-confirmed CIN 1 (BII recommendation).
3. Diagnostic excisional procedures are preferred when colposcopy is unsatisfactory in women with biopsy-confirmed CIN 1 (AII recommendation). Follow-up without treatment is acceptable in pregnant and immunosuppressed women and adolescents with biopsy-confirmed CIN 1 and an unsatisfactory colposcopy (CIII recommendation).
4. Application of podophyllin to the cervix or vagina, ablative treatment in women with unsatisfactory colposcopy, and hysterectomy as the primary treatment for biopsy-confirmed CIN 1 are unacceptable treatment options (EII recommendation).

CIN 2–3

Approximately 43% of untreated CIN 2 and 32% of CIN 3 will regress spontaneously; 35% of CIN 2 and 56% of CIN 3 will persist; and 22% of CIN 2 and 14% of CIN 3 will progress to carcinoma-in-situ or invasive cancer. Therefore, except in special circumstances, women with biopsy-confirmed CIN 2–3 should be treated.

Effective treatment of biopsy-confirmed CIN 2–3 requires the removal of the entire transformation zone rather than just the removal of the lesion. When colposcopy is satisfactory, any ablative or excisional modality will treat CIN effectively. However, because excisional modalities allow for the pathologic identification of unanticipated microinvasive or occult invasive cancer, these methods are preferred to treat biopsy-confirmed CIN 2–3.

Management of Biopsy-Confirmed CIN 2–3 (Fig. 19.31)

Because a small number of women with biopsy-confirmed CIN 2–3 and unsatisfactory colposcopy (Figs 19.30 and 19.32) have occult invasive cancer, excisional procedures should be performed. Cold knife and LEEP conizations effectively diagnose and treat these women. The pathologic margin of specimens from cold knife conization is less frequently involved and is easier to interpret than the margin of LEEP conizations, although the complication rate of cold knife conization is greater (Fig. 19.32).

Positive conization margins or positive endocervical curettage performed at the time of a diagnostic excisional procedure is predictive of recurrent or persistent CIN, which occurs in up to 7% of women with negative endocervical margins and 30% of women with positive endocervical margins. Therefore, it is recommended that women with positive margins be counseled about the relative risks of observation versus

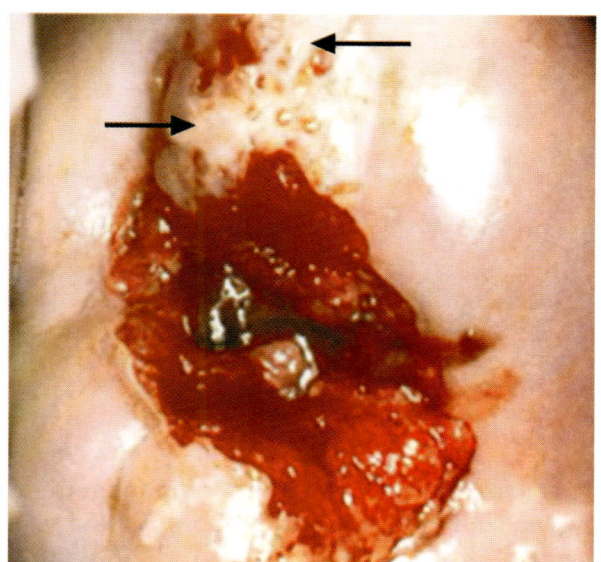

Fig. 19.30: Colposcopic image of a cervical intraepithelial neoplasia 3 lesion with dense acetowhite changes, coarse mosaic *(long arrow)*, and punctuation *(short arrow)*. The image represents satisfactory colposcopy (i.e. the entire squamocolumnar junction and lesions are visualized)

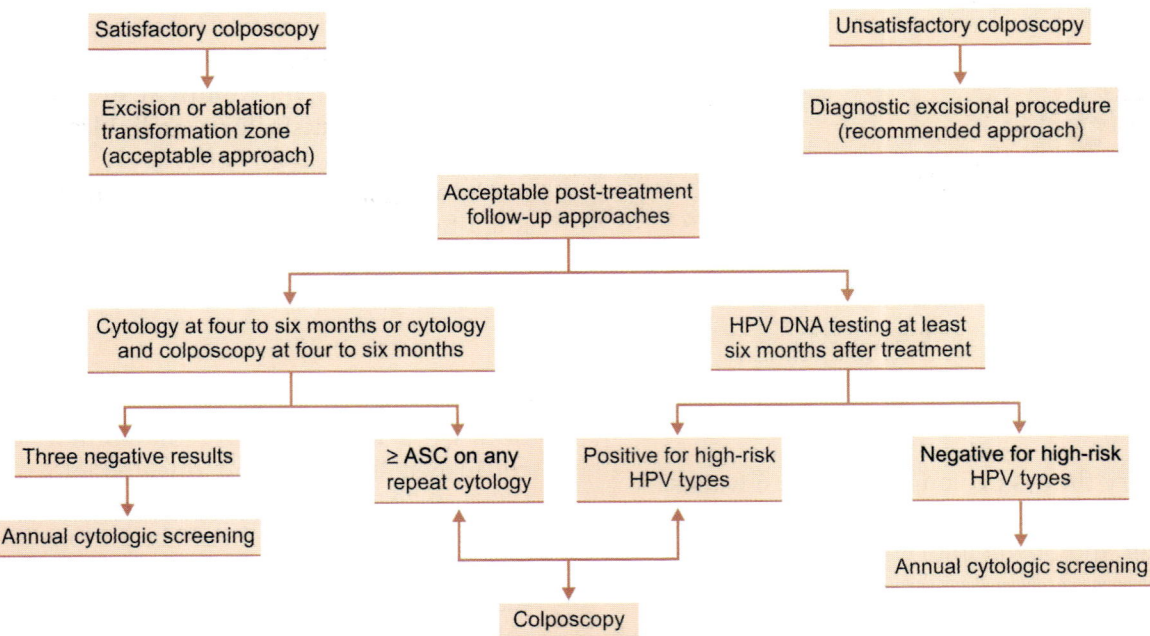

Management options may vary if the woman is pregnant, immunosuppressed, or an adolescent.
Excisional modalities are preferred for women with recurrent CIN 2–3.

Fig. 19.31: Algorithm for the management of biopsy-confirmed cervical intraepithelial neoplasia (CIN) 2–3. (HPV = human papillomavirus; ASC = atypical squamous cells)

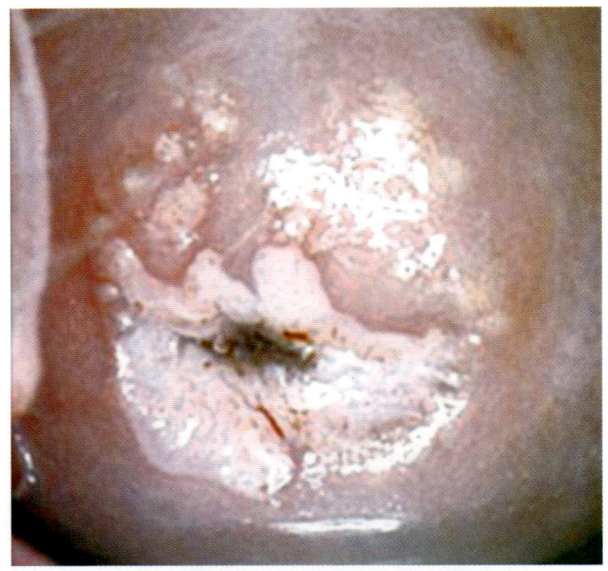

Fig. 19.32: Colposcopic image of a cervical intraepithelial neoplasia 3 lesion with dense acetowhite changes and sharp margins. The image represents unsatisfactory colposcopy (i.e. the entire squamocolumnar junction is not visualized)

further treatment and that their management be individualized. Hysterectomy is appropriate in selected patients.

Recommendation of Management of CIN 2–3

- Excision and ablation of the transformation zone are acceptable treatments for women with biopsy-confirmed CIN 2–3 and satisfactory colposcopy (AI recommendation)
- Excisional modalities are preferred in women with recurrent CIN 2–3 (AII recommendation).
- A diagnostic excisional procedure is recommended in women with biopsy-confirmed CIN 2–3 and unsatisfactory colposcopy (AII recommendation).
- Observation of CIN 2–3 without treatment is unacceptable except in special circumstances (EII recommendation).
- Hysterectomy is unacceptable as a primary therapy for women with CIN 2–3 (EII recommendation).

Follow-Up after Treatment for Biopsy-Confirmed CIN 2–3

- Acceptable follow-up protocols after treatment of CIN 2–3 include cytology or a combination of cytology and colposcopy at four- to six-month intervals until three negative evaluations have been performed (AII recommendation). Annual cytologic follow-up is recommended thereafter (AII recommendation).
- A cytologic result of ASC is the recommended threshold for referral to colposcopy during follow-up (AII recommendation).
- Surveillance with HPV DNA testing performed no sooner than six months after treatment is acceptable (BII recommendation).

- A positive test for high-risk HPV types is the recommended threshold for referral to colposcopy (BIII recommendation).
- If HPV testing is negative, annual cytologic screening is recommended (BIII recommendation).
- Repeat conization or hysterectomy based on a single positive HPV test that is not corroborated by other findings (e.g. cytology, colposcopy, histology) is unacceptable (DIII recommendation).

- When CIN 2–3 is identified at the endocervical margin or in the endocervical sampling obtained after the diagnostic excisional procedure, a repeat diagnostic excisional procedure is acceptable (AII recommendation).
- Hysterectomy is acceptable when repeat diagnostic excision is not feasible (BII recommendation) or for women with recurrent or persistent CIN 2–3 (BII recommendation).

19B. INVASIVE CANCER CERVIX

Cervical cancer is the third most common malignancy in women worldwide, and it remains a leading cause of cancer-related death for women in developing countries. India represents 26.4% of all women dying of cervical cancer globally, with China, Bangladesh, Pakistan, Indonesia and Thailand also showing high death incidence. Cervical cancer kills an estimated 275,000 women every year and 500,000 new cases reported worldwide.

Epidemiology

The global cervical cancer incidence has increased from 378,000 cases per year in 1980 to 454,000 cases per year in 2010 (annual rate of increase, 0.6%). Cervical cancer death rates have been decreasing, but the disease still account for 200,000 deaths in 2010. Indeed, rates of cervical adenocarcinoma have been increasing in women under 40 years of age. These cases are less easily detected with Pap test screening, and survival is low because cases tend to be detected at a late stage. Moreover, the HPV types causing adenocarcinoma are different from the types causing squamous carcinoma. HPV 16, which is a stronger carcinogen than other HPV types, has been found more frequently in younger women than in older ones.

Pathophysiology

Human papillomavirus (HPV) infection must be present for cervical cancer to occur. HPV infection occurs in a high percentage of sexually active women. However, approximately 90% of HPV infections clear on their own within months to a few years and with no sequelae, although cytology reports in the 2 years following infection may show a low-grade squamous intraepithelial lesion.

On average, only 5% of HPV infections will result in the development of CIN grade 2 or 3 lesions within 3 years of infection. Only 20% of CIN 3 lesions progress to invasive cervical cancer within 5 years, and only 40% of CIN 3 lesions progress to invasive cervical cancer within 30 years.

Because only a small proportion of HPV infections progress to cancer, other factors must be involved in the process of carcinogenesis. The following factors have been postulated to influence the development of CIN 3 lesions:

- The type and duration of viral infection, with high-risk HPV type and persistent infection predicting a higher risk for progression; low-risk HPV types do not cause cervical cancer
- Host conditions that compromise immunity (e.g. poor nutritional status, immunocompromise, and HIV infection)
- Environmental factors (e.g. smoking and vitamin deficiencies)
- Lack of access to routine cytology screening

In addition, various environmental factors significantly increase the risk of HPV infection. These include early age of first intercourse and higher number of sexual partners.

Although use of oral contraceptives for 5 years or longer has been associated with an increased risk of cervical cancer, the increased risk may reflect a higher risk for HPV infection among sexually active women. However, a possible direct interaction between oral contraceptives and HPV infection has been disproved.

Genetic Susceptibility

Genetic susceptibility to cervical cancers caused by HPV infection has been identified. Women who have an affected first-degree biologic relative have a 2-fold relative risk of developing a cervical tumor. Genetic susceptibility accounts for fewer than 1% of cervical cancers.

Genetic changes in several classes of genes have been linked to cervical cancer. Tumor necrosis factor (TNF) is involved in initiating the cell commitment to apoptosis, and the genes *TNFα-8*, *TNFα-572*, *TNFα-857*, *TNFα-863*, and *TNF γ-308A* have been associated with a higher incidence of cervical cancer. Polymorphisms in another gene, *Tp53*, is also associated with an increased rate of HPV infection progressing to cervical cancer.

Human leukocyte antigen (HLA) genes are involved in various ways. Some HLA gene anomalies are associated with an increased risk of HPV infection progressing to cancer others with a protective effect. The chemokine receptor-2 (*CCR-2*) gene on chromosome 3p21 and the *Fas* gene on chromosome 10q24 influence genetic susceptibility to cervical cancer, perhaps by disrupting the immune response to HPV.

Human Papillomavirus

HPV comprises a heterogeneous group of viruses that contain closed circular double-stranded DNA. The viral genome encodes 6 early open reading frame proteins (i.e. E1, E2, E3, E4, E6, and E7), which function as regulatory proteins, and 2 late open reading frame proteins (i.e. L1 and L2), which make up the viral capsid.

To date, more than 115 different genotypes of HPV have been identified and cloned. A large multinational cervical cancer study found that more than 90% of all cervical cancers worldwide are caused by 8 HPV types: 16, 18, 31, 33, 35, 45, 52, and 58. Three types—16, 18, and 45—cause 94% of cervical adenocarcinomas. HPV type 16 poses a higher risk of cancer than that posed by other high-risk HPV types.

The HPVs that infect the human cervix fall into 2 broad risk categories. The low-risk types (e.g. HPV 6 and 11) are associated with condylomata and a very small number of low-grade squamous epithelial lesions (SILs) but are never found in invasive cancer. The high-risk types (e.g. HPV 16) vary in prevalence according to the cervical disease state.

Upon integration into the human genome, the linearization of high-risk HPV DNA places the E6 and E7 genes in a position of enhanced replication. E7 binds and inactivates the Rb protein while E6 binds p53 and directs its degradation, and the functional loss of the *Tp53* and *Rb* genes leads to resistance to apoptosis, causing uncensored cell growth after DNA damage. This ultimately results in progression to malignancy.

Human Immunodeficiency Virus

The role of HIV infection in the pathogenesis of cervical cancer is not fully understood. However, HIV infection is known to suppress the already low level of immune recognition of HPV infection, allowing HPV to cause more damage than it would in immunocompetent women.

Cervical cancer is at least 5 times more common in HIV-infected women, and this increased prevalence has remained essentially unchanged with the use of highly active antiretroviral therapy. Studies have shown a higher prevalence of HPV infection in HIV-seropositive women than in seronegative women, and the HPV prevalence being directly proportional to the severity of immunosuppression as measured by CD4+ T cell counts.

Etiology

With rare exceptions, cervical cancer results from genital infection with HPV, which is a known human carcinogen. Although HPV infections can be transmitted via nonsexual routes, the majority result from sexual contact. Consequently, major risk factors identified in epidemiologic studies are as follows:

- Sex at a young age
- Multiple sexual partners
- Promiscuous male partners
- History of sexually transmitted diseases
- HIV infection is associated with a 5-fold increase in the risk of cervical cancer, presumably because of an impaired immune response to HPV infection.
- Exposure to diethylstilbestrol *in utero* is associated with an increased risk of CIN grade 2 or higher.

History

Because many women are screened routinely, the most common finding is an abnormal Papanicolaou (Pap) test result. Typically, these patients are asymptomatic.

Clinically, the first symptom of cervical cancer is abnormal vaginal bleeding, usually postcoital. Vaginal discomfort, malodorous discharge, and dysuria are often the initial presenting symptoms.

The tumor grows by extending along the epithelial surfaces, both squamous and glandular, upward to the endometrial cavity, throughout the vaginal epithelium, and laterally to the pelvic wall. It can invade the bladder and rectum directly, leading to constipation, hematuria, fistula, and ureteral obstruction, with or without hydroureter or hydronephrosis. *The triad of leg edema, pain, and hydronephrosis suggests pelvic wall involvement*. The common sites for distant metastasis include extrapelvic lymph nodes, liver, lung, and bone.

Other risk factors for cervical cancer include:
- Having sex at an early age
- Multiple sexual partners
- Sexual partners who have multiple partners or who participate in high-risk sexual activities
- Women whose mothers took the drug DES (diethylstilbestrol) during pregnancy in the early 1960s to prevent miscarriage
- Weakened immune system
- Poor economic status

Symptoms

Most of the time, early cervical cancer has no symptoms. Symptoms that may occur can include:
- Continuous vaginal discharge, which may be pale, watery, pink, brown, bloody, or foul-smelling
- Abnormal vaginal bleeding between periods, after intercourse, or after menopause
- Periods become heavier and last longer than usual
- Any bleeding after menopause

Symptoms of advanced cervical cancer may include:
- Loss of appetite
- Weight loss
- Fatigue
- Pelvic pain
- Back pain
- Leg pain
- Single swollen leg
- Heavy bleeding from the vagina
- Leaking of urine or feces from the vagina
- Bone fractures

Physical Examination

I. General Examination

a. Poor general condition with cachexia
b. Increasing pallor
c. Unilateral/bilateral leg edema, lymphedema
d. Evidence of lung, bone, liver, spine metastases

II. Abdominal Examination

a. Enlarged liver
b. Enlarged hydronephrotic kidneys, distended bladder
c. Enlarged uterus due to hematometra following cervical stenosis due to growth
d. Co-existing pathology like uterine fibroid, ovarian tumor
e. Rarely, ascites

III. Pelvic Examination

A. *Per speculum examination:* Cusco's bivalve speculum is used to inspect the cervical growth from a distance without touching it. It observes the following findings:
   a. Origin of the growth from the portion of the cervix
   b. Size of the growth (<4 cm or >4 cm)
   c. Surface—hemorrhagic, necrotic
   d. Type of the growth—cauliflower, ulcerative, infiltrative
   e. Area of involvement—vaginal walls (upper part, vault, lower third or only limited to cervix); anterior vagina involved or not
   f. Growth is bleeding on touch or not
B. *Per vaginal examination:* It gives the following informations:
   Confirm the speculum findings:
   a. Size
   b. Feel of the growth (Fig. 19.33)
   c. Feel of the cervix—hard, friable, barrel-shaped

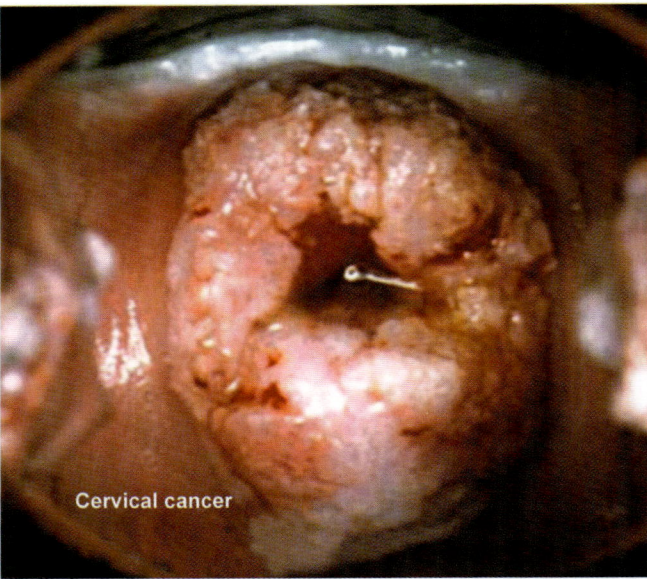

Fig. 19.33: Exfoliation growth in cervix

   d. Surface, mobility and fixity of the growth
   e. Size of the uterus, mobility, endocervical involvement
   f. Adnexal pathology
   g. Pouch of Douglas—any pathology
   h. Feel and the extension of growth in the vaginal wall
   i. Enlarged pelvic lymph nodes
C. *Per rectal examination:* It assess the following:
   a. Involvement of parametrium
   b. Any tumor free space in the lateral pelvic wall
   c. Any involvement of the rectum
   d. Involvement of the pelvic bones

Confirmation of Diagnosis

This is always done by histopathology for which cervical biopsy is taken. This is of the following types:
a. Surface biopsy
b. Cone biopsy
c. Four quadrant punch biopsy
d. Colposcopy directed cervical biopsy
e. Endocervical curettage

Histological Types of Cervical Cancer

The World Health Organization (WHO) recognises two main histological types of invasive cancer:
- **Squamous carcinoma** (which constitute about 85% of all cases)
- **Adenocarcinoma** (which constitute about 10–12% of all cases)

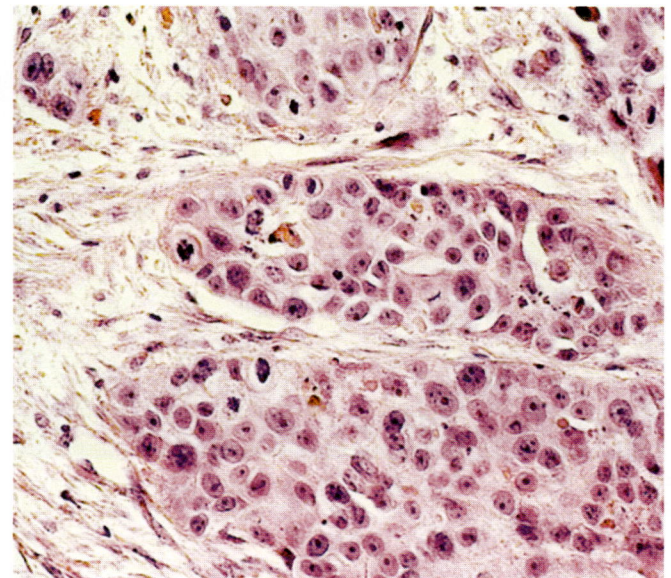

Fig. 19.34: Nonkeratinizing invasive squamous cell carcinoma (histology)

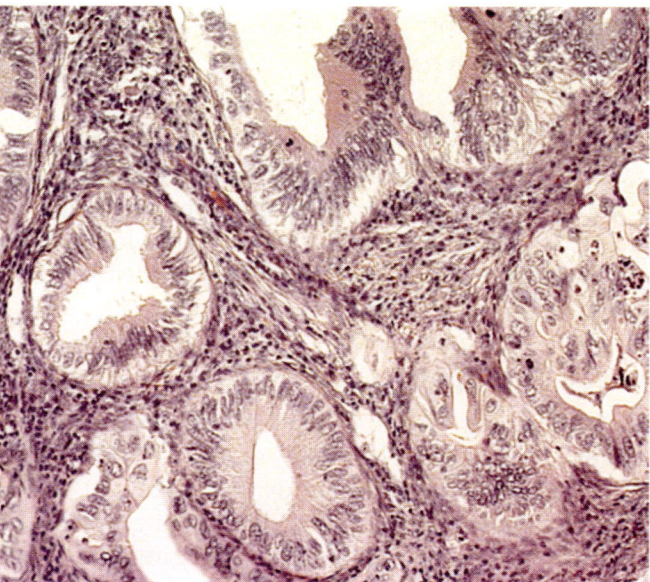

Fig. 19.35: Adenocarcinoma of cervix—well differentiated (histology). Note tumor cells are forming glands. The glands are crowded and penetrate beyond the stroma of the cervical epithelium into the fibromuscular wall of the cervix. The tumor cells lining the glands are abnormal showing loss of polarity of the nuclei which are large, hyperchromatic and irregular. Mitotic figures are often present

- Several other types of carcinoma—adenosquamous carcinoma, adenoid cystic carcinoma, metastatic carcinoma, make up the remaining 3–5% of all cases.

Squamous carcinomas are further typed according to whether they are keratinizing or non-keratinizing carcinomas (Fig. 19.34). Keratinizing carcinomas may be well differentiated or moderately differentiated and are composed of large tumor cells. The non-keratinizing carcinomas (poorly differentiated carcinomas) may be of large cell or small cell type.

Adenocarcinomas (Fig. 19.35) are less commonly found and although each type is histologically distinct. It is not uncommon for two or more histological forms of adenocarcinoma to be present in a single tumor. The frequent cooexistence of glandular and squamous carcinomas suggests that they may have a common origin in the reserve cells of the cervix as well as a common etiology. The most frequent type of adenocarcinoma to be found in the cervix is the endocervical type of mucinous adenocarcinoma. Three grades of endocervical carcinoma are recognised—well differentiated, moderately differentiated and poorly differentiated–depending on the similarity of the tumor cell to the glandular epithelial lining of the endocervix.

Histological Types of Carcinoma Cervix (WHO Classification—Extended)

- Squamous cell carcinoma (epidermoid carcinoma)
  - Keratinizing (well differentiated and moderately differentiated)
  - Non-keratinizing (large and small cell types)
  - Spindle cell carcinoma
- Adenocarcinoma endocervical type
  - *Variant*: Adenoma malignum (minimal deviation carcinoma)
  - *Variant*: Villoglandular papillary adenocarcinoma
- Endometrioid adenocarcinoma
- Clear cell adenocarcinoma
- Serous adenocarcinoma
- Mesonephric adenocarcinoma
- Intestinal type (signet ring) adenocarcinoma
- Other epithelial tumors
  - Adenosquamous carcinoma
  - Adenoid cystic carcinoma
- Small cell carcinoma
- Undifferentiated carcinoma
  - Metastatic tumors (breast, ovary, colon, and direct spread of endometrial carcinoma)

Once the diagnosis is established, a complete blood count (CBC) and renal and hepatic function should be ordered to look for abnormalities from possible metastatic disease, and imaging studies should be performed for staging purposes.

In the International Federation of Gynecology and Obstetrics [FIGO]) guidelines for staging, procedures are limited to the following:

- Colposcopy
- Cystoscopy
- IVU

- Proctosigmoidoscopy
- Barium enema
- Chest X-ray
- USG

Cystoscopy and proctoscopy should be performed in patients with a bulky primary tumor to help rule out local invasion of the bladder and the colon. Barium enema studies can be used to evaluate extrinsic rectal compression from the cervical mass.

Special Investigations

The pretreatment evaluation of patients with cervical cancer includes physical examination, chest radiography, and intravenous urography (IVU) or cross-sectional imaging (computed tomography [CT] scanning or magnetic resonance imaging [MRI]). In early stage disease with a small tumor confined to the cervix, IVU and cross-sectional imaging are not routinely performed because of their relatively low yield.

Barium enema examination, radioisotope bone scanning, cystoscopy, and proctosigmoidoscopy have a low yield, particularly in early disease, and these procedures are performed for only specific indications that are based on the symptoms or clinical findings.

MRI has excellent soft-tissue contrast resolution, which exceeds that of CT scanning and ultrasonography. Consequently, MRI is significantly more valuable than CT and US in the assessment of the size of the tumor, the depth of the cervical invasion, and the regional extent of the disease (direct invasion of the parametrium, pelvic sidewall, bladder, or rectum) and detection of enlarged lymph nodes. Despite the advantages of MRI, the gynecology literature mostly recommends the use of CT scanning for the pretreatment evaluation of cervical cancer because the additional information provided with the excellent soft-tissue contrast resolution of MRI often has no significant effect on clinical decision making or on the choice of therapy.

In general, CT scanning and MRI are not warranted in patients with small-volume, early disease (stage Ib disease and a cervical tumor diameter <2.0 cm) because of the low probability of parametrial invasion and nodal metastasis. Imaging with CT scanning or MRI (Fig. 19.36) is appropriate when the cervical tumor is larger than 2.0 cm, when the size of the tumor cannot be adequately evaluated during the clinical examination, or when the tumor is endocervical.

CT scan of cervical cell carcinoma demonstrates markedly enlarged lymph node at left pelvic sidewall.

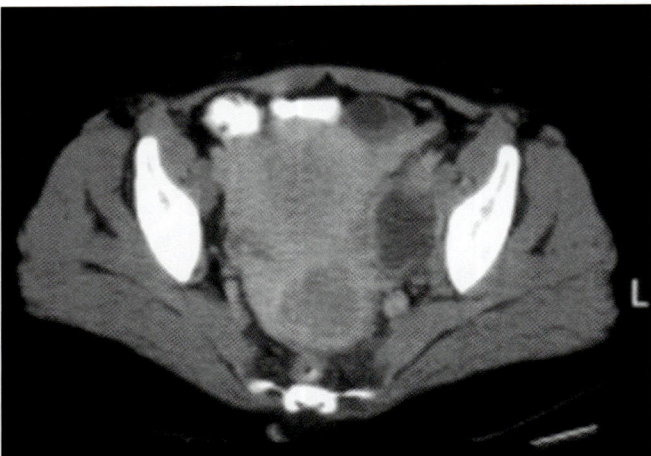

Fig. 19.36: CT demonstrates enlarged lymph node at left pelvic side wall

A CT scan of the abdomen and pelvis is performed to look for metastasis in the liver, lymph nodes, or other organs (Fig. 19.36) and to help rule out hydronephrosis or hydroureter. MRI or positron-emission tomography (PET) scanning is an alternative to CT scanning; in fact, PET scanning is now recommended for patients with stage IB2 disease or higher.

Differential Diagnoses

- Cervicitis
- Endometrial carcinoma
- Pelvic inflammatory disease
- Vaginitis
- Cervical endometriosis
- Cervical tuberculosis

FIGO (International Federation of Gynecology and Obstetrics) Staging of Cervical Cancer (Figs 19.37 to 19.39)

- *Stage 0:* Carcinoma in situ, or CIN grade III
- *Stage I:* Confined to the cervix (uterine spread not evaluated)
- *Stage IA:* Invasive carcinoma diagnosed by biopsy
  - Stage IA1: Invasion depth <3 mm or lateral extension <7 mm
  - Stage IA2: Invasion depth 3 to 5 mm, extension <7 mm.
- *Stage IB:* Visible lesion
  - Stage IB1: 4 cm or less
  - Stage IB2: More than 4 cm.
- *Stage II:* Cancer invades beyond the cervix but not to the pelvic sidewall, or the distal third of the vagina
  - Stage IIA: Vaginal involvement without obvious parametrial involvement

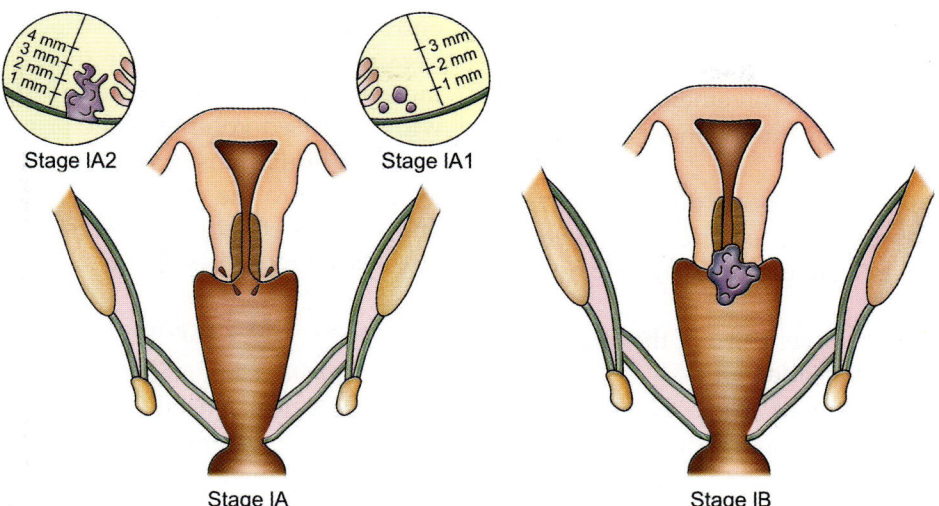

Fig. 19.37: Cervical cancer stage I

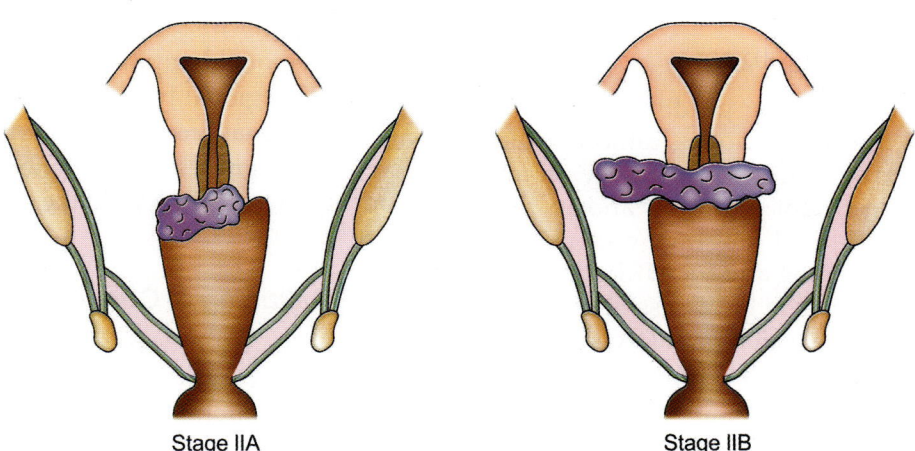

Fig. 19.38: Cervical cancer stage II

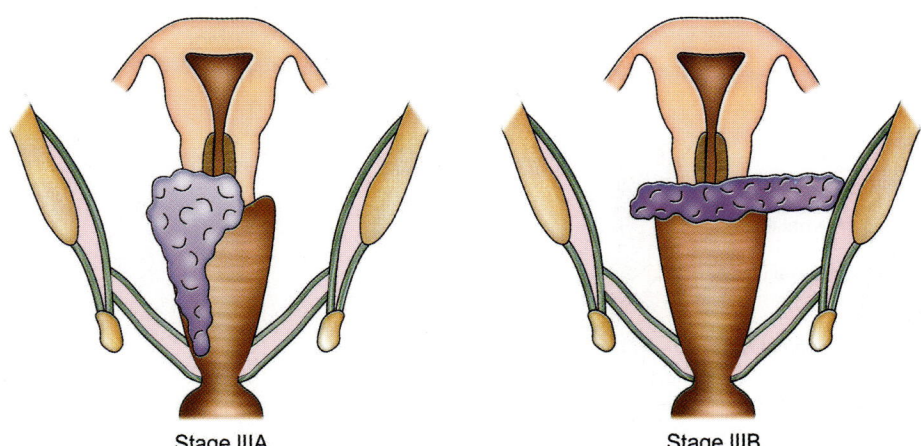

Fig. 19.39: Cervical cancer stage III

IIA1: Clinically visible lesion <4 cm

IIA2: Clinically visible lesion >4 cm

- Stage IIB1: Parametrial involvement, 4 cm or less.
- Stage IIB2: Parametrial involvement, more than 4 cm.
- *Stage III:* Tumor affixed to pelvic sidewall, or involving the lower third of the vagina, or is associated with a nonfunctioning kidney or hydronephrosis
  - Stage IIIA: Involves lower third of the vagina but no extension to pelvic sidewall
  - Stage IIIB: Extension to the pelvic sidewall, nonfunctioning kidney, or hydronephrosis.
- *Stage IV:* Carcinoma has extended out of the pelvis, involving the mucosa of bladder, or rectum.
  - Stage IVA: Spread to adjacent pelvic organs— locally advanced disease
  - Stage IVB: Spread to distant organs—extra-pelvic metastases.

Lymph Node Evaluation (Fig. 19.40)

The strict FIGO clinical staging guidelines do not include the status of the lymph nodes, although the presence of metastatic lymphadenopathy is an important factor in treatment planning and in the prognosis. Extended clinical staging with cross-sectional imaging (CT scanning and/or MRI) includes the status of the lymph nodes in the assessment of the extent of the disease. The detection of enlarged pelvic lymph nodes is considered equivalent to pelvic sidewall tumor extension (stage III), and the detection of enlarged lymph nodes in the para-aortic, paracaval, or inguinal regions is considered extrapelvic tumor spread (stage IV).

The major limitations of the FIGO clinical staging system are encountered in the estimation of the size of the primary tumor, particularly when the tumor is endocervical. The size of the tumor is significant because, in each stage, the incidence of lymph node metastases increases and the prognosis deteriorates with increased volume of the primary tumor.

Other limitations occur in the evaluation of tumor extension into the parametrium and pelvic sidewalls and in the detection of metastatic lymphadenopathy or distant metastasis.

FIGO and TNM Staging

There are two major staging systems that are frequently used in cervical cancer.

- The TNM system, developed by the International Union Against Cancer (UICC) and the American Joint Committee on Cancer (AJCC).

  In the UICC/AJCC system, regional lymph node (N) involvement—including paracervical, parametrial, hypogastric (obturator), common, internal and external iliac, and presacral and sacral nodes—is graded as follows.
  - NX: Regional lymph nodes cannot be assessed
  - N0: No regional lymph node metastasis
  - N1: Regional lymph node metastasis

The T and N grades are combined with the grade for distant metastasis (M) to yield the staging for the cancer (Tables 19.4 and 19.5).

New FIGO Staging of Cancer Cervix

IA1   Confined to the cervix, diagnosed only by microscopy with invasion of <3 mm in depth and lateral spread <7 mm

IA2   Confined to the cervix, diagnosed with microscopy with invasion of >3 mm and <5 mm with lateral spread <7 mm

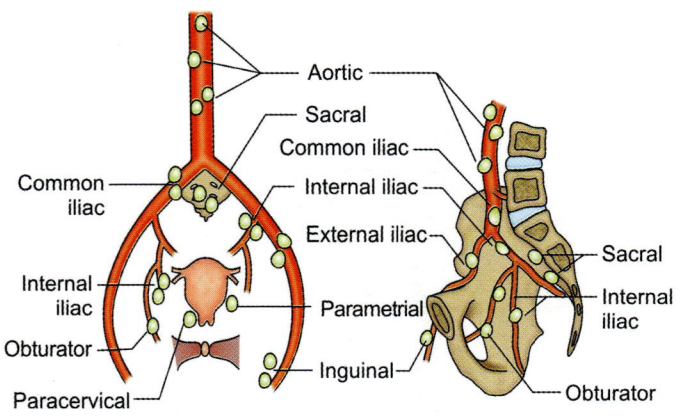

Fig. 19.40: Lymph node spread in cancer cervix

Table 19.4: UICC/AJCC staging for cervical cancer			
Stage	*Tumor*	*Node*	*Metastasis*
0	Tis	N0	M0
IA1	T1a1	N0	M0
IA2	T1a2	N0	M0
IB1	T1b1	N0	M0
IIA	T2a	N0	M0
IIB	T2b	N0	M0
IIIA	T3a	N0	M0
IIIB	T1	N1	M0
—	T2	N1	M0
—	T3a	N1	M0
—	T3b	Any N	M0
IVA	T4	Any N	M0
IVB	Any T	Any N	M1

Table 19.5: TNM and FIGO staging combined

TNM stage	FIGO stage	
TX	—	Primary tumor cannot be assessed
T0	—	No evidence of primary tumor
Tis	0	Carcinoma in situ
T1	I	Cervical carcinoma confined to uterus (extension to corpus should be disregarded)
T1a	IA	Invasive carcinoma diagnosed only by microscopy. All macroscopically visible lesions—even with superficial invasion—are T1b/1B. Stromal invasion with a maximal depth of 5.0 mm measured from the base of the epithelium and a horizontal spread of 7.0 mm or less. Vascular space involvement, venous or lymphatic, does not affect classification.
T1a1	IA1	Measured stromal invasion 3 mm or less in depth and 7 mm or less in lateral spread
T1a2	IA2	Measured stromal invasion more than 3 mm but not more than 5 mm with a horizontal spread 7 mm or less
T1b	IB	Clinically visible lesion confined to the cervix or microscopic lesion greater than IA2
T1b1	IB1	Clinically visible lesion 4 cm or less in greatest dimension
	IB2	Clinically visible lesion more than 4 cm
T2	II	Cervical carcinoma extends beyond the cervix but not to the pelvic sidewall or to the lower third of vagina
T2a	IIA	Tumor without parametrial invasion
T2b	IIB	Tumor with parametrial invasion
T3	III	Tumor extends to the pelvic wall and/or involves the lower third of the vagina and/or causes hydronephrosis or nonfunctioning kidney
T3a	IIIA	Tumor involves lower third of vagina; no extension to pelvic sidewall
T3b	IIIB	Tumor extends to pelvic sidewall and/or causes hydronephrosis or nonfunctioning kidney
—	IV	Cervical carcinoma has extended beyond the true pelvis or has involved (biopsy proven) the bladder mucosa or rectal mucosa. Bullous edema does not qualify as a criteria for stage IV disease.
T4	IVA	Spread to mucosa of adjacent organs (bladder, rectum, or both)
M1	IVB	Distant metastasis

IB1	Clinically visible lesion or greater than A2, <4 cm in greatest dimension
IB2	Clinically visible lesion, >4 cm in greatest dimension
IIA1	Involvement of the upper two-thirds of the vagina, without parametrial invasion, <4 cm in greatest dimension
IIA2	>4 cm in greatest dimension
IIB	With parametrial involvement
IIIA/B	Unchanged
IVA/B	Unchanged

STAGE-BASED THERAPY

Stage 0 Cancer

Carcinoma in situ (stage 0) is treated with local ablative or excisional measures such as cryosurgery, laser ablation, and loop excision. Surgical removal is preferred in that it allows further pathologic evaluation to rule out microinvasive disease. After treatment, these patients require lifelong surveillance.

Stage IA1 Cancer

The treatment of choice for stage IA1 disease is surgery. Total hysterectomy, radical hysterectomy, and conization are accepted procedures. Lymph node dissection is not required, if the depth of invasion is less than 3 mm and no lymphovascular invasion is noted.

Selected patients with stage IA1 disease but no lymphovascular space invasion who desire to maintain fertility may undergo therapeutic conization with close follow-up, including cytology, colposcopy, and endocervical curettage. Patients with comorbid medical conditions who are not surgical candidates can be successfully treated with radiation.

According to National Comprehensive Cancer Network (NCCN) guidelines, pelvic radiation therapy is currently a category 1 recommendation for women with stage IA disease and negative lymph nodes after surgery who have high-risk factors (e.g. a large primary tumor, deep stromal invasion, or lymphovascular space invasion).

Stage IA2, IB, or IIA Cancer

For patients with stage IB or IIA disease, there are two treatment options:

1. Combined external beam radiation with brachytherapy
2. Radical hysterectomy with bilateral pelvic lymphadenectomy

Radical vaginal trachelectomy with pelvic lymph node dissection is appropriate for fertility preservation in women with stage IA2 disease and those with stage IB1 disease whose lesions are 2 cm or smaller. The principal problems with pregnancy after trachelectomy are premature labor and the need to undergo cesarean section for delivery.

Current surgical guidelines for stage IA2 to IIA cervical cancers allow for minimally invasive techniques, such as traditional laparoscopic and robotically assisted laparoscopic techniques, in the surgical management of these tumors. Indeed, it has been shown that these less morbid procedures are equally effective in achieving adequate surgical margins and lymph node dissection while possessing the added advantage of shorter postoperative recovery times.

Postoperative combination of cisplatin-containing chemotherapy and pelvic irradiation of the pelvis reduces the risk of local recurrence in patients with high-risk factors (i.e. positive pelvic nodes, positive surgical margins, and residual parametrial disease). Postoperative radiation therapy is also recommended in patients who have at least 2 intermediate risk factors (including tumor size greater than 2 cm, deep stromal invasion, or lymphovascular space invasion). For patients with IB2 or IIA cancer and tumors larger than 4 cm, radiation and chemotherapy is selected in most cases.

Stage IIB, III, or IVA Cancer

For locally advanced cervical carcinoma (stages IIB, III, and IVA), radiation therapy was the treatment of choice for many years. Radiation therapy begins with a course of external beam radiation to reduce tumor mass and thereby enable subsequent intracavitary application. Brachytherapy is delivered by means of afterloading applicators that are placed in the uterine cavity and vagina.

Additionally, a dramatic improvement in survival when chemotherapy is combined with radiation therapy. Consequently, the use of cisplatin-based chemotherapy in combination with radiation has become the standard of care for primary management of patients with locally advanced cervical cancer.

Stage IVB and Recurrent Cancer

Individualized therapy is used on a palliative basis. Radiation therapy is used alone for control of bleeding and pain, whereas systemic chemotherapy is used for disseminated disease.

Treatment of pelvic recurrences after primary surgical management should include single-agent chemotherapy and radiation, and treatment for recurrences elsewhere should include combination chemotherapy. For central pelvic recurrence after radiation therapy, modified radical hysterectomy (if the recurrence is smaller than 2 cm) or pelvic exenteration should be undertaken. For disease recurring after chemotherapy and radiation therapy, a disease-free interval of more than 16 months is considered to designate the tumor as platinum-sensitive. The standard of care in these cases is chemotherapy with a platinum-based doublet of paclitaxel and cisplatin.

The NCCN also recommends bevacizumab, docetaxel, gemcitabine, ifosfamide, 5-fluorouracil, mitomycin, irinotecan, and topotecan as possible candidates for second-line therapy (category 2B recommendation), as well as pemetrexed and vinorelbine (category 3 recommendation).

According to National Cancer Institute (NCI) and Gynecologic Oncology Group (GOG), bevacizumab at a dose of 15 mg/kg in conjunction with chemotherapy, 1 day every 3 weeks extend survival by almost 4 months in patients with advanced, recurrent, or persistent cervical cancer that had not responded to standard surgery or radiotherapy.

Classification of Radical Hysterectomy (Rutledge Classification)

1. *Type I or simple extra-fascial hysterectomy*
2. *Type II or modified radical hysterectomy:* Here, the uterus, cervix, medial half of the cardinal and uterosacral ligament, upper vagina of 1–2 cm are removed. Here the superior layer of ureteric tunnel (vesicouterine ligament) is removed which contains the uterine artery. The uterine artery is ligated at the level of the ureter thus preserving the ureteric branch to the ureter. Along with this, bilateral pelvic lymphadenectomy is done which can be done intraperitoneal (in Wertheim's) or extraperitoneal (in Mitra's operation which is combined with radical vaginal hysterectomy).
3. *Type III radical hysterectomy or Meig's radical hysrterectomy:* Here, en block removal of the uterus, parametrium, upper third of the vagina along with bilateral pelvic lymphadenectomy is done. The uterine vessels are ligated at its origin from anterior

division of internal iliac artery and the cardinal and uterosacral ligament is removed from the pelvic sidewall. The both superior and inferior layers of the vesicouterine ligament (ureteric tunnel) is removed.

4. *Type IV radical hysterectomy:* Here the periureteral tissue, superior vesical artery, and as much as three-fourths of the vagina are removed.

5. *Type V radical hysterectomy:* In anterior type (anterior exanteration), the portion of the distal ureter and the bladder is removed whereas in the posterior type, the portion of the rectosigmoid is removed followed by colostomy.

Removal of the tubes and ovaries is not part of radical hysterectomy.

A. Wertheim's (Radical Hysterectomy with Bilateral Intraperitoneal Pelvic Lymphadenectomy)

1. The abdomen is opened by either a low transverse incision (Pfannestiel or muscle cutting Maylard) or by midline vertical incision. The transverse incision gives better exposure to lateral pelvic space.

2. The vagina can be packed with antisceptic soaked Roller gauge to sterilize, paint and elevate the vagina for better dissection.

3. The stomach, liver, omentum, kidneys, intestines and para-aortic lymph nodes are evaluated.

4. The pelvic lymphadenectomy can be done after hysterectomy or before hysterectomy. The round ligament and the infundibulopelvic ligament containing the ovarian vessel are clamped, cut and ligated. The retroperitoneal space is created through broad ligament and the external iliac vessel is identified. The lateral and medial chain of external iliac lymph nodes, and lymphatic cannels are removed and collected for histology. Next, the common iliac lymph glands are looked for and removed till the bifurcation of common iliac vessels. The ureter over the bifurcation is identified and mobilized till the crossing over of the uterine vessels. The uterine artery is traced up to its origin at the anterior division of internal iliac artery or the superior vesical artery where it is ligated. The obliterated hypogastric artery which is the continuation of internal iliac artery in the lower part is identified and the external iliac vein is reflected medially to reach the obturator space which is freed till the obturator nerve entering into the obturator canal is identified. The whole pelvic sidewall is cleared where the obturator lymph glands (rat-tail-shaped) and the hypogastric

lymphatics are removed and collected for histology. **The presacral lymph nodes are never removed** (Fig. 19.41).

5. The **paravesical space** is created which is bounded by:
   a. The obliterated umbilical artery running along the bladder medially
   b. The obturator internus muscle along the pelvic sidewall laterally.
   c. The cardinal ligament posteriorly.
   d. The pubic symphysis anteriorly.

6. The similar step is done on the opposite side

7. The bladder is dissected down below the upper third of the vagina.

8. Similarly, the posterior reflection below the uterosacral ligament is dissected down to separate the posterior vagina from the rectum and **pararectal space** is created which is bounded by:
   a. Rectum medially
   b. Cardinal ligament anteriorly
   c. Hypogastric artery laterally
   d. Sacrum posteriorly.

9. The terminal part of ureter is dissected through the urteric tunnel, the roof of which contains the uterine vessels which are cut and ligated to release the ureter further lateral and down away from the lateral side of the vagina till it enters the bladder. Caution is exercised not to skeletonize the ureter and preserve the blood supply to avoid vascular necrosis and ureteric fistula.

10. The uterosacral ligament (medial half) and then the cardinal ligament (medial half) is clamped, cut and ligated.

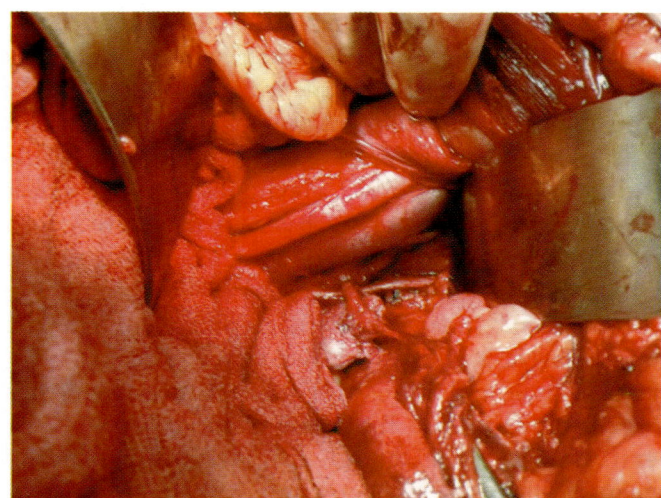

Fig. 19.41: Dissected lateral pelvic space to show big vessels with obturator nerve

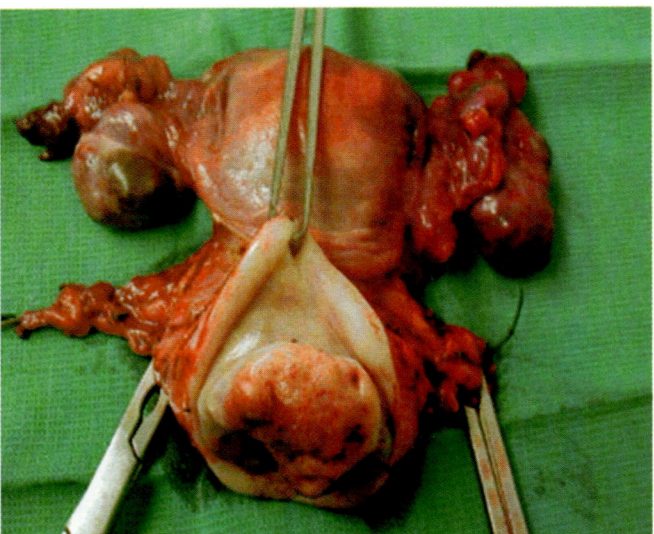

Fig. 19.42: Radical hysterectomy specimen

11. The vagina is entered anteriorly and suitable >2 cm proximal vaginal wall is removed along with the uterus and cervix with the growth.
12. The vault is closed with the open technique suturing the vaginal margins but without closing the vagina keeping a gap to maintain a natural drainage for 48 hours to prevent any postoperative collection.
13. The whole of the specimen along with the lymph nodes are sent for histology (Fig. 19.42).

B. Mitra's Operation (Radical vaginal hysterectomy with bilateral extraperitoneal pelvic lymphadenectomy)

Dr. Subodh Mitra, professor in RG Kar Medical College developed a technique in the surgery of *cervical cancer*. His technique was well appreciated world over. The technique developed by Dr. S Mitra for cancer cervix operation namely *Extended Radical Vaginal Hysterectomy with Extraperitoneal Lymphadenectomy* was officially announced in British, American and German gynecological conferences. He demonstrated this technique in Vienna in 1952. He did the extraperitoneal pelvic lymphadenectomy by two separate groin incisions parallel to inguinal ligament at the junction of lateral 1/3rd and medial 2/3rd of the line joining the umbilicus and anterior iliac spine. The external oblique fascia is incised followed by the muscle belly of transversus abdominis and internal oblique which is cut through to reach the extraperitoneal space. The peritoneum is reflected medially to reach the retroperitoneal space where round ligament, ovarian vessels are identified and cut. The ureter is identified and the lymph nodes are removed along the major

vessels and uterine artery is ligated at the origin. The layers are closed. The vaginal part begins with the circumferential incision in the vagina 2–3 cm below the cervical growth. The proximal inner layers are separated from the distal layers and the dissection is carried till the peritoneum is opened. The parametrium and the uterosacral ligament are clamped, cut and removed maximum and the uterus is removed vaginally.

C. Radical Vaginal Hysterectomy with Bilateral Intraperitoneal Lymphadenectomy

The pelvic lymph nodes are removed through intraperitoneal approach. The round ligament, ovarian ligament, uterine vessels are ligated intraperitoneal with long tie attached to the proximal end of the pedicles. The ureter is identified and dissected to make it free till the terminal end. The anterior and posterior space is created. The abdomen is closed in layers. The vaginal approach begins with circumferential incision in the vaginal wall 2–3 cm below the cervical growth. The proximal vaginal wall with the growth is dissected out from the distal layer of the vagina till the peritoneum is reached. The parametrium and the uterosacrals are clamped, cut and excised at will and the uterus with all the proximal sutures is delivered and removed. The vaginal vault is closed with open cuff closure method.

The vaginal approach has the following advantages over the abdominal approach:
1. The more than two-thirds of the vagina can be removed.
2. The parametrium is also removed more from the lateral pelvic wall.
3. No ureteric dissection is necessary.
4. The complication like bleeding, ureter and bladder injury is less.
5. Postoperative morbidity is much less.

D. Laparoscopic-vaginal Radical Hysterectomy

laparoscopic-vaginal radical hysterectomy (LVRH) for the treatment of FIGO IB disease appears to be a safe and effective alternative to conventional abdominal RH. The lymph node yield after laparoscopic lymph node dissection is comparable to open surgery. There is no significant difference in recurrence rate following LVRH compared to RH (8.5% and 2% respectively). The mean duration of surgery is longer for LVRH compared to abdominal RH. The patients' hospital stay is shorter after LVRH than after RH. The laparoscopic-vaginal radical hysterectomy should not be offered to patients with tumor diameter greater than 2 cm.

Surgical Complications

The most frequent complication of radical hysterectomy is:

1. Urinary dysfunction like retention, overflow incontinence resulting from partial denervation of the detrusor muscle.
2. Shortened vagina.
3. Vesicovaginal or ureterovaginal fistula.
4. Hemorrhage from pelvic vessels
5. Sepsis
6. Bowel obstruction, stricture and fibrosis of the intestine or rectosigmoid colon
7. Rectovaginal fistulas.

Invasive procedures (e.g. nephrostomy or diverting colostomy) sometimes are performed in this group of patients to improve their quality of life.

Radiation Therapy for Cervical Cancer

Radiation therapy, or radiotherapy, is a common way to treat cervical cancer. During radiation therapy, high-energy X-rays are used to kill cancer cells. Radiation therapy can be administered by a machine that aims X-rays at the body (external beam radiation) or by placing small capsules of radioactive material directly into the cervix (internal or implant radiation or brachytherapy). Many patients receive both kinds of radiation therapy. In stage I cervical cancer, radiation therapy may be used instead of surgery, or it may be used after surgery to destroy remaining cancer cells. In stages IB–IVA cervical cancer, radiation therapy is administered concurrently with chemotherapy.

External beam radiation therapy (EBRT) for cervical cancer is administered on an outpatient basis, 5 days a week for 4 to 6 weeks. EBRT begins with a planning session, or simulation, where marks are placed on the body and measurements are taken in order to line up the radiation beam in the correct position for each treatment.

Brachytherapy (Fig. 19.43)

Brachytherapy involves the temporary placement of intrauterine tandem and intravaginal ovoid that are loaded with radioactive material. The devices are placed with the patient under general anesthesia or heavy sedation. Radiopaque vaginal gauze is applied to secure the devices in place and fix their position relative to the bladder and rectum. Intraoperative radiographs or digital fluoroscopic images document appropriate device positioning. Contrast material in a Foley catheter and a rectal tube can be used to identify the International Commission of Radiological Units (ICRU) reference points.

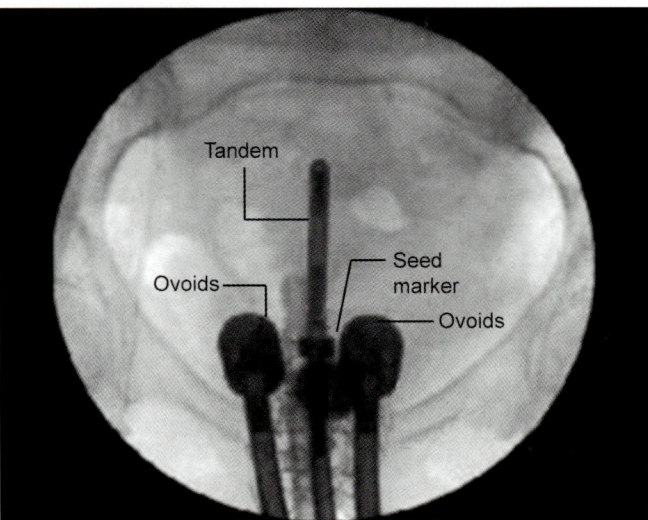

Fig. 19.43: Anteroposterior view of an intrauterine tandem and vaginal ovoids used for low-dose rate brachytherapy. A rectal tube is also seen. A nonradioactive gold seed marker was placed near the cervical os to help in verifying that the flange is in contact with the exocervix

ICRU reference points for gynecologic brachytherapy doses are as follows:

- Point A = 2 cm cephalic to the external os along the tandem and 2 cm perpendicular to the plane of the tandem
- Point B = 2 cm cephalic to the os and 5 cm lateral to the patient's midline
- Bladder point = Most posterior point in the bulb of the Foley catheter along a direct AP line through the center of the bulb
- Rectal point = 0.5 cm posterior to the vaginal mucosa in the patient's midline at the level of the posterior aspect of the ovoid

Doses are prescribed to ICRU points A and B. The reference point of origin for points A and B is the cervical os, which is identified by using a radiopaque flange adjusted and fixed at the time of tandem placement.

Brachytherapy may be performed with low dose rate (LDR) or high dose rate (HDR) applications. LDR is defined as a dose of 0.4–2 Gy per hour and HDR is defined as a dose of greater than 12 Gy per hour. HDR brachytherapy typically involves 5–7 weekly outpatient procedures in which the radioactive source is iridium-192 (^{192}Ir) of high activity. Point A is given a dose of 5–7 Gy during each treatment, which is typically accomplished in less than an hour. LDR brachytherapy usually involves 1 or 2 placement procedures in which the radioactive source is cesium-137 (^{137}Cs). Each time, the sources are left in place for approximately 2 days, during which a dose of 20–40 Gy is administered to point A.

Total combined external-beam and HDR brachytherapy to point A usually is 75–80 Gy, somewhat lower than the total dose of LDR brachytherapy. In the latter, the biologically equivalent total dose to point A is 85–90 Gy.

The advantages of LDR brachytherapy include more than 100 years of safety and efficacy data; standardization of treatment plans, times, and radiation doses; and a requirement for just 2 cesium insertions. Disadvantages of LDR include the need for regional or general anesthesia and inpatient treatment with prolonged bedrest (with a concomitant risk of venous thromboembolism), radiation exposure to staff, and limitations of source strengths.

The advantages of HDR include ease of outpatient treatment with shortened administration times, minimization of staff exposure, the ability to reassess tumor size with each application, and the ability to perform the procedure with the patient under conscious sedation. Disadvantages of HDR, on the other hand, include a higher risk of amplifying dosimetry errors, expense, a need to replace iridium sources frequently, and the need for multiple applications.

Intracavitary brachytherapy devices are sometimes difficult to position because of anatomic distortion due to tumoral infiltration into surrounding structures. In high-stage disease, the vaginal fornices are commonly effaced because tumor erodes the cervix. The lateral distribution of the radiation dose to the parametrium is compromised when ovoids cannot be placed to a level near the cervical os. The net result can be that the devices cannot be appropriately arranged to avoid excessive doses to the bladder and rectal reference points while giving an adequate dose to point A.

One solution is to administer pelvic XRT and brachytherapy in moderately high doses and then perform extrafascial hysterectomy to resect the residual cervical tumor. However, this option is generally not feasible for disease of stage IIB or higher. An alternative is to use interstitial brachytherapy, wherein blind-ended catheters are placed through the perineum into areas of tumor infiltration in the lower pelvis lateral to the cervix.

When the right parametrial tissues are retracted, penetration of the catheter into the peritoneal cavity can be observed. The catheter is then repositioned to avoid exposing its sharp end to the mobile bowel in the low pelvis (Fig. 19.44).

Treatment Combining XRT and Brachytherapy

Comprehensive radiotherapy for stages IB–IVA cervical cancer involves both XRT and brachytherapy. Initial

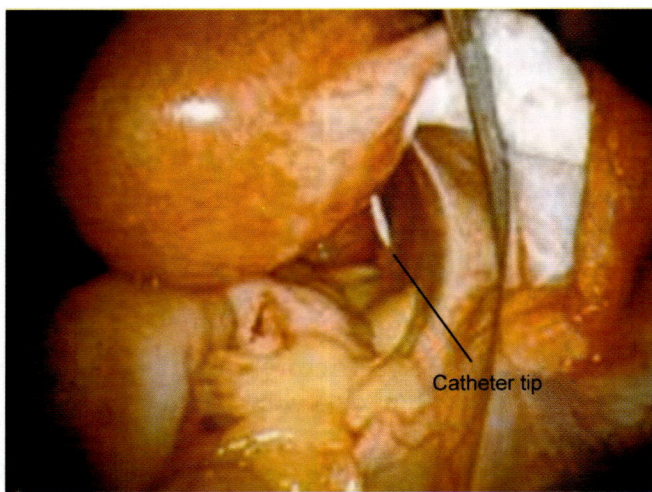

Catheter tip

Fig. 19.44: Laparoscopic view of the pelvis during application of the device for interstitial brachytherapy

external-beam fields encompass a clinical target volume including the primary tumor and the adjacent areas at risk for direct occult invasion or regional lymph node metastases. The superior border is typically placed at L4–L5 interspace.

A typical regimen includes an initial external-beam dose of 40–45 Gy to the pelvis in fractions of 1.8–2 Gy. Cisplatin is usually given weekly at a dose of 40 mg/m² of body surface area, with a maximum weekly dose of 70 mg.

Newer radiation techniques: EBRT can be delivered more precisely to the cervix by using a special CT scan and targeting computer. This capability is known as three-dimensional conformal radiation therapy, or 3D-CRT. The use of 3D-CRT appears to reduce the chance of injury to nearby body structures, such as the bladder or rectum. Since 3D-CRT can better target the area of cancer, radiation oncologists are evaluating whether higher doses of radiation can be given safely and improve the chance of cure.

Preservation of ovarian function: A new procedure that involves the permanent placement of a section (cortical strip) from a patient's ovaries into her forearm may preserve fertility and normal ovarian function in premenopausal women who are treated with radiation to the pelvic area or undergo the removal of their ovaries.

Complications of Therapy

Radiation-related Complications

During the acute phase of pelvic radiation therapy, the surrounding normal tissues (e.g. intestines, bladder, and perineal skin) often are affected. Acute adverse gastrointestinal (GI) effects include diarrhea, abdominal cramping, rectal discomfort, and bleeding. Diarrhea can usually be controlled by giving either loperamide or atropine sulfate. Small steroid-containing enemas are prescribed to alleviate symptoms from proctitis.

Cystourethritis also can occur, leading to dysuria, frequency, and nocturia. Antispasmodics often are helpful for symptom relief. Urine should be examined for possible infection. If urinary tract infection (UTI) is diagnosed, therapy should be instituted without delay.

Proper skin hygiene should be maintained for the perineum. Topical lotion should be used, if erythema or desquamation occurs.

Late sequelae of radiation therapy usually appear 1–4 years after treatment. The major sequelae include rectal or vaginal stenosis, small bowel obstruction, malabsorption, radiation enteritis, and chronic cystitis.

Chemotherapy for Cervical Cancer

1. *As a part of the main treatment:* For some stages of cervical cancer, chemotherapy is given to help the radiation work better. When chemotherapy and radiation therapy are given together, it is called *concurrent chemoradiation*. One option is to give a dose of the drug cisplatin every week during radiation. This drug is given into a vein (IV) about 4 hours before the radiation appointment. Another choice is to give cisplatin along with 5-fluorouracil (5-FU) every 4 weeks during radiation.
2. *To treat cervical cancer that has recurrence after treatment:* Chemotherapy may be used to treat cancers that have spread to other organs and tissues.

Drugs most often used to treat cervical cancer include:
- Cisplatin
- Carboplatin
- Paclitaxel
- Topotecan
- Gemcitabine

Often combinations of these are used.

Some other drugs can be used as well, such as docetaxel, ifosfamide, 5-fluorouracil (5-FU), irinotecan, and mitomycin.

Side Effects

Chemotherapy drugs kill cancer cells but also damage some normal cells, which can lead to certain side effects. Side effects depend on the type of drugs, the amount taken, and the length of time treated. Common side effects of chemotherapy include:
- Nausea and vomiting
- Loss of appetite
- Loss of hair
- Mouth sores
- Fatigue

Because chemotherapy can damage the blood-producing cells of the bone marrow, the blood cell counts might become low. This can result in:
- An increased chance of infection due to leukopenia
- Bleeding or bruising after minor cuts or injuries because of thrombocytopenia
- Shortness of breath due to anemia

Most side effects are short-term and go away after treatment is finished.

Menstrual changes: For younger women, premature menopause and infertility may occur and may be permanent. Patients who have finished treatment with chemotherapy can safely try for pregnancy after 2 years, but it is not safe to get pregnant while on treatment.

Neuropathy: Paclitaxel and cisplatin damage nerves outside of the brain and spinal cord. This *peripheral neuropathy* can sometimes lead to symptoms like numbness, pain, burning or tingling sensations, sensitivity to cold or heat, or weakness. In most cases, this gets better or even goes away once treatment is stopped, but it might last a long time in some women.

Increased risk of leukemia: Very rarely, certain drugs can permanently damage the bone marrow, leading to a disease called *myelodysplastic syndrome* or even acute myeloid leukemia, a life-threatening cancer of white blood cells. It usually occurs within 10 years after treatment.

Prevention of Human Papillomavirus Infection

Human papillomavirus (HPV) infection is usually transmitted sexually, though rare cases have been reported in virgins. Condom use may not prevent transmission.

Evidence suggests that HPV vaccines prevent HPV infection. PATRICIA (PApilloma TRIal against Cancer In young Adults) found HPV 16/18 vaccine to be efficacious against cervical intraepithelial neoplasia (CIN) grade 2 or 3 and adenocarcinoma in situ, irrespective of the HPV type in the lesion. Use of an HPV 6/11/16/18 vaccine reduced the risk of any high-grade cervical lesions by 19.0% overall, irrespective of causal HPV type.

The following 2 HPV vaccines are approved by the US Food and Drug Administration (FDA):
- *Gardasil:* This quadrivalent vaccine is approved for girls and women 9 to 26 years of age to prevent cervical cancer (and also genital warts and anal

cancer) caused by HPV types 6, 11, 16, and 18; it is also approved for males 9 to 26 years of age.

- *Cervarix:* This bivalent vaccine is approved for girls and women 9 through 25 years of age to prevent cervical cancer caused by HPV types 16 and 18.

The Advisory Committee on Immunization Practices (ACIP) recommends routine HPV vaccination of girls aged 11–12 years with 3 doses of either HPV vaccine. The vaccination series can be started as young as age 9 years. Catch-up vaccination is recommended for females aged 13–26 years who have not been previously vaccinated.

Screening for cervical cancer should continue in vaccinated women, following the same guidelines as in unvaccinated women. These vaccines do not provide complete protection against cervical cancer; oncogenic HPV types other than 16 and 18 account for about 30% of cases, and cross-protection may be only partial. In addition, not all vaccinated patients may mount an effective response to the vaccine, particularly if they do not receive all 3 doses or if they get the doses at time intervals that are not associated with efficacy.

Finally, the duration of protection with these vaccines has not yet been determined. The available evidence suggests that immunity from infection with the HPV types covered by these vaccines will persist for at least 6–8 years, but continuing follow-up will be required to determine whether revaccination will be necessary.

The safety of HPV vaccines is a deeply controversial topic. Follow-up of large patient populations who participated in phase 3 clinical trials has documented that both FDA-approved HPV vaccines are extremely safe. Articles in the popular media, however, have detailed cases of young women with devastating illness attributed to the vaccines.

In post-licensure safety surveillance for the quadrivalent HPV vaccine, 6.2% of all reports to the Vaccine Adverse Event Reporting System (VAERS) have described serious adverse events, including neurologic injury (e.g. Guillain-Barré syndrome) and 32 reports of death. In comparison with other vaccines, rates of most of these adverse events are no greater than the background rates, but there are disproportional reporting of syncope and venous thromboembolic events.

Human Papillomavirus Vaccine, Quadrivalent (Gardasil)

The quadrivalent recombinant HPV vaccine is indicated to prevent disorders secondary to infection from HPV types 6, 11, 16, and 18, including cervical cancer, genital warts (condylomata acuminata), and the following precancerous genital lesions:

- Cervical adenocarcinoma in situ
- Cervical intraepithelial neoplasia (CIN) grades 1, 2, and 3
- Vulvar intraepithelial neoplasia grades 2 and 3
- Vaginal intraepithelial neoplasia grades 2 and 3

The efficacy of the vaccine is mediated by humoral immune responses following the immunization series.

Dose

9–26 years: 0.5 mL IM × 3 doses administered at 0, 2, and 6 months.

Human Papillomavirus Vaccine, Bivalent (Cervarix)

The bivalent recombinant HPV vaccine is prepared from the L1 protein of HPV types 16 and 18. It is indicated for girls and women (ages 9–25 years) to prevent the following diseases caused by oncogenic HPV types 16 and 18:

- Cervical cancer
- CIN grade 2 or higher
- Cervical adenocarcinoma in situ
- CIN grade 1

CDC Recommendations

- Girls and women aged 9–26 years: 0.5 mL IM for 3 doses administered at schedule of 0, 2, and 6 months.
- CDC recommends routine vaccination for females at age 11 or 12 years with either HPV2 or HPV4; may begin vaccination series as early as age 9 years.
- CDC recommends routine vaccination for females at age 13–26 years with either HPV2 or HPV4, if not previously vaccinated.
- If age 26 years is reached before vaccination series completed, remaining doses can be administered after age 26 years.

Scottish Guidelines (NHS) of Cancer Cervix

1. *Signs and symptoms* of cancer cervix are: (a) Intermenstrual bleeding, (b) postcoital bleeding, (c) postmenopausal bleeding, (d) abnormal cervix, (e) vaginal discharge, (f) pelvic pain.
2. *Tumor markers:* Squamous cell carcinoma antigen (SCCA) belongs to a family of serine and cysteine protease inhibitors. The antigen is present in normal squamous cervical epithelium and its expression is increased in cervical squamous

cancers. Pre-treatment levels of SCCA are related to tumor volume but are not reliable to identify patients at risk of having pelvic node metastasis or parametrial involvement.

3. *Primary tumor assessment:* There is consistent evidence that MRI is more accurate than CT for radiological staging of cervical carcinoma and both are more accurate than clinical staging. USG is not generally reliable in either assessment of primary tumor size or nodal status. PET-CT can assess both the primary tumor and detect metastatic spread. It has potential for more accurately selecting patients for surgery than PET imaging alone in addition to contributing to more accurate treatment planning.

4. *Bladder and rectal invasion:* Assessment of bladder and rectal invasion is more accurate with CT and MRI than clinical staging with the specificity of MRI considerably greater than CT. A normal appearance of bladder and rectum on MRI obviates the need for cystoscopy or sigmoidoscopy. Intravenous urography (IVU) is a stand-alone investigation and is as accurate as CT/MRI in determining ureteric obstruction secondary to parametrial invasion. Barium enema is not routinely indicated.

5. *Pelvic and para-aortic lymph nodes:* Although not a part of FIGO staging criteria, the involvement of pelvic or para-aortic lymph nodes is the greatest single predictor of long-term survival. Lymphangiography is not routinely available in many radiology and is probably less sensitive than CT/MRI for assessment of lymph node involvement. PET-CT scan is perhaps the most accurate imaging method of detecting involved lymph nodes with the sensitivity of 75% and 100% respectively.

6. *Chest X-ray:* CT scan is more accurate than chest X-ray in identifying pleural effusion, thoracic nodal status and parenchymal metastases. Routine chest X-ray is not indicated in women with operable disease (FIGO 1A,1A2,1B1)

7. Cystoscopy and sigmoidoscopy should not be routinely performed for staging purpose. It is done only when imaging cannot exclude bladder or bowel involvement. USG, IVU, lymphangiography are not recommended for staging.

8. *Radical hysterectomy(RH):* Radical surgery is recommended for FIGO IB1 disease, if there is no contraindication to surgery. RH is not recommended, if tumor measures more than 4 cm to reduce the likelihood of using post-surgery chemoradiation.

9. *Treatment of cervical cancer after subtotal hysterectomy:* The incidence of cervical cancer in women who have had subtotal hysterectomy is no different to that in women with an intact cervix. And, therefore, it is managed in the same way a cervical cancer arising from intact cervix. (Grader C)

10. *Treatment of early stage (FIGOIA1/IA2):* Removal of pelvic lymph nodes is not recommended during treatment for FIGO IA1 disease. Pelvic lymph nodes should be removed, if FIGO IA2 disease is present. In FIGOIA2 with LVSI, decision for lymphadenectomy should be individualized taking into account of the pattern and extent of invasion.

11. *Fertility conservation surgery:* Standard treatment for IA1 disease is simple hysterectomy, if fertility is not an issue. For IA2 it is simple hysterectomy with pelvic node dissection. For IB2 it is radical hysterectomy with pelvic lymphadencetomy. In women where preservation of fertility is desirable, an alternative is radical trachelectomy. This involves vaginal resection of cervix, upper 1–2 cm of the vaginal cuff and medial portion of the cardinal and uterosacral ligaments. The cervix is transected at the lower uterine segment and a prophylactic encirclage is placed at the time of surgery. Radical trachelectomy does not appear to increase the rate of recurrence provided the tumor diameter is not greater than 2 cm and there is no evidence of LVSI (Grade C). It must be combined with pelvic lymph node dissection for IA2 and IB1 disease. Following radical trachelectomy, patient can conceive spontaneously and deliver near term. Women with early stage disease with no LVSI requesting fertility cold knife conization ot LLETZ combined with pelvic node dissection is recommended.

12. *Laparoscopic vaginal radical hysterectomy:* LVRH for treatment of FIGO IB1 disease appears to be safe and effective alternative to conventional abdominal RH. Its lymph node yield is comparable to open surgery. It should not be offered to patients with tumor diameter greater than 2 cm.

13. *Concurrent chemoradiation:* Any patient with cervical cancer considered suitable for radical radiotherapy treatment should have concurrent chemoradiation with cisplatin. Patients who have undergone surgery for cervical cancer and have positive nodes should be considered for concurrent chemoradiation with cisplatin.

14. *Negative lymph nodes:* Patients who have undergone surgery for cervical cancer with negative nodes but

with the risk factors like (a) greater than one-third stromal invasion, (b) evidence of LVSI, (c) tumor diameter of >4 cm should be considered for adjuvant treatment with radiotherapy.

15. *Radiation-induced cystitis and proctitis:* Patients with late radiation affected cystitis should be treated symptomatic under supervision of urologist. Rectal sucralfate may be considered to reduce late radiation-induced proctitis.

16. *Hormone replacement therapy:* HRT is recommended for women who have lost ovarian function as a result of treatment for cervical cancer.

17. *Treatment of cancer cervix with pregnancy:* For pregnant women diagnosed with cervical cancer before 16 weeks immediate treatment is recommended. For pregnant women with early stage disease (FIGO IA1,IA2,IB) diagnosed after 16 weeks of gestation treatment may be delayed to allow fetal maturity to occur. For advanced disease (FIGO IB2 or greater) diagnosed after 16 weeks consideration for delay must be based on gestational age at the time of diagnosis. (Grade C)

18. *Lymphedema:* It presents as a swelling of one or both lower limbs as a complication of lymphatic obstruction in cancer cervix. Hysterectomy with pelvic node dissection for early stage cancer is associated with 7–14% incidence of swelling. It can occur following radiotherapy treatment alone. The incidence of lymphedema following pelvic node dissection and radiotherapy for FIGO IB/IIA is around 19% at one year and 12% at five years. Diagnosis is made by (a) increase in circumference of the limb, (b) feeling of sensations like fullness, tightness, heaviness, throbbing, shooting pains, (c) reduced flexibility in the limb and (d) palpable changes in the skin or subcutaneous tissue such as fibrosclerosis that may be pitting or nonpitting. Lymphedema often occurs in the first two years following cancer treatment. Swelling subsides on elevation at early stage but may become chronic with skin and tissue changes including thickening, skin folds and fat deposits. Cancer recurrence should be considered in patients with new onset lymphedema. The possibility of deep venous thrombosis should also be kept in mind. Expert opinion supports the use of conservative physical therapy in lymphedema management. This includes decongestive lymphatic therapy (DLT) with compression bandaging, and manual lymphatic drainage (MLD) massage combined with lymphedema hosiery, skin care and exercise. Patients with lymphedema should be trained to self-management under supervision of an expert. These are: (a) taking care of skin and nails and avoiding fungal infection, (b) maintaining optimal body weight, (c) avoiding injury to affected limbs including scratches and insect bites, (d) avoiding temperature extremes, (e) protecting limbs from the skin and (f) wearing comfortable supportive shoes.

19. *Follow-up:* History taking and clinical examination should be carried out during follow-up of patients with cervical cancer to detect symptomatic and asymptomatic recurrence. Cervical cytology or vault smears are not indicated to detect asymptomatic recurrence of cervical cancer. Patients should be followed up every four months for at least two years. Patients with early stage disease who have had fertility conserving surgery should have a smear at six months, 12 months and annually for four years before being returned to cervical screening program. MRI/CT should be considered initially to assess potential clinical recurrence in symptomatic patients. A whole body PET scan or PET-CT should be performed on all patients in whom recurrent or persistent disease has been demonstrated on MRI or CT in whom salvage therapy is being considered. A PET-CT scan at nine months of follow-up is recommended in women who have had chemoradiotherapy. The routine use of SCCA to determine disease recurrence is not recommended.

20. *Management of recurrent disease:* The survival period for patients with recurrent disease is six months to two years. Therapeutic options for those patients with cervical cancer whose first-line treatment has failed include: (a) surgery (salvage), (b) chemotherapy and (c) palliative treatment only if further surgery or chemotherapy is not appropriate. Pelvic exanteration should be reserved a salvage therapy for women with recurrent cervical cancer in the central pelvis whose chemotherapy has failed. Palliative chemotherapy should be offerd to women with FIGO stage IVB or recurrent cervical carcinoma with (i) Cisplatin 50 mg/m^2 on day 1 plus Topotecan 0.75 mg/m^2 on days 1 to 3 every 3 weeks or (ii) Cisplatin 50 mg/m^2 on day 1 plus Paclitaxel 135 mg/m^2 every 3 weeks.

Complications and Management

1. *Fistula:* It may occur as a late complication of radiotherapy with a mean latency period of 17 months to 5 years or as a result of progressive disease. Radiation dose and dose distribution are the main

risk factors for the development of post-radiation rectovaginal fistula. The symptoms include: (a) persistent continuous watery discharge, (b) continuous feculant discharge with pneumaturia. Patients with advanced disease RVF are seldom able to undergo surgery to attempt repair due to incurable nature of the condition. The appropriate non-surgical treatments include: (a) octreotide or glycopyrronium to reduce volume of discharge, (b) loperamide to firm stool, (c) barrier cream to protect the perineal skin, (d) topical steroid like prednisolone foam enema administered vaginally for local effect, (e) vaginal moulds, (f) tampons and (g) low residue diet.

2. *Pain control:* In advanced cancer cervix, it is appropriate to (a) have nerve-blocking procedures along with analgesic drugs, (b) spinal therapy using opioids, local anesthetics, clonidine to provide regional blockade for neuropathic pain from metastatic disease in the spine or pelvis, (c) percutaneous cementoplasty for painful lytic bone metastatic disease of the pubic ramus or acetabulum, if pain is refractory to conservative treatment.

3. *Renal failure:* In advanced cancer, cervix has post-renal etiology from lymphadenopathy or direct tumor invasion. Ureteric obstruction may initially produce no biochemical evidence of impaired renal function but if left untreated will lead to renal failure. Therefore, the initial management include (a) initial no treatment, (b) percutaneous nephrostomy (PCN), (c) retrograde stenting. PCN can substitute a peaceful uremic death for a painful poor quality life with minimal improved survival. Internal stent fails in at least one-third of patients within six months. Stent failure is indicated by 50% rise in creatinine level, pain, infection or hydronephrosis. If retrograde stent is unsuccessful, PCN/or antegrade stent may be a successful alternative. Retrograde ureteric stent should be changed according to the level of ureteric obstruction ranging from 3–12 months. Urinary diversion may be considered in suitable patients.

4. *Deep venous thrombosis:* Risk factors for thrombosis include: (a) presence of pelvic masses which compress large veins, (b) impaired mobility, (c) effect of treatment. The diagnosis of DVT is usually made clinically but in mobile patient whole blood D-dimer testing or USG scanning may be appropriate but this should not delay the initiation of anti-thrombolysis therapy in clinically diagnosed cases. Treatment with LMWH is shown to be more effective than oral anticoagulant in reducing risk of recurrent thromboprophylaxis without increasing ther risk of bleeding. The duration of therapy should be considered on individual basis. Compression garments in conjunction with LMWH and early walking exercises should be considered in patients with DVT.

5. *Hemorrhage:* Relapsed cervical cancer can present with vaginal bleeding and massive hemorrhage. Bladder or bowel invasion may cause hematuria or rectal bleeding.

   i. If a minor hemorrhage occurs, (a) systemic cause of bleeding like thrombocytopenia, antiplatelet drug effect must be excluded, (b) to stop any offending drugs whick can excite bleeding, (c) fibrinolytic inhibitors like tranexamic acid or aminocaproic acid can be administered, (d) antibiotics should be considered, if sepsis is present and (e) hemostatic dose of radiotherapy.

   ii. The aim of treatment is to relieve patient distress by (a) midazolam or dimorphine to sedate the mother from anxiety and (b) adequate blood component replacement therapy.

6. *Malodorous discharge:* This reflects advanced cancer cervix with adverse impact on body image, sense of worth and self as a social being. This is usually due to breakdown of cancerous tissue causing loss of fluid from a necrotic tumor along with superadded infection or from erosion of the bowel or urinary tract causing leakage of feces or urine. Management should be tailored to treat infection, reduce fluid loss, colostomy or urinary diversion as the case may require to maximize the quality of life.

7. *Mental depression:* Psychological support must be offered throughout the management. Women should be assessed for support needs in relation to dependants in their care.

Ovarian Lesions

20A. BENIGN OVARIAN NEOPLASM

WHO Classification of Ovarian Neoplasms

The World Health Organization histological classification for ovarian tumors separates ovarian neoplasms according to the most probable tissue of origin: Surface epithelial (65%), germ cell (15%), sex cord-stromal (10%), metastases (5%), miscellaneous.

Ovarian epithelial tumors are classified according to the following histological subtypes:

- Serous
- Mucinous
- Endometrioid
- Clear cell
- **Brenner**
- Transitional cell
- Small cell
- Mixed mesodermal
- Undifferentiated.

Usually each subtype can be classified as benign, borderline (low malignant potential, LMP), or malignant (invasive).

Serous tumors are further subdivided into the following:
- Serous cystadenoma
- Borderline serous tumor
- Serous cystadenocarcinoma
- Adenofibroma
- Cystadenofibroma

Mucinous tumors are further classified as:
- Mucinous cystadenoma
- Borderline mucinous tumor
- Mucinous cystadenocarcinoma
- Adenofibroma

Endometrioid tumors
- Benign (cystadenoma)
- Borderline tumors (endometrioid borderline tumor)
- Malignant (endometrioid adenocarcinoma)

Clear cell tumors
- Benign
- Borderline tumors
- Malignant (clear cell adenocarcinoma)

Transitional cell tumors
- Brenner tumor
- Brenner tumor of borderline malignancy
- Malignant Brenner tumor
- Transitional cell carcinoma (non-Brenner type)

Epithelial-stromal tumors
- Adenosarcoma
- Carcinosarcoma (formerly mixed müllerian tumors)

Sex cord-stromal tumors
Granulosa tumors:
- Fibromas
- Fibrothecomas
- Thecomas

Sertoli cell tumors
- Leydig cell tumors
- Sex cord tumor with annular tubules

- Gynandroblastoma
- Steroid (lipid) cell tumors

Germ cell tumors
Teratoma:
- Immature
- Mature
- Solid
- Cystic (dermoid cyst)

- Monodermal (e.g. struma ovarii, carcinoid)
- Dysgerminoma
- Yolk sac tumor (endodermal sinus tumor)
- Mixed germ cell tumors

Malignant, not otherwise specified
Metastatic cancer from nonovarian primary:
- Colonic, appendiceal
- Gastric
- Breast

Embryogenesis

Cells from adjacent transient embryonic structures, known as mesonephros, concurrently invade the mesenchyme and the primordial germ cells arrive after a long journey that starts at their place of origin in the yolk sac and takes the cells along the distal embryonic intestine and the posterior wall of the embryonic body cavity. The different tumor types that arise in the ovary are linked to the different cell types that are present at this stage of development—coelomic epithelial, mesenchymal, mesonephric, and germ cells (Fig. 20.1).

The coelomic epithelium remains at the periphery, enwrapping the developing ovary. In the adult, the ovaries are flat, nodular, oval structures that measure between 3 and 5 cm in their greatest dimension and weigh between 2 and 4 g. They are suspended by peritoneal folds and ligaments on either side of the uterus and attached to the back of the broad ligament of the uterus, behind and below the uterine tubes. A single layer of cells, the surface epithelium, which is derived from the coelomic epithelium, lines their external surface. A dense, fibrous tissue, the stroma, which is derived from the mesenchyme, makes up most of their internal substance. The germ cells, also known as oocytes, are located near the periphery of the stroma. The granulosa cells, specialized cells of probable mesonephric origin that are derived from the sex cords, surround the germinal cells that form the follicles. The stroma immediately surrounding the follicles differentiates into plum elongated cells known as theca cells. When stimulated, theca cells accumulate abundant lipids in their cytoplasm by a process known as luteinization. The ovary also contains hilus cells (which are identical to a type of testicular cells known as Leydig cells) that specialize in hormone production. The rete ovarii, a network of cellular cords and tubes, is similar to a testicular structure known as the rete testis.

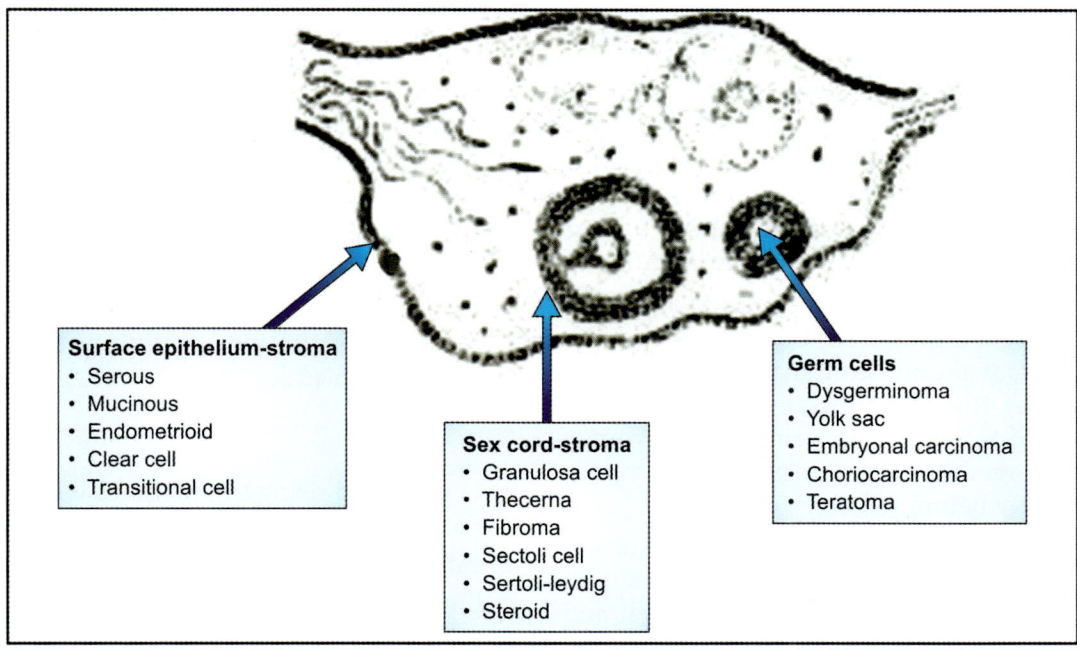

Fig. 20.1: Origins of the three main types of ovarian tumors

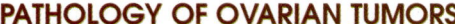

PATHOLOGY OF OVARIAN TUMORS

Most tumors of the ovary can be placed into one of three major categories—surface epithelial-stromal tumors, sex cord-stromal tumors, and germ cell tumors according to the anatomic structures from which the tumors presumably originate (Fig. 20.1).

The ovarian surface epithelium is histologically similar to the mesothelium, which is the epithelium that lines the interior of the pelvic and abdominal cavities. This similarity, as well as the close morphologic resemblance of ovarian epithelial-stromal tumors to some epithelial tumors arising elsewhere within the pelvis and abdomen, may be explained by the shared origin (i.e. the primitive coelomic epithelium) of the ovarian surface epithelium and the mesothelium.

The sex cord-stromal group includes tumors of mesenchymal and mesonephric origin. Some of these tumors, namely fibromas and thecomas, have a fibrous appearance, and some appear to be derived from the granulosa cells or their testicular sex cord counterparts, the Leydig and Sertoli cells.

The ovarian germ cells are the origin of a number of tumors that are identical to testicular germ cell tumors. Germ cells that are stranded or have gone astray during their migration between the yolk sac and the developing gonads may develop into germ cell tumors outside the gonads.

Surface Epithelial-Stromal Tumors

Surface epithelial-stromal tumors are believed to originate from the surface epithelium of the ovary. They are classified as **benign** if they lack exuberant cellular proliferation and invasive behavior; as **borderline** (also known as atypically proliferating or of low malignant potential) if there is exuberant cellular proliferation but no invasive behavior; and as **malignant** if there is invasive behavior. Surface epithelial-stromal tumors account for approximately 60% of all ovarian tumors and approximately 90% of malignant ovarian tumors.

Most borderline tumors behave clinically as benign tumors and have good prognosis, but some may recur after surgical removal and some may seed extensive implants within the abdominal cavity. Surface epithelial-stromal tumors occur primarily in women who are middle-aged or older and are rare in young adults, particularly before puberty.

Five major subtypes are included within the surface epithelial-stromal group. They are designated as follows: Serous, mucinous, endometrioid, clear cell, and transitional cell (or Brenner type). Highly malignant epithelial-stromal tumors lacking any specific differentiation are classified as undifferentiated. Epithelial stromal tumors that are not designated as having a specific subtype commonly are recorded as adenocarcinomas not otherwise specified (NOS).

Serous or mucinous tumors identical to those occurring in the ovary may arise in multiple locations within the pelvic and abdominal cavities. They sometimes coincide with ovarian tumors of identical type. When they do so, it may be difficult to establish whether the extraovarian sites represent seedlings or implants originating from the ovarian tumor or *de novo* malignancies. By convention, when the ovaries appear to be incidentally involved and do not appear to be the primary origin of the tumor, the tumor is recorded as an extraovarian peritoneal carcinoma.

Clinical Features of Benign Ovarian Neoplasm

Symptoms

a. Majority the patients remain asymptomatic in the initial stages unless the tumour mass is very enlarged.
b. Vague GI symptoms like nausea, dyspepsia, bloating sensation, loss of appetite, indigestion.
c. Pain abdomen due to enlargement of the cyst or tumor or pressure effects. Pain may be acute and severe in case of complications like torsion, intracystic hemorrhage, infection, adhesion, perforation and malignancy.
d. Pressure symptoms like retention of urine, frequency, urgency, stress incontinence or bowel disturbances like constipation, intestinal obstruction.

Signs

a. General condition may be cachectic in very large mucinous cystadenomas.
b. Pallor may be related to hemorrhage, malignancy.
c. Tachycardia due to torsion, hemorrhage, perforation, adhesion pain and malignancy.
d. Any other intra-abdominal mass like hepato-splenomegaly, GB lump, ileocecal lump, mesenteric lump, lymphadenopathy, enlarged kidneys, distended bladder, etc.

Examination of the Ovarian Mass

a. Leg or head rising test to assess whether the mass is parietal or intra-abdominal
b. Bilateral or unilateral
c. Oval in shape
d. Smooth surface
e. Cystic or solid in feel

f. Mobile in all directions
g. Tender or nontender
h. Well-defined margins
i. Easily can reach lower pole of the mass
j. Any fluid thrill or shifting dullness to assess for ascites.

On PV Examination

a. Uterus is normal in size and separate from the mass; fixity to the mass is assessed   and the Hingorani's groove is diagnostic.
b. Ovarian mass unilateral or bilateral is felt through the respective fornices.
c. Assess surface, mobility, size, shape, volume, feel of the mass.
d. Pouch of douglas-nodule/fixity of the mass to the vault/anterior or posterior vagina/fullness/tenderness/ shallowness.

PR examination or rectovaginal examination to rule out rectal involvement or any possibility of retroperitoneal mass.

Serous Tumors (Fig. 20.2)

Serous tumors are epithelial-stromal tumors formed by cells that resemble those of the internal lining of the fallopian tube. Benign serous tumors are thin-walled cysts formed by a single chamber filled with a watery, straw-colored fiuid. The internal lining of the cyst is usually flat but may display a few coarse papillary projections (Fig. 20.3). Benign serous tumors account for approximately one-quarter of all benign ovarian neoplasms and two-thirds of all ovarian serous tumors.

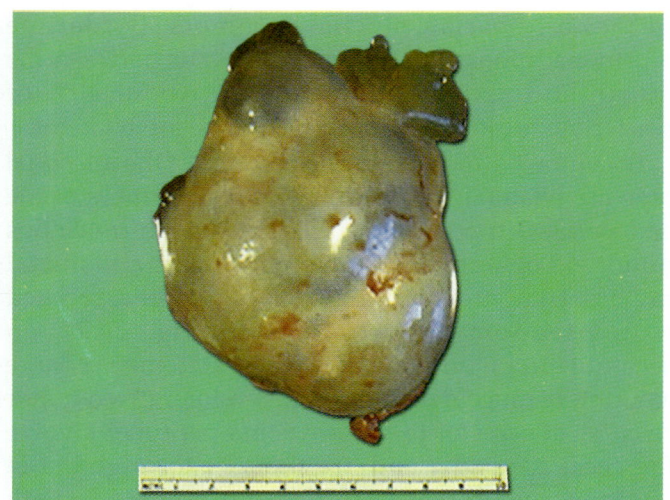

Fig. 20.2: Serous cystadenoma, filled with pale yellow serous fluid in a single cavity

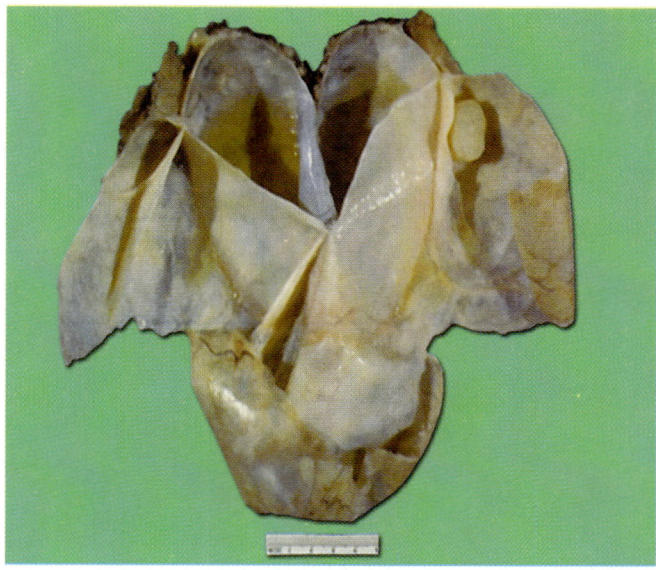

Fig. 20.3: Benign serous cystadenoma that demonstrates multiloculation. Note that the inner surf ace is, for the most par t, smooth, with only a solitary papillation at the upper right

Benign serous tumors most frequently occur between the fourth and fifth decades of life. In up to 20% of patients, benign serous tumors are bilateral, occurring simultaneously in both ovaries.

Pathogenesis

Serous tumors are characterized by a proliferation of epithelium resembling that lining the fallopian tubes. They are virtually all cystic, are most commonly seen in women in their 40s and 50s, and are bilateral in 15–20% of cases.

Compared with benign tumors, borderline serous tumors have more exuberant and finer papillary projections within the cyst cavity (Fig. 20.4). Similar projections also may occur on the external surface of the tumor. Small tumorlets with similar features may be found elsewhere on the internal lining of the pelvic and abdominal cavities in up to 40% of patients. In most cases, these tumorlets do not progress, but they occasionally display invasive behavior. Borderline serous tumors account for 10–15% of all ovarian serous tumors. Most studies show that on average, borderline serous tumors are diagnosed in the fifth decade of life. Up to one-third of these tumors are bilateral.

The malignant counterpart of this type of cyst is termed serous cystadenocarcinoma.

Mucinous Tumors

Mucinous tumors are epithelial ovarian tumors formed by cells that resemble either those of the endocervical epithelium (endocervical or müllerian type) or, more

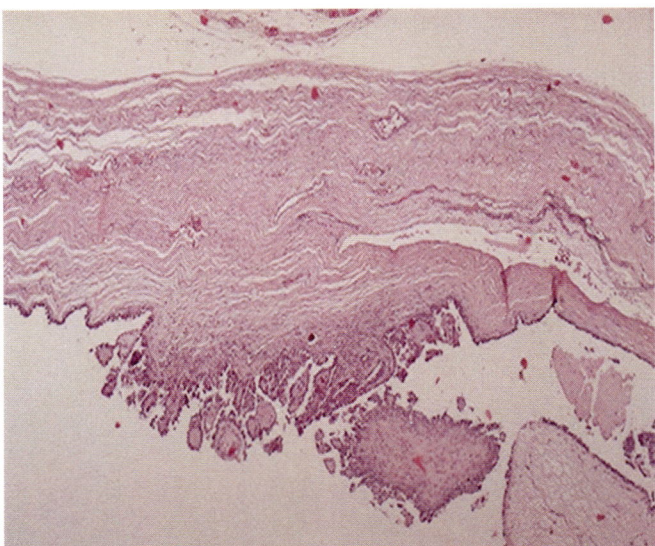

Fig. 20.4: Microscopically, a borderline serous cystadenoma is seen here with papillary projections of epithelium extending into the lumen of the tumor. There is no invasion of the stroma or capsule

frequently, those of the intestinal epithelium (intestinal type).

Benign mucinous tumors are multiloculated cysts (Fig. 20.5) that are filled with opaque, thick, mucoid material. They account for up to one-fourth of all benign ovarian neoplasms and 75–85% of all mucinous ovarian tumors. Benign mucinous tumors most frequently occur between the third and fifth decades of life. They often present as a huge mass covering whole of the abdomen making the patient grossly cachectic (Fig. 20.6).

- Somewhat less common, it accounts for about 25% of all ovarian neoplasms.
- Occur principally in middle adult life and are rare before puberty and after menopause.
- 80% are benign or borderline and about 15% are malignant.

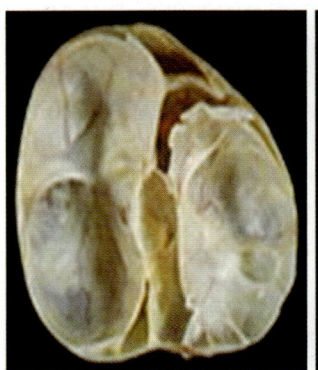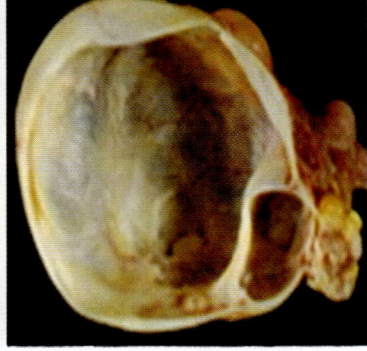

Fig. 20.5: Macroscopic picture of benign mucinous multiloculated cyst

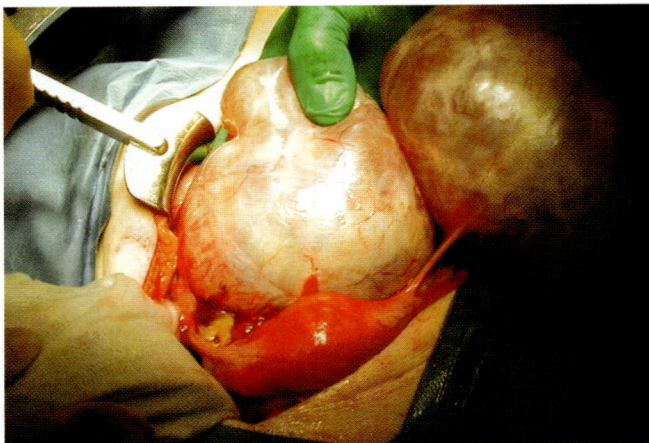

Fig. 20.6: Benign mucinous cystadenoma

- Mucinous cystadenocarcinomas (the malignant form of this tumor) are relatively uncommon and account for only 10% of all ovarian cancers.
- Mucinous tumors are characterized by more cysts of variable size and a rarity of surface involvement as compared to serous tumors.
- Also in comparison to serous tumors, mucinous tumors are less frequently bilateral, approximately 5% of primary mucinous tumors are bilateral.
- May form very large cystic masses, with recorded weights exceeding 25 kg.
- Appear as multiloculated tumors filled with sticky, gelatinous fluid.

Brief Features

Upon gross pathologic examination, borderline mucinous tumors are similar to benign mucinous tumors but may have solid regions and exhibit papillae projecting into the cyst chambers. They make up 10–14% of all ovarian mucinous tumors. Borderline mucinous tumors most frequently occur between the fourth and sixth decades of life. About 40% of borderline tumors of endocervical type are bilateral.

In contrast, 10% of borderline tumors of the intestinal type are bilateral. Borderline mucinous tumors of the endocervical type may be associated with mucinous tumorlets or implants in the pelvic and abdominal cavities. Tumors of the intestinal type may be associated with **pseudomyxoma peritonei** (Fig. 20.7), an accumulation within the pelvis and abdomen of large amounts of mucoid material with few intermixed tumor cells. Most cases of pseudomyxoma peritonei involve the cecal appendix and are thought to originate in mucinous tumors that are primary to the appendix with secondary involvement of the ovaries. Pseudomyxoma peritonei also may be associated with malignant

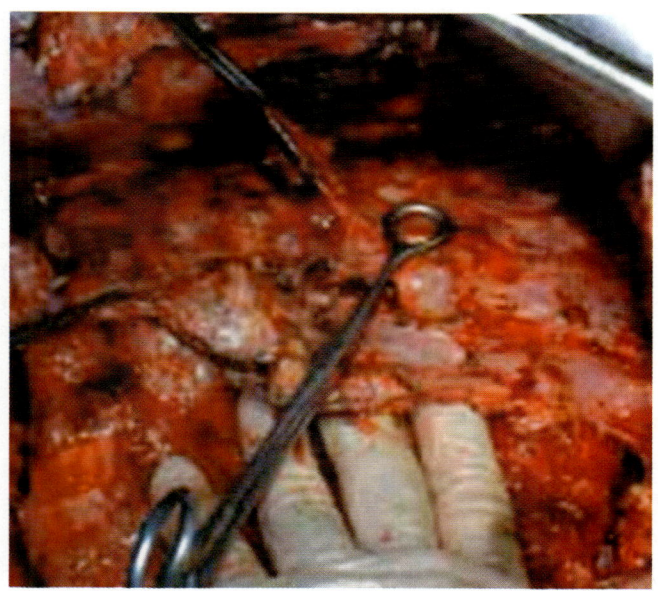

Fig. 20.7: Pseudomyxoma peritonei

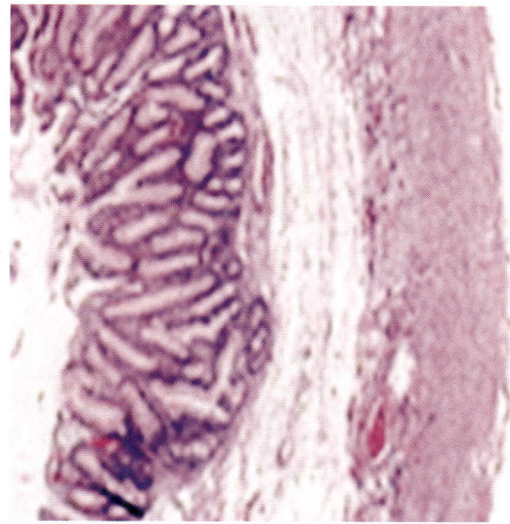

Fig. 20.8: The epithelial lining of ovarian mucinous tumors may resemble that seen in endocervix, gastric pylorus, or intestine. The glands in this mucinous cystadenoma are lined by a single layer of intestinal epithelium

ovarian mucinous neoplasms, and its presence does not indicate dissemination. Treatment of borderline mucinous tumors is surgical. Tumor recurrence and metastatic disease are rare. Five-year survival rates are reported to be between 51 and 92%, depending on disease stage. Pseudomyxoma peritonei follows a relentless and protracted course. Treatment involves the removal of as much tumor as possible followed by abdominal taps to remove fluid and alleviate symptoms. Sometimes this may need chemotherapy to prevent recurrences and is considered a tumor of low malignant potential.

Compared with borderline tumors, malignant mucinous tumors may contain more papillary projections within the cyst cavities, larger solid areas, and larger areas of necrosis and hemorrhage. Malignant mucinous tumors (mucinous cystadenocarcinoma) represent 5–10% of all malignant ovarian neoplasms.

Endocervical-like mucinous borderline tumors (EMBT) account for approximately 15% of mucinous borderline tumors. They are seen in some-what younger age-group than intestinal type and often associated with endometriosis. They show papillary architecture with atypical cells lining stromal papillae.

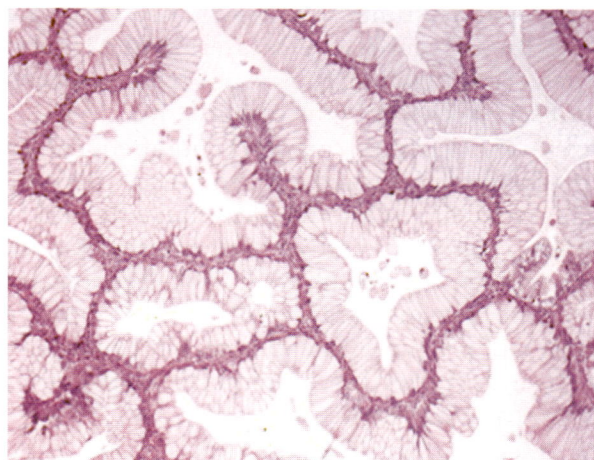

Fig. 20.9: Glandular lumens are complex sho wing papillary infoldings in mucinous cystadenoma of intestinal type

Microscopic Picture (Figs 20.8 to 20.10)

1. Tall, columnar, nonciliated cells, basal nuclei, abundant intracellular mucin.
2. Usually endocervical type; also intestinal type (picket fence architecture with Paneth cells) or mixed
3. Stroma may be fibrous or mimic ovarian stroma.

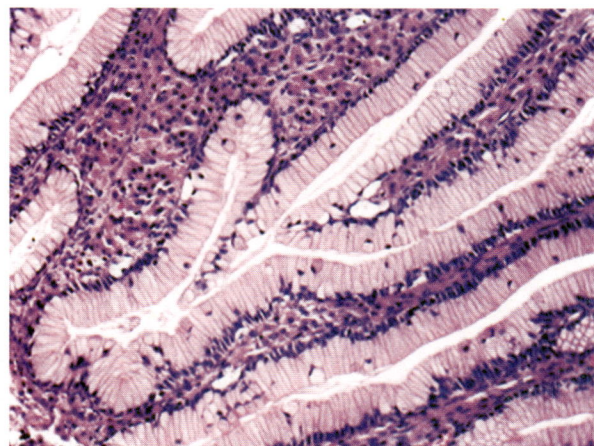

Fig. 20.10: Case of mucinous borderline tumor of the o vary. The focus with borderline morphology shows moderate nuclear atypia and occasional mitotic figures

4. Tumor may be hypercellular or luteinized, often with calcifications.
5. May have microscopic rupture of cysts with inflammatory reaction including histocytes and necrosis.
6. Small bland papillae may be present, and mild, focal cytologic atypia may be present.
7. Adenofibroma may have crowded glands with atypia.

Endometrioid Tumors (Fig. 20.11)

Endometrioid tumors account for approximately 20% of all ovarian cancers and are mostly malignant (endometrioid carcinomas). They are made of tubular glands bearing a close resemblance to benign or malignant endometrium. 15–30% of endometrioid carcinomas occur in individuals with carcinoma of the endometrium, and these patients have a better prognosis. They appear similar to other surface epithelial-stromal tumors, with solid and cystic areas. 40% of these tumors are bilateral. They may be associated with endometriosis and with endometrial hyperplasia or cancer of the endometrium.

Benign endometrioid tumors occur infrequently and are predominantly cystic and unilateral. Borderline endometrioid tumors also are predominantly cystic and unilateral, but they often exhibit internal papillary projections. They represent one-fifth of all endometrioid ovarian neoplasms. Treatment of these tumors is surgical and prognosis is excellent. On average, both benign and borderline endometrioid tumors are diagnosed in the sixth decade of life.

Pathology

- Glands bearing a strong resemblance to endometrial-type glands:
  - Benign tumors have mature-appearing glands in a fibrous stroma.
  - Borderline tumors have a complex branching pattern without stromal invasion.
  - Malignant tumors have invasive glands with crowded, atypical cells, frequent mitoses and with poorer differentiation, the tumor becomes more solid.

Prognosis

Prognosis is dependent on the spread and differentiation of the tumor. The overall prognosis is somewhat worse than for serous or mucinous tumors, and the 5-year survival rate for patients with tumors confined to the ovary is approximately 75%.

Clear Cell Tumors (Fig. 20.12)

Clear cell tumors are epithelial ovarian tumors that are formed by clear, peg-like or hobnail-like cells. Benign and borderline clear cell tumors are quite rare. They are characterized by large epithelial cells with abundant clear cytoplasm and may be seen in association with endometriosis or endometrioid carcinoma of the ovary, bearing a resemblance to clear cell carcinoma of the endometrium. They may be predominantly solid or cystic. If solid, the clear cells tend to be arranged in sheets or tubules. In the cystic variety, the neoplastic cells make up the cyst lining.

Most clear cell ovarian tumors are malignant. Clear cell tumors represent 4–5% of all malignant ovarian epithelial tumors. On average, diagnosis occurs in the fifth decade of life. Two-thirds of all women with malignant clear cell tumors have never given birth and 50–70% have endometriosis.

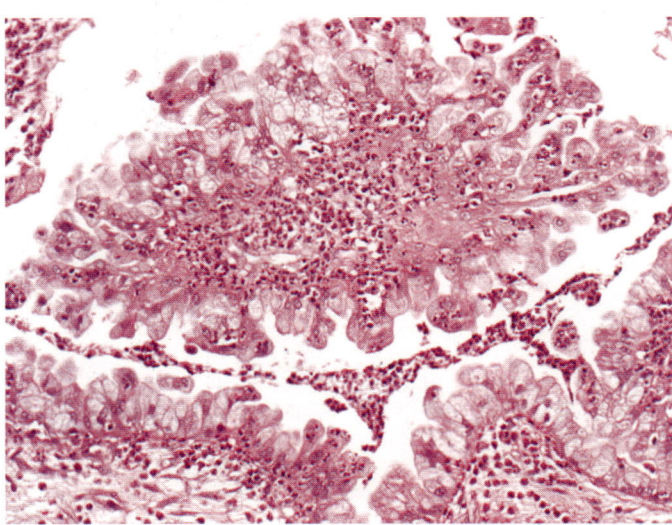

Fig. 20.11: Endometrioid borderline tumour (EMBT)—microscopic picture

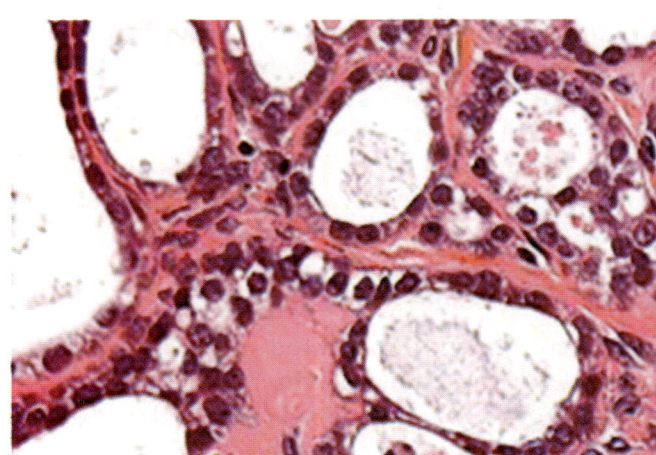

Fig. 20.12: Clear cell tumor of the ovarey

Transitional Cell (Brenner) Tumors (Fig. 20.13)

Transitional cell tumors are epithelial ovarian tumors formed by cells that resemble transitional epithelium or urothelium of the urinary bladder. These tumors presumably are derived from surface ovarian epithelium that undergoes urothelium like transformation (e.g. urothelial metaplasia, Walthard nests). They are rare and may occur in association with similar tumors in the urinary bladder.

Most benign transitional cell ovarian tumors are very small, asymptomatic, incidentally discovered, and clinically irrelevant. They are solid and nodular, and most are unilateral. Benign transitional cell ovarian tumors often arise in association with endocervical-type mucinous and serous tumors, and they most frequently occur between the fifth and sixth decades of life. Surgical excision is curative. Borderline transitional cell tumors characteristically contain solid and cystic areas, with papillary or polypoid projections within the cyst lumen. Borderline transitional cell tumors, most of which are unilateral, most often occur between the sixth and seventh decades of life. They are believed to behave in a benign manner and seldom recur after surgical treatment.

Histologically, the tumor consists of nests of transitional cells within surrounding tissue that resembles normal ovary. Brenner tumors may be benign or malignant, depending on whether the tumor cells invade the surrounding tissue. Brenner tumors are solid or cystic, yellow-tan color and firm upon gross examination. Histological examination of Brenner tumor reveals epithelial nests or cysts of cells, resembling urothelium, separated by a cellular, fibrous stroma composed of spindle-like cells. The nuclei are relatively uniform, lacking pleomorphism, hyper-

chromasia or macronucleoli, and mitoses are not identified. There is a moderate amount of eosinophilic cytoplasm.

Diagnosis of Benign Ovarian Lesions

I. Diagnostic Imaging

Ultrasonography, both transabdominal and transvaginal, plays a very important role in assessing ovarian masses in all age groups—neonates, children, and virginal adolescents. Color-coded Doppler ultrasonography improves the diagnostic accuracy of B-mode ultrasonography.

Ultrasonography helps determine whether the mass is ovarian or extraovarian, solid or cystic, simple or complex, and vascular or avascular. It can be used to evaluate material or fluid contained in a mass, as well as to assess the surface of the ovarian capsule. Color-flow Doppler ultrasonography is useful for distinguishing between benign and potentially malignant lesions. In most cases, computed tomography (CT) and magnetic resonance imaging (MRI) are unnecessary in the evaluation of an adnexal mass.

Ultrasonographic findings suggestive of malignancy include the following:

- Ovarian mass with solid or complex components
- Septations
- Evidence of surface nodularity or papillae
- Increased vascular flow
- Heterogeneous echotexture

Furthermore, serial or foll ow-up ultrasonograms are helpful in monitoring the progression of an ovarian mass by repeating at interval of 6 weeks to 6 months.

The presence of pelvic or abdominal ascites or lymphadenopathy on CT or MRI further raises the index of suspicion for ovarian malignancy.

II. Laboratory Studies

CA-125 screening does not add useful information for specific diagnosis of benign adnexal tumors (except in the case of endometrioma). An elevated level significantly increases the probability of such a lesion.

Alpha-fetoprotein (AFP) is another tumor marker that is elevated in the setting of endodermal sinus tumors, mixed germ cell tumors, immature teratomas, and embryonal carcinomas. The lactate dehydrogenase (LDH) level may be elevated in women with dysgerminomas, whereas the human chorionic gonadotropin (hCG) level may be elevated in women with choriocarcinomas, germ cell tumors, or embryonal cell tumors.

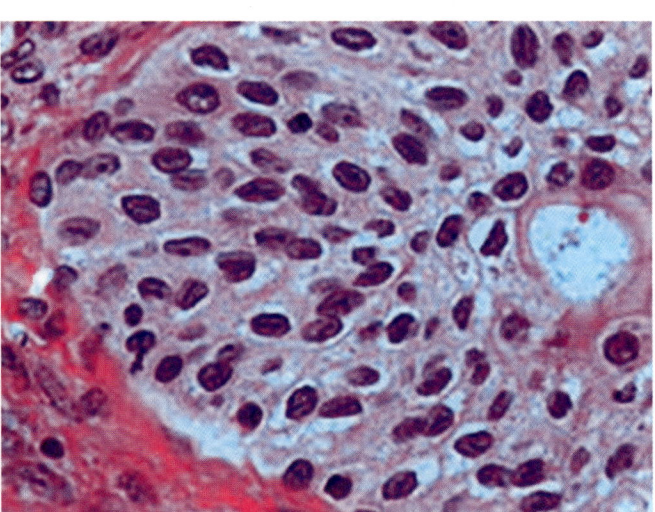

Fig. 20.13: Brenner tumor

Testosterone levels may be elevated in patients with fibromas and Sertoli-Leydig tumors, and estradiol levels may be elevated in patients with thecomas or dysgerminomas. Often, these patients present with symptoms of rapidly virilizing clinical signs of elevated testosterone, such as male-pattern baldness, voice deepening, clitoromegaly, and increased hirsutism. In the setting of a suspicious ovarian mass, tumor markers should be evaluated, and if the results are abnormal, the patient should be referred for a complete evaluation by a gynecologic oncologist.

Treatment

It is always surgical. In young patients, unilateral ovarian cystectomy or unilateral ovariotomy or salpingo-oophorectomy is appropriate treatment. In elderly patient with completed family, often hysterectomy with bilateral salpingo-oophorectomy is done. All these operations can be perfomed by conventional laparotomy or by laparoscopy.

Ovarian cystectomy (Fig. 20.14): An incision is given over the capsule on laparotomy or a scissor incision is given over the capsule by laparoscopy. The cyst is dissected out and removed. The rest of the ovarian tissue is preserved. Bleeding if occur in the hilar region is arrested easily by both the routes.

Ovariotomy (Fig. 20.15): The clamps are placed medial to the ovary over the appendages comprising of ligament of ovary and broad ligament containing anastomosing ovarian and uterine vessels after dissecting out the stretched fallopian tube from the surface of the mass. The lateral clamp is placed over the infundibulopelvic ligament containing ovarian vessels, lymphatics and nerves. The same principle is

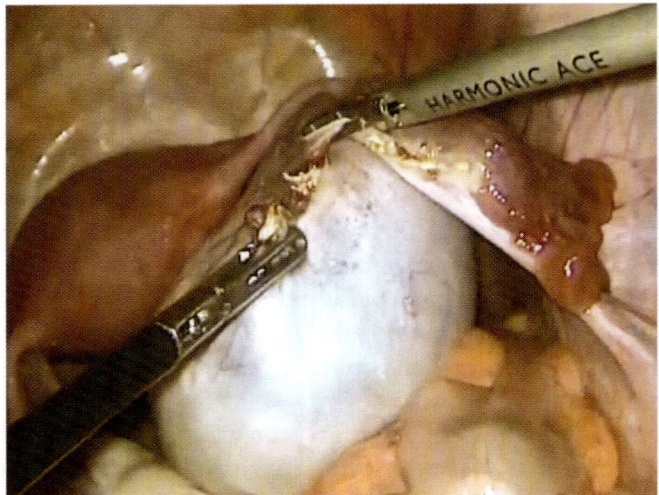

Fig. 20.15: Laparoscopic ovariotomy

followed on laparoscopy also except that the diathermy coagulation current is used in the pedicles to remove the mass.

Salpingo-oophorectomy: The medial pedicle will be composed of structures like Fallopian tube with mesosalpinx, broad ligament and ligament of ovary along with anastomosing ovarian and uterine vessels. The lateral pedicle is composed of infudibulopelvic ligament.

Maternal Ovarian Cysts during Pregnancy

Maternal ovarian cysts during pregnancy are fairly common and arise largely as a result of excessive stimulation of human chorionic gonadotropin (hCG) by the corpus luteum. The corpus luteum itself may then become quite large and undergo ovarian torsion. Additionally, because pregnancy is a time of frequent ultrasonographic evaluation, the other common ovarian cysts seen in the childbearing age group are (serous cysts, dermoid cysts, endometriomas, and, occasionally, malignant epithelial tumors) tend to be diagnosed more frequently during pregnancy. About 12% dermoid cysts are seen in pregnancy though serous tumors and luteal functional cysts may be more commonly found in pregnancy.

Fetal Cysts

In the fetal and neonatal period, both the maternal and fetal ovaries are exposed to excessive stimulation by human chorionic gonadotropin. In addition, the fetal pituitary gland is also producing follicle-stimulating hormone (FSH), which increases the size and number of fetal ovarian follicles. These factors may contribute to the formation of fetal ovarian cysts.

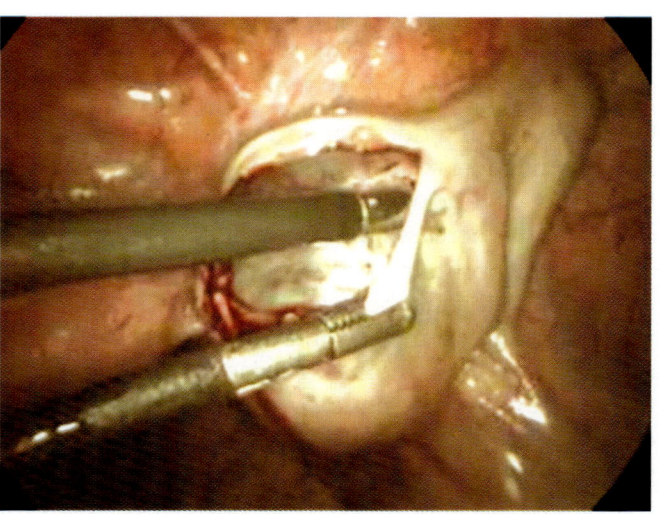

Fig. 20.14: Laparoscopic ovarian cystectomy

Often diagnosed in the third trimester during routine ultrasound surveillance, these lesions are typically cystic (99%) and can be either simple or complex. The contralateral ovary also may be cystic. Of all fetal cysts, 97% are functional, and the average size is approximately 3.4 cm. Half of these cysts spontaneously resolve, and of the remainder, 25–40% undergo torsion.

The differential diagnosis of an adnexal mass detected in utero includes neoplastic lesions (e.g. cystic teratomas, cystadenomas, granuloblastomas); mesenteric cysts; and gastrointestinal, genitourinary, or enteric duplication. In the antenatal period, a conservative approach is recommended because many spontaneously resolve. Although antenatal aspiration is an option, it has not shown any significant benefit and is not the standard of care.

Ovarian Lesions in Childhood and Adolescence

Childhood is a time of busy activity for the ovaries, a fact that may be underrecognized by both gynecologists and pediatricians. Histologically, the ovarian stroma is growing, causing the ovaries to enlarge. When cysts manifest, they are usually small and simple. The incidence of simple cysts increases with age, and most are caused by a failure of the follicle to undergo involution. Not surprisingly, in this age group, most cysts are diagnosed incidentally after radiographic studies. When smaller than 5 cm, these lesions may be followed conservatively.

Intervention should be considered for cysts larger than 5 cm, lesions demonstrating solid components, those accompanied by pain, those associated with systemic endocrinologic signs, and those with complex components or internal septations. When ovarian neoplasms are encountered in girls of this age group, they fall into the germ cell, epithelial cell, and stromal/sex chord familial classification. The vast majority of ovarian lesions of childhood are of the germ cell variety, but only about 8% of ovarian tumors of childhood are malignant.

The most common germ cell tumor of this age group is the benign cystic teratoma. These lesions also known as dermoid cysts have a characteristic radiographic appearance. Commonly described as complex, with an enhancing rim and often with visible calcifications (teeth), these cysts are unilateral in greater than 90% of children. Although surgery is not always necessary, ovarian cystectomy with preservation of the ovary is the standard of care.

Benign Solid Ovarian Tumors

Common benign solid tumors include fibromas and thecomas, solid mature teratomas (tumors consisting of differentiated tissue from all 3 germ layers), Brenner tumors and solid epithelial tumors.

Fibroma

The most common benign solid tumor of the ovary is the fibroma. These tumors occur most commonly in women of postmenopausal age. They are often unilateral and are minimum 3 cm in size. Fibromas are derived from connective tissue and arise from the solid ovarian cortical stroma. Histologically, spindle cells are seen. Ultrasonographically, these tumors appear hypoechoic with attenuation of the ultrasound beam.

On magnetic resonance imaging (MRI), fibromas demonstrate low-signal intensity on T2-weighted images relative to the myometrium, secondary to their mostly fibrous composition. On computed tomography (CT), ovarian fibromas appear as well-defined, solid masses with mild heterogeneity.

These tumors may undergo calcification and degeneration. More than 90% are unilateral, and approximately 10–15% are found in association with ascites. Fewer than 1% undergo malignant transformation to fibrosarcomas. About 1% of cases are associated with Meigs syndrome, characterized by ovarian fibroma, ascites, and pleural effusion.

These tumors occur most commonly in women of postmenopausal age. They are unilateral and are often at least 3 cm in size. Fibromas are connective-tissue tumors that arise from the ovarian cortical stroma. If the stroma is estrogenic or luteinized, the tumors are actually thecomas.

Ovarian Thecoma

It is a benign ovarian tumor of sex cord—stromal (mesenchymal) origin. It accounts for approximately 0.5–1% of all ovarian tumors. It secretes estrogen and therefore, is described as functional ovarian tumor. It typically presents in older women with over 80% presenting in the post-menopausal period.

Clinical Presentation

Clinical manifestations of thecomas are similar to those of granulosa cell tumors, with uterine bleeding predominating in 60% of cases. Occurrences of hyperestrogenism secondary to a thecoma or fibrothecoma are less common than those secondary to a granulosa cell tumor (GCT).

Pathology

The tumor belongs to the same histopathologic spectrum as a fibroma/fibrothecoma. A typical thecoma consists of swollen lipid-laden stromal cells with a variable component of fibroblasts.

The tumor can be divided into two main types:

- Typical
- Luteinized: A thecoma containing steroid-type cells resembling luteinized theca and luteinized stromal cells are called a luteinized thecoma.
  - Occurs in a younger age group than a typical thecoma.
  - 50% estrogenic
  - 40% non-functioning
  - 10% androgenic

On gross examination, they appear as solid masses of varying sizes, cystic changes may be occasioanlly be seen. Most thecomas appear as a mixture of fibroma and thecoma components and are called ovarian fibrothecoma. More than 20% thecomas have concurrent endometrial carcinoma.

Radiographic Features

I. *Ultrasound:* Sonographic features are generally non-specific. Thecoma may manifest as:

- An echogenic mass with distal acoustic attenuation
- A well-defined hypoechoic mass, or
- An anechoic lesion with through-transmission

Secondary features of hyperestrogenism, such as endometrial thickening, also may be seen.

II. CT: Typically appear as unilateral, solid ovarian masses.

III. *Pelvic MRI*

- *T2:* Usually hyperintense (often from edema and cystic degeneration) and may mimic more common malignant ovarian tumors. However, the signal characteristics at T2-weighted imaging may vary in the presence of edema or cystic degeneration.
- *Chemical shift:* Intratumoral lipid may give a chemical shift artefact.
- *Dynamic contrast imaging:*
  - The degree of contrast enhancement varies with the amount of fibrous tissue within the tumor.
  - While theca cells in the normal ovary are highly vascularized, the fibrous tissue is known for delayed weak enhancement at dynamic contrast-enhanced imaging.
  - If the tumor has an significant fibroma component (i.e. fibrothecoma), the abundant fibrous

tissue may produce predominantly low signal intensity on both T1- and T2-weighted sequences.

Treatment and Prognosis

Thecomas are almost always benign and have low malignant potential, although there have been isolated reports of malignant thecomas.

Mature (Cystic) Ovarian Teratoma

Ovarian dermoid cyst and **mature cystic teratoma** are terms often used interchangeably to refer to the most common ovarian neoplasm. Although they have very similar imaging appearances, the two have a fundamental histological difference: Dermoids are composed only of dermal and epidermal elements, whereas teratomas have mesodermal and endodermal elements.

Mature cystic teratomas account for 10–20% of all ovarian neoplasms. They tend to be identified in young women, typically around the age of 30 years and are also the most common ovarian neoplasm in patients younger than 20 years.

Clinical Presentation

Uncomplicated ovarian dermoids tend to be asymptomatic and are often discovered incidentally. They do, however, predispose to ovarian torsion, and may then present with acute pelvic pain.

Pathology

Mature cystic teratomas are encapsulated tumors with mature tissue or organ components. They are composed of well-differentiated derivations from at least two of the three germ cell layers (ectoderm, mesoderm, and endoderm). They, therefore, contain developmentally mature skin complete with hair follicles and sweat glands, clumps of long hair, and often pockets of sebum, blood, fat, bone, nails, teeth, eyes, cartilage, and thyroid tissue. Typically their diameter is smaller than 10 cm, and rarely more than 15 cm. Real organoid structures (teeth, fragments of bone) may be present in 30% of cases.

They can be bilateral in 10–15% of cases.

Variants

Struma ovarii tumor: Contains thyroid elements, however, sometimes these are seperately classified as *specialised teratomas* of the ovaries.

Radiographic Features

Plain film: May show calcific and tooth components with the pelvis.

Pelvic ultrasound: Ultrasound is the preferred imaging modality. Typically, an ovarian dermoid is seen as a cystic adnexal mass with some mural components. Most lesions are unilocular.

The spectrum of sonographic features includes:
- *Rokitansky nodule—dermoid plug*
- Diffusely or partially echogenic mass with posterior sound attenuation owing to sebaceous material and hair within the cyst cavity—the *tip of the iceberg sign.*
- Echogenic, shadowing calcific or dental (tooth) components.
- Presence of fluid—fluid levels
- Multiple thin, echogenic bands caused by hair in the cyst cavity—the *dot-dash pattern*

CT: CT has high sensitivity in the diagnosis of cystic teratomas, though is not routinely recommended for this purpose in view of ionizing radiation.

Typically, CT images demonstrate fat, *fat fluid level*, calcification, *Rokitansky protuberance* and tufts of hair. The presence of most of the above tissues is diagnostic of ovarian cystic teratomas in 98% of cases. Whenever the size exceeds 10 cm or shows soft tissue plugs and cauliflower appearance with irregular borders is seen, *malignant transformation* should be suspected which is termed epidermoid carcinoma (squamous cell carcinoma).

When ruptured, the characteristic hypo-attenuating fatty fluid can be found as ante-dependent pockets, typically below the right hemidiaphragm, a pathognomonic finding. The escaped cyst content also leads to a chemical peritonitis and the mesentery may be stranded and the peritoneum thickened, which may mimic *peritoneal carcinomatosis.*

Pelvic MRI: MR evaluation usually tends to be reserved for difficult cases, but is exquisitely sensitive to fat components. Both fat suppression techniques and chemical shift artefact can be used to confirm presence of fat.

Enhancement is also able identify solid invasive components, and as such can be used to accurately locally stage malignant variants.

Complications

Recognised complications include:
- *Ovarian torsion:* 3–16% of ovarian teratomas on general: Considered the most common complication
- *Rupture:* 1–4%
- *Malignant transformation*: 1–2%: Usually into *squamous cell carcinoma* (adults) or rarely into *endodermal sinus tumors* (child).

- *Suprimposed infection:* 1%
- *Autoimmune hemolytic anemia:* <1%.

Treatment

They are slow growing (1–2 mm a year) and, therefore, some advocate non-surgical management. Larger lesions are often surgically removed. Many recommend initial serial follow for lesions under 7 cm to monitor growth, beyond which a resection is advised (ovariotomy).

Functional Cysts of the Ovary

1. Follicular cysts
2. Luteal cysts
3. Endometriotic cysts
4. Polycystic ovary

1. Follicular Cyst of Ovary

The **follicular cyst of ovary**, or *graafian follicle* cyst, or *follicular* cyst is a type of functional simple cyst, and is the most common type of *ovarian cyst*.

Pathophysiology

This type can form when ovulation doesn't occur, and a follicle doesn't rupture or release its egg but instead grows until it becomes a cyst, or when a mature follicle *involutes* (collapses on itself). It usually forms during ovulation, and can grow to about 7 cm in diameter. It is thin-walled, lined by one or more layers of *granulosa* cell, and filled with clear fluid.

Presentation

Its rupture can create sharp, severe pain on the side of the ovary on which the cyst appears. This sharp pain (sometimes called *mittelschmerz*) occurs in the middle of the *menstrual cycle*, during ovulation. About one-fourth of women with this type of cyst experience pain. Follicular cyst enlarges in anovulatory cycles when it does not rupture particularly in association with PCOS and with fibroids. They are bilateral and often do not increase more than 5 cm in size and resolute spontaneously or with treatment with OC pills by 3 months.

2. Luteal Cysts

It is a type of *ovarian cyst* which may rupture about the time of *menstruation*, and take up to three months to disappear entirely. A corpus luteum cyst rarely occurs at age 50+, because eggs are no longer being produced in menopausal women.

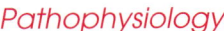

Pathophysiology

This type of functional cyst occurs after an egg has been released from a follicle. The follicle then becomes a secretory gland that is known as the *corpus luteum*. The ruptured follicle begins producing large quantities of *estrogen* and *progesterone* in preparation for conception. If a pregnancy doesn't occur, the corpus luteum usually breaks down and disappears. It may, however, fill with fluid or blood, causing the corpus luteum to expand into a cyst, and stay in the ovary. Usually, this cyst is on only one side, and does not produce any symptoms.

In women of reproductive age, cysts with a diameter of less than 5 cm are common, clinically inconsequential, and almost always a physiological condition.

Presentation

It can, however, grow to almost 10 cm (4 inches) in diameter and has the potential to bleed into itself or twist the ovary, causing pelvic or abdominal pain. If it fills with blood, the cyst may rupture, causing internal bleeding and sharp pain. This pain disappears within a few days of the rupture. Rarely, it may cause the ovary to twist around the ovarian ligament and can cut off the blood flow to the ovary. This is known as ovarian torsion and causes pain and other symptoms.

3. Endometriomas (Endometriotic Cysts)

With the high prevalence of endometriosis currently observed in women of childbearing age, it is not surprising that endometriomas are commonly encountered in clinical practice. An estimated 1–10% of reproductive age women may have endometriosis to some degree.

The primary pathologic definition of endometriosis requires the presence of endometrial glandular tissue outside the cavity of the uterus. Histologically, endometrial glands, stroma, or hemosiderin pigment must be detected in these lesions. When this tissue invades the ovaries, endometriomas frequently form. These are cystic, blood-filled spaces that contain "chocolate" blood (i.e. old blood).

On pelvic ultrasonography, endometriomas may appear multilocular and quite large and may appear solid or cystic (simple or complex). Sonograms typically show a cystic mass with diffuse low-level echoes. On MRI, their appearance is variable, depending on the quantity of blood present in the cyst. Most endometriomas, however, show multiple high-signal intensity on T1-weighted images and very low-signal intensity on T2-weighted images.

4. Polycystic Ovary

The normal adult ovary measures 1 cm in thickness, 2 cm in width, and 3 cm in length, and it usually weighs 5–8 g. In females with polycystic ovary syndrome (PCOS), the ovaries are usually bilaterally enlarged, contain multiple follicles, and demonstrate increased stromal echogenicity.

The diagnosis of PCOS has been simplified. Currently, 2 of the following 3 criteria are required to establish the diagnosis of PCOS:

- Polycystic ovaries (multiple small cysts, often around the periphery of the ovary—the classic "string of pearls" appearance)
- Signs of androgen excess (e.g. acne, hirsutism, temporal balding, male pattern hair loss, or clitoromegaly)
- Menstrual irregularities (oligomenorrhea or polymenorrhea)

Ultrasonographic findings suggestive of PCO commonly include the following:

- Ovarian enlargement
- Increased follicle count (4–8 follicles of diameter 2–4 mm arranged peripherally)
- Stromal echogenicity

The ovaries are usually bilaterally enlarged and spherical rather than ovoid in shape. However, 30% of patients with PCOS may show no increase in ovarian volume. Typically, multiple small (<1 cm) follicles are present, and no dominant follicle is observed. These follicles are usually arranged along the periphery of the ovarian parenchyma, in a "string of pearls" configuration. The ovaries may have increased echogenicity in relation to the myometrium.

Many women with PCOS has anovulatory subfertility secondary to anovulation or oligo-ovulation. Fortunately, most women with PCOS respond favorably to oral ovulation induction medications (clomiphene citrate), with or without progestin regulation of menses.

RCOG Guidelines 2016

The Management of Ovarian Cysts in Postmenopausal Women

1. *Diagnosis and significance of ovarian cysts in postmenopausal women*

How are ovarian cysts diagnosed in postmenopausal women and what initial investigations should be performed?

Clinicians should be aware of the different presentations and significance of ovarian cysts in postmenopausal women. [New 2016]

In postmenopausal women presenting with acute abdominal pain, the diagnosis of an ovarian cyst accident should be considered (e.g. torsion, rupture, haemorrhage). [New 2016]

It is recommended that ovarian cysts in postmenopausal women should be initially assessed by measuring serum cancer antigen 125 (CA125) level and transvaginal ultrasound scan.(A)

2. What is the role of history and clinical examination in postmenopausal women with ovarian cysts?

A thorough medical history should be taken from the woman, with specific attention to risk factors and symptoms suggestive of ovarian malignancy, and a family history of ovarian, bowel or breast cancer. [New 2016]

Where family history is significant, referral to the Regional Cancer Genetics service should be considered. [New 2016]

Appropriate tests should be carried out in any postmenopausal woman who has developed symptoms within the last 12 months that suggest irritable bowel syndrome, particularly in women over 50 years of age or those with a significant family history of ovarian, bowel or breast cancer. [New 2016] [C]

A full physical examination ofthe woman is essential and should include body mass index, abdominal examination to detect ascites and characterise any palpable mass, and vaginal examination. [New 2016] [C]

3. What blood tests should be performed in postmenopausal women with ovarian cysts?

CA125 CA125 should be the only serum tumour marker used for primary evaluation as it allows the Risk of Malignancy Index (RMI) of ovarian cysts in postmenopausal women to be calculated. [New 2016] [B]

CA125 levels should not be used in isolation to determine if a cystis malignant.While a very high value may assist in reaching the diagnosis, a normal value does not exclude ovarian cancer due to the nonspecific nature of the test. [New 2016][B]

There is currently not enough evidence to support the routine clinical use of other tumour markers, such as human epididymis protein 4 (HE4), carcinoembryonic antigen (CEA), CDX2, cancer antigen 72-4 (CA72-4), cancer antigen 19-9 (CA19-9), alphafetoprotein (-FP), lactate dehydrogenase (LDH) or beta-human chorionic gonadotrophin (-hCG), to assess the risk of malignancy in postmenopausal ovarian cysts. [New 2016] [B]

4. What imaging should be employed in the assessment of ovarian cysts in postmenopausal women? What is the role of ultrasound scanning in categorising cysts?

A transvaginal pelvic ultrasound is the single most effective way of evaluating ovarian cysts in postmenopausal women. [New 2016][C]

Transabdominal ultrasound should not be used in isolation. It should be used to provide supplementary information to transvaginal ultrasound particularly when an ovarian cyst is large or beyond the field of view of transvaginal ultrasound. [New 2016] [B]

On transvaginal scanning, the morphological description and subjective assessment of the ultrasound features should be clearly documented to allow calculation of the risk of malignancy. [New 2016] [B]

Transvaginal ultrasound scans should be performed using multifrequency probes by trained clinicians with expertise in gynaecological imaging. [New 2016] [B]

What is the role of Doppler and three-dimensional ultrasound studies?

Colour flow Doppler studies are not essential for the routine initial assessment of ovarian cysts in postmenopausal women. Spectral and pulse Doppler indices should not be used routinely (resistive index, pulsatility index, peak systolic velocity, time-averaged maximum velocity) to differentiate benign from malignant ovarian cysts, as their use has not been associated with significant improvement in diagnostic accuracy over morphologic assessment by ultrasound scan. Three-dimensional ultrasound morphologic assessment does not appear to improve the diagnosis of complex ovarian cysts and its routine use is not recommended in the assessment of postmenopausal ovarian cysts. [New 2016] [B]

What is the role of computed tomography (CT) scan, magnetic resonance imaging (MRI) and other cross-sectional imaging?

CT, MRI and positron emission tomography (PET)-CT scans are not recommended for the initial evaluation of ovarian cysts in postmenopausal women. CT scan CT should not be used routinely as the primary imaging tool forthe initial assessment of ovarian cysts in postmenopausal women because of its low specificity, its limited assessment of ovarian internal morphology and its use of ionising radiation. [New 2016] [B]

If, from the clinical picture, ultrasonographic findings and tumour markers, malignant disease is suspected, a CT scan of the abdomen and pelvis should be arranged, with onward referral to a gynaecological oncology multidisciplinary team. [New 2016]

MRI: MRI should not be used routinely as the primary imaging tool for the initial assessment of ovarian cysts in postmenopausal women. MRI should be used as the second-line imaging modality for the characterisation of indeterminate ovarian cysts when ultrasound is inconclusive. [New 2016]

PET-CT Scan: Current data do not support the routine use of PET-CT scanning in the initial assessment of postmenopausal ovarian cysts. Data suggest there is no clear advantage over transvaginal ultrasonography. Initial assessment and estimation of the risk of malignancy.

Which RMI should be used? The 'RMI I' is the most utilised, widely available and validated effective triaging system for women with suspected ovarian cancer. [New 2016] [A]

Although an RMI I score with a threshold of 200 (sensitivity 78%, specificity 87%) is recommended to predict the likelihood of ovarian cancer and to plan further management, some centres utilise an equally acceptable threshold of 250 with a lower sensitivity (70%) but higher specificity (90%). [New 2016][A]

CT of the abdomen and pelvis should be performed for all postmenopausal women with ovarian cysts who have a RMI I score greater than or equal to 200, with onward referral to a gynaecological oncology multidisciplinary team. [New 2016] [B]

What other scoring systems are available and when should they be used?
Other scoring systems are described.OVA1 and Risk of Malignancy Algorithm require specific assays which may make routine use impractical. The International Ovarian Tumor Analysis (IOTA) classification, which is based on specific ultrasound expertise, has comparable sensitivity and specificity to RMI and forms an alternative for those experienced in this technique. [New 2016] [A]

5. *How do you manage ovarian cysts in post-menopausal women? Do all postmenopausal women with ovarian cysts require surgical evaluation and is there a role for conservative management?*
Asymptomatic, simple, unilateral, unilocular ovarian cysts, less than 5 cm in diameter, have a low risk of malignancy. In the presence of normal serum CA125 levels, these cysts can be managed conservatively, with a repeat evaluation in 4–6 months. It is reasonable to discharge these women from follow-up after 1 year if the cyst remains unchanged or reduces in size, with normal CA125, taking into consideration a woman's wishes and surgical fitness. [D]

If a woman is symptomatic, further surgical evaluation is necessary [New 2016]

A woman with a suspicious or persistent complex adnexal mass needs surgical evaluation. [New 2016]

What is the role of aspiration of ovarian cysts in postmenopausal women?
Aspiration is not recommended for the management of ovarian cysts in postmenopausal women except for the purposes of symptom control in women with advanced malignancy who are unfit to undergo surgery or further intervention.

Could postmenopausal ovarian cysts be managed by laparoscopy?
Women with a RMI I of less than 200 (i.e. at low risk of malignancy) are suitable for laparoscopic management. [New 2016][B]

Laparoscopic management of ovarian cysts in postmenopausal women should be undertaken by a surgeon with suitable experience. Laparoscopic management of ovarian cysts in postmenopausal women should comprise bilateral salpingo-oophorectomy rather than cystectomy. [C]

Women undergoing laparoscopic salpingo-oophorectomy should be counselled preoperatively that a full staging laparotomy will be required if evidence of malignancy is revealed. [New 2016] [C]

Where possible, the surgical specimen should be removed without intraperitoneal spillage in a laparoscopic retrieval bag via the umbilical port. This results in less postoperative pain and a quicker retrieval time than when using lateral ports of the same size. Transvaginal extraction of the specimen is also acceptable, if the surgeon has the available expertise. [New 2016] [B]

When should laparotomy be undertaken?
All ovarian cysts that are suspicious of malignancy in a postmenopausal woman, as indicated by an RMI I greater than or equal to 200, CT findings, clinical assessment or findings at laparoscopy, require a full laparotomy and staging procedure. If a malignancy is revealed during laparoscopy or from subsequent histology, it is recommended that the woman be referred to a cancer centre for further management. [D]

Who should manage ovarian cysts in postmenopausal women?
While a general gynaecologist might manage women with a low risk of malignancy (RMI I less than 200) in a general gynaecology or cancer unit, women who are at higher risk should be managed in a cancer centre by a trained gynaecological oncologist, unless the

multidisciplinary team review is not supportive of a high probability of ovarian malignancy. [*New 2016*][D]

Management of Ovarian Cysts (Flowchart 20.1)

Conservative Management

Simple, unilateral, unilocular ovarian cysts less than 5 cm in diameter have a low risk of malignancy. It is recommended that in presence of a normal serum CA125 levels, they can be managed conservatively.

Surgical Management

Those women who do not fit the above criteria for conservative management should be offered surgical management which include aspiration of the cyst, laparoscopy and laparotomy.

1. *Aspiration:* Aspiration is not recommended for the management of ovarian cysts in postmenopausal women.

2. *Laparoscopy:* It is recommended that 'risk of malignancy index' should be used to select women for laparoscopic surgery to be undertaken by a suitably qualified surgeon. The main purpose for operating is to exclude ovarian malignancy. If ovarian malignancy is present, the appropriate management in postmenopausal women is to perform laparotomy and a total abdominal hysterectomy, bilateral salpingo-oophorectomy and full staging procedure. It is recommended that laparoscopic management of ovarian cysts in postmenopausal women should involve bilateral oophorectomy rather than cystectomy. If malignancy

Flowchart 20.1: Management of ovarian cyst in postmenopausal women

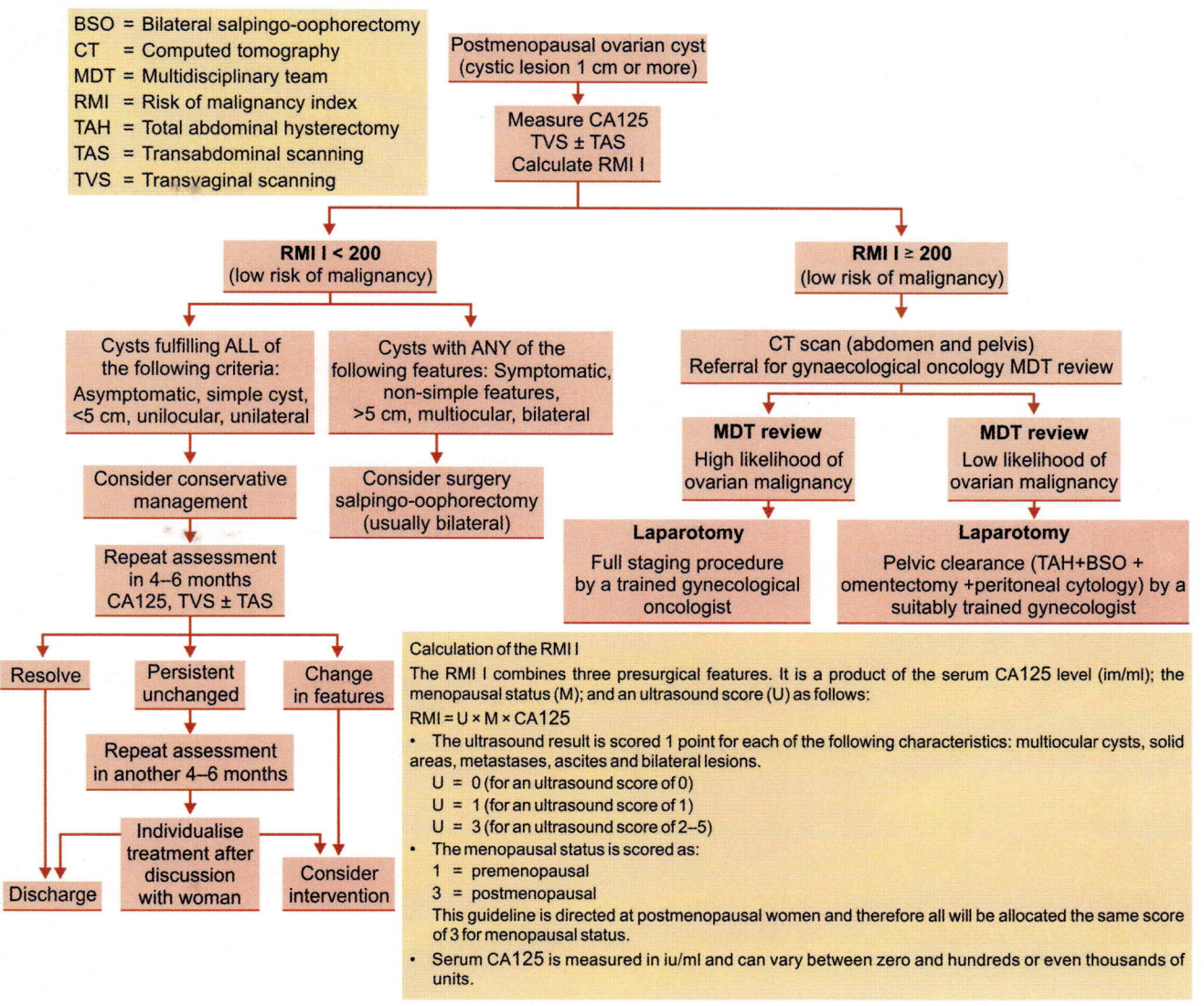

is revealed on subsequent histology, relaparotomy or referral to cancer center is done for further management.

3. *Laparotomy:* This includes (in case of ovarian cancer):
   a. Collection of ascetic fluid or peritoneal wash for cytology
   b. Biopsy from different adhesion and suspicious sites
   c. TAH/BSO and infracolic omentectomy
   d. Bilateral selective pelvic and para-aortic lymphadenectomy

Summary of Suggested Management Protocol

I. **Low risk:** Less than 3% risk of cancer:
- Simple cysts less than 5 cm and CA125 less than 30 may be managed conservatively.
- Conservative management should include repeat ultrasound scans and serum CA125 measurement every 4 months for one year.
- Laparoscopic oophorectomy is an acceptable treatment, if surgery is decided.

II. **Moderate risk:** Approximately 20% risk of cancer:
- Management in a cancer unit.
- Laparoscopic oophorectomy is acceptable in selected cases.
- If malignancy is discovered, then a full staging procedure should be undertaken

III. **High risk:** Greater than 75% risk of cancer
- Management in a cancer center
- Full staging procedure

20B. EPITHELIAL OVARIAN CANCER

Introduction

Ovarian cancer is the most common cause of cancer death from gynecologic tumors in the developed country. Malignant ovarian lesions include primary lesions arising from normal structures within the ovary and secondary lesions from cancers arising elsewhere in the body. Primary lesions include epithelial ovarian carcinoma (70% of all ovarian malignancies), germ-cell tumors, sex-cord stromal tumors, and other more rare types. Metastases to the ovaries are relatively frequent; the most common are from the endometrium, breast, colon, stomach, and cervix.

Epidemiology

Ovarian cancer has emerged as one of the most common malignancies affecting women in India. Epithelial ovarian cancer is the sixth most common cancer in women and is the second most common female genital tract malignancy after cervical cancer in developing country like India. They are usually found in postmenopausal women though no age is immune to ovarian cancers. The age specific incidence rate (ASIR) for ovarian cancer revealed that the disease increases from 35 years of age and reaches a peak between the ages 55–64. There is an increasing trend in the incidence of ovarian cancer rise, with a mean annual percentage increase in ASIR ranges from 0.7 to 2.4%. The annual lifetime risk for ovarian cancer is 1.4 per 100 women. Epithelial ovarian cancer can occur in females as young as 15, however, the mean presentation age is 56 years. The age-specific incidence gradually rises and peaks at 70 years of age. The median age for ovarian adenocarcinoma (which accounts for 85–90% of all malignant tumors) is between 60 and 65 years.

Pathophysiology

Most theories of the pathophysiology of ovarian cancer include the concept that it begins with the dedifferentiation of the cells overlying the ovary. During ovulation, these cells can be incorporated into the ovary, where they then proliferate. Ovarian cancer typically spreads to the peritoneal surfaces and omentum.

Ovarian carcinoma can spread by local extension, lymphatic invasion, intraperitoneal implantation, hematogenous dissemination, and transdiaphragmatic passage. Intraperitoneal dissemination is the most common and recognized characteristic of ovarian cancer. Malignant cells can implant anywhere in the peritoneal cavity but are more likely to implant in sites of stasis along the peritoneal fluid circulation. In contrast, hematogenous spread is clinically unusual early on in the disease process, although it is not infrequent in patients with advanced disease.

Epithelial tumors represent the most common histology (90%) of ovarian tumors. Other histologies include the following:
- Sex-cord stromal tumors
- Germ cell tumors
- Primary peritoneal carcinoma
- Metastatic tumors of the ovary

Epithelial ovarian cancer is thought to arise from epithelium covering the ovaries, which is derived from the coelomic epithelium in fetal development. This coelomic epithelium is also involved in formation of the müllerian ducts, from which the fallopian tubes, uterus, cervix, and upper vagina develop.

Five main histologic subtypes, which are similar to carcinoma, arise in the epithelial lining of the cervix, uterus, and fallopian tube, as follows:
- Serous (from fallopian tube)
- Endometrioid (endometrium)
- Mucinous (cervix)
- Clear cell (mesonephros)
- Brenner

Epithelial tumors are found as partially cystic lesions with solid components. The surface may be smooth or covered in papillary projections (Fig. 20.16) and the cysts contain fluid ranging from straw-colored to opaque brown or hemorrhagic.

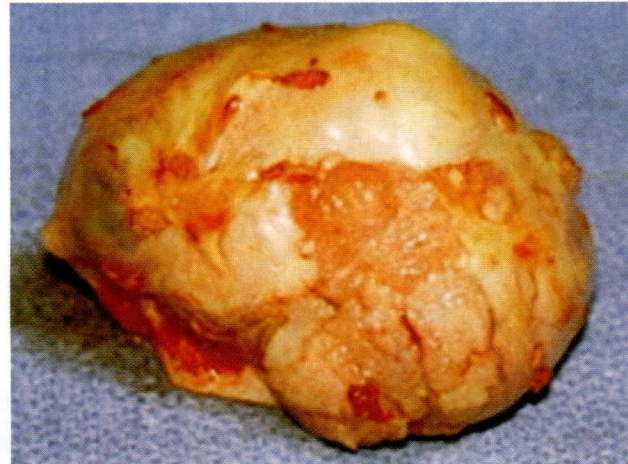

Fig. 20.16: An enlarged ovary with a papillary serous carcinoma on the surface

Epithelial ovarian cancer most often spreads initially within the peritoneal cavity. Metastatic disease often is found on the peritoneal surfaces, particularly on the undersurface of the diaphragms, the paracolic gutters, the bladder, and the cul-de-sac. Other common sites are the surface of the liver, the mesentery and serosa of the large and small bowel, in the omentum, the uterus, and para-aortic and pelvic lymph nodes (Figs 20.17 to 20.19).

Outside the peritoneal cavity, epithelial ovarian cancer may spread to the pleural cavity, lungs, and groin lymph nodes. Presence of pleural effusion does not necessarily indicate disease in the chest, and malignancy can be diagnosed only cytologically. Mucinous tumors tend to form large dominant masses, while papillary serous tumors have a more diffuse distribution and are more commonly bilateral.

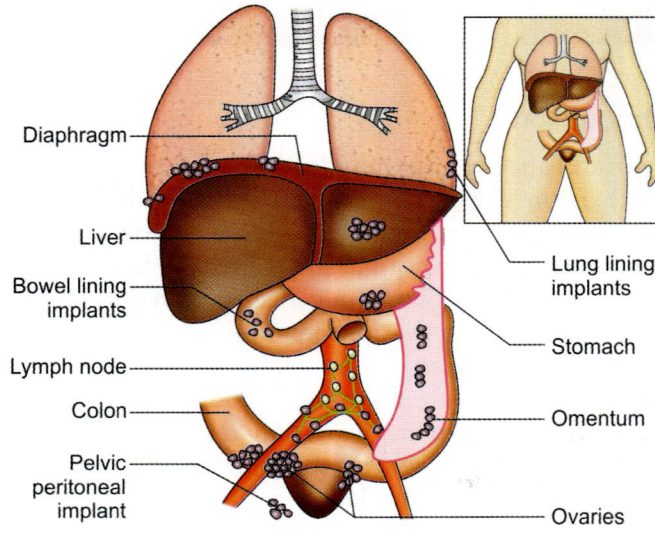

Fig. 20.19: Metastatic spread of cancer of ovary

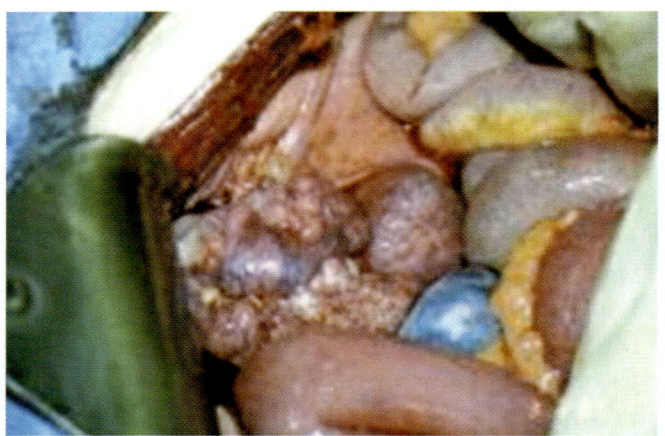

Fig. 20.17: A loop of sm all bowel is adherent to a poor ly differentiated primary epithelial ovarian carcinoma

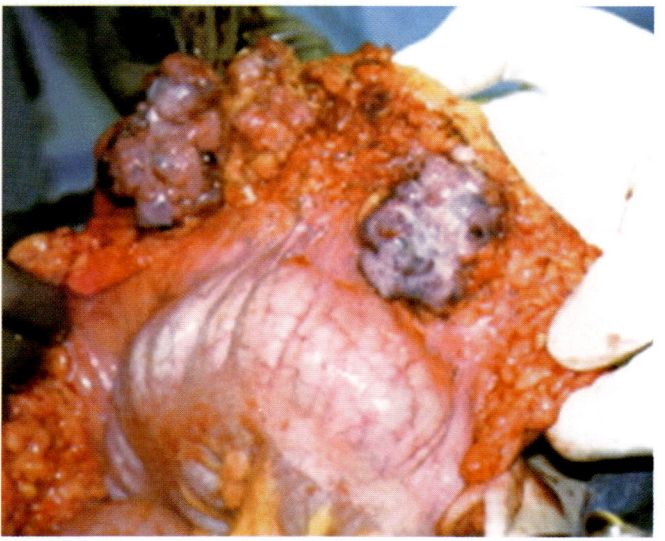

Fig. 20.18: Metastases from epithelial ovarian carcinoma involving the omentum

Endometrioid and clear-cell variants more commonly exhibit local invasion, retroperitoneal disease, and hepatic metastases.

Etiology

The precise cause of ovarian cancer is unknown, but several risk and contributing factors have been identified.

Epidemiology studies have shown increased risk for ovarian cancer with greater numbers of ovulation cycles. There are two theories explaining for the association of decreased risk with decreased number of ovulation cycles:

1. *Theory of incessant ovulation:* Repeated ovarian follicular rupture and subsequent repair results in increased likelihood of genetic alterations within the surface epithelium.
2. *Gonadotropin theory hypothesis:* Persistent stimulation of the ovaries by gonadotropins, together with local effects of endogenous hormones, results in increased proliferation and mitotic activity of the surface epithelium. This is consistent with ovarian cancer being associated with high gonadotropin states such as the menopause, and less commonly associated with low gonadotropin states such as oral contraceptive use and high parity.

Epithelial ovarian carcinoma develops sporadically in about 90–95% of patients. Environmental and dietary factors are thought to have a role. These include use of talc on the perineum and vulva, asbestos, pelvic irradiation, viruses (particularly mumps), high-fat diet, and lactose consumption. Other factors are associated with an increased number of ovulation cycles: low parity, delayed childbearing, early menarche and late menopause. However, genetic factors are the most important risk factors for ovarian epithelial carcinoma.

Factors that decrease the risk for ovarian cancer predominantly reduce the number of ovulation cycles a women encounters—such as the use of oral contraceptives, breastfeeding and multiparity. Long-term use of oral contraceptives has reduced the risk of ovarian cancer by more than 50% in unselected women. Decreased risk of ovarian cancer has also been associated with tubal ligation and hysterectomy.

Genetic Factors

Family history plays an important role in the risk of developing ovarian cancer. The lifetime risk for developing ovarian cancer is 1.6% in the general population. This compares with a 4–5% risk when 1 first-degree family member is affected, rising to 7% when 2 relatives are affected. About 5–10% of cases of ovarian cancer occur in an individual with a family history of the disease. Hereditary epithelial ovarian cancer occurs at a younger age (approximately 10 years younger) than nonhereditary epithelial ovarian cancer, but the prognosis may be somewhat better.

Integrated genomic analyses by the Cancer Genome Atlas Research Network have revealed that high-grade serous ovarian cancer is characterized by *Tp53* mutations in almost all tumors. At least 2 syndromes of hereditary ovarian cancer are clearly identified, involving either (1) disorders of the genes associated with breast cancer, *BRCA1* and *BRCA2*, or (2) more rarely, genes within the Lynch II syndrome complex. Breast/ovarian cancer syndrome is associated with early onset of breast or ovarian cancer. Inheritance follows an autosomal dominant transmission. It can be inherited from either parent. Most cases are related to the *BRCA1* gene mutation. *BRCA1* is a tumor suppressor gene that inhibits cell growth when functioning properly; the inheritance of mutant alleles of *BRCA1* leads to a considerable increase in risk for developing ovarian cancer.

Approximately 1 person in 4000 in the general population carries a mutation of *BRCA1*. Some populations have a much higher rate of *BRCA1* and *BRCA2* mutations, especially Ashkenazi Jews. In families with 2 first-degree relatives (mother, sister, or daughter) with premenopausal epithelial ovarian cancer, the likelihood of a female relative having an affected *BRCA1* or *BRCA2* gene is as high as 40%.

Individuals with a *BRCA1* gene mutation have a 50–85% lifetime risk of developing breast cancer and a 15–45% risk of developing epithelial ovarian cancer. Those with a *BRCA2* gene mutation have a 50–85% lifetime risk of developing breast cancer and a 10–20% risk of developing epithelial ovarian cancer. Families with *BRCA2* mutations are at risk for developing cancer of the prostate, larynx, pancreas, and male breast.

Families with Lynch II syndrome or hereditary non-polyposis colorectal cancer are characterized by high risk for developing colorectal, endometrial, stomach, small bowel, breast, pancreas, and ovarian cancers. This syndrome is caused by mutations in the mismatch repair genes like *MSH2, MLH1, PMS1,* and *PMS2.*

Previous Hormone Therapy in Menopause

Risk for ovarian cancer is increased with hormone therapy, regardless of duration of use, formulation, estrogen dose, regimen, progestin type, and administration route. Incidence rates in current and never users of hormones are 0.52 and 0.4 per 1000 years, respectively.

Other Factors

Lactose consumption and the use of talcum powder on the vulva and perineum may be associated with increased risk of epithelial ovarian cancer.

History

Assessment of women for their risk of ovarian cancer necessitates obtaining a careful family history of cancers in both male and female relatives. Age, parity, duration of symptoms, loss of weight, previous treatment all are taken into account to assess the progress of the disease.

Signs and Symptoms

Early ovarian cancer causes minimal, nonspecific, or no symptoms. The patient may feel an abdominal mass. Most cases are diagnosed in an advanced stage because of lack of proper screening possible.

Epithelial ovarian cancer presents with a wide variety of vague and nonspecific symptoms, including the following:
- Bloating; abdominal distention or discomfort
- Pressure effects on the bladder and rectum
- Constipation
- Vaginal bleeding
- Indigestion and acid reflux
- Shortness of breath
- Tiredness
- Weight loss
- Early satiety

Symptoms independently associated with the presence of ovarian cancer include pelvic and

Findings suspicious for ovarian malignancy		
Malignant cachexia	Pallor	Enlarged Virchow's gland
bilateral rales	evidence of lung metastasis	Breast lump
Hepatomegaly	Hard GB lump	Discrete intestinal metastatic lump
Ascites	pedal edema	Bilateral mass in fornices, separate from uterus
		Ovarian lump—Irregular hard surface/ restricted mobility/tender mass
		Hard tender fixed nodule in POD

abdominal pain, increased abdominal size and bloating, and difficulty eating or feeling full. Presentation with swelling of a leg due to venous thrombosis is not uncommon.

Physical Examination

Physical findings are uncommon in patients with early disease. Patients with more advanced disease may present with ovarian or pelvic mass, ascites, pleural effusion, or abdominal mass or bowel obstruction.

Most early ovarian carcinomas and the serous and mucinous cystadenomas are asymptomatic. Two-thirds of patients present with extensive intra-abdominal metastases. Pelvic examination revealing firmness, fixation, nodularity, lack of tenderness, or cul-de-sac nodules are indicative of malignancy. 50% of all ovarian carcinomas are bilateral. Malignant serous tumors constitute over 40% of invasive epithelial carcinomas. Both borderline and malignant serous tumors are often bilateral. Mucinous carcinomas are diagnosed at stage I in approximately half of patients, whereas serous tumors are usually diagnosed at advanced stages.

Diagnosis Considerations

Presence of advanced ovarian cancer is often suspected on clinical grounds but can be confirmed only pathologically by ovarian biopsy after removal of the ovaries.

Pelvic ultrasound or CT scan of the abdomen and pelvis is always warranted for confirmation of diagnosis.

Chest radiographs are common and considered routine. CT scan of the chest is seldom indicated.

MRI can increase the specificity of imaging evaluation in cases where the ultrasound appearance of the lesion is indeterminate. MRI is not definitive, however. On MRI, endometriotic cysts with enhanced mural nodules are a hallmark of ovarian cancer, but they may also be a feature of benign neoplasms and even inflammatory diseases. Large contrast-enhanced nodules on large endometriotic cysts in an elderly patient are more likely to indicate malignancy.

When imaging studies demonstrate an adnexal mass, the decision whether to observe the patient with repeat imaging or to proceed to surgical evaluation must take into account not only the imaging characteristics but also the patient's medical history, physical examination results, and cancer antigen 125 (CA125) level. CA125 is not good discriminator of benign lesions from malignant lesions in premenopausal women but have better accuracy in postmenopausal women.

In patients with diffuse carcinomatosis and GI symptoms, **a GI tract workup** may be indicated, including one of the following:
- Upper GI endoscopy
- Barium enema
- Colonoscopy and sigmoidoscopy

Fine-needle aspiration (FNA) or percutaneous biopsy of an adnexal mass is not routinely recommended. In most cases, this approach may only serve to delay diagnosis and treatment of ovarian cancer. Instead, if a clinical suggestion of ovarian cancer is present, the patient should undergo a laparotomy for diagnosis and staging. An FNAC or diagnostic paracentesis should be performed in patients with diffuse carcinomatosis or ascites without an obvious ovarian mass.

Screening of Ovarian Cancer

No approved screening method is available for ovarian cancer because it has a relatively low prevalence within the general population and no proven precursor lesion exists that can be detected and treated to prevent the cancer from occurring.

Currently, the National Cancer Institute (NCI) recommends that high-risk women should be identified and consider having annual ultrasonographic examination, annual CA125 testing, and be considered for oophorectomy. The NCI recommends no screening methodology for women at normal risk for epithelial ovarian cancer (Table 20.5).

1. Tumor Markers

Tumor markers are glycoproteins that are usually detected by monoclonal antibodies. Each tumor marker has a variable profile of usefulness for screening, determining diagnosis and prognosis, assessing response to therapy, and monitoring for cancer recurrence. They are produced by tumor cells in response to cancer or certain benign conditions and indicate biological changes that signal the existence of malignancy. These soluble molecules can usually be detected in elevated quantities in the blood, urine, or body tissues of patients with certain types of cancer (Table 20.1).

The levels of tumor marker are not altered in all cancer patients, especially in early stage cancer. The level of some tumor markers can be elevated in patients with noncancerous conditions.

CA125 is a glycoprotein antigen detected by using mouse monoclonal antibody OC125 raised from an ovarian cancer cell line. CA125 is not specific for epithelial ovarian cancer and is elevated in other benign and malignant conditions, including menstruation; endometriosis; pelvic inflammation; liver, renal, and lung disease; and cancer of the endometrium, breast, colon, pancreas, lung, stomach, and liver. It is also elevated in 6% of women who do not have epithelial ovarian cancer. Although CA125 is elevated in 83% of women with epithelial ovarian cancer, it is elevated in only 50% of those with stage I disease.

Besides CA125, other markers have been investigated, including lysophosphatidic acid, tumor-associated glycoprotein 72 (TAG 72), OVX1, and macrophage colony-stimulating factor (M-CSF). Newer experimental markers have been identified through various laboratory techniques. These markers include mesothelin, human epididymis protein 4, kallikrein, and haptoglobin-alpha.

Alpha-fetoprotein (AFP) is another tumor marker that is elevated in the setting of endodermal sinus tumors, mixed germ cell tumors, immature teratomas, and embryonal carcinomas. The lactate dehydrogenase (LDH) level may be elevated in women with dysgerminomas, whereas the human chorionic gonadotropin (hCG) level may be elevated in women with choriocarcinomas, germ cell tumors, or embryonal cell tumors.

Testosterone levels may be elevated in patients with fibromas and Sertoli-Leydig tumors, and estradiol levels may be elevated in patients with thecomas or dysgerminomas. Often, these patients present with symptoms of rapidly virilizing clinical signs of elevated testosterone, such as male-pattern baldness, voice deepening, clitoromegaly, and increased hirsutism. In the setting of a suspicious ovarian mass, tumor markers should be evaluated, and if the results are abnormal, the patient should be referred for a complete evaluation by a gynecologic oncologist.

2. Mammography

The preoperative workup should also include mammography for women older than 40 years who have not had one in the preceding 6–12 months. This is especially important in women with estrogen-producing tumors because these may increase the risk of breast malignancies.

Additionally, breast cancers can metastasize to the ovaries and are often bilateral. Mammography can help rule out the possibility of a nongynecologic primary neoplasm in the breast.

3. USG

- *Ovarian volume on TVS:* >20 cm^3 in premenopausal women and >10 cm^3 in postmenopausal women is abnormal.
- Any solid or papillary projection from the tumor wall is suspicious.

A. RMI (Risk of Malignancy Index)

The risk of malignancy index (RMI) was introduced for discriminating ovarian cancer from other ovarian mass in 1990. The RMI score is calculated from menstruation status, ultrasonographic result and CA125 level. RMI cut-off level of 200 has 85% sensitivity and 97% specificity to identify ovarian cancer (Table 20.2 and Fig. 20.20).

RMI is a product of the ultrasound scan score (U), menopausal status (M) and serum CA125 level.

- The ultrasound result is scored 1 point for each of the following characteristics: Multilocular cysts, solid areas, metastases, ascites, bilateral lesions. U = for

Table 20.1: Serum markers in ovarian cancers	
Tumor histology	*Serum markers*
• Epithelial ovarian cancers	• CA 125
	• CEA
	• AFP
	• hCG, AFP
	• hCG
	• LDH-1, LDH-2
	• Inhibin
• Mucinous cystadenoma carcinoma	CEA
• Endodermal sinus tumour	AFP
• Embryonal cell carcinoma	hCG, AFP
• Choriocarcinoma	• hCG
• Dysgerminoma	• LDH-1,LDH-2
• Granulosa cell tumor	• Inhibin

Table 20.2: Risk-of-malignancy index according to ultrasound findings, absolute values of CA-125 serum levels and menopausal status

Ultrasound findings	Score
Unilocular simple cysts with regular fine wall or lesion suggesting dermoid cyst.	
Multilocular cyst with regular and smooth wall (<3 mm) or thick (>3 mm) or solid homogeneous tumor with hyperechogenic and well-defined wall.	1
Unilocular cyst or multilocular cyst with fine wall, with irregularity in the wall or septa (>3 mm).	2
Multilocular cyst with thick and irregular wall (irregularity <3 mm), and/or irregular septa; or cyst with papillary irregularity over 3 mm.	4
Complex lesion, with predominance of cystic or solid area, without irregularity in surface.	5
Complex lesion with irregularity in surface (<3 mm) or bodly-defined and irregular wall; or solid heterogeneous lesion.	10
Multiplicity—unilateral lesion or bilateral lesions.	0
Associated lesions: Ascites	1
wall expansive involvement greater than 3 mm	2
CA-125 serum level	0.00
Premenopausal	1
Postmenopausal	3

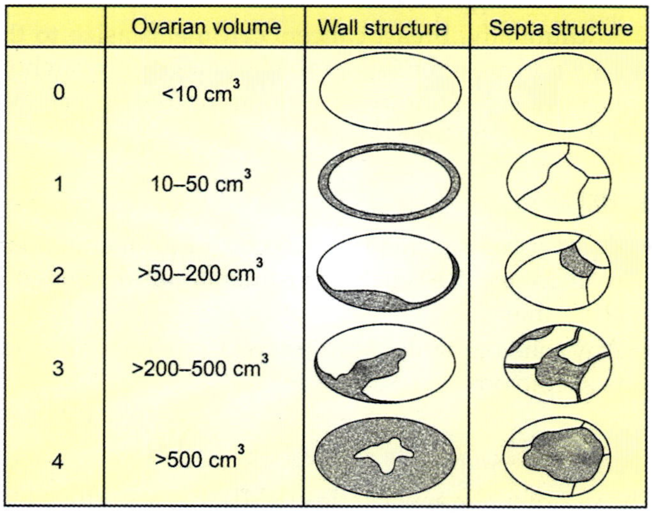

Fig. 20.20: Morphology index

an ultrasound score of points, U=1 for an ultrasound score of 1 point, U=3 for an ultrasound score of 2–5 points.

- Menopausal status is scored as 1 = pre-menopausal and 3 = post-menopausal. The classification of 'post-menopausal' is a woman who has had no period for more than 1 year or a woman over 50 who has had a hysterectomy.
- Serum CA125 is measured in IU/mL.

B. ROMA (Risk of Ovarian Malignancy Algorithm)

ROMA is intended to aid in assessing whether a premenopausal or postmenopausal woman who presents with an ovarian adnexal mass is at high or low likelihood of finding malignancy on surgery. ROMA is indicated for women who meet the following criteria: over age 18; ovarian adnexal mass present for which surgery is planned, and not yet referred to an oncologist. ROMA must be interpreted in conjunction with an independent clinical and radiological assessment. The test is not intended as a screening or stand-alone diagnostic assay.

HE4 (human epididymis protein 4) is a new FDA approved biomarker for use in managing women with an ovarian adnexal mass. It is a protease inhibitor expressed by malignant epithelial ovarian cells that is measurable in the serum of women with ovarian cancer. This HE4 value in combination with CA125 and menopausal status evaluates women with an adnexal mass regarding predictability of epithelial ovarian malignancy. The ROMA score is calculated from the Predictive Index.

Demonstration of stages in pictures (Fig. 20.21): UICC (Union for International Cancer Control) advocated TNM classification for ovarian tumors and correlates with FIGO staging in Tables 20.3 to 20.5.

Stage I: Growth limited to ovaries

IA
T1a

IB
T1b

IC
T1c

—Malignant
cells in
ascites

Tumors previously staged as IAII, IBII as stage IC

Stage II: Spread to pelvic tissues

IIB
T2b

IIA
T2a

IIC
T2c

—Malignant
cells in
ascites

Rectum

Aorta

Aorta

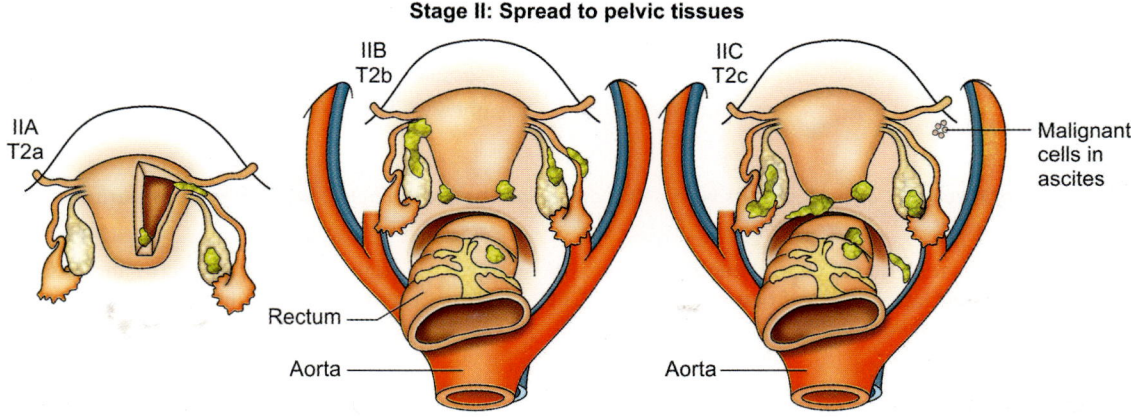

Stage III: Spread to retroperitoneal nodes, peritoneum, abdominal organs
Stage IV: Distant metastases—pleural effusion, liver parenchyma

Stage III

T3

IIIC/3c
Peritoneal
metastases
>2 cm

IIIA/3a
Microscopic only

IIIB/3b
Macroscopic
peritoneal
metastases
≤2 cm

Stage III

T3

Stage IV

MI

—Parenchymal

Liver capsule—

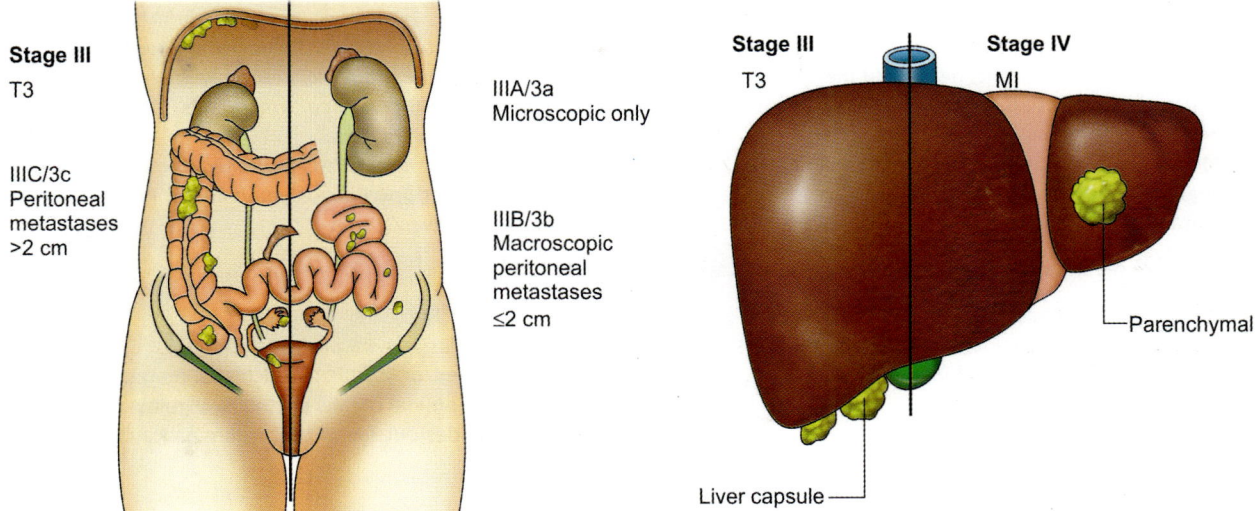

Fig. 20.21: UICC advocated TNM classification for ovarian tumors correlates with FIGO staging

Table 20.3: ROMA predictive index

Premenopausal	Predictive index (PI) = .120 + 2.38 LN(HE4) + 0.0626 LN (CA-125)
Postmenopausal	PI = −8.09 + 1.04 LN (HE4) + 0.732 LN(CA 125)
	Predicted probability exp(PI)/[1 + exp(PI)]
Cut-off values:	
Premenopausal	>7.4% High risk of finding EOC
	<7.4% Low risk of finding EOC
Postmenopausal	>24.3% High risk of finding EOC
	<25.3% Low risk of finding EOC

Table 20.4: FIGO Ovarian Cancer Staging
Effective Jan. 1, 2014 (changes are in Italics)
STAGE I: Tumor confined to ovaries

Old		New	
IA	Tumor limited to 1 ovary, capsule intact, no tumor on surface, negative washings/ascites.	IA	Tumor limited to 1 ovary, capsule intact, no tumor on surface, negative washings.
IB	Tumor involves both ovaries otherwise like IA.	IB	Tumor involves both ovaries otherwise like IA.
IC	Tumor involves 1 or both ovaries with any of the following: capsule rupture, tumor on surface, positive washings/ascites.	IC	*Tumor limited to 1 or both ovaries*
		IC1	*Surgical spill*
		IC2	*Capsule rupture before surgery or tumor on ovarian surface. Malignant cells in the ascites or peritoneal washings.*

STAGE II: Tumor involves 1 or both ovaries with pelvic extension (below the pelvic brim) or primary peritoneal cancer

Old		New	
IIA	Extension and/or implant on uterus and/or fallopian tubes	IIA	Extension and/or implant on uterus and/or fallopian tubes
IIB	Extension to other pelvic intraperitoneal tissues	IIB	Extension to other pelvic intraperitoneal tissues
IIC	IIA or IIB with positive washings/ascites.		

STAGE III: Tumor involves 1 or both ovaries with cytologically or histologically confirmed spread to the peritoneum outside the pelvis and/or metastasis to the retroperitoneal lymph nodes

	Old		New
IIIA	Microscopic metastasis beyond the pelvis.	*IIIA*	*Positive retroperitoneal lymph nodes and/or microscopic metastasis beyond the pelvis*
		IIIA1	*Positive retroperitoneal lymph nodes only*
			IIIA1(i) Metastasis <10 mm
			IIIA1(ii) Metastasis >10 mm
		IIIA2	*Microscopic, extrapelvic (above the brim) peritoneal involvement ± positive retroperitoneal lymph nodes*
IIIB	Macroscopic, extrapelvic, peritoneal metastasis <2 cm in greatest dimension.	IIIB	*Macroscopic, extrapelvic, peritoneal metastasis <2 cm ± positive retroperitoneal lymp nodes. Includes extension to capsule of liver/spleen.*
IIIC	Macroscopic, extrapelvic, peritoneal metastasis >2 cm in greatest dimension and/or regional lymph node metastasis.	IIIC	*Macroscopic, extrapelvic, peritoneal metastasis >2 cm ± positive retroperitoneal lymph nodes. Includes extension to capsule of liver/spleen.*

STAGE IV: Distant metastasis excluding peritoneal metastasis

	Old		New
IV	Distant metastasis excluding peritoneal metastasis. Includes hepatic parenchymal metastasis.	*IVA*	*Pleural effusion with positive cytology*
		IVB	*Hepatic and/or splenic parenchymal metastasis, metastasis to extra-abdominal organs (including inguinal lymph nodes and lymph nodes outside of the abdominal cavity)*

Other major recommendations are as follows:
• Histologic type including grading should be designated at staging
• Primary site (ovary, fallopian tube or peritoneum) should be designated where possible
• Tumors that may otherwise qualify for stage I but involved with dense adhesions justify upgrading to stage II, if tumor cells are histologically proven to be present in the adhesions.

Table 20.5: Carcinoma of the ovary—stage grouping

FIGO Stage	T	UICC N	M
IA	T1a	N0	M0
IB	T1b	N0	M0
IC	T1c	N0	M0
IIA	T2a	N0	M0
IIB	T2b	N0	M0
IIC	T2c	N0	M0
IIIA	T3a	N0	M0
IIIB	T3b	N0	M0
IIIC	T3c	N0	M0
Any T	N1	M0	
IV	Any T	Any N	M1

Regional Nodes (N)

Nx	Regional lymph nodes cannot be assessed
N0	No regional lymph node metastasis
N1	Regional lymph node metastasis

Distant Metastasis (M)

Mx	Distant metastasis cannot be assessed
M0	No distant metastasis
M1	Distant metastasis (excluding peitoneal metastasis)

Treatment

I. Sequelae and Impact of Ovarian Cancer

1. Suffer from gut obstruction and malnutrition, renal failure, liver failure, respiratory failure, severe chronic pain, infection and sepsis.
2. Direct sequelae from cancer and metastases:
   • Primary tumor: Intractable pain
   • Secondary tumor: Brain, bone, lung, liver, KUB system, GI system, lymph nodes
3. Indirect sequelae from treatments and complications:
   • *Surgery:* Hemorrhage, internal organ injury, gut obstruction.
   • *Chemotherapy:* Leukopenia, thrombocytopenia, sepsis, renal failure, cardiotoxicity, hypersensitivity reaction.
   • *Molecular therapy:* Hypertension, bowel perforation.

II. Challenges of Ovarian Cancer

1. Pre-cancer lesion has not yet been identified.
2. Most cases are diagnosed in advanced stage. 85% patients with ovarian cancer are diagnosed when the cancer cells already metastasize out of the ovary to the whole abdomen.
3. Survival and prognosis directly relate to extent of disease. Women with early ovarian cancer remain largely asymptomatic.
4. Symptoms are non-specific: 90% patients with ovarian cancer had non-specific symptoms which mostly are misdiagnosed and, therefore, result in delay to start proper treatment.
5. Difficulty in palpation by either patients or physicians: Neither the patient nor the non-gynecologic physicians can feel abdominal mass before it is enlarged to beyond pubic symphysis.
6. Result of the treatment is poor in advanced stage since the most reliable prognosis depends on the residual tumor after every attempted surgery.
7. The present tumor markers are non-specific: Currently, CA125 is widely used as the most promising tool. But only 50% of patients with FIGO stage I and 60% of patients with FIGO stage II have shown an increased CA125 level.

Surgery in Ovarian Cancer

 i. Total abdominal hysterectomy with bilateral salpingo-oophorectomy
 ii. With infracolic/total omentectomy with or without appendicectomy
 iii. With bilateral para-aortic and pelvic node dissection
 iv. Delayed primary surgery
 v. Primary debulking or cytoreductive surgery
 vi. Secondary debulking surgery
 vii. 2nd look laparoscopy
 viii. 2nd look laparotomy
 ix. Random biopsy of abdominal peritoneum in early-stage disease

Choosing Appropriate Surgery

Appropriate surgery depends on whether or not disease is visible outside the ovaries. It is essential that where no disease is visible outside the ovaries, the patient must be adequately surgically staged because the incidence of microscopic metastases is significant. Surgery for patients with advanced stage disease should be individualized, particularly when disease is in the liver and above the diaphragm. Patients who are in stage IV because of small-volume disease in the liver, abdominal wall, or lung should undergo cytoreductive surgery, if medically fit.

Surgical Staging

The standard care for ovarian cancer includes surgical exploration for primary staging and for cytoreduction or debulking. If the disease appears to be confined to the pelvis, comprehensive surgical staging is indicated.

The staging procedure should include the following:
- Peritoneal cytology
- Multiple peritoneal biopsies
- Omentectomy
- Pelvic and para-aortic lymph node sampling.

I. Staging Laparotomy (Primary Definitive Surgery)

a. Incision is always midline vertical.
b. After entering peritoneal cavity, ascitic fluid of 100 mL is collected for cytology.
c. If ascites is absent, peritoneal wash is given in the peritoneal cavity and returning fluid is collected and sent for cytology.
d. This is followed by detailed examination of the abdominal contents including the peritoneal surface. Random biopsy is taken from all the suspicious sites. The whole peritoneal surfaces, paracolic gutters, ascending, transverse and descending colons, undersurface of diaphragm, liver, gallbladder, greater and lesser sac, epiploic foramen, stomach, pylorus, DJ flexure, pelvic side walls, pouch of Douglas, rectosigmoid areas, appendix, superior surface of bladder are explored and biopsy taken.
e. The greater and lesser omentum, pelvic and para-aortic lymph nodes are looked for enlarged metastases.
f. The primary ovaries, uterus are next explored and watched for unilateral or bilateral involvement, rupture of capsules, adhesions to surrounding areas, uterine position, its surfaces, anterior reflection of vesicouterine fold of peritoneum, uterosacral ligaments, parametrium are looked for involvement.
g. Total hysterectomy and bilateral salpingo-oophorectomy along with removal of all the tumor sites are completed. Total or infracolic omentectomy along with appendicectomy is also done, if mucinous tumor is suspected.

In younger patients where fertility preservation is an issue, the prognosis according to the extent of the tumor should be discussed and conservative surgery is considered with informed consent.

Conservative surgery should include the following:
a. Assessment of the whole intraperitoneal areas.
b. Removal of the affected ovary with tube, if there is unilateral ovarian involvement with capsule intact (stage IA).
c. Normal examination of the opposite ovary and *contralateral wedge biopsy is not recommended as it can affect the subsequent fertility*.

II. Cytoreductive Surgery

This should be performed by a gynecologic oncologist at the time of initial laparotomy. The volume of residual disease at the completion of surgery represents one of the most powerful prognostic factors. According to the 2011 National Comprehensive Cancer Network (NCCN) ovarian cancer guidelines (Table 20.6), residual disease of less than 1 cm is evidence of optimal cytoreduction and, therefore, greatest possible effort should be made to remove all obvious disease. According to this guideline, distal pancreatectomy may be considered in all stages for optimal surgical cytoreduction.

Patients with advanced ovarian cancer are classified in 3 groups as follows, based on the postoperative residual tumor:
- *Low risk:* Microscopic disease outside the pelvis (stage IIIA) or macroscopic disease less than 2 cm outside the pelvis (stage IIIB).
- *Intermediate risk:* Macroscopic disease less than 2 cm outside the pelvis only after surgery.
- *High risk:* Macroscopic disease more than 2 cm after surgery or disease outside the peritoneal cavity.

III. Interval Debulking

Interval debulking is performed in patients who were not adequately debulked at the time of initial primary surgery. It should also be considered in those patients

Table 20.6: Treatment plans (NCCN guidelines)		
1A: Cancer only in one ovary	Unilateral salpingo-oophorectomy or total abdominal hysterectomy with bilateral salpingo-oophorectomy	+ Surgical staging
1B: Cancer confined to both ovaries	Total abdominal hysterectomy with bilateral salpingo-oophorectomy	+ Surgical staging
1C: Cancer in one or both ovaries with cancer cells on ovarian surface or in peritoneal fluid	TAH+BSO+ infracolic omentectomy	+ Surgical staging
II: Cancer in one or both ovaries with spread into pelvis	TAH & BSO+ infracolic omentectomy+ remove as much tumor as possible	
III & IV: Cancer involving one or both ovaries spread to distant sites	If all cancer can be removed, debulking surgery, if all cancer cannot be removed, take biopsy, start chemotherapy for 3 cycles and then remove all lesions	

in whom an initial debulking surgery was not attempted. Patients usually receive 3 cycles of postoperative chemotherapy. Approximately 60% of patients are then able to undergo optimal resection. Surgical treatment is followed by 3 more cycles of chemotherapy.

A meta-analysis found no conclusive evidence regarding the possible survival benefit of interval debulking but noted apparent benefit only in patients whose primary surgery was not performed by gynecologic oncologists or was less extensive.

IV. Laparoscopic Surgery

According to guidelines developed by the American College of Obstetricians and Gynecologists, laparoscopy may be used for diagnostic purposes in a patient with low risk for ovarian cancer and to remove cystic masses.

a. The mass must be 10 cm or smaller
b. Must have a distinct border and no solid parts
c. Must not be associated with ascites.
d. The serum CA125 level must be normal (<35 U/mL).
e. Early stage lesions (stage I).

As part of initial treatment of epithelial ovarian cancer, laparoscopic surgery may be performed for early stage disease when no disease is visible outside of the ovaries. Its use in more advanced disease (when spread is visible outside the ovaries) is more limited due to disseminated intraperitoneal metastatic deposits, need for extensive cytoreduction necessary and the risk of port-site recurrence. Laparoscopy also has a role in second-look inspection in treatment follow up and in the staging of apparently early-stage disease found by chance during another surgery.

V. Secondary Surgery

Secondary cytoreductive surgery is safe and effective in patients with platinum-sensitive recurrent ovarian cancer. The surgery was most beneficial in patients who had remained disease free for more than 24 months after primary treatment and in those who achieved optimal cytoreduction.

Stage I and Stage II Ovarian Epithelial Cancer Treatment

Treatment Options

1. If the tumor is well differentiated or moderately well differentiated, surgery alone may be adequate treatment for patients with stages IA and IB disease. Surgery should include hysterectomy, bilateral salpingo-oophorectomy, and omentectomy. Additionally, the undersurface of the diaphragm should be visualized and biopsied; pelvic and abdominal peritoneal biopsies and pelvic and para-aortic lymph node biopsies are required and peritoneal washings should be obtained routinely. In selected patients who desire childbearing and have grade I tumors, unilateral salpingo-oophorectomy may be associated with low risk of recurrence.

2. If the tumor is grade III, densely adherent, or stage IC, the chance of relapse and death from ovarian cancer is almost 30%. The following treatment approaches have been performed:
   - Intraperitoneal P-32 or radiation therapy.
   - Systemic chemotherapy based on platinum compounds alone or in combination with alkylating agents.
   - Systemic chemotherapy based on platinums with paclitaxel. Chemotherapy is given for at least 6 cycles.

Stage III

First, the cancer is surgically *staged* and the tumor is debulked. The uterus, both fallopian tubes, both ovaries, and omentum (fatty tissue from the upper abdomen near the stomach and intestines) are removed. The goal is to leave behind no tumor larger than 1 cm. When this goal is reached, the cancer is said to have been *optimally debulked*.

Sometimes tumor is growing on the intestines, and in order to remove the cancer, part of the intestine will have to be removed. Sometimes pieces of other organs (like the bladder or liver) may have to be removed to remove the cancer.

After recovery from surgery, combination chemotherapy is given. The combination used most often is carboplatin (or cisplatin) and a taxane, such as paclitaxel, given IV for 6 cycles.

Another option is to give intra-abdominal (intraperitoneal or IP) chemotherapy after surgery. IP chemotherapy means giving the drug paclitaxel IV along with cisplatin and paclitaxel into the abdomen (IP); women who get IP chemotherapy are actually receiving both IV and IP chemotherapeutic drugs. This is only considered, if the cancer is optimally debulked but because of its worse side effects, it is not favored always.

After surgery, and during and after chemotherapy, blood tests for CA125 will be done to determine to assess the therapeutic response. A CT scan, PET-CT scan, or MRI can be done to evaluate response to treatment.

Patients who are too weak to have full staging they are treated with chemotherapy as the first line of treatment. If the tumor respond to chemotherapy and the patient becomes stronger, surgery to debulk the cancer may be done, often followed by more chemotherapy. Most often, 3 cycles of chemotherapy are given before surgery with at least 3 more after surgery for a total of at least 6 cycles.

Second look surgery: In the past, many experts recommended this operation (laparoscopy/laparotomy) to assess the tumor response to chemotherapy. This is known as a *second look surgery*. These operations haven't been shown to have any real benefit, and so are no longer a standard part of ovarian cancer care. Still, they may be done as part of a clinical trial. In a clinical trial of new treatments, the second-look operation may be worthwhile to help determine how effective the new treatment is.

In 2nd look laparoscopy, one can inspect the abdominal cavity to see how successful treatment has been.

Stage IV Ovarian Epithelial Cancer Treatment

Treatment options for patients with all stages of ovarian epithelial cancer consist of surgery followed by chemotherapy.

Surgery

Patients diagnosed with stage IV disease are treated with surgery and chemotherapy; however, the outcome is generally less favorable for patients with stage IV disease. The role of surgery for patients with stage IV disease is unclear, but in most instances, the bulk of the disease is intra-abdominal, and surgical procedures are optimal cytoreduction before or after chemotherapy. The options for intraperitoneal (IP) regimens are less likely to be effective in patients with stage IV disease.

Surgery has been used as a therapeutic modality and also to adequately stage the disease. It includes total abdominal hysterectomy, bilateral salpingo-oophorectomy with omentectomy and debulking of as much gross tumor as can safely be performed. Despite primary cytoreductive surgery, considerable evidence indicates that the volume of disease left at the completion of the primary surgical procedure is the major prognostic factor related to patient survival.

Treatment Options for Patients with Suboptimally Cytoreduced Stage IV Disease

Cytoreductive surgery: The value of interval cytoreductive surgery has been the subject of two large phase III trials. In the first study, performed by the European Organisation for Rasearch Treatment of Cancer (EORTC), patients subjected to debulking after four cycles of cyclophosphamide and cisplatin (with additional cycles given later) have an improved survival rate compared with patients who completed six cycles of this chemotherapy without surgery.

Systemic chemotherapy: First-line treatment of ovarian cancer is cisplatin, given IV, or its second-generation analog, carboplatin, given either alone or in combination with other drugs. Clinical response rates from these drugs regularly exceed 60%, and median time-to-recurrence usually exceeds 1 year in this subset of suboptimally debulked women. Agents used include pegylated liposomal doxorubicin, docetaxel, paclitaxel, topotecan, gemcitabine, etoposide, and bevacizumab. The order, schedule and dosing are quite variable, depending on many factors.

With the introduction of the taxane paclitaxel, two trials confirmed the superiority of cisplatin combined with paclitaxel to the previous standard of cisplatin plus cyclophosphamide. Two important trials on combination chemotherapy are listed in Table 20.7.

Recurrent or Persistent Ovarian Cancer

Cancer is called *recurrent* when it relapses after treatment. Recurrence can be local (in or near the same place where it originated) or distant (spread to organs like the lungs or bone). Persistent tumors are those that never go away completely after treatment. Sometimes, more *surgery* is recommended. Most patients with recurrent or persistent ovarian cancer are treated with alternate form of *chemotherapy*. The longer it takes for the cancer to come back after treatment, the better the chance that additional chemotherapy will work. If it has been at least 6 months since any chemothearpy, the

Table 20.7: Combination chemotherapy—two important trials		
Trial	*Treatment regimens*	*Overall Survial (mth)*
GOG-132	Paclitaxel (135 mg/m², 24 h) and cisplatin (75 mg/m²)	26.6
	Cisplatin (100 mg/m²)	30.2
	Paclitaxel (200 mg/m², 24 h)	26
MRC-ICON3(20)	Paclitaxel (175 mg/m², 3 h) and carboplatin AUC 6	36.1
	Carboplatin AUC 6	35.4
	Paclitaxel (175 mg/m², 3 h) and carboplatin AUC 6	40
	Cyclophosphamide (500 mg/m²) and doxorubicin (50 mg/m²) and cisplatin (50 mg/m²)	40

patient may be treated with carboplatin and paclitaxel (even if these drugs were given before).

If the cancer comes back in less than 6 months or in case of persistent disease, different chemotherapy drugs usually are tried. In addition, some patients benefit from *hormonal treatment* with drugs like anastrozole, letrozole, or tamoxifen.

High-dose chemotherapy with stem cell rescue (*stem cell transplant*) has been used for women with recurrent or persistent ovarian cancer.

Palliative treatment: A common problem that can occur in women with ovarian cancer is the development of ascites. When it becomes huge producing cardio-respiratory emberassment. It is treated with repeated paracentesis. Treatment with bevacizumab may also be an option. These treatments can relieve symptoms for some patients and, rarely, might extend life.

Ovarian cancer can also result in intestinal obstruction and can cause abdominal pain, nausea, and vomiting. This is overcome by nasogastric suction, colostomy or resection anastomosis.

Consolidation and/or Maintenance Therapy

Trials of consolidation and/or maintenance therapy have been carried out with drugs that contribute to the treatment of recurrent ovarian cancer. Presently, none of the treatments given after the initial platinum/paclitaxel induction has been shown to improve survival; these treatments include the following:

- Intraperitoneal cisplatin for four cycles.
- Yttrium-labeled radioimmunoconjugate plus IP chemotherapy.
- IV topotecan for four cycles.
- Oregovomab vaccination.
- Monthly paclitaxel for 12 cycles.
- Olaparib, an oral (adenosine diphosphate [ADP]-ribose) polymerase (PARP) inhibitor can be used in advanced ovarian cancer linked to BRCA mutation.

Chemotherapy for Ovarian Cancer

Chemotherapy is administered through different routes like oral, parenteral, thecal and intraperitoneal. For some cases of ovarian cancer, chemotherapy may also be injected through a catheter directly into the abdominal cavity. This is called *intraperitoneal (IP) chemotherapy*.

Chemotherapy for Epithelial Ovarian Cancer

Chemotherapy for ovarian cancer most often is a combination of 2 or more drugs, given IV every 3- to 4-weeks. Giving 2 or more drugs in combination seems to be more effective in the initial treatment of ovarian cancer than giving just one drug alone.

The standard approach is the combination of a platinum compound, such as *cisplatin* or *carboplatin*, and a taxane, such as *paclitaxel* or *docetaxel*. For IV chemotherapy, most doctors favor carboplatin over cisplatin because it has fewer side effects and is just as effective.

The typical course of chemotherapy for epithelial ovarian cancer involves 3 to 6 cycles. A cycle is a schedule of regular doses of a drug, followed by a rest period.

Some of the other drugs that are helpful in treating ovarian cancer include:

- Altretamine, capecitabine
- Cyclophosphamide
- Etoposide
- Gemcitabine
- Ifosfamide
- Irinotecan, camptosar
- Liposomal doxorubicin
- Melphalan
- Pemetrexed
- Topotecan
- Vinorelbine

Chemotherapy drugs has some serious side effects, which depend on the type of drugs, the amount taken, and the length of treatment. Common side effects include:

- Nausea and vomiting
- Loss of appetite
- Loss of hair
- Hand and foot rashes
- Mouth sores
- Leucopenia
- Thrombocytopenia
- Fatigue caused by anemia

Most side effects disappear once treatment is stopped. Hair will grow again after treatment ends, although it may look different.

Some chemotherapy drugs may have long-term or even permanent side effects. For example, cisplatin can cause kidney damage, ototoxicity. Both cisplatin and the taxanes can cause peripheral neuropathy causing numbness, tingling, or even pain in the hands and feet.

Chemotherapeutic drugs can also cause early menopause and permanent infertility. Therefore, in young patient, cryopreservation of eggs is currently being considered in IVF center for those who are willing to have future pregnancy before start of treatment.

Rarely, some drugs can permanently damage bone marrow resulting in myelodysplastic syndrome or even acute myeloid leukemia. This is called **secondary malignancy.**

Intraperitoneal Chemotherapy

In intraperitoneal (IP) chemotherapy for ovarian cancer, in addition to giving the chemotherapeutic drug systemetically, the drugs cisplatin and paclitaxel are injected into the abdominal cavity through a catheter . The tube can be placed during the staging/debulking surgery, but sometimes it is placed later. If it is done later, it can be placed by a surgeon using laparoscopy, or by an interventional radiologist under X-ray guidance. The catheter is usually connected to a port which is placed under the skin against a bony structure of the abdominal wall, such as a rib or pelvic bone. A needle can be placed through the skin and into the port to give anticancer. Problems may rarely occur with the catheter become plugged or infected or even damage the bowel.

This gives the most concentrated dose of the drugs to the cancer cells in the abdominal cavity. This drug also gets absorbed into the bloodstream and so can reach cancer cells outside the abdominal cavity. IP chemotherapy works well, but the side effects are often more severe than with regular route.

IP chemotherapy currently is only given to some of the women with ovarian cancer that has spread to the inside of the abdomen. They are not very effective in presence of lot of adhesions or scar tissue inside their abdomen because this can prevent the drugs from spreading well.

Epithelial Cancers

I. Serous Cystadenocarcinoma/Carcinoma
(Fig. 20.22)

General

- 65% bilateral.
- May arise from tubal intraepithelial carcinoma.
- Recommended to classify as high grade or low grade.
- May present as lymphadenopathy (usually inguinal (supraclavicular), has similar survival by stage as classic presentation.
- Rarely metastasizes to breast or axillary nodes, associated with advanced stage disease; usually have papillary features but only occasionally psammoma bodies.
- 5-year survival of 70%, if confined to ovary; drops to 25%, if involves peritoneum.
- Rarely produces AFP.

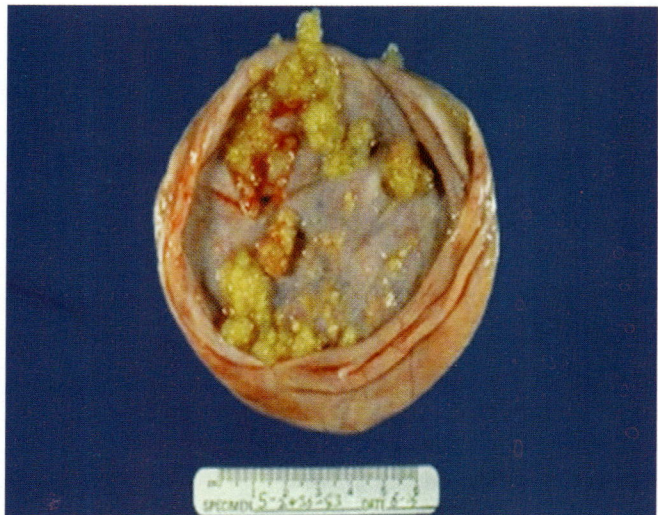

Fig. 20.22: Serous cystadenocarcinoma. The tumor is solid, hemorrhagic, necrotic with papillary growth inside or protruding outside. High grade tumors often have extreme drug resistance

II. Mucinous Cystadenocarcinoma
(Figs 20.23 and 20.24)

- 77% of ovarian mucinous carcinomas are metastases, 23% are ovarian primaries.
- Of the ovarian primaries, most arise in a benign or borderline tumor; only 5–10% are pure.
- Features favoring primary ovarian carcinoma vs. metastasis are: unilateral, "expansile" pattern of invasion, complex papillary pattern, size >10 cm; metastatic tumors have smooth external surface, microscopic cystic glands, necrotic luminal debris, mural nodules and accompanying teratoma, adenofibroma.

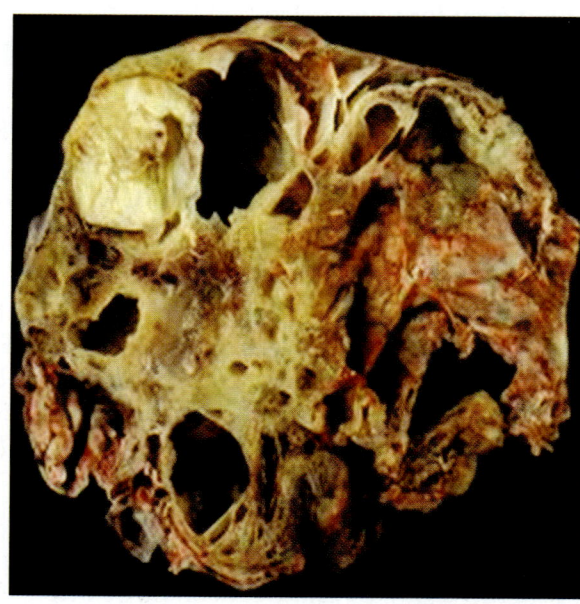

Fig. 20.23: Mucinous cystadenocarcinoma

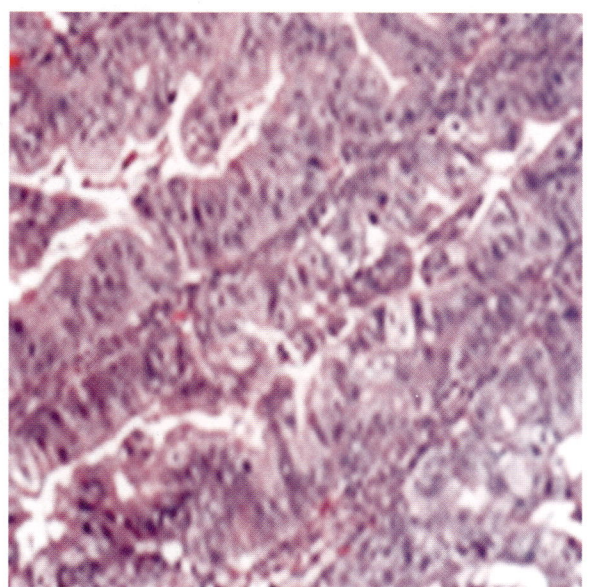

Fig. 20.24: Histologic picture of mucinous cystadenocarcinoma

- Stromal invasion >10 mm² distinguishes these tumors from borderline tumors.
- Two types of invasion—expansile or infiltrative:
  - Expansile tumors are usually stage I and behave "benign".
  - Infiltrative tumors may demonstrate malignant behavior and cause death even if stage I.

Clinical Features

Distant metastases are rare.
Survival: 95% for stage I vs. 32% for stages II or greater.

Micro Description

- Stromal invasion with solid growth, atypia, stratification, papillae, loss of glandular architecture, necrosis (resembles colon carcinoma), greater complexity of glands than borderline tumors.
- Stromal invasion may be *infiltrative* with disorderly penetration of stroma by neoplastic glands, single cells or cell clusters, may have desmoplastic response or *expansile (confluent)* with complex arrangement of glands, cysts or papillae lined by malignant epithelium with minimal or no intervening stroma with a broad, sharply defined border.
- Glands are almost always intestinal type.
- Endocervical type usually has other epithelial components (serous, endometrioid, squamous).
- Carcinoma often merges with borderline or benign mucinous tumors.
- Rarely has signet ring cells, but differs from Krukenberg tumor.

Grading

- Not standardized, and does not predict prognosis
- Grade 1—no solid areas
- Grade 2—up to 50% solid foci
- Grade 3—more than 50% solid foci
- Severe nuclear atypia can increase grade 1 or 2 carcinomas by one grade.

III. Endometrioid Carcinoma (Fig. 20.25A and B)

General

- 10–25% of primary ovarian carcinomas.
- 15% coexist with endometriosis; tumors may arise from endometriotic cysts.
- 15–30% of patients have synchronous endometrial hyperplasia or carcinoma; these tumors are often well differentiated with squamous metaplasia.
- Associated with keratin granulomas of peritoneum, which are devoid of viable cells; may contain ghosts of squamous cells or keratin debris.
- Search for viable tumor cells; but granulomas alone do not change stage or prognosis.
- Mean age 51 years, range 26–87 years.
- Grading: Similar to primary carcinomas in the endometrium.

Gross Description

- Cystic, solid, hemorrhagic
- Papillary formations are absent or inconspicuous
- 5% bilateral
- Mean 11 cm, range 3–22 cm

Micro Description

- It has either non-cystic villoglandular pattern, glandular confluence or stromal disappearance.
- Stromal invasion is seen with confluent glandular growth or stromal disappearance.
- Resembles endometrioid adenocarcinoma of endometrium, usually well differentiated.
- 50% have squamous metaplasia (morules or keratin pearls, formerly called adenoacanthomas), 40% of

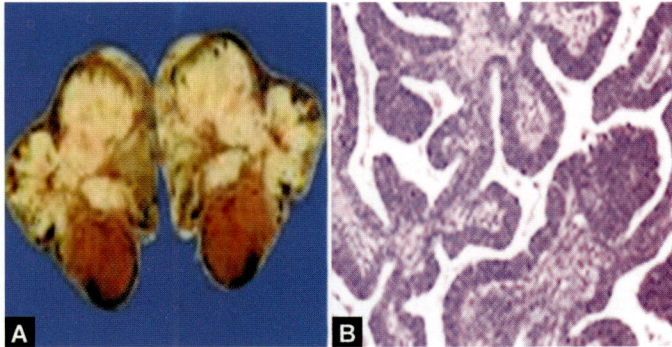

Fig. 20.25: (A) Endometrioid adenocarcinoma of ovary, (B) Microscopic picture of endometrioid adenocarcinoma

well-differentiated tumors have adenofibromatous component.
- 10% are associated with luteinized stroma cells.
- May contain luminal but not cytoplasmic mucin, may have clear cells but lacks the architecture of clear cell carcinoma.
- Vascular invasion rare.

Prognostic Factors

- Better than serous/mucinous tumors because it is usually stage I and well differentiated, but when matched for age, stage and grade, prognosis is similar to serous type.
- Cytologic atypia and microinvasion do not appear to affect prognosis.
- Prognosis not as good as borderline tumors; may have malignant behavior, if limited destructive stromal invasion.
- Mixed variety with serous or undifferentiated carcinoma component lowers 5-year survival from 63% (pure) to 8%. Tumors with yolk sac component are unusually aggressive.

IV. Malignant Brenner Tumor

General

Ovarian masses are bossilated, soft to firm and relatively rare tumor. Cut section shows yellowish white, homogenous, smooth surfaces with peripheral cyst. The tumor contains predominately malignant transitional cells. The malignant cells are arranged in nests and sheets, inflitrating and replacing the fibrous stroma. The tumor cells display moderate degree of anaplasia with high mitotic activity and necrosis.

Microscopic Appearance (Fig. 20.26)

The cysts show glandular pattern and contain necrotic tumor cells. Benign Brenner tumor components are also seen in the sections. The peripheral cysts have transitional cell lining. The malignant counterpart has atypical cytology and stromal invasion. It may be bilateral and has better prognosis than urothelial (transitional cell) carcinoma.

V. Clear Cell Adenocarcinoma

General

This is also called mesonephroid adenocarcinoma. It is associated with endometriosis or endometrioid carcinoma of the ovary. This is common in ages 40–59 years. Stage for stage, it has similar prognosis to other ovarian carcinomas. It is characterized by resistance to conventional platinum-based chemotherapy, and new therapeutic strategies are urgently required.

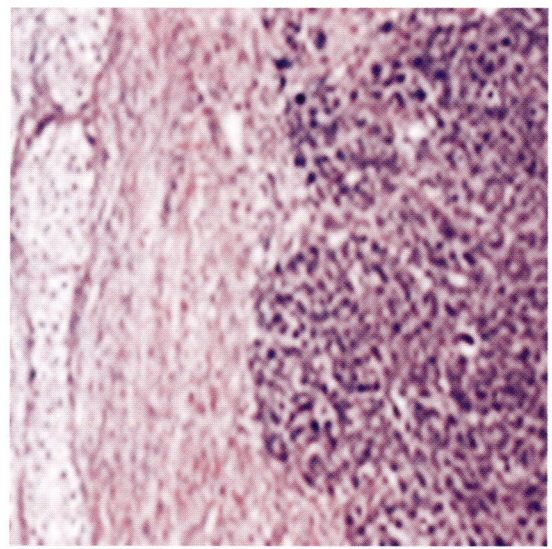

Fig. 20.26: Microscopic picture of Malignant Brenner tumor

Gross Description

Clear cell ovarian *tumors* are part of the *surface epithelial-stromal tumor* group of *ovarian cancers*, accounting for 6% of these cancers. Typically, they are cystic neoplasms with polyploid masses that protrude into the cyst.

Micro Description (Fig. 20.27)

On *microscopic pathological* examination, they are composed of cells with clear *cytoplasm* (that contains *glycogen*) and ***hobnail* cells** (from which glycogen is secreted). The pattern may be glandular, papillary or solid. Papillary cores have prominent hyalinization. Large tumor cells, some with nuclei that protrude into lumina (hobnail), clear cytoplasm (glycogen, mucin, fat). It resembles mucinous tumor on frozen section.

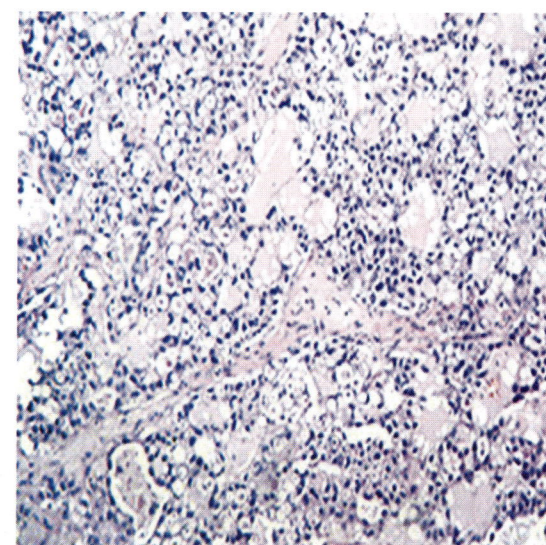

Fig. 20.27: Microscopic picture of clear cell adenocarcinoma

20C. OVARIAN GERM CELL TUMORS

Ovarian germ cell tumor is a disease in which malignant cells form in the germ cells of the ovary. Ovarian germ cell tumors usually occur in teenage girls or young women and most often affect just one ovary.

Incidence

Ovarian germ cell tumors (OGCT) are a type of ovarian neoplasm principally affecting young women. Germ cell neoplasms are thought to be derived from primitive germ cells of the embryonic gonad. They constitute the second largest group of ovarian neoplasms (15–20%). These tumors can occur in women at any age, but peak incidence is seen during the early 20s. In children and adolescents, >60% of ovarian neoplasms are of germ cell origin, of which one-third are malignant. In adults, the vast majority of germ cell tumors are benign (nearly all mature cystic teratomas). Dysgerminoma is the most common germ cell tumor, accounting for 50% of all germ cell tumor cases. About 20% of cases are diagnosed during pregnancy, and 80% occur in women under 30. Yolk sac tumors (endodermal sinus tumors) are the second most common germ cell tumor, accounting for 20% of all cases, and are common in girls and young adults (Table 20.8).

Clinical Features (Table 20.9)

Ovarian germ cell tumors can be difficult to diagnose in early stage since there are no symptoms in the early stages. The tumors may be found during routine gynecologic checkups. The young age, family

Table 20.8: Cellular classification of ovarian germ cell tumors

The following histologic subtypes have been described.
- Dysgerminoma
- Endodermal sinus tumor (rare subtypes are hepatoid and intestinal)
- Embryonal carcinoma
- Polyembryoma
- Choriocarcinoma
- Teratoma
- Immature
- Mature
- Solid

Cystic:
- Dermoid cyst (mature cystic teratoma)
- Dermoid cyst with malignant transformation

Monodermal and highly specialized:
- Struma ovarii
- Carcinoid
- Struma ovarii and carcinoid
- Others (e.g. malignant neuroectodermal and ependymoma)
- Mixed forms

history, association with pregnancy along with the following symptoms are suggestive of germ cell tumor:
- Swelling of abdomen in a very short duration
- Short history of onset of GI symptoms.
- Bleeding from the vagina after menopause
- Pain abdomen

Physical examination: Low general condition, anemia, enlarged lymph glands, evidence of lung metastases,

Table 20.9: Features of different types of germ cell tumors

Subtype	Frequency of OGCT	Benign/Malignant	Uni- or bilateral	Tumor markers expressed	Metastasis route
Dysgerminoma	35–50%	Malignant	10–15% are bilateral	Serum lactic dehydrogenase and serum hCG	Lymphatic system
Endodermal sinus tumor (EST)	20%	Malignant	Usually unilateral	AFP (commonly), apha1-antitypsin (rarely).	Intraperitoneally and hematogenously
Embryonal carcinoma	Rare	Malignant	Usually unilateral	AFP and hCG	Intraperitoneally
Polyembryoma	Rare			AFP and hCG	
Choriocarcinoma	Very rare	Malignant	Usually unilateral	hCG	
Teratoma	Immature account for 20% of v malignant GCT	Benign or malignant	12–15% are bilateral	Immature teratomas sometimes secrete AFP, Serum LDH and CA-125	
Mixed GCT	10–15%	Dependent upon the cell types present		Dependent upon the cell types present	

enlarged liver, omental cakes, discrete intra-abdominal metastases, presence of tender ovarian lumps with variegated partially solid, partially cystic feel with irregular borders, ascites are suggestive of malignancy in advanced stage.

Pelvic examination: Bilateral or unilateral solid enlarged ovarian SOL felt through fornices, separate from uterus with restricted mobility, tender, irregular surface and nodular metastases are diagnostic of ovarian malignancy. The germ cell origin of the tumor is only ascertained by its histological examination.

Investigations

- *USG* (Fig. 20.28): This is the primary investigation of choice to assess the origin of the mass, its internal structures, involvement of one or both ovaries, its vascularity, evidence of extra ovarian metastases, ascites, etc.
- *CT scan/MRI:* A procedure that makes a series of detailed pictures of areas inside the body, taken from different angles. A dye may be injected into a vein or swallowed to help the organs or tissues show up more clearly (Figs 20.29 and 20.30).
- *PET scan (positron emission tomography scan):* A procedure to find malignant tumor cells in the body. A small amount of radioactive glucose (sugar) is injected into a vein. The PET scanner rotates around the body and makes a picture of where glucose is being used in the body. Malignant tumor cells show up brighter in the picture because they are more active and take up more glucose than normal cells do.
- *Serum tumor marker test:* Blood is checked to measure the amounts of certain substances released

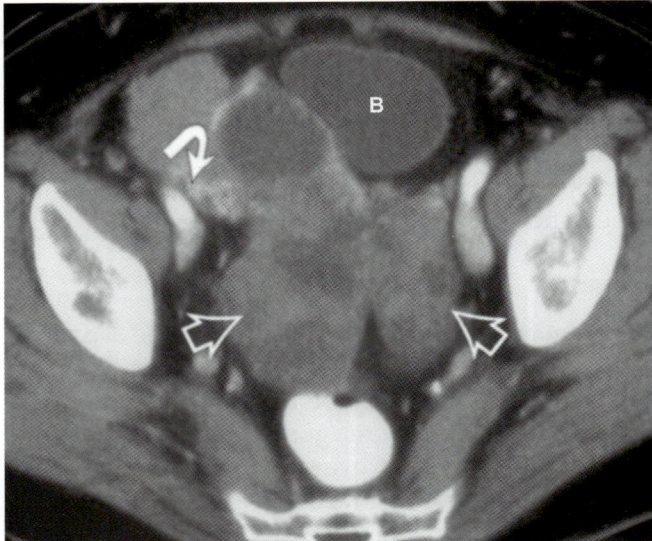

Fig. 20.29: CT scan shows bilateral complex solid and cystic adnexal tumors (open arrows)

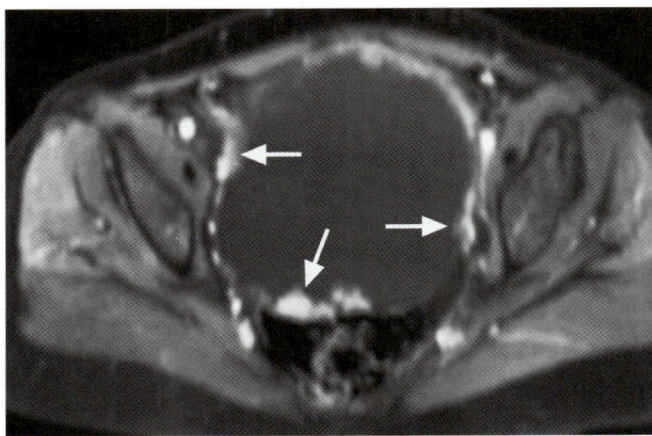

Fig. 20.30: T2-weighted and fat suppressed T1-weighted images after intravenous gadolinium enhancement show a large predominantly cystic ovarian mass with nodular vegetation seen on its internal surface (arrows)

into the blood by organs, tissues, or tumor cells in the body, which are linked to specific types of cancer when found in increased levels in the blood. These are called tumor markers. An increased level of alpha fetoprotein (AFP) or human chorionic gonadotropin (hCG) in the blood may be a sign of ovarian germ cell tumor.

TNM and FIGO Staging of Germ Cell Tumors

The American Joint Committee on Cancer (AJCC) TNM classification and the International Federation of Gynecology and Obstetrics (FIGO) staging system for germ cell tumors are listed in Tables 20.10 and 20.11.

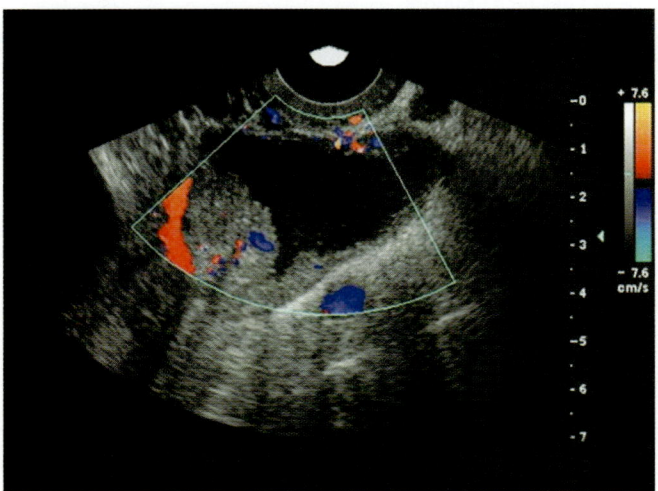

Fig. 20.28: Solid component within an ovarian malignancy with internal vascular flow

Table 20.10: FIGO staging of carcinoma of the ovary

Stage	
I	Growth limited to the ovaries.
IA	Growth limited to one ovary; no ascites present containing malignant cells. No tumor on the external surface; capsule intact.
IB	Growth limited to both ovaries; no ascites present containing malignant cells. No tumor on the external surfaces; capsules intact.
IC	Tumor either stage Ia or Ib, but with tumor on surface of one or both ovaries, or with capsule ruptured, or with ascites present containing malignant cells, or with positive peritoneal washings.
II	Growth involving one or both ovaries with pelvic extension.
IIA	Extension and/or metastases to the uterus and/or tubes.
IIB	Extension to other pelvic tissues.
IIC	Tumor either stage IIa or IIb, but with tumor on surface of one or both ovaries, or with capsule(s) ruptured, or with ascites present containing malignant cells, or with positive peritoneal washings.
III	Tumor involving one or both ovaries with histologically confirmed peritoneal implants outside the pelvis and/or positive regional lymph nodes. Superficial liver metastases equals stage III. Tumor is limited to the true pelvis, but with histologically proven malignant extension to small bowel or omentum.
IIIA	Tumor grossly limited to the true pelvis, with negative nodes, but with histologically confirmed microscopic seeding of abdominal peritoneal surfaces, or histologic proven extension to small bowel or mesentery.
IIIB	Tumor of one or both ovaries with histologically confirmed implants, peritoneal metastasis of abdominal peritoneal surfaces, none exceeding 2 cm in diameter; nodes are negative.
IIIC	Peritoneal metastasis beyond the pelvis >2 cm in diameter and/or positive regional lymph nodes.
IV	Growth involving one or both ovaries with distant metastases. If pleural effusion is present, there must be positive cytology to allot a case to stage IV. Parenchymal liver metastasis equals stage IV.

Table 20.11: TNM and FIGO staging of ovarian cancer

Primary tumor (T)

TNM	FIGO	Definition
TX		Primary tumor cannot be assessed
T0		No evidence of a primary tumor
T1	I	Tumor confined to the ovaries
T1a	IA	Tumor limited to one ovary, without capsular or surface involvement; cytology from peritoneal washings or ascites negative
T1b	IB	Tumor limited to both ovaries, without capsular or surface involvement; cytology from peritoneal washings or ascites negative
T1c	IC	Tumor limited to one of both ovaries, with any of the following: capsule ruptured, tumor on ovarian surface, malignant cells on cytology of ascites or peritoneal washings
T2	II	Tumor extends beyond ovaries but is limited to the pelvis
T2a	IIA	Extension and/or implants to uterus or tubes; cytology negative
T2b	IIB	Extension and/or implants to other pelvic tissue; cytology negative
T2c	IIC	Pelvic extension and/or implants; malignant cells on cytology of ascites or peritoneal washings
T3	III	Tumor extends to peritoneal cavity outside the pelvis or to regional lymph nodes
T3a	IIIA	Microscopic peritoneal metastasis beyond the pelvis
T3b	IIIB	Macroscopic peritoneal metastasis beyond the pelvis but = 2 cm in greatest dimension
T3c	IIIC	Peritoneal metastasis beyond pelvis = 2 cm in greatest dimension and/or regional lymph node metastasis

Regional lymph nodes (N)

TNM	FIGO	
NX		Regional lymph nodes cannot be assessed
N0		No regional lymph node metastasis
N1	IIIC	Regional (pelvic, para-aortic, inguinal) lymph node metastasis

Distant metastasis (M)

TNM	FIGO	
M0		No distant metastasis
M1	IV	Distant metastasis

Description of Germ Cell Tumors

Dysgerminoma (Fig. 20.31)

General

- 3–5% of ovarian malignant tumors and most common malignant ovarian germ cell tumor.
- Typically occurs in 2nd and 3rd decades (80% under 30 yrs)
- A unilateral, solid, firm to fleshy tumor.
- Composed of malignant germ cells, similar to primordial germ cells, admixed with non-neoplastic chronic inflammatory cells and occasionally granulomatous inflammation.
- Counterpart of testicular seminoma.

- Usually occur in young patients (81% under age 30).
- 5% associated with gonadal dysgenesis (Swyer syndrome), androgen insensitivity or pseudohermaphroditism; rarely associated with hypercalcemia.
- Metastasize to opposite ovary, retroperitoneal nodes and peritoneal cavity.
- Rarely transforms to yolk sac tumor.
- Mixture with choriocarcinoma, yolk sac or embryonal carcinoma worsens prognosis.
- It is highly sensitive to radiation and/or chemotherapy.

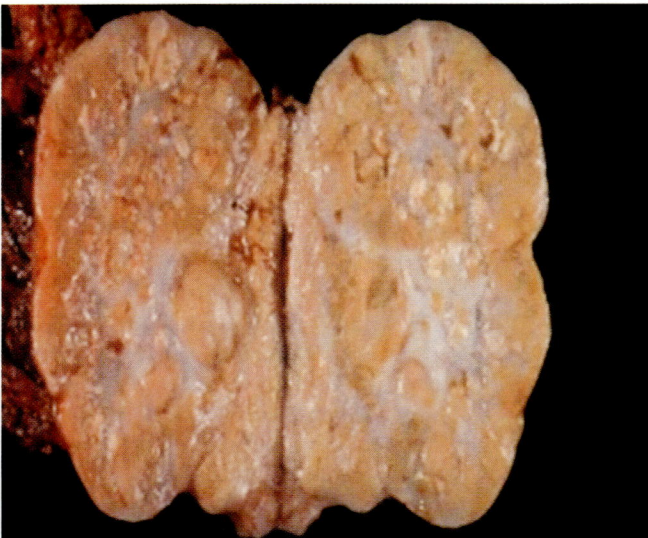

Fig. 20.31: Dysgerminoma

Gross Description

- 15% are bilateral.
- Solid, nodular, small to huge and gray-pink (resembles cerebral cortex).
- Hemorrhage and necrosis common, but less prominent than other malignant tumors.

Micro Description (Fig. 20.32)

- Nests of tumor cells separated by fibrous stroma with T lymphocytes.
- Large vesicular cells with well-defined cell borders, cleared cytoplasm containing glycogen and central nuclei.
- 1+ prominent nucleoli; occasional granulomas.

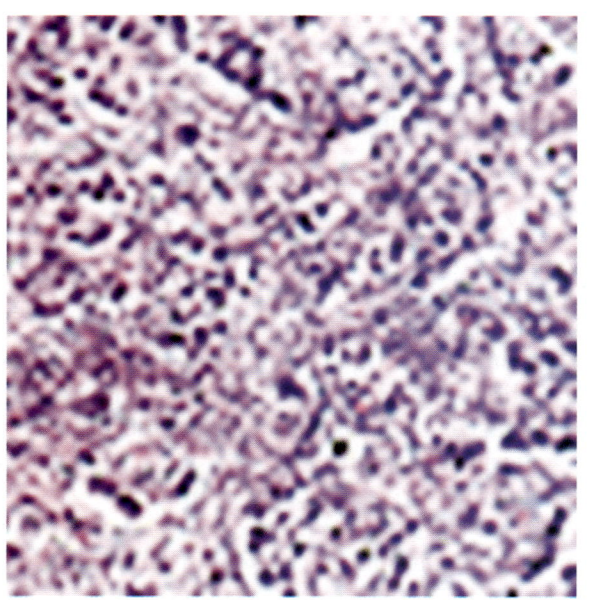

Fig. 20.32: Microscopic picture of dysgerminoma

- May have hCG+ve syncytiotrophoblastic cells close to blood vessels or hemorrhagic foci with increased serum hCG.
- May have abortive yolk sac elements with increased serum AFP.
- May be present in wall of mature teratoma; may have pseudotubular or cord-like architecture.
- **Early carcinomatous differentiation:** 30+ mitoses per 10 high power fields, may worsen prognosis.

Prognosis

- 10-year survival rate of 88.6% following conservative surgery for patients with dysgerminoma confined to the ovary; less than 10 cm in size; with an intact, smooth capsule unattached to other organs; and without ascites.
- Number of patients do have one or more successful pregnancies following unilateral salpingo-oophorectomy.
- Even patients with incompletely resected dysgerminoma can be rendered disease-free following chemotherapy with bleomycin, etoposide, and cisplatin (BEP) or a combination of cisplatin, vinblastine, and bleomycin, also known as PVB.

II. Yolk Sac Tumor (Endodermal Sinus Tumor—EST)

General

- Second most common malignant ovarian germ cell tumor.
- Occurs in childhood, adolescence, and adult life (most <30 years). Usually children or young adults (median age 19 years) present with abdominal pain and rapidly growing mass and fever.
- Can be pure or a component of a mixed germ cell tumor.
- Almost always a unilateral solid or solid and cystic tumor.
- Displays wide range of histologic patterns (microcystic, endodermal sinus, solid, alveolar-glandular, papillary, myxomatous, macrocystic, hepatoid, primitive endodermal, polyvesicular vitelline).
- Classic pattern shows perivascular formations (**Schiller-Duval bodies**) and eosinophilic globules that contain AFP.
- Associated with elevated serum AFP and alpha-1-antitrypsin levels and normal hCG levels.
- Highly malignant neoplasm that is radioresistant but responds to combination chemotherapy.
- Fatal without chemotherapy since most have subclinical metastases at presentation.

Gross Description

- Mean 15 cm, smooth and glistening external surface, cystic cut surface with hemorrhage and necrosis
- Often has benign teratoma component; rarely is found in pelvis unattached to ovary

Micro Description

- Numerous patterns
- **Schiller-Duval body** (Fig. 20.33) is pathognomonic—central blood vessel enveloped by germ cells within a space similarly lined by germ cells, resembles glomerulus.
- Hyaline droplets present in all tumors (positive for AFP, PAS and alpha-1-antitrypsin).
- **Patterns:**
  - Reticular or microcystic patterns formed by a loose network of flat/cuboidal cells.
  - Polyvesicular vitelline pattern: In 25%; vesicular structures with eccentric constrictions surrounded by dense spindle cell stroma; may have better prognosis in pure form.
  - Other patterns: Endometrioid (rare), hepatoid (large polyhedral cells with hyaline bodies but no bile, resembling metastatic hepatocellular carcinoma), glandular (may be cribriform or resemble endometrioid carcinoma), intestinal differentiation, parietal (thick layers of basement membrane), solid, undifferentiated.

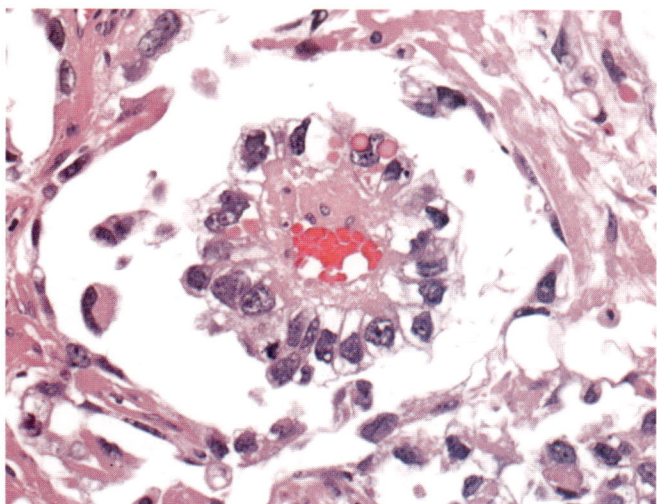

Fig. 20.33: Schiller–Duval body is EST

III. Embryonal Carcinoma (Fig. 20.34)

In the ovary, embryonal carcinoma is quite rare, amounting to approximately 3% of ovarian germ cell tumors.

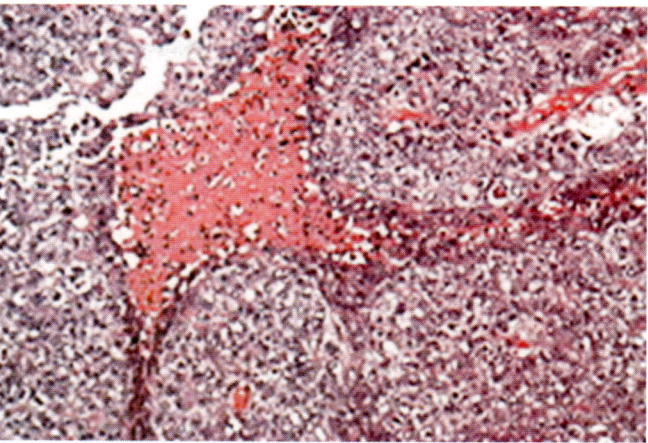

Fig. 20.34: Microscopic appearance of embryonal cell carcinoma

- It occurs in children and young adults. The median age at diagnosis is 15 years.
- Symptoms and signs are varied, and may include sexual precocity and abnormal (increased, reduced or absent) uterine bleeding.
- It usually occurs in combination with yolk sac tumor
- It is typically a unilateral, solid tumor with hemorrhage and necrosis composed of undifferentiated, pleomorphic, large cells.
- It is highly malignant neoplasm that is radioresistant but responds to combination chemotherapy.
- There may be elevations in serum **human chorionic gonadotropin** (**hCG**) and **alpha-fetoprotein** (**AFP**) levels but it would be in association with other tumors (e.g. yolk sac tumor), because they themselves do not produce the serum markers.
- At surgery, there is extension of the tumor beyond the ovary in 40% of cases. They are generally large tumors with a median diameter of 17 cm.
- Long-term survival has improved following the advent of chemotherapy.
- The *gross* and *histologic* features of this tumor are similar to that seen in the testis.

Pathologic Features

The *gross examination* usually shows 2–3 cm pale grey, poorly defined tumor with associated *hemorrhage* and *necrosis*.

The microscopic features include—indistinct cell borders, mitoses, variable architecture (tubulopapillary, glandular, solid, **embryoid bodies**—ball of cells surrounded by empty space), nuclear overlap, and necrosis.

An important key to distinguish it from other tumors, such as seminoma (vacuolated), *teratocarcinoma* (3 differentiated germ layers), *yolk sac tumor (Schiller-*

Duval bodies), and the *Sertoli-Leydig cell tumor* (strings of glands), is that the embryonal carcinoma cells are "trying" to evolve into their next stage of development.

IV. Choriocarcinoma (Fig. 20.35)

General

- Rare primary ovarian tumor that account for less than 1% of primitive ovarian germ cell tumors.
- Ovarian choriocarcinomas may develop from ovarian pregnancy (gestational choriocarcinoma) or as a germ cell tumor (pure or mixed, non-gestational choriocarcinoma) or as a surface epithelial tumor with choriocarcinomatous differentiation.

Epidemiology

- Primary ovarian choriocarcinomas are more common in children and adolescents.
- After puberty, origin from an ovarian ectopic pregnancy cannot be excluded.

Clinical Features

- Abdominal enlargement
- Pain, and sometimes hemoperitoneum
- Iso-sexual precocity
- Menstrual abnormalities
- Androgenic changes
- Presentation similar to ectopic or tubal pregnancy
- Markedly elevated serum beta-hCG
- Monitoring serum levels of hCG is helpful in predicting recurrence and response to therapy
- Occurs in children and young adults

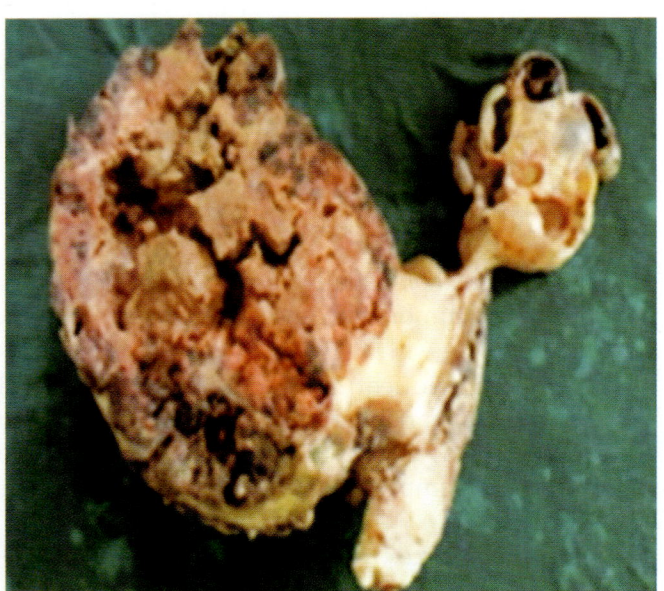

Fig. 20.35: Cut specimen of choriocarcinoma

- Associated with elevated serum hCG levels
- Typically a unilateral, solid, hemorrhagic tumor
- Composed of malignant cytotrophoblast and syncytiotrophoblast
- Nongestational choriocarcinoma is a highly malignant neoplasm that responds to combination chemotherapy.

Radiology

On imaging, choriocarcinomas appear as vascular solid tumors with cystic, hemorrhagic, and necrotic areas.

Gross Description

Hemorrhagic, soft, and tan with necrosis.

Microscopic Appearances (Fig. 20.36)

- Composed of cytotrophoblasts, intermediate trophoblasts, and multinucleated syncytiotropho-blasts which are arranged around the periphery of blood channels.
- The cytotrophoblasts are mononucleated with vesicular nuclei, distinct nucleolus, and clearly defined cytoplasmic borders.
- The syncytiotrophoblasts contain mutliple nuclei within a basophilic to amphophilic cytoplasm.

Treatment is basically surgery followed by chemotherapy.

Prognostic Factors

- In contrast to gestational choriocarcinomas, non-gestational choriocarcinomas are difficult to treat, generally unresponsive to chemotherapy.
- Metastases to lungs, liver, bone and viscera are common at diagnosis.

V. Polyembryoma

- Embryonal carcinoma is composed primarily of embryoid bodies.
- Embryoid body has amniotic cavity-like structure and is continuous with intestinal duct, and rarely has squamous cell nests, while "yolk sac" is continuous with hepatic tissue.
- Embryoid body is a product of divergent differentiation into intestine and liver from the plastic epithelium derived from embryonic gut.

VI. Teratoma—Mature (Fig. 20.37)

General

- Mature, if only contains adult tissues.

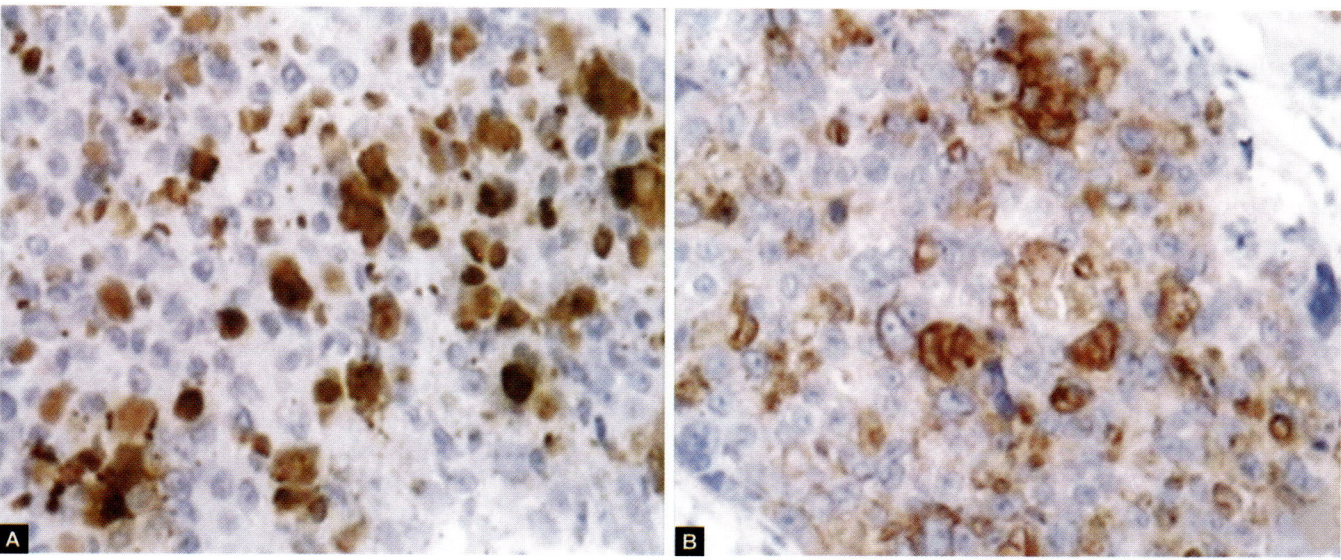

Fig. 20.36: Pure choriocarcinoma with widespread necrosis

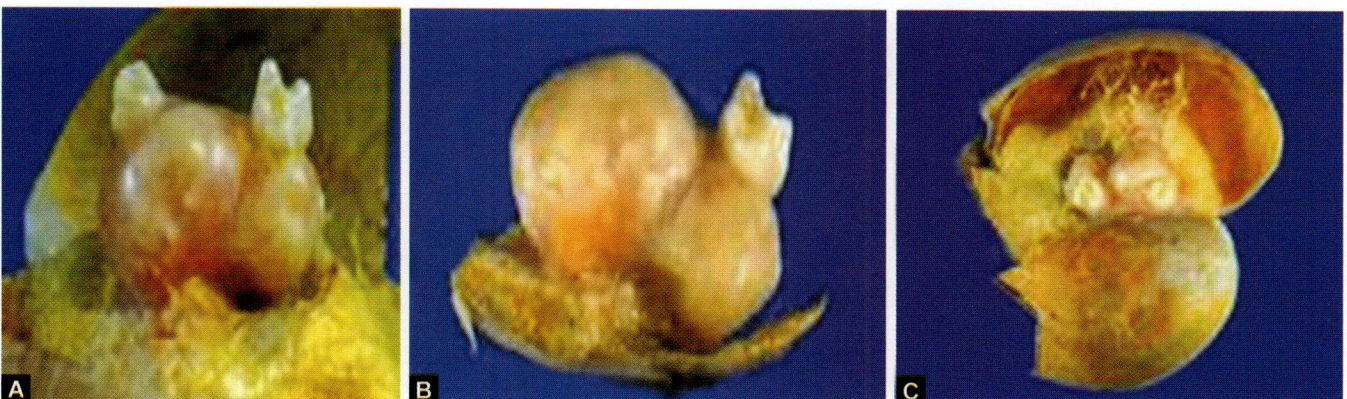

Fig. 20.37: (A, B) Dermoid cyst with teeth elements; (C) Dermoid cyst with hairs and sebum

- Usually presents in teenage women (solid) or children (cystic).
- Excellent prognosis, even if peritoneal implants are present.
- Rarely associated with hemolytic anemia.
- May rupture into peritoneal cavity causing foreign body reaction that simulates metastatic carcinoma or miliary tuberculosis.
- Tumors arise from a single germ cell after first meiotic division.

Gross Description

- Cystic tumors may contain squamous cell carcinoma, carcinoid tumor or adenocarcinoma.
- **Dermoid cyst:** Usually mature teratoma which contains ectodermal elements.

- **Gliomatosis peritonei:** Peritoneal implants exclusively composed of mature glial tissue; benign if all tissue is mature and other teratomatous elements are absent.
- **Bilateral in 12% cases and most common germ cell tumor associated with pregnancy.**
- **It is susceptible to undergo torsion mostly in puerperium because of long pedicle with heavy tumor.**
- Solid or cystic
- Cystic content may contain greasy material composed of keratin, hair and teeth.
- Rarely is "fetiform" (partial human body-like structure) or contains partial mandible.
- Teeth may be found in Rokitansky's protuberance—a well-defined, nipple-like structure covered with hair.

Micro Description (Fig. 20.38A)

- Ectodermal structures in 100%, mesodermal in 93% and endodermal in 71%.
- Skin and glial tissue common; prostate tissue in 10%.
- Still considered mature, if microscopic foci of immature tissue is present.

Dermoid Cyst (Malignant Change) (Fig. 20.38B)

- Tumor is apparently derived from germ cell elements of teratoma, but behavior is based on phenotype.

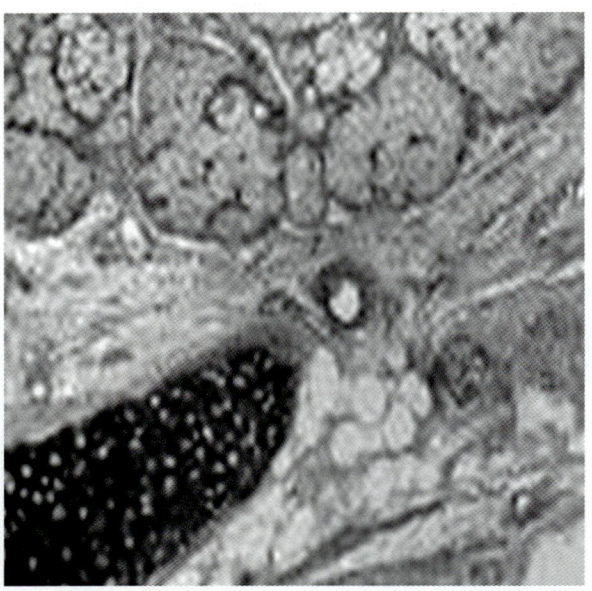

Fig. 20.38A: Sebaceous glands and cartilage

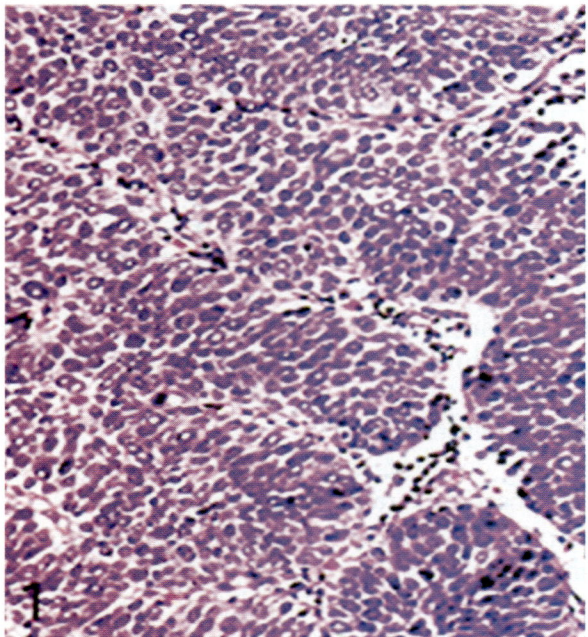

Fig. 20.38B: Malignant change in cystic teratoma

- **Squamous cell carcinoma:** Most common malignant change in cystic teratoma; 5-year survival is 52%, dependant on histologic grade and vascular invasion; appears to arise from columnar epithelium.

Teratoma—Immature

General

- Malignant tumor, whose tissue resembles embryonal or fetal tissue.
- Usually prepubertal or young women (mean 18 years).
- Most recurrences occur within 2 years; presence of yolk sac component is best predictor of recurrence in pediatric tumors (Fig. 20.39).

Treatment

- Surgery followed by multiagent chemotherapy.
- Better prognosis if only mature teratoma found after chemotherapy, although abnormal karyotype is maintained in mature teratoma.

Gross Description

Bulky, solid or cystic with necrosis, hemorrhage.

Micro Description

- Usually neurogenic and mesodermal elements common; some tumors are derived primarily of esophageal, liver and intestinal structures (endodermal).
- *Grading:* Histologic grade is based on proportion of tissue containing immature neuroepithelium.

  Norris grading system (correlates best with extraovarian spread, survival)
1. Abundant mature tissue, loose mesenchymal tissue with occasional mitoses, immature cartilage and tooth anlage.

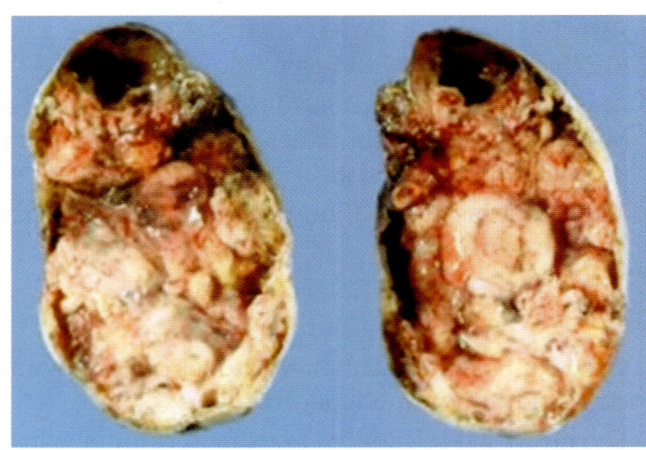

Fig. 20.39: Teratoma with yolk sac component

2. Less mature tissue than grade 1, rare foci of neuroepithelium with mitoses, <4 low power fields in any one slide (Fig. 20.40).
3. Little/no mature tissue; numerous neuroepithelial elements merging with cellular stroma occupying low power fields.

Struma Ovarii

- Rare monodermal teratoma composed predominantly of mature thyroid tissue (Fig. 20.41).
- May show pathologic changes of thyroid gland including hyperfunctioning; malignancies are usually papillary thyroid carcinoma.
- May be associated with mucinous cystadenoma, Brenner tumor, carcinoid tumor and dermoid cyst.
- On gross description, it resembles red-brown thyroid tissue but usually multilocular cystic; usually unilateral.

Microscopic Appearances (Fig. 20.42)

- Thyroid follicles with colloid; other teratomatous elements may be present.

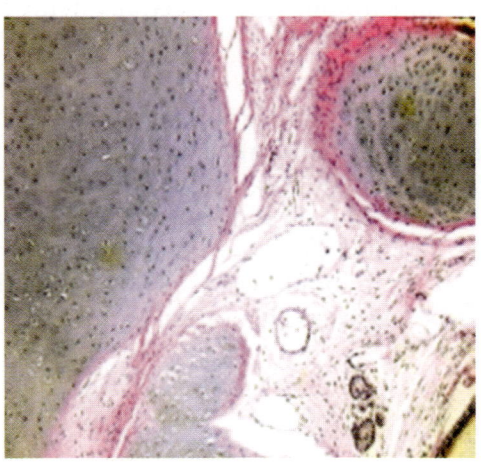

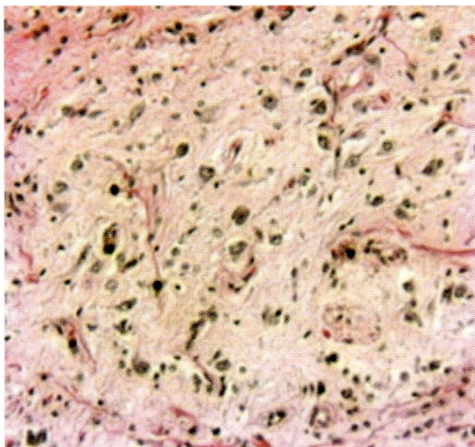

Fig. 20.40: Neural tissue

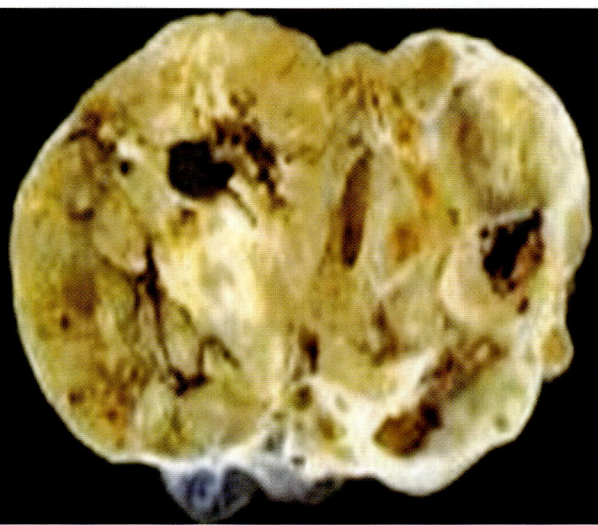

Fig. 20.41: Partially cystic tumor resembling thyroid

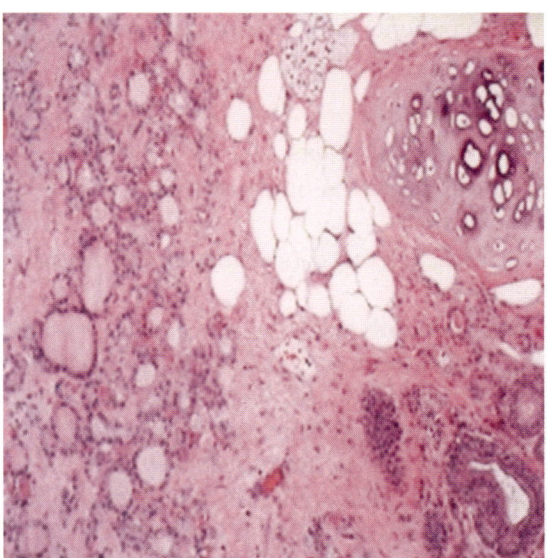

Fig. 20.42: Thyroid-like follicles

- Rarely has solid or pseudotubular patterns, microfollicles, abundant eosinophilic clear cytoplasm with minimal thyroid follicles.

National Cancer Institute Guideline

Stagewise Treatment of Germ Cell Tumors

Stage I Dysgerminomas

Standard treatment options:

1. Unilateral salpingo-oophorectomy followed by observation.
2. Unilateral salpingo-oophorectomy with adjuvant radiation therapy or chemotherapy.

For patients with stage I dysgerminoma, unilateral salpingo-oophorectomy conserving the uterus and opposite ovary is accepted treatment of the younger patient who wants to preserve fertility. Postoperative lymphangiography or CT is indicated before treatment decisions are made for patients who have not had adequate surgical and pathological examination of pelvic and para-aortic lymph nodes during surgery.

Patients who have been completely staged and have stage IA tumors may be observed after surgery without adjuvant treatment. About 15 to 25% of these patients will relapse, but they can be treated successfully at the time of recurrence with a high likelihood of cure.

Incompletely staged patients or those with higher stage tumors should receive adjuvant treatment. Options include radiation therapy or chemotherapy. The main disadvantage of radiotherapy is loss of fertility resulting from ovarian failure. In advanced stage dysgerminoma, adjuvant chemotherapy is likely to be very effective and allow recovery of reproductive potential in patients with an intact ovary, fallopian tube, and uterus.

Other germ cell tumors

Standard treatment options:

1. Unilateral salpingo-oophorectomy with adjuvant chemotherapy.
2. Unilateral salpingo-oophorectomy followed by observation.

For patients with stage I germ cell tumors, unilateral salpingo-oophorectomy should be performed when fertility is to be preserved. For all patients with tumors other than pure dysgerminoma and low-grade (grade I) immature teratoma, chemotherapy is usually given postoperatively, although excellent survival has been demonstrated for patients with all types of stage I tumors managed by surveillance, reserving chemotherapy for cases in which postsurgery recurrence is documented.

There is considerable experience with a combination of vincristine, dactinomycin, and cyclophosphamide (VAC) given in an adjuvant setting; however, combinations containing cisplatin, etoposide, and bleomycin (BEP) are now preferred because of a lower relapse rate and shorter treatment time.

BEP regime

Cisplatin	20 mg/m^2 on days 1–5
Etoposide (VP16)	100 mg/m^2 on days 1–5
Bleomycin	40 mg IV weekly

Evidence suggests that second-look laparotomy is not beneficial in patients with initially completely resected tumors who receive cisplatin-based adjuvant treatment.

Stage II Ovarian Germ Cell Tumors

Dysgerminomas

Standard treatment options:

1. Total abdominal hysterectomy and bilateral salpingo-oophorectomy with adjuvant radiation therapy or chemotherapy.
2. Unilateral salpingo-oophorectomy with adjuvant chemotherapy.

For patients with stage II dysgerminoma, total abdominal hysterectomy and bilateral salpingo-oophorectomy are usually performed. For the younger patient who wants to preserve fertility, a unilateral salpingo-oophorectomy is done followed by adjuvant chemotherapy. The chemotheapy is likely to be effective to allow recovery of reproductive potential in patients with an intact ovary, fallopian tube, and uterus. Thus, adjuvant chemotherapy with the combination of bleomycin, etoposide, and cisplatin (BEP) has replaced radiation therapy though the tumor is very radiosensitive.

Other germ cell tumors

Standard treatment options:

1. Unilateral salpingo-oophorectomy with adjuvant chemotherapy (BEP).
2. Second-look laparotomy.

Evidence suggests that second-look laparotomy is not beneficial in patients with initial completely resected tumors who receive cisplatin-based adjuvant treatment. Second-look surgery may be of benefit for a minority of patients whose tumor was not completely resected at the initial surgical procedure and is now made resectable after chemotherapy.

Stages III and IV Ovarian Germ Cell Tumors

Dysgerminomas

Standard treatment options:

1. Total abdominal hysterectomy and bilateral salpingo-oophorectomy with adjuvant chemotherapy.
2. Unilateral salpingo-oophorectomy with adjuvant chemotherapy.

For patients with stage III and IV dysgerminoma, total abdominal hysterectomy and bilateral salpingo-oophorectomy are recommended with removal of as much gross tumor as can be done safely without resection of portions of the urinary tract or large segments of the small or large bowel. Patients who want to preserve fertility may be treated with unilateral salpingo-oophorectomy followed by chemotherapy.

Combination chemotherapy with bleomycin, etoposide, and cisplatin (BEP) can cure the majority of such patients or cisplatin, vinblastine, and bleomycin (PVB) with a disease free interval of 26 months. When there is bulky residual disease, it is common to give three to four courses of PVB or BEP. Because chemotherapy with BEP appears to be less sterilizing than wide-field radiation, combination chemotherapy is the preferred treatment in the patient who wants to preserve fertility.

PVB regime

Cisplatin	20 mg/m^2 on days 1–5
Vinblastine	0.15 mg/kg on days 1 and 2
Bleomycin	30 mg on days 2, 9 and 16

Stage IV dysgerminoma is not treated with radiation therapy, but rather with chemotherapy, preferably with three to four courses of cisplatin-containing combination chemotherapy such as BEP. A second-look operation following treatment is rarely beneficial.

Other germ cell tumors (stage III & IV)

Standard treatment options:

1. Total abdominal hysterectomy and bilateral salpingo-oophorectomy with adjuvant chemotherapy, with or without neoadjuvant chemotherapy.
2. Unilateral salpingo-oophorectomy with adjuvant chemotherapy, with or without neoadjuvant chemotherapy.
3. Second-look laparotomy.

Recurrent Ovarian Germ Cell Tumors

Dysgerminomas

Standard treatment options:

Cisplatin-based chemotherapy has been used effectively for patients with recurrent dysgerminoma with and without adjuvant radiation therapy.

Other germ cell tumors

Standard treatment options:

- Patients with recurrent germ cell tumors of the ovary other than pure dysgerminoma should be treated with chemotherapy, the type of which is determined by previous treatment. Radiation therapy is not effective in this setting. Cisplatin-based combination chemotherapy is effective. Patients who do not respond to a cisplatin-based combination may still attain a durable remission with VAC or ifosfamide/cisplatin as salvage therapy.
- Newer potential treatments include an ifosfamide combination or high-dose chemotherapy and autologous marrow rescue.
- Although the role of secondary cytoreductive surgery for patients with recurrent or progressive ovarian germ cell tumors remains controversial, it may have some benefit for a select group of patients, particularly those with immature teratoma. After maximal effort for surgical cytoreduction, chemotherapy should be considered.

20D. SEX CORD-STROMAL TUMORS OF OVARY

Definition

Sex cord-stromal tumors are groups of tumors composed of granulosa cells, theca cells, Sertoli cells, Leydig cells and fibroblasts of stromal origin, singly or in various combinations.

According to the WHO, sex cord-stromal tumors are classified into the following categories:

I. Granulosa-stromal cell tumors
- Adult
- Juvenile

II. Thecoma-fibroma group
- Thecoma
  1. Typical
  2. Luteinized
- Fibroma
  1. Cellular fibroma
  2. Fibrosarcoma
     i. Stromal tumor with minor sex cord elements
     ii. Sclerosing stromal tumor
     iii. Signet ring cell stromal tumor
     iv. Unclassified (fibrothecoma)

III. Sertoli-stromal cell tumors
- Sertoli-Leydig cell tumors group (androblastomas)
  i. Well differentiated
  ii. Of intermediate differentiation
  iii. Poorly differentiated (sarcomatoid)
  iv. Retiform
  v. Sertoli cell tumors
  vi. Stromal-Leydig cell tumor

IV. Sex cord-stromal tumors of mixed or unclassified cell types
- Sex cord tumor with annular tubules
- Gynandroblastoma
- Sex cord-stromal tumor, unclassified

V. Steroid cell tumors
- Stromal luteoma
- Leydig cell tumor group
  1. Hilus cell tumor
  2. Leydig cell tumors nonhilar type
  3. Leydig cell tumors, not otherwise specified
- Steroid cell tumors, not otherwise specified
  1. Well differentiated
  2. Malignant

Epidemiology

Sex cord-stromal tumors account for approximately 8% of all ovarian tumors. Most of them are solid ovarian tumors. Table 20.12 lists solid tumors of ovary.

Table 20.12: Solid ovarian tumors	
• Fibroma	• Dysgerminomas
• Thecoma	• Sertoli-Leydig tumor
• Granulosa cell tumors	• Sclerosing stromal tumor
• Brenner tumors	• Fibrosarcoma

Immunohistochemistry

CD56 is a sensitive marker of ovarian sex cord-stromal tumors and is useful in the diagnosis of this group of neoplasms, especially in cases that are inhibin or calretinin negative.

Tumor Spread and Staging

The International Federation of Gynecology and Obstetrics (FIGO) staging of ovarian tumors is as follows:

I. *Growth Limited to the Ovaries*

- A: Growth limited to one ovary; no ascites. No tumor on the external surface; capsule intact.
- B: Growth limited to both ovaries; no ascites. No tumor on the external surface; capsule intact.
- C: Tumor either Stage IA or Stage IB, but with tumor on the surface of one or both ovaries, or with capsule ruptured, or with ascites containing malignant cells or with positive peritoneal washings.

II. *Growth involving One or both Ovaries with Pelvic Extension*

- A: Extension and/or metastases to the uterus and/or tubes
- B: Extension to other pelvic tissues
- C: Tumor is either Stage IIA or IIB but with tumor on the surface of one or both ovaries; or with capsule ruptured; or ascites present containing malignant cells or with positive peritoneal washings.

III. *Tumor involving One or both Ovaries with Peritoneal Implants Outside the Pelvis and/or Positive Retroperitoneal or Inguinal Nodes . Superficial Liver Metastasis Equals Stage III*

- A: Tumor grossly limited to the true pelvis with negative nodes but with histologically confirmed microscopic seeding of abdominal peritoneal surfaces.

- B: Tumor of one or both ovaries with histologically confirmed implants of abdominal peritoneal surfaces, none exceeding 2 cm in diameter. Nodes are negative.
- C: Abdominal implants more than 2 cm in diameter and/or positive retroperitoneal or inguinal nodes.

IV. Growth involving One or Both Ovaries with Distant Metastasis

If pleural effusion is present, positive cytology must be present to allot a case to stage IV. Parenchymal liver metastasis equals stage IV.

Granulosa Cell Tumor Group

Definition

WHO defines granulosa cell tumor (GCT) as a neoplasm composed of pure or at least 10% population of granulosa cells, often in a fibroatheromatous background. Two major subtypes are recognized, an adult (AGCT) and a juvenile type (JACT).

Epidemiology

Granulosa cell tumors account for about 1.5% of all ovarian tumors and occur in a wide age range, from newborn to postmenopausal women.

Adult Granulosa Cell Tumor

Epidemiology

Adult granulosa cell tumor (AGCT) accounts for more than 95% of granulosa cell tumors and occurs more often in postmenopausal than premenopausal women, with a peak incidence between 50 and 55 years.

Etiology

The etiology as well the molecular genetic events involved in the pathogenesis of granulosa cell tumor are unknown; however, amplification and/or over expression of the ERBB genes like erb B2, B3, B4 are found in a number of granulosa cell tumors. Several studies suggest that infertile women and those exposed to ovulation induction agents have an increased risk for granulosa cell tumor.

History

any patients with GCTs present with manifestations of hyperestrogenism. Approximately 70% of these tumors are hormonally active. Hormonal influences can cause different presenting symptoms depending on patient age and menstrual status.

Most patients have a palpable mass found during examination. Abdominal symptoms may be due to enlargement of the mass but also can be due to the production of ascites, which occurs in approximately 10% of patients. Increasing size of the mass can lead to symptoms associated with compression of adjacent structures, such as abdominal pain, dysuria, urinary frequency and constipation.

Acute onset of abdominal pain also can occur, although rarely. Acute abdominal or pelvic pain may be observed in combination with nausea, vomiting, dizziness, and shoulder pain. These symptoms may be due to adnexal torsion, rupture of a partially cystic GCT, or hemorrhage either within the tumor or into the peritoneum.

- **Prepubertal girls**
  - Patients usually present with precocious pseudopuberty (70–80%) and have secondary sex characteristics at a very early age. These may include increased linear growth, breast enlargement, clitoral enlargement, pubic hair development, increased vaginal secretions, and vaginal bleeding.
  - These virilizing symptoms develop as a result of testosterone production by the tumor cells. Many of these hormone-induced symptoms abate following resection of the tumor.
- **Premenopausal women**
  - Apart from increasing abdominal girth related to an enlarging adnexal mass menstrual irregularities such as oligomenorrhea, menorrhagia, and secondary amenorrhea tend to be the hallmark of these tumors in reproductive-aged women.
- **Postmenopausal women**
  - The most common endocrine manifestation of GCTs in postmenopausal women is abnormal uterine bleeding. This is caused by endometrial proliferation due to estrogen production by the tumor. Therefore, endometrial hyperplasia and/or endometrial adenocarcinoma may be a concomitant finding in women with GCT.
  - Patients also can have breast tenderness and increased vaginal secretions from estrogenic stimulation of the breast and vaginal tissues, respectively.
  - Rarely, a patient may present with virilizing symptoms such as acne, hirsutism, deepening of the voice, and clitoral enlargement. This is due to testosterone and/or androstenedione production in a minority of these tumors.

Physical Examination

- Pelvic mass is the most consistent finding on pelvic and rectal examination in patients of all ages with GCT. A palpable mass can be found in 85–97% of patients. A bimanual examination and a rectovaginal examination should be performed to evaluate the pelvis and lower abdomen for masses, size of the uterus, the posterior cul-de-sac for nodularity.
- For patients presenting with acute abdominal pain, a careful speculum examination should be performed to help rule out infectious etiologies.

Laboratory Studies

Tumor markers

- In patients who are prepubertal or younger than 30 years, especially if the mass has solid components present, blood is checked for levels of βhCG, AFP, LDH and CA125.
- In reproductive-aged women older than 30 years, CA125 level and serum inhibin levels are measured. Inhibin is now the most specific marker for GCTs that is currently clinically available. Inhibin is a peptide hormone produced by ovarian granulosa cells that plays a role in regulation of FSH secretion by the pituitary. It is composed of an alpha subunit and 1 of 2 beta subunits (BA or BB). Although inhibin A and inhibin B levels can both be elevated in patients with granulosa cell tumors, inhibin B level is usually elevated in a higher proportion of these tumors. Normal inhibin levels in postmenopausal women are less than or equal to 5 ng/L and 15 ng/L for inhibin A and B, respectively.
- Serum levels for estrogen, testosterone, and dehydroepiandrosterone is also tested if elevation of these hormones is suspected on the basis of clinical findings. GCTs are the most common estrogen-producing neoplasms in females and are found to produce estradiol in approximately 40–60% of patients. This estradiol production is dependent on stimulation by testosterone secreted by the theca cells. However, not all GCTs are hormonally active or have theca cells that secrete testosterone, and this type of testing lacks sensitivity and specificity.
- In postmenopausal women, CA125 level higher than 60 U/mL has a good positive predictive value for malignancy.

Antimüllerian hormone (AMH) or Müllerian inhibiting substance (MIS)

- This hormone is produced exclusively by granulosa cells in postnatal females and both prenatally and postnatally by the Sertoli cells in the male testis.

Serum MIS/AMH may be a marker of ovarian reserve and typically disappears from the serum after menopause or bilateral oophorectomy. However, in patients with GCTs, levels have been shown to parallel the extent of disease.
- Serum MIS/AMH levels correlate well with tumor presence in patients with GCTs. This marker is highly specific for GCT in postmenopausal women. It may also be elevated in women with Sertoli-Leydig cell tumors of the ovary. This is in sharp contrast to inhibin and estradiol levels, both of which may be elevated in a variety of other extraovarian disorders. This makes AMH/MIS attractive as a marker for diagnosis and prospective follow-up of patients with GCTs.

Imaging Studies

- **Transvaginal sonography (TVS)** is by far the best primary modality for imaging pelvic structures. This may allow for delineation between ovarian, tubal, uterine, and other pelvic masses. If an adnexal mass is identified, the presence of cystic or solid components, the internal architecture like septations, excrescences should be made. Free pelvic fluid also can be identified readily on TVS images. The presence of solid, complex, cystic, or bilateral masses, with or without free fluid, increases the possibility of malignancy.
- **Roentgenography**
  - Chest radiography is useful in helping exclude pulmonary spread of malignant diseases of the ovary.
  - Abdominopelvic CT scanning or MRI may help in diagnosing intraperitoneal spread or involvement of other organ systems prior to surgery.
  - IVP, barium enemas, and upper GI series also can be useful adjuncts in patients with symptoms involving the GI or genitourinary tracts.
  - Barium enema or colonoscopy prior to surgical intervention help rule out colonic involvement, colon cancer, or both as the primary tumor in women older than 40 years. However, if abdominopelvic CT scanning with oral and intravenous contrast already has been performed, IVP, colonoscopy, and barium enema are not required.
- **Mammography:** The preoperative workup also should include mammography for women older than 40 years who have not had one in the preceding 6–12 months. This is especially important in women with estrogen-producing tumors because these may

increase the risk of breast malignancies. Additionally, breast cancers can metastasize to the ovaries and are often bilateral. Mammography can help rule out the possibility of a nongynecologic primary neoplasm in the breast.

Clinical Features

Granulosa cell tumor may present as an abdominal mass with symptoms suggestive of functioning ovarian tumor. In approximately 5–15% of patients, hemoperitoneum may develop secondary to rupture of a cystic lesion. 10% of patients may remain asymptomatic though the patients may present with ascites in 10% cases.

Granulosa cell tumors are the most common estrogenic ovarian tumors clinically. The symptoms and clinical manifestation vary according to the age of the patient and reproductive state. In prepubertal girls, granulosa cell tumor often induces **isosexual pseudoprecocious puberty**. In women of reproductive age, the tumor may be associated with heavy menstrual bleeding due to hyperestrogenism. In postmenopausal women, **irregular uterine bleeding** is the most common manifestation due to endometrial hyperplasia or, rarely well-differentiated adenocarcinoma.

Gross Findings (Fig. 20.43)

Granulosa cell tumors (GCTs) vary from tiny lesions to huge masses filling the abdomen, with a mean diameter of about 13 cm. GCTs are bilateral in only 2%. The external surface may be smooth or bosselated. The cut surface is solid, partly solid and partly cystic, or rarely, entirely cystic. Cystic tumors may be unilocular or multilocular. Solid areas may be hard and rubbery or soft in consistency and tend to be yellowish or gray in color; the cystic spaces may contain proteinaceous fluid or old altered blood. Hemorrhage and necrosis are common.

Microscopic Findings

Granulosa cells are small, usually round to polygonal- or spindle-shaped with scanty amphophilic cytoplasm and indistinct cell borders. Their round, oval or angular nuclei often show a deep longitudinal grooves and may exhibit a small, variably prominent nucleolus. The nuclear chromatin may be compact and dense or loose and vesicular. The luteinized granulosa cells, seen particularly in the diffuse, multicystic, and "juvenile" types of granulosa cell tumors, have larger, more rounded and generally ungrooved nuclei and abundant pale eosinophilic lipid-laden cytoplasm.

The tumor cells grow in a variety of patterns, including **microfollicular** (Fig. 20.44), **macrofollicular, trabecular, insular, tubular, diffuse and gyriform**. The microfollicular variant is characterized by multiple small rounded spaces formed by cystic degeneration in small aggregates of granulosa cells, containing eosinophilic PAS-positive material (chondroitin 6-sulphate) and often fragments of nuclear debris or pyknotic nuclei. These spaces, known **as Call–Exner bodies**, are found in 30–50% of tumors. The granulosa cell nuclei are oriented somewhat radially around these structures.

The macrofollicular variant comprises cysts of differing sizes lined by multilayered well-differentiated granulosa cells (Fig. 20.45), often cuffed by a layer of theca like cells and apparently also formed by cystic

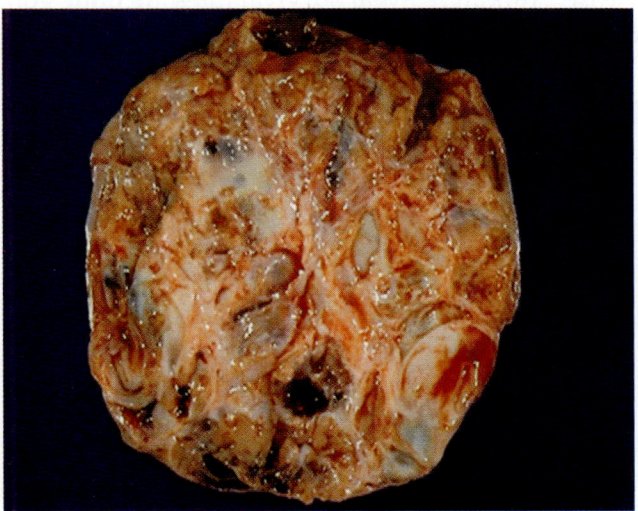

Fig. 20.43: Granulosa cell tumor of ovary

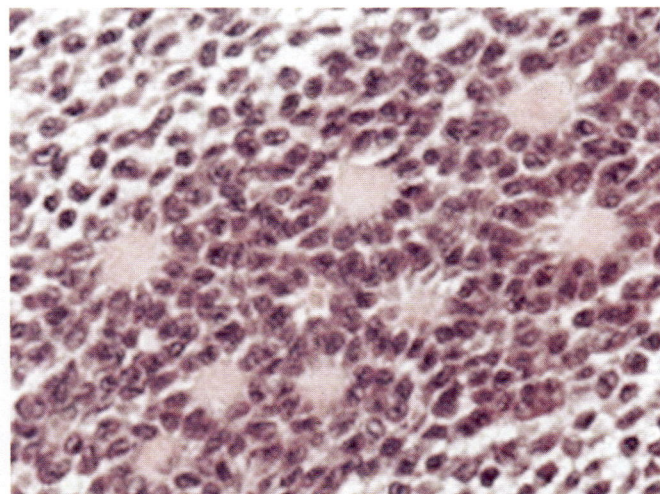

Fig. 20.44: Granulosa cell tumor, microfollicular pattern Call-Exner bodies are formed by a discrete array of granulosa cells with angular grooved nuclei and central inspissated eosinophilic material

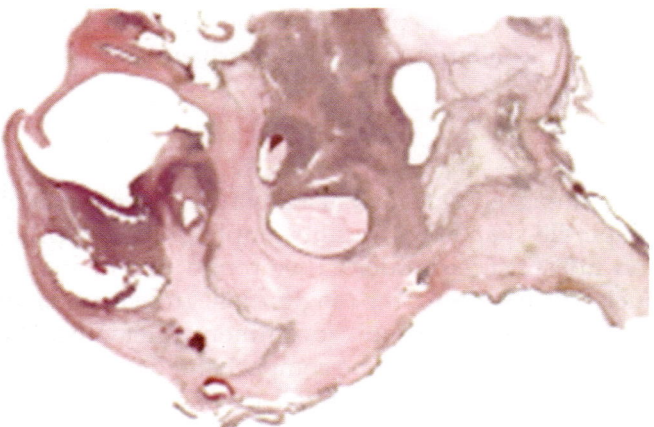

Fig. 20.45: Granulosa cell tumor, macrofollicular pattern

degeneration in large masses of granulosa cells. Either or both of these cell layers may be luteinized.

Insular and trabecular variants (Fig. 20.46) exhibit islands and bands of granulosa cells with peripherally palisaded nuclei separated by a fibroma-like or thecoma-like stroma.

The gyriform patterns (Fig. 20.47) are characterized by undulating parallel rows and zigzag cords of granulosa cells, respectively. The diffuse pattern (Fig. 20.48) is characterized by a monotonous sheet like cellular proliferation .

Immunohistochemistry

Granulosa cell tumors are positive for **inhibin and calretinin** but negative for **cytokeratin 7 and epithelial membrane antigen.** Epithelial membrane antigen immunoreactivity is present in many of the histologic mimics of GCTs, such as metastatic or primary carcinoma. The absence of staining in GCT has diagnostic value. CD56 is useful in distinguishing between granulosa cell tumor and normal ovarian follicles or endometrioid adenocarcinoma.

A single, recurrent somatic mutation (402C → G) in **FOXL2 gene** has been identified in 80% of SCCTs and 95% of adult and Juvenile granulose cell tumors studied. It is one of the earliest markers of ovarian differentiation, and its expression persists into adulthood. *FOXL2* plays a major role in cell cycle regulation and is required for the normal development and function of granulosa cells. Therefore, diagnostic testing for the *FOXL2* mutation can be used to distinguish AGCT from sex cord-stromal tumors.

Prognosis and Predictive Factors

Granulosa cell tumors of all patterns have a malignant potential, with the capacity to extend beyond the ovary or recur after surgical removal; recurrent disease sometimes presents within 8–9 years of removal of the primary tumor. Distant metastases are rare but have been reported in the lungs, brain, bones, and liver. All granulosa cell tumors are considered as low-grade malignancies.

The most important prognostic factor is the stage of the tumor; nearly 90% of patients with GCT have stage I disease. Factors related to a relatively poor prognosis include age over 40 years at the time of diagnosis, large tumor size (>5 cm), bilaterality, tumor rupture, mitotic activity, and atypia. Serum inhibin levels are used to monitor patients for tumor recurrence.

Mortality/Morbidity

AGCTs and JGCTs have very good cure rates due to the early stage of disease at diagnosis. More than 90% of AGCTs and JGCTs are diagnosed before spread occurs outside the ovary. Five-year survival rates usually are 90–95% for stage I tumors compared to 25–50% for patients presenting with advanced-stage disease. Although 5-year survival rates are quite good, AGCTs have a propensity for late recurrence.

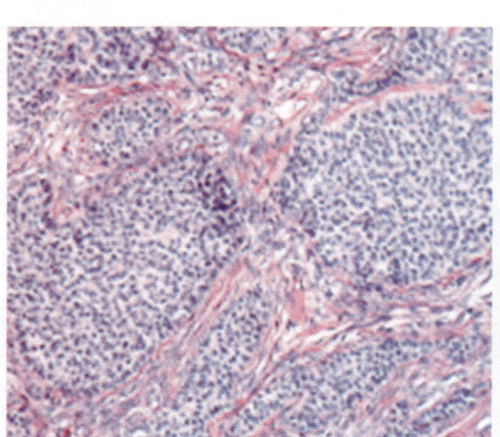

Fig. 20.46: Insular pattern

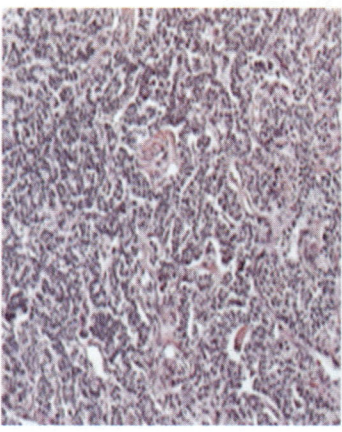

Fig. 20.47: Gyriform pattern

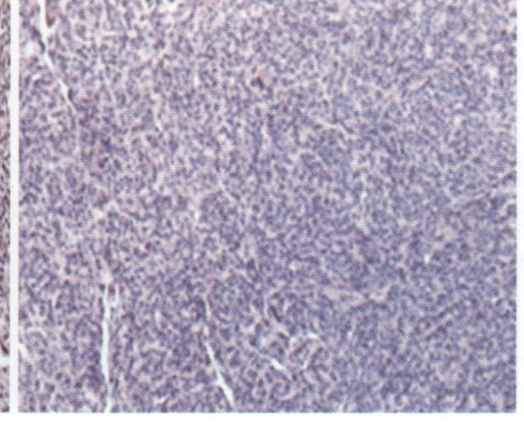

Fig. 20.48: Diffuse pattern

Juvenile Granulosa Cell Tumor

Epidemiology

Juvenile granulosa cell tumor (JGCT) accounts for approximately 5% of all granulosa cell tumors. The neoplasm occurs mainly during the first 3 decades of life.

Clinical Features

About 80% of JGCT occur in children, who typically present with isosexual pseudoprecocity. When JGCT occurs after puberty, patients usually present with abdominal pain, swelling, menstrual irregularities, or amenorrhea.

Gross Findings

The appearance of juvenile granulosa cell tumor is solid and almost similar in appearances to the adult variant.

Microscopic Findings (Fig. 20.49)

JGCT is typically a solid cellular neoplasm, with focal follicle formation. The follicles generally do not reach the large size of the follicles in the macrofollicular variant of adult granulosa cell tumor. Their lumens contain basophilic or eosinophilic fluid. Variable layers of granulosa cells line the follicles and occasionally surrounded by theca cells. The neoplastic cells in the solid areas may be arranged diffusely or divided into nodules by fibrous septae. The neoplastic granulosa cells have abundant eosinophilic and/or vacuolated cytoplasm and rounded hyperchromatic nuclei. Nuclear grooves are rare. Nuclear atypia in JGCTs varies from minimal to marked. The mitotic rate is also

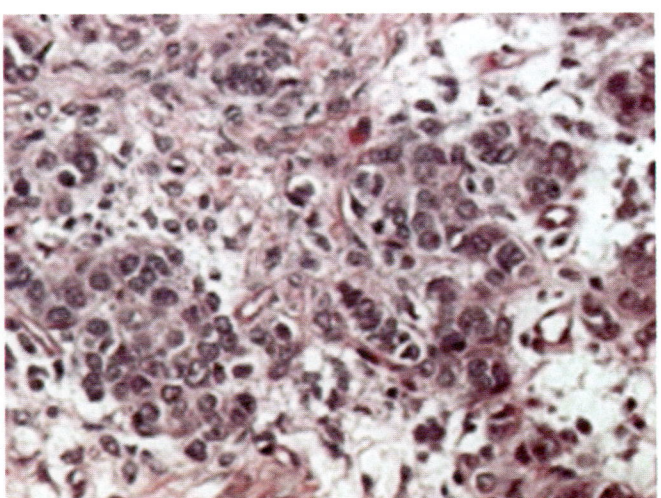

Fig. 20.49: Juvenile granulosa cell tumor. The cells have abundant eosinophilic cytoplasm; their nuclei are hyperchromatic and lack grooves

variable but is generally higher than adult granulosa cell tumor.

Molecular and Genetics

An association between tuberous sclerosis and juvenile granulosa cell tumor of the ovary has been reported. JGCT may present as a component of a variety of nonhereditary congenital syndromes, including Ollier disease (enchondromatosis) and Maffucci syndrome (enchondromatosis and hemangiomatosis). Bilateral JGCT may develop in infants with features suggestive of Goldenhar (craniofacial and skeletal abnormalities) or Potter syndrome.

Prognosis and Predictive Factors

Most JGCTs are clinically benign. The most important prognostic factor is the stage of the tumor and almost all clinically malignant JGCT recur within 3 years.

Thecoma–Fibroma Group

Thecoma (Fig. 20.50)

Thecoma is a benign tumor composed of plump spindle cells with obvious lipid-containing cytoplasm and resembling cells of the ovarian theca interna.

Epidemiology

Thecoma occurs at any age but predominantly over the age of 40 years and rarely in children. Luteinized variants are more likely to occur in younger women.

Clinical Features

Estrogenic manifestations are the commonest mode of clinical presentation for thecoma and usually take the form of menstrual irregularities or postmenopausal bleeding. Androgenic thecomas are rare.

Gross Findings

Thecomas range in size from small nodules to large, solid, firm or rubbery tumors several centimeters in diameter. The cut surface is characteristically bright yellow to orange. They are usually unilateral.

Microscopic Findings (Fig. 20.50)

Thecoma has 1 of 2 patterns. Typical thecomas consist of large, ill-defined, nodular masses of plump eosinophilic or vacuolated cells with small, pale, round, or ovoid, central, nongrooved nuclei, interspersed between less conspicuous bands of fibrous connective tissue, which often exhibit hyalinized plaques. Edema

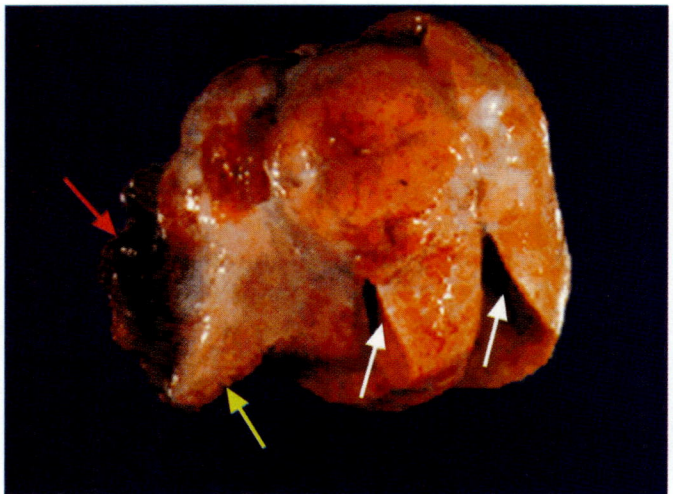
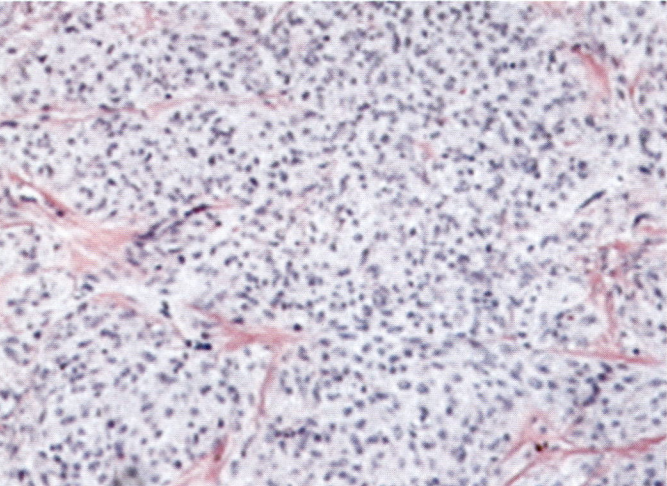

Fig. 20.50: Thecoma: Tumor cells have abundant pale cytoplasm

or myxoid change is often prominent and some tumors show an occasional focus of dystrophic calcification. Occasional small nests of granulosa cells may be found; such tumors are called "thecomas with minor sex cord elements.

The second histological pattern, designated luteinized thecoma, is a typical thecoma throughout which clusters of large eosinophilic, lipid-laden lutein cells are scattered. Microscopic examination of this lesion reveals alternating hypercellular and hypocellular areas, with edema and microcystic changes. The mitotic count is usually elevated; however, no evidence exists that this lesion has the ability to metastasize.

Prognosis and Predictive Factors

Thecomas are benign. Luteinizing thecoma with sclerosing peritonitis requires more extensive surgery due to the associated adhesions and obstructive symptoms.

Fibroma

Epidemiology

Fibromas are the most commonly encountered subtype of the sex cord-stromal tumors, accounting for almost two-thirds of neoplasms in this group. The mean age of incidence is about 48 years. Ascites is the most frequent general abdominal symptom associated with ovarian fibromas, being present in over 10% of cases.

Gross Findings

Fibromas are bilateral in 5% of cases and of average 6 cm in diameter. Larger tumors have a smooth or slightly bosselated serosal surface, are solid, and vary from edematous and somewhat rubbery to rock-hard in consistency. The cut surface is white and faintly whorled, often with areas of cystic degeneration.

Microscopic Findings (Fig. 20.51)

The basic architectural pattern of fibroma comprises variably cellular bundles and intersecting collagenous fibrous tissue, occasionally with a striking storiform pattern resembling ovarian cortex. The elongated fibroblastic tumor cells have spindle-shaped nuclei and may contain small amounts of lipid in their cytoplasm. Dystrophic calcification may be occasionally seen. Nuclear atypia and mitoses are rarely seen.

Occasional fibromatous tumors are hypercellular and show appreciable mitotic activity. These tumors are designated as cellular fibromas, mitotically active cellular fibromas (Fig. 20.52), or fibrosarcomas,

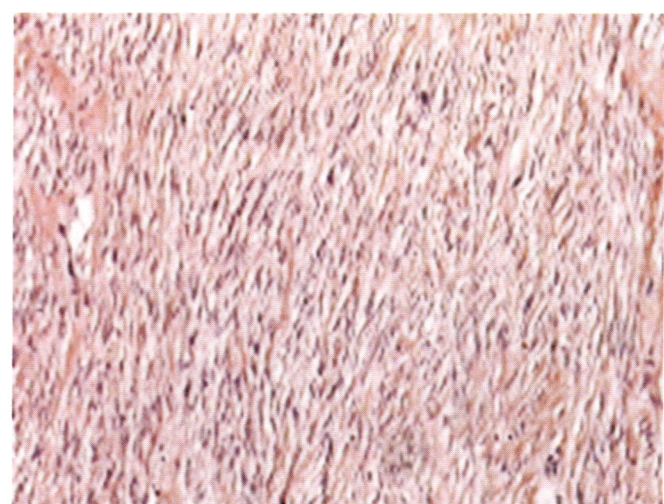

Fig. 20.51: Fibroma: The cells have small spindle-shaped nuclei lacking, atypia or mitotic activity

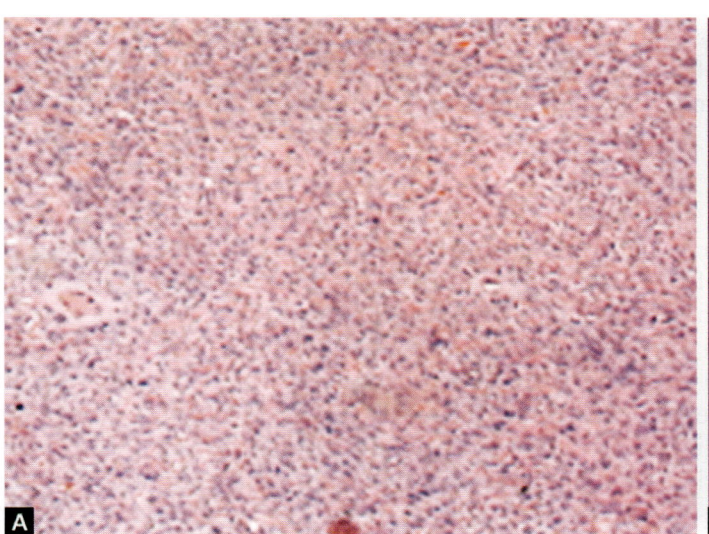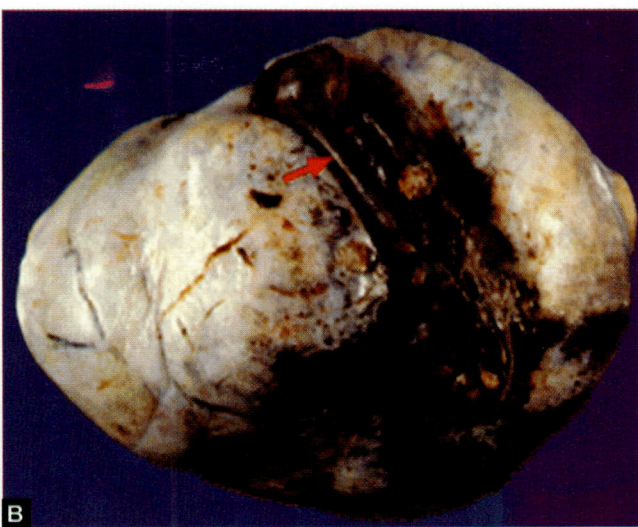

Fig. 20.52A and B: (A) Cells have no cytological atypia, (B) Cellular fibroma

depending on the degree of mitotic activity and nuclear atypia. Cellular fibromas contain 1–3 mitotic figures per 10 high-power fields but display bland nuclei. Mitotically active cellular fibromas contain 4–19 mitotic figures per 10 high-power fields. Both variants may exhibit foci of necrosis, but nuclear atypia is minimal or absent.

Fibrosarcomas have increased cellularity, often a high mitotic rate, and diffuse nuclear hyperchromasia with atypia. The latter tumors tend to be large, solid tumor masses accompanied by dense adhesions.

Molecular and Genetics

Trisomy 12 is a common finding in benign and cellular fibromas, while trisomy 8 has been identified in cases of clinically malignant fibrosarcomas.

Prognosis

Fibromas are benign. Cellular and mitotically active fibromas are also clinically benign, although tumor rupture and/or adhesions may be associated with local recurrence. Fibrosarcoma often has a malignant clinical course.

Sclerosing Stromal Tumor

Definition

Sclerosing stromal tumor (SST) of the ovary is a very rare sex cord stromal tumor occurring in a younger age group than other types of stromal tumors and most commonly accompanied by menstrual irregularity and characterized by several unique histologic features including pseudolobulation, sclerosis, and prominent vascularity.

Gross Findings

Sclerosing stromal tumor is usually unilateral, rarely bilateral, and well-circumscribed. The cut section is solid and white with areas of edema, cyst formation, and yellowish discoloration.

Microscopic Findings

Sclerosing stromal tumor is characterized by the presence of pseudolobular pattern in which cellular nodules were separated by areas of densely collagenous or edematous connective tissue, which contained fewer cells. The nodules are composed of an admixture of fibroblasts and rounded vacuolated cells, with prominent thin-walled blood vessels.

Sertoli-Stromal Cell Tumors

Definition

Sertoli-stromal cell tumors are tumors in pure form or in various combinations of Sertoli cells, resembling rete epithelial cells, fibroblasts, and Leydig cells in variable degree of differentiation.

Sertoli Cell Tumors

Sertoli cell tumors typically occur in young patients with a mean of 30 years; however, a wide age range exists. The tumors are more commonly estrogenic than androgenic.

Gross Findings

Sertoli cell tumors vary markedly in size, but most are smaller than 10 cm in diameter. They tend to be solid, firm, encapsulated and lobulated masses, typically yellow or tan in color. Small cystic areas are infrequently present. They are typically unilateral, but may be bilateral in phenotypic females with testicular feminization.

Microscopic Findings (Fig. 20.53)

Sertoli cell tumors are composed of lobules of uniform, solid, or hollow tubules, lined by one or more layers of cuboidal to columnar benign-appearing cells with eosinophilic or vacuolated cytoplasm and dark, oval, basal nuclei. Mitoses are rare. Sertoli cells usually contain lipid droplets but, in some tumors, they are greatly distended by fat, giving rise to lipid-rich Sertoli cell tumor. Intervening stroma is usually represented by a few bands of acellular connective tissue that is either edematous or hyalinized and contains few or no Leydig cells. If Leydig cells are present, the diagnosis of well-differentiated Sertoli-Leydig cell tumor should be made.

Sertoli cell tumor shows closely packed hollow and solid tubules lined by well-differentiated cuboidal-to-columnar epithelial cells. Leydig cell are absent.

Prognosis and Predictive Factors

Well-differentiated Sertoli cell tumors are benign, whereas those exhibiting atypical features frequently present with advanced stage disease and exhibit aggressive behavior. The histologic features of ovarian Sertoli cell tumors that best correlate with adverse outcome are nuclear atypia, 5 or more mitotic figures per 10 high power fields, and tumor necrosis.

Sertoli-Leydig Cell Tumor Group

Epidemiology

Sertoli-Leydig cell tumors are uncommon benign tumors, accounting for less than 0.5% of all ovarian

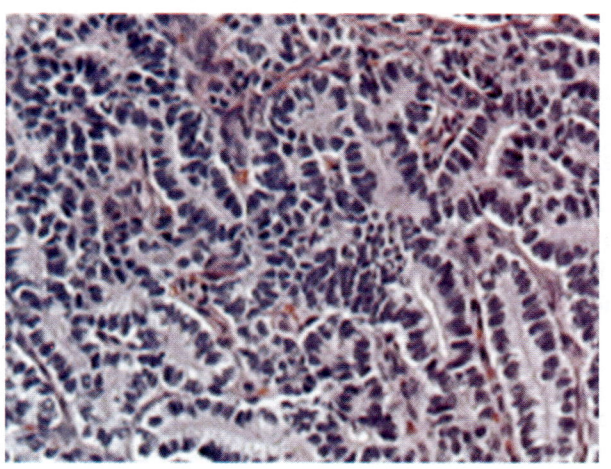

Fig. 20.53: Sertoli cell tumor

tumors. The mean age of incidence is 23–25 years. The well-differentiated tumors occur at an average age of 35 years and retiform tumors at an average age of 15 years.

Clinical Features

About one-third of patients with Sertoli-Leydig cell tumor have androgenic manifestations including: oligomenorrhea that may proceed into amenorrhea, hirsutism, hoarseness, breast atrophy, and clitoral hypertrophy. Approximately half of patients with Sertoli-Leydig cell tumor have no endocrine manifestation and mainly experience abdominal swelling and pain. Occasionally patients have been represented with estrogenic manifestation, including irregular menstruation or menorrhagia in women in the reproductive age group and postmenopausal bleeding in older women.

Pathology

Well-differentiated Sertoli-Leydig cell tumors account for about 10% of all Sertoli-Leydig cell tumors. There is a statistical association with congenital anomaly of the internal genitalia in otherwise normal women and with the testicular feminization syndrome.

Gross Findings

These tumors are usually unilateral, solid, well-circumscribed, yellow, firm, and lobulated masses of 5–6 cm in average size. The cut surface shows hemorrhage and cystification. Moderately differentiated and poorly differentiated tumors are bilateral in less than 2% of cases, circumscribed, partly solid, and partly cystic with a bosselated outer surface. The mean diameter is about 15 cm. Solid portions of the tumor are lobulated, firm or fleshy in consistency, and usually yellow-gray in color. Necrosis and hemorrhage are often prominent.

Microscopic Findings

Well-differentiated Sertoli-Leydig cell tumor consists of uniform solid or hollow tubular structures lined by Sertoli-type cells. The intervening stroma contains variable numbers of Leydig cells. The latter tend to be packed in nests between the Sertoli cell tubules but may form more solid sheets in some tumors. Mitoses are rare in these tumors. Moderately differentiated Sertoli-Leydig cell tumors usually exhibit cellular nodules or "lobules" separated by zones of loose fibrous or fibromyxoid mesenchymal stroma. Immature Sertoli-type cells, with small oval or angular nuclei and pale cytoplasm are arranged in short, thin cords resembling the sex cords of the immature testes. Nuclei are relatively bland and mitoses, average about 5 mitotic figures per 10 high-power fields.

Mature Leydig cells are usually apparent in the stroma, particularly around the periphery of the tumor as sheets, clusters, or single cells within the cellular zones The poorly differentiated tumors show spindle-shaped immature Sertoli cells that may exhibit nuclear atypia and mitotic activity admixed, with clusters of Leydig cells with abundant eosinophilic cytoplasm (Fig. 20.54).

Sertoli-Leydig Cell Tumour with Heterologous Elements

These tumors are characterized by the presence of heterologous elements, the most common of which is gastrointestinal mucin-secreting epithelium. Mucinous heterologous elements are seen in about 20% of Sertoli-Leydig cell tumors. Approximately, 5% of cases contain immature skeletal muscle and/or cartilage.

Gross Findings

Part or the entire cystic component of a Sertoli-Leydig cell tumor may be mucinous in type; however, heterologous elements are only occasionally diagnosed macroscopically.

Microscopic Findings (Fig. 20.55)

Heterologous mesenchymal elements usually consist of mucinous epithelium, cartilage, skeletal muscle or rhabdomyosarcoma. The mucinous epithelium is

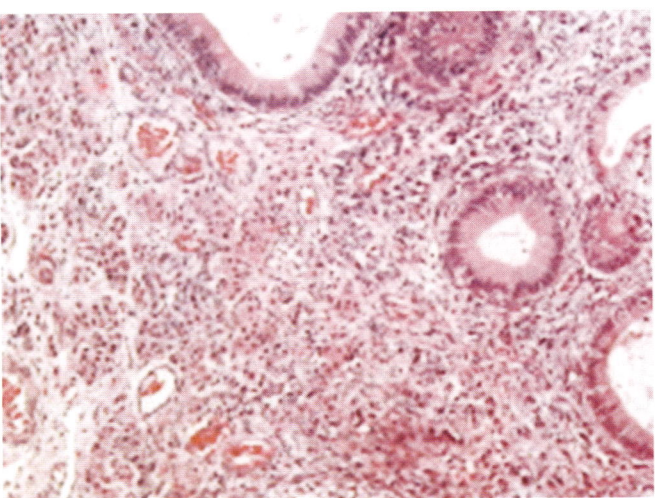

Fig. 20.55: Moderately differentiated Sertoli-Leydig cell tumor with heterologous elements shows admixture of glands lined b y well-differentiated mucinous epithelial cells with inter spersed goblet cells, Sertoli cells, and Leydig cells

usually intestinal, or gastric-type epithelium, but sometimes shows borderline or malignant changes.

Retiform Variants (Fig. 20.56)

14% of moderately and 30% of poorly differentiated ovarian Sertoli-Leydig cell tumors exhibit retiform foci because of a resemblance to the rete testis. Tumors with this pattern occur at a slightly younger age (mean age of 15 years) and are less likely to produce clinical signs of virilization.

Microscopically, this pattern is typified by an irregular network of slit-like spaces and cysts, often containing papillae of various shapes. The cystic and compressed tubular spaces and the papillae are lined

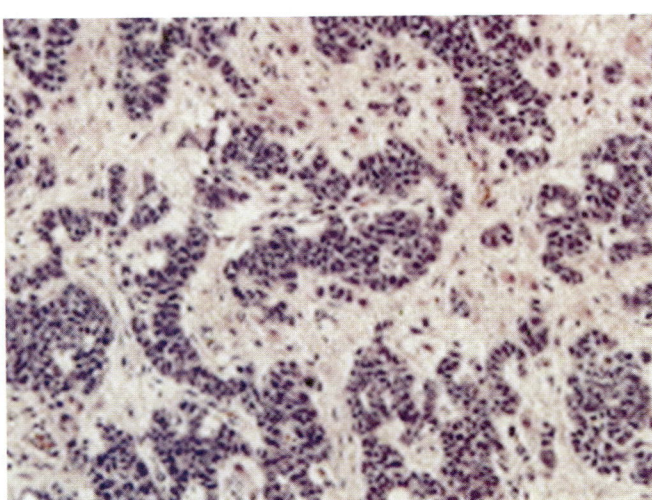

Fig. 20.54: Poorly differentiated Sertoli-Leydig cell tumor sho ws nests and cord of immature Sertoli cells and occasional Le yding cells with eosinophilic cytoplasm

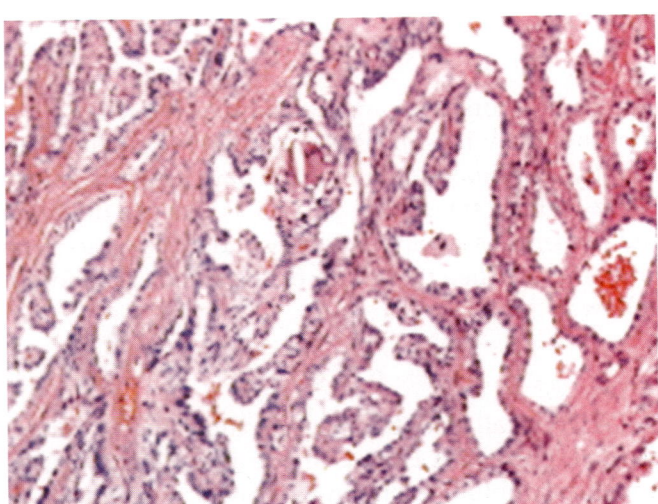

Fig. 20.56: Retiform Sertoli-Leydig cell tumor sho ws admixtures of branching retiform tubules and pa pillary areas with pr ominent hyalinized cores

by flattened or cuboidal cells resembling immature Sertoli cells.

Prognosis and Predictive Factors

The incidence of clinical malignancy in Sertoli stromal cell tumors is 10–30%. The most reliable indication of malignancy is evidence of local extraovarian spread or metastases at the time of staging laparotomy. Histological grade correlates to the likely clinical outcome; 11% of moderately differentiated tumors are clinically malignant, while 20% of those with heterologous mesenchymal elements and 60% of poorly differentiated tumors are clinically malignant.

Sex Cord Tumor with Annular Tubules

Definition

Sex cord tumor with annular tubules (SCTAT) is a tumor composed of sex cord (Sertoli) cells arranged in simple and complex annular tubules.

Epidemiology

Sex cord tumors with annular tubules occur in 2 clinical settings. Firstly, they occur in almost all female patients with the Peutz-Jeghers syndrome (generalized hamartomatous intestinal polyposis and melanin spots of the oral mucosa, lips and digits). The tumors may occur at almost any age, but the mean age at presentation is 27 years. Secondly, cases not associated with the Peutz-Jeghers syndrome (PJS) occur at mean age of 34 years. Over one-half of patients give a history of postmenopausal bleeding, menstrual irregularities or isosexual pseudopuberty, suggesting hyperestrogenism.

Gross Findings

Sex cord tumors with annular tubules, which occur in conjunction with the Peutz-Jeghers syndrome, are usually multifocal, bilateral. In patients without the Peutz-Jeghers syndrome, SCTAT is usually unilateral and presents as a solitary, large solid mass up to 33 cm in diameter. The cut section of the tumor is solid and yellow.

Microscopic Picture (Fig. 20.57)

SCTAT typically exhibits well circumscribed, rounded or oval, epithelial islands made up of ring-shaped, lumenless tubules encircling glassy, acidophilic, PAS-positive, basement membrane-like material. The cytoplasm is abundant, pale, and vacuolated or slightly granular. Regular, rounded, occasionally grooved

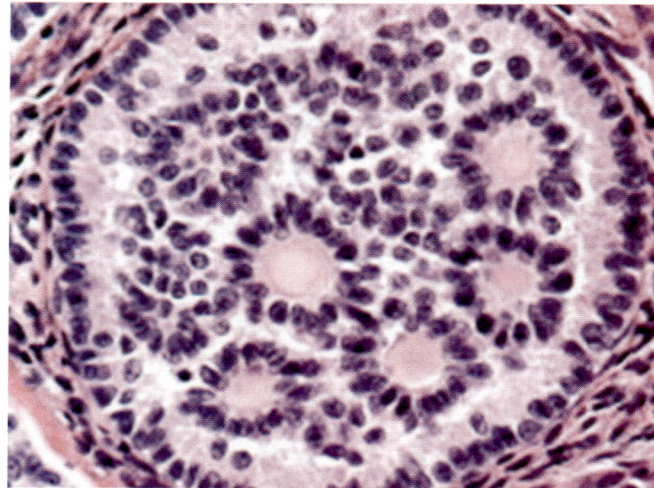

Fig. 20.57: Sex cord-stromal tumor with annular tubules sho ws complex annular tubular pattern consisting of pale cells arranged around multiple hyaline bodies

nuclei, often with a single small nucleolus, are generally arranged in a double row: one row at the periphery of the cell nests and the second around the hyaline deposits. Mitoses are rare.

Prognosis

All Peutz-Jeghers syndrome-associated tumorlets are benign, while up to 25% of sex cord tumors with annular tubules that occur in the absence of the Peutz–Jeghers syndrome are clinically malignant. Tumors with an infiltrative growth pattern and mitotic figures beyond the usual 3–4 MF/10 HPF are more likely to recur or behave aggressively.

Gynandroblastoma

The term gynandroblastoma should be used only for those tumors that show admixture of well-differentiated Sertoli cell and granulosa cell components with the second cell population comprising at least 10% of the lesion.

Gynandroblastoma is very rare and occurs in a wide age range but more commonly in young adults.

Gross Findings

Gynandroblastomas are variable in size with predominantly solid cut section.

Microscopic Picture (Fig. 20.58)

The ovarian elements are seen as nests of mature granulosa cells in which Call–Exner bodies may be found. Male or testicular components are in the form of well-formed hollow tubules lined by typical Sertoli cells or Leydig cells containing Reinke crystals.

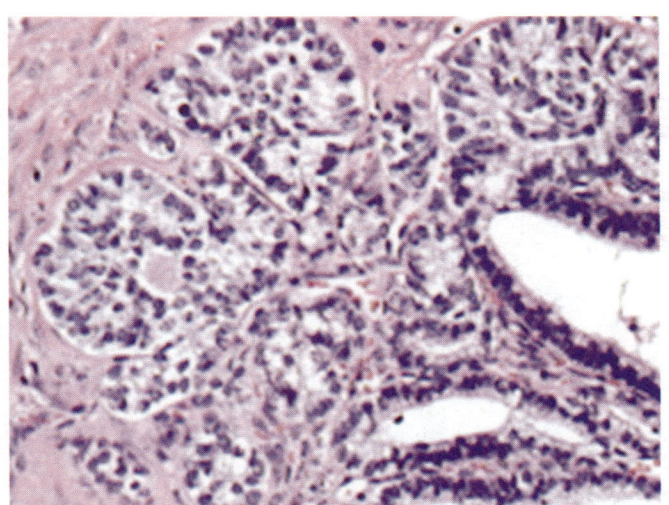

Fig. 20.58: Gynandroblastoma shows granulosa cell with well-formed Call-Exner body on the left admixed with well-differentiated Sertoli cell tubules on the right

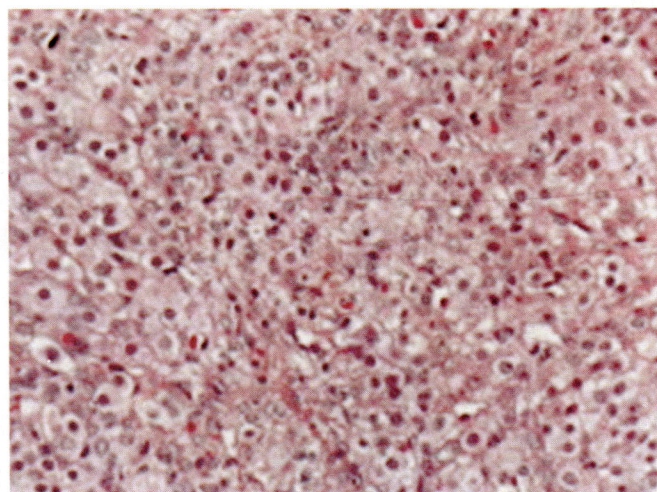

Fig. 20.59: Steroid cell tumor showing steroid cells with abundant eosinophilic cytoplasm

Steroid Cell Tumors

Definition

Steroid cell tumors are tumors composed entirely or predominantly of cells resembling steroid hormone secreting cells.

Steroid Cell Tumors, Not Otherwise Specified

Epidemiology

Steroid cell tumors not occur most often in women of reproductive age, particularly during the third and fourth decades, and rarely in postmenopausal women or children. They are clinically androgenic in 40% of cases and regularly secrete androstenedione, α-hydroxyprogesterone, and testosterone.

Gross Findings

Steroid cell tumors are usually well circumscribed, unilateral, and solid with cystification due to degeneration and hemorrhage. They vary greatly in size from 0.5 to 45 cm in diameter. The cut surface, is frequently lobulated and ranges in color from bright yellow through red-brown to dark green-brown.

Microscopic Findings (Fig. 20.59)

Steroid cell tumors consist of rounded or polygonal vacuolated cells arranged in nests or columns and separated by a rich network of capillaries and vascular sinusoids. The tumor cell cytoplasm is moderate to abundant in amount and can be clear, granular or eosinophilic. Varying degrees of nuclear pleomorphism and mitotic activity have been observed, but a definitive diagnosis of malignancy can only really be made by the presence of local invasion.

Prognosis and Predictive Factors

About 30% of cases are clinically malignant and have an extraovarian spread of tumor at the time of operation. Pathological findings associated with malignant behavior include two or more mitotic figures/10 high power fields, necrosis, hemorrhage, diameter greater than 7 cm, moderate-to-marked nuclear atypia.

Stromal Luteoma

Definition

Stromal luteomas are defined as small steroid cell tumors that are confined to the ovarian stroma and do not have crystals of Reinke.

Stromal luteoma usually occurs in postmenopausal women and is associated with estrogenic effects commonly in the form of abnormal vaginal bleeding. Rarely, androgenic manifestations may be present.

Gross Findings

These tumors are usually unilateral, small (rarely exceed 3 cm), circumscribed, gray-white, or yellow masses.

Microscopic Findings

Stromal luteoma appears as nodules of luteinized stromal cells that may be arranged diffusely or in nests and cords. The cytoplasm is pale or eosinophilic, the nuclei are bland, and mitoses are rare. Foci of degenerative change, lipochrome pigment, and

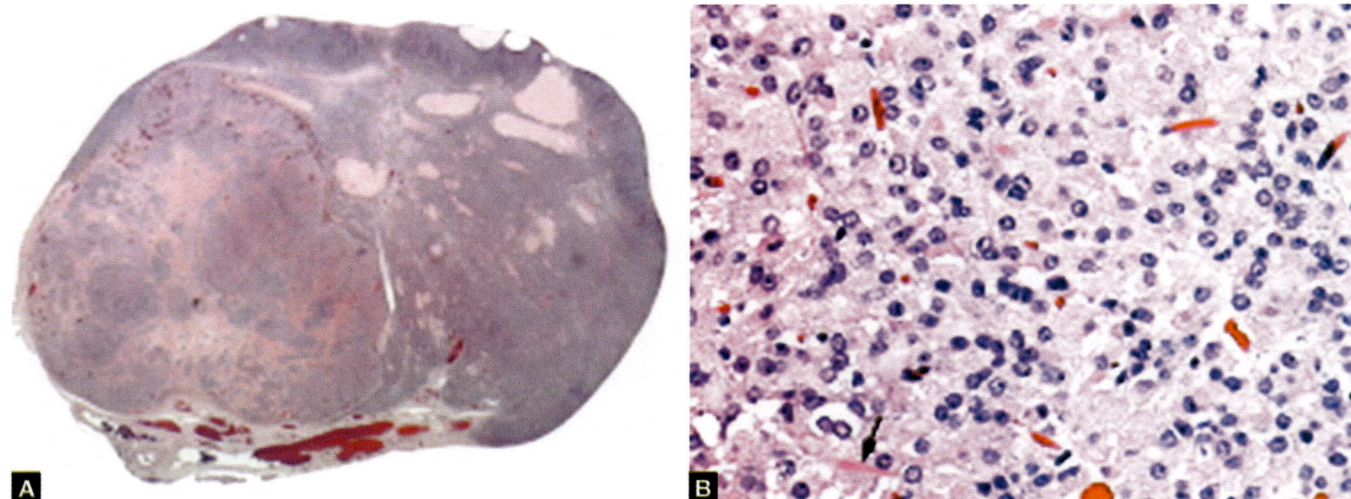

Fig. 20.60: Hilus cell tumor showing Leydig cells with abundant eosinophilic cytoplasm and characteristic nuclear-rich zones separated by nuclear-free zones. The arrows point to crystals of Reinke

hyalinized stroma may be present. Stromal luteomas are usually associated with stromal hyperthecosis in the same or contralateral ovary in 90% of cases.

Leydig Cell Tumors

Leydig cell tumors are rare ovarian steroid cell neoplasms composed of Leydig cells that contain Reinke crystals. Depending on their location, they are divided into hilus cell tumors and Leydig cell tumors of nonhilar type.

Hilus Cell Tumors (Fig. 20.60)

Definition: A hilus cell tumor is a Leydig cell tumor of the ovary that arises in the ovarian hilus.

Gross findings: Leydig cell tumor, hilar cell type, is unilateral, small, mostly microscopic, yellow-to-brown, soft, fleshy, circumscribed masses in the hilar region of the ovary and adjacent mesovarium.

Microscopic findings: Leydig cell tumors are composed of closely packed sheets or solid cords of uniform, polyhedral, and eosinophilic cells. Nuclei are round, central, and vary in size. They frequently give an

appearance of being unevenly distributed in the tumor with "nuclear-rich" and "nuclear-poor" zones, a feature regarded as almost pathognomonic of Leydig cell differentiation, even in the absence of Reinke crystals . Leydig cell cytoplasm is densely eosinophilic and finely granular with small lipid-containing cytoplasmic vacuoles. PAS-positive yellow-brown lipochrome pigment is seen in many cells.

Reinke crystals are slender rods with square or tapered ends, within an incomplete "halo," and best seen when stained bright red with Mallory trichrome stain. They are found in just over 50% of these tumors, but are irregularly distributed in the tumor and thus may require extensive searching to locate them.

Leydig Cell Tumor, Nonhilar Type

A Leydig cell tumor originates from the ovarian stroma and contains Reinke crystals. Leydig cell tumor, nonhilar type, is composed of steroid cells containing Reinke crystals and surrounded by ovarian stroma that often shows stromal hyperthecosis, and except for their location, the clinical and pathological features of the nonhilar type is similar to that of the hilar type.

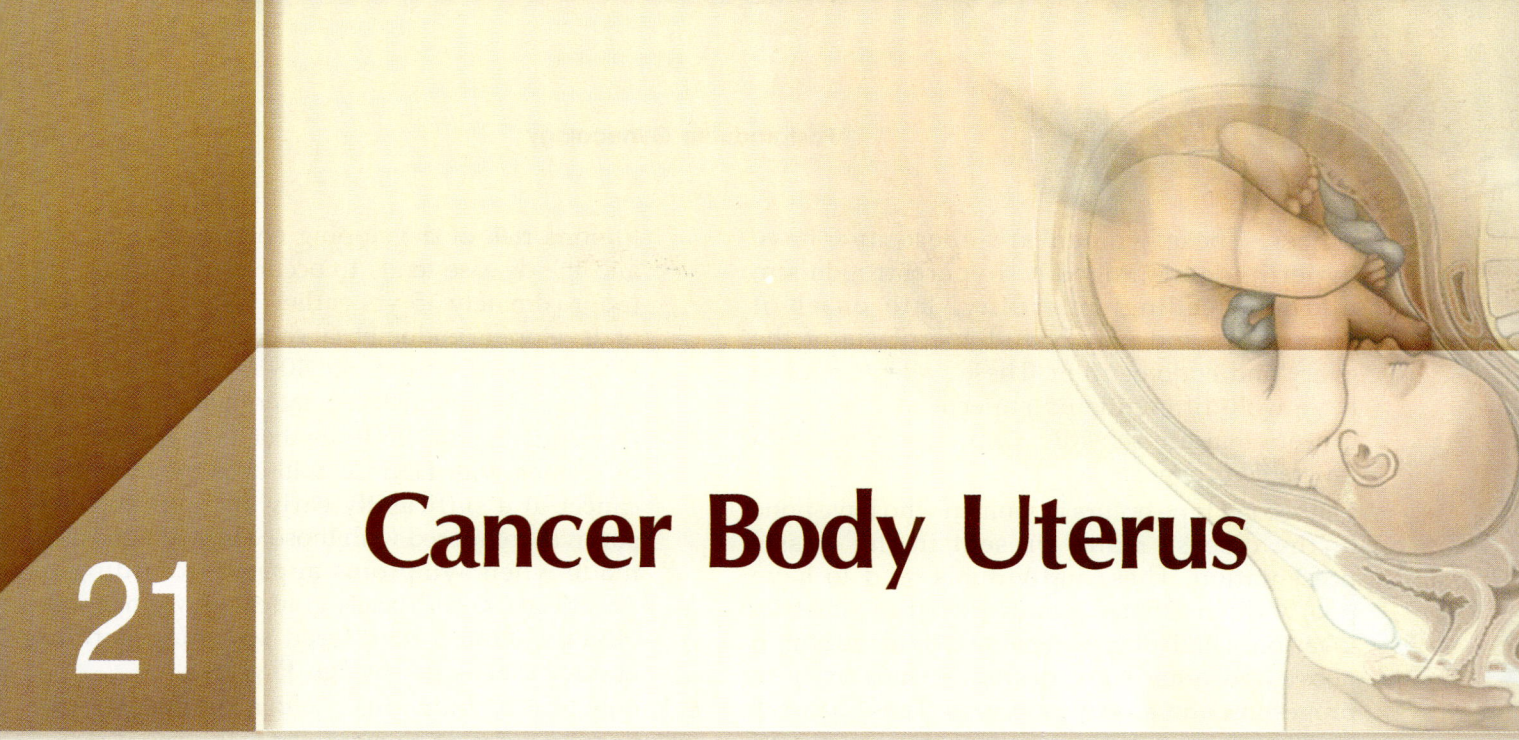

21 Cancer Body Uterus

Corpus cancer is the most frequently occurring female genital cancer. It is the fourth most common cancer among women. In developed countries, adenocarcinoma of the endometrium is the most common gynecological cancer; however, in developing countries, it is much less common than carcinoma of the cervix.

Frequency

The latest Surveillance, Epidemiology, and End Results (SEER) data note a total age-adjusted incidence of 24.4 cases per 100,000 people and the incidence in black women is 22.6 cases per 100,000 persons.

Race

Mortality is higher in black women than in white women, with a mortality ratio of 7.3 deaths per 100,000 persons in black women and only 3.8 deaths per 100,000 persons in white women.

Age

Endometrial adenocarcinoma occurs primarily in postmenopausal years. The median age of persons with this malignancy is early in the seventh decade of life, although most patients are aged 50–59 years. Approximately 5% of women younger than 40 years have adenocarcinoma, and 20–25% of women are diagnosed before menopause.

Incidence and Epidemiology

Endometrial cancer is the seventh most common cause of death from cancer in women in western Europe every year. More than 75% of cases occur in women older than 50 years of age, with a median age of 63 years.

Multiple risk factors have been identified		
Early onset of menstruation	Obesity	Nulliparity
late menopause infertility	Diabetes mellitus	Hypertension
	Unopposed estrogen and tamoxiphen exposure	Atypical endometrial hyperplasia

- **Endogenous factors**
  - Obesity increases the risk for developing endometrial cancer, and some data suggest that a 2- to 3-fold increase in risk occurs, if an individual is more than 50 lb heavier than the ideal weight for that person.
  - Nulliparity also increases risk 2- to 3-fold compared with parity.
  - An individual who has had a late menopause >52 yrs also appears to have an increased risk.
- **Unopposed estrogen**
  - Unopposed estrogen, either as replacement therapy or endogenously produced (e.g., granulosa cell tumor, polycystic ovarian disease), increases the risk of endometrial cancer several times.
  - Obesity is known to increase endogenous estrogen due to peripheral aromatization of fats from androstenedione to estrogen compounds at a much higher rate than if fat is not present.
  - Anovulation, which may be secondary to unopposed estrogen, also appears to contribute to this situation.
- **Phenotype characteristics**
  - A classic phenotypic characteristic is thought to exist for a woman who may develop endometrial

cancer. These women are obese and have hyperlipidemia, signs of hyperestrogenism, uterine bleeding, infertility, late onset of menopause and may have hyperplasia of the ovary and endometrium. These patients tend to have well-differentiated superficially invasive cancers that are sensitive to progesterone with favorable prognosis.

– The second type occurs in women who have none of the disease states present in the classic presentation. These individuals tend to have poorly differentiated tumors, deep myometrial invasion, a high degree of metastasis to the lymph nodes and other sites, decreased sensitivity to progestins, and a poor prognosis. These patients tend to be thin, multiparous women.

• **Tamoxifen:** The most widely used anticancer drug is tamoxifen, and this drug has been suggested by some studies to cause an increased incidence of adenocarcinoma of the endometrium.

• **Combined oral contraceptives:** Women who use OCs at some time have a 0.5 relative risk of developing endometrial cancer compared with women who have never used OCs. This protection occurs in women who have used OCs for at least 12 months, and the protection continues for at least 10 years after OC use. Protection is most notable for nulliparous women.

• **Cigarette smoking:** Smoking apparently decreases the risk of developing endometrial cancer. The effects of smoking are related to body weight. Heavier women who smoke have the greatest reduction in risk. Women who smoke are known to undergo menopause 1–2 years earlier than women who do not smoke.

Associated Medical Conditions

Some associated medical conditions have been found to increase the incidence of endometrial cancer.

• Breast, colon, and ovarian cancers are frequently observed in women with endometrial cancer.

• Women who have had breast cancer have a 2- to 3-fold increased risk of subsequently developing endometrial cancer.

• Women who have hereditary nonpolyposis colon cancer (HNPCC) appear to have a markedly increased risk for developing endometrial cancer.

– Women with HNPCC account for only 2–10% of all female cases of colon cancer, but approximately 5% of all endometrial cancers occur in women with this risk factor. These women have a 22–50%

lifetime risk of developing endometrial cancer, and the disease tends to occur at a younger age (approximately 15 yrs earlier). The greatest risk of developing endometrial cancer in women with HNPCC occurs from age 40–60 years, at which time the absolute risk is greater than 1% per year.

– Currently, no data indicate that annual screening of women with HNPCC will detect endometrial cancer at a sufficiently early stage to improve survival compared with those whose diagnosis is made when symptoms appear. According to American Cancer Society guidelines, women with HNPCC should be offered screening with an endometrial biopsy by age 35 years.

• Family history: Individuals with a family history of endometrial cancer appear to be at increased risk.

The risk of endometrial hyperplasia progressing to carcinoma is related to presence and severity of cytologic atypia. It is found that progression to carcinoma occurs in 1% of patients with simple hyperplasia, 3% of patients with complex hyperplasia, 8% with atypical simple hyperplasia and 29% with atypical complex hyperplasia.

Table 21.1: Causes of postmenopausal uterine bleeding

Cause of bleeding	Percentage
Endometrial atrophy	60–80
Estrogen replacement therapy	15–25
Endometrial polyp	2–12
Endometrial hyperplasia	5–10
Endometrial cancer	10

History

• Because approximately 75% of women with endometrial cancer are postmenopausal, the most common symptom is postmenopausal bleeding and abnormal vaginal discharge (90%). The patient may present with heavy frequent menstrual periods or intermenstrual bleeding.

• Less than 5% women may remain asymptomatic.

• Associated pain abdomen may be due to coexisting infection in the uterus due to fungating growth or local extrauterine metastases.

• All bleeding during menopause must be investigated unless the patient is on cyclic replacement therapy with normally anticipated withdrawal bleeding. The duration or amount of bleeding does not make any difference. The fact that approximately 12% of postmenopausal bleeding may be due to cancer is appreciated the diagnosis must be eliminated in these patients. The idea that any type of bleeding during the perimenopausal period is probably due to menopausal transition is a common misconception. This irregular bleeding is often ignored by the patient and health care providers.

Physical Examination

- Obesity, hypertension and diabetes may be the coexisting morbid condition found in these women. Pathology in breast, ascites and enlarged liver and lymph nodes must be looked for.
- Because bleeding usually occurs from the endometrium, pelvic examination findings may be:
  a. Entirely normal.
  b. Uterus appears bulky, soft, often tender with no gross evidence of disease on the cervix.
  c. Can present with pyometra.
  d. In Stage II, cervix may appear bulky with endocervical involvement.
  e. In stage III & IV, ovaries are involved with bilateral mass in fornices and POD.
  f. Vagina or periurethral area may show signs of metastases.

Imaging Studies

Transvaginal Ultrasonography (Figs 21.1 and 21.2)

The increased use of vaginal ultrasonography to evaluate the endometrial thickness appears to be the first diagnostic procedure for detection of endometrial cancer. Any increased endometrial thickness with SOL and irregular margin and myometrial invasion is diagnostic.

Postmenopausal women with ET ≥5 mm are at an increased risk of cancer. It is often difficult to

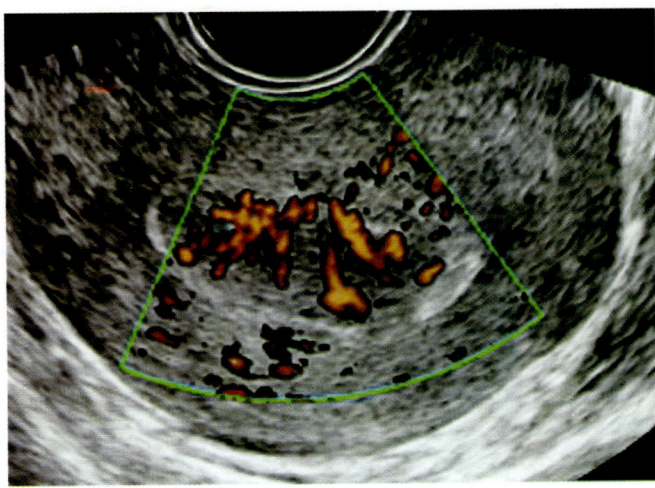

Fig. 21.2: Multiple vessels in women with endometrial cancer

differentiate between benign and malignant endometrium based on endometrial grayscale morphology assessment especially in women with an ET <15 mm. Endometrial echogenicity and border in combination with ET has been shown to be a better predictor of endometrial cancer than ET measurement alone. Assessment of vascular morphology of endometrial vessels can also be used to estimate the risk of endometrial cancer. The presence of multiple vessels with irregular vascular branching and areas of densely packed vessels has a sensitivity of around 80% for the detection of cancer at a specificity of 54–100%.

Hydroultrasonography (Fig. 21.3)

If a thickened endometrium is present, this is very effective to diagnose intrauterine SOL. This is accomplished by placing a small volume of saline into

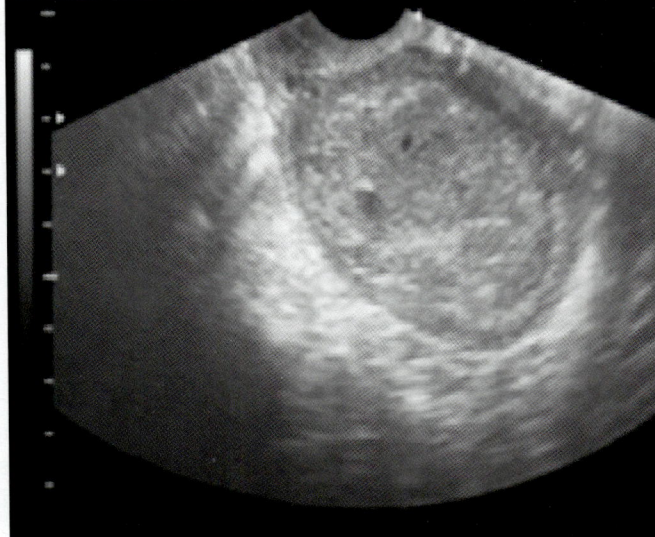

Fig. 21.1: Myometrial invasion by endometrial cancer: Invasion of the external third of the myometrium

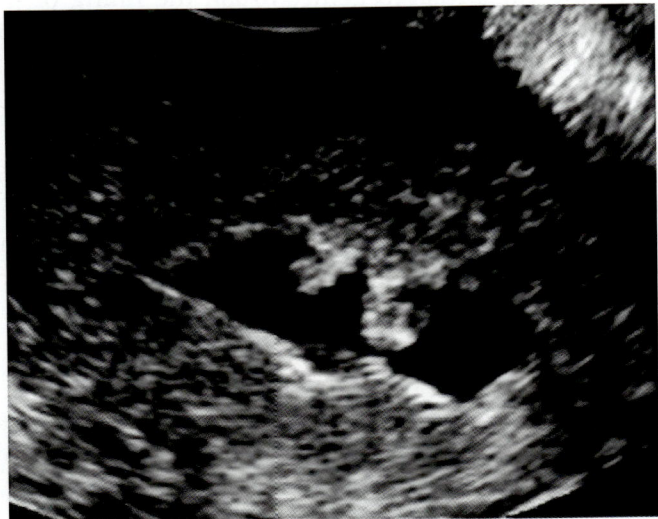

Fig. 21.3: Irregular focal lesion in women with endometrial cancer on SIS

the endometrial cavity and then repeating the vaginal ultrasonogram. In many instances in which the original vaginal ultrasonogram shows significant endometrial thickness, hydroultrasonogram helps differentiate other pathology from true endometrial thickness.

Invasive Procedures

Endometrial Biopsy

- Although fractional dilatation and curettage was historically the definitive diagnostic procedure to rule out endometrial cancer, in current practice endometrial biopsy as an office procedure is quick, well tolerated, and sensitive for making the diagnosis.
- If endometrial pathology is not present on biopsy specimens and the patient has no further bleeding, no additional diagnostic tests need to be performed.
- If the patient continues to be symptomatic, then further evaluation of the endometrial cavity is necessary.

Biopsy Instruments

A number of biopsy instruments are in use. The **Novak curette** is a thin metallic tube with a side opening at the tip; suction with attached syringe can be applied to help to remove tissue. The **Pipelle** is a more flexible plastic tube with a side opening at the tip. A smaller tube (internal piston) inside the Pipelle will be withdrawn to create suction. The pipelle will be rotated and moved in and out to collect small pieces of endometrial tissue. Recently, the **TruTest** has been introduced as an alternative method of endometrial biopsy. Rather than using a suction tube, this method uses the Tao Brush to gently brush the lining of the uterus. Generally, this method has been found to be less painful than the traditional suction method.

Risks

While procedure is generally considered safe, cramps or pelvic pain is a common, if short-lived side effect. After the procedure, the patient may experience some bleeding. *Uterine perforation* or an infection are rare complications.

Endometrial Biopsy Procedure

1. The patient is placed in dorsal lithotomy position. Asceptic dressing and draping is done followed by pelvic examination after emptying the bladder.
2. A Sims posterior vaginal *speculum* is inserted into the vagina to expose the *cervix*. The cervix will then be cleansed with an antiseptic solution.

3. A *tenaculum*, hold the anterior lip of cervix steady for the biopsy.
4. The cervix is dilatated with Hegar's dilators up to maximum 10–14 mm.
5. The biopsy curette is inserted into the uterine cavity till the fundus and with a scraping and rotating motion endometrium from all its walls are removed.
6. The removed tissue is placed in *formalin* or equivalent for preservation and sent for a histologic diagnosis.

Contraindications

The procedure is contraindicated in pregnancy. Other contraindications are pelvic inflammatory disease and coagulopathies.

An endometrial biopsy usually cannot be done as an office procedure in children, young women, women with *vaginismus*, or women with *cervical stenosis*. If necessary, an examination under *anesthesia* could be performed at which time a biopsy could be taken.

Pipelle Biopsy

- Pipelle endometrial biopsy is a cost-effective and safe procedure that is well-tolerated by patients.
- There is less pain and a lower risk of perforation with the pipelle than with the Novak curette.
- The pipelle is more portable than the Novak curette and the Vabra aspirator, both of which require external suction.
- The detection rates for endometrial carcinoma using the pipelle device are 99.6% in postmenopausal women and 91% in premenopausal women.
- In postmenopausal women, the combined use of pipelle sampling and ultrasound has a high detection rate for endometrial carcinoma.
- The pipelle is poor at detecting endometrial pathologies such as polyps and submucosal myomas.
- However, sampling error is greater with the pipelle and the device samples only 4% of the endometrium compared with 42% with the Vabra aspirator.

Procedure (Fig. 21.4)

- Bimanual examination to assess the uterus.
- The cervix is then visualized and cleaned.
- A tenaculum is applied to the anterior lip of the cervix, and is used to provide gentle traction whilst a sound is inserted though the cervical os. This minimizes the risk of perforation.
- Dilators may be required, if there is difficulty in passing the sound.

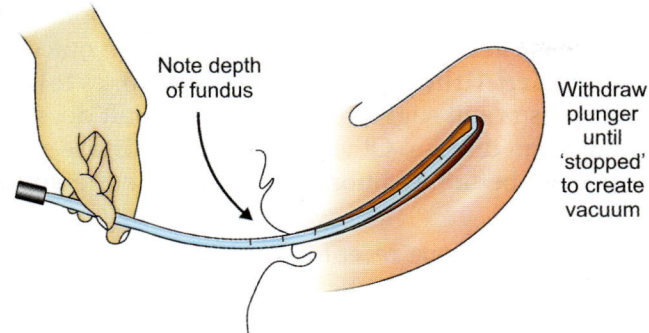

Fig. 21.4: Endometrial aspiration

- When the position and size of the uterine cavity have been assessed, the pipelle is inserted through the cervical os and advanced until gentle resistance is felt.
- The inner piston of the device is then withdrawn to create suction and the endometrial sample is obtained by moving the pipelle up and down within the uterine cavity by approximately 2–3 cm but not beyond the cervical os.
- This procedure should be repeated at least four times and the device is rotated 360° to ensure adequate coverage of the area.
- The pipelle is then withdrawn from the cervical os and the endometrial sample expelled into a solution of formalin for transport to the laboratory.

Tao Brush

The Tao Brush method uses a small, flexible brush to gently brush the entire inside of the uterus. The Tao Brush is theoretically able to gather a more complete sampling of the uterus lining, removes less tissue and is less painful.

Procedure

1. The cervix is fixed with usual tenaculum after similar preparation of the patient placed in dorsal lithotomy position.
2. The brush is inserted into the uterus. The covering sheath protects the brush from collecting any contaminating tissue from the cervix.
3. Once the brush is in place, the sheath is removed.
4. The brush is then rotated 4–5 times, collecting tissue from the entire uterine lining.
5. The sheath is then replaced, ensuring that the tissue samples are trapped on the brush.
6. The brush is removed and placed directly in the fixative solution.

Hysteroscopy Directed Biopsy

The more accurate way of determining the status of the endometrium is hysteroscopically directed biopsy. At hysteroscopy, the disease shows polypoid, either sessile or pedunculated and is composed of irregularly heaped up tissue that often has a granular surface. It appears opaque, dry pale yellow or white, and friable. Areas of necrosis or the accumulation of lipid-filled cells of stromal origin between the neoplastic glands appear as dark yellow areas. When the tumor is poorly differentiated hemorrhage, ulcerations and abnormal vascular patterns may be seen.

Microscopic Spread

The most debatable issue is perhaps the potential risk of microscopic extrauterine spread of endometrial cancer through hysteroscopy. Concern has often been expressed that the increase in intrauterine pressure during hysteroscopy may lead to dissemination of malignant cells into the abdominal cavity.

Histological Classification of Endometrial Cancer

The most common endometrial cancer cell type is endometrioid adenocarcinoma, which is composed of malignant glandular epithelial elements; an admixture of squamous metaplasia is not uncommon. Adenosquamous tumors contain malignant elements of both glandular and squamous epithelium; clear cell and papillary serous carcinoma of the endometrium are tumors that are histologically similar to those noted in the ovary and the fallopian tube, and the prognosis is worse for these tumors. Mucinous, squamous, and undifferentiated tumors are rarely encountered. The mixed müllerian tumors originally thought to be a sarcoma are actually epithelial in origin and should be included here instead of a primary sarcoma.

Frequency of endometrial cancer cell types is as follows:

   i. Endometrioid (75–80%).
      a. Ciliated adenocarcinoma.
      b. Secretory adenocarcinoma.
      c. Papillary or villoglandular.
      d. Adenocarcinoma with squamous differentiation.
         1. Adenoacanthoma.
         2. Adenosquamous.
   ii. Uterine papillary serous (<10%).
  iii. Mucinous (1%).
   iv. Clear cell (4%).
    v. Squamous cell (<1%).
   vi. Mixed (10%).
  vii. Undifferentiated.

The pattern of spread is partially dependent on the **degree of cellular differentiation**. Well-differentiated tumors tend to limit their spread to the surface of the endometrium; myometrial extension is less common. In patients with poorly differentiated tumors, **myometrial invasion** occurs much more frequently. Myometrial invasion is frequently a harbinger of lymph node involvement and distant metastases and is often independent of the degree of differentiation. Metastatic spread occurs in a characteristic pattern. Spread to the pelvic and para-aortic nodes is common. When distant metastasis occurs, it most commonly involves the following:

- Lungs
- Inguinal and supraclavicular nodes
- Liver
- Bones
- Brain
- Vagina

Another factor found to correlate with extrauterine and nodal spread of tumor is **involvement of the capillary-lymphatic space** on histopathologic examination. Three prognostic groupings of clinical stage I disease become possible by careful operative staging.

Patients with grade 1 tumors involving only endometrium and no evidence of intraperitoneal disease (i.e. adnexal spread) have a low risk (<5%) of nodal involvement.

Patients with grade 2 or 3 tumors and invasion of less than 50% of the myometrium and no intraperitoneal disease have a 5 to 9% incidence of pelvic node involvement and a 4% incidence of positive para-aortic nodes.

Patients with deep muscle invasion and high-grade tumors and/or intraperitoneal disease have a significant risk of nodal spread, 20 to 60% to pelvic nodes and 10 to 30% to para-aortic nodes. Therefore, the following are significant adverse prognostic factors:

- Myometrial invasion
- Vascular invasion
- Eight or more mitoses per ten high-power fields
- An absence of progesterone receptors

A gynecologic oncology group study has related surgical-pathologic parameters and postoperative treatment to recurrence-free interval and recurrence site. For patients without extrauterine spread, the greatest determinants of recurrence are grade 3 histology and deep myometrial invasion. The frequency of recurrence is greatly increased with positive pelvic nodes, adnexal metastasis, positive peritoneal cytology, capillary space involvement, involvement of the isthmus or cervix, and positive para-aortic nodes.

When the only evidence of extrauterine spread is positive peritoneal cytology, the influence on outcome is unclear. Although the collection of cytology specimens is still suggested, a positive result does not upstage the disease. Other extrauterine disease must be present before additional postoperative therapy is considered.

The progesterone receptor levels may be the single most important prognostic indicator in clinical stages I and II disease. Patients with progesterone receptor levels higher than 100 has a 3-year disease-free survival of 93% compared with 36% for a level lower than 100. Therefore, progesterone and estrogen receptors, assessed either by biochemical or immunohistochemical methods, should be included in the evaluation of stages I and II patients.

FIGO Staging of Carcinoma of the Endometrium, 2009

FIGO recommended that corpus cancer be staged surgically. Previously, clinical evaluation was used for staging, and multiple studies noted the inaccuracy of clinical staging compared with surgical pathological findings. Therefore, once the diagnosis of endometrial cancer has been made, routine presurgical evaluation is performed to assess operability.

- Special studies, such as CT scans of the abdomen and pelvis or MRIs, are not routinely performed.
- The preoperative evaluation includes: Chest X-ray, clinical and gynecological examination, transvaginal ultrasound, blood counts, and liver and renal function profiles. Abdominal computed tomography (CT) scan is indicated for investigating extrapelvic disease. Dynamic contrast-enhanced magnetic resonance imaging (MRI) is the best tool to assess the cervical involvement. Fluorodeoxyglucose-positron emission tomography (FDG-PET)/CT could be useful to detect distant metastases accurately.
- Once preoperative evaluation results are found, the patient is deemed a surgical candidate. Then, an exploratory laparotomy, total abdominal hysterectomy, bilateral salpingo-oophorectomy, peritoneal cytology, and pelvic and para-aortic lymphadenectomy are performed.
- Obviously, if intraperitoneal disease is identified at the time of surgery, attempts are made at surgical removal.
- Staging is then determined based on surgical pathologic findings. Subsequent therapy, if needed, is then determined, depending on the surgical pathological findings of the operative procedure.

FIGO Staging

Stage	
I	Tumor confined to the corpus uteri.
IA	No or less than half myometrial invasion.
IB	Invasion equal to or more than half of the myometrium.
II	Tumor invades cervical stroma but does not extend beyond the uterus.
III	Local and/or regional spread of the tumor.
IIIA	Tumor invades the serosa of the corpus uteri and/or adnexae.
IIIB	Vaginal and/or parametrial involvement.
IIIC	Metastases to pelvic and/or para-aortic lymph nodes.
IIIC1	Positive pelvic nodes.
IIIC2	Positive para-aortic lymph nodes with or without positive pelvic lymph nodes.
IV	Tumor invades bladder and/or bowel mucosa, and/or distant metastases.
IVA	Tumor invasion of bladder and/or bowel mucosa.

*Adapted from FIGO Committee on Gynecologic Oncology
*Either G1, G2 or G3 (G = grade).
*Endocervical glandular involvement only should be considered as stage I and no longer as stage II
*Positive cytology has to be reported separately without changing the stage.

- Cases of carcinoma of the corpus should be classified (or graded) according to the degree of histologic differentiation. The histopathology and degree of differentiation is as follows:
  - Class G1: Nonsquamous or nonmorular solid growth pattern of 5% or less.
  - Class G2: Nonsquamous or nonmorular solid growth pattern of 6–50%.
  - Class G3: Nonsquamous or nonmorular solid growth pattern of more than 50%.

TNM Classification for Endometrial Cancer

Primary Tumor (T)

TNM	FIGO stages	Surgical-pathologic findings
TX		Primary tumor cannot be assessed
T0		No evidence of primary tumor
Tis*		Carcinoma in situ (preinvasive carcinoma)
T1	I	Tumor confined to corpus uteri
T1a	IA	Tumor limited to endometrium or invades less than one-half of the myometrium
T1b	IB	Tumor invades one-half or more of the myometrium
T2	II	Tumor invades stromal connective tissue of the cervix but does not extend beyond uterus**
T3a	IIIA	Tumor involves serosa and/or adnexa (direct extension or metastasis)

TNM	FIGO	Surgical-pathologic findings
T3b	IIIB	Vaginal involvement (direct extension or metastasis) or parametrial involvement
	IIIC	Metastases to pelvic and/or para-aortic lymph nodes
	IV	Tumor invades bladder mucosa and/or bowel mucosa, and/or distant metastases
T4	IVA	Tumor invades bladder mucosa and/or bowel mucosa (bullous edema is not sufficient to classify a tumor as T4)

*FIGO no longer includes stage 0 (Tis)
**Endocervical glandular involvement should only be considered as stage I and no longer as stage II

Regional Lymph Nodes (N)

TNM	FIGO stages	Surgical-pathologic findings
NX		Regional lymph nodes cannot be assessed
N0		No regional lymph node metastasis
N1	IIIC1	Regional lymph node metastasis to pelvic lymph nodes
N2	IIIC2	Regional lymph node metastasis to para-aortic lymph nodes, with or without positive pelvic lymph nodes

Distant Metastasis (M)

TNM	FIGO stages	Surgical-pathologic findings
M0		No distant metastasis
M1	IVB	Distant metastasis (includes metastasis to inguinal lymph nodes, intraperitoneal disease, or lung, liver, or bone metastases; it excludes metastasis to para-aortic lymph nodes, vagina, pelvic serosa, or adnexa)

AJCC (American Joint Committee on Cancer) Stage Grouping and FIGO Stages

Information about the tumor, lymph nodes, and any cancer spread is then combined to assign the stage of disease. This process is called *stage grouping*. The stages are described using the number 0 and Roman numerals from I to IV. Some stages are divided into substages indicated by letters and numbers.

Stage 0

Tis, N0, M0: This stage is also known as *carcinoma in situ*. Cancer cells are only found in the surface layer of cells of the endometrium, without growing into the layers of cells below. The cancer has not spread to nearby lymph nodes or distant sites. This is a precancerous lesion. This stage is not included in the FIGO staging system.

Stage I

T1, N0, M0: The cancer is only growing in the body of the uterus. It may also be growing into the glands of the cervix, but is not growing into the supporting connective tissue of the cervix. The cancer has not spread to lymph nodes or distant sites.

- ***Stage IA (T1a, N0, M0):*** In this earliest form of stage I, the cancer is in the endometrium (inner lining of the uterus) and may have grown from the endometrium less than halfway through the underlying muscle layer of the uterus (the myometrium). It has not spread to lymph nodes or distant sites.
- ***Stage IB (T1b, N0, M0):*** The cancer has grown from the endometrium into the myometrium, growing more than halfway through the myometrium. The cancer has not spread beyond the body of the uterus.

Stage II

T2, N0, M0: The cancer has spread from the body of the uterus and is growing into the supporting connective tissue of the cervix (called the cervical stroma). The cancer has not spread outside of the uterus. The cancer has not spread to lymph nodes or distant sites.

Stage III

T3, N0, M0: Either the cancer has spread outside of the uterus or into nearby tissues in the pelvic area.

- ***Stage IIIA (T3a, N0, M0):*** The cancer has spread to the outer surface of the uterus (called the serosa) and/or to the fallopian tubes or ovaries (the adnexa). The cancer has not spread to lymph nodes or distant sites.
- ***Stage IIIB (T3b, N0, M0):*** The cancer has spread to the vagina or to the tissues around the uterus (the parametrium). The cancer has not spread to lymph nodes or distant sites.
- ***Stage IIIC1 (T1 to T3, N1, M0):*** The cancer is growing in the body of the uterus. It may have spread to some nearby tissues, but is not growing into the inside of the bladder or rectum. The cancer has spread to pelvic lymph nodes but not to lymph nodes around the aorta or distant sites.
- ***Stage IIIC2 (T1 to T3, N2, M0):*** The cancer is growing in the body of the uterus. It may have spread to some nearby tissues, but is not growing into the inside of the bladder or rectum. The cancer has spread to lymph nodes around the aorta (periaortic lymph nodes) but not to distant sites.

Stage IV

The cancer has spread to the inner surface of the urinary bladder or the rectum (lower part of the large intestine), to lymph nodes in the groin, and/or to distant organs, such as the bones, omentum or lungs.

- ***Stage IVA (T4, any N, M0):*** The cancer has spread to the inner lining of the rectum or urinary bladder (called the mucosa). It may or may not have spread to nearby lymph nodes but has not spread to distant sites.
- ***Stage IVB (any T, any N, M1):*** The cancer has spread to distant lymph nodes, the upper abdomen, the omentum, or to organs away from the uterus, such as the bones, omentum, or lungs. The cancer can be any size and it may or may not have spread to lymph nodes.

Uterine sarcomas were staged previously as endometrial cancers, which did not reflect clinical behavior. Therefore, a new corpus sarcoma staging system is developed based on the criteria used in other soft tissue sarcomas.

Uterine Sarcomas (Leiomyosarcoma, Endometrial Stromal Sarcoma and Adenosarcoma)

IA	Tumor limited to uterus <5 cm
IB	Tumor limited to uterus >5 cm
IIA	Tumor extends to the pelvis, adnexal involvement
IIB	Tumor extends to extrauterine pelvic tissue
IIIA	Tumor invades abdominal tissues, one site
IIIB	More than one site
IIIC	Metastasis to pelvic and/or para-aortic lymph nodes
IVA	Tumor invades bladder and/or rectum
IVB	Distant metastasis

Treatment Option

Patients with endometrial cancer who have localized disease are usually curable by hysterectomy and bilateral salpingo-oophorectomy. Best results are obtained with either of two standard treatments—hysterectomy or hysterectomy and adjuvant radiation therapy (when deep invasion of the myometrial muscle [50% of the depth] or grade 3 tumor with myometrial invasion is present). The use of external-beam radiation therapy (EBRT) in patients with stage I disease does not show improved survival but shows reduced locoregional recurrence (3–4% vs 12–14%) after 5–6 years' median follow-up.

Vaginal cuff brachytherapy is associated with less radiation-related morbidity than is EBRT and has been shown to be equivalent to EBRT in the adjuvant setting for patients with stage I disease. A subset of patients with stage I disease are at a high risk of recurrence and are eligible for adjuvant therapy. Most patients will do well with surgery alone.

Some patients have regional and distant metastases that, though occasionally responsive to standard hormone therapy, are rarely curable. Progestational agents as adjuvant therapy in stage I disease have been shown to be of no benefit. Determination of progesterone receptors in the primary tumor is encouraged and adjuvant trial with progesterone should be considered in those cases with high progesterone receptor level.

Stage I Endometrial Cancer

Standard treatment options: The standard surgical approach for stage I endometrial cancer consists of total hysterectomy and bilateral salpingo-oophorectomy with or without lymphadenectomy [IA]. This is justified, if the tumor:

- Is well or moderately differentiated.
- Involves the upper 66% of the corpus.
- Has negative peritoneal cytology.
- Is without vascular space invasion.
- Has less than a 50% myometrial invasion.

Procedures

1. Abdomen is opened by midline vertical incision.

2. Any peritoneal fluid or 100 mL peritoneal wash is collected and sent for cytology.

3. Whole abdomen including liver, under surface of diaphragm, right paracolic gutter, transverse colon, mesentery, left paracolic gutter, small and large intestines, pelvis, pouch of douglas are explored. Any possible areas are biopsied.

4. During hysterectomy, uterine corneal ends are clamped and total extrafascial abdominal hysterectomy with bilateral salpingo-oophorectomy is done. No additional vaginal cuff is removed nowadays and vault is closed without opening the vaginal cuff.

The role of systematic pelvic lymphadenectomy is an issue of current debate. Selected pelvic lymph nodes may be removed. If they are negative, no postoperative treatment is indicated. *Efficacy of Systemic Pelvic Lymphadenectomy in Endometrial Cancer (ASTEC) trial* concluded that routine systematic pelvic lymphadenectomy cannot be recommended in women with stage I endometrial cancer. Lymphadenectomy is highly important in determining patient's prognosis and in tailoring adjuvant therapies. Hence, many authors suggest a complete surgical staging for intermediate-, high-risk endometrioid cancer (stages IA G3 and IB). Therefore, in these cases, a pelvic and selective periaortic node sampling should be combined with the total hysterectomy and bilateral salpingo-oophorectomy.

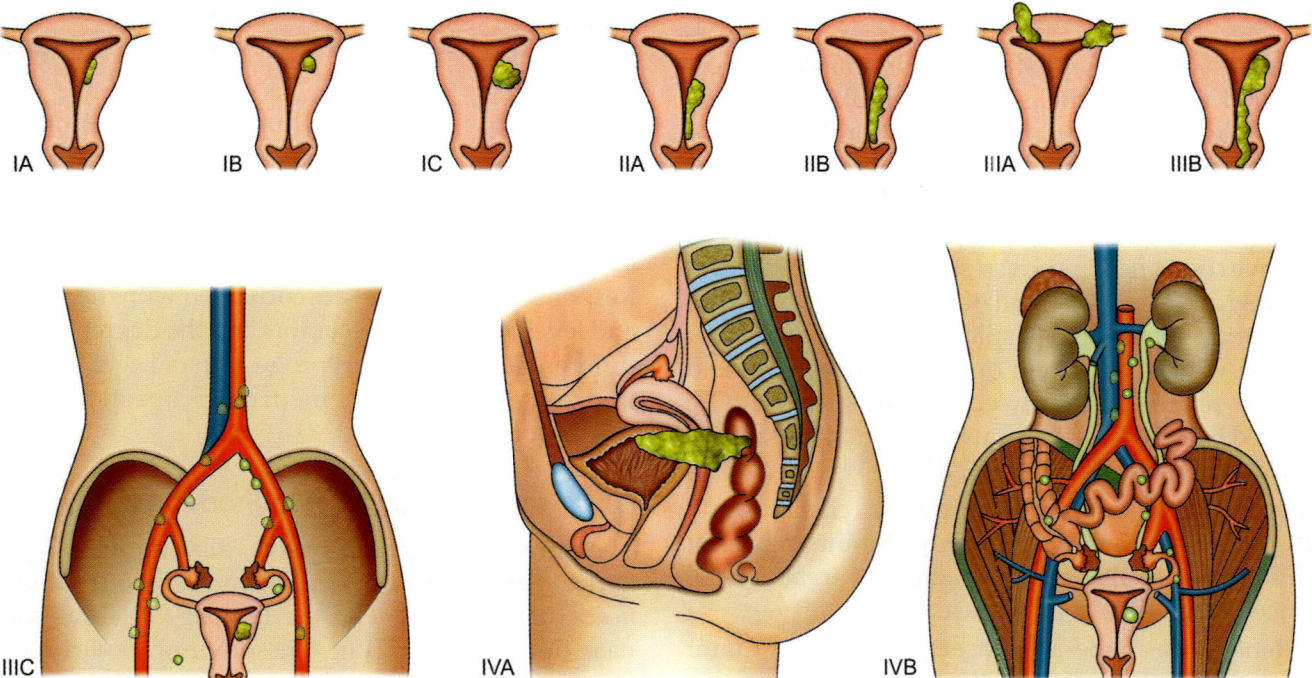

Fig. 21.5: Stages of cancer endometrium

Patients who have medical contraindications to surgery should be treated with radiation therapy alone, but the result is inferior cure rates below those attained with surgery.

Total laparoscopic hysterectomy (TLH) for patients with early-stage endometrial cancer is associated with a longer operative time but is claimed to have an improved or similar adverse event profile and a shorter hospital stay when compared with TAH. TLH is definitely associated with less pain and quicker resumption of daily activities.

Stage II Endometrial Cancer

Standard Treatment Options

Traditionally, the surgical approach consists of radical hysterectomy with bilateral salpingo-oophorectomy and systematic pelvic lymphadenectomy with or without para-aortic lymphadenectomy. In stage II, lymphadenectomy is essential to guide surgical staging and adjuvant therapy.

1. If cervical involvement is documented, options include radical hysterectomy, bilateral salpingo-oophorectomy and pelvic and para-aortic lymph node dissection.
2. If the cervix is clinically uninvolved but extension to the cervix is documented on postoperative pathology, radiation therapy should be considered.

Stage III Endometrial Cancer

Standard Treatment Options

In general, patients with stage III endometrial cancer are treated with maximal surgical debulking surgery, followed by chemotherapy, or radiation therapy, or both. For many years, radiation therapy was the standard adjuvant treatment for patients with endometrial cancer. However, several randomized trials have confirmed improved survival when adjuvant chemotherapy is used instead of radiation therapy. The use of the combination of cisplatin and doxorubicin or paclitaxel with doxyrubicin or use of carboplatin and paclitaxel results in improved overall survival (OS) compared with whole-abdominal radiation therapy (5-year survival rates of 55% vs. 42%).

The three-drug regimen (doxorubicin, cisplatin, and paclitaxel) with granulocyte colony-stimulating factor (G-CSF) is also considered for adjuvant treatment of advanced stage III and IV disease.

Patients with inoperable disease caused by tumor that extends to the pelvic wall may be treated with a combination of chemotherapy and radiation therapy.

The usual approach is to use a combination of intracavitary radiation therapy and external-beam radiation therapy. Patients who are not candidated for either surgery or radiation therapy may be treated with progestational agents.

Stage IV Endometrial Cancer

Standard Treatment Options

Treatment of patients with stage IV endometrial cancer is dictated by the site of metastatic disease and symptoms related to disease sites. For bulky pelvic disease, radiation therapy consisting of a combination of intracavitary and external-beam radiation therapy is used. When distant metastases, especially pulmonary metastases, are present, hormonal therapy is indicated and useful.

When possible, patients with stage IV endometrial cancer are treated with debulking surgery, followed by chemotherapy, or radiation therapy, or both. For many years, radiation therapy was the standard adjuvant treatment for patients with endometrial cancer. However, improved survival is observed when adjuvant chemotherapy is used instead of radiation therapy. In a trial conducted in a subset of patients with stage III or IV disease with residual tumors smaller than 2 cm and no parenchymal organ involvement, the use of the combination of cisplatin/paclitaxel and doxorubicin or three-drug regime of doxorubicin, cisplatin, paclitaxel (TAP) with G-CSF resulted in improved overall survival (OS) compared with whole-abdominal radiation therapy (5-year survival rates of 55% vs 42%).

The most common hormonal treatment is progestational agents, which produce good antitumor responses in as many as 15 to 30% of patients. Progesterone and estrogen hormone receptors have been identified in endometrial carcinoma tissues. Responses to hormones are correlated with the presence and level of hormone receptors and the degree of tumor differentiation. Standard progestational agents include hydroxyprogesterone, medroxyprogesterone, and megestrol.

Pelvic and Para-aortic Lymphadenectomy

The **para-aortic lymph nodes** (also known as **para-aortic**, **periaortic** and **lumbar**) are a group of *lymph nodes* that lie in front of the lumbar vertebral bodies near the *aorta* (Fig. 21.6). These lymph nodes receive drainage from the lower *gastrointestinal tract* and the *pelvic* organs.

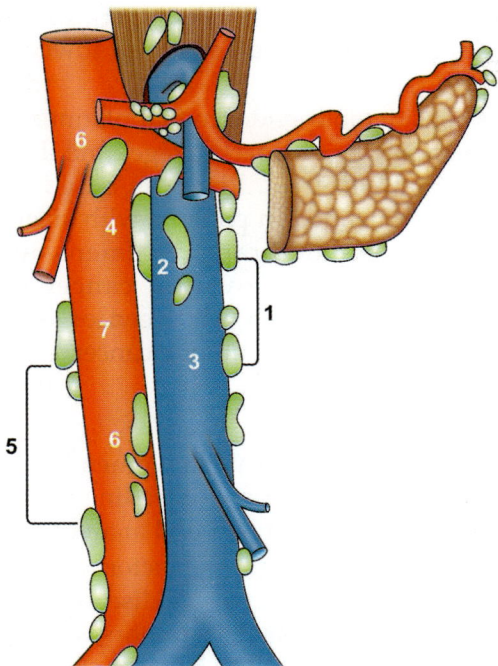

Fig. 21.6: Types of para-aortic lymph nodes

Left Lumbar Lymph Nodes
(Para-aortic Lymph Nodes)

1. Lateral aortic
2. Preaortic
3. Postaortic
4. Intermediate lumbar

Right Lumbar Lymph Nodes
(Paracaval Lymph Nodes)

5. Lateral caval
6. Precaval
7. Postcaval

The para-aortic lymph node group is divided into three subgroups—preaortic, retroaortic, and right and left lateral aortic.

- The *preaortic group* drains the abdominal part of the gastrointestinal tract above the mid-rectum.
- The *retroaortic group* drains from the lateral and preaortic glands.
- The *lateral group* drains the *iliac lymph nodes*, the *ovaries*, and other pelvic organs. The lateral group nodes are located adjacent to the *aorta*, anterior to the spine, extending laterally to the edge of the *psoas major muscles*, and superiorly to the *crura of the diaphragm*.

The Gynecologic Oncology Group (GOG) has adopted as their standard both right- and left-sided aortic lymph node sampling in staging gynecologic malignancies.

Pelvic and Para-aortic Lymph Node Sampling Procedure

Content of Procedure—Pelvic Node Sampling

Removal of the nodal tissue contained within the following boundaries:

1. Identify the bifurcation of the common iliac, external iliac, hypogastric arteries and veins and the ureter.
2. Any enlarged or suspicious nodes will be excised or biopsies, if unresectable.
3. Nodal tissue from the distal one-half of each common iliac artery should be removed.
4. The nodal tissue from the anterior and medial aspect of the proximal 1/2 of the external iliac artery and vein will be excised.
5. The distal 1/2 of the obturator fat pad anterior to the obturator nerve is excised.
6. Ligation of the proximal and distal attachments of the nodal tissue and retroperitoneal suction drainage is recommended.

Aortic Node Sampling

Removal of the nodal tissue within the following boundaries:

1. The bifurcation of the aorta, the inferior vena cava, the ovarian vessels, the inferior mesenteric artery, the ureters and duodenum should be identified.
2. Any enlarged or suspicious nodes will be excised or biopsied, if unresectable.
3. The nodal tissue between the aorta and the left ureter from the inferior mesenteric artery to the left mid-common iliac artery is removed.
4. Ligation of the proximal and distal nodal tissue is recommended.
5. Dissection cephalad to the inferior mesenteric artery is restricted to those cases with palpably suspicious nodes above that level.

Laparoscopic Para-aortic Lymphadenectomy

In 1989, Dargent used the laparoscope to perform limited pelvic lymphadenectomy on women with cervical cancer. Subsequently, additional observational studies have established the feasibility, oncologic validity, and safety of laparoscopic pelvic and para-aortic node dissection in women with a variety of gynecologic cancers. A transperitoneal incision directly over the aorta is used. Initially, only the right-side infra-inferior mesenteric artery nodes are removed. Then left-side low para-aortic nodes are removed. This is followed by removal of right- and left-side nodes above the transverse duodenum.

General advantages of the laparoscopic approach are a decrease in operative time, less blood loss, shorter hospital stay, and reduction in total cost.

Recurrent Endometrial Cancer

Systemic treatment for metastatic and relapsed disease may consist of endocrine therapy or cytotoxic chemotherapy. Hormonal therapy is recommended for endometrioid histologies only and involves mainly the use of progestational agents; tamoxifen and aromatase inhibitors are also being used. The main predictors of response in the treatment of metastatic disease are well-differentiated tumors, a long disease-free interval and the location and extent of extrapelvic (particularly pulmonary) metastases. The overall response to progestins in progesterone receptor positive tumors is 25%. Megestrol acetate, 80 mg twic daily or medroxyprogesterone acetate, 50–100 mg thrice daily should continue at least for 2–3 months to assess response. If response is favorable, progestin should continue as long as disease is static or in remission. Patients positive for estrogen and progesterone receptors respond best to progestin therapy to the extent of 75% compared with only 7% without detectable progesterone receptors. Tamoxifen, 20 mg twice daily is also recommended where progesterone use is contraindicated.

Single cytotoxic agents have been reported to achieve a response rate up to 40% in chemotherapy—naïve patients with metastatic endometrial cancer. Among those, platinum compounds, anthracyclines and taxanes are most commonly used alone and in combination.

For patients with localized recurrences (pelvis and periaortic lymph nodes) or distant metastases in selected sites, radiation therapy may be an effective palliative therapy. In rare instances, pelvic radiation therapy may be curative in pure vaginal recurrence when no prior radiation therapy has been used. Patients positive for estrogen and progesterone receptors respond best to progestin therapy to the extent of 75% of those with detectable progesterone receptors in their tumors compared with only 7% without detectable progesterone receptors.

Papillary Serous Carcinoma and Clear Cell Carcinoma

Papillary serous and clear cell carcinomas require complete staging with total hysterectomy, bilateral salpingo-oophorectomy, pelvic and para-aortic lymphadenectomy, omentectomy, appendicectomy and peritoneal biopsies. They are more aggressive with higher rates of metastatic disease and lower 5-year survival rates.

There is considerable evidence that platinum-based adjuvant chemotherapy for early (stage I and II) disease improves overall survival. Platinum-based chemotherapy is recommended in patients with stage III or IV. The same chemotherapy regimens usually employed for epithelial ovarian cancer can be considered in women with advanced or recurrent papillary serous or clear cell uterine cancer.

Prognosis

The overall 5-year survival rate in women with endometrial cancer is 83%. A key factor leading to this high rate is that most cases are diagnosed at an early stage.

The most important prognostic factors at diagnosis are: Stage, grade, depth of invasive disease, LVSI and histological subtype. Endometrial tumors have a 5-year survival of 83% compared with 62% for clear cell and 53% for papillary carcinomas. Five-year overall survival is 64% and 88% with or without LVSI, respectively.

Follow-up

Most recurrences will occur within the first 3 years after treatment. Patients should undergo follow-up every 3–4 months with physical and gynecological examination for the first 2 years, and then with a 6-month interval until 5 years. The utility of PAP smears for detection of local recurrences has not been demonstrated.

Mortality/Morbidity

Mortality is higher in black women than in white women, with a mortality ratio of 7.3 deaths per 100,000 persons in black women and only 3.8 deaths per 100,000 persons in white women.

5-year survival rate according to stages are given in Table 21.2.

Table 21.2: Endometrial adenocarcinoma	
Stage	*5-year survival*
Stage 0	90%
Stage IA	88%
Stage IB	75%
Stage II	69%
Stage IIIA	58%
Stage IIIB	50%
Stage IIIC	47%
Stage IVA	17%
Stage IVB	15%

Scope of HRT

Twenty-five percent of women with endometrial cancer are premenopausal and 5% may be under 40 years where ovaries are sacrificed in surgical management since in 23% of these women ovaries are involved. Therefore, though systemic estrogen replacement appears safe in terms of possible recurrence in some reports, its safety profile is not fully established. That is why, topical estrogen alone in vaginal dryness and dyspareunia is advocated. Symptomatic relief of hot flushes is achieved by prescribing progestins like medroxyprogesterone acetate, 10 mg orally daily or 150 mg IM every 3 months or with nonhormonal agents like clonidine and venlafaxine.

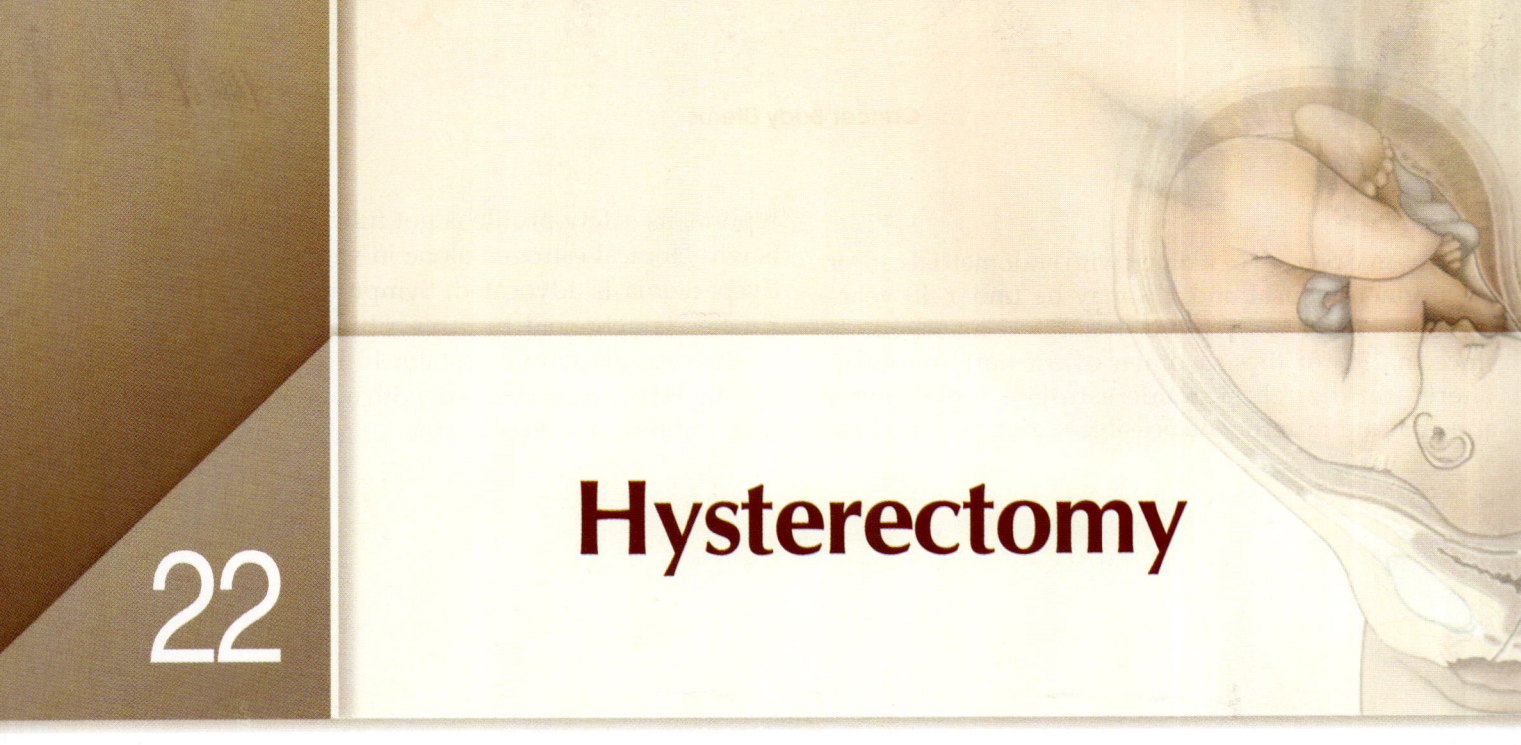

Hysterectomy

22A. TOTAL ABDOMINAL HYSTERECTOMY

Hysterectomy is the most common gynecological major surgery performed on women. This surgical procedure involves removal of the uterus and cervix, and for some conditions, the fallopian tubes and ovaries. Hysterectomy (Greek *'hystera'* = womb; *'ektomia'* = cutting out) refers to the surgery performed by gynecologists to remove the uterus in women.

Incidence

Compared to a higher frequency of hysterectomy (10–20%) of gynecological operations in other countries, a lower rate (4–6%) has been reported from India.

Is Abdominal Hysterectomy Obsolete?

It will never be obsolete. There still are situations in which an abdominal hysterectomy is appropriate, such as a large uterus suspicious of malignancy where morcellation is not an option. In addition, if a surgeon in a remote area does not have the skills or referral availabilities, an abdominal approach may be the safest option and the long-term outcome between different routes of hysterectomy remains same. Nevertheless, with more training, available subspecialists, and patient awareness, a 90% minimally invasive hysterectomy rate is a realistic goal for the foreseeable future.

Different Types of Hysterectomy

Various hysterectomy procedures are available, including the following:
- Total abdominal hysterectomy involves removal of the uterus and cervix through an abdominal incision.

- Supracervical or subtotal hysterectomy is removal of the uterus through an abdominal incision, while sparing the cervix.
- Radical hysterectomy is extensive surgery that, in addition to removal of the uterus and cervix, includes removal of pelvic lymph nodes, parametrium, loose areolar tissue near major blood vessels, and upper vagina.
- Oophorectomy and salpingo-oophorectomy: Oophorectomy is the surgical removal of the ovary and salpingo-oophorectomy is the removal of the ovary and the fallopian tube.
- Vaginal hysterectomy is removal of the uterus and the cervix through the vagina.
- Laparoscopy-assisted vaginal hysterectomy is vaginal hysterectomy with the help of laparoscopy.
- Total laparoscopic hysterectomy is removal of uterus, tubes, ovaries through laparoscopic instruments.

Surgical Approaches to Hysterectomy: Relevant Factors in Decision Making

The American College of Obstetricians and Gynecologist's (ACOG) guidelines for hysterectomy are probably the most widely accepted and most employed of those found in the literature. The most determinant factors for choosing one or another approach are surgeon skill, uterus size, uterine mobility, nulliparity and previous pathological conditions (Box 22.1).

Box 22.1. Comparison of different approaches to hysterectomy

Vaginal hysterectomy compared with abdominal hysterectomy
- Shorter duration of hospital stay
- Faster return to normal activity
- Fewer febrile episodes or unspecified infections

Vaginal hysterectomy compared with laparoscopic hysterectomy
- Shorter operating time

Laparoscopic hysterectomy compared with abdominal hysterectomy
- Faster return to normal activity
- Shorter duration of hospital stay
- Smaller drop in hemoglobin
- Lower intraoperative blood loss
- Fewer wound or abdominal wall infections
- Longer operating time
- Higher rate of lower urinary tract (bladder and ureter) injuries

Surgeon Skill

Age, parity, uterine size, vaginal anatomy, pelvic mobility and any pelvic disease or previous pelvic surgery are among the most important factors to take into account when considering a hysterectomy. Yet, an even more important aspect is the quality of the surgeon's training with respect to the different possible approaches. This is why continuous training programs must be offered to residents and gynecologic surgeons with the intention of developing effective guidelines for the determination of the route of hysterectomy.

Uterine Size

ACOG and other researchers assert that VH should be indicated in women with mobile uteri of less than 12-week gestational size (i.e. 280 gm) because uterine size reduction is usually the principal problem confronting surgeons, and morcellation technique skills are a limiting factor. In that situation, TAH or TLH is mostly favored depending on the surgeon's expertise.

Uterine Mobility

Uterine mobility is another important relevant factors in determining the route of a hysterectomy. A vaginal route is usually indicated in cases of vaginal prolapse (degree ≥1), a wide vaginal apex and a nonadhered uterus. On the other hand, fixed retroversion, shallow POD, pelvic inflammation, and suspected malignancy favor either laparoscopy or abdominal route.

Pathological Condition

If the clinical history or pelvic examination indicates possible extrauterine disease or adhesions (e.g. endometriosis, pelvic inflammatory disease, ovarian disease, previous pelvic surgery or cesarean delivery), laparoscopy should be performed. This allows the pelvic pathology to be treated correctly and can be of assistance in performing or finalizing the hysterectomy.

Nulliparity

Nulliparity usually leads to decision in favor of AH as a general consensus among health professionals though there are no differences between the complication rates of AH and LH in nulliparous women. Because even if the vaginal route is chosen, the uterosacral and Mackenrodt's ligaments can be dissected even in nulliparous women to restore the uterine mobility.

Indications of Hysterectomy

- Premenopausal woman with symptomatic leiomyoma.
- Pre- or postmenopausal woman with persistent or recurrent abnormal uterine bleeding (DUB).
- Adenomyosis in elderly.
- Endometriosis of Grade 3 and 4 in elderly.
- Chronic tubo-ovarian mass.
- Benign ovarian tumours in elderly.
- Early stages of cancer cervix or uterine cancer.
- Cancer ovary of all stages.
- Uterine sarcoma

Additional Situations

- Premenopausal or postmenopausal woman with cervical intraepithelial neoplasia grade III.
- Septic uterus.
- Repeated hematometra with cervical stenosis particularly when repeated dilatation following hysterovaginoplasty fails.
- Irrepairable uterine perforation.
- Gestational trophoblastic tumor.

Preoperative Evaluation

- Complete history and physical examination to evaluate in detail any comorbid conditions such as diabetes mellitus, hypertension, cardiac disease, or asthma.
- Medication history such as use of aspirin, oral hypoglycemics, heparin, or warfarin.
- PAP smear, endometrial sampling, ultrasonography, CBC, blood type and crossmatch, and depending upon age and risk factors, ECG and chest radiograph.
- In case of malignancy, preoperative staging can be determined with the help of biopsies, CT scans, IVP, cystoscopy, barium enema, etc.

Abdominal Hysterectomy

In 1843, Charles Clay performed the first hysterectomy in Manchester, England. The earliest hysterectomies were supracervical, or subtotal, hysterectomies. The body of the uterus was removed while the cervix remained intact. In 1929, Richardson performed the first TAH, in which the entire uterus was removed. In general, the modified Richardson technique of intrafascial hysterectomy is used.

Technique

Step 1

The patient is placed in the dorsal lithotomy position under regional or general anesthesia. A Foley catheter is placed in the bladder for continuous drainage. In general, midline incisions are preferred for malignant disease, uncertain diagnosis and supraumbilical lump since they allow accurate staging and exposure to the upper abdomen and aortic lymph nodes. However, for benign disease, the Pfannenstiel incision is the incision of choice.

After the abdomen is entered, it should be thoroughly explored; including the liver, gallbladder, stomach, kidneys, and aortic lymph nodes.

Step 2

Self-retaining retractors are placed in the abdominal incision, and the bowel is packed off with warm, moist gauze packs. A 0 synthetic absorbable suture is placed in the fundus of the uterus and used for uterine traction. The uterus is deviated to the patient's right. The left round ligament is placed on stretch and incised between clamps.

Step 3 (Figs 22.1 and 22.2)

The distal stump of the round ligament is ligated with 0 synthetic absorbable suture. The proximal stump is held with a straight Ochsner clamp. At this point, the leaves of the broad ligament are opened both anteriorly and posteriorly. This is performed by delicate dissection with the Metzenbaum scissors.

Step 4 (Fig. 22.3)

While retracting the uterus cephalad, the surgeon opens the anterior leaf of the broad ligament to the vesicouterine fold. Steps 2–4 are carried out on the opposite side.

Step 5 (Fig. 22.4)

If the tube and ovary are to be removed, a finger is placed under the infundilbulopelvic ligament on that

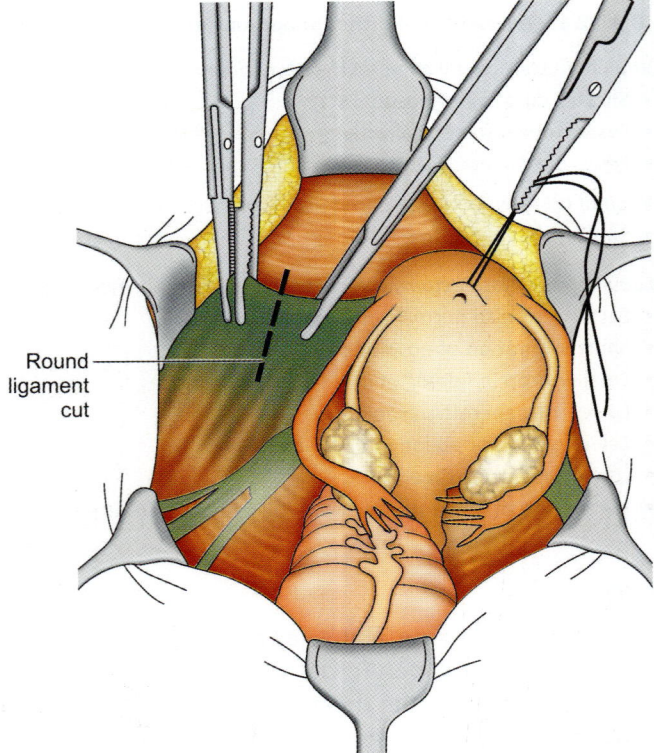

Fig. 22.1: Abdominal hysterectomy: Step 3a

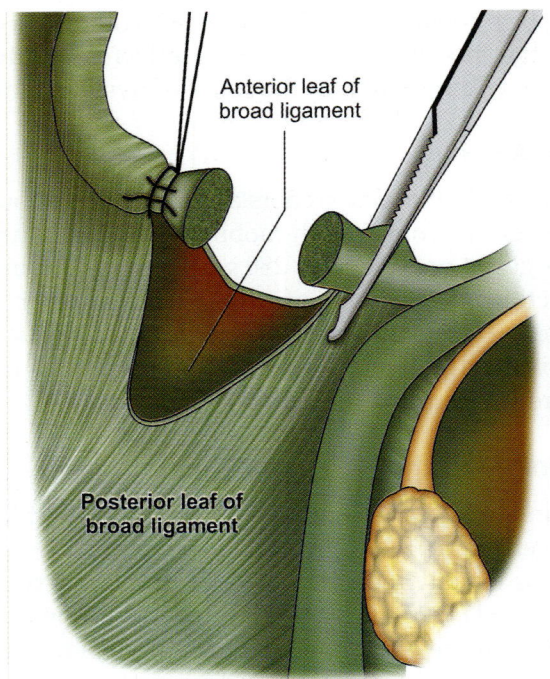

Fig. 22.2: Abdominal hysterectomy: Step 3b

side. Care is taken to ensure that the ureter is not included. In various forms of pelvic disease (endometriosis, pelvic inflammatory disease, etc.), the ureter can be deviated close to the infundibulopelvic ligament.

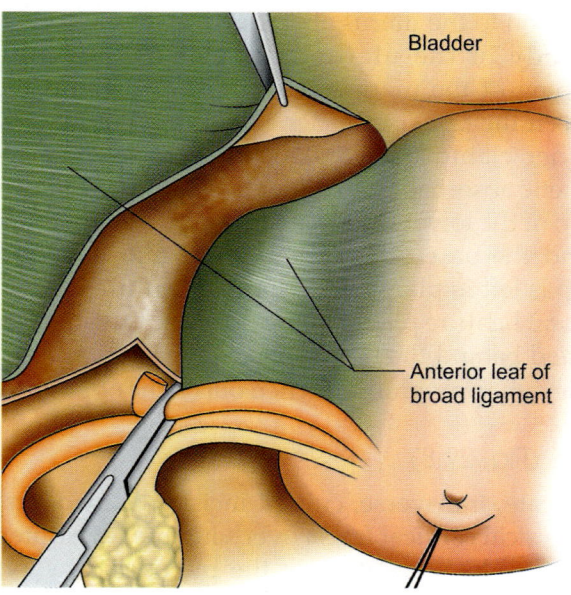

Fig. 22.3: Abdominal hysterectomy: Step 4

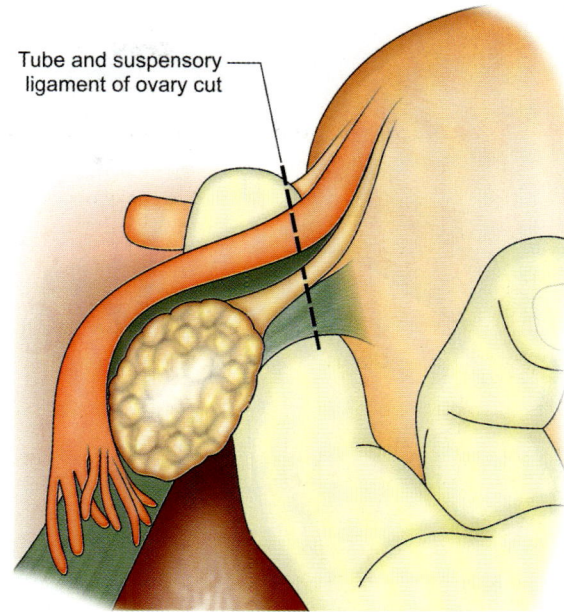

Fig. 22.5: Abdominal hysterectomy: Step 6

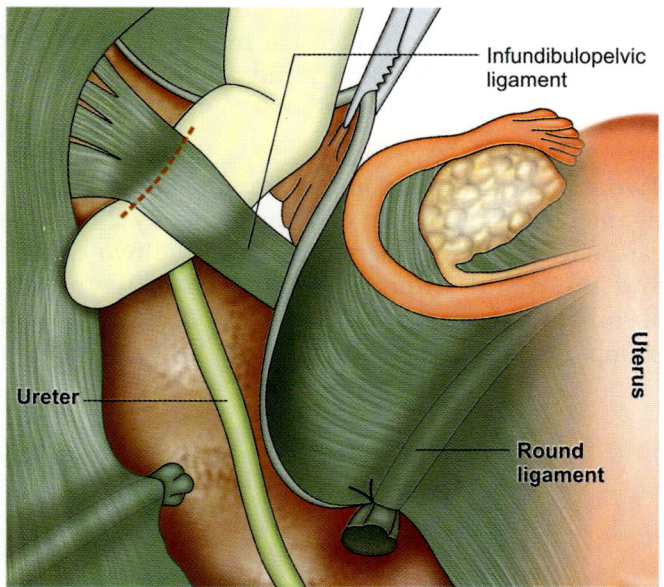

Fig. 22.4: Abdominal hysterectomy: Step 5

The infundibulopelvic ligament is doubly clamped and incised, and the distal stump of the ligament is doubly ligated with a tie of 0 synthetic absorbable suture plus a ligature of 0 synthetic absorbable suture.

For a bilateral salpingo-oophorectomy, the same procedure is carried out on the opposite infundibulo-pelvic ligament.

Step 6 (Fig. 22.5)

If the ovaries are to be preserved, the uterus is retracted toward the pubic symphysis and deviated to one side with the infundibulopelvic ligament, tube, and ovary

on tension. A finger should be inserted through the peritoneum of the posterior leaf of the broad ligament under the suspensory ligament of the ovary and fallopian tube. The tube and suspensory ligament are doubly clamped, incised, and tied with 0 synthetic absorbable suture. Currently tubes are removed when healthy ovaries are preserved if fertility preservation is not the issue; because it has been reported that removing fallopian tubes reduce incidence of neoplasm of left out ovaries. The distal stump of this structure is best doubly tied, first with a single tie of 0 synthetic absorbable suture and then with a ligature of 0 synthetic absorbable suture. The same procedure is carried out on the opposite side.

Step 7 (Fig. 22.6)

The vesicoperitoneal fold is elevated, and the fine filmsy attachments of the bladder to the pubovesicocervical fascia are visible. The bladder can be dissected off the lower uterine segment of the uterus and cervix by either blunt or sharp dissection. If there has been extensive lower segment adhesion due to adhesions, previous cesarean sections, or pelvic irradiation, blunt dissection of the bladder off the cervix is dangerous, and a sharp dissection technique should be performed. Often a window is made from the lateral sides to reach the midline areas of adhesion and sharp dissection is done to achieve the bladder plane.

Step 8 (Fig. 22.7)

The uterus is then retracted cephalad and deviated to one side of the pelvis with the lower broad ligament

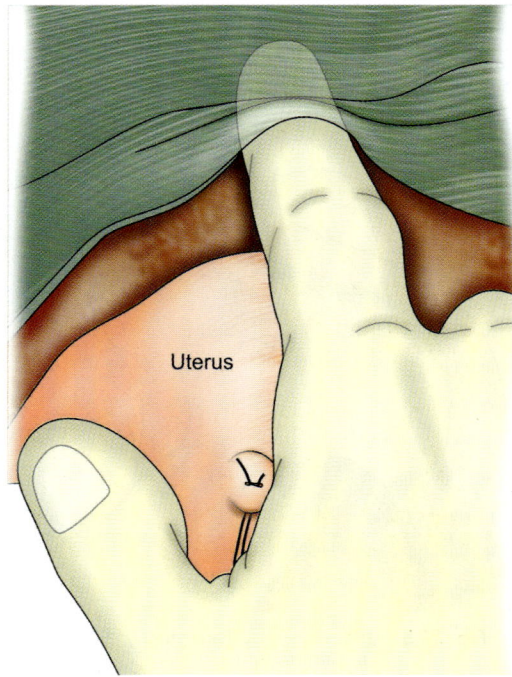

Fig. 22.6: Abdominal hysterectomy: Step 7

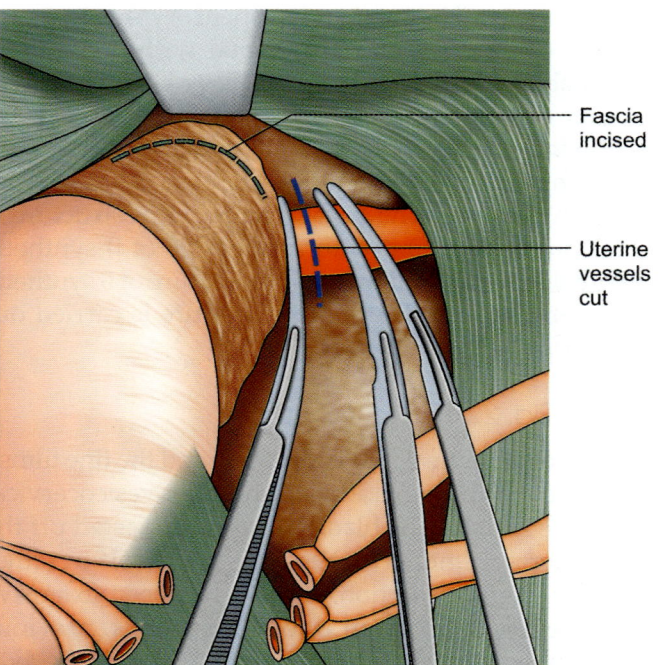

Fig. 22.7: Abdominal hysterectomy: Step 8

clamps on to the uterus and allowing them to slide off the body of the uterus, thus ensuring complete clamping of the uterine vessels. An incision is made between the upper Ochsner clamp and the two lower Ochsner clamps. This is suture-ligated with two 0 synthetic absorbable sutures, placing the first suture at the tip of the lower Ochsner clamp and tying the suture behind the base of the clamp. The middle Ochsner clamp is left in place and is similarly suture-ligated by a second ligature placed at the tip of the Ochsner clamp and tied behind the base of the clamp.

The same procedure is carried out on the opposite side.

Step 9 (Fig. 22.8)

A delicate, transverse, curved incision is made in the pubovesical cervical fascia overlying the lower uterine segment. The separation of the pubovesical cervical fascia from the underlying cervical stroma is facilitated by placing traction on the uterus in the cephalad position. The uterus is held in traction in the cephalad position, and the handle of the knife is used to dissect the pubovesical cervical fascia inferiorly. This step mobilizes the ureter laterally and caudally.

Step 10 (Fig. 22.9)

Two straight Ochsner clamps are applied to the cardinal ligament for a distance of approximately 2 cm. The cardinal ligament is incised between the two clamps, and the distal stump is ligated with 0 synthetic absorbable suture. The suture is tied at the base of the clamp; no attempt is made to place this suture within

on stretch. The filmsy tissue surrounding the uterine vessels is skeletonized by elevating the round ligament and dissecting the tissue away from the uterine vessels. Three curved Ochsner clamps are placed at the junction of the lower uterine segment perpendicular to the uterine wall on the uterine vessels. This is best performed by placing the tips of the curved Ochsner

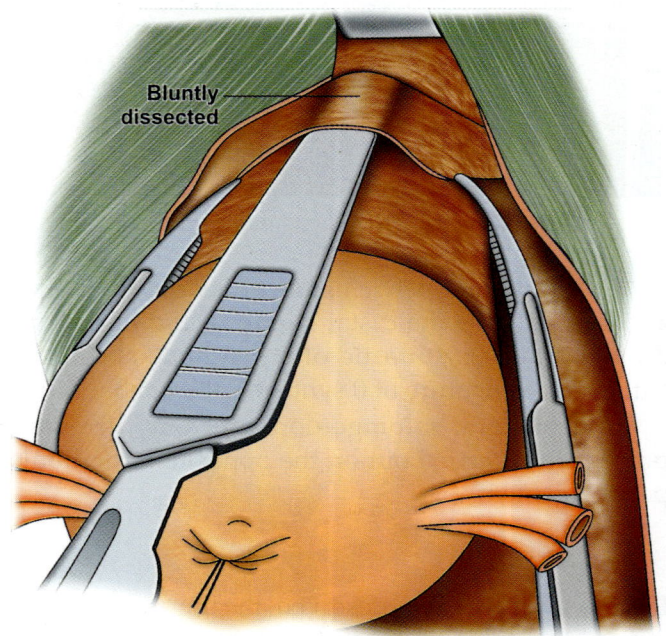

Fig. 22.8: Pubovesicocervical fascia bluntly dissected: Step 9

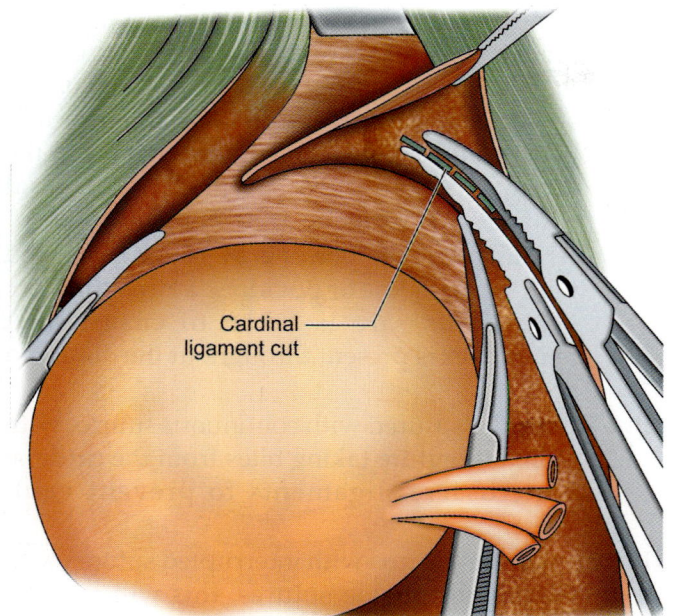

Fig. 22.9: Abdominal hysterectomy: Step 10

the body of the pedicle because vessels can be torn and hematomas created.

The same procedure is carried out on the opposite cardinal ligament.

Step 11 (Fig. 22.10)

The posterior leaf of the broad ligament is incised down to the uterosacral ligaments and across the posterior lower uterine segment between the rectum and cervix.

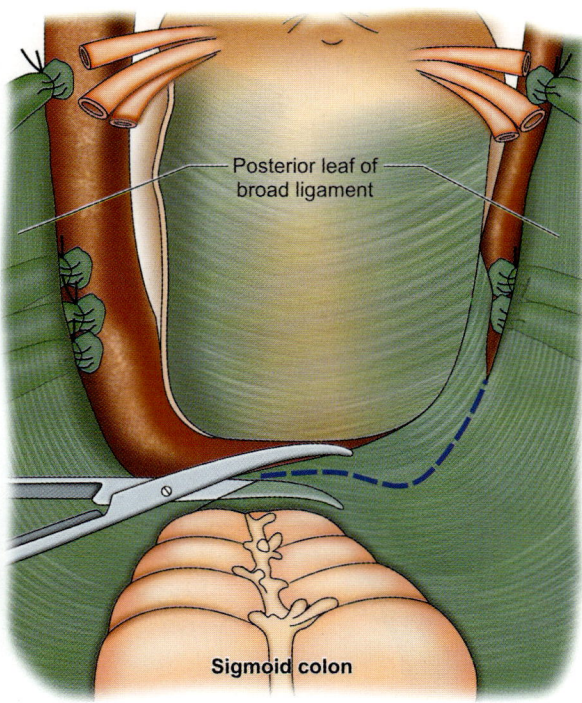

Fig. 22.10: Abdominal hysterectomy: Step 11

Step 12 (Fig. 22.11)

The uterosacral ligaments on both sides are clamped between straight Ochsner clamps, incised, and ligated with 0 synthetic absorbable suture.

Step 13 (Fig. 22.12)

The uterus is placed on traction cephalad, and the lower uterine segment and upper vagina are palpated to

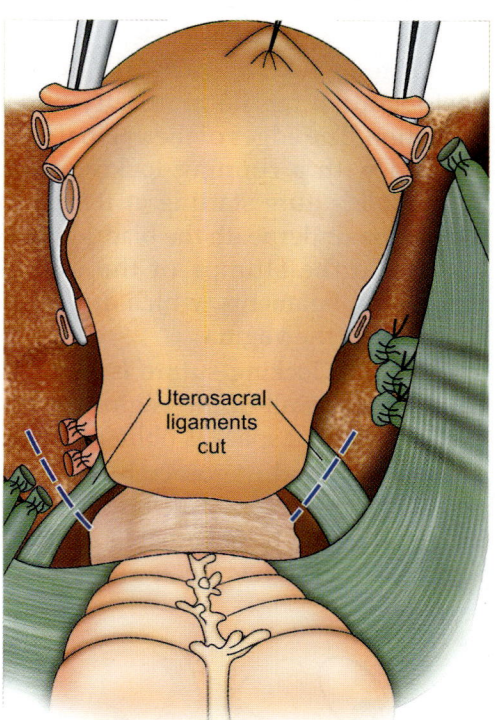

Fig. 22.11: Abdominal hysterectomy: Step 12

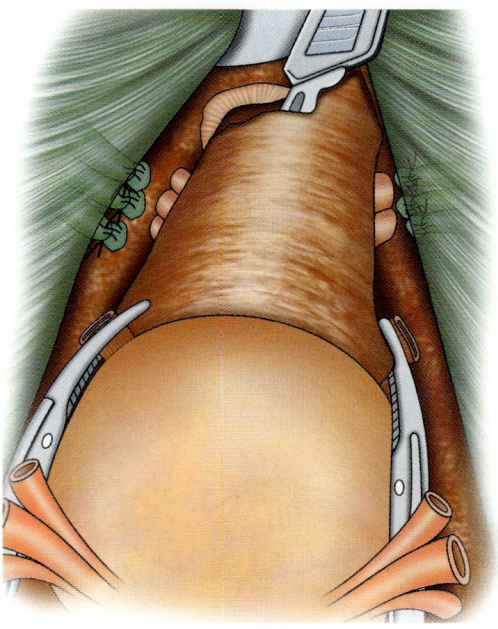

Fig. 22.12: Abdominal hysterectomy: Step 13

ensure that the ligaments have been completely incised. The vagina is entered by a stab wound with a scalpel and is cut across with either a scalpel or scissors. The uterus is removed. The edges of the vagina are picked up with straight Ochsner clamps all over the corners.

Step 14—Vault Closure

Three different techniques can be followed.

I. Open cuff method (Fig. 22.13)

  a. The vaginal cuff is not closed. This alone has accounted for a radical decrease in postoperative febrile morbidity and abscess formation. The edges of the vaginal mucosa are sutured with a running locking 0 synthetic absorbable suture starting at the midpoint of the vagina underneath the bladder and carried around to the stumps of the cardinal and uterosacral ligaments, which are sutured into the angle of the vagina.

  b. The running locking suture is carried around the posterior wall of the vagina ensuring that the rectovaginal space is obliterated.

  c. The cardinal and uterosacral ligaments of the opposite side have been included in the running locking 0 synthetic absorbable suture, and the reefing process has been completed to the midpoint of the anterior vaginal wall. At this point, meticulous care should be taken to ensure that the lateral angle of the vagina is adequately secured and that hemostasis is complete between the lateral angle of the vagina and the stumps of the cardinal and uterosacral ligaments. This can be a site of hemorrhage.

At this point, the pelvis is thoroughly washed with sterile saline or povidone iodine solution. Meticulous care is taken to ensure that hemostasis is present throughout the dissected area.

  II. Vault can be sutured with continuous sutures with 0 absorbable suture taking bites from the cardinal and uterosacral ligaments to prevent vault prolapse.

  III. Vault can be sutured with interrupted sutures with 0 delayed absorbable sutures; this will prevent shortening of vagina and vaginal necrosis maintaining good blood supply.

Step 15 (Fig. 22.14)

The pelvic peritoneum is not reperitonealized nowadays as there is no extra advantage with this step; rather there is spontaneous peritonization within 48 hours.

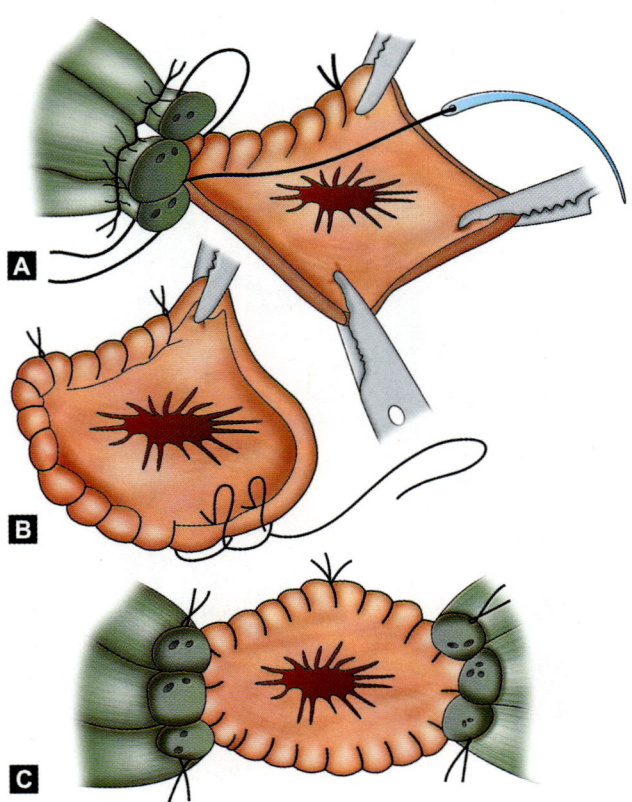

Fig. 22.13: Abdominal hysterectomy: Step 14

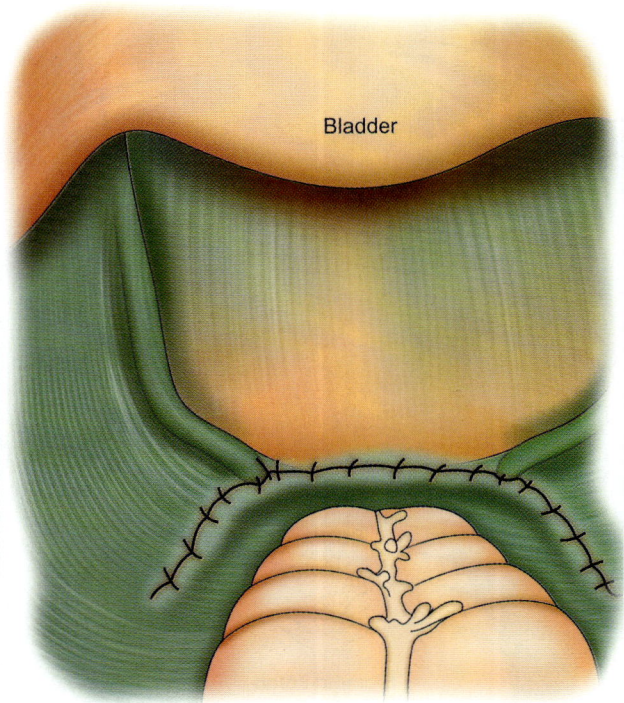

Fig. 22.14: Abdominal hysterectomy: Step 15

Step16

Drains are rarely needed. Hemostasis is checked and abdomen is closed in layers. The parietal peritoneum closure is debatable as many do not recommend its routine closure as it may increase postoperative pain, intraperitoneal adhesions. The parietal peritoneum is found closed spontaneously within 48 hours.

Postoperative Details

1. Early feeding (oral intake of fluids or food within 24 hr of surgery, irrespective of appearance of bowel sounds) after major abdominal gynecological surgery is safe and associated with reduced length of hospital stay but increased nausea.
2. Antibiotics: Peroperative single dose of 2 gm cephalosporines and metronidazole is useful. The postoperative 5 days of routine antibiotic with combination of cephalosporines, aminoglycosides and metronidazole is prescribed to combat postopearative sepsis.
3. Routine analgesics like paracetamol infusion, tramadol hydrochloride is useful in 1st two postopertve days.
4. Bladder catheterization is removed after 48 hours and bowel is cleared on 3rd postoperative day.
5. The patient becomes fit for discharge on day 5.

Follow-up

- After the surgery, it takes 4–6 weeks to recover.
- Lifting of anything heavy for 6 weeks after the surgery is to be avoided.
- In case of oophorectomy in premenopausal women, patients experience menopausal symptoms like hot flashes, vaginal dryness, and mood disturbances. This can be discussed with the patient regarding need of HT in some cases.
- Return to normal sexual activities is expected after 6 weeks of surgery.
- Biopsy report should be tallying with the clinical findings and advise accordingly.
- The patient is allowed to resume sexual intercourse 4 weeks after examination in the clinic and is allowed to resume work 5 weeks postoperatively.

Complications

I. *Peroperative*

a. Hemorrhage due to injury to major vessels like uterine, ovarian artery, pelvic veins.
b. Injury to bladder, ureter, bowel

II. *Immediate Postoperative*

a. Postoperative fever
b. Abdominal distension—paralytic ileus, sepsis, band obstruction
c. Shock—hypotension, cardiac decompensation, dehydration, internal hemorrhage, rectus sheath hematomas
d. Urinary retention, UTI, anuria
e. Nerve damage
f. Urinary incontinence—urge, true incontinence like VVF, ureteric fistula
g. Severe sepsis—pyoperitoneum, left out foreign body
h. Thromboembolism: Routine thromboprophylaxis with LMWH is indicated in case of prolonged surgery, previous history of thromboembolism, obesity, operations with pelvic dissections.
i. Wound dehiscence, burst abdomen.

IIi. *Late Postoperative*

a. Secondary hemorrhage
b. Vault sepsis—persistent vaginal discharge
c. Dysparunia—prolapse of ovary, vault granulation
d. Incisional hernia
e. Vault prolapse.

Management of Secondary Hemorrhage

Hemorrhage after hysterectomy is a rare but life-threatening complication. The incidence ranges between 0.23 and 0.45%.

Possible factors that may play a role in secondary hemorrhage are vaginal vault infection, vault hematoma, poor surgical technique including excessive thermal injury by electrocoagulation, and early resumption of physical activity.

Another possible reason for the higher rate of secondary hemorrhage is technique of preserving the arch of the uterosacral ligaments, which includes more cervical tissue and may have a greater chance of bleeding.

The source of bleeding in secondary hemorrhage can be from the uterine vessels or descending cervical/vaginal vessels. The source of bleeding is from the sloughed out necrosed tissues and eroded uterine vessels. Occasionally, uterine artery pseudoaneurysm can cause delayed heavy vaginal bleeding after hysterectomy. The use of thermal energy may result in increased tissue damage to the vaginal cuff. Vaginal vault dehiscence is one of the rare complications after hysterectomy.

The time interval between hysterectomy and the onset of secondary hemorrhage range between 3 and 22 days.

Steps of Management

1. Assess the amount of blood loss. Fresh bleeds are alarming. Darkish spotting is due to oozing from nonhealing vault tissues. Vaginal packing should be tight enough to stop the bleeding.
2. Start high dose of antibiotics. It is always ideal to send vaginal swab.
3. Local treatment with Betadine vaginal tablets are often effective.
4. If bleeding does not subside, vaginal vault is explored under general anesthesia and interrupted stitches are given, if local vaginal cuff oozes.
5. Often bleeding is heavy; in that case abdomen is reopened and vault is separated from adhered tisssue, bladder and rectum separated. The vault resutured, uterine vessels and parametrial tissues are freshly sutured. Often the tissues are fragile and anterior divisions of internal iliac artery are ligated on both sides. Blood transfusion may be necessary.
6. Emergency therapeutic arterial embolization is a safe and effective minimally invasive procedure—sometimes can be effective where facilities are available.

22B. VAGINAL HYSTERECTOMY

In the United States, hysterectomy is one of the most frequently performed surgical procedures. Even with the increased use of conservative therapies, approximately 600,000 hysterectomies are performed each year.

Hysterectomy may be performed vaginally, abdominally, laparoscopically, or with robotic assistance, with the route depending primarily on physician choice. Most of the literatures support the view that vaginal hysterectomy, when feasible, is the safest and most cost-effective procedure for removal of the uterus. Nevertheless, the abdominal route is the one most commonly chosen: 66% of hysterectomies are performed abdominally, 22% are performed vaginally, and 12% are performed laparoscopically.

Types of Vaginal Hysterectomy

1. Total vaginal hysterectomy (nondescent vaginal hysterectomy)
2. Total vaginal hysterectomy with bilateral salpingo-oophorectomy
3. Radical vaginal hysterectomy
4. Vaginal hysterectomy with pelvic floor repair
5. Laparoscopy assisted vaginal hysterectomy

Indications

1. Abnormal uterine bleeding in elderly
2. Adenomyosis
3. Symptomatic fibroid uterus preferably <12 weeks
4. CIN III on biopsy
5. Early stage endometrial cancer
6. Uterine prolapse—vaginal hysterectomy with pelvic floor repair
7. Early cancer cervix—radical vaginal hysterectomy with bilateral pelvic lymphadenectomy

Contraindications

There are no absolute contraindications for vaginal hysterectomy. However, there are some factors that may influence the surgeon's choice of a route for hysterectomy like:
- Surgeon training and experience
- Accessibility of the uterus
- Extent of extrauterine disease
- Size and shape of the uterus
- Need for concurrent procedures
- Patient preference

Therefore, the following may be considered contraindications for vaginal hysterectomy:
- Enlarged uterus >12 weeks
- Nulliparity
- Previous cesarean delivery
- Narrow vagina
- Narrow pubic arch (<90°)
- Restricted mobility
- Extrauterine disease (e.g. adnexal pathology), severe endometriosis, adhesions, and an indication for salpingo-oophorectomy. When these concerns arise, many surgeons choose to visualize the pelvis laparoscopically before deciding on the route for hysterectomy.
- The decision to perform a salpingo-oophorectomy should not be influenced by the chosen route for hysterectomy and is not a contraindication for vaginal hysterectomy.

One algorithm (Fig. 22.15) has been proposed by Kovac et al that aids the clinician in choosing the route by which hysterectomy will be performed.

i. In practice, most vaginal surgeons individualize the choice of a hysterectomy route. Many nulliparous women and many women who have undergone cesarean delivery do in fact have sufficient vaginal capacity to allow a vaginal hysterectomy. As long as the surgeon can obtain adequate access for division of the uterosacral and cardinal ligaments, the uterus can be mobilized sufficiently to allow vaginal extraction.

ii. Even when the uterus is enlarged, vaginal hysterectomy often can be accomplished safely by means of morcellation, uterine bisection, wedge debulking, or intramyometrial coring.

Outcomes

A Cochrane review found that the vaginal route, compared with all other routes for hysterectomy, yields better outcomes and fewer complications.

The authors also noted that when vaginal hysterectomy is not possible, laparoscopic vaginal hysterectomy has advantages over abdominal hysterectomy (e.g. faster return to normal activity, shorter hospital stay, reduced intraoperative blood loss, and fewer wound infections) but also disadvantages (e.g. longer operating time and higher rate of urinary tract injury).

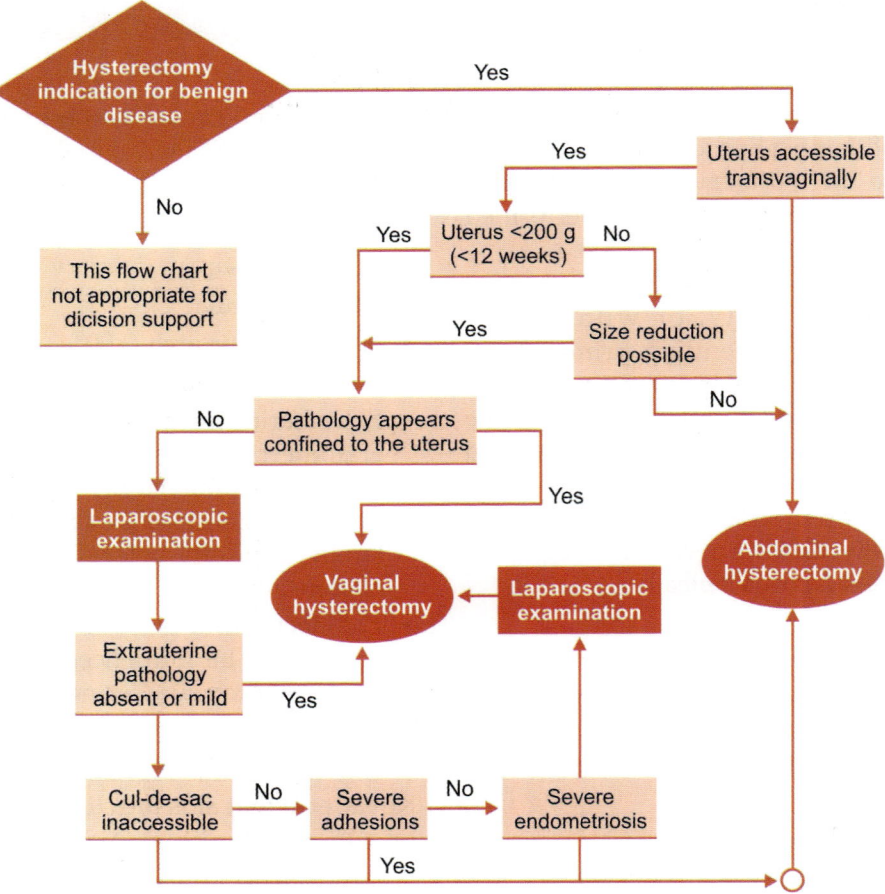

Fig. 22.15: Kovac algorithm for decision for routes of hysterectomy

Conversion to Abdominal Route

1. Uterine size appears bigger than what is expected
2. Restricted mobility
3. Unable to deliver the uterus
4. Very narrow pelvic angle
5. Slipping of uterine and ovarian vessels and cannot be secured
6. Failure to open the peritoneum
7. Suspected bowel injury
8. Accidental adnexal mass

Preprocedural Planning

For optimal surgical outcome, a preoperative health/risk assessment is critical. This assessment should always include a complete history and physical examination. Some preoperative laboratory tests, like CBC, KFT, blood glucose, are routinely recommended, screening laboratory tests, like thyroid tests, chest X-ray, ECG, should be ordered as indicated by the patient's underlying medical problem.

Informed consent should include discussion of oophorectomy and sexual function after surgery. Perioperative care includes the following:

- H_2 blockers and tranquilizers, mild laxatives are given overnight.
- Prophylactic providone iodine or estrogen cream in the vagina for 6 preoperative nights.
- Prophylactic antibiotics like first- or second-generation cephalosporins within 1 hour before incision.
- Discontinuance of antibiotics within 24 hours after surgery.
- Prophylaxis for venous thromboembolism—Unfractionated heparin (5,000 U every 12 hours, beginning 2 hours before incision) or low-molecular-weight heparin (e.g. enoxaparin 40 mg or dalteparin 2500 U, beginning 2 hours before incision) or intermittent pneumatic compression devices before incision.

Patient Preparation

Vaginal hysterectomy can be performed with either general anesthesia or regional anesthesia.

Placing the patient in the dorsal lithotomy position is critical for obtaining optimal exposure. The surgeon must be careful to protect the vulnerable neurologic, vascular, and bony points of the lower extremities. The buttocks should be positioned at the end of the table, with the table level with the floor. Hyperflexion of the hips should be avoided because it can cause femoral neuropathy. Padding should be used at all potential pressure points.

Once the patient has been properly positioned and appropriate anesthesia has been provided, a bimanual pelvic examination should be performed to assess uterine mobility and descent, to confirm the findings of the office examination, and to determine whether unsuspected adnexal pathology is present. This step affords the surgeon a final opportunity to decide whether to proceed with a vaginal or an abdominal approach.

The patient is then prepared and draped, with the stirrups positioned so that assistants can place themselves inside them to visualize the operative field. A bladder catheter may be inserted. Alternatively, some surgeons believe that a distended bladder facilitates recognition of urogenital injuries and therefore do not drain the bladder at all.

Technique of Non-descent Vaginal Hysterectomy

Once the patient has been properly positioned, a weighted speculum is placed into the posterior vagina, and a right-angle retractor is positioned anterior to the cervix while the anterior and posterior lips of the cervix are grasped with a single- or double-toothed tenaculum. Some surgeons inject vasopressin (10–20 U in 50 mL of saline) or lidocaine 0.5% into the cervical, paracervical, and submucosal tissues to help identify tissue planes and reduce blood loss.

Vaginal Incision and Opening of Posterior Peritoneum

The initial vaginal incision is made circumferentially, beginning at the level of the vaginal rugae through the full thickness of the vagina, just below the bladder reflection—not on the cervix (Fig. 22.16). The vaginal epithelium is dissected bluntly or sharply to the underlying tissue with an open sponge over the index finger and Mayo scissors.

Aquadissection (Fig. 22.16) is one method where around 150–200 mL normal saline is instilled in the vaginal mucosa all over the cervix to make it distended and avascular. This reduces the hemorrhage as well as pushes the bladder up and help in achieve easy plane to work on.

The posterior peritoneum (Fig. 22.17) is then identified where rugae are not present and where the

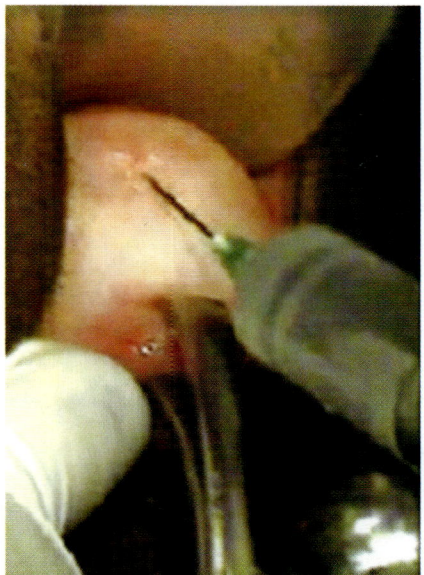
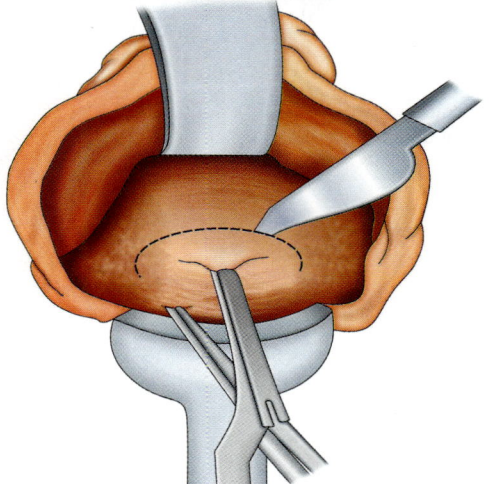

Fig. 22.16: Aquadissection and initial vaginal incision

uterosacral ligaments join the cervix. The peritoneum is grasped with tissue forceps and incised with Mayo scissors in a generous bite and a Steiner-Anvard weighted speculum is inserted into the posterior cul-de-sac.

Division and Ligation of Uterosacral Ligaments

The uterosacral ligaments are identified and clamped, with the tip of the clamp incorporating the lower portion of the cardinal ligaments. The clamp is placed perpendicular to the uterine axis, and the pedicle is cut so that approximately 0.5 cm of tissue is distal to the clamp. A transfixion suture is placed at the tip of the clamp and tied. This suture may be held with a hemostat to facilitate location of any bleeding at the completion of the procedure and to aid in vaginal vault support.

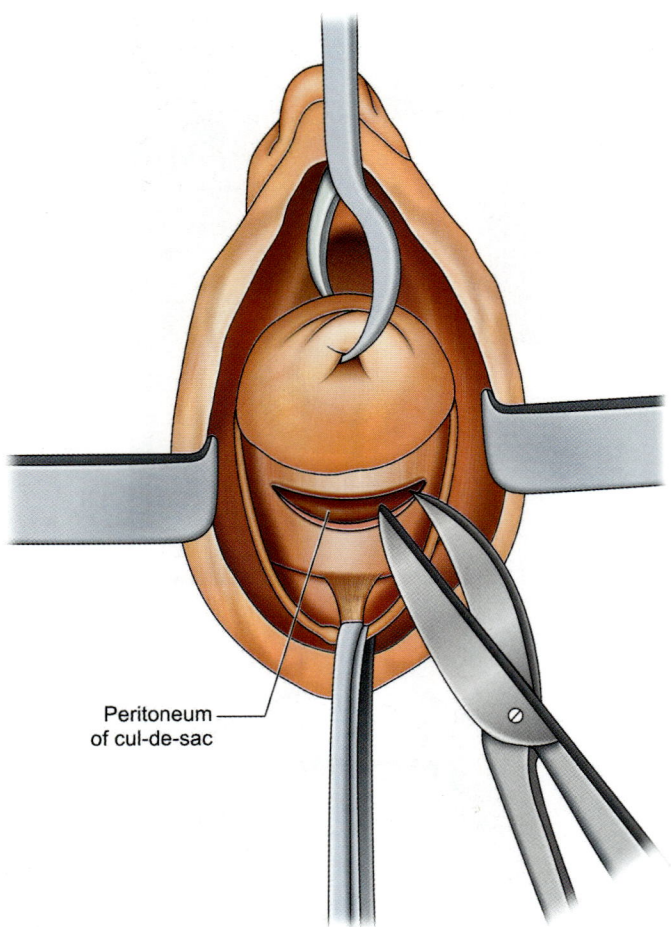

Fig. 22.17: Peritoneum is incised with Mayo scissors

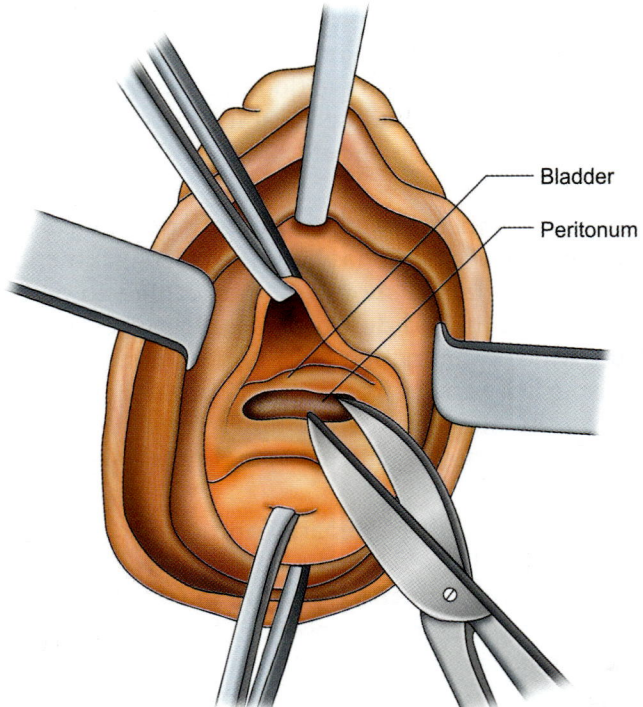

Fig. 22.18: Peritoneal reflection is grasped with tissue forceps, tented, and opened

Opening of Anterior Peritoneum

Attention is then directed to opening the anterior peritoneum. The anterior peritoneal fold appears as a crescent-shaped line. The peritoneal reflection is grasped with tissue forceps, tented, and opened with scissors that have their tips pointed toward the uterus (Fig. 22.18). A Heaney or Deaver retractor is placed into this space to protect the bladder and to facilitate visualization of the abdominal contents.

If the peritoneal reflection is not readily identified, one can wait to make the entry, as long as the bladder has been safely advanced cranially. A Deaver or Heaney retractor is placed in the midline to keep the bladder out of the operative field. Blunt or sharp advancement of the bladder should continue before each clamp placement until the vesicovaginal space is entered. Once this space is entered, the Heaney or Deaver retractor is placed into the peritoneal cavity.

Division and Ligation of Cardinal Ligaments (Fig. 22.19)

Next, the cardinal ligaments are identified, clamped, cut, and suture-ligated in a manner similar to that previously described for the uterosacral ligaments. Alternatively, newer electrocauterization devices can be used in vessels up to 7 mm in diameter to accomplish the same task.

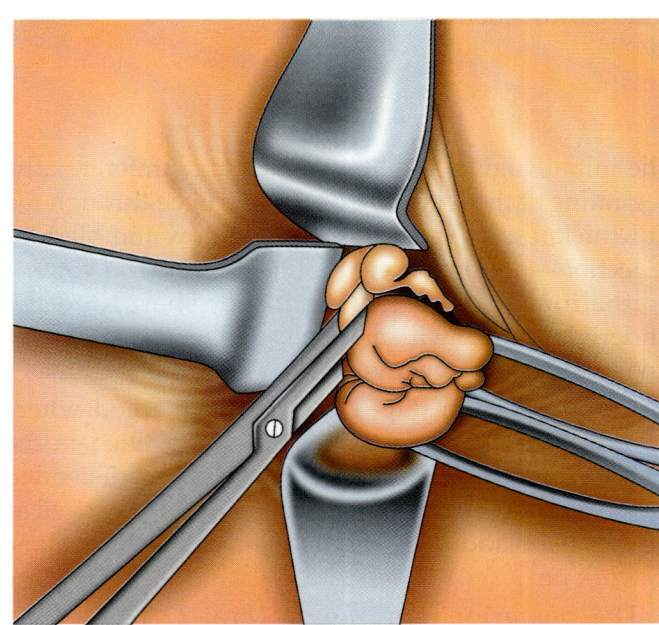

Fig. 22.19: Cardinal ligaments are clamped

The uterine vessels are then clamped in such a way as to incorporate the anterior and posterior leaves of the visceral peritoneum. A single-clamp technique reduces the risk of ureteral injury (Fig. 22.20).

Delivery of Surgical Specimen (Fig. 22.21)

The uterine fundus is delivered posteriorly by placing a tenaculum or towel clip on the uterine fundus in successive bites. The utero-ovarian ligament is identified with the surgeon's finger, then clamped and cut. The pedicles are double-ligated, first with a suture tie and then with a suture ligature medial to the first tie. A hemostat is placed on the second suture to assist in the identification of any bleeding.

If the adnexa are to be removed, round ligaments are cut separate. Traction is placed on the ovary by grasping it with a Babcock clamp. A Heaney clamp is placed across the infundibulopelvic ligament with the help of a retractor, and the ovary and tube are excised. Both a suture tie and a transfixion suture ligature are placed on this pedicle (Fig. 22.21).

To remove adnexa, traction is placed on ovary by grasping it with Babcock clamp. Heaney clamp is placed across infundibulopelvic ligament, and ovary and tube are excised. Both suture tie and transfixion suture ligature are placed on this pedicle.

Management of Enlarged Uterus

For enlarged uteri, the following techniques may be employed to facilitate removal of the uterus: Morcellation, intramyometrial coring, uterine bisection, and wedge debulking.

Morcellation can be used in cases involving uterine enlargement, uterine fixation, or limited vaginal exposure. It should not be performed, if the uterine arteries cannot be secured or if malignancy is suspected.

Intramyometrial coring (Fig. 22.22) is accomplished by circumferentially incising the outer myometrium beneath the uterine serosa with a scalpel while placing

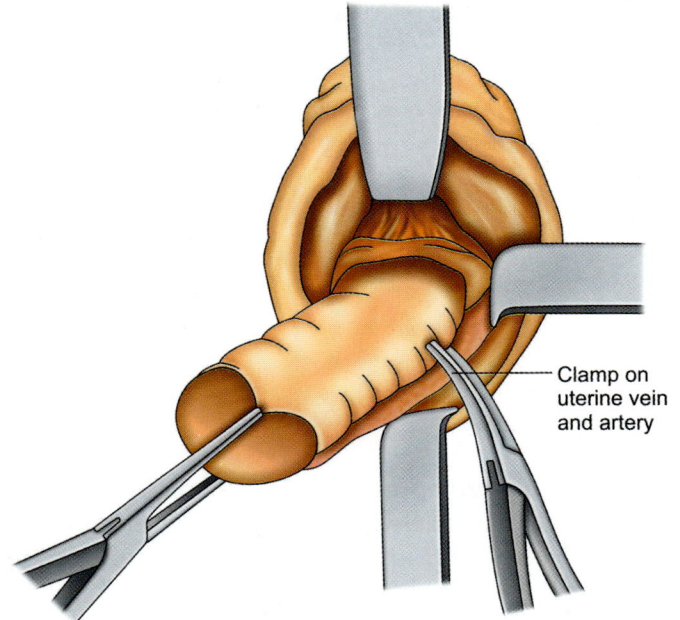

Clamp on uterine vein and artery

Fig. 22.20: Uterine vessels are clamped with single clamp so as to incorporate anterior and posterior leaves of visceral peritoneum

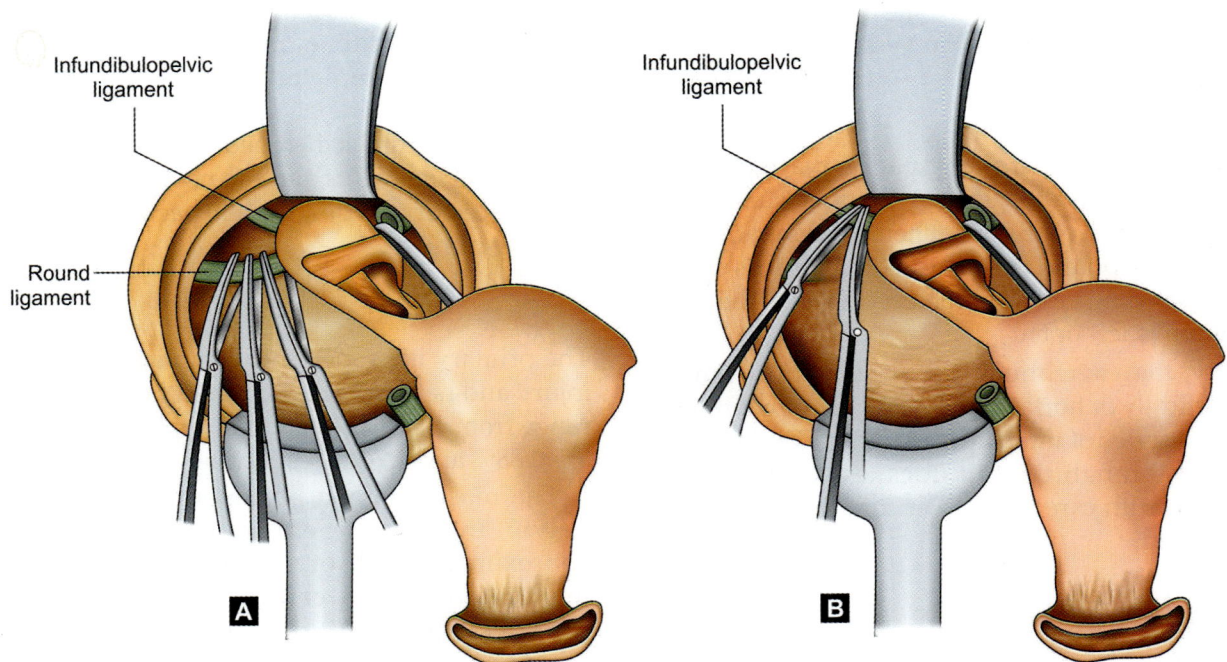

Infundibulopelvic ligament

Round ligament

Infundibulopelvic ligament

A

B

Fig. 22.21: Placing highest clamp to remove uterus

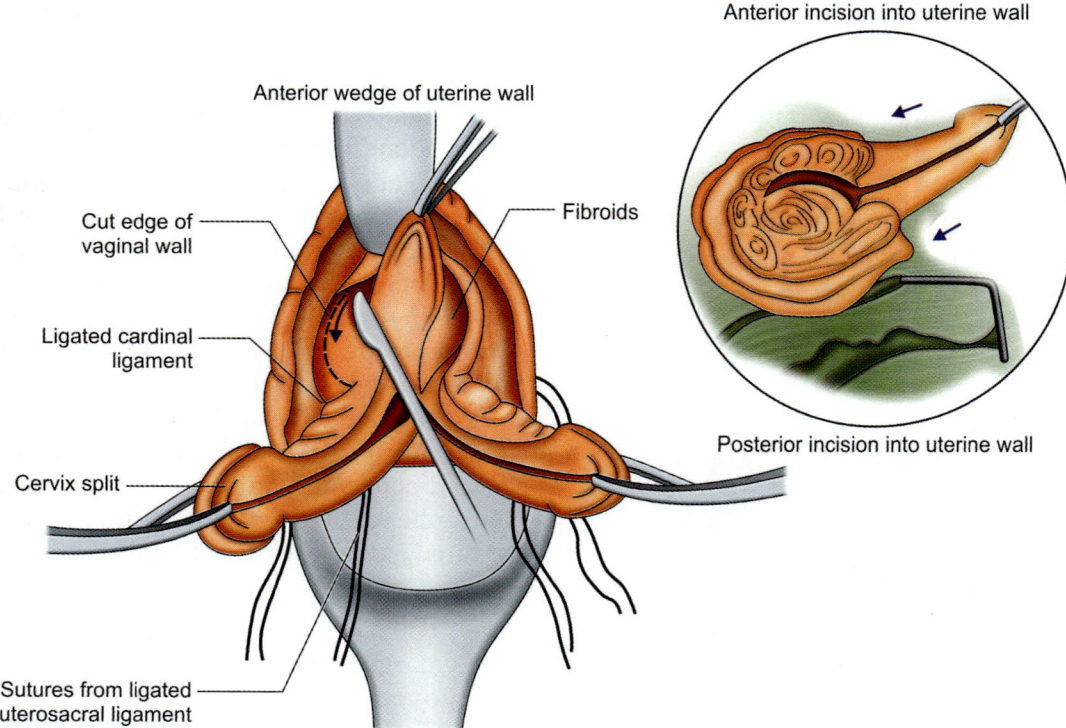

Anterior wedge of uterine wall

Cut edge of vaginal wall

Ligated cardinal ligament

Cervix split

Sutures from ligated uterosacral ligament

Fibroids

Anterior incision into uterine wall

Posterior incision into uterine wall

Fig. 22.22: Intramyometrial coring technique

the cervix on traction. The incision should be kept as close to the uterine serosa as possible. The enlarged uterus is delivered as an elongated mass inverting the uterine fundus.

Uterine bisection is performed by cutting the cervix and the uterine fundus in the sagittal plane. This technique is often combined with myomectomy or wedge morcellation to reduce the bulk of the uterine halves so that the tubo-ovarian vessels can be ligated.

Completion and Closure

A sponge-stick or laparotomy pad is placed into the peritoneal cavity to allow the surgeon to visualize each of the pedicles and confirm that hemostasis is adequate. If any bleeding points are identified, a suture is used to ligate the bleeding vessel under direct vision. The pelvic peritoneum is left open.

Finally, the vaginal epithelium is reapproximated either vertically or horizontally with either a continuous suture or a series of interrupted sutures. These sutures are placed through the full thickness of the vaginal epithelium, with care taken to ensure that the bladder is not entered.

Culdoplasty for Prevention of Enterocele

A culdoplasty is generally recommended to reduce the risk of subsequent enterocele formation and potential

vaginal vault prolapse. The McCall culdoplasty (i.e. obliterating the cul-de-sac, plicating the uterosacral-cardinal complex, and elevating any redundant posterior vaginal apex) is commonly practised.

In this procedure, an absorbable suture is placed through the full thickness of the posterior vaginal wall at the apex of what will be the vaginal vault. This suture is passed through the left uterosacral ligament pedicle, the posterior peritoneum, and the right uterosacral ligament and completed by being passed from the inside to the outside at the same point where it was begun. The suture is then tied, thus approximating the uterosacral ligaments and the posterior peritoneum. It is not necessary to use a vaginal pack or leave a bladder catheter in place.

Complications of Procedure

The primary intraoperative complications are visceral injury and hemorrhage. Reported rates of hemorrhage range from 1.4 to 2.6% and ureteral and bladder injury are 0.88% and 1.76%, respectively.

The most common postoperative complication is pelvic infection. Febrile morbidity occurs in approximately 15% of women who undergo vaginal hysterectomy and can be reduced by means of prophylactic antibiotics. Infections after vaginal hysterectomy include vaginal cuff cellulites, hemorrhage, secondary pelvic cellulitis, and pelvic abscess. These infections occur in approximately 4% of women.

Complications of Vaginal Hysterectomy

Hemorrhage: It can be primary, reactionary and Secondary type. The secondary hemorrhage mainly results due to sepsis and manifests in day 7–14 postoperative. It may need exploration sometimes. The management of the different hemorrhage is as follows:

a. *Primary hemorrhage:* This hemorrhage mainly happens during surgery producing preoperative hypotension and collapse. This can be due to slipped ovarian or uterine vessels or in the vesicovaginal space. This need to be secured to restore hemostasis. If ovarian vessel slips, the technique is to pull the stump medially and grasp the bleeding pedicles with Allis tissue forceps under vision with the help of lateral retractor. The clamps are placed lateral to the bleeding tissues and resutured. In case of uterine stump bleeding, the retracted tissues are grasped and reclamped lateral to the bleeding site and resutured. In case of bleeding in vesicovaginal space, electrocautery or separate ties are given to arrest bleeding.

b. *In case of secondary hemorrhage, the following steps are adopted:*
   1. Quick assessment of the condition.
   2. Correct hypotension with ringer lactate/colloids to maintain circulation in vital organs.
   3. Vaginal swab collected and sent for bacteriological study.
   4. High dose of parenteral antibiotics like third-generation cephalosprins, metronidazole and aminoglycosides.
   5. Replacement of blood loss by fresh RBC.
   6. Vaginal wash is given with povidone iodine lotion.
   7. Tests for full blood count, blood glucose, kidney function, coagulation profile, electrolytes are done.
   8. Exploration of the vaginal wound under GA; most of the time, continuous oozing surfaces are detected and interrupted sutures may be required over the necrotic sloughed out tissues and tight vaginal pack is given for 48 hours.
   9. Sometimes, bleeding may be profuse with features of internal vessel hemorrhage with hemoperitoneum. This may need urgent laparotomy for bilateral intraperitoneal or extraperitoneal ligation of anterior division of internal iliac artery.

Infection: Low-grade fever is common after hysterectomy. It is not always caused by infection, and usually resolves without treatment. However, a high or persistent fever may signal an infection. Serious infection occurs in less than 5% of women, and can usually be treated with intravenous antibiotics. Any retrovesical hematoma may produce sepsis and pelvic collection requiring drainage.

Constipation: Constipation occurs in most women following hysterectomy, and can usually be controlled with a regimen of stool softeners, dietary fiber, and laxatives.

Urinary retention: Urinary retention, or the inability to pass urine, can occur after vaginal hysterectomy. Urine can be drained using a catheter until retention resolves, usually within 24 to 48 hours.

Thromboembolism: Pelvic surgery increases the risk of developing blood clots in the large veins of the leg or lung. The risk is increased for approximately six weeks after surgery.

Damage to adjacent organs: The urinary tract (bladder, ureters) and bowel (large and small intestines) injury can occur during vaginal hysterectomy. Bladder injury may occur in steps: (a) Bladder dissection, (b) cardinal ligament suturing, (c) during uterine artery ligations, (d) ovarian vessel ligations in 1–2% of women who have vaginal hysterectomy.

Bowel injury occurs in <1% of women during steps: (a) Posterior pouch opening, (b) uterosacral ligament suturing, (c) during delivery of uterus with bowel adhesions not expected. Injury can usually be detected and corrected at the time of surgery. If detected with VVF/ureteric or bowel fistula after surgery, appropriate surgery with the help of urosurgeons or general surgeon respectively may be needed after 3 months.

Early surgical menopause: Women who have undergone hysterectomy only may experience menopause earlier than the average age of menopause (age 51). This may be due to an interruption in blood flow to the ovaries as a result of removing the uterus.

Outcomes

A Cochrane review found that the vaginal route, compared with all other routes for hysterectomy, yields better outcomes and fewer complications.

In cases when vaginal hysterectomy is not possible, laparoscopic vaginal hysterectomy has advantages over abdominal hysterectomy like faster return to normal activity, shorter hospital stay, reduced intraoperative blood loss, and fewer wound infections but also have disadvantages like longer operating time, steep learning curve and higher rate of urinary tract injury.

22C. LAPAROSCOPIC HYSTERECTOMY

Minimally Invasive Procedure for Hysterectomy

There are several approaches that can be used for an MIP hysterectomy:

- *Nondescent vaginal hysterectomy:* This is an unique approach where mobile uterus is removed through vaginal orifice leaving no visible scar and provide very fast recovery.
- *Laparoscopic hysterectomy:* This surgery is done using a laparoscope and three to four 5 mm portals under magnified camera vision and the instruments are played through the portals. The uterus and adnexal masses can be removed through vagina from above.
- *Laparoscopic-assisted vaginal hysterectomy:* Using laparoscopic approach, surgeon performs hysterectomy and removes the uterus through an incision in the vagina.
- *Robot-assisted laparoscopic hysterectomy:* This procedure involves a sophisticated robotic system of surgical tools from outside the body. Advanced technology allows the surgeon to use natural wrist movements and view the hysterectomy on a three-dimensional screen.

Cervix Removal

Laparoscopic supracervical hysterectomy (LSH) has been associated with a shorter operating time, decreased trauma, and less technical difficulty. However, a small proportion of these patients continue to have cyclical bleeding until menopause and there is 2.2% small risk of developing cervical cancer, if the cervix is retained. In addition, comparing total to subtotal abdominal hysterectomy, there is no significant differences in sexual function, urinary tract symptoms, bowel symptoms or in development of pelvic organ prolapse.

Steps of Total Laparoscopic Hysterectomy

1. Preparation and Positioning

Patients are admitted one day prior to the day of surgery and informd consent is taken. The patient is put on H_2 blockers and gut is well prepared with enema or Peglec solution so that gut remains collapsed during surgery. The surgeon must assess the pathology of the pelvic organs and plan his surgery beforehand. All the hardware equipment and the hand instruments are thoroughly checked before start of the surgery.

2. Insertion of a Uterine Manipulator

Uterine manipulator (Fig. 22.23) with a colored vaginal tube fixes at the cervix and the manipulator within the uterus rotates and pushes the uterus to facilitate surgery and the exact site of colpotomy can be assessed. Ideally, the manipulator should have the following characters:

- Easy to assemble
- Inexpensive
- Does not breakdown during procedure
- Should have a wide range of movement and mobilizes the uterus in different directions (anteversion, retroversion, lateral movement)
- Can be easily placed inside the uterus and stay in place all throughout the procedure.
- Vaginal tube of different sizes should be available appropriate to vaginal length available.

Functions

A uterine manipulator performs the following functions:

- Raises the uterus and brings it close to the instruments to facilitate surgery.
- Manipulates the uterus and stretches the side being operated upon.
- Increases the distance between the uterus and the bladder, ureters, and rectum thus reducing chance to injury.
- Can be used to pull the uterus vaginally after its complete detachment.
- Facilitates identification of the uterovesicle peritoneum, the cul-de-sac and the vaginal cuff just below the cervical attachment.
- Maintain the pneumoperitoneum following colpotomy.

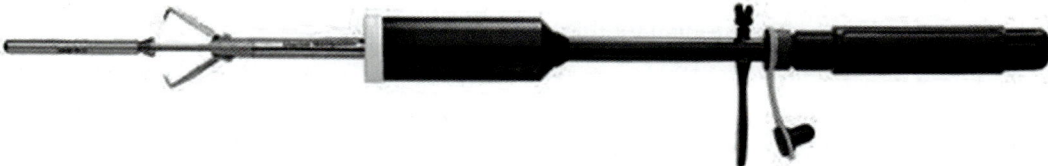

Fig. 22.23: Vaginal manipulator

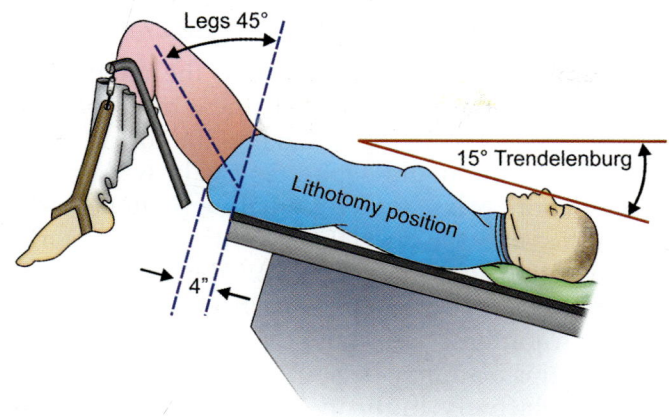

Fig. 22.24: Position of patient

The cervix is initially dilated under anesthesia and uterine manipulator is placed through the cervix inside the uterus with the colored vaginal tube of appropriate length pushed high in the vagina and held by the vaginal assistant. A Foley catheter is inserted into the bladder before start of the surgery.

3. *Positioning of the Patient* (Fig. 22.24)

The patient is placed in the dorsal lithotomy position. The legs are not placed in the standard 90° flexion, as in the classic dorsal lithotomy position, but are positioned at 45° flexion from the hip. The body surface and the thigh surface is almost at the same plane for surgeon on both sides to have adequate space to operate. The table should be placed low for surgeon to operate instruments freely without any strain.

The monitor is placed on the footend of the patient. It is extremely important to have the buttocks at least 4 inches off the end of the operating table to facilitate manipulation of the cervical instruments for maximum anteversion of the uterus. The operating table should be placed low for surgeon to operate instruments freely without any strain and slanted to 15° Trendelenburg position to displace the intestines out of the pelvis and into the upper abdomen. It is more comfortable for the operating surgeon to have the patient's arms down at her sides than extended on an arm board.

4. *Abdominal Entry and Trocar Placement* (Fig. 22.25)

A 5 mm skin incision is made at the supraumbilical or intraumbilical site using a #15 blade. The skin around the umbilicus is elevated and a Veress needle is inserted into the peritoneal cavity. The gas tubing is already connected to the needle to reduce manipulation following insertion. An easy way to confirm intraperitoneal entry is to look for a negative pressure reading on the insufflator. Once intraperitoneal pressure has reached 15 mm Hg, an optical trocar is inserted through the umbilicus or supraumbilical port under direct vision and a complete survey of the

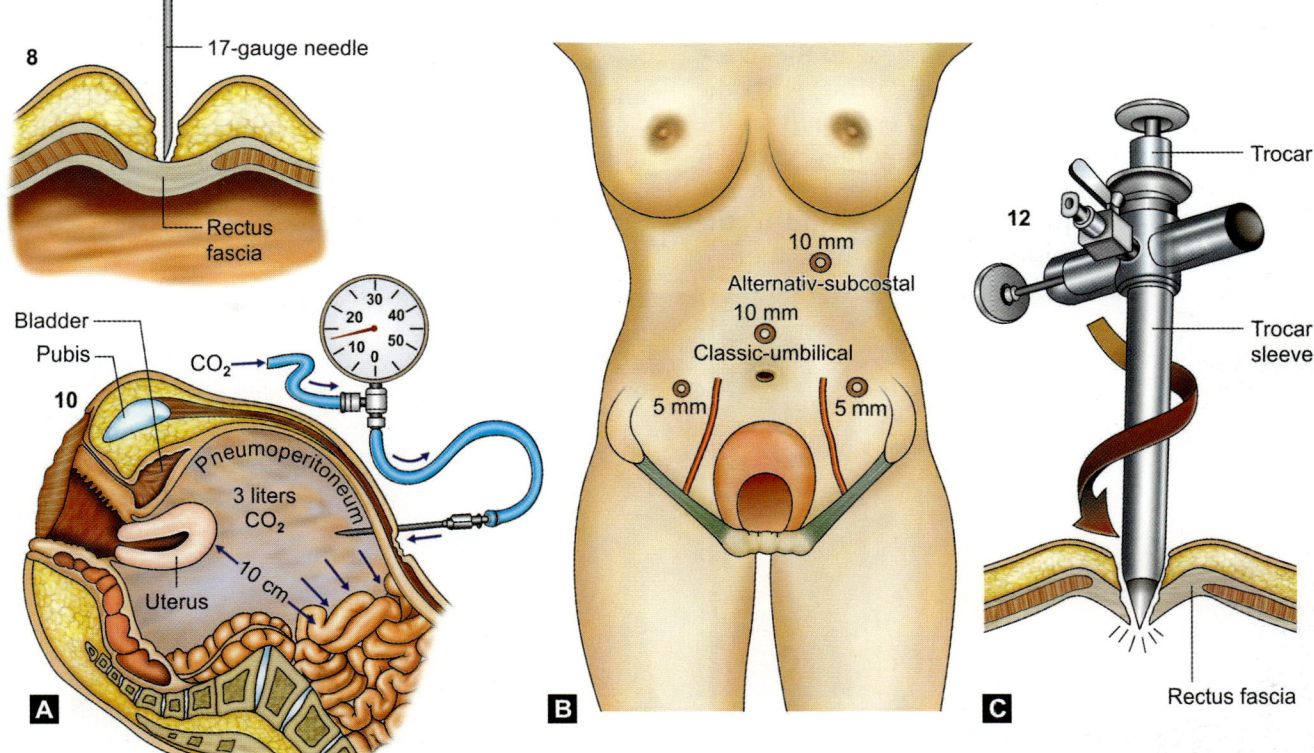

Fig. 22.25: Different ports of abdominal entry. (A) Veress needle placement, (B) Different parts of abdominal entry; (C) Trocar placement

abdomen is done to rule out any visceral injury at the time of entry.

The lower quadrant trocar sleeves are placed under direct vision. These trocars are placed lateral to the rectus abdominis muscles, 2 cm above and 2 cm medial to the anterior superior iliac spine. Usually, 5 mm trocar is placed on both the sites. In addition, a 5 mm trocar is placed approximately 8 cm above and parallel to the lower left trocar site below the subcostal arch. The 2 ports on the left greatly facilitate suturing and help to maintain an ergonomic position for the surgeon throughout the procedure. The port at the palmar point (3 cm below the left costal arch) may need to increase to 12 mm port to facilitate morcellation procedure and retrieval of specimen. On occasions, palmar point is used for pneumoperitoneum in cases of suspected midline bowel adhesions.

5. To remove the Ovaries (Fig. 22.26)

The infundibulopelvic ligament or the utero-ovarian ligament is initially desiccated with a reusable bipolar grasper. It is important to stay close to the ovary as this helps to avoid the pelvic sidewall during ovarian removal and the ascending uterine vessel during ovarian conservation.

The surgeon should take special care to desiccate the parametrial veins that run between the ovary and the round ligament as these can be quite tortuous and tend to bleed, if left unattended. The IP ligament or utero-ovarian ligament is then transected close to the ovary using the bipolar grasper prior to cutting with the scissor. Bleeding can be encountered especially in the setting of an enlarged uterus with engorged vascular plexuses. During this step of the procedure, the uterine manipulator is being pushed upwards and to the contralateral side to provide maximal visualization.

6. Mobilization of the Bladder (Fig. 22.27)

The round ligament is transected and the anterior and posterior leaves of the broad ligament are separated with the blade. It is important to find the correct plane where the peritoneum separates easily with gentle manipulation. Next, the vesicouterine peritoneal fold is identified and the dissection is continued anteriorly, thereby mobilizing the bladder off the lower uterine segment. It is important to stay in the loose areolar tissue. In patients who have had a prior cesarean delivery, this area may be scarred and it is important to stay relatively high on the uterus during the dissection. A reevaluation of the route of dissection is advised, if fat is encountered because the fat belongs to the bladder; this may indicate that the dissection is moving too close to the bladder.

The dissection of the anterior leaf of the broad ligament continues anteriorly and the bladder is dissected from the lower uterine segment.

7. Secure the Uterine Vessels (Fig. 22.28)

Due to a wide variety in anatomy and in the course of the uterine vessels, it is helpful to initially skeletonize them with the Harmonic scalpel or scissor. The ascending uterine vessels are then dessicated with the bipolar grasper at the level of internal cervical os. During the procedure, the uterine manipulator is pushed cephalad to move the uterine vessels away from the ureter. Complete desiccation of the vessels can be assessed visually by observing the bubbles coming and going during this process; when the bubbles stop forming, the vessel is desiccated and safe to transect with the Harmonic scalpel or scissor.

An inverted V-shape cut is made on the anterior and medial and posterior and medial to the vascular pedicle.

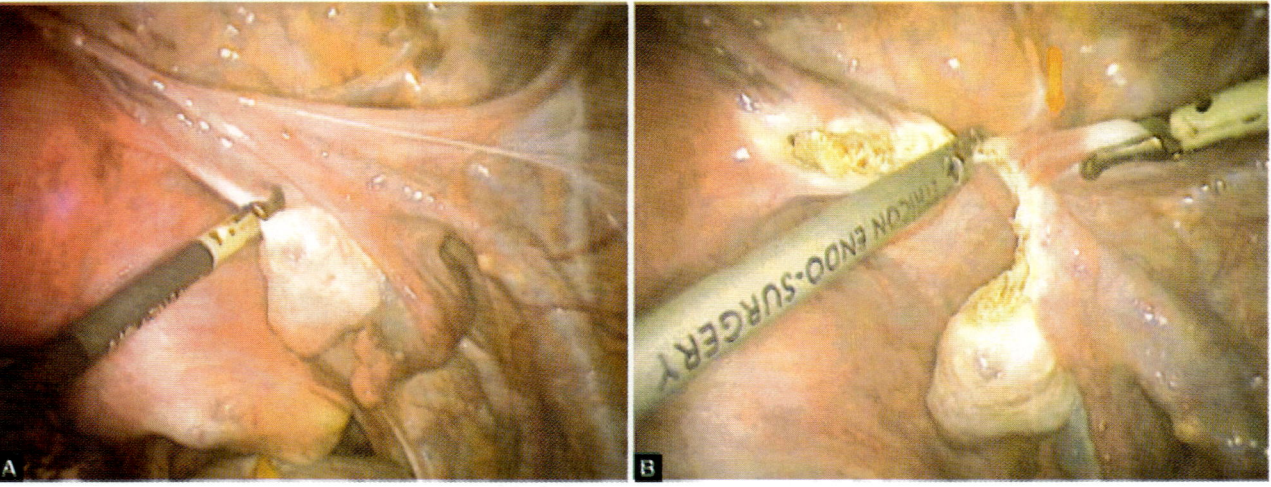

Fig. 22.26: Cauterizing the ligament of ovary

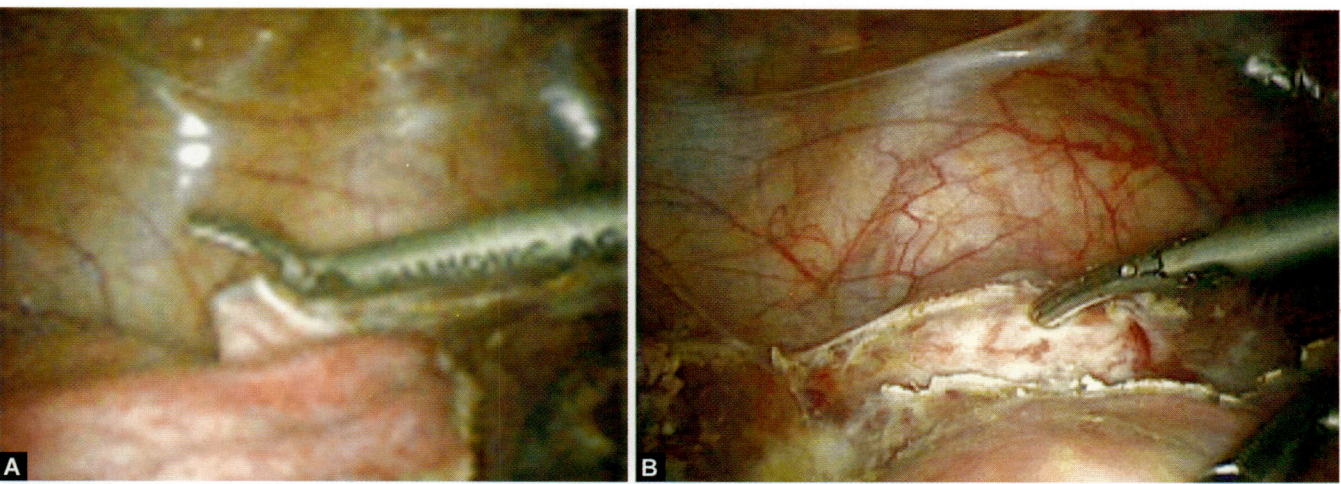

Fig. 22.27: Mobilizing the bladder

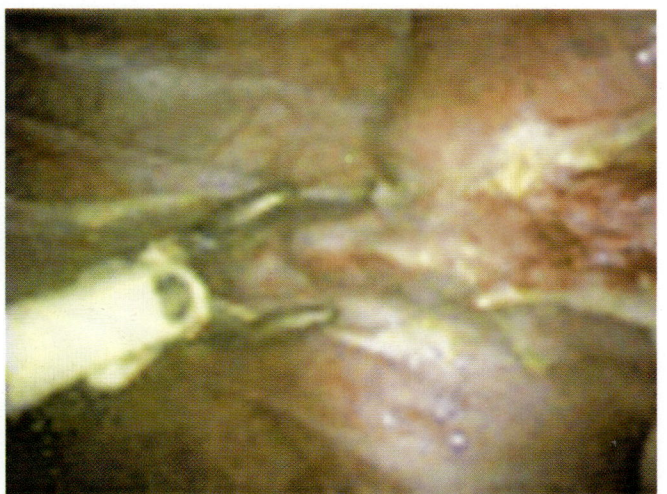

Fig. 22.28: Securing the uterine vessels

This enables the vascular pedicle to fall out laterally, thereby providing easy and avascular access to the cervical cup. It is important to take the uterine vessels high and then dissect medially to the uterine vessels down to the cup. This averts ureteral injury and provides a healthy vascular pedicle that can be safely desiccated further in the event of bleeding.

8. *Separate the Uterus and Cervix from the Vaginal Apex* (Fig. 22.29)

The vaginal fornices is identified while pushing cephalad with the uterine manipulator. The surgeon can either see the indentation or be able to palpate it with a laparoscopic instrument. The Harmonic scalpel or monopolar hook is then used to cut circumferentially around the cup.

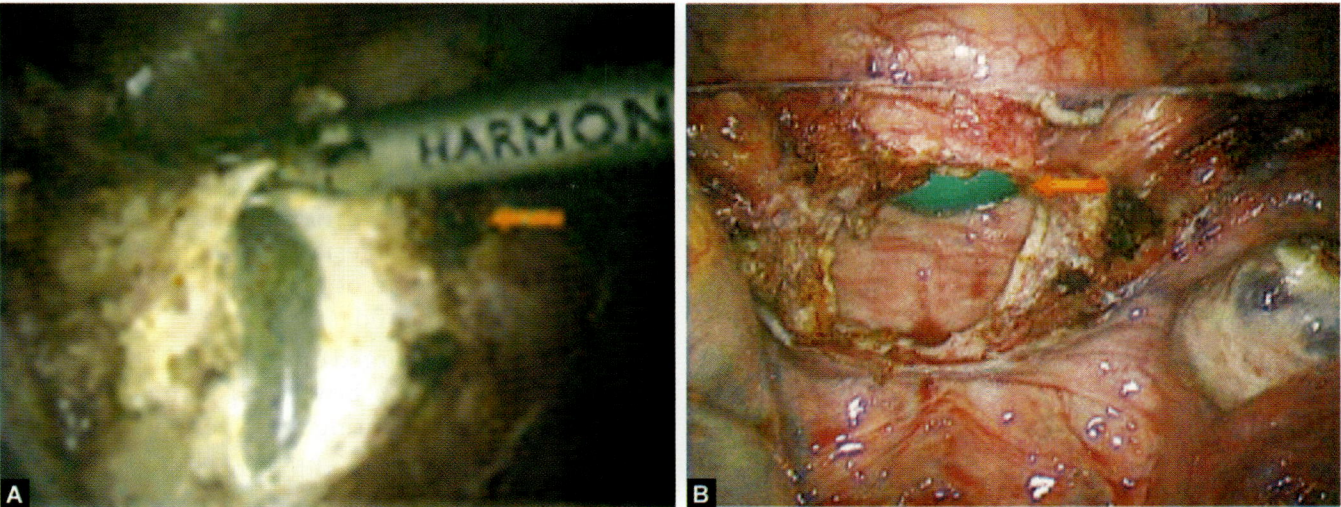

Fig. 22.29: Separating uterus from the vault

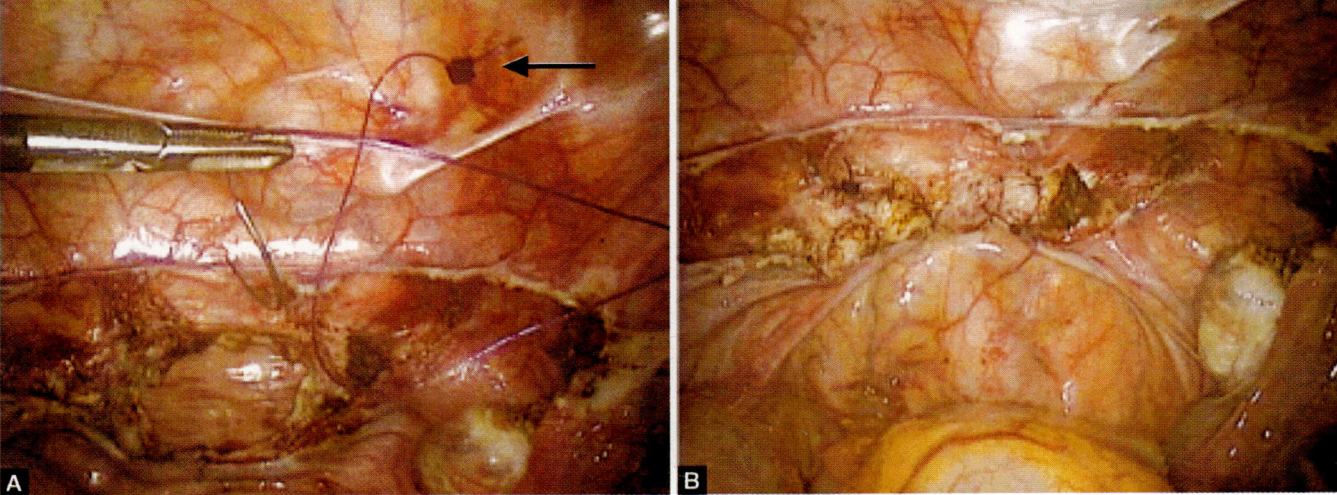

Fig. 22.30: Vault closure

9. Removal of the Uterus

The uterus made free is pulled into the vagina, if it fits. The uterus can remain there to maintain pneumo-peritoneum during suturing. Alternatively, the uterus is removed and a glove with a pair of 4 × 4 sponges is placed into the vagina to maintain pneumoperitoneum. If the uterus is too large to fit through the vagina, it can be carefully morcellated transvaginally by using a 10-blade scalpel and triple hooks for retraction. In patients with limited vaginal access, the uterus can be morcellated using an electronic morcellator. It is important to keep the tip of the morcellator in clear view at all times.

10. Vault Closure (Figs 22.30 and 22.31)

One-half of a 14 × 14 cm 1-0 vicryl suture is cut in the middle and it is secured with a Merryland forceps to put the niddle in the abdomen. Closure begins at the distal angle of the vaginal cuff and proceeds in a running fashion, making sure to include the vaginal mucosa and the pubocervical and rectovaginal fascia. Each bite should be approximately 1 cm in thickness and continued from one corner to the opposite corner of the vault and is completed with placing knot. The needle is cut free and removed through the 12 mm port. The pelvis can now be irrigated and hemostasis at all sites is assured.

11. Port Site Closure

The fascia at the 12 mm incision in the left lower quadrant is closed using 0 vicryl sutures with a fascia closure device. The skin is closed with 4-0 monocryl suture in a continuous subcutaneous fashion. The 5 mm incisions are closed with fast absorbable suture.

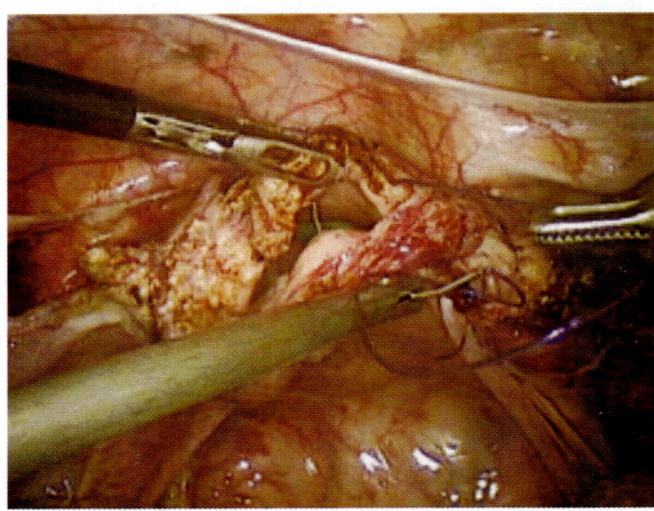

Fig. 22.31: Steps of vault closure

Postoperative Management

1. The patient is kept on NPM for 6 hours normally and can start consuming oral sips after 6 hrs.

2. After 12 hrs, she starts liquid and in the next 24 hrs she is given solid diet.

3. Usual antibiotic, antiemetic, H_2 blockers and postoperative analgesia with IV paracetamol and sedation with narcotics are given in immediate postoperative period.

4. Patients are discharged on 2nd or 3rd day depending on her recovery, bowel clearance and vitals remaining stable during these periods.

5. Port site areas are asked to keep clean.

6. Patients resume their normal activities on average within 2 to 3 weeks following surgery.

Additional Practical Tips for Challenging Cases

- If the uterus is large and requires manipulation with a tenaculum, consider injecting dilute vasopressin subserosally prior to applying traction to the uterus. This can reduce bleeding associated with pulling and tearing of the uterine serosa.
- In cases with poor exposure, sutures are used to retract organs away from the surgical field. A distended sigmoid can be retracted by taking a series of bites with a 0 prolene suture through the epiploica and pulling the suture through the lower quadrant port. The port is removed to get the sutures out and then reinserted. The sutures are then secured to the skin with a hemostat. Take care to include a number of epiploica to avoid tearing.
- Alternatively, ovaries or other structures can be tacked away using a 6-inch 0 vicryl suture with a LapraTy on the end. The needle is passed through the structure and then a bite is taken through the inside of the anterior abdominal wall. This end of the suture is then secured with another LapraTy and the needle is cut away and removed.
- If access to the uterine vessels is difficult, take the uterine vessels up high initially to secure the blood supply to the upper uterus and then gradually work down, staying medially to the vessels.
- The combination of a prior cesarean delivery and a large uterus is a case at risk for bladder injury—surgeon has to stay high on the vesicouterine peritoneum, respect any fat that may indicate proximity of bladder wall and watch out for the Foley balloon.
- In severely distorted anatomy, the retroperitoneum is entered sooner rather than later. The easiest starting point is usually at the round ligament.

22D. RADICAL HYSTERECTOMY FOR CANCER CERVIX

I. Pelvic Lymph Node Dissection and with Extension of the Vagina

Radical Wertheim hysterectomy is performed predominantly for stage IB and early stage IIA carcinoma of the cervix and for stage I carcinoma of the vagina. It is also appropriate for stage II adenocarcinoma of the endometrium. The operation essentially includes removal of the uterus, cervix, ovaries, upper vagina, and all the parametrial tissues to the pelvic side wall as well as bilateral pelvic lymphadenectomy.

There are several surgical procedures that can be used in treating women with early stage cervical cancer. The majority of the gynecological surgeons have adopted five classes of the Piver-Rutledge-Smith classification of radical hysterectomy published in 1974. However, the Surgery Committee of the Gynecological Cancer Group(GCG) approved and adopted a revised version of the original Piver classification of radical hysterectomy. The goal of this new classification is to make it more practical, clinically more relevant.

Classification of Radical Hysterectomy

1. **Simple extrafascial hysterectomy (Type I)**
2. **Modified radical hysterectomy (Type II):** The uterus, paracervical tissues, and upper vagina (1–2 cm) are removed after dissection of the ureters to the point of their entry to the bladder. The uterine arteries are ligated, and the medial half of the parametrium and proximal uterosacral ligaments are resected.
3. **Radical hysterectomy (Type III):** En bloc uterus with the upper third of the vagina along with the paravaginal and paracervical tissues are removed. The uterine vessels are ligated at their origin and the entire width of the parametria and uterosacral ligaments is resected bilaterally.
4. **Extended radical hysterectomy (Type IV):** As in class III and in addition three-fourth of the vagina and paravaginal tissue are excised.
5. **Partial exanteration (Type V):** The terminal ureter or a segment of the bladder or rectum is removed along with the uterus and parametrium.

Types II–V hysterectomies are combined with bilateral pelvic lymphadenectomy removing all the lymphofatty tissue along the common iliac artery including both-sided external, internal, common iliac

and the obturator nodes (at least to the level of the obturator nerve).

Removal of the tubes and ovaries is not part of radical hysterectomy per se. The ovaries are preserved in young patients.

History

Ernst Wertheim (1864-1920) was an Austrian gynecologist born in Graz. In 1898, Wertheim performed the first radical abdominal hysterectomy for cervical cancer. This operation involved removal of the uterus, parametrium, tissues surrounding the upper vagina, and pelvic lymph nodes.

Radical Wertheim Hysterectomy Technique

Surgical Steps

Patient Positioning

The patient is placed in the modified dorsal supine lithotomy position (15° Trendelenburg). The bladder is emptied with a Foley catheter. A thorough bimanual examination is performed. The abdomen, perineum, and vagina are surgically prepared.

An abdominal incision is made in the midline and extended around the umbilicus. A Foley catheter is left in the bladder and connected to straight drainage. Alternatively, Cherney or Maylard transverse incisions allow good access to lateral pelvis.

Exploration

The abdomen is thoroughly explored. The peritoneum between the cecum and terminal ileum is opened, the common iliac and aortic areas are exposed, and any suspicious lymph nodes are removed for biopsy. The intestine is packed off in the upper abdomen.

Entering Retroperitoneal Space (Fig. 22.32)

A large clamp is placed on the uterine fundus and used as an elevator. Alternatively, two cornu are fixed with silk sutures and tied together for traction.The round ligaments are clamped at both pelvic walls, incised, and tied. The anterior leaf of the broad ligament is opened along with the vesicouterine peritoneal fold.

The posterior leaf of the broad ligament is opened, exposing the infundibulopelvic ligament in the area of the pelvic brim. A finger is inserted under the infundibulopelvic ligament. The ureter is identified and dissected free of the infundibulopelvic ligament. Three

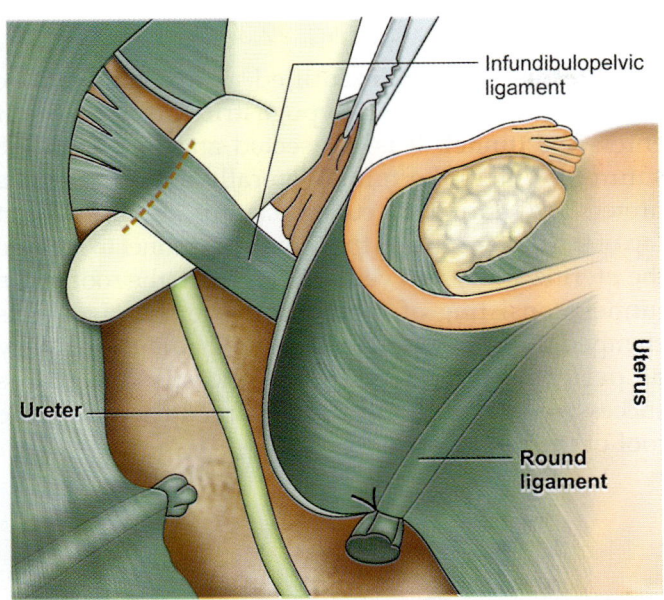

Fig. 22.32: Clamping infundibulopelvic ligament

clamps are applied to the infundibulopelvic ligament, and it is transected and doubly tied. The same procedure is carried out on the opposite side.

Ovarian Transposition (Fig. 22.33)

In young women, one or both ovaries can be preserved by dissecting out the infundibulopelvic ligament with its ovarian artery and vein and suspending the ovary to the psoas muscle high in the abdomen under the

inferior pole of the kidney. This removes the ovary from any potential field of radiation that may be utilized postoperatively.

The round ligaments have been cut and divided. The anterior leaves of the broad ligament have been opened, and the vesicouterine peritoneum has been transected. The vesical peritoneum is grasped with two forceps and elevated. Scissors are used to dissect the vesicovaginal space between the bladder and the anterior vaginal wall (Fig. 22.34). Elevation of the bladder can be facilitated by the placement of two sutures through the vesicoperitoneum to the skin incision above the symphysis pubis.

The infundibulopelvic ligament, tubes, ovaries, and round ligaments are all tied to the thyroid clamp placed on the middle of the fundus. The surgical field is kept free of excessive instruments.

Entering Retroperitoneal Space (Fig. 22.34)

The uterus is retracted caudal and medially. The base of the aorta is exposed, and the lymphatic tissue surrounding the common iliac artery and vein is removed with sharp dissection. The ureter is identified, dissected free of the artery, and retracted laterally. Blunt dissection with a finger or suction tip is used in a sweeping motion from top to bottom along the medial peritoneal leaf to identify and sufficiently mobilize the lateral surface of the ureter at this site. All lymphatic tissue surrounding the external iliac and common iliac blood vessels is removed from the bifurcation of the aorta to the inguinal ligament at the femoral canal. The lymph nodes are carefully isolated in individual specimen containers for precise pathologic analysis.

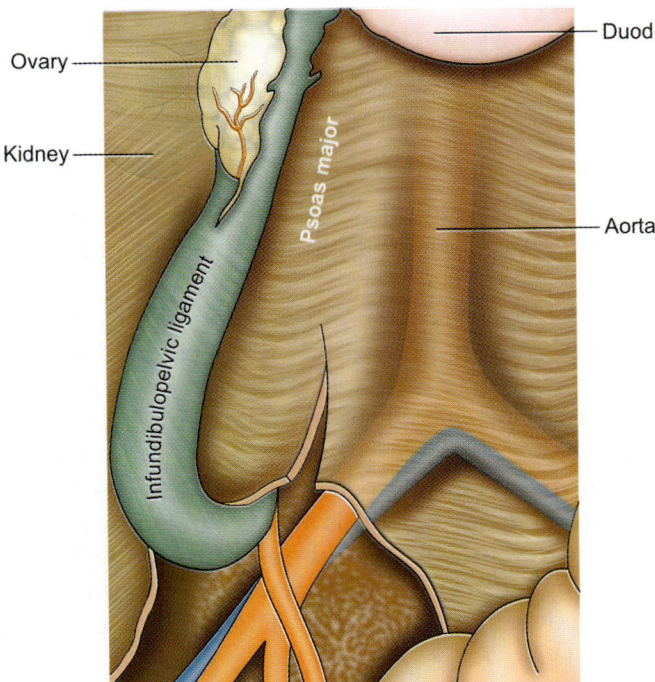

Fig. 22.33: Ovarian transposition

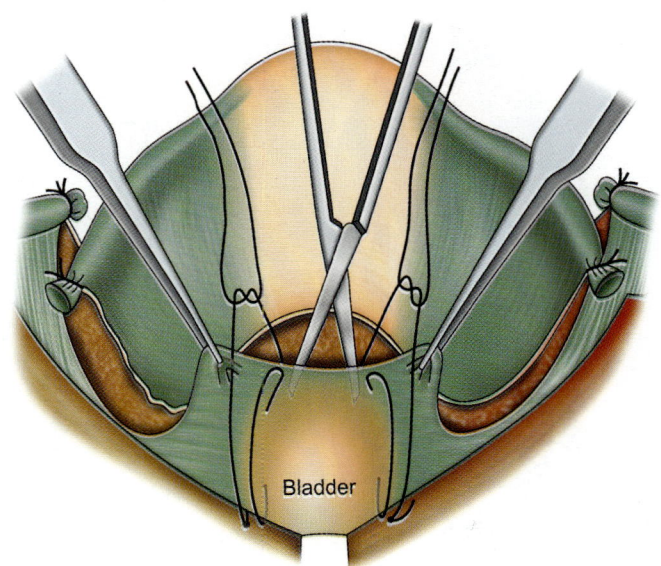

Fig. 22.34: Entering posterior retroperitoneal place

The common iliac, external iliac and upper hypogastric vessels have been stripped of all lymphatic-bearing tissue (Fig. 22.35). The obturator fossa and the lower branches of the hypogastric artery are dissected. A vein retractor is used to retract the external iliac artery and vein laterally and all lymphatic tissues are removed from behind these vessels and from the obturator fossa. The obturator nerve is preserved. Vessels deep in the obturator fossa may be ligated with hemoclips (Fig. 22.36).

The same procedure is carried out on the left side.

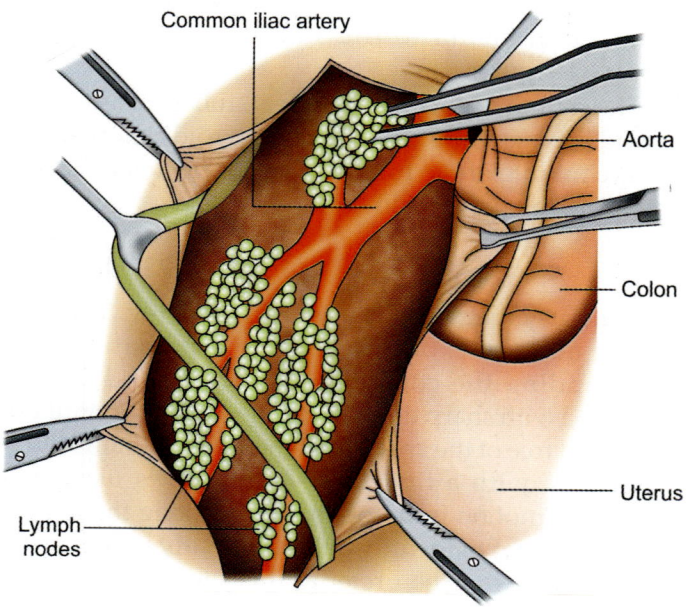

Fig. 22.35: Pelvic lymphadenectomy

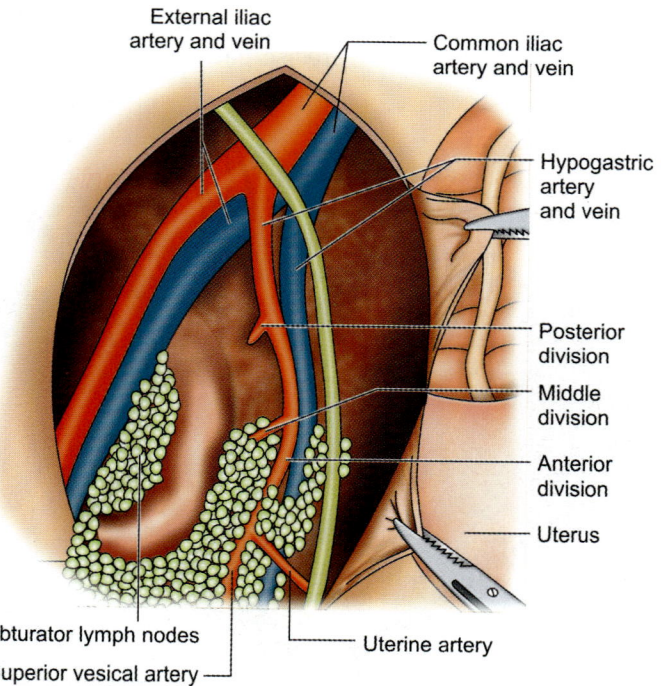

Fig. 22.36: Obturator space dissection for lymphadenectomy

Uterine Artery Ligation (Fig. 22.37)

The uterine artery is identified as it comes off the anterior division of the hypogastric artery before it enters the tunnel. It is transected and tied with 2-0 suture. It enters the tunnel laterally and crosses the ureter. Two horizontal curved clamps are inserted on top of the ureter beneath the roof of the tunnel to include the uterine artery and vein. The tissue in the roof of the tunnel, consisting of the uterine artery and vein, is clamped, incised, and tied. In some patients, this may be performed in one step; in others, two to three successive bites with horizontal curved clamps on the roof of the tunnel are needed.

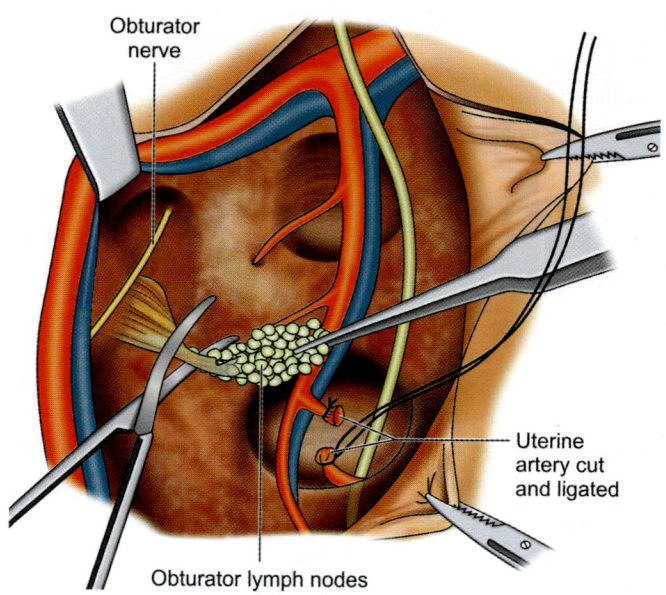

Fig. 22.37: Uterine artery cut and ligated

Creating Spaces (Fig. 22.38)

Prior to performing the next step, the surgeon must completely dissect the paravesical and pararectal spaces.

The presacral space (*PSS*) is at the top. Advancing anteriorly, the surgeon finds the rectum(*R*) and the pararectal spaces (*PRS*). The surgeon can enter this space by displacing the ureter and moving between the ureter and internal iliac artery.

The rectovaginal space (*RVS*) is the next space anterior to the rectum. This area is entered by incising the peritoneum in the cul-de-sac of Douglas and dissecting the posterior vaginal wall from the perirectal fascia covering the rectum. The next space is the vagina (*V*).

The vesicovaginal space (*VVS*) is entered by retracting the bladder (*B*) anteriorly and dissecting this

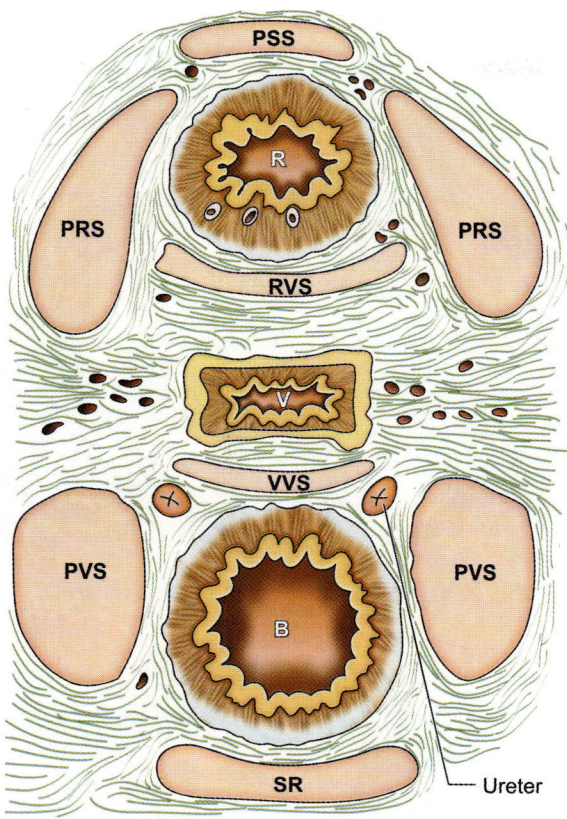

Fig. 22.38: Peritoneal spaces

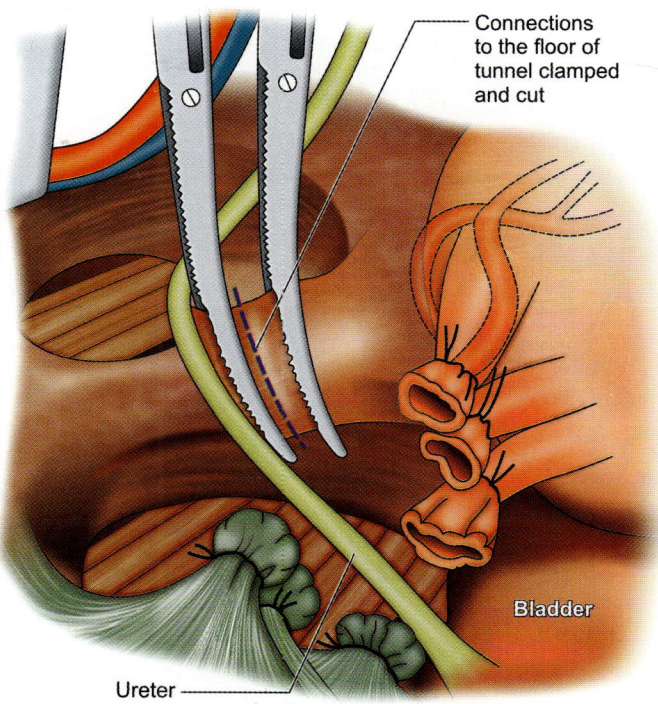

Fig. 22.39: Medial 3rd parametrial resection and deroofing the tunnel

space with sharp dissection along the pubovesical cervical fascia.

The next significant space is the paravesical space *(PVS)*. Between the pararectal space and the paravesical space is the lateral extent of the cardinal ligament, originally described as the "web" by Wertheim. The web contains the venous network of the internal iliac vein. The superior portion of the web contains the sympathetic nerve fibers to the bladder along with the venous plexus. The inferior portion of the web contains the parasympathetic nerve fibers to the bladder. In between the paravesical space is the bladder. Anterior to the bladder is the space of Retzius, the retropubic space.

Uniting Paravesical and Pararectal Spaces (Fig. 22.39)

The external iliac artery and vein and the hypogastric artery and vein are retracted medially. The pararectal and the paravesical spaces are exposed. The parametrial resection to unite the spaces can be performed by several methods: (a) by clamping, cutting and suturing, (b) by electrosurgical blade dissection to the pelvic sidewalls using a right-angle clamp to elevate and isolate parametrial tissue. The ureter is detached from the medial leaf of the peritoneum by tip of a right-angle

clamp placed perpendicular to and just above the ureter. The right index finger carefully sweeps the ureter downwards and laterally till the floor of the tunnel can be visualized.

Unroofing the Ureteric Tunnel (Fig. 22.40A and B)

The uterus is placed on lateral traction and the proximal ureter is held on traction to straighten it by gently pulling on the penrose drain. On reaching the tunnel, one right-angle clamp is inserted with the tips directed upward while direct visualization of the ureter is confirmed. The tips are directed medially towards the cervix and popped through the paracervical tissue. A second clamp is placed through the opening. The ureter is bluntly dissected and pushed posteriorly towards the tunnel floor. It should be visible below before cutting the overlying paracervical tissue. Delayed absorbable 3-0 suture tie is used to secure the paracervical tissue pedicles held by the right-angle clamps. The same procedure may be repeated several times to completely deroof the tunnel and expose the ureter under direct vision to prevent ureter injury. This can happen when sometimes significant bleeding occur at this site. This completely frees the ureter from any attachment to the web.

Exposing the Rectovaginal Space (Fig. 22.41)

The uterus is retracted upward and in front. The incision in the posterior leaf of the broad ligament is

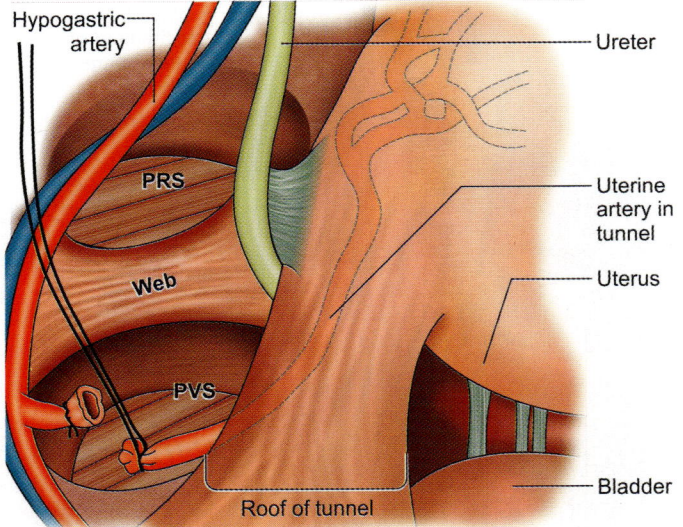

Fig. 22.40A: Ureteric tunnel

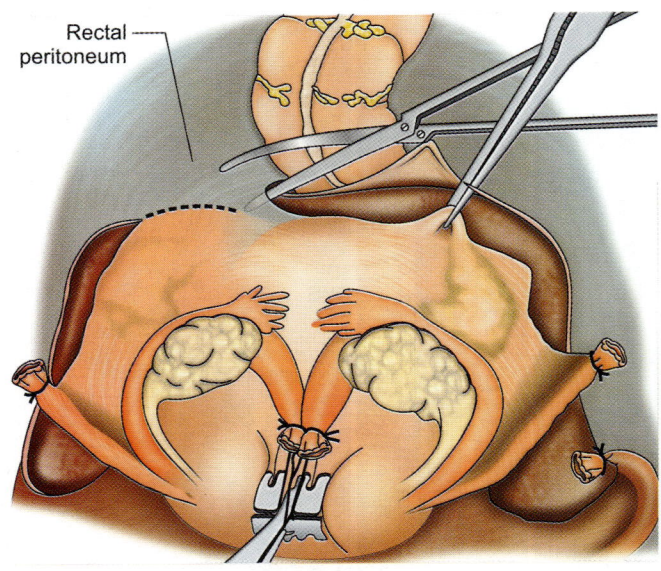

Fig. 22.41: Rectovaginal space being entered

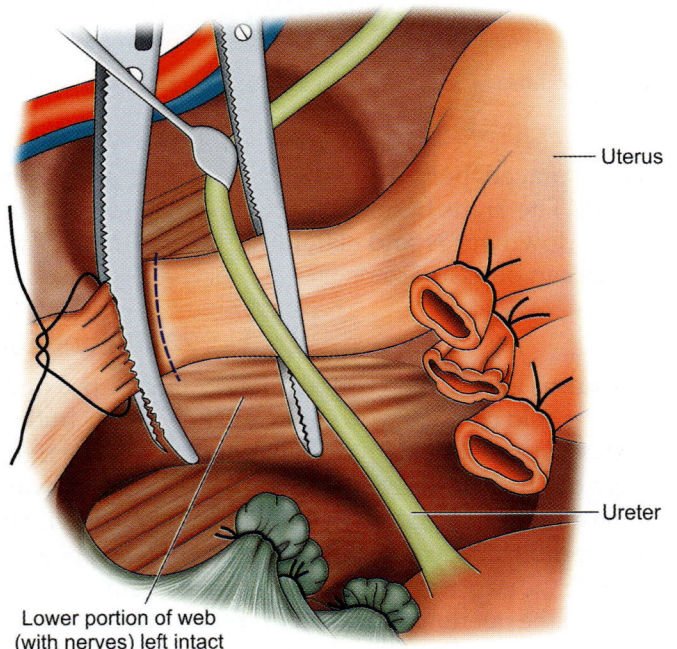

Fig. 22.40B: Total parametrial resection and deroofing the tunnel

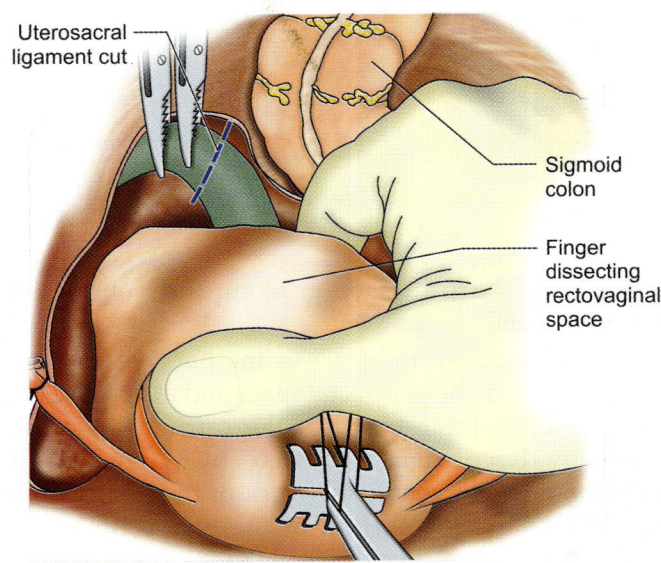

Fig. 22.42: Rectovaginal space created

extended across the cul-de-sac and peritoneum overlying the cul-de-sac between the cervix and rectum.

The uterus is retracted cephalad, a finger is inserted between the uterosacral ligaments, and the posterior wall of the vagina is dissected off the anterior rectal wall. Retraction on the uterus is changed to the anterior caudal position, placing the uterosacral ligaments on tension. The upper portion of the uterosacral ligaments is clamped, incised, and tied (Fig. 22.42). The lower portion of the uterosacral ligaments, containing the parasympathetic nerves to the bladder, is left.

Vaginal Resection (Fig. 22.43)

The lateral, posterior, and anterior attachments of the uterus and its parametria have all been transected and tied. Two right-angle Heaney clamps are placed on the paravaginal tissue on each side, and a scalpel is used to transect the remaining paravaginal tissue and vagina between these clamps. The paravaginal tissue pedicle is tied with a 0 synthetic absorbable suture. Approximately 5 cm of vagina should be removed.

Vaginal Cuff Closure (Fig. 22.44)

This is mainly done by open technique method. In this method, the uterosacral and cardinal pedicles are

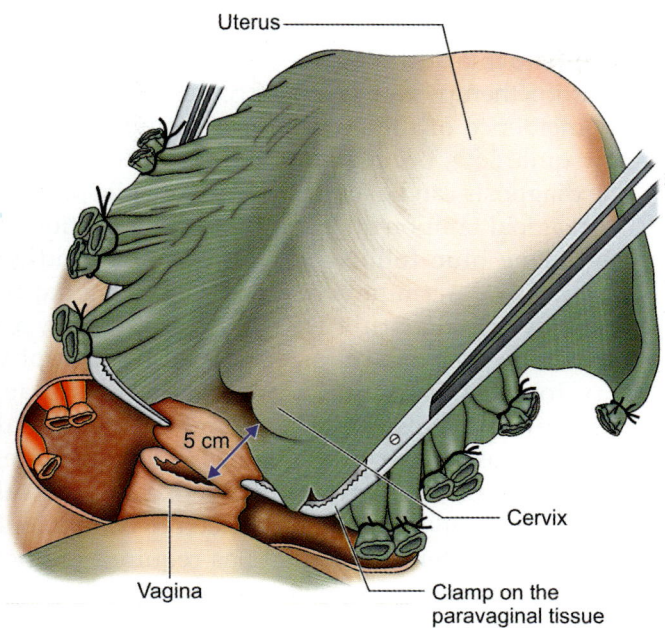

Fig. 22.43: Vaginal resection

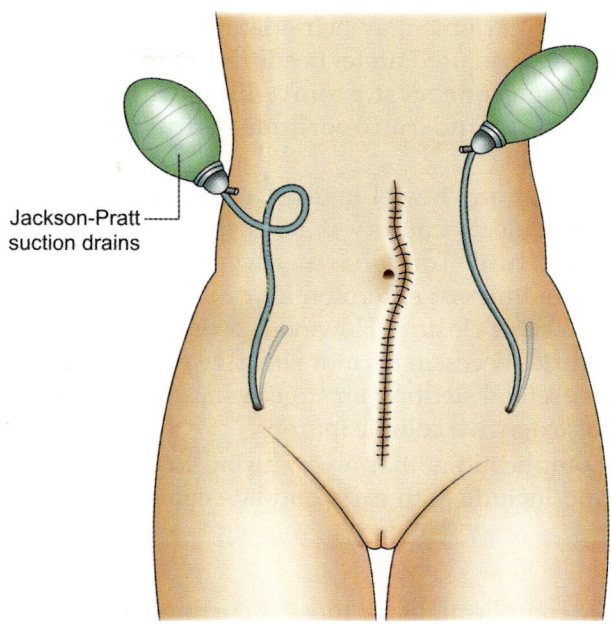

Fig. 22.45: Suction drains

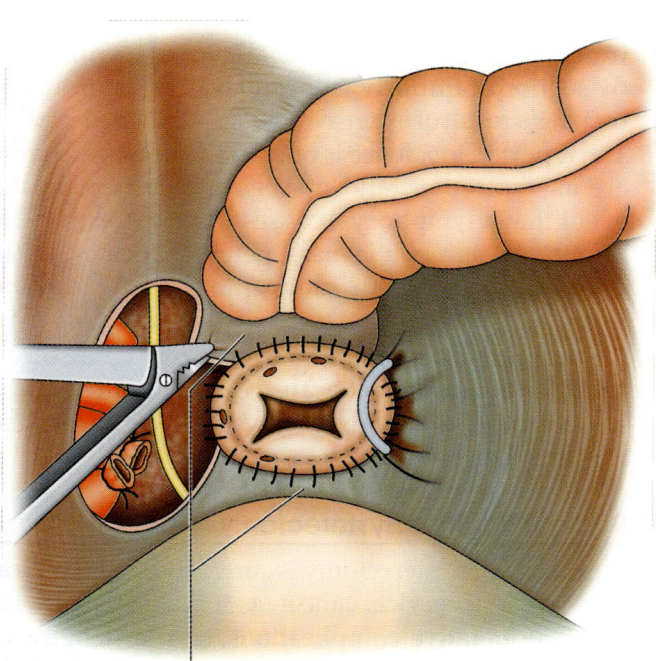

Fig. 22.44: Vault closure—open technique

sutured with the vaginal angles and the anterior and posterior margins are sutured separately keeping the vagina open for natural drainage. This proves superior to closed cuff closure as it prevents collection of tissue exudates, blood collection and thus prevent cuff cellultitis, infection. If in younger patients during radical Wertheim hysterectomy in which a longer vagina is desired, the following steps can be performed.

The vesical peritoneum coming off the bladder can be sutured to the anterior vaginal cuff. The serosa from the rectosigmoid colon can be sutured to the posterior vaginal cuff.

Silastic Jackson-Pratt closed suction drains (Fig. 22.45) are inserted into the paravesical and pararectal spaces on each side. These are brought retroperitoneally to the anterior abdominal wall. The Silastic closed suction drains are brought out, respectively, through the right and left lower quadrants of the abdominal wall. The midline incision, extended around the umbilicus, is closed in layers.

Complications of Radical Hysterectomy

Radical hysterectomy can be accomplished with acceptable morbidity (<5%) in the hands of an experienced surgeon. Nevertheless, complications do occur. Predisposing factors include previous pelvic surgery or radiation, endometriosis, pelvic inflammatory disease, anatomic anomalies, obesity, and pregnancy.

Intraoperatively, the most common complication of radical hysterectomy is:

1. Hemorrhage—the average blood loss is from 600 to 1900 mL. Injured vessels can be repaired with hemoclips or suture ligatures, although hypogastric artery ligation is sometimes required to control hemorrhage.
2. Ureteral injury is recognized intraoperatively in less than 1% of cases, however, it may occur more frequently and go unnoticed. The use of intravenous

Indigo carmine may help identify the site of injury. When an injured ureter needs repair, techniques such as ureteroneocystostomy, ureteroureterostomy, stenting, and retroperitoneal drainage may be required.

3. Bladder and bowel injuries also occur, particularly when electrocautery is used inappropriately as a substitute for sharp dissection. Typically, cystotomies or enterotomies can be repaired with a two-layer closure. However, proper repair of some injuries necessitates more involved procedures such as ureteral stenting for trigone injuries or colostomy for extensive colonic injuries.

Complications that arise during the postoperative period include both early and late complications.

Early Complications

Early complications, or those occurring within the first 30 postoperative days, may vary.

1. Infectious and febrile morbidity is the most common postoperative complication. Prophylactic use of broad-spectrum antibiotics reduces the frequency of this complication.

2. Postoperative bleeding may require reoperation; however, most cases are self-limited and can be treated conservatively with close observation for hemodynamic instability and blood transfusions.

3. Clinically significant thromboembolic complications occur in approximately 5% of cases. Early diagnosis requires a high index of suspicion because clinical findings are frequently subtle or nonspecific.

4. Prolonged ileus or intestinal obstruction occurs occasionally, but both conditions usually resolve with conservative management. Postoperative mortality is less than 1%.

5. Voiding dysfunction in the immediate postoperative period is nearly universal; denervation of the bladder during the operation results in transient hypertonia that is gradually replaced by hypotonia. Bladder drainage can be achieved with intermittent self-catheterization, or indwelling urethral catheterization. For most patients, the ability to void returns within 2–3 weeks; however, voiding dysfunction may persist in approximately 5% of patients. In addition, a substantial number of patients develop persistent urinary incontinence postoperatively.

Late Complications

1. Urinary tract fistulas are the most dreaded postoperative complications. Interruption and mobilization of the vasculature of the bladder and ureters predisposes to ischemia that lends itself to fistula formation. The need for postoperative radiation therapy worsens this problem. Fortunately, the incidence of this troublesome complication is now quite low, occurring in less than 2% of cases. The diagnosis can be made by sequential inspection of a vaginal tampon after intravesical instillation of methylene blue followed by intravenous Indigo carmine to determine whether a vesicovaginal or ureterovaginal fistula exists. Alternatively, an intravenous pyelogram or computed tomography may locate the fistula. Vesicovaginal fistulas, particularly those that are small, may heal spontaneously with prolonged bladder drainage; however, larger defects and those that fail to heal with conservative management need to be repaired surgically. Ureterovaginal fistulas require stenting; if a retrograde stent cannot be passed, percutaneous nephrostomy with anterograde stenting is required.

2. Lymphedema develops insidiously over time, making its true incidence difficult to determine. It occurs more frequently when pelvic lymphadenectomy is followed by radiation or groin node dissection. Similarly, lymphocyst formation can occur as a result of extensive pelvic lymphadenectomy. The reported incidence is only 2–3%; however, many are asymptomatic and may go undetected. In the event that a lymphocyst causes ureteral obstruction or presents as a pelvic mass, percutaneous drainage or reoperation with marsupialization may be necessary.

3. Sexual dysfunction and surgical menopause can result in difficult life because quality of life will be important to the many survivors of early cervical cancer.

II. Radical Vaginal Hysterectomy

Radical vaginal hysterectomy is currently a valid option for treatment of cervical cancer, as it is associated with fewer postoperative complications, shorter lengths of hospital stay and consequently, lower cost, particularly in the public health care settings.

The advent of laparoscopy has made it possible to perform pelvic lymphadenectomy, which was previously performed using the Mitra technique (extraperitoneal pelvic lymphadenectomy). Both approaches provide an excellent method for disease staging, with the number of nodes sampled comparable to that of open dissection.

Schauta's operation (radical vaginal hysterectomy) thus constitutes a good option for the treatment of cervical cancer, as it provides cost reductions, decreased operative time, earlier discharge, and a lower complication rate compared with the Wertheim/Meigs procedure (radical abdominal hysterectomy).

Indications

Indications for Schauta's operation overlap with those of Wertheim/Meigs hysterectomy:

1. Stages IA2, IB1, and IIA cervical tumors <4.0 cm in size;
2. Patients at high surgical risk, including those with obesity, diabetes mellitus, and chronic hypertension, among other conditions (a particular indication for the procedure);
3. Young patients who request improved cosmesis.

Historical Aspects

The use of radical vaginal hysterectomy in the treatment of neoplastic disease of the uterus was first proposed by Karl August Schuchardt in the late 18th century. In 1893, Schuchardt performed the first such procedure in a patient with cervical cancer, using the incisional approach to the vagina, perineum, and levator ani muscles which allows opening of the apex of the vaginal fornix for complete resection of the parametria.

Around the same time, Friedrich Schauta, a young Viennese gynecologist, took Schuchardt's ideas to the next level, perfecting the latter's approach even further and showing that survival rates after radical vaginal hysterectomy were dramatically superior to those obtained with simple vaginal hysterectomy.

In 1958, Dr. Subodh Mitra introduced a new technique to gynecologic practice—*extraperitoneal pelvic lymphadenectomy*. The relatively challenging nature of vaginal surgery, which requires above average dexterity and experience due to the constraints of the surgical field curtailed wider use of the Mitra procedure.

Operative Technique of Schauta-Amreich Radical Vaginal Hysterectomy

The patient is placed in the lithotomy position with the legs suspended in high stirrups. Bladder catheterization is done to ensure the bladder remains empty intraoperatively.

A. Schuchardt incision and Preparation of the Left Pararectal Space

The procedure begins with a mediolateral perineal incision on the patient's left side, through skin and vaginal mucosa and extending as high and deep as the perineal muscles and levator ani; this is known as the Schuchardt incision (Fig. 22.46).

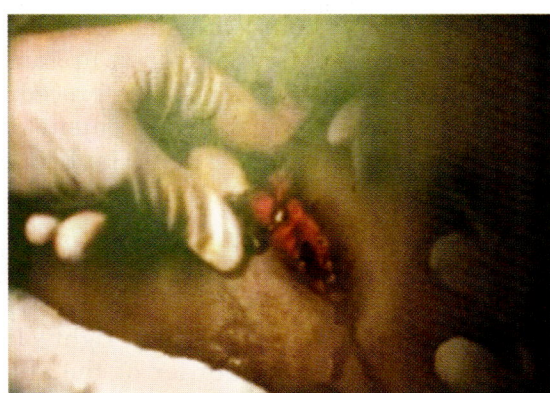

Fig. 22.46: Schuchardt's incision

In recent years, the Schuchardt incision is no longer used as it is considered inordinately invasive and unnecessary. The left pararectal space is dissected and Breisky retractors are used to displace the rectum medially until the inferior border of the left cardinal ligament presents itself.

B. Cervical Incision and Preparation of the Vaginal Vault

One of the advantages of radical vaginal hysterectomy is that it enables more precise demarcation of the amount of vaginal mucosa to be removed, guiding circular incision of the cervix according to tumor size, location, and extension. The anterior vaginal mucosa is pulled downward and incised perpendicularly all the way with a scalpel. This incision must be performed above the anterior sulcus of the vagina, permitting dissection of enough vaginal tissue to invaginate the tumor. The posterior vaginal mucosa is then pulled upward; a circular incision is performed with a scalpel and the tissue is dissected with scissors as in the anterior mucosa. After the vaginal cuff has been created, the cervix is invaginated, enclosing the tumor, to prevent seeding of tumor cells and facilitate manipulation of the uterus (Fig. 22.47).

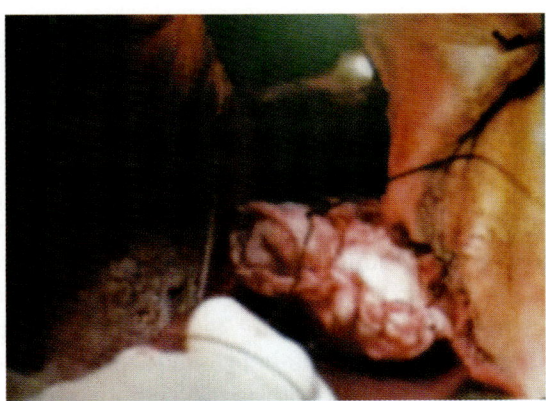

Fig. 22.47: Preparation of vaginal cuff

The supravaginal septum is divided with scissors, the vesicouterine excavation is opened up, and the bladder is retracted cranially. The same procedure is performed posteriorly, with displacement of the rectum, although the rectouterine pouch is not opened.

C. *Opening of the Paravesical Space, Dissection of the Ureter and Resection of the Anterior Parametrium*

The uterus is retracted downward and rightward by the first assistant while the border of the anterior mucosal incision is grasped by two Kocher clamps at the 1 and 3 o' clock positions. The left paravesical space is entered with scissors; the incision thus made is expanded bluntly with the operator's finger and a Breisky retractor is introduced. Traction on the retractors introduced into the vesicouterine excavation and left paravesical space distends the bladder pillar, which contains the ureter. The left ureter can be palpated between two fingers, allowing the surgeon to determine exactly where the anterior parametrium is to be incised. Three structures must be identified at this point—the ureter, the vascular bundle, and the dome of the bladder. The surgeon should know the exact location of the ureter, because the radical nature of the procedure is dependent upon how much of the anterior parametrium (vesicouterine ligament) is resected. The ureter can then be further dissected cranially to the level of the tunnel, where it crosses the cardinal ligament. The uterine artery is located near a bend or elbow in the ureter, and should then be protected and displaced cranially with Breisky retractors.

The ureter and pedicle of the uterine artery are then retracted cranially, exposing the upper border of the cardinal ligament. The same procedure is repeated on the right side after development of the right pararectal space. Ureteral dissection allows safe resection of the cardinal ligaments (lateral parametria) (Fig. 22.48).

D. *Opening of the Rectouterine Pouch and Resection of the Posterior Parametrium* (Fig. 22.49)

The uterus is retracted upward by an assistant and the posterior peritoneum is opened with scissors. The next step is resection of the posterior parametrium, which requires broad dissection of the rectovaginal space, exposing the full extent of the uterosacral ligaments. A Breisky retractor is introduced into the peritoneal cavity to provide upward traction on the uterus, while another retractor is placed into the left pararectal space. Simultaneously, a forceps-held gauze swab is used to depress the lateral portion of the rectum, distending the left uterosacral ligament. The base of the ligament

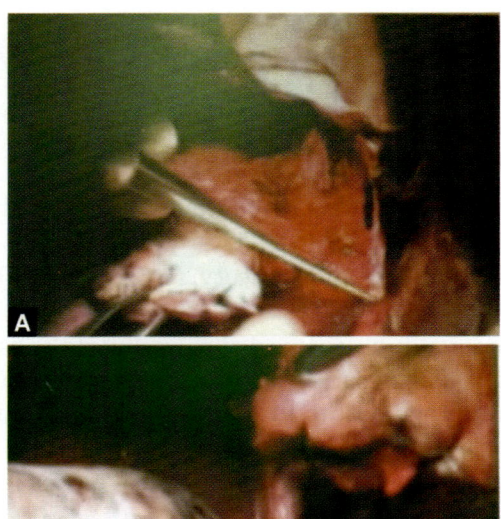

Fig. 22.48: (A) Opening of paravesical space parametrium; (B) Dissection of ureter and resection of anterior parametrium

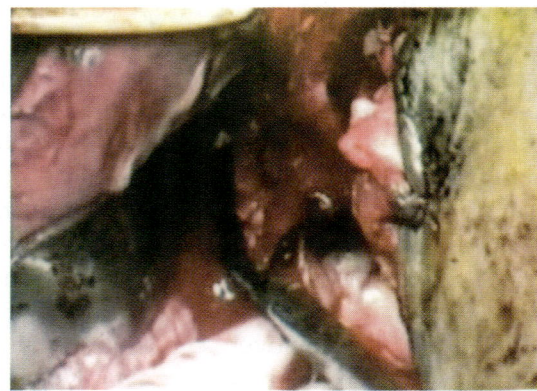

Fig. 22.49: Opening of the rectouterine pouch and resection of the posterior parametrium

is clamped with a slightly curved Z-clamp, cut, and ligated. The same procedure is repeated contralaterally.

E. *Opening of the Anterior Peritoneum and Removal of the Uterus and Adnexae* (Fig. 22.50)

The peritoneum is opened and a Breisky retractor is introduced into the anterior portion of the rectouterine pouch. The index finger of the operator's left hand is advanced under the peritoneal leaf until it reaches the left round ligament, which is clamped, cut, and sutured; this brings the uterus further downward and broadens exposure of the suspensory ligament of the left ovary. The ovaries and Fallopian tubes are removed or preserved depending on patient age. The same

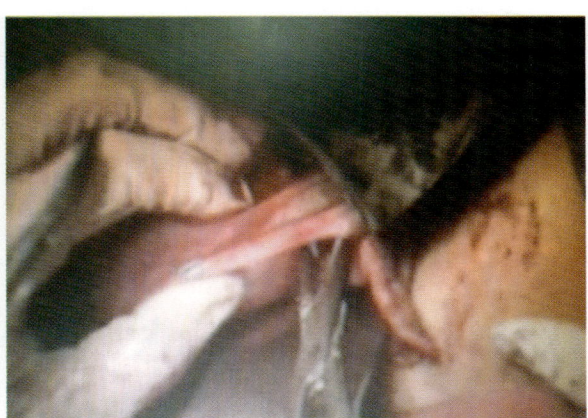

Fig. 22.50: Opening of the anterior peritoneum and removal of the uterus and adnexae

procedure is repeated on the right, again resecting or preserving the adnexa as appropriate.

F. Resection of the Cardinal Ligament (Fig. 22.51)

Adequate resection of the lateral parametrium away from the uterus and near the pelvic wall requires complete exposure of the surgical field with Breisky retractors and lateral traction on the uterus. One retractor is placed in the pararectal fossa while a wider one retracts the bladder and ureter upward. The cardinal ligament and adjacent paravaginal tissues are clamped laterally with a strongly curved Z-clamp. The precise location of clamping in relation to the pelvic wall will depend on the desired radicality of the procedure. Clamping, section, and suture of the right cardinal ligament follow the same sequence; the uterus will then easily deliver through the introitus, attached solely to the infundibulopelvic ligament.

G. Closure of the Vaginal Dome and Schuchardt Incision

The vaginal dome is closed with slow absorption sutures. Finally, the Schuchardt incision is closed in a

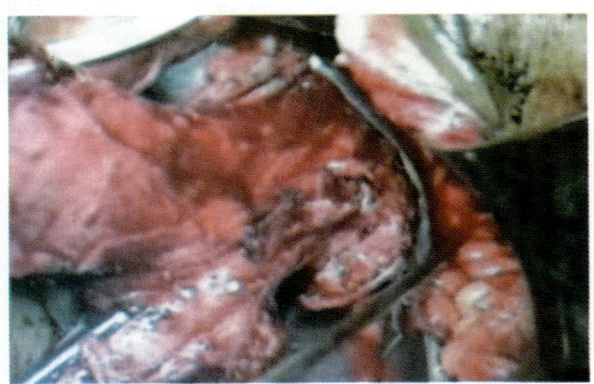

Fig. 22.51: Resection of the cardinal ligament

layered fashion (levator ani muscles, subcutaneous tissue, vaginal mucosa and skin).

Classes of Radical Vaginal Hysterectomy

The term "radical" hysterectomy is used to refer to any procedure in which the uterus is removed with its surrounding connective tissue, the anterior, posterior, and lateral parametria are resected, the uterine artery is ligated at its source, and the distal ureter is mobilized.

Massi et al. suggested three classes of radical vaginal hysterectomy, also according to the amount of vaginal tissue and parametrium removed, namely:

1. *Vaginal hysterectomy (Class I):* The parametria are dissected near the uterus. No ureteral dissection is performed.
   Indications: Recurrent cervical carcinoma in situ, unclear margins after conization/LEEP, selective cases of microinvasive carcinoma (stage IA1).

2. *Schauta-Stoeckel operation (Class II):* The initial stages are similar to those of the classical Schauta-Amreich operation ; however, the ureter is dissected not completely, but only far enough to enable ligation of the uterine artery a few centimeters from the uterus and resection of the proximal portion of the anterior parametrium. The distal half of the posterior parametrium is left intact, whereas resection of the lateral parametrium is identical to that performed in class III surgery (near the pelvic wall).
   Indications: Invasive stage IA2 and IB cervical tumors <2 cm in size.

3. *Schauta-Amreich surgery (Class III).*
   Indications: Alternative to the Wertheim/Meigs radical abdominal hysterectomy. Schauta's operation is chiefly indicated in obese or high-risk patients with stage IB or IIA cervical cancer. However, augmentation of this procedure with extraperitoneal or laparoscopic pelvic lymphadenectomy allows safe expansion of these indications to include all operable cases of cervical cancer.

   Available options for lymphadenectomy (Mitra vs. laparoscopic)→Pelvic lymphadenectomy may be performed by various approaches: Intraperitoneal abdominal (Wertheim/Meigs), extraperitoneal abdominal (Mitra), or laparoscopically. The advantages of laparoscopy include the absence of scars on the lower abdomen, the lower rate of surgical site complications.

Complications

A. The mortality rate of radical vaginal hysterectomy ranges from 0.27 to 2.5%.
B. Morbidity is related to the underlying indication for the procedure, and includes:

1. Urinary and bowel complications (injury, fistulas, and infection). The main urinary tract complication is bladder atony; all patients experience this adverse effect to some extent after radical vaginal surgery. The incidence of major bladder atony may exceed 50%.
2. Ureteral dilatation occurs in 87% of patients in the first postoperative week. In most cases, the dilatation has resolved and ultrasonographic assessment of the urinary tract is within normal limits on the sixth postoperative week. Peristalsis along the distal ureter returns to normal within 1 month of the procedure.
3. The incidence of vesicovaginal, ureterovaginal, and rectovaginal fistula is 2.0%, 3.0%, and 0.7%, respectively.
4. Other complications include surgical site infection of the Schuchardt incision, dehiscence of the vaginal vault, and, on rare occasions, bowel evisceration.

III. Mitra's Operation

Dr. Subodh Mitra (1896-1961) was an eminent obstetrician and gynecologist in India. He is the founder of the "Mitra operation" for cervical cancer. Dr. Mitra developed a technique in the surgery of cervical cancer. His technique was well appreciated world over. The technique developed by Dr. S. Mitra for cancer cervix operation, namely *Extended Radical Vaginal Hysterectomy with Extraperitoneal Lymphadenectomy*, was officially announced in British, American and German gynecological conferences. He demonstrated this technique in Vienna in 1952.

Mitra's Opration Procedure

This is performed in two stages: Extraperitoneal abdominal approach for pelvic lymphadenectomy and vaginal approach for radical vaginal hysterectomy.

I. *Extraperitoneal Lymphadenectomy*

The lateral pelvic space is approached extraperitoneally by using two separate inguinal incisions one on each side. The incision extends downwards and medially from a point at a junction of medial two-thirds and lateral one-third of spinoumbilical line. The incision extends below at the pubic tubercle (Fig. 22.52).

The subcutaneous tissues are excised and the external oblique aponeurosis is excised along the same line up to the superficial inguinal ring. The inguinal canal is opened and the conjoined tendon formed by the internal oblique and the transversus abdominis muscles

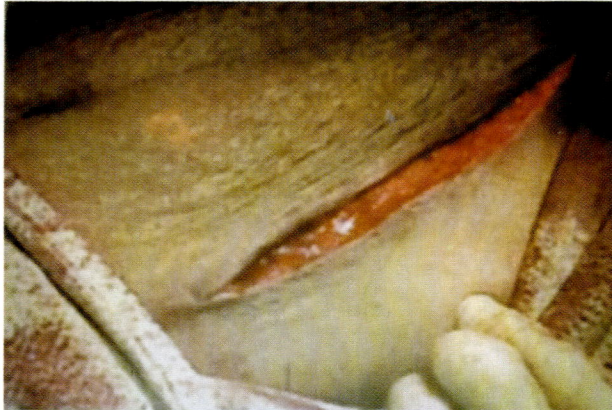

Fig. 22.52: The inguinal incision

is exposed. A tunnel is made by introducing a finger below the conjoined tendon to separate the muscles from the underlying peritoneum. The muscles are cut along the line of incisions (Fig. 22.53).

The peritoneum is gently retracted from the pelvic sidewalls exposing the retroperitoneal space and completed till the full extent of the incison. The round ligament is found as a band entering the inguinal canal after piercing the peritoneum. The round ligament is cut between clamps and ligated. The peritoneum is pushed medially till the common iliac vessels with its bifurcation into external and internal iliac vessels are exposed. The paravesical and pararectal spaces are dissected out. The pelvic lymph node dissection is started by incising the lymphoareolar tissues around the external iliac artery to remove the lateral and medial chains of external iliac lymph nodes. All the lymphatic tissues are removed along the course of the vessels on both sides. The internal iliac nodes are seen at the bifurcation of the common iliac artery and are removed. The common iliac nodes are usually found towards the lateral and posterior aspect of the common iliac artery and are removed (Fig. 22.54).

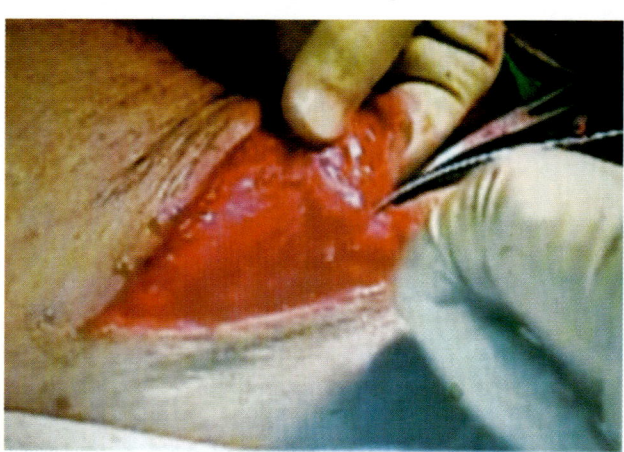

Fig. 22.53: Internal oblique, transversus abdominis muscles are cut

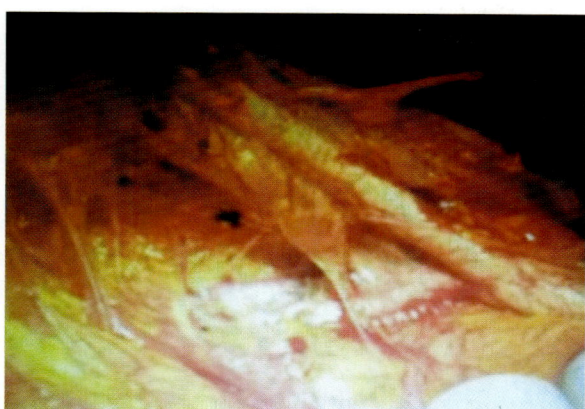

Fig. 22.54: External and internal iliac vessels are debrided of lymphatic tissues

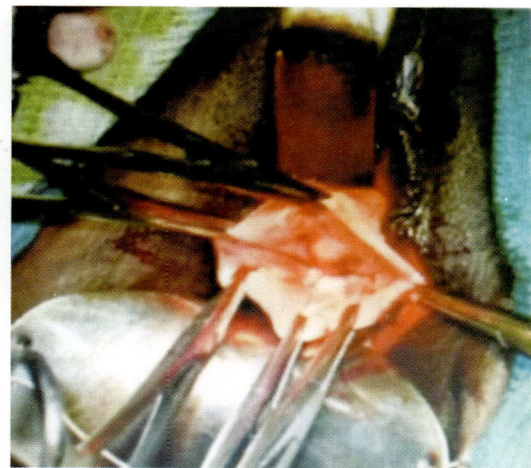

Fig. 22.55: Vaginal cuff formed by holding vaginal flap with Kocher's forceps

The uterine artery is seen arising from the anterior division of the internal iliac artery as a tortuous vessel and is cut and ligated at its origin. The distal part of the artery is dissected further medially till the ureteric crossing is reached and the artery forms the roof of the tunnel, the vesicouterine ligament. The lower part of the ureter is exposed and rest of the dissection is done during the vaginal part of the surgery.

The ovarian vessels are seen in the retracted peritoneal flap and running parallel and above the ureter. The vascular pedicles are cut and ligated.

Afetr confirming proper hemostasis, abdomen is closed in layers. The entire procedure is repeated on the other side.

II. *Vaginal Approach for Radical Hysterectomy*

The patient is placed in lithotomy position. The adequate vaginal exposure is obtained by adequate posterior and anterior retraction with Auvard's speculum and anterior vaginal retractor respectively and the Schuchardt's incision on the perineum.

The vaginal cuff is developed by grasping the mucosa overlying the cervix circumferentially with six long Kocher's clamps producing a circular fold just below the part of the vagina that is to be excised. The cuff should be adequate to cover the cervical growth. A deep circular incision is made through the vagina and the incision is extended into the vesicovaginal space anteriorly, rectovaginal space posteriorly and the paravaginal space laterally. The vaginal flap is dissected down and closed over the cervical growth using series of figure of eight sutures to be used for traction (Fig. 22.55).

The bladder is dissected up from the vagina, cervix and the anterior part of the uterus by sharp dissection. The dissection continues till the glistening uterovesical fold of peritoneum is visible. The bladder is also mobilized from the sides and the anterior surface of Mackenrodt's ligament to create paravesical fossa (Fig. 22.56).

The bladder pillars (vesicouterine ligaments) are clearly exposed between the uterovesical space medially and the paravesical space laterally. The vesicouterine ligment is firmly attached to the Mackenrodt's ligament with the ureter as its content felt through fingers. The layers of the ligament is gradually dissected from the lateral side till the ureteric tunnel is opened and ureter is exposed. The ureter is displaced laterally and upwards. This will facilitate adequate removal of parametrium. The uterine vessels seen adherent to the uterus and are brought down.

The posterior pouch of Douglas is opened and rectovaginal and pararectal space is formed. The uterus is retracted up and anterior to make the uterosacrals prominent and the ligaments are divided as posteriorly as possible up to the level of the Mackenrodt's ligaments.

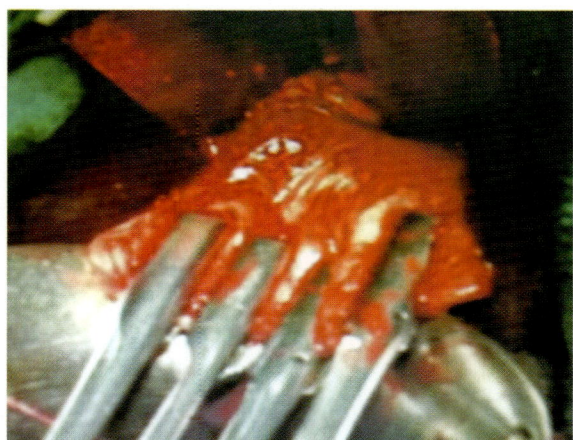

Fig. 22.56: Bladder dissected up from cervix and vagina

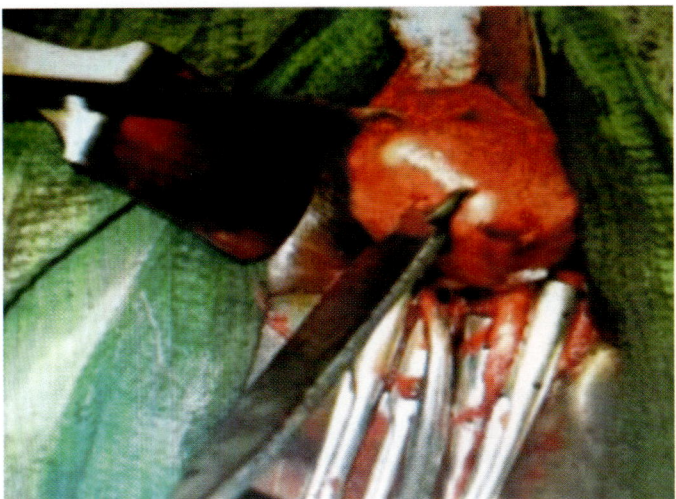

Fig. 22.57: Uterus is delivered through vagina

The uterus is now brought down by traction on the vaginal cuff and uterovesical fold is cut open. The whole of the adnexal structures are gradually delivered releasing the ovarian stump from the infundibulopelvic ligament (Fig. 22.57). The uterus is now attached to the pelvic wall by Mackenrodt's ligaments which are cut as lateral as possible. The uterus with adnexae is now removed and sent for histology. The peritoneum and the vaginal opening is closed by interrupted stitches.

Conclusion

Radical hysterectomy with bilateral pelvic lymphadenectomy, therefore, is the operation of choice in early stage carcinoma cervix and the route of radical hysterectomy is the surgeon's choice based on patients profile and the surgeon's expertise.

Endoscopy Procedures

23

Hysteroscopy is the process of viewing and operating in the endometrial cavity from a transcervical approach. The basic hysteroscope is a long, narrow telescope connected to a light source to illuminate the area to be visualized. With a patient in the lithotomy position, the cervix is visualized by placing a speculum in the vagina. The distal end of the telescope is passed into a dilated cervical canal, and, under direct visualization, the instrument is advanced into the uterine cavity. A camera is commonly attached to the proximal end of the hysteroscope to broadcast the image on to a large video screen. Hysteroscopy is a minimally invasive intervention that can be used to diagnose and treat many intrauterine and endocervical problems. Given their safety and efficacy, diagnostic and operative hysteroscopy have become modern standard form of care in gynecologic practice.

Equipment

Hysteroscopes (Fig. 23.1)

The telescope consists of three parts—the eyepiece, the barrel, and the objective lens. The focal length and angle

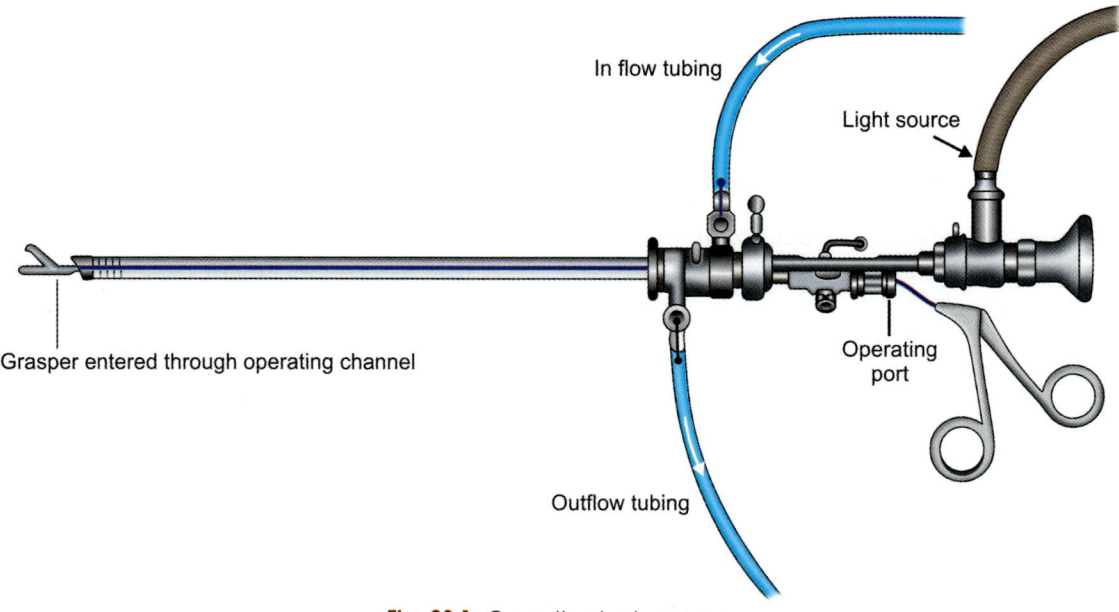

Fig. 23.1: Operative hysteroscope

of the distal tip of the instrument are important for visualization.

Angle options include 0°, 12°, 15°, 25°, 30°, and 70°. A 0° hysteroscope provides a panoramic view, whereas an angled one might improve the view of the ostia in an abnormally shaped cavity.

Hysteroscopes are available in different styles, including rigid and flexible hysteroscopes, contact hysteroscopes, and microcolpohysteroscopes. The diameter of each instrument varies. The requirement of a sheath for input-outflow of distention media increases the size of the hysteroscope.

Rigid Hysteroscopes

Rigid hysteroscopes are the most commonly used instruments. Their wide range of diameters allows for in-office and complex operating-room procedures. Of the narrow options (3–5 mm in diameter), the 4 mm scope offers the sharpest and clearest view. It accommodates surgical instruments and is small enough to require minimal cervical dilatation and can be done under paracervical block anesthesia.

Rigid scopes larger than 5 mm in diameter (commonly 8–10 mm) require increased cervical dilatation for insertion and therefore are mostly used in the operating room with intravenous (IV) sedation or general anesthesia. Large instruments include an outer sheath to introduce and remove media and to provide ports to accommodate large and varied surgical instruments.

Flexible Hysteroscopes

The flexible hysteroscope is most commonly used for office hysteroscopy. It is notable for its flexibility, with a tip that deflects over a range of 120–160°. Its most appropriate use is to accommodate the irregularly shaped uterus and to navigate around intrauterine lesions. It is also used for diagnostic and operative procedures.

During insertion, the flexible contour accommodates to the cervix more easily than does a rigid scope of a similarly small diameter. The view was initially described as having a ground-glass quality, which was markedly less desirable than the view obtained with rigid scopes. New, digitally enhanced scopes now offer similar image quality to a rigid hysteroscope lens.

Light Source

Each hysteroscope is attached to an internal or external light source for illumination at the distal tip. Energy sources include tungsten, metal halide, and xenon. A xenon light source with a liquid cable is considered the superior option.

Surgical Instruments

Surgical instruments are available in both rigid and flexible forms to be inserted through the operating channels of the scopes.

Examples of surgical instruments and their uses are listed below:

- Scissors — to incise a septum, excise a polyp, or lyse synechiae.
- Biopsy forceps—to perform directed biopsy for pathologic review.
- Grasping instruments—to remove foreign bodies.
- Roller ball, barrel, or ellipsoid with resectoscope—to perform endometrial ablation and/or desiccation.
- Loop electrode—to resect a fibroid or polyp or endometrium.
- Scalpel—to cut or coagulate tissue, with high power density at its tip.
- Vaporizing electrodes—to destroy endometrial polyps, fibroids, intrauterine adhesions, and septa; also used for endometrial ablation.
- Morcellator—to cut and remove endometrial polyps or fibroids. It requires cervical dilatation up to 9 mm.

Energy Sources and Uses

Monopolar and bipolar electricity, as well as laser energy, all have used in hysteroscopy.

Monopolar Cautery

The resectoscope is a specialized instrument often used with a monopolar, double-armed electrode and a trigger device for use in hypotonic, nonconductive media, such as glycine. It cuts and coagulates tissue by means of contact desiccation with resistive heating. The depth of thermal damage is based on several factors like endometrial thickness, duration of contact during motion and power setting.

A thin electrode can cut tissue, whereas one with a large surface area, such as a ball or barrel, is best suited for coagulation.

Bipolar Cautery

The Versa Point system uses bipolar circuit for electrosurgery, which can be performed in isotonic conductive media. This system includes a spring tip for hemostatic vaporization of large areas, a ball tip for precise vaporization, and a twizzle tip for hemostatic resection and morcellation of tissue.

Laser Techniques

Several fiberoptic lasers are available for gynecologic use, including potassium-titanyl-phosphate (KTP), argon, and Nd:YAG lasers. They all have different wavelengths, though the KTP and argon lasers have similar properties.

Media

The use of media is critical for panoramic inspection of the uterine cavity. The medium opens the potential space of the otherwise narrow uterine cavity. Intrauterine pressures needed to adequately view the endometrium are proportional to the muscle tone and thickness of the uterus. The refractive index of each medium affects magnification and visualization of the endometrium.

Gases

Carbon dioxide (CO_2) is rapidly absorbed and easily cleared from the body by respiration. The refractory index of CO_2 is 1.0, which allows for excellent clarity and widens the field of view at low magnification. The gas easily flows through narrow channels in small-diameter scopes, making it useful for office-based diagnostic hysteroscopy.

With CO_2, a hysteroscopic insufflator is required to regulate flow and limit maximal intrauterine pressure. A flow rate to 40–60 mL/min at a maximum pressure of 100 mm Hg is generally accepted as safe. Pressures and rates higher than this can result in cardiac arrhythmias, embolism, and arrest.

Fluids

The advantage of fluid over gas is the symmetric distention of the uterus with fluid and its effective ability to flush blood, mucus, bubbles, and small tissue fragments out of the visual field. Both low-viscosity and high-viscosity fluid media can be used for distention. A pressure of 75 mm Hg is usually adequate for uterine distention; rarely is more than 100 mm Hg required, and pressures higher than this can increase the risk of intravasation of medium.

Various delivery systems are designed to suit the many media used for uterine distention and to accurately record volumes of inflow and outflow. This recording is important because fluid can leave the uterus by means of intended efflux systems, cervical or tubal leakage, or intravasation. Preventing excess absorption of hypotonic fluids is essential for patient safety. Hanging, gravity-fed containers to deliver low-viscosity fluids can be raised or compressed with a cuff;

however, these can be unreliable in estimating intrauterine pressures. Media then usually flow into the uterine cavity through an inner sheath around the hysteroscope. A perforated outer sheath is used for collection or efflux of media. This design creates laminar flow, which keeps the visual field clear.

There are many new, sophisticated efflux mechanisms which have been designed to improve the clearance of both blood and particulate matter from the operating space. Closed systems actively return fluid to a pump reservoir, whereas open systems allow free flow of the medium out the cervix into a collection bag for volume monitoring.

0.9% sodium chloride solution and lactated Ringer solution: Normal sodium chloride solution and lactated ringer solution are isotonic, conductive, low-viscosity fluids that can be used for diagnostic hysteroscopy and for limited operative procedures. Surgical procedures using mechanical, laser, monopolar (only with the ERA sleeve) and bipolar energy (Versa Point system) are safe.

Two major disadvantages associated with these solutions include (1) their miscibility with blood, which obscures visibility with bleeding, leading to the need for increased volumes to clear the operative field, and (2) their excellent conductivity, which precludes procedures that use standard monopolar electrosurgery.

5% mannitol, 3% sorbitol, and 1.5% glycine: These hypotonic, nonconductive, low-viscosity fluids improve visualization when bleeding occurs. They can be used in diagnostic as well as operative hysteroscopy. All impose a risk of volume overload and hyponatremia from intravascular absorption (particularly >2 L). Therefore, careful fluid monitoring is required during their use. When intravasation of 5% mannitol occurs, it stays in the extracellular compartment; treatment of this condition is discontinuing the procedure and administering diuretics. 3% sorbitol is broken down into fructose and glucose and, therefore, has an added risk of hyperglycemia when absorbed in excess. 1.5% glycine should be used with caution in patients with impaired hepatic function because glycine is metabolized to ammonia.

Dextran 70: Dextran 70 is a nonelectrolytic, nonconductive fluid that can be used in all types of procedures. It is immiscible with blood and minimally leaks through the cervix and tubes, allowing for excellent visibility during surgical procedures. It is monitored to prevent absorption of more than 500 mL to avoid fluid overload. With each 100 mL of Dextran 70 absorbed, the intravascular volume increases by

800 mL. Allergic reactions and anaphylaxis, fluid overload, disseminated intravascular coagulopathy, and destruction of instruments are adverse effects of this medium for which it has become out of favor now.

History of the Procedure

The development of hysteroscopy is rooted in the work of Pantaleoni, who first reported uterine endoscopy in 1869. However, at that time, instrumentation was elementary, and expansion of the uterine cavity was insufficient. In 1925, Rubin first used CO_2 to distend the uterus.

Hysteroscopy did not become popular until the 1970s, when technology afforded more practical and usable instruments than before. The use of liquid distention media became routine by the 1980s. Initially used by urologists for transurethral resection of the prostate, the resectoscope was modified for hysteroscopic procedures, allowing for resection of intrauterine pathology with monopolar cautery. By the mid-1980s, hysteroscopic procedures had nearly replaced dilatation and curettage (D&C) for diagnosing intrauterine pathology.

Indications

Abnormal Uterine Bleeding

Hysteroscopy allows direct visualization and make a diagnosis of intrauterine abnormalities, benign lesions, premalignant and malignant pathology and it often offers an opportunity for simultaneous treatment.

Uterine sampling can now be done by endometrial biopsy under direct visualization with hysteroscopy. Evaluation of the uterine cavity with sonohysterography or diagnostic hysteroscopy is up to 88% effective in identifying polyps and submucosal fibroids.

For patients with AUB for whom fertility is not an issue, and endometrial atypia or malignancy is ruled out, endometrial ablation has become an acceptable alternative to hysterectomy and ablation for a benign disorder results in amenorrhea in approximately 30% of patients though reoperation rates after endometrial ablation have been reported to be as high as 38% at 5 years.

Infertility

Hysteroscopy is not part of the routine workup for infertility, but when compared with hysterosalpingography, hysteroscopy is equivalent for evaluating the uterine cavity, and it increases accuracy in diagnosing the cause of intrauterine filling defects. In unexplained infertility, hysteroscopy may be performed simultaneously with laparoscopy to evaluate the uterine cavity and cervix for any evidence of synechia, endometrial preparation for implantation (Fig. 23.2).

Intracavitary lesions are implicated as causes of infertility, and their removal may increase fertility. Overall, pregnancy rates of 50–78% in previously infertile women have been reported after hysteroscopic polypectomy. The effect of hysteroscopic polypectomy on IVF also remains unclear. In general, hysteroscopic removal of lesions <2 cm does not adversely affect an IVF cycle.

The incidence of myomas in women without another obvious etiology for infertility is small, estimated to be 1–2.4%. The effect of myomas on reproduction is not definitive but it is generally accepted that fibroids causing distortion of the endometrial cavity may adversely influence fertility. Surgical management with hysteroscopic myomectomy has been reported to yield pregnancy rates of around 45% in infertile women. For patients with recurrent miscarriage and intracavitary fibroids, surgery increases rates of viable pregnancy outcomes.

Intrauterine Adhesions

The intrauterine adhesions (IUA) are often associated with amenorrhea or infertility. The prevalence rate of IUAs in the general population is 1.5%, with adhesions noted in up to 30% of women undergoing hysteroscopy following 3 or more spontaneous abortions treated with dilatation and curettage. Hysteroscopy is the gold standard used to diagnose and treat these adhesions. Filmy adhesions are often lysed by distention alone, whereas the dense adhesions often require cutting or excision with blunt, sharp, electrocautery, or laser techniques.

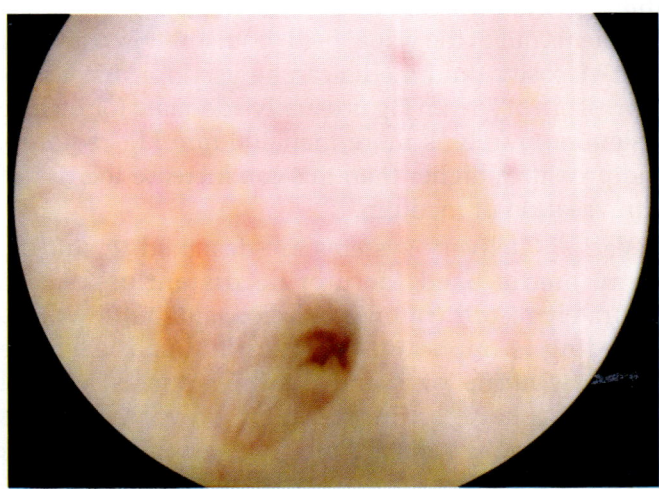

Fig. 23.2: Cornual opening of tube

In case of abnormal bleeding, hysteroscopic treatment results in 88–98% return to normal menstrual cycles. If no other infertility issues are present, 75% of those with mild disease and 30% with severe adhesions achieve normal pregnancy. But conception rates in women with recurrence of adhesions after initial hysteroscopic adhesiolysis have been found to be significantly lower. Hysteroscopic treatment may also increase the risk of abnormal placentation in the resulting pregnancy (e.g. accreta, percreta, increta, previa).

Müllerian Anomalies

Approximately 1–2% of all women, 4% of infertile women, and 10–15% of patients with recurrent miscarriage have müllerian anomalies. These anomalies range from didelphys to müllerian agenesis. Patients with a bicornuate uterus have a >50% live birth rate compared with those with a uterine septum, who have a <30% live birth rate. Patients with *in utero* DES exposure are likely to have a T-shaped uterus with pretubal bulges, lower uterine segment dilatation, and a small and irregular cavity with borders resembling adhesions. Hysteroscopy can be used to confirm but not always to treat these findings.

Septate uterus is the most common structural uterine anomaly, accounting for 35% of anomalies, and is associated with the highest incidence of reproductive failure. Division of uterine septum is now most commonly performed via a hysteroscopic approach. Live birth rates after excision of septum is as high as 80% although 20% may have dysmenorrhea after surgery. Significant improvements are seen in pregnancy outcomes following hysteroscopic metroplasty in women with recurrent miscarriage. Pregnancy rates increase from 3% prior to surgery to approximately 80% after hysteroscopic correction with a significant decrease in miscarriage rates. Metroplasty should also be considered for women who plan to undergo IVF.

Polyps and Fibroids (Fig. 23.3)

Polyps and submucosal fibroids can be definitively diagnosed and effectively treated with hysteroscopy with 87–94% sensitivity and 92–95% specificity. When AUB is present, polypectomy can successfully alleviate symptoms in 75–100% of cases. Hysteroscopy can successfully remove fibroids in 85–95% of cases, with additional surgery required in approximately 5–15%.

The advantages of hysteroscopic resection are numerous and include avoiding laparotomy, uterine incision, and prolonged hospital stays. The uterine thinning induced by use of GnRHa or danazole can sometimes be useful in making the fibroid submucus and more approachable to hysteroscopic myomectomy. Recently hysteroscopic morcellation is also available to reduce the size of the myoma hysteroscopically.

In patients desiring to maintain fertility, hysteroscopic myomectomy is a reasonable option and minimal cauterization should be used to decrease damage to otherwise healthy endometrium.

Proximal Tubal Obstruction

This diagnosis is difficult to make and is most often suggested by the failure of contrast to enter the fallopian tube on HSG. It may be due to infection, intraluminal debris, salpingitis isthmica nodosum, or endometriosis. Many cases may simply be due to spasm. Up to 85% of occlusions can be treated with cannulation, but reocclusion occurs in approximately one-third of cases. Tubal perforation is rare but can occur leading to further tubal complication.

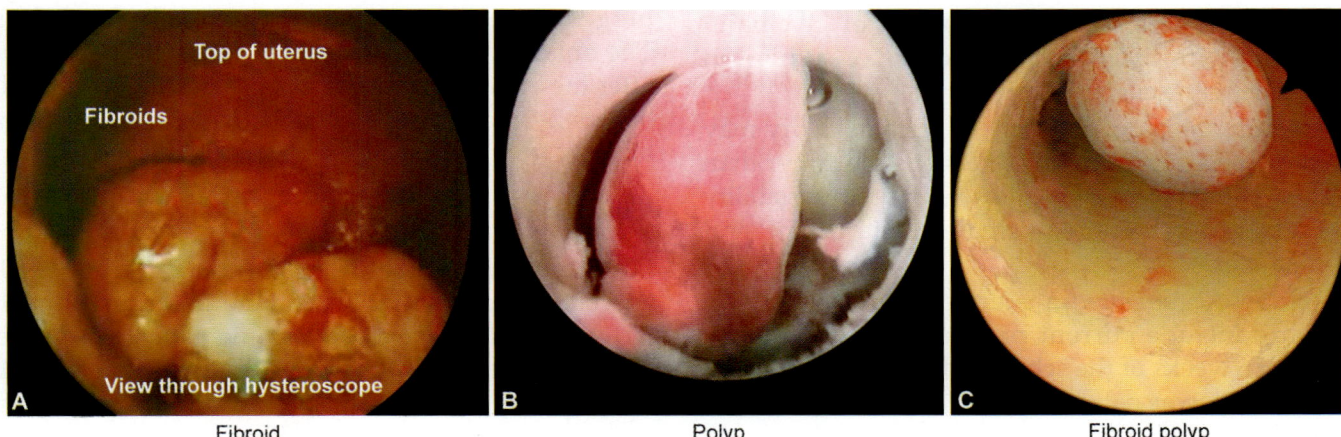

| Fibroid | Polyp | Fibroid polyp |

Fig. 23.3: Fibroid and polyp in uterine cavity

Intrauterine Devices

Hysteroscopy can be applied to remove an intrauterine device (IUD) under direct visualization after sonography-guided retrieval fails.

Relevant Anatomy

For any hysteroscopic procedure, the surgeon must understand the thickness of the uterine wall. Table 23.1 lists the wall thicknesses for each area of the uterus. Remember that the uterus is longer and thicker in reproductive-aged women than in postmenopausal women.

Table 23.1: Thickness of the uterine wall

Location	Mean (mm)	Range (mm)
Anterior wall	22.5	17–25
Posterior wall	21	15–25
Fundus	19.5	15–22
Isthmus	10	8–12
Corpus	5.5	4–7

Contraindications

In general, hysteroscopy is avoided in patients with the following findings:

- Active cervical or uterine infection
- A large uterine cavity, i.e. longer than 10 cm in length (clinically similar to a 12 wk pregnant uterus)
- Severe medical conditions precluding surgery
- Pregnancy

Concerns and contraindications for hysteroscopy depend on the procedure planned.

a. For endometrial ablation, contraindications are desire for future fertility, atypical endometrial hyperplasia or endometrial cancer, and undiagnosed abnormal bleeding.

b. For polypectomy and myomectomy, contraindications are transmural lesions, use of hypotonic media in patients with hyponatremia, use of glycine in patients with liver disease, and use of sorbitol in patients with severe diabetes.

c. If the uterus is deeper than 12 cm, the cavity may not distend appropriately. If lesions are larger than 2 cm, patients must be counseled about possibility of a staged procedure, increased fluid deficit, and blood loss.

d. Contraindications to transcervical sterilization with Essure include current pregnancy or pregnancy within 6 weeks of the scheduled procedure, current or recent lower pelvic infection, allergy to contrast, hypersensitivity to nickel, or tubal occlusion or uterine abnormalities.

Preoperative Details

Appropriate surgical management always begins with accurate history taking, physical examination, and careful workup of the suspected problem. In preparation for hysteroscopic procedures, the following considerations may be useful.

Antibiotic Prophylaxis

For hysteroscopy, prophylactic antibiotics are not indicated unless the patient has clinically significant valvular disease or a history of tubal occlusion due to pelvic inflammatory disease.

Cervical Stenosis

In patients with known cervical stenosis or tortuous cervical canals, preoperative vaginal or oral misoprostol, or intraoperative vasopressin 1% administered paracervically may be used to assist in cervical dilatation. This increases the ease of dilatation, reduces the need for mechanical cervical dilatation, and lowers the rate of cervical laceration.

Endometrial Preparation for Ablation

Before ablation procedures are performed, the administration of a GnRH agonist in the luteal phase of the previous menstrual cycle in ovulating women improves visibility and provides a smooth, pale, hypovascular surface 3–4 weeks later. These changes make the procedure easier to perform and improve its success rate.

For those who do not want a GnRH agonist, the simultaneous use of a GnRH antagonist with progesterone at any point in the menstrual cycle creates a similar surface with fewer adverse effects.

A single 3 mg dose of cetrorelix is administered subcutaneously every 4 days along with medroxyprogesterone acetate 10 mg taken orally for 5 days. The ablation procedure is then typically performed after the patient completes her menses, which usually begins 2–3 days after she takes the last progesterone tablet.

Fibroids

For large submucosal fibroids, the use of a GnRH agonist decreases uterine volume by approximately 30%. It may decrease blood loss and allow for an easier and more complete resection, though the change in tissue quality may make the procedure technically more difficult. There is currently no consensus on their use prior to hysteroscopic myomectomy.

Large Uterus

During ultrasonography or sonohysterogram, measurements of the uterine dimensions are helpful. In particular, a uterus longer than 10 cm makes the case difficult because of the length of the hysteroscope (typically 35 cm) since it must traverse the length of the uterus, cervix, and vagina while maintaining a position outside the introitus with enough distance to attach the camera and manipulate the fluid inflow-outflow valves and the surgical instruments. Also, maintaining intrauterine pressures with large cavities is more difficult than with small cavities.

Intraoperative Details

Anesthesia

The type of anesthesia used depends on the procedure, the patient's level of anxiety, and the anesthesiologist's expertise. Simple diagnostic procedures can be completed without anesthesia, with a paracervical block alone, or with mild sedation on day care basis. For extensive procedures, general or regional anesthesia is indicated. If electrosurgery is to be performed, sufficient anesthesia must be given to ensure that the patient does not move with uterine stimulation because of the risk of uterine perforation and intraperitoneal injury.

Positioning

The patient is placed in the dorsal lithotomy position then prepared and draped in a sterile manner. Unless a laparoscopy is also planned, the patient's thighs should be positioned at a 90° angle to the pelvis to create enough space for the surgeon to manipulate the hysteroscope. The patient's perineum should be just past the edge of the table, with the coccyx and sacrum well supported on the flat surface of the table. The patient's legs should be secured in the leg stirrups to avoid any abrupt movements, which can cause nerve or muscle injury to the patient or potential injury to the surgeon. The surgeon should be seated with the operative field and hysteroscope at the level of his or her abdomen. If it is positioned higher, the surgeon's shoulders become fatigued, and, if it is positioned lower, the instrument is hard to maneuver and is likely to become contaminated.

Hemostasis

Attempts are to be made to reduce blood loss and fluid deficits during surgery. Use of cold (5°C) distention medium causes vasoconstriction and reduces blood loss and distention fluid deficits. However, the patient's core body temperature substantially decreases and may interfere with the anesthesia process. Vasopressin in dilute solution (i.e. 1%) can be injected paracervically to help constrict the cervical and lower uterine branches of the uterine artery and its collaterals, reducing blood loss and fluid deficits.

Placing the Hysteroscope

a. *Bladder catheterization:* The bladder may need to be emptied with a straight, red rubber catheter by using sterile technique.

b. *Examination under anesthesia:* Bimanual examination should always be performed before the endocervix and uterus are dilated and entered. This examination aids the surgeon in assessing angles and preventing perforation.

c. *Cervical dilatation:* Using the standard approach, the cervix is manually dilated with metal dilators to the same diameter as the outer diameter of the outer sheath of the hysteroscope. A tenaculum is placed on the anterior lip of the cervix while dilating to help straighten the cervix and uterus. However, office hysteroscope 2.5 mm do not need dilatation.

d. *Visualization of the uterine cavity:* After the cervix is dilated, the hysteroscope is inserted into the endocervical canal and advanced into the uterine cavity (with the distention medium flowing) under direct visualization to limit the risk of perforation. The tenaculum on the cervix is left in place to help in manipulating the uterus, and the vaginal speculum is removed to increase maneuverability of the hysteroscope. If the cervix is dilated too much and fluid is leaking extensively, a purse-string suture can be placed around the cervix using 0-Vicryl to limit this leakage. The suture should be removed at the end of the procedure.

Alternatively, a **vaginoscopic approach** has also been defined. Distention media is introduced into the vagina at the same pressure used for dilatation of the uterine cavity (around 30–40 mm) to distend the vaginal cavity. The hysteroscope is then used to visualize the cervix and facilitate its entry into the cervical canal. The use of a speculum and tenaculum is not needed with this approach.

Techniques

Procedures are individually described below with regard to the type and width of the hysteroscope, the type of medium, and the use of surgical instrumentation and energy sources, depending on the indications and desired outcomes.

Diagnostic Hysteroscopy

A small 5 or 7 mm hysteroscope can be used with isotonic sodium chloride distention medium. A 30° scope is preferable to clearly visualize the tubal ostia. The ability to introduce small surgical instruments through an operating channel is optimal. Office procedures can be performed with 2.5 to 3 mm flexible or rigid hysteroscopes that are attached to isotonic sodium chloride solution in a bag or 30 mL syringe. Some models have a small operating channel through which a thin-wired biopsy forceps can be placed. This channel is enough to sample suspected areas or to remove small polyps.

Endometrial Ablation

First-generation endometrial ablation using the roller-ball or roller-barrel method, resection method, and laser method are described below.

The Roller-ball or Roller-barrel Method

- The cervix must typically be dilated to 7–9 mm depending on the resectoscope used. A 12° scope is suggested because it provides a panoramic view of the uterine cavity. A coagulation mode of 50–100 watts is used.
- A roller barrel improves the uniformity of contact with the endometrium compared with the roller ball, but it may inadequately ablate the cornua and fundus. A 2 mm roller ball is more effective than a 4 mm ball because it has more current density for a given power level.
- On occasion, the roller ball or barrel may become coated with tissue, and it may have to be removed and cleaned with a sterile gauze. If the endometrium is not thinned, resection may be preferred. The uterine cornua and tubal angles are ablated first because of their difficulty. Starting at the 9 o'clock position, the lateral and anterior walls are ablated next because blood, debris, and bubbles rise, making later ablation attempts more difficult. The posterior wall is then ablated by continuing in a clockwise fashion. Ablation is not repeated over areas that have already been treated because of the risk of uterine perforation.

The Resection Method

The cervix is typically dilated to the size of the resectoscope. A blended current of 70–100 watts is preferred. A 5 or 7 mm loop electrode is used and extended. The electrode is allowed to return passively at 1.0–1.5 mm/s. A methodical approach should be used, with a plan to uniformly continue around the cavity. The same place is not resected twice. The angles of the tubal ostia are difficult to ablate with the loop electrode, so a small rollerball is preferable. Depending on the system used, the strips of resected tissue may require removal intermittently with polyp forceps. All tissue is sent to the pathologist for histologic evaluation.

The Laser Method

- The neodymium-yttrium-aluminium-garnet laser (Nd:YAG laser) can be used for ablation. Laser energy is delivered to the tissues via a fiber inserted through an operating hysteroscope. The laser energy provides a tissue penetration of 5–6 mm. Two techniques are commonly described.
- The dragging technique requires the laser fiber to be in constant contact with the endometrium, which ultimately results in vaporization of the tissue.
- Alternatively, coagulation can be induced with the blanching technique in which the fiber does not come in direct contact with the endometrium. Both techniques require constant motion to minimize risk of perforation. Choice of distention media includes normal saline or Dextran 70.

Second-generation Endometrial Ablation, Hydrothermal Method

The HydroThermAblator System is the second generation ablation device that uses direct visualization with the hysteroscope. A single-use 3 mm hysteroscope coated with polycarbonate is inserted into the endometrial cavity. Saline is instilled at low intrauterine pressures of < 45 mm Hg and then heated to 90°C. This low pressure is used to prevent flow of heated saline through the fallopian tubes. After the treatment is complete, cool saline is used to replace the heated saline prior to removal of the device from the cavity. Endomyometrial necrosis to a depth of 2–4 mm is achieved after 10 minutes of treatment. The endometrial cavity is uniformly ablated with this method, including both cornua.

Hysteroscopic Myomectomy for Submucosal Fibroids

This include the resectoscope, scissors, the laser, and the morcellator. Some gynecologists inject vasopressin into the cervical stroma before the procedure to decrease blood loss and surgical time.

Resection

- This is similar to resection of the endometrium, but the resectoscopic method results in resection of only the fibroid rather than the surface layer of endometrium. The fibroid can be resected to the level of only the endometrium. After some is removed, any remaining intramural portion of the fibroid may begin to invert into the endometrial cavity. Surgeons should apply their skill and experience to estimate how many passes they will continue to resect while aiming to avoid uterine perforation. The loop can often be used to separate the fibroid from the pseudocapsule, often called cold-loop resection, facilitating its removal and helping to identify normal myometrium and endometrium to avoid coagulation, especially in young women desiring to conceive.

- For resection of a submucosal fibroid, high cutting power is required. Using the cutting mode at 80–100 watts provides clean cuts through the fibroid and facilitates a rapid technique. Power settings lower than this do not allow for easy resection and only delay completion of the procedure, with resulting fluid deficits.
- Resectoscopes historically relied on monopolar currents to cut tissue and thus require the use of hypotonic electrolyte-free distention media like Glycin. Strict fluid monitoring is an obvious need. Fortunately, bipolar resectoscopes are now in use.
- Obstructed visualization due to floating tissue fragments during resection can prove difficult and may necessitate catching the loose tissue with the loop electrode or small ovum forceps, removing the hysteroscope to grab the tissue, followed by reintroduction of the scope. To address this problem, the Bipolar Chip E-Vac System has been introduced. The system uses a traditional resectoscope with an automatic chip aspirator and can be used with monopolar or bipolar current to aspirate chips out through an operative channel in the hysteroscope while preventing fluid losses and uterine collapse. But the problem is that the aspiration system is prone to becoming clogged if tissue chips are too large. This system requires the surgeon to remove smaller tissue fragments with each pass of the resectoscope.

Vaporization

- Vaporization of a fibroid can also be performed through the use of a variety of different shaped electrodes. The chosen electrode is dragged along the surface of the myoma to directly vaporize the tissue. Perforation from prolonged use at one point can occur. Using this method, tissue is destroyed and thus unavailable for pathologic examination.
- Versapoint bipolar electrosurgery system provides the opportunity to use both a vaporizing electrode

and resecting loop electrode with normal saline distention media for a variety of operative needs. Vaporizing electrode options include a ball or spring electrode for rapid vaporization and desiccation.

Laser Ablation

Fibroids less than 2 cm in diameter can also be ablated with the use of the Nd:YAG laser. The laser fiber is dragged over the surface of the fibroid until it is flat. As with its use for endometrial ablation, continuous movement is required and tissue is destroyed and not available for pathology evaluation.

Morcellation

- Hysteroscopic morcellation may also be used for resection of submucosal fibroids, as well as, endometrial polyps. The intrauterine morcellator (IUM) provides a nonelectrosurgical removal option. The morcellator consists of an inner rotating or reciprocating tube electronically controlled by a foot pedal and a 4.5-mm outer tube. Only a single insertion through a 9-mm rigid hysteroscope is required, followed by saline inflation of the uterus. After the fibroid or polyp is visualized, the morcellator is placed against the lesion and rotation or reciprocation of the inner tube cuts the lesion as controlled suction is used for continuous tissue removal and outflow.
- Advantages of morcellation include the use of physiologic saline for distention and irrigation and the availability of tissue fragments for histologic analysis after morcellation. This system is not designed to be used for submucosal fibroids with greater than 50% intramural penetration. Mean operating time has been demonstrated to be shorter in comparison to resectoscope.

Fibroids with an Intramural Component

In general, nonhysteroscopic myomectomy should be considered for fibroids with greater than 50% myometrial extension (type II, G2 fibroids), which are technically the most difficult resections to perform through the hysteroscope. In addition, resection of a completely intramural fibroid poses the risk of intravasation of media due to prolonged procedure time.

Resection

- After initial excision of the intracavitary portion of the fibroid, the intramural component will typically expel into the cavity, but the volume of the remaining intramural fibroid will subsequently increase. Thus, excising only the intracavity portion can prove futile.

- One surgical option is complete electrosurgical excision of the fibroid, including the intramural component. This technique is associated with increased risk of perforation, bleeding, thermal damage, and fluid absorption.

- Another suggested resection technique involves using a resectoscope to cut the capsule of the myoma away from myometrium to prevent the fibroid from sinking into the muscular layer, followed by grasping of the myoma with graspers. Rotation can then be used to pull the myoma into the intrauterine cavity. This is accomplished under ultrasonographic guidance.

- *Cold-loop:* Alternatively, the cold-loop myomectomy can be used. The surgeon first excises the intracavitary portion of the fibroid and then uses a loop, not connected to an electrical source, for blunt dissection. The loop is used to mechanically create a plane between the fibroid and myometrium. Once the fibroid is detached from the myometrium, it can then be removed in pieces.

- *Total enucleation:* An elliptic incision is made in the endometrial mucosa covering the fibroid until the cleavage zone of the myoma and myometrium is reached. Tissue bridges between the myoma and muscle fibers are resected with electrocautery, resulting in protrusion of the fibroid into the uterine cavity. Myomectomy can then be completed by slicing. This technique is successful in women with myomas less than 4 cm in diameter.

Intrauterine Adhesions

- The standard treatment of intrauterine adhesions is hysteroscopic resection. The operative hysteroscope is introduced into the uterine cavity and centrally located synechiae are lysed first. Progression is then made to the margins of the cavity. Thin, filmy adhesions can often be lysed with blunt dissection, but thicker adhesions require excision or transection. This can be accomplished with scissors, vaporization with bipolar electrocautery, or fiberoptic laser. Concurrent use of laparoscopy or ultrasonography may be useful with extensive adhesive disease to reduce the risk of perforation.

- Intraoperative fluoroscopic guidance during synechiolysis has also been proposed. With this technique, a 16-gauge, 80 mm needle is used to introduce contrast transcervically along side the hysteroscope. As contrast is injected, pockets of endometrium are identified and the needle is used

to create a passageway in the surrounding adhesions. Subsequent sharp resection with the needle or hysteroscopic scissors then follows. Advantages of this technique may include early detection of false passage and capability to concurrently assess tubal patency.

Transection and Resection of the Uterine Septum (Fig. 23.4)

This can be accomplished by three different methods. A 12° scope is preferred with this procedure. If extensive lysis is indicated, laparoscopy can be used as an aid to decrease the risk of perforation by visualizing the illuminated cavity intra-abdominally.

The first method involves the use of resectoscope, a straight, 5 mm loop electrode, and a blended current of 70–100 watts. The septum is transected until small areas of bleeding are observed; these indicate that myometrium is reached. The intrauterine fluid pressure is not allowed to become higher than the patient's mean arterial pressure because this may prevent these bleeders from being observed easily.

In the second method, a 5 to 7 mm operative hysteroscope and small scissors are used to transect the septum until the important, small bleeding areas are observed. The intrauterine pressure helps in expanding the septum as it is cut.

With the third method, an operative hysteroscope and vaporizing electrode (i.e. Versapoint system) is used with 0.9% sodium chloride solution. By vaporizing the septum distally toward the fundus, it is completely removed rather than just transected.

Resection of uterine septum can be performed with scissors, a laser, or the resectoscope (Fig. 23.5). When the septum is narrower than 3 cm at the fundus, incising it from distal to cephalic may allow the fibroelastic band to retract; this usually results in minimal bleeding. A broad septum requires a different approach. The first step is a lateral, alternating technique of side-to-side resection up to 0.5 cm from the fundus. Then, the

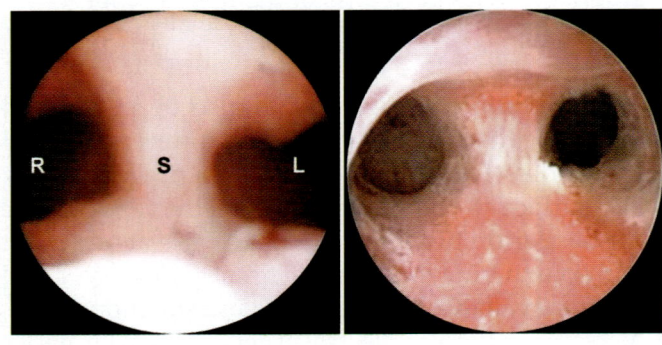

Fig. 23.4: Hysteroscopic view of septum

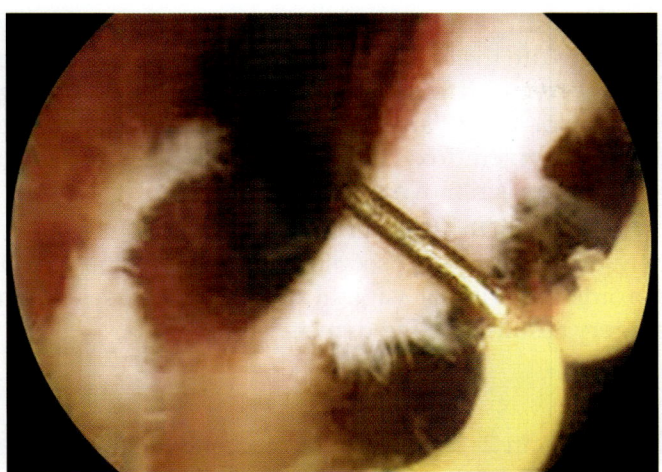

Fig. 23.5: Hysteroscopic resection of septum

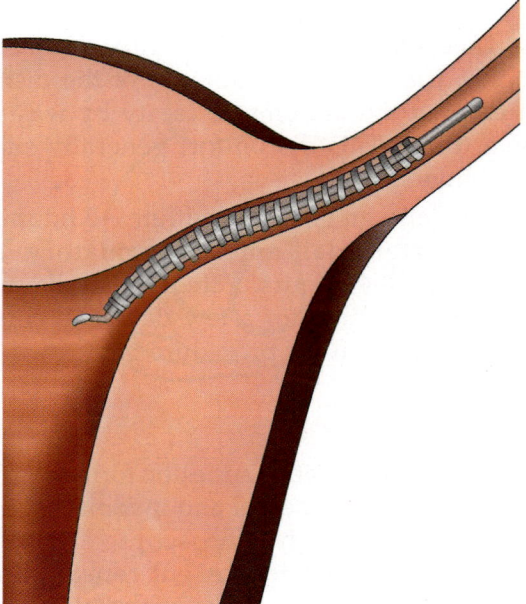

Fig. 23.6: Essure sterilization

remainder is removed from cornua to cornua to avoid damage to this area and to decrease bleeding. Laparoscopy or transabdominal ultrasonography may be useful to evaluate the external uterus during resection. If ultrasonography is used, the bladder should be left full to best visualize the uterus.

Although the septum is usually contained within the uterine cavity, a cervical septum may be present. The cervical septum can be incised with the use of scissors followed by hysteroscopic resection of the corporal portion. Recent studies have demonstrated improved outcomes after resection of cervical septum with decreased operating times, use of less distending media and favorable reproductive outcomes.

Transcervical Tubal Sterilization

With the Essure system (Fig. 23.6), a 5 mm hysteroscope is used to introduce a delivery catheter that contains a 3.85 cm flexible coil called a microinsert into the proximal portion of the fallopian tube. The inserts are made of a stainless steel inner coil wound in polyethylene fibers and an outer coil of nickel titanium. After a microinsert is placed at the uterotubal junction, the delivery catheter is removed and the outer coil of the insert expands. Three to eight trailing coils of the insert should remain visible at the tubal ostia. The inner polyethylene fibers induce tissue in-growth into the insert, facilitating occlusion of the tubal lumen by 12 weeks. The procedure can be performed without any anesthesia with acceptable pain scores.

IUD Removal

By using a 5 to 7 mm hysteroscope and a 12° scope, the IUD is grasped with a toothed grasper. The IUD is pulled toward the hysteroscope sheath. Pulling the IUD

through the operating channel of the hysteroscope is not possible. Instead, the grasper is held closed, and both hysteroscope and the IUD are pulled out together.

Proximal Tubal Cannulation

A 5- to 7-mm hysteroscope is used with a 30° scope. The occluded tubal ostia is cannulated approximately 1–2 cm with a flexible tubal catheter, and indigo carmine is injected through the cannula and observed for its spillage through the fimbriated end by laparoscopy. If no patency is documented, the laparoscopy surgeon straightens the fallopian tube as the hysteroscopic surgeon slides a guide wire with a soft, flexible tip through the initial catheter and into the isthmic area of the fallopian tube. The wire is then withdrawn and patency is evaluated again.

Operative Office Hysteroscopy

Small, more sophisticated instruments and improved flow systems now allow an operative therapy to be performed at the same time as initial diagnosis. Procedures performed in the office setting include targeted endometrial biopsy, polypectomy, myomectomy, adhesiolysis, metroplasty, and tubal sterilization.

Postoperative Details

General Posthysteroscopy Care

Patients typically report cramping after the procedure. A single dose of diclofenac injection reduces postoperative discomfort. Opioid derivatives can be added, if needed, for severe pain. Peritoneal discomfort may occur, if a substantial amount of the distention media entered the abdominal cavity by way of the fallopian tubes. This discomfort generally subsides within 24 hours.

Most patients can go home within 1–2 hours. They require nonsteroidal anti-inflammatory drugs (NSAIDs) for 24–48 hours. Patients may have some light-to-heavy spotting for a few days to a couple of weeks, depending on the procedure performed.

Intrauterine Adhesiolysis

Prevention of postoperative adhesion formation begins with minimizing endometrial and myometrial trauma during the initial hysteroscopic procedure. Postoperative stenting to prevent repeat adhesion formation with an IUD has been suggested, but copper IUDs may induce an excessive inflammatory reaction and the LNG IUD may be too small to achieve adequate results.

A Foley catheter placed into the uterine cavity with estrogen supplementation (conjugated estrogen 5 mg for 25 days with medroxyprogesterone 10 mg for the last 5 days) also has been used for stenting the cavity. The purpose of the estrogen is to limit the amount of postoperative bleeding due to vasoconstriction of small blood vessels and to rapidly rejuvenate the endometrial lining, which is less prone to form adhesions than a persistently raw, cut surface. If any sort of intrauterine stent is used, antibiotic prophylaxis should be considered for the duration of the stent placement. Oral doxycycline 100 mg twice daily is typically used.

Follow-up hysterosalpingography or diagnostic hysteroscopy after withdrawal bleeding is recommended. Intrauterine use of auto-crosslinked hyaluronic acid gel has also been examined in prevention of intrauterine adhesions after hysteroscopic surgery. Administration of 10 mL of gel after adhesiolysis or hysteroscopic surgery for intrauterine lesions may be associated with a significant reduction in the development and severity of *de novo* adhesions.

Resection of Fibroids

If a fibroid resection is performed, the patient may pass small pieces of tissue, which may cause cramping. Many surgeons advocate the use of high-dose estrogen to encourage endometrial growth over any denuded areas. Conjugated estrogen 2.5–5 mg daily or estradiol velarate 2 mg twice daily for 25 days, followed by progesterone for 5 days is typically sufficient.

Many surgeons prefer to use a pediatric Foley catheter with the balloon filled with 15–20 mL of sterile water because it has the added benefit of providing tamponade to any areas that may be bleeding and the patient is given doxycycline 100 mg twice daily until the catheter is removed 7 days later.

Vaginal birth is generally an accepted means of delivery after hysteroscopic resection of type 0 or 1 fibroids. But risk of vaginal delivery increases when surgery results in large defects.

Follow-up

Follow-up in 2–4 weeks is recommended to evaluate the patient and to probe the cervix particularly when ablation is performed to break up any scar tissue that may have developed near the internal os. For simple diagnostic hysteroscopy, no postoperative visit is usually necessary.

After resection of fibroids or polyps or transection of a septum, sonohysterography should be performed to confirm a normal uterine cavity. If adhesions are removed, diagnostic hysteroscopy in the office or operating room is likely to be most sensitive.

Complications

The most common complications after hysteroscopy are bleeding and uterine trauma. An accepted rate for all complications during surgical hysteroscopy is 3.8%.

Mechanical Complications

Perforation and cervical trauma are two of the most common complications of hysteroscopy, with uterine perforation rates of approximately 0.7–0.8%. Risk factors for perforation include cervical stenosis, severe uterine anteflexion or retroflexion, infection, myomas of lower uterine segments, and synechiae. Most cervical traumas and uterine perforations occur during dilatation of the cervix.

Cervical lacerations can occur from tearing of the single-toothed tenaculum from the cervix. Some authors suggest using a relatively atraumatic instrument, such as a double-toothed tenaculum or a ringed forceps, to prevent this complication. Using medical or mechanical preoperative cervical dilators may help to decrease resistance during dilatation. The vaginoscopic entry approach, when appropriate, eliminates the need for a tenaculum entirely.

Uterine perforations can occur during operative maneuvers as well. Care should be taken during procedures in the cornua because this is the thinnest portion of the myometrium. In general, a small midline or fundal injury with a blunt instrument does not have clinically significant sequelae, if bleeding is minimal, but large rents and lateral perforation involving risk of vessel injury caused by sharp or electrosurgical instruments should be inspected with laparoscopy.

Whenever electrical or laser injury to the bowel or bladder is suspected, laparoscopy or laparotomy is required for complete evaluation. The risk of peritonitis, sepsis, and death are most often associated with unrecognized and untreated thermal injuries to the viscera.

Media-related Complications

The risk of gas embolism is the primary complication associated with the use of CO_2 as the distention medium. Because of its solubility in plasma, CO_2 has a wide margin of safety. Trendelenburg positioning, cervical trauma, and overdilation of the cervix should be avoided to help prevent embolus formation. Intrauterine pressures should be maintained below 100 mm Hg, with maximal flow rates less than 100 mL/min.

When gas embolism occurs, results can be devastating, and circulatory collapse can occur. If an embolus is suspected in presence of hypotension, tachycardia, tachypnea, desaturation, decreased end-tidal CO_2 value, the hysteroscope should be removed, the patient positioned on her left side, and an IV bolus of isotonic sodium chloride solution should be delivered as a first-line treatment as well as echocardiography, cardiopulmonary resuscitation, percutaneous aspiration of embolus may be indicated.

The risk of absorption of media is minimal under normal operative conditions. Risk factors for clinically significant intravasation of fluid include prolonged operative procedures, the use of large volumes of low-viscosity media, or the resection of fibroids or myometrial trauma that results in open uterine venous channels or unidentified perforations. Intravasation can occur when the intrauterine pressure is greater than the patient's mean arterial pressure.

Fluid overload is rare with electrolyte-containing fluids. When excessive intravasation occurs, isotonic fluid overload occurs. This is relatively easy to treat. However, these fluids are uncommonly used in operative procedures.

On the contrary, nonelectrolyte, hypotonic media, which are nonconductive, are most often used for the prolonged, complicated electrosurgical procedures. These media have relatively serious adverse effect profiles. When large volumes of these solutions are absorbed, subsequent hyponatremia, hypervolemia, hypotension, pulmonary edema, cerebral edema, and cardiovascular collapse can occur. Absorption (or deficit) of nonelectrolyte solutions must be closely monitored throughout operative hysteroscopy.

For every liter of hypotonic media absorbed, the patient's serum sodium decreases by 10 mEq/L. If the patient's sodium level is less than 120 mEq/L, she is at increased risk for generalized cerebral edema, seizures, and even death. In general, if a fluid deficit is greater than 1500 mL or if sodium level is less than 125 mEq/L, the procedure should be terminated. Out of all nonelectrolyte media, 5% mannitol has the safest adverse effect profile because it can maintain a patient's osmolality despite hyponatremia, improving neurologic outcomes.

If the patient's sodium osmolality is less than 125 mOsm, forced diuresis with furosemide (Lasix) 40 mg IV, fluid restriction, and administration of 3% sodium chloride at a rate to correct hyponatremia by 1.5–2.0 mOsm/L/h is required. To limit any cerebral effects, do not correct the osmolality to more than 135 mOsm. Frequent assessments of the patient's sodium levels every 30 minutes may be appropriate to follow up this titration.

Dextran 70 can cause clinically significant overload in long surgical procedures; maximal absorption should not exceed 500 mL. This type of overload does not respond to diuretic treatment because the kidneys poorly excrete Dextran 70. Therefore, plasmapheresis may be required. Pulmonary edema and diffuse intravascular coagulation are other adverse effects associated with the use of Dextran 70.

Anaphylaxis is another complication of Dextran 70, though very rare, treatment of which includes diphenhydramine, epinephrine, steroids, and possible fluid and ventilatory support.

Bleeding

Bleeding during or after surgery is the second most common complication of hysteroscopy (0.25% of all cases). Myomectomy is the procedure with the highest complication rate (2–3%). The operative blood loss can be substantially reduced when patients are pretreated with GnRH agonists or oral contraceptives. Distention media themselves may yield enough pressure to cause hemostasis during a procedure. In addition, the coagulating effects of surgical instruments can aid in controlling bleeding during surgery.

If bleeding persists after surgery, a 30 mL Foley catheter balloon filled with 15–30 mL of fluid can be inserted into the cavity. This balloon can easily be removed 24 hours later. Antibiotic prophylaxis should be given, if a foreign body is placed in the uterus. Vasopressin and misoprostol are alternate medications that can help with vasoconstriction and uterine contractions. As a last resort, embolization of the uterine artery or hysterectomy is an option for definitive management.

Infection

Infection is an uncommon complication of hysteroscopy. If a patient has a preoperative infection or a significant history of pelvic inflammatory disease, treatment before surgery is recommended, but prophylactic antibiotics do not reduce the risk of infection after surgery. Cystitis and endometritis are the most common infections associated with hysteroscopic procedures which should be treated appropriately.

Future Developments

A variety of nonhysteroscopic instruments and techniques are now available for endometrial ablation. In general, these techniques are safe, effective, quick, and easy to learn.

The thermal balloon used for menorrhagia has effects equal to those of hysteroscopic ablation, though amenorrhea is not as common with the thermal balloon as with hysteroscopic ablation. The balloon method is fast and simple to complete.

Cryoablation of the endometrium is also used with success. The procedure is performed to desiccate and coagulate the endometrium and a superficial layer of myometrium by using radiofrequency energy delivered through a bipolar array.

The microwave endometrial ablation system offers excellent rates of amenorrhea but requires increased dilatation of the cervix to introduce the mechanism.

An area of current interest is the feasibility and safety of simultaneous nonhysteroscopic endometrial ablation and Essure tubal sterilization. Many women of reproductive age require ablation. Reproductive outcomes can be adversely affected should a women become pregnant after an ablation. Thus, it seem a reasonable option to offer permanent sterilization at the time of endometrial ablation.

In addition to the innovative Essure sterilization system, a second hysteroscopic transcervical sterilization method is currently seeking FDA approval. The **Adiana sterilization method** (Fig. 23.7) combines controlled thermal damage to the endosalpinx and insertion of a nonabsorbable silicone elastomer matrix. The hysteroscope which is inserted into the fallopian

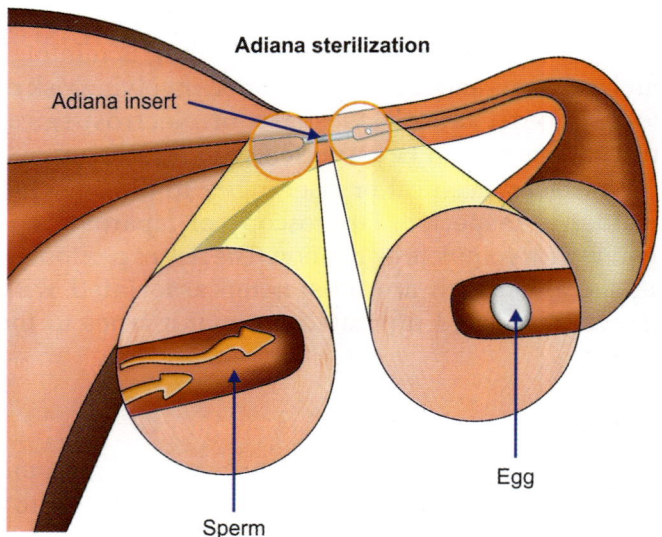

Fig. 23.7: Adiana sterilization

tubes through the vaginal opening. A small amount of heat is applied to each fallopian tube to removed thin layer of cell on the inside of each fallopian tube. Adiana is a soft flexible implant about the size of a grain of rice is inserted into both tubal opening. Natural tissue grows around the implant to create blockage between sperm and egg.

As sonohysterography becomes common, MRI-guided ultrasonic destruction of fibroids has completed initial phase I and II trials. The trials have shown the treatment to be highly acceptable to patients, safe, and effective at 24 months of follow-up. Patient demand for safe and minimally invasive treatments will continue to drive research and development.

RCOG Guidelines

1. *What is the ideal setting for performing hysteroscopy?* All grynecology units should provide a dedicated outpatient hysteroscopy service to aid management of women with abnormal uterine bleeding.

2. Analgesia

2.1 Do analgesics given before diagnostic hysteroscopy reduce the pain felt by women during the procedure? Routine use of opiate analgesia before outpatient hysteroscopy should be avoided as it may cause adverse effects.

Women without contraindications should be advised to consider taking standard doses of non-steroidal anti-inflammatory agents (NSAIDs) around 1 hour before their scheduled outpatient hysteroscopy appointment with the aim of reducing pain in the immediate postoperative period.

3. Cervical preparation

3.1 Does cervical preparation reduce uterine trauma, failure to access the uterine cavity or pain associated with outpatient hysteroscopy? [A]

Routine cervical preparation before outpatient hysteroscopy should not be used in the absence of any evidence of benefit in terms of reduction of pain, rates of failure or uterine trauma.

4.1 What size and angle of heteroscope should be used in the outpatient setting?

Miniature hysteroscopies (2.7 mm with a 3–3.5 mm sheath) should be used for diagnostic outpatient hysteroscopy as they significantly reduce the discomfort experienced by the woman. [A]

There is insufficient evidence to recommend 0° or fore-oblique optical lenses (i.e. 12°, 25° or 30° off-set lenses) for routine outpatient hysteroscopy. Choice of hysteroscope should be left to the discretion of the operator. ✓

4.2 Should rigid or flexible heteroscopies be used routinely in the outpatient setting? [B]

Flexible hysteroscopies are associated with less pain during outpatient hysteroscopy compared with rigid hysteroscopies. However, rigid hysteroscopies may provide better images, fewer failed procedures, quicker examination time and reduced cost. Thus, there is insufficient evidence to recommend preferential use of rigid or flexible hysteroscopies for diagnostic outpatient procedures. Choice of hysteroscope should be left to the discretion of the operator.

5.1 Which uterine distension medium should be during outpatient hysteroscopy? [A]

For routine outpatient hysteroscopy, the choice of distension medium between carbon dioxide and normal saline should be left to the discretion of the operator as neither is superior in reducing pain, although uterine distension with normal saline appears to reduce the incidence of vasovagal episodes.

Uterine distension with normal saline allows improved image quality and allows outpatient diagnostic hysteroscopy to be completed more quickly compared with carbon dioxide. [A]

Operative outpatient hysteroscopy, using bipolar electrosurgery, requires the use of normal saline to act as both the distension and conducting medium.

5.6 Which distension medium should be used for operative procedures?

Normal saline should be used as the distension medium when bipolar intrauterine equipment is used for hysteroscopic surgery. Thus, it is more practical to perform diagnostic procedures with normal saline in units offering simultaneous diagnosis and treatment as this avoids having to swap distension media should operative procedures need to be carried out. Hysteroscopic sterilization requires fluid distension medium, the choice of normal saline or glycine depends upon the specific technology adopted.

6.1 Should routine dilatation of the cervical canal be used before insertion of the hysteroscope in an outpatient setting? [C]

Blind cervical dilatation to facilitate insertion of the miniature outpatient hysteroscope is unnecessary in the majority of procedures. Routine cervical dilatation is associated with pain, vasovagal reactions and uterine trauma and should be avoided.

6.2 Should topical local anesthetic be administered before outpatient hysteroscopy?

Instillation of local anesthetic into the cervical canal does not reduce pain during diagnostic outpatient hysteroscopy but may reduce the incidence of vasovagal reactions.

Topical application of local anesthetic to the ectocervix should be considered where application of a cervical tenaculum is necessary.

6.3 Should injectable local anesthetic be administered to the cervix and/or paracervix before outpatient hysteroscopy? [A]

Application of local anesthetic into or around the cervix is associated with a reduction of the pain experienced during outpatient diagnostic hysteroscopy. However, it is unclear how clinically significant this reduction in pain is. Miniaturization of hysteroscopies and increasing use of vaginoscopy approach avoid use of intracervical or paracervical anesthesia.

7.1 Does a vaginoscopies approach to outpatient hysteroscopy reduce pain and increase the feasibility of the procedure?

Vaginoscopy reduces pain during diagnostic rigid outpatient hysteroscopy.

Vaginoscopy should be the standard technique for outpatient hysteroscopy especially where successful insertion of vaginal speculum is anticipated to be difficult and where blind endometrial biopsy is not required.

23B. LAPAROSCOPY IN GYNECOLOGY

During the last 40 years, laparoscopy has evolved from a limited gynecologic surgical procedure used only for diagnosis and tubal ligations to a major surgical tool used for a multitude of gynecologic and nongynecologic indications. Today, laparoscopy is one of the most common surgical procedures performed in many parts of the world. Laparoscopic techniques have also continued to evolve, primarily as a result of technological advances. In addition to better cameras and instruments, technology has resulted in the development of robotically assisted laparoscopy, and most recently single-port laparoscopy.

History of the Procedure

Laparoscopy was first performed in dogs in the early 1900s by Dr. Georg Kelling, a German surgeon, who called his procedure *koelioskopie*. While experimenting with the use of air for pneumoperitoneum to stop intra-abdominal bleeding, he introduced a cystoscope into the abdomen to view the effects of increased pressure on abdominal organs.

Dr. Hans Christian Jacobaeus, a Swedish surgeon, was the first to publish a description of *laparothorako-skopie* in humans in 1910. He used air pneumoperitoneum and a cystoscope to evaluate the peritoneal cavity of tuberculosis patients with ascites. Shortly thereafter, Dr. Bertram M. Bernheim of the Johns Hopkins Hospital, reported a series of the first human laparoscopy performed in the United States, which he called *organoscopy*.

Early in the 20th century, diagnostic laparoscopy was used by a limited number of general surgeons in place of diagnostic laparotomy, but had a substantial complication rate. Throughout the 1920s and 1930s, advocates of the procedure continued to develop improved laparoscopic equipment, such as pyramidal trocars for port introduction and lenses with a wider angle of view than the 90° afforded by the cystoscope. During this period, Dr. Janos Veress, a Hungarian internist, developed a spring-loaded needle with an inner stylet that automatically converted the sharp cutting edge to a rounded end. The Veress needle continues to be used today to create a pneumoperitoneum.

A major step forward in the development of laparoscopy was the development of a safer laparoscopic lighting system in the 1950s. Up until that time, intra-abdominal light was produced by a small electric light bulb at the distal tip of the laparoscope analogous to a bronchoscope. The use of a quartz light rod to transmit light from an external source to the tip of the laparoscope increased brightness and decreased the risk of intra-abdominal burns. This was soon followed by the application of fiberoptic technology still used in modern laparoscopes.

Dr. Raoul Palmer, a French gynecologist, in 1961, described the first laparoscopic retrieval of oocytes, and in 1974 he described the point 3 cm below the last rib in the left mid-clavicular line. Palmer's point is often used today for left upper quadrant laparoscopic entry.

Dr. Kurt Semm, a German gynecologist invented the automatic insufflator, and laparoscopic instruments, including a thermocoagulator, loop ligature, and devices for extracorporeal and intracorporeal endoscopic knot tying. He was one of the first proponents of video monitoring for laparoscopy, using a series of lenses and mirrors in an articulated arm to connect the laparoscope to a ceiling-mounted video camera.

A major breakthrough came with the introduction of the solid state video camera for laparoscopy in 1982. With the widespread application of these compact cameras, both laparoscopist and assistants could simultaneously view the operative field on a video screen. By the end of the decade, video-laparoscopy had become standard and operative laparoscopy became widely accepted as a safe and effective surgical approach.

In recent years, 3 innovations that have been introduced or reintroduced to the field of laparoscopy: 1) robotic surgery, 2) natural orifice transluminal surgery (NOTES), and 3) single incision laparoscopic surgery (SILS). All 3 have their advantages and disadvantages compared to traditional laparoscopy. Of these 3 developing technologies, robotic surgery is having the largest impact on clinical care.

Frequency

Laparoscopy currently is one of the most common surgical procedures performed in all over the globe. In addition to diagnostic laparoscopy and sterilization, operative gynecological endoscopy is used to perform common procedures like removal of ectopic pregnancies, treatment of endometriosis, and lysis of pelvic adhesions. Almost one-third of hysterectomies are performed annually with the aid of a laparoscope. Although the ideal role of laparoscopy in gynecologic surgery continues to be defined, it has become a standard approach for a large number of gynecologic procedures.

The laparoscopic approach has been gaining popularity for several reasons:
- Usually can be performed in the outpatient setting.
- Shorter hospitalization when admission is necessary.
- Better cosmetics.
- Faster recovery and earlier return to normal activity.
- Less risk of postoperative adhesion formation

Indications

Almost any gynecologic surgery can be performed laparoscopically in carefully selected patients and in the hands of a skilled minimally invasive surgeon. Advancement in technology and the availability of a wide spectrum of laparoscopic equipment and energy sources have allowed a large variety of surgery to be performed laparoscopically, ranging from simple tubal ligation to complex urogynecologic and oncologic procedures. Reasons for diagnostic laparoscopy are:
- Unexplained pelvic pain
- Unexplained infertility, tubal disease
- Pelvic infection
- Unexplained vaginal bleeding
- Endometriosis
- Uterine fibroids
- Ovarian cysts or tumors
- Ectopic pregnancy
- Infertility
- Pelvic inflammatory disease
- Reproductive cancers

Indications for operative laparoscopy include:
- Hysterectomy
- Ovarian cystectomy/ovariotomy/salpingo-oophorectomy
- Myomectomy
- Endometrial tissue ablation in endometriosis
- Adhesion removal
- Reversal of tubal ligation, tuboplasty, tubectomy
- Burch colposuspension for USI
- Colposacropexy for vault prolapse

Contraindications

Absolute contraindications for operative laparoscopy include the following:
- Surgeon's lack of skills
- Inadequately equipped operating room
- Shock
- Markedly increased intracranial pressure
- Retinal detachment

Relative contraindications include:
- Compromised cardiopulmonary status
- Ventriculoperitoneal shunt
- Pregnancy
- Large pelvic masses

Equipment

Camera

The current laparoscopic cameras use three chips, each detecting one of the primary colors—red, green, and blue. The mixture of these primary colors in different proportions allows the camera to capture all colors. Three-chip cameras generally provide the highest fidelity. The camera head attaches to the laparoscope and a cable connects to the camera control unit. The signal is then transmitted to the monitor, which converts the electric signal to an analog image (Fig. 23.8).

Light Source (Fig. 23.9)

Light sources most commonly use xenon bulbs, which provide the highest light intensity and are long lasting.

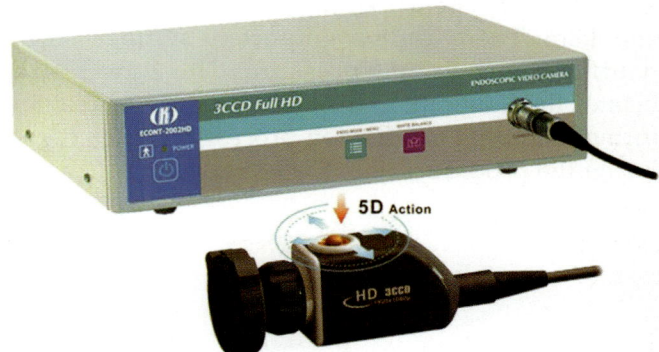

Fig. 23.8: Camera control unit

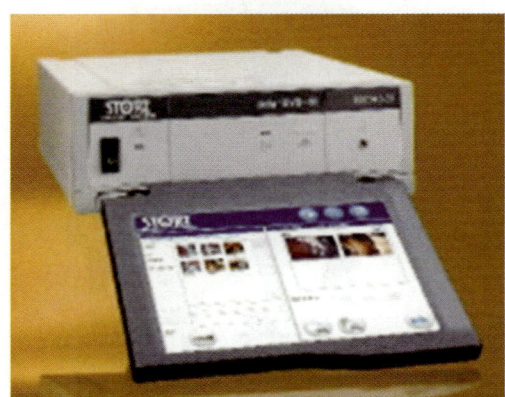

Fig. 23.9: Light source

The light cable connects the source to the scope. There are two types of cables—fiberoptic and liquid crystal gel cables. The fiberoptic cable is composed of a bundle of optical fiberglass threads swaged at both ends. The liquid crystal cable consists of a sheath filled with a clear optical gel and made rigid by a metal sheath, making it more difficult to store and maintain. The liquid crystal gel cable transmits more heat and more light than the fiberoptic cable. Both cables are fragile and need to be handled with care. Twisting of the cable should be avoided. A damaged cable will provide a suboptimal image.

Once turned on, the surgeon has to adjust the focus and the white balance. Focusing the camera is performed at a distance of 5 cm from an object. Then white balance is performed to adjust the color. A white surface, typically clean gauze, is used. During this process, the white color becomes a reference against which to adjust the three primary colors.

Insufflator

The insufflator delivers CO_2 gas into the peritoneal cavity (Fig. 23.10).

CO_2 gas is preferred because it is noncombustible, soluble, and cheap. Being soluble prevents air embolism. There are two important settings on the insufflator—flow and pressure. The flow setting dictates the flow rate in liters per minute; it is set low during the initial insufflation process and then higher during the procedure.

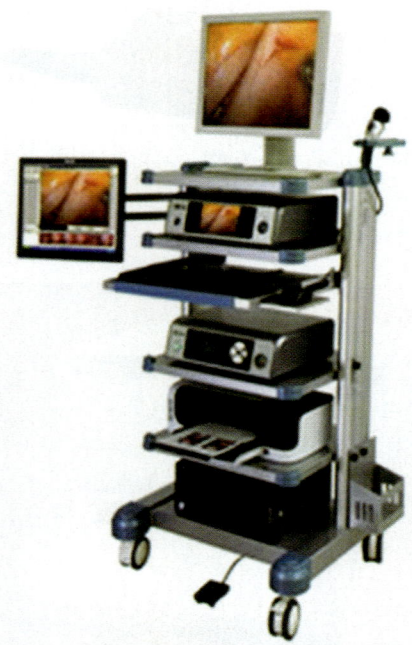

Fig. 23.10: Instrument trolley from top to bottom: Recorder, light source, insufflator, and energy source

During operative laparoscopy, CO_2 gas is typically lost through leakage of the multiple ports and suctioning. In these cases, the flow rate can be set high. The pressure setting sets the upper limit of the intra-abdominal pressure. This is typically set at 15 mm Hg. The insufflator is automatic and delivers the flow of CO_2 as needed to maintain the desired intra-abdominal pressure. The following points can help with troubleshooting:

- A low flow and low pressure indicates an empty gas tank.
- A low flow and high pressure indicates an obstruction, typically kinked tubing, turned-off valve, or preperitoneal insufflation.
- A high flow and low pressure indicates a gas leak; this is typically associated with a hissing sound.

The CO_2 gas is usually delivered cold at a temperature of 21°C and dry with 0% humidity though cold, dry CO_2 may cause peritoneal cell desiccation, acidify the peritoneal surface, and impair the mesothelial lining immune response. The heated and humidified CO_2 is associated with less postoperative pain, lower risk of hypothermia, and lower analgesic requirements.

Veress Needle

The Veress needle consists of a cannula with a needle point (Fig. 23.11).

Inside the cannula there is a blunt stylet loaded with a spring. When faced with resistance, the stylet is pushed inward, compressing the spring and allowing the cutting edge of the outer cannula to pierce the skin. Once the resistance is lost, the spring pushes the stylet forward and a click is heard. The click heard is used to indicate the level of penetration. The blunt tip extends past the cutting edge, protecting it. The Veress needle has lateral holes at its distal ends to deliver the CO_2. It comes in three different lengths—80 mm, 100 mm and 120 mm. The Veress needle is used in a closed-entry technique to obtain pneumoperitoneum. The goal of the stylet is to prevent injury to soft tissue, which has lower resistance than the fascia and peritoneum.

Trocars (Fig. 23.12)

Trocars come in different sizes and lengths; they also have different tips and can be disposable or reusable. They range from 2 to 15 mm and can be sharp or blunt.

The Hasson-type trocar is a blunt-tip trocar used in an open-entry technique.

The new optical trocars have clear conical tips and hollow cannula through which a scope can be placed

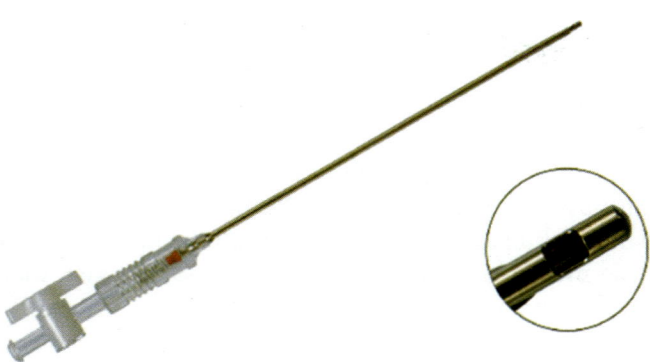

Fig. 23.11: Veress needle

to visualize the different tissue layers during insertion. Although the tip is not sharp, its shape allows tissue separation with twisting and countertwisting motions. Trocars were initially designed to limit injury to underlying structures. These trocars can be used during a closed-entry technique.

The radially expanding trocar is bladeless and consists of a radially expanding sleeve, which is first inserted as Veress needle. Once in place, the needle is removed and a blunt trocar is inserted, which enlarges the sleeve and accommodates instruments up to 15 mm in diameter. It creates a smaller fascial defect than conventional trocars, potentially making fascial closure unnecessary and causing less postoperative wound pain. The reported incidence of trocar-site hernia is 0.66% in patients without fascial closure after using 12 mm radially expanding trocars.

Laparoscopes

Laparoscopes vary in size from 1.5 to 12 mm; the 5 mm and 10 mm laparoscopes are most commonly used in gynecology. The degree of the scope also varies; the most commonly used are 0-degree and 30-degree laparoscopes. The 0-degree laparoscope has the greatest application range because of the panoramic view it provides. However, the 30-degree laparoscope is often preferred in operative laparoscopy because it permits seeing anatomic structures better, especially during hysterectomy of a large uterus. The 45-degree laparoscope can also be used when dealing with a very large uterus.

Laparoscopic Hand Instruments (Fig. 23.13)

These instruments are essential for surgical maneuvers. The main hand instruments are:

1. Graspers—toothed and non-toothed
2. Merryland
3. Scissors
4. Babcock
5. Needle holders (Fig. 23.14)
6. Suction-irrigation
7. Electrocautery—bipolar/monopolar forceps with cable and electrosurgical source
8. Vessel sealing systems—Harmonics, Ligasures, N-SEAL
9. Myomectomy hook
10. Morcellation systems
11. Uterine elevators
12. Port closure needle

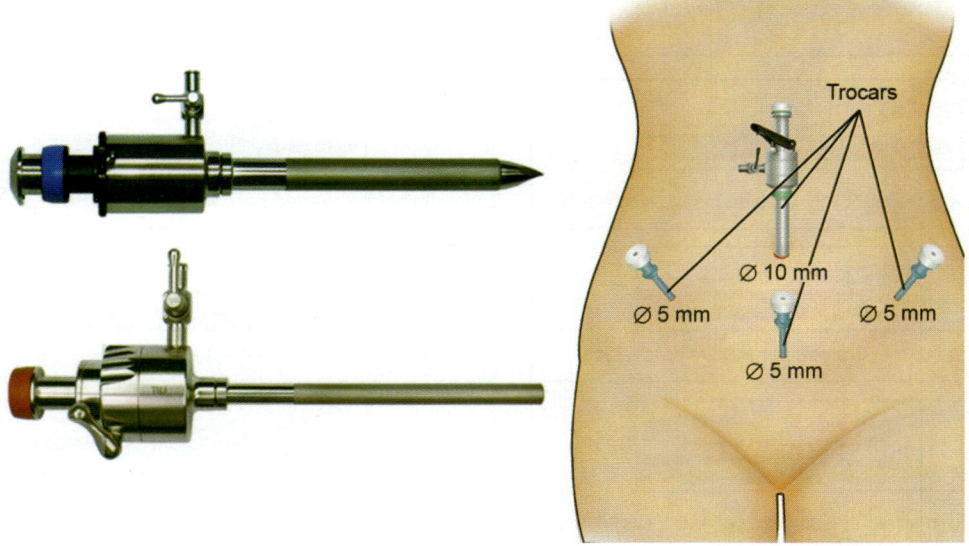

Fig. 23.12: Trocar with different ports of entry

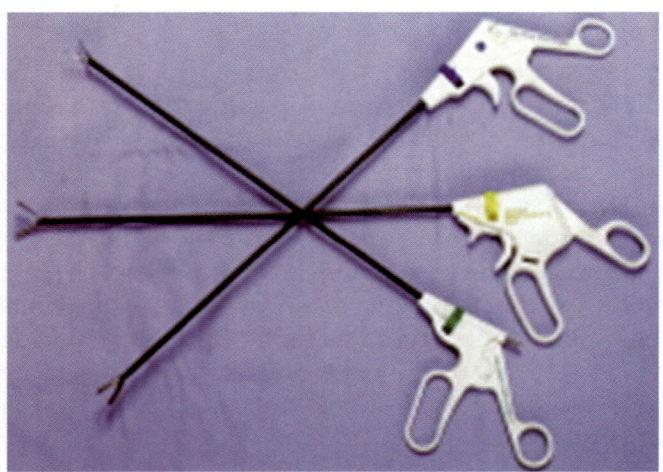

Fig. 23.13: Laparoscopic hand instruments

Relevant Anatomy

Anterior abdominal wall anatomy should receive special attention prior to laparoscopy because many laparoscopic complications result from trocar placement.

Abdominal Scars

Previous surgery is associated with a greater than 20% risk of adhesions of bowel or omentum to the anterior abdominal wall. For this reason, many laparoscopists adjust their techniques in these patients to minimize the risk of bowel injury. Of special concern are incisional scars immediately adjacent to the umbilicus because bowel adherent underneath the umbilicus may be at risk for injury regardless of the technique used. Although Pfannenstiel and abdominal incisions distant to the umbilicus may also be associated with adhesions, these incisions appear to represent less of a risk than incisions near the umbilicus.

Abdominal Wall Thickness

Although abdominal thickness correlates with patient weight, short stature or truncal obesity may increase abdominal wall thickness out of proportion to patient weight. Routine evaluation of the abdominal wall prior to laparoscopy is important because the success of trocar insertion may depend on altering the technique based on abdominal wall thickness.

Umbilicus

The umbilicus should be examined for signs of umbilical hernia. Techniques for trocar insertion should be adjusted, and closure of the defect should be

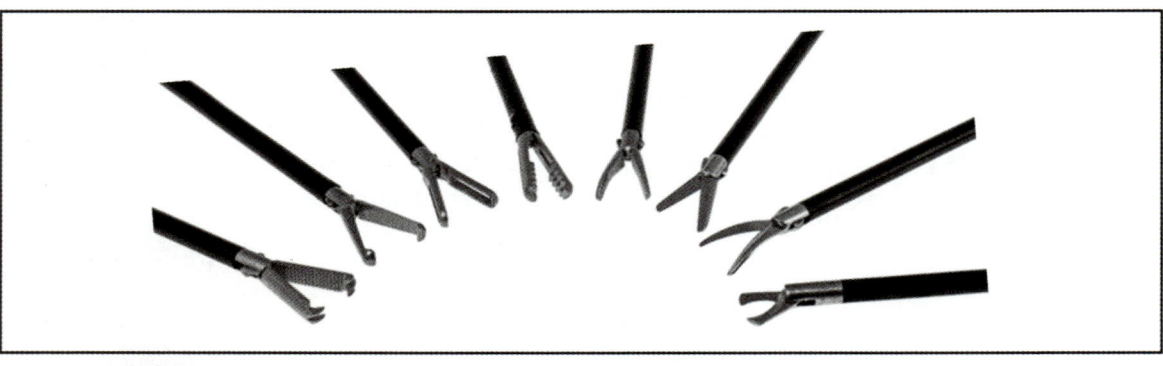

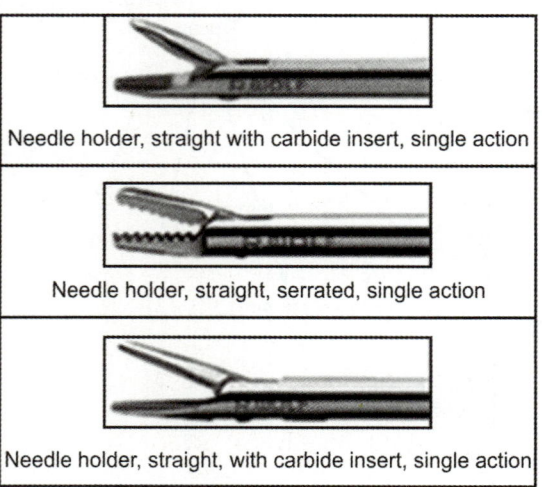

Needle holder, straight with carbide insert, single action	Needle holder, curved right with carbide insert, single action
Needle holder, straight, serrated, single action	Needle holder, curved left with carbide insert, single action
Needle holder, straight, with carbide insert, single action	Needle holder, straight, with carbide insert, single action

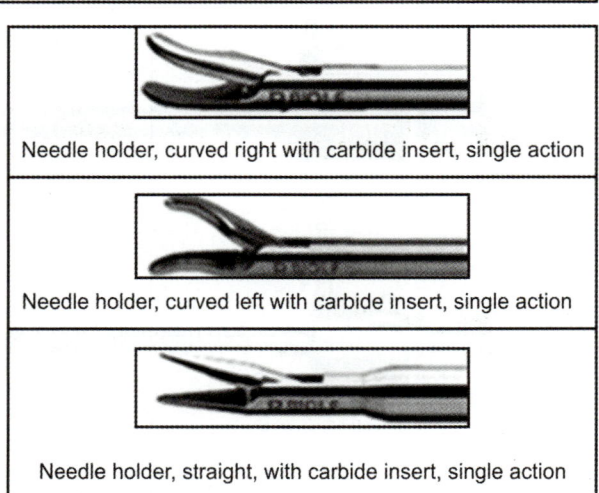

Fig. 23.14: Needle holders

considered. In the absence of incarcerated bowel, the skin over the hernia can be carefully incised and the peritoneal cavity entered using an open technique. Closure of a small defect can be performed with interrupted sutures at the completion of the laparoscopic procedure.

Abdominal Wall Vessels

The anterior abdominal wall contains two sets of bilateral vessels—the superficial and the inferior (deep) epigastric vessels. These arteries originate from the femoral and external iliac arteries, respectively, and are accompanied by large vein in most cases. Immediately above the symphysis pubis, they are both located at around 5.5 cm from the midline and course slightly more laterally at points more cephalad. In order to avoid injuring these vessels during lateral trocar placement, the superficial vessels should be visualized by transillumination and the inferior vessels should be laparoscopically visualized whenever possible. The use of conical trocars (as opposed to pyramidal tipped trocars) can also decrease the risk of injury to these vessels.

Patient Risk Factors

Obesity

Obesity is a well-recognized factor that increases the risk of any abdominal surgery. Women with a body mass index (BMI) greater than 25 kg/m^2 are classified as overweight, and those with a BMI greater than 30 kg/m^2 are considered obese. Placement of laparoscopic instruments becomes much more difficult and often requires special techniques. Bleeding from abdominal wall vessels may be more common because these vessels become difficult to locate. Many intra-abdominal procedures become increasingly difficult because of a restricted operative field secondary to retroperitoneal fat deposits in the pelvic sidewalls and increased bowel excursion into the operative field. This second problem is probably related to increased volume of bowel, decreased elevation of a heavier anterior abdominal wall by the pneumoperitoneum, and the inability to place many patients who are obese in steep Trendelenburg position because of anesthetic problems.

Age

- Older patients are at increased risk of having concomitant disease processes that affect their perioperative morbidity and mortality. Intra-operative cardiac stress related to anesthesia and the surgery itself may result in sudden cardiac decompensation based on arrhythmia, ischemia, or infarct.
- Of special importance is the increased susceptibility of elderly persons to hypothermia because the vast majority of patients experience some degree of hypothermia during laparoscopy. In older patients, even mild degrees of hypothermia may increase the risk of cardiac arrhythmia and prolong recovery time.

Previous Abdominal Surgery

- As far as laparoscopic complications are concerned, one of the most important risk factors is a history of previous abdominal surgery. The risk of adhesions of omentum and/or bowel to the anterior abdominal wall after previous abdominal surgery is greater than 20%. Because laparoscopy requires the insertion of sharp instruments into the abdominal cavity, a reasonable assumption is that previous surgery would increase the risk of bowel injury. Thus, strategies have been developed to decrease the risk of bowel injury in patients with previous abdominal surgery.
- The most common of these strategies is the use of an open technique for laparoscopic trocar placement, as first advocated by Hasson. Open laparoscopy techniques almost certainly decrease the risk of bowel injury distant to the umbilicus. To avoid bowel injury at the site of entry, modifications of the open technique have employed blunt entry of the peritoneal cavity with a hemostat to avoid inadvertently grasping and incising the bowel. In patients with previous laparotomy in which the scar is located at the umbilicus, use of an alternative location for trocar insertion (usually in the left upper quadrant Palmer's point) has been recommended to avoid injury of bowel adherent immediately beneath the umbilicus. The closest organ to the left upper quadrant is the stomach (therefore, an oral gastric tube is recommended before insertion) and the left lobe of the liver.
- Despite the potential for increased risk of bowel injury after previous laparotomy, some laparo-scopists advocate the use of a closed periumbilical trocar insertion techniques in all patients, regardless of a history of previous surgery. One justification is that bowel injury is uncommon (approximately 3 cases per 10,000 procedures) and open laparoscopy does not completely avoid the risk of bowel injury.

Anesthetic Risk Factors

I. Time Since Last Oral Intake

- Because both general anesthesia and increased intra-abdominal pressure may increase the risk of regurgitation and resultant aspiration, approximately 6 hours be allowed to elapse between the last intake of solid food and the elective induction of anesthesia. In patients with conditions associated with decreased gastric emptying (e.g. diabetes-induced autonomic dysfunction) or in the presence of predisposing factors for regurgitation (e.g. sliding hiatal hernia, known reflux), a longer period of fasting may be indicated.

- Unfortunately, in emergency cases such as ectopic pregnancy or ovarian torsion, general anesthesia may be required despite a period of fasting of less than 6 hours. In these cases, steps can be taken to decrease the incidence of aspiration pneumonia, by administration of antacids and metoclopramide.

II. Cardiopulmonary Disease

- Patients with ischemic heart disease who undergo anesthesia may have decreased cardiac blood return coupled with an increased heart rate that may result in infarction. Laparoscopic-associated metabolic acidosis, respiratory acidosis, and hypothermia may result in arrhythmia in predisposed patients. Finally, patients at risk for congestive heart failure should be evaluated carefully prior to laparoscopy because a decrease in cardiac output may be related to decreased venous return and increased peripheral vascular resistance.

- The relatively decreased postoperative pain following laparoscopy may result in less ventilatory compromise than laparotomy and thus, fewer problems with atelectasis or pulmonary failure in those with borderline pulmonary function.

- Special care should be taken during laparoscopy in patients with pulmonary disease. Hypercarbia and decreased ventilation associated with laparoscopy may be especially deleterious in pulmonary patients with chronic respiratory acidosis. In patients with compromised pulmonary function, even a small intravasation of carbon dioxide could result in significant pulmonary decompensation.

Preoperative Details

Preoperative Medications

- *Gonadotropin-releasing hormone agonists:* The most common situation in which this is helpful in the presence of a large leiomyoma when size alone makes surgery difficult. This is most common when hysteroscopic resection of a large submucosal leiomyoma is to be attempted or when LAVH is planned for a markedly enlarged uterus. In general, uterine volume can be decreased by up to 50% with 2–3 months of administration of a long-acting GnRH agonist. This may also be helpful in some cases of laparoscopic myomectomy.

- *Prophylactic antibiotics:* The use of prophylactic antibiotics are well-established method of decreasing risk of postoperative infections.

- *Oral contraceptives:* The risk of postoperative thromboembolism appears to be increased by the preoperative use of high-dose oral contraceptives (50 µg ethinyl estradiol) in women undergoing major gynecologic surgery. Therefore, women undergoing laparoscopic hysterectomy should probably discontinue oral contraceptives 1 month prior to surgery unless the patient decides that the risk of inadvertent pregnancy is greater than the small, but uncertain, increased risk of thromboembolism associated with preoperative oral contraceptives.

Preoperative Gastrointestinal Preparation

Bowel preparation

- If significant enterolysis is planned and either endometriosis or pelvic adhesions are known or suggested to be present, preoperative bowel preparation is commonly used in an effort to decrease the risk of serious postoperative sequelae though a recent Cochrane database has questioned the entire concept of a bowel preparation.

- The most common oral agents are either magnesium citrate or a polyethylene glycol solution. Unfortunately, a thorough bowel preparation is often uncomfortable for the patient. However, in high-risk patients, preoperative bowel preparation may allow primary closure of an unplanned enterotomy; in the presence of an unprepared colon, a temporary diverting colostomy may be required.

- *Oral intake:* Nothing by mouth after 12:00 midnight remains a sound approach in most patients undergoing early morning surgery to avoid the risk of aspiration. In patients whose cases are scheduled later, clear liquids until 6 hours prior to surgery may make the patient more comfortable and also decrease the degree of preoperative dehydration.

Other Preoperative Considerations

- *Intravenous access:* A balanced salt solution is administered at a moderate rate to hydrate the patient prior to administering regional or general anesthesia.

- **Bladder catheterization:** Traditionally, complete emptying of the urinary bladder with a catheter immediately prior to Veress cannula or trocar placement is performed to minimize the risk of bladder injury. For procedures of longer duration, indwelling catheter is used to avoid bladder refilling, although this probably increases the risk of infection.

Deep Vein Thrombosis Prophylaxis

About 14% of patients who undergo gynecologic surgery for benign conditions can develop thromboembolism. The decision to provide thromboprophylaxis should be made based upon patient risk factors and the type of surgery performed. The American Academy of Chest Physicians (ACCP) suggests that low-risk patients do not need prophylaxis. Patients at moderate and high risk undergo thromboprophylaxis with sequential compression devices (SCD) (lower extremity) or unfractionated heparin 5,000 units bid or low molecular weight heparin such as enoxaparin 40 mg daily. Low-risk patients include those younger than 40 years with no additional risk factors whose surgery duration is less than 30 minutes. Patients at moderate risk include those aged 40–60 years with no additional risk factors undergoing surgery of any duration. High-risk patients include those aged 60 years or aged 40 years with one additional risk factor, such as prior DVT, varicose veins, infection, malignancy, obesity, estrogen therapy, or surgery lasting longer than 5 hours.

Patient Positioning (Fig. 23.15)

- Gynecologic laparoscopy procedures are usually performed with the patient in the dorsal lithotomy position to allow vaginal access for uterine manipulation.
- Most laparoscopists now use boot stirrups specially designed for laparoscopy. These have a footplate and also support the popliteal fossa. This avoids pressure on the lateral or posterior aspect of the calf and permits easy positional changes from low lithotomy for laparoscopy to high lithotomy for vaginal procedures, such as hysteroscopy or vaginal hysterectomy.
- The patient's thighs should be in the same plane as the body, hence the low lithotomy position. This will prevent the instruments from bumping into the patient's thigh and allows more space for the surgeon, especially when accessory trocars are placed low in the pelvis. The legs should be well supported and padded to prevent injury to the peroneal nerve. The hips should be minimally abducted and not more than 45°. When access to the vagina is required, the thighs can be flexed (but not to more than 90°) to avoid injury to the femoral, obturator, and sciatic nerves.
- Once the primary trocar is placed, the patient is usually placed in no more than 25° Trendelenburg position to help keep the bowel out of the pelvis. The use of steep Trendelenburg position for prolonged periods has been associated with Erbs palsy, especially with the use of shoulder braces.

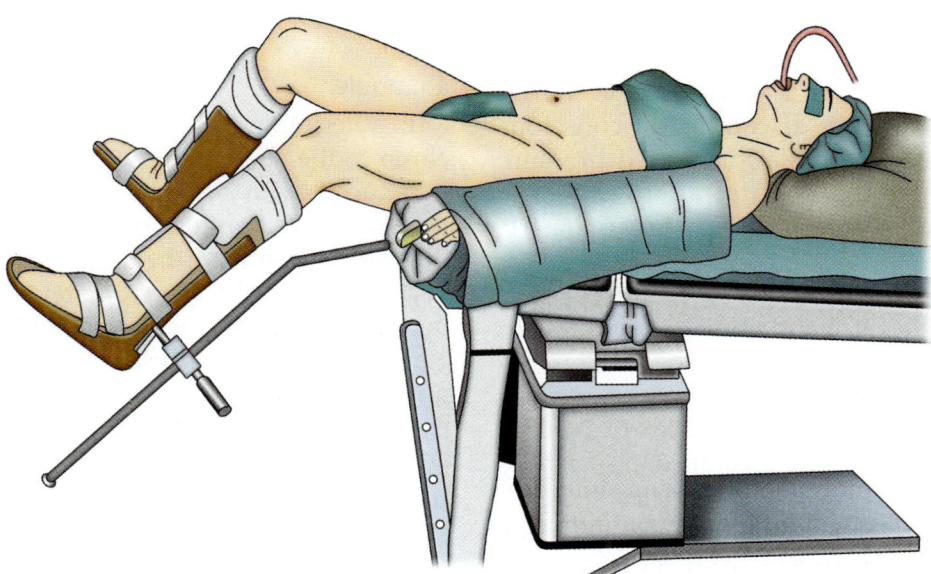

Fig. 23.15: Position of patient during laparoscopy

Skin Preparation

- Clipping the pubic hair above the symphysis may be required, if hair extends to the intended site of ancillary trocar placement, usually 3–4 cm above the symphysis pubis. Standard antiseptic preparation of the abdominal skin and the vagina are followed by placement of specially designed fenestrated laparoscopy drapes. Vaginal instruments are placed for uterine manipulation and then draped to keep the abdominal field separate from the lower vaginal field.
- After changing gloves, avoid contamination of both the abdominal field and instruments placed into the abdominal cavity. Nevertheless, the risk of infection involving the wound or the peritoneal cavity after laparoscopy is extremely low, most likely because of the small incisions and decreased opportunity for intra-abdominal contamination.

Type of Anesthesia

Because of two unique aspects of gynecologic laparoscopy, (1) abdominal insufflation and (2) routine use of the Trendelenburg position, general anesthesia is the most common technique used today.

Abdominal insufflation, usually with carbon dioxide at a pressure of 15–20 mm Hg, has significant physiologic effects. Transperitoneal absorption of carbon dioxide results in a relative acidosis that plateaus after approximately 15 minutes of insufflation. Acidosis can be corrected by increasing ventilation 10–25% and usually has minimal effect on healthy patients. However, in susceptible patients, these changes in acid-base status may increase the risk of cardiac arrhythmia. Probably a more significant effect of abdominal insufflation and stiff Trendelenburg position is increased pressure on abdominal structures and diaphragm. While associated with significant discomfort in conscious patients (in regional anesthesia), increased pressure can also result in passive regurgitation of gastric contents, even in patients without a history of gastric reflux.

Abdominal insufflation can also have direct cardiac effects. Pressure on the intra-abdominal venous system can decrease the venous return to the heart. Pressure transmitted to the right atrium decreases preload further. This may be of minimal consequence in healthy patients, but it may lead to cardiac compromise in those with borderline cardiac function.

During laparoscopy, both the discomfort and the risk of aspiration may be decreased by using the least intra-abdominal pressure possible for insufflation (usually <14 mm Hg) and using the least amount of Trendelenburg position necessary to visualize the pelvis.

Technique

General techniques for laparoscopy are described as follows:

Primary Trocar Placement

Numerous techniques exist for creating a pneumoperitoneum and placing a laparoscopic port into the abdomen. Each is purported to offer a unique advantage. Five common approaches are: 1) Veress needle insertion followed by a primary trocar insertion, 2) direct trocar insertion, 3) open laparoscopy, 4) expanding-access cannulas, and 5) left upper quadrant insertion. Physician experience significantly contributes to the safety of the individual technique.

1. Veress Needle and Primary Trocar Insertion

When the Veress needle is placed through the umbilicus and into the peritoneal cavity, avoidance of both the retroperitoneal vessels and the intestinal tract is of paramount importance. The patient must be in the complete horizontal position and the patient's body habitus should be carefully assessed.

The abdominal wall (Fig. 23.16) is elevated by manually grasping the skin and subcutaneous tissue to maximize the distance between the umbilicus and the retroperitoneal vessels. An alternative method for elevation is to place penetrating towel clips at the base of the umbilicus (Fig. 23.17).

In persons of average weight, the lower anterior abdominal wall is grasped and elevated and the Veress needle is inserted toward the hollow of the sacrum at a 45° angle.

In a very thin patient, the vital structures are much closer to the abdominal wall and the margin for error is reduced, with sometimes as little as 4 cm between the skin and large retroperitoneal vessels. In patients who are obese (BMI of 30 kg/m² or more), a more vertical approach, approximately 70–80°, is required because of the increased thickness of the abdominal wall. Without the vertical insertion, the trocar would not be long enough to penetrate the layers and enter the peritoneal cavity.

Correct placement of the Veress needle may be confirmed by a number of methods, such as the hanging drop test, injection and aspiration of fluid through the Veress needle, or measurement of intra-abdominal pressure with carbon dioxide insufflation. After a

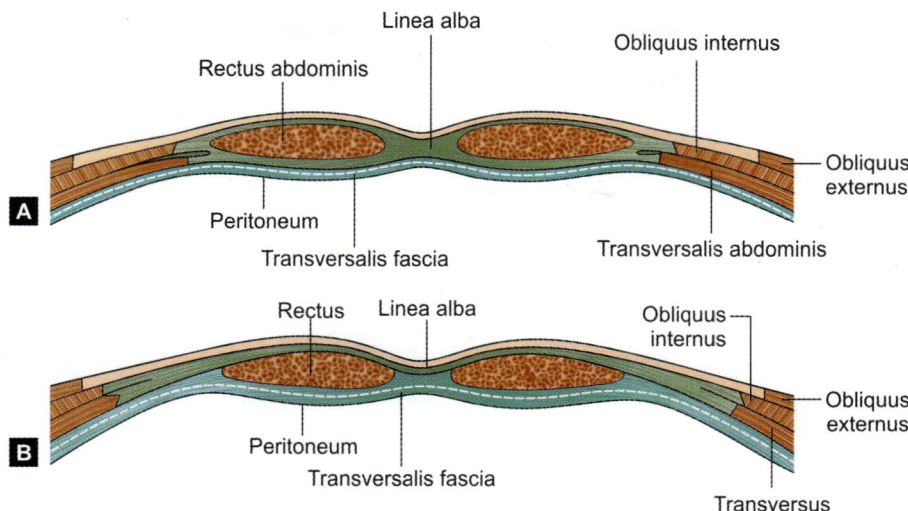

Linea alba
Rectus abdominis — Obliquus internus
— Obliquus externus
Peritoneum — Transversalis abdominis
Transversalis fascia

Rectus — Linea alba — Obliquus internus
— Obliquus externus
Peritoneum
Transversalis fascia — Transversus

Fig. 23.16: Transverse sections through anterior abdominal wall, traditional view: (A) immediately above umbilicus; (B) below arcuate line

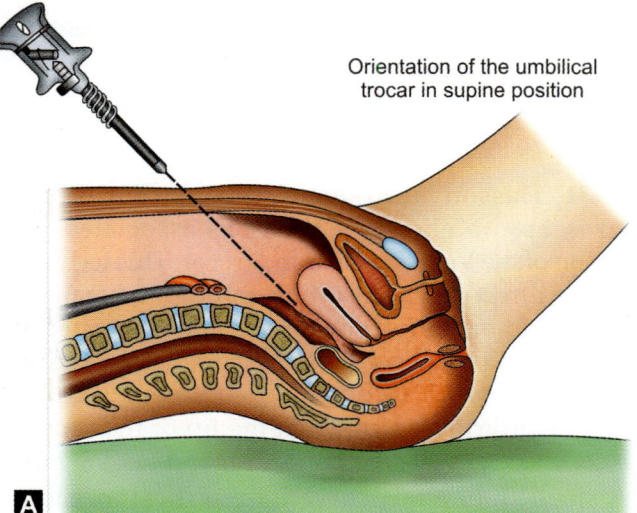

Orientation of the umbilical trocar in supine position

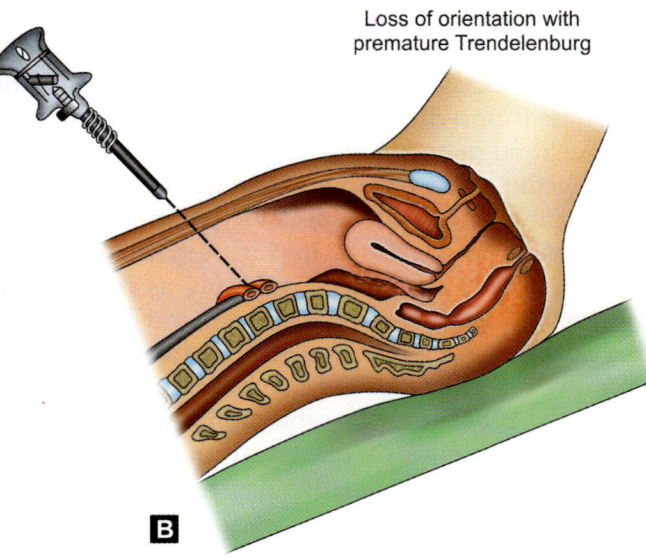

Loss of orientation with premature Trendelenburg

Fig. 23.17: Direction of Veress needle enty

pneumoperitoneum has been achieved with a Veress needle, the primary trocar with sleeve (most commonly 5 or 10 mm in diameter) is placed at a similar angle to the Veress needle (Table 23.2).

Placement of the primary trocar: The sharp primary trocar is aimed toward the sacral promontory. Dull trocars require increased force during insertion, and

Table 23.2: Most common tests used to ensure correct entry using the Veress needle	
Tests	*Description*
Double click	The operator listens to the needle as it passes through the rectus sheath (first click) and the peritoneum (second click); three clicks may be heard at Palmer's point because of the posterior fascia.
Aspiration	A 5 cc syringe filled with normal saline is attached to the Veress needle. The syringe is aspirated to confirm no fecal material or blood and then a few milliliters are injected. The flow should be without resistance, and then respiration should fail to draw back any fluid.
Hanging drop	After injecting a few mL, the syringe is removed and the column of saline is monitored. The saline column should move freely down the needle due to positive pressure between atmospheres and the negative pressure of the intra-abdominal space.
Serial intra-abdominal gas pressure measurement	After priming the gas tubing with CO_2, the tube is attached to the Veress needle and the flow is set at 1 L/minute, with the pressure recorded every 5 seconds for 5 readings. Initial pressures should be around 3–4 mm Hg.

excessive instrument manipulation. The insertion of a disposable-shielded trocar in the presence of a pneumoperitoneum requires half the force needed for the insertion of a reusable sharp trocar. A pneumoperitoneum reduces the proximity of the abdominal wall to the spine and the potential for damage to bowel and vessels.

Conventional technique: The direction of trocar insertion is 90° to the abdominal wall plane toward the sacral promontory. Control of the laparoscopic trocar is essential as it penetrates each layer of the anterior abdominal wall. The trocar is inserted with the patient in a horizontal position because viscera tend to slide away from the advancing trocar. A premature Trendelenburg position does not prevent visceral injury even if significant adhesions are present. Altering the patient's position affects the surgeon's view of important landmarks, such as the sacral promontory and hollow of the sacrum. The major anatomic landmarks include the umbilicus located at the level of L3 and L4. The abdominal aorta bifurcates between L4 and L5.

With all trocar insertions, the surgeon must hold the instrument properly with the patient in a supine position at the height of the surgeon's waist or slightly below it. The trocar and its sleeve are held with the index finger extended to the level of the maximal planned penetration to prevent the sharp trocar tip from thrusting too deeply. The trocar is held in the palm of the dominant hand. It is rotated in a semicircular fashion with its long axis as controlled, firm downward pressure is applied. As the trocar is advanced, the operator senses when the fascia is traversed; the force is reduced as the trocar is advanced slowly to enter the peritoneum. Disposable pyramidal tip trocars are preferable. Flat dilating tip trocars leave a smaller fascial defect, but require more force pressure with less control.

2. Direct Trocar Insertion (Fig. 23.18)

Direct trocar insertion refers to inserting the primary trocar without having previously inserted the Veress needle and insufflating the abdomen with carbon dioxide. The primary trocar is inserted in a manner similar to the Veress needle. The sleeve from the trocar is then used to insufflate the abdomen with carbon dioxide. The advantage of this is that it avoids extraperitoneal insufflation. Several studies suggest that the safety of this technique is equal to the Veress needle technique, i.e. complications for bowel injury is between 0.06 and 0.09%.

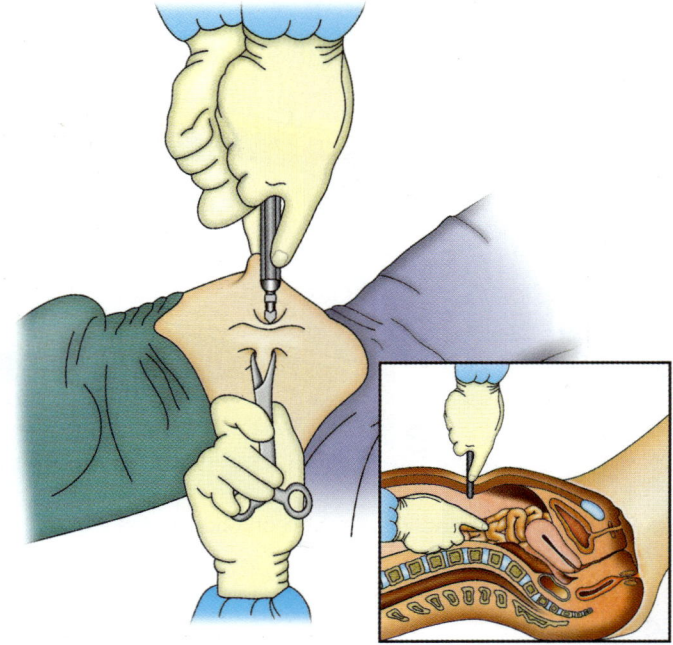

Fig. 23.18: Direct trocar insertion

3. Open Laparoscopy

In 1971, Hasson introduced the concept of open laparoscopy to eliminate the risks associated with insertion of the Veress needle and trocar. This technique involves direct trocar insertion through a small skin incision without prior pneumoperitoneum. Specially designed equipment consists of a cannula and trumpet valve fitted with a cone-shaped sleeve. A blunt obturator protrudes 1 cm from the tip of the cannula. The cone sleeve seals the peritoneal and fascial gap.

A small transverse, curved, or vertical incision is made at or just above the umbilicus. As the incision is made, Allis clamps or a self-retaining retractor is used to provide adequate exposure. Once the fascia is cut, a 1 cm incision is made in the peritoneum. One suture of 0 polydioxanone is passed through each peritoneal edge and fascia and tagged. The cannula carrying the blunt obturator is inserted through the opening into the peritoneal cavity. The obturator is withdrawn, and CO_2 is insufflated through the cannula, which is inserted as deeply as required to prevent leakage. The previously placed sutures are used to fix the trocar sleeve so that the laparoscope can move freely within the abdominal cavity. At the end of the procedure, the abdominal wall is closed, by using the previously placed sutures.

Open laparoscopy usually takes about 5 to 10 min longer than closed laparoscopy performed by operators with comparable expertise. Incidence of minor wound infection is 0.6% and that of small bowel injury is 0.1%.

4. Left Upper Quadrant Insertion

Left upper quadrant insertion of the primary cannula is especially useful for patients with large pelvic masses, patients with suspected abdominal wall adhesions, or in patients in the second trimester of pregnancy. Relative contraindications include ascites, hepatomegaly, and splenomegaly. After induction of general anesthesia with the patient in a horizontal supine position, a gastric drainage tube is placed to empty the stomach.

The skin incision is made 3 cm below the costal margin (4 cm for thin patients with BMI < 20 kg/m^2) in the left midclavicular line. The abdominal skin is tented anteriorly and a 5 mm cannula is advanced at a 45° angle from the horizontal directly into the peritoneal cavity in the sagittal plane. After proper placement is confirmed with the laparoscope, pneumoperitoneum is obtained.

Placement of secondary trocars (Figs 23.19 and 23.20): Secondary trocars are used for most gynecologic laparoscopy procedures, with the exception of some diagnostic laparoscopies. After identifying the epigastric vessels by transillumination and intraperitoneal observation, 1–3 secondary trocars are placed, depending on the procedure and the number of trocars required for the operation.

The trocars are placed either in the midline, 3 cm above the pubic symphysis, or laterally, approximately

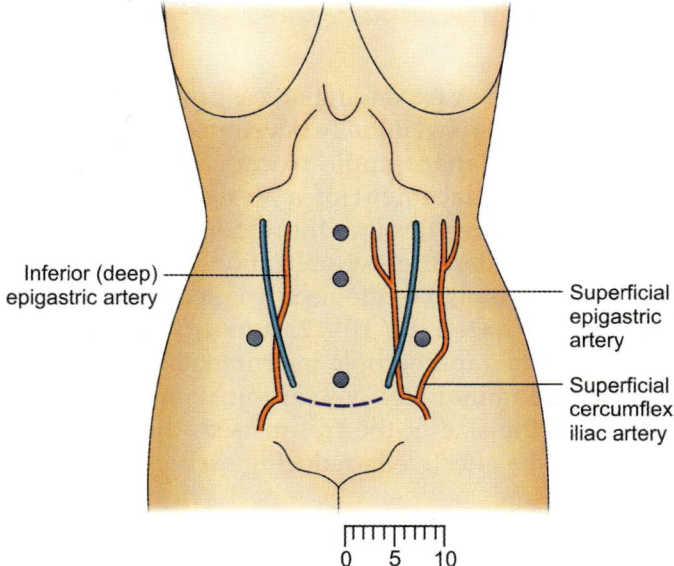

Fig. 23.19: Gynecologic laparoscopy. Location of deep and superficial vessels of the anterior abdominal wall. Blue circles indicate recommended locations for trocar placement

8 cm from the midline and 8 cm above the pubic symphysis to avoid the inferior epigastric vessels, which is 5.5 cm from the midline at this level.

Insertion of the trocar and removal of the sleeves are performed under direct laparoscopic visualization while observing for signs of hemorrhage. If the trocar is larger than 8 mm, the fascia is closed with suture after removal of the sleeve to reduce risk of hernia.

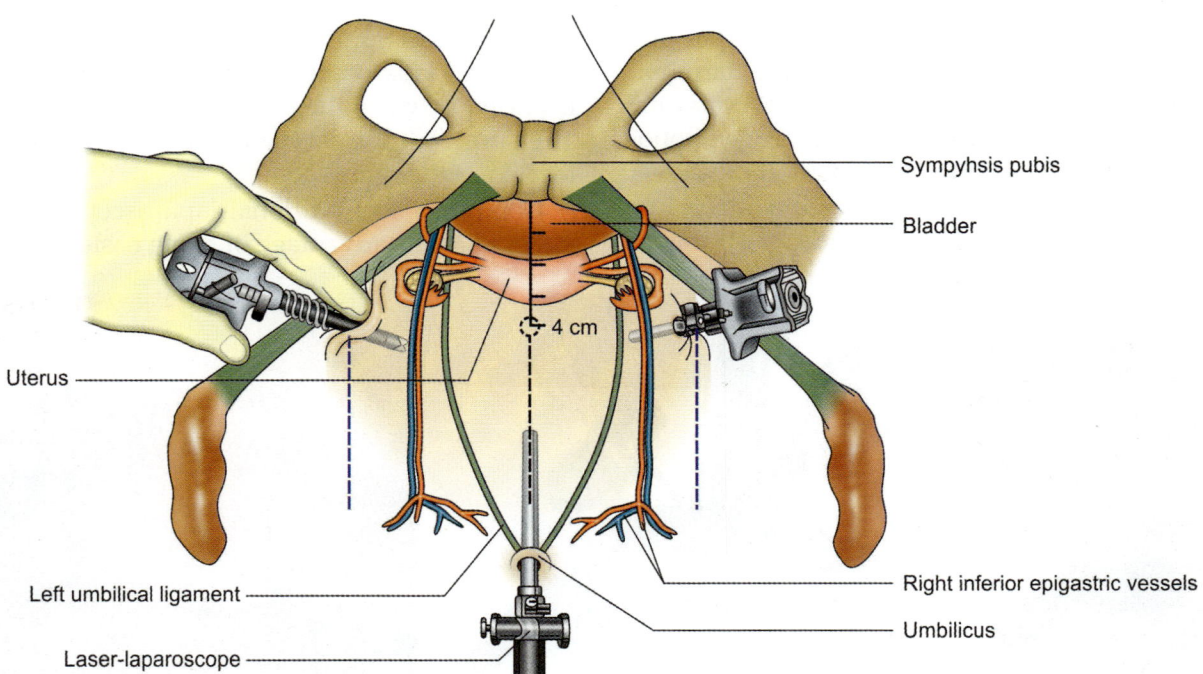

Fig. 23.20: Secondary trocars entry points

5. Radially Expanding-access (REA) Cannulas for Secondary Trocar Placement

The relatively new expanding-access cannula technique described above was initially developed for placement of secondary laparoscopic trocars. This technique involves the placement of a Veress needle in an expandable sleeve through the abdominal wall at the desired site under direct visualization. Once the needle and sleeve are placed, the needle is removed and the sleeve is dilated to 10–12 mm in diameter to accommodate laparoscopic instruments. Because the risk of abdominal wall vessel injury appears to be related to the size of the trocar used, this technique appears to be effective in reducing such injuries.

Power Instruments

Monopolar electrosurgery was the first methodology used for laparoscopic coagulation. In the past 20 years, other methodologies have been developed to minimize the risk of inadvertent injury to adjacent tissue, particularly the bowel. Bipolar electrosurgery offers a greater margin of safety because damage is limited by thermal spread rather than by electrical current; however, cutting ability is reduced. The laser offers a precise, rapid, and accurate method of thermally destroying the tissue, although hemostatic effects are less and the cost is more. Scissors, hook, and ball accessories are available.

Newer energy sources are available that decrease lateral thermal spread of energy while providing hemostasis and the ability to cut tissue. Among these newer instruments are the Harmonic scalpel and impedance-controlled bipolar devices. The Harmonic scalpel uses vibration at the rate of 55,000 cycles per second as an energy source to break hydrogen bonds in tissue, resulting in cutting or coaptation of vessels. It is available as a 5 mm rounded scalpel with a blunt or hooked edge or as a 5 to 10 mm shear or Harmonic

ACE, which can also be used to grasp tissue. The impedance-controlled devices include Enseal, Plasma Kinetic dissection forceps, and LigaSure. They use pressure and pulsed current to seal vessels with minimal lateral thermal spread.

Techniques for Large Vessel Occlusion

As laparoscopy has become more prominent in gynecology, techniques have been designed to offer efficient means of tying and cutting large vessels, such as ovarian and uterine vessels. Traditional suturing with intracorporal or extracorporal knot-tying has been used effectively; however, for most surgeons, these techniques are relatively difficult and slow. The first technique developed to assist in occluding large vessels was the pretied suture loop (Endoloop). Although simple and quick, these types of loops can loosen in the immediate postoperative period.

More recently, new instruments have become available to aid in the suturing process. In addition, linear stapling devices have been used for occluding vessels during removal of adnexal. Finally, one of the best and least expensive approaches for occluding large vessels is bipolar electrocautery, although care must be taken to avoid damage to adjacent structures secondary to lateral heat spread. The newer impedance-controlled bipolar devices are able to seal and divide vessels up to 7 mm in diameter.

Robotic Surgery (Fig. 23.21)

The only robotic system commercially available today is the da Vinci Surgical System. Robotic tools attach to traditional laparoscopic ports and the robotic system is placed between the patient's legs for hysterectomy. The surgeon controls the instruments from a console located in the same room.

Compared to traditional laparoscopy, the robotic system has the advantage of being easier for surgeons

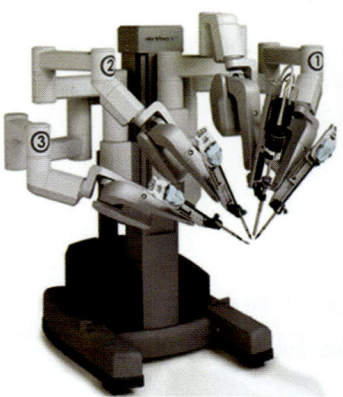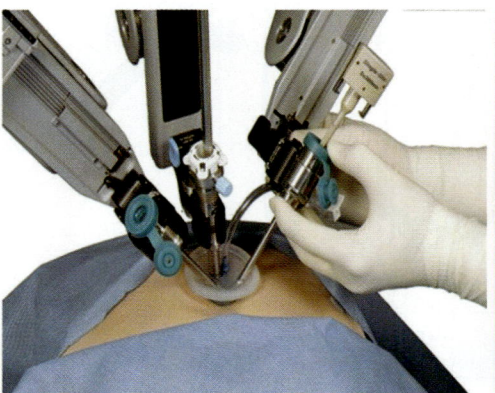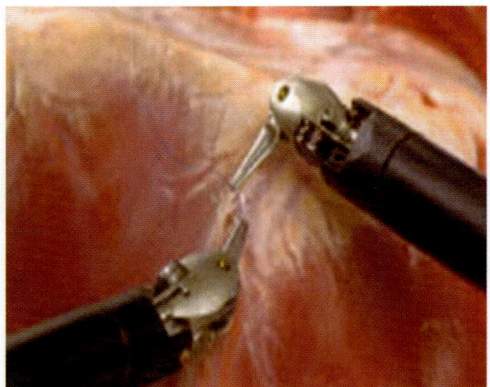

Fig. 23.21: Robotic surgery

to acquire the new skills necessary to operate safely and effectively with this system. Another advantage is direct correlation between hand movements and instrument movements. This is in contrast to traditional laparoscopy, where hand movements are translated into grasping or cutting movements in different flat planes, and gross movements of laparoscopic instrument handles result in mirror image movements of the instrument tips. As a result, surgeons can become proficient in robotic surgery in a matter of months. It appears that robotic technology is allowing the more widespread application of laparoscopy for complicated gynecologic procedures.

Natural Orifice Transluminal Surgery

Natural orifice transluminal surgery (NOTES) refers to using an endoscope to access the abdominal cavity through existing body openings, most notably the mouth, rectum, and vagina. However, the ability to perform complex operative procedures has so far been limited. So far, the role of NOTES in gynecologic practice has been relatively limited as a result of the relative advantages and low complication of traditional laparoscopy.

Single Incision Laparoscopic Surgery

Single incision laparoscopic surgery (SILS) refers to performing laparoscopy through a single incision. This approach is also referred to as single port laparoscopy (SPL) and one port umbilical surgery (OPUS). Gynecologists have performed SILS for decades, using single channel 10 mm operating laparoscopes to perform diagnostic laparoscopy and tubal ligations.

The potential benefit of SILS is similar to NOTES in that it minimizes the number of incisions. This in turn results in decreased pain, improved cosmetics, and reduces the risks associated with a secondary port placement.

The disadvantages of SILS are also similar to NOTES: visibility, depth perception, maneuverability, reach, and the ability to create countertraction are all limited. Articulating instruments are being developed to improve maneuverability; however, these tools have yet to be in common use.

Few gynecologists use the SILS approach because these disadvantages clearly outweigh the potential advantages.

Obtaining Pneumoperitoneum

The next step of the surgery is obtaining the pneumoperitoneum. This step is critical because more than 50% of laparoscopic complications occur during this stage. The insufflation is commenced at 1 liter per minute. Initial pressure should be less than 8 mm Hg. The volume insufflated should be sufficient to increase the distance of inner peritoneal layer 10 cm above the vital intra-abdominal contents for safe entry of trocars. Therefore, initially intra-abdominal pressure may be increased to 25 mm Hg and once ports have been inserted pressure is reduced to maintain at 15 mm Hg.

Closing 5 mm Incisions

Traditionally, the fascia is not closed when incisions are smaller than 10 mm, owing to the low risk of fascial dehiscence and bowel herniation. To avoid this potential problem, all accessory trocars are removed under direct visualization before releasing the pneumoperitoneum, the fascial incision is explored though the scope to notice any bleeding or tissue shredding, and then the abdomen is deflated slowly through the umbilical site. The anterior abdominal wall is then gently pulled outward and gently shaken to release any omental adhesions to the accessory sites. Closing the 5-mm lateral trocar sites depends on whether the fascia is too thinned out, or if the portsite is bleeding or if extensive manipulation or multiple reinsertions of the accessory ports occurred during the procedure. However, umbilical port is routinely closed with Vicryl 2-0 where the fascia and posterior sheath are commonly absent.

Operative Procedures

I. Tubal Sterilization (Fig. 23.22)

Trocar placement is similar to diagnostic laparoscopy. Bipolar electrosurgery, clips, or silastic bands may be used to occlude the tubes at the mid-isthmic portion, approximately 2–3 cm from the cornua. Bipolar surgery desiccates the tube with 3 adjacent passes to occlude approximately 2 cm of tube. However, sialistic band loop closure is most commonly practised method of sterilization with the best possible success rate and reversal rate following tubal reanastomosis. Pregnancy rates vary by patient age, ranging from 1–3% after 10 years.

II. Lysis of Adhesion

Adhesions may form due to prior infection, such as a ruptured appendix or pelvic inflammatory disease (PID), endometriosis, or previous surgery. Adhesions may contribute to infertility or chronic pelvic pain. The chances of pregnancy after lysis of adhesions is relatively low for most patients, and this type of surgery

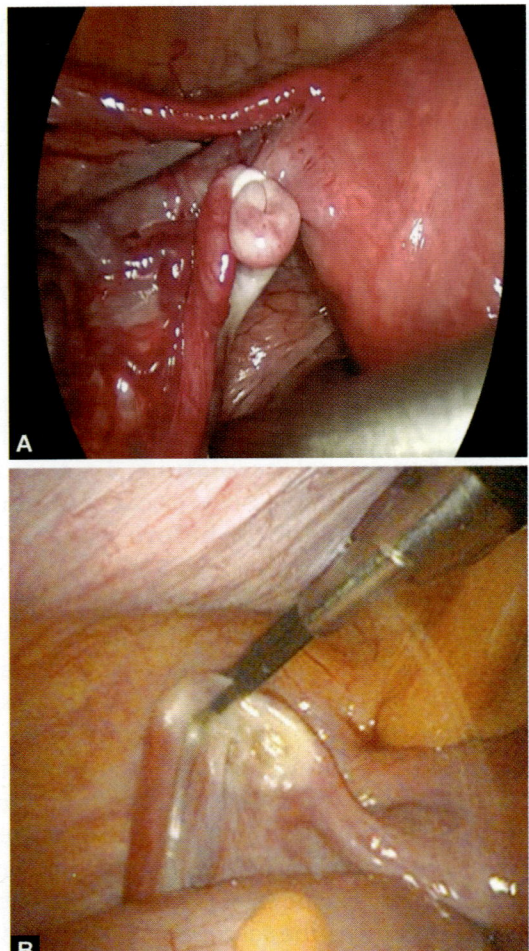

Fig. 23.22: (A) Sialistic band and (B) Tubal coagulation

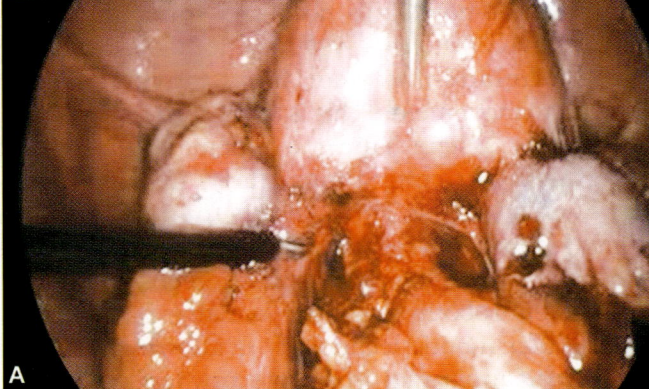

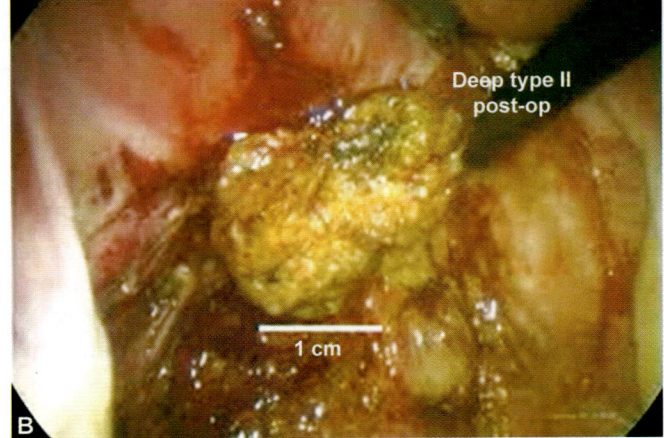

Fig. 23.23: Endometrial peritoneal lesions of laparoscopy

has been largely replaced by in vitro fertilization and embryo transfer. Likewise, adhesiolysis is often ineffective in curing chronic pelvic pain, in part because most adhesions rapidly reform after surgery.

Adhesions may be lysed by blunt or sharp dissection. Aquadissection may aid in the development of planes prior to lysing. Any of the power instruments may be used for cutting and coagulation although use of unipolar electrosurgery is generally recommended to be limited to adhesions 1–2 cm from the ureter and bowel due to the unpredictable nature of current arcing. Other power techniques may be safer choices for adhesiolysis near the bowel.

Adhesions may reform after lysis, although this can be reduced with good hemostasis and minimal use of electrocautery. Recently, 4% icodextrin solution has been shown to decrease adhesion reformation.

III. Treatment of Endometriosis (Fig. 23.23)

Laparoscopy is the most common procedure used to diagnose and treat endometriosis. Endometriotic lesions may be resected or ablated using any of the power instruments. Both of these techniques have shown to improve fertility and decrease pelvic pain.

Several surgical treatments are available for endometriomas. They are:

- *Simple puncture:* This procedure is completed by draining the fluid from the cyst. Endometriomas have been shown to recur in more than 50% of the patients treated with simple puncture.
- *Ablation:* Another approach is to drain the cyst and remove its base with laser or electrosurgery. However, heat can also damage the ovary.
- *Excision of the cyst wall:* This is the procedure of choice to decrease recurrence of disease. This procedure can also damage the outer layer of the ovary that contains the eggs.
- *Draining, drug therapy, and surgery:* Endometriomas can also be drained, treated with medication, and later removed by surgery.

IV. Treatment of Ectopic Pregnanc y

Laparoscopy is the surgical approach of choice for most ectopic pregnancies. A salpingostomy or salpingectomy is performed to remove the embryo and gestational sac.

In salpingostomy, initially a linear slit is made in the fallopian tube over the ectopic with a monopolar cautery. Then the ectopic gestation sac is teased out of the tube intact and hemostatsis is done by forceful irrigation and bipolar cautery. No suture is given on the tube.

V. Ovarian Cystectomy (Fig. 23.24)

If a simple ovarian cyst of 6 cm or larger size persists for 2 or more cycles in a premenopausal, nonpregnant female, cystectomy is indicated. The cyst can be removed by a number of techniques. If the cyst is complex, malignancy needs to be excluded by looking for signs of ascites; excrescences on the ovary; or implantations on the peritoneal, liver, or diaphragmatic surfaces. If malignancy is not apparent, the cyst is dissected out, making an effort to remove the cyst intact. A bag may be used to transfer the cyst out of the peritoneal cavity through a 10 mm port, draining the cyst prior to removal of the bag. If any doubt exists, the cyst wall should be sent for frozen section to confirm a benign cyst. If malignancy is found, a laparotomy should be performed.

If the cyst ruptures during removal, the peritoneal cavity is rinsed liberally with Ringer lactate solution. A dermoid cyst is particularly concerning because of contamination of the peritoneal cavity with sebaceous material, causing a chemical peritonitis. Fear of seeding the cavity with a malignant tumor has always been present, although recent data suggest that spilling does not alter the prognosis if a staging laparotomy is performed immediately.

Ovariotomy (Fig. 23.25)

An oophorectomy may be more appropriate in postmenopausal women with a growing or persistent cyst. The power instruments, pretied loops, or stapling devices may be used to occlude the infundibular ligament and safely remove the ovary. Because of ovary

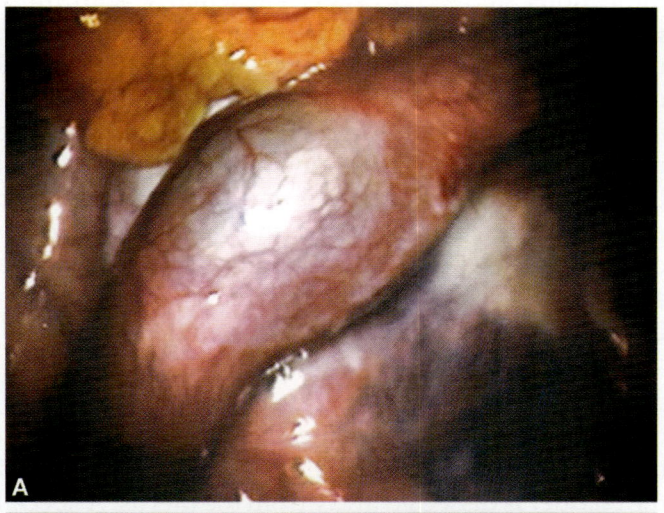

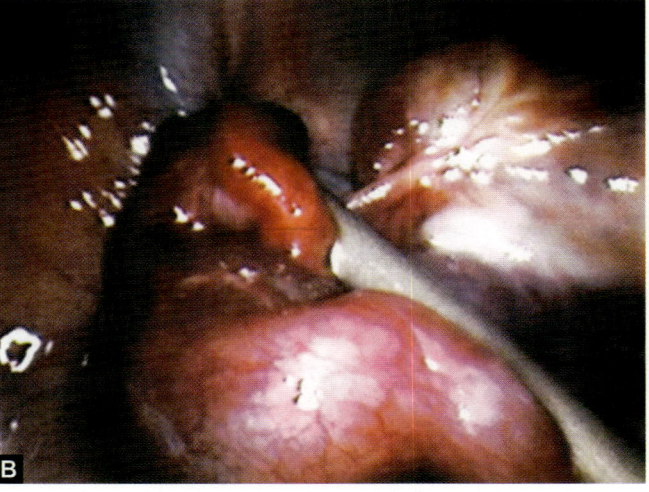

Fig. 23.24: Ovarian cystectomy

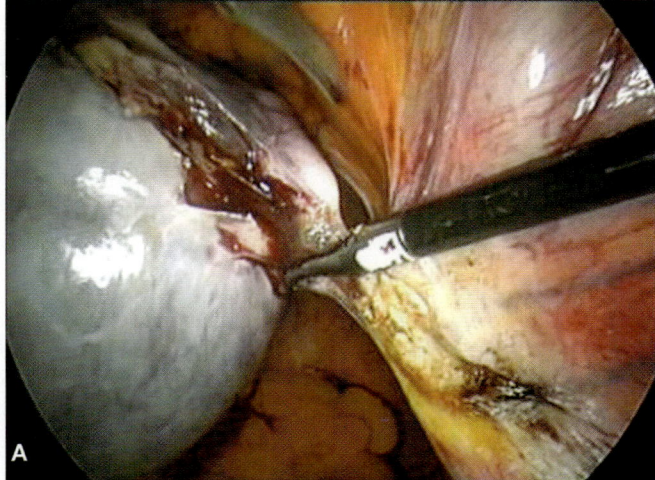

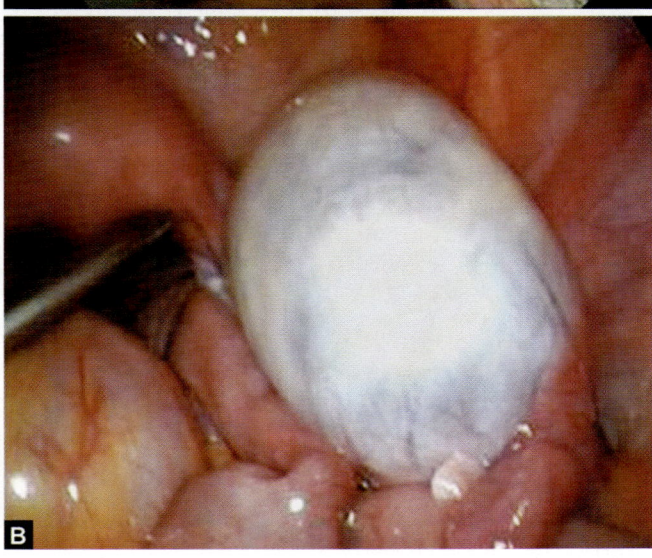

Fig. 23.25: Ovariotomy

size, a retrieval bag is needed to remove the tissue. Options for removing the ovary from the peritoneal cavity include (1) using a 12-mm port and removing the sleeve with the bag or (2) performing a minilaparotomy or colpotomy.

Myomectomy (Fig. 23.26)

Many women with symptomatic fibroid uterus prefer myomectomy to hysterectomy in order to preserve fertility and the uterus. If the patient has a pedunculated fibroid, the stalk may be easily incised. However, for intramural fibroids, the risk of bleeding increases. The use of preoperative gonadotropin-releasing hormone (GnRH) agonist may be considered in patients who are anemic. However, this results in longer operative times and higher conversion rate to laparotomy due to difficult cleavage planes. An injection of vasopressin into the uterus may help maintain hemostasis. The defect left by the fibroid are sutured with delayed absorbable suture (vicryl) in layers or Barbed sutures which do not require tying knots. Barrier techniques may be used to decrease adhesion formation.

The fibroid may be removed by morcellation or colpotomy. Some concern exists that the risk of subsequent uterine rupture during pregnancy may be greater after myomectomy performed by laparoscopy compared with laparotomy. However, recent studies do not confirm this.

Hysterectomy

Currently, laparoscopic hysterectomy is done in all indicated cases even in malignant condition of cervix and uterus in early stages. It is often used to assess feasibility of a vaginal hysterectomy when adhesions, endometriosis, or a large fibroid uterus is supected. The three basic laparoscopic approaches for hysterectomy are laparoscopic-assisted vaginal hysterectomy (LAVH), total laparoscopic hysterectomy (TLH), and laparoscopic supracervical hysterectomy (LSH).

LAVH is the most commonly employed and technically straight forward of the three techniques. Using 3–4 ports, the peritoneal cavity is surveyed and lysis of adhesions is performed, if necessary. The infundibular or utero-ovarian ligaments are occluded and divided, depending on whether the ovaries will be removed. The round ligament is cut in a similar fashion, and the uterovesical peritoneum is incised. Depending on surgeon's preference, the proximal uterine blood supply is occluded and divided laparoscopically. The posterior cul-de-sac is also excised. The surgeon then proceeds vaginally for the remainder of the case, dissecting the vesicovaginal septum anteriorly to enter the peritoneal cavity, ligating the uterine vessels, removing the uterus and ovaries (if appropriate), and closing the vaginal cuff.

TLH (Figs 23.27 and 23.28) is performed initially like the LAVH, except that the entire hysterectomy is performed laparoscopically. The surgeon would choose indications similar to LAVH particularly with those with lack of uterine descent. After the infundibular, utero-ovarian, and round ligament are occluded and divided, the bladder is dissected off the uterus anteriorly. The ureter is identified and dissected along its entire course, and the uterine vessels and uterosacral ligaments are then occluded and divided. After the posterior cul-de-sac is incised, the vault is made open over a vaginal tube, uterus is made free from vagina and is removed vaginally. The cuff is closed with intracorporeal sutures.

LSH is rarely promoted for benign indications with gross adhesions. The technique begins as for LAVH, but proceeds with separating the entire fundus from the cervix after the proximal vessels are divided and the bladder is dissected away from the uterus. A special instrument is used to core-out or cauterize the

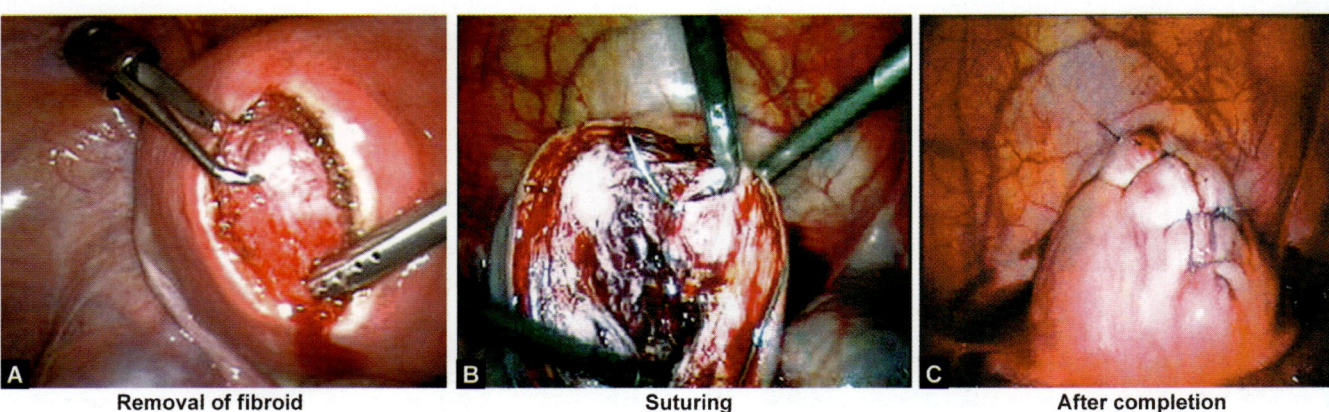

A   **Removal of fibroid**   B   **Suturing**   C   **After completion**

Fig. 23.26: Laparoscopy myomectomy

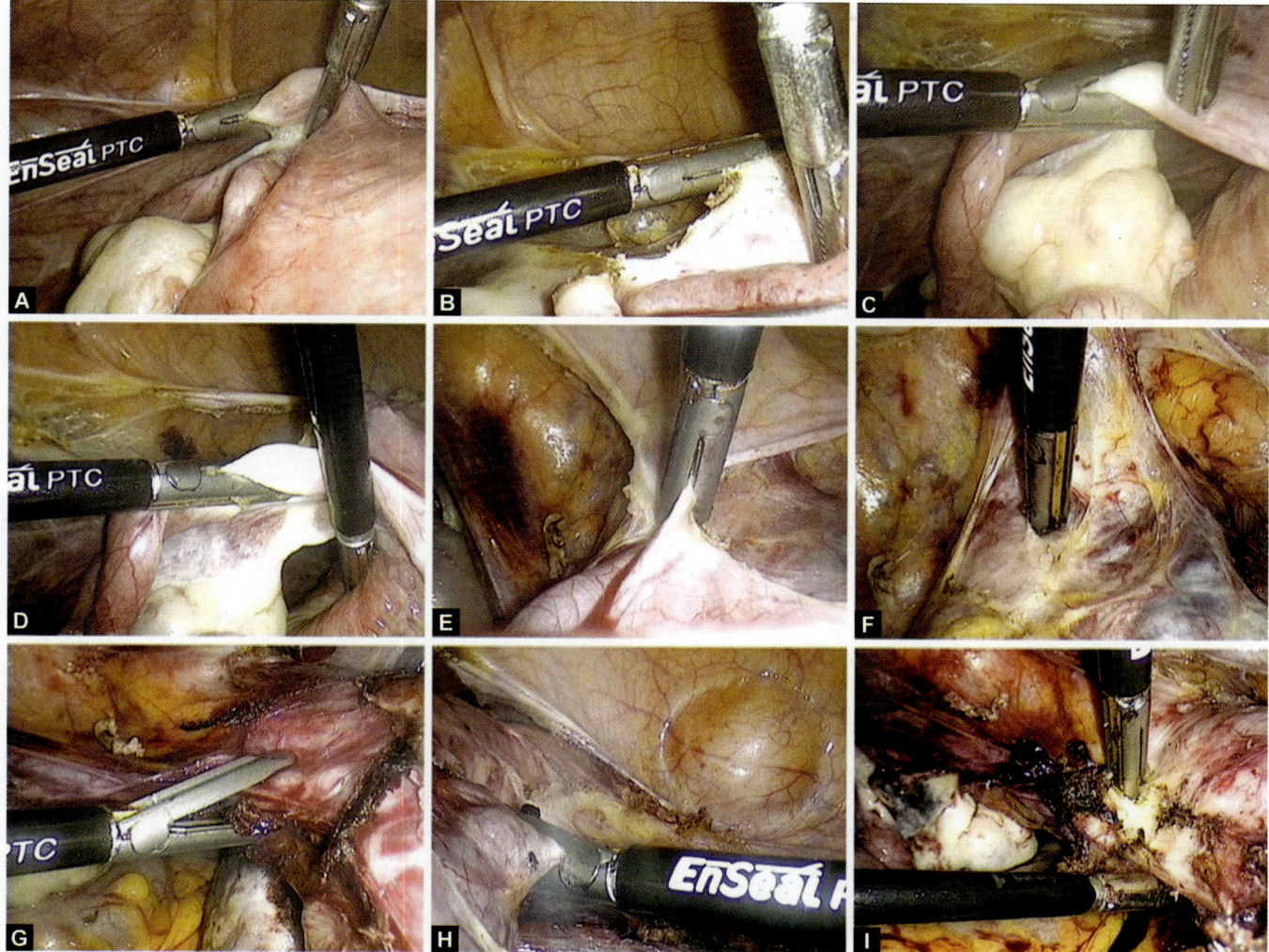

Fig. 23.27: Steps of TLH: (A, B) Ovarian vessel ligation; (C, D) Round ligament cut; (E) Uter ovesical fold being cut; (F) Bladder dissected down; (G, H) Uterine vessels ligation; (I) Parametrium cardinal ligament being cut

endocervix, and the uterus is then removed through a 12 mm port abdominally by morcellation. This approach eliminates vaginal and abdominal incisions, with no need to dissect near the uterine artery or ureter. Proponents of LSH advocate that the operating room and recovery time are decreased and risk of both infection and ureteral injury are minimized. However, an increased risk exists for reoperation for cervical bleeding and prolapse. Furthermore, patients must follow the recommendations for regular cervical cytology.

Oncologic Procedures

Laparoscopy has long been used in oncology for second-look procedures following surgery and chemotherapy. More recently, laparoscopy has also been used for staging, including peritoneal washes with biopsy, partial omentectomy, and pelvic and periaortic lymphadenectomy. Procedures such as laparoscopic radical hysterectomy with bilateral lymphadenectomy are performed regularly for operable cancer cervix (Fig. 23.29).

Robotic laparoscopic surgery have changed the approach to many gynecologic cancer cases. The robotic system has the advantages of three-dimensional, high-definition imaging and magnification that improve the topography of the pelvis and the cervicovaginal plane. Fully articulated instruments emulate the full range of motion of a surgeon's wrists and hands. This enhances the surgeon's ability to remotely perform fine motor skills such as intricate dissections and intracorporeal suturing that remain difficult during traditional laparoscopy.

Postoperative Care

After any gynecologic laparoscopic procedure, progressive resolution of symptoms is expected 3–7 days postoperatively. With major procedures, return

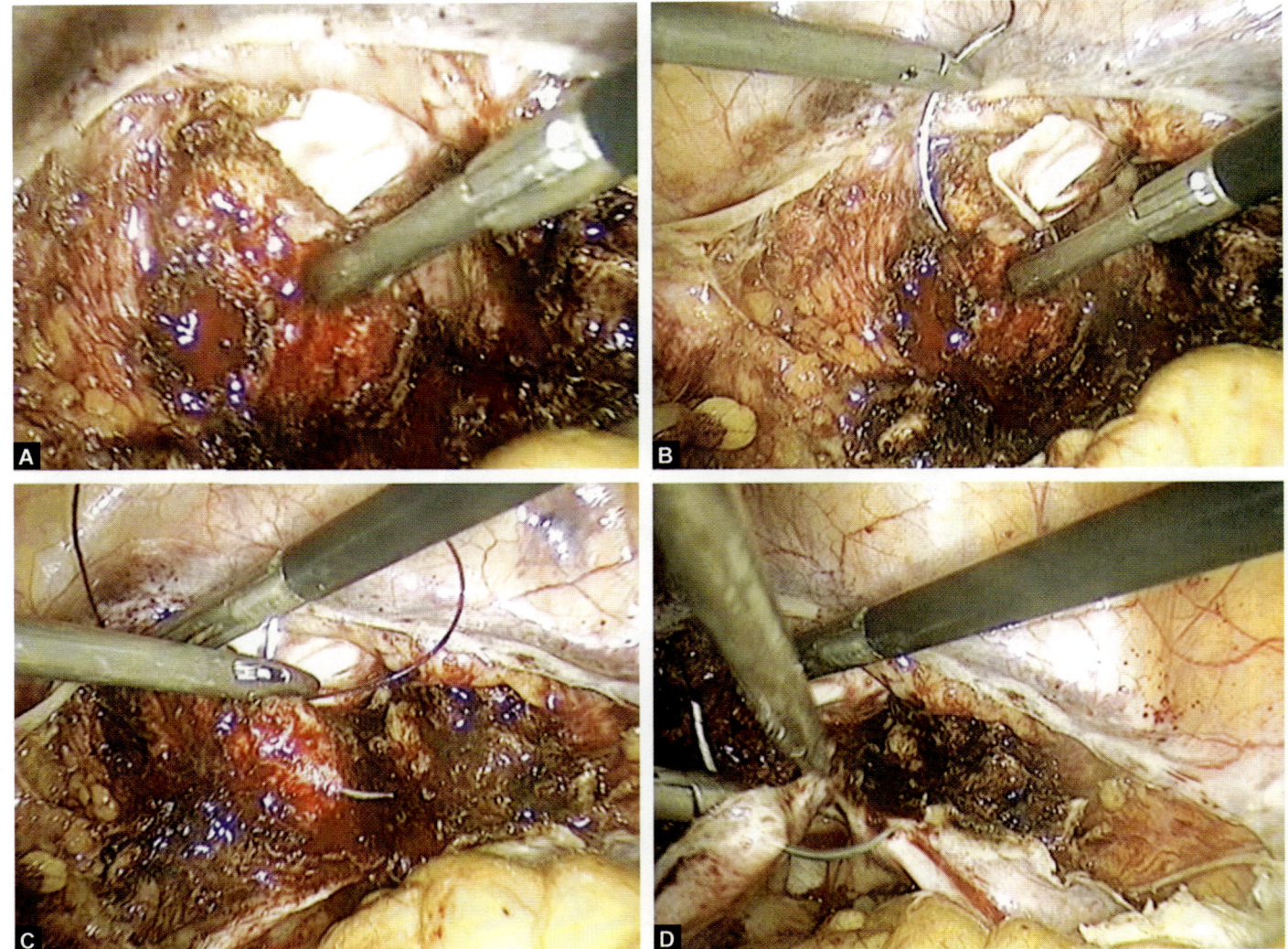

Fig. 23.28: Vault suturing in TLH

to completely normal bowel function may take several days. For any procedure, pain may be perceived as slightly worse on the day following the procedure but should improve after this point. Likewise, the incision should appear healthy and become almost painless within the first week.

Probably the most concerning postoperative symptom is worsening abdominal pain, especially in the presence of distension. Signs of an occult injury of bowel or bladder may take hours or days to develop (Fig. 23.30).

An unusual cause of abdominal pain is an entrapped incisional hernia that can occur after laparoscopy. Herniation is rare at the site where the laparoscope is placed through the umbilicus. However, bowel herniation has been reported to occur when larger trocars (>5 mm) are used in locations lateral to the midline. Apparently, this is not related to herniation through a fascial defect, but rather entrapment of bowel that has herniated through the peritoneum into the preperitoneal space.

Follow-up

In the absence of complications, the patient should be able to return to full activity within 72 hours after most gynecologic laparoscopic procedures other than hysterectomy. Because complete healing of fascial defects takes several weeks, the patient should avoid lifting anything heavier than 15 pounds for the first month.

Recovery from laparoscopic hysterectomy can be expected within 2–3 weeks. Again, because healing continues to take place for the first month, heavy lifting should be delayed for 4 weeks. Follow-up visits in patients without complications are usually scheduled 2–4 weeks after surgery.

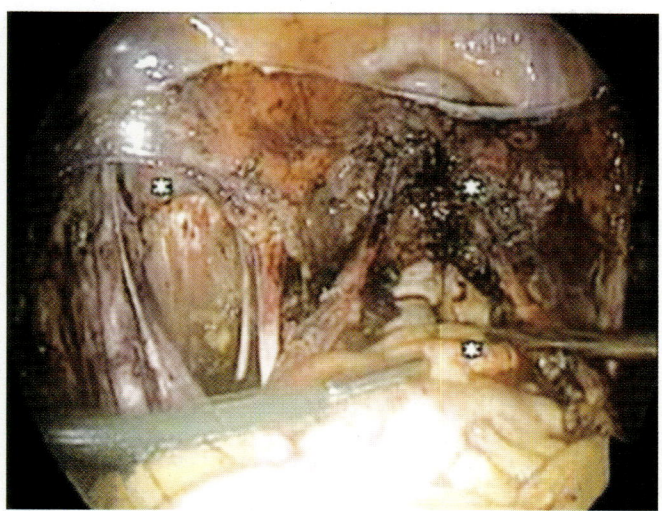

Fig. 23.29: Laparoscopic view of the field after radical hysterectomy and pelvic lymphadenectomy

Complications of Laparoscopic Gynecologic Surgery (Table 23.3)

Despite rapidly improving technical equipment and surgical skill, complication rates and preventable injuries still persist. The overall complication rates range from 0.2 to 10.3%. Major laparoscopic procedures are associated with a higher rate of complications compared with minor procedures, 0.6 to 18% and 0.06 to 7.0%, respectively.

The majority of complications occur during entry of instruments into the abdomen used to create pneumoperitoneum. The incidence of many complications decreases with open-entry technique.

Other reasons for complications are thermal and energy source injuries, operative manipulations, and suturing, and the presence of CO_2 out of the peritoneum. Because some complications result from more than one cause, clear classification of complications is challenging.

Intestinal Injury (Fig. 23.30)

The incidence of bowel injury is reported to be 0 to 0.5%. Approximately half of bowel injuries occur during entry, and the rest occur during the operation.

Entry-related bowel injuries are mostly lacerations, and intraoperative injuries are mostly thermal. Most bowel injuries are not diagnosed during surgery. Delayed intervention may be life-threatening. Therefore, this complication is reported to be the most common cause of laparoscopy-related mortality. If the diagnosis is delayed more than 72 hours, the mortality rate significantly increases.

When bowel is entered via Veress needle or trocar, bowel content or gas passage may be observed, or may

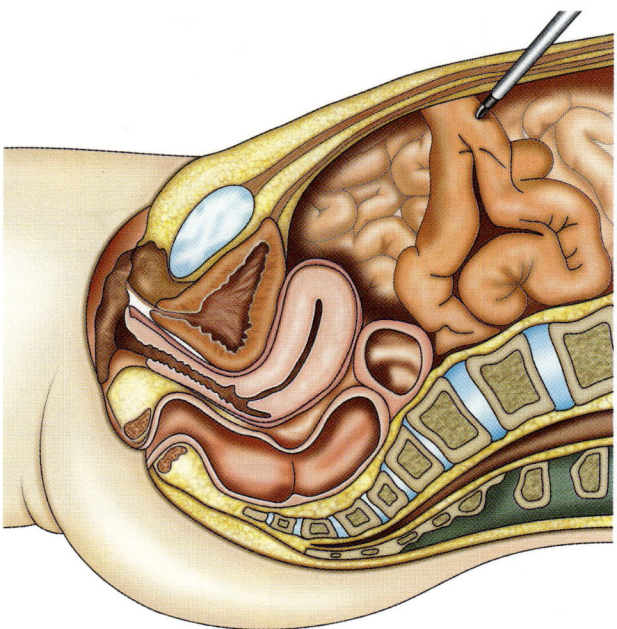

Fig. 23.30: Entry related bowel injury

be controlled with a syringe, if suspected. A laparoscope will show bowel lumen in such a case. If intraoperatively unrecognized, patients present with nonspecific complaints not exactly pointing to peritonitis, such as mild abdominal pain, fever, diarrhea, and abdominal distension, further delaying the diagnosis. Late consequences may be generalized peritonitis, abscess formation, and septic shock.

Between 52.4 and 90.0% of intestinal injuries are repaired laparotomically. Injury caused by the Veress needle may be managed expectantly. However, trocar injuries deserve laparotomic repair according to the size and location of the injury. Primary closure in 2 layers is adequate in small bowel injuries. If the large bowel is involved, the treatment options include primary repair, colostomy, or segmental resection. Resection is mandatory in thermal injuries. Intraoperative lacerations may be repaired laparoscopically according to the size of the lesion, surgeon experience, and preoperative bowel preparation.

Urinary Tract Injury

Incidence varies between 1.4 and 0.7%. Of all urinary injuries, 64.7% occur with laparoscopic-assisted vaginal hysterectomy, 18.0% during operations for endometriosis, and 12.3% during diagnostic or sterilization procedures.

Ureteral Injury

Pelvic surgery is the most common cause of iatrogenic ureteral injury. It is becoming more common as a result

Table 23.3 Summary of complications of laparoscopic gynecologic surgery

Complication	Rate (%)	Cause of complication	Clinical presentation	Management
Abdominal wall vascular injury	0.5	Entry related	Intraoperative blood dropping to operation field Postoperative hemorrhage and hematoma	Coagulation tamponade suturing
Intestinal injury	0-0.5	Entry related (laceration) Operative (thermal)	Usually diagonsed postoperatively with peritonitis-like findings.	Most cases require conversion to laparotomy. Thermal injury: bowel resection Tracar injury: Primary repair or resection is related to site of injury and bowel preparation. Veress injury: can be managed expectantly
Ureteral injury	0.025–2	Electrocautery (leading cause) Other (i.e. trocar, laser, dissection, staples, suturing)	Intraoperative diagnosis is very rare. Presentation may be delayed by several weeks especially in thermal injury. Symptoms are variable.	Intraoperative diagnosed patients: Intraoperative laparoscopic repair, double J-shaped catheter for focal injury Postoperative diagnosed patients: Laparotomic end-to-end anastomosis, ureteral implantation, ureteral reconstruction or ureteroneocystostomy
Bladder injury	0.02–8.3	Entry related Thermal during dissection	Most of cases diagnosed intraoperatively. Abdominal discomfort and oliguria are major findings postoperatively.	Based on localization, extension and type of injury; conservative management or surgical repair
Major vascular injury	0.04–0.5	Entry related Energy source Operative	Bleeding from trocar or Veress observation via laparoscope Retroperitoneal hematoma	Laparotomic vessel repair without removing Veress or trocar Laparoscopic repair also reported.
Hernia at trocar site	0.17–0.2	Entry related	Bowel obstruction findings, incarceration	Laparoscopic or laparotomic hernia repair. Bowel resection in incarcerated cases
Subcutaneous emphysema	2.3	CO_2 presence in subcutaneous tissue	Subcutaneous emphysema	Resolve spontaneously
Hypercarbia	5.5	Longer operative times, high end-tidal CO_2, old age	Acidosis	Ventilation
Cardiac arrhythmia	27	—	Sinus tachycardia, bradycardia, ventricular, tachycardia, and asystole	Stoppping gas in-flow, anticholinergic agent for bradycardia Reinsufflation after arrhythmia settles down
Pneumothorax/ pneumomediastinum	0.2–1.9	Pneumoperitoneum, diaphragmatic defect	Respiratory related symptoms	Discharging CO_2 from peritoneal cavity Inhalation with 100% O_2, thorax tube
Port-site metastasis	1.1–2.3	Pneumoperitoneum and CO_2 related	Postoperative port-site tumor	Resection, chemotherapy, radiotherapy

of the increasing number of laparoscopic hysterectomies and retroperitoneal laparoscopic procedures that are being performed. The majority of patients with ureteral injuries have no identifiable predisposing risk factors. Estimated incidence of ureteral injury during laparoscopic hysterectomy is 0.2 to 6% (2.6 to 35 times more common than in abdominal hysterectomy) and account for 4.3 to 7% of total laparoscopy complications.

Electrocautery (unipolar or bipolar) is identified as the leading cause of laparoscopic ureteral injury. Injuries with loop suturing, trocars, laser devices, staples, and sharp dissection are also described. In particular, the three locations carry the risk for ureteral injury during laparoscopic surgeries: At the pelvic brim, where the ureters lie beneath the insertions of the infundibulopelvic ligaments; deep ovarian fossa where the ureter passes; and the place of crossing over of uterine vessels.

Injuries may include transection, ligation, avulsion, crush injury, devascularization, resection, fulguration, and perforation. The injuries mainly occur in LAVH (20%), 11% during oophorectomy, 10% during laparoscopic pelvic lymphadenectomy, 7% during laparoscopic sterilization, 7% during excision and ablation of endometriosis, and 4% during each of the following—drainage of lymphoceles, electrocoagulation, and laparoscopic adhesiolysis.

These injuries are frequently undetected. Depending on the type of injury, patients may present in the early postoperative period (first 3 days), or presentation of the thermal or laceration injuries may be delayed by several days or weeks.

There are five methods for identifying ureteral injury: (1) retrograde ureteral dye injection; (2) 5 to 10 mL intravenous Indigo carmine injection; (3) intraoperative ureteral catheterization; (4) intravenous excretory urography; and (5) dissection of the ureter. A coagulated or ligated ureter may not demonstrate an intraperitoneal urine leak when tested intraoperatively. The lack of ureteral jet at cystoscopic examination will indicate the problem clearly in such a case.

Postoperative presentation is variable and nonspecific, such as acute pelvic pain, nausea, vomiting, malaise, leakage of fluid via the trocar sites, abdominal distension and an inflammatory reaction in the serum (elevated CRP and leukocytosis), elevated creatinine level, costovertebral angle tenderness, ileus, fever, flank pain, and peritonitis. X-ray of the abdomen may reveal a ground-glass appearance indicative of fluid collection. A computed tomography scan reveal the presence of urine in the peritoneal cavity after intravenous contrast medium injection. Ligation of the ureter, with stapling or stricture resulting from thermal injury may lead to obstructive uropathy and superimposed pyonephrosis. The diagnosis should be confirmed by an intravenous urogram.

Laparoscopic repair is frequently used in cases recognized intraoperatively, while the laparotomic approach is performed in patients diagnosed postoperatively. Focal ureteral injuries can be treated using a double J-shaped catheter allowing for spontaneous healing. However, more extensive damage may require laparotomy to perform an end-to-end anastomosis or ureteral implantation. In delayed recognition of ureteral injury, initial treatment with ureteral stenting may not be useful, and early open repair (ureteral reconstruction, ureteroneocystostomy) for these injuries is advocated.

To minimize ureteral injury, use of sutures should be preferred instead of staplers or electrocautery in close proximity to ureters. Visualization of ureters during the operation, use of ureteral catheters, and creating hydroprotection by injection of saline to parietal peritoneum are the other protective measures.

Bladder Injury

The most common type of urinary injury during laparoscopy is bladder entry with an incidence of 0.02 to 8.3%. Most injuries occur during hysterectomy operations. Endometriosis, previous surgery, an inexperienced surgeon, overdistended bladder, and pelvic adhesions are proposed risk factors for bladder injury.

Bladder injury may occur during insertion of trocars, especially suprapubic ones, dissection of the bladder during gynecologic operations, or as a result of thermal energy. Of bladder injuries, 90% occur at the bladder dome, and the rest at the base. Of these injuries, 33% follow sharp electrocautery dissections, 21% by blunt and 15% by scissors. Five percent of thermal injuries may lead to fistula formation. More than half of trocar-related injuries occur via 5 mm and the rest via 10 mm trocars.

Only 9.2% of bladder injuries are not recognized intraoperatively, in contrast to ureteral injuries; therefore, morbidity is lower. In suspected cases, filling the bladder with methylene blue dye to observe dye leakage will help in diagnosis. Patients with unrecognized cases present with abdominal discomfort and oliguria as a cardinal sign. According to type, size, and localization of injury, conservative or surgical management via laparoscopic, laparotomic, or vaginal approaches may be considered.

To prevent bladder injures: (1) Perform a very careful dissection of the vesicovaginal pouch and use uterine cannulation; (2) fill the bladder with a methylene blue dye solution to visualize its limits in case of difficult dissection, such as previous surgery (cesarean delivery, endometriosis surgery, conization, and others.); (3) perform very careful and restricted use of bipolar coagulation in the vesicovaginal space for hemostasis; and (4) follow the safety rules of introduction, in particular avoiding the Pfannenstiel scar.

Abdominal Wall Vascular Injury

Injuries involving the inferior epigastric vessel are the most common type of vascular complication. The incidence of abdominal wall bleeding is 0.3 to 0.5%. Epigastric and less commonly muscular vessels may be the origin of bleeding. These injuries usually occur in relation to the positioning of accessory ports, used principally to allow the insertion of the hand instruments necessary for dissecting and manipulating tissue. Blood dripping into the operative field may indicate intraoperative bleeding, and postoperatively if not detected early patient may go into shock.

Postoperative hematoma and abscess may be other consequences.

The most rapid and practical technique for hemostasis is coagulation. If bleeding is not controlled in this way, tamponade and suturing may be used. Suturing may be either laparoscopic or through an enlarged incision at the trocar site. Minilaparotomy may also be used. The site of bleeding should be re-evaluated under low pneumoperitoneal pressure after coagulation, tamponade, and suturing. Transillumination of the anterior abdominal wall, insertion of the trocar lateral to the sheath of the rectus muscle, and use of smaller trocars in lateral ports may help avoid vascular injury. It is good practice to inspect all secondary trocar sites for active bleeding before the laparoscope is finally withdrawn.

Hernia at the Site of the Abdominal Wall Trocar

Up to one-third of all trocar injuries cause incisional hernia formation. It is a preventable complication with an incidence of 0.17 to 0.2%. Generally, extraumbilical and >5 mm trocar sites are prone to herniation. Intestines, colon, and omentum may be involved. Signs of intestinal obstruction, increased bowel sounds, diarrhea, nausea, and vomiting may indicate a hernia.

Although repairing the hernia is enough in most of these cases, 19% require intestinal resection secondary to incarceration. Hernias are repaired laparotomically or less commonly, laparoscopically. Trocar sites > 10 mm should be sutured for prevention. To minimize the risk of herniation, secondary trocars should be removed under supervision before the primary one, valves should be kept closed to prevent a sucking effect, and 5 mm trocars should be preferred.

Pneumoperitoneum Related Complications

Hypercarbia and, therefore, acidosis develop due to absorption of CO_2 in prolonged operations with an incidence of 5.5%.

Subcutaneous emphysema, pneumomediastinum, and pneumothorax may result from preperitoneal insufflation or leakage of CO_2 around the cannula sites. Prolonged operations, higher maximum measured end-tidal CO_2, a greater number of surgical ports, and old, obese patient increase the risk.

Subcutaneous emphysema means the subcutaneous presence of CO_2. Its incidence is 2.3%. Generally, it has no significant clinical outcome and resolves spontaneously. Subcutaneous emphysema may be extensive involving the extremities, the neck the

mediastinum, and even the pericardium, and can result in hypercapnia and cardiovascular collapse.

Preperitoneal emphysema results from preperitoneal insufflation, especially in obese patients when the Veress needle cannot reach the peritoneal cavity. The Veress needle can be inserted at a 90° angle in obese patients. However, this application may increase the risk of other complications. Alternatively, open-entry may be preferred. Some authors advocate direct trocar entry that may prevent preperitoneal emphysema without increasing other complications.

Pneumomediastinum results from migration of preperitoneal gas to the mediastinum. In the presence of a congenital diaphragmatic defect or intraoperative diaphragm injury, pneumomediastinum and **pneumothorax** may occur. The incidence is 0.2 to 1.9% for pneumothorax/pneumomediastinum. Inhalation of 100% O_2 and application of a thorax tube after discharging CO_2 from the peritoneal cavity must be done. **Pneumopericardium** has also been reported to occur in association with pneumomediastinum and subcutaneous emphysema.

Persistence of Pneumoperitoneum

Because CO_2 is more rapidly absorbed than air, less intra-abdominal air persistence is observed postoperatively than in laparotomic operations. It is even less in obese patients than in lean patients. Generally, it does not persist after the seventh day.

Gas Embolism

This is a rare but life-threatening complication. It results from introduction of CO_2 through the Veress needle into the large veins. Its earliest sign is a drop in end-tidal carbon dioxide concentration, due to diminished blood flow to the lungs. The diagnostic features include sudden circulatory collapse, cyanosis, and raised jugular venous pressure. Blood coming from the Veress needle is an alert, and the needle should not be removed. It necessitates cardiopulmonary resuscitation. The patient lies on her left side. Aspiration of intracardiac gas may be tried. To prevent room-air embolism, which is more dangerous than CO_2, the air in the insufflation tube should be flushed out.

Postoperative Shoulder Pain

Secondary to irritation of the diaphragm, shoulder pain is felt through phrenic nerves. Also a stretched falciform ligament due to the Trendelenburg position adds to the shoulder pain. Careful discharge of intraperitoneal gas after the operation is necessary.

Vulvar Edema

This occurs especially in patients in whom adhesion barrier solution is used; therefore, its leakage to the vulva is thought to be the cause. The method of the leakage could be either through patent canal of Nuck, or a fistulous tract originating in a lower trocar puncture wound and dissecting downward subcutaneously by the force of gravity, as supported by others.

Complications Related to Anesthesia and Patient Position

Nerve Injury

Transient nerve injuries may occur during any procedure with incorrect positioning, affecting brachial plexus, common peroneal nerve, and also the saphenous nerve.

Cardiac Arrhythmia

Cardiac arrhythmias including bradycardia, sinus tachycardia, ventricular tachycardia, and arrest related to anesthesia have been reported in laparoscopy. The incidence of cardiac and respiratory arrest is 0.02%.

Port Site Infection (Fig. 23.31)

Infections at the port sites of laparoscopic surgery can be of two types. The first type occurs immediately within a week of surgery. It is caused by gram-negative or positive bacteria derived from infection acquired during surgery from the infected gallbladder or from the skin or the surgical procedure itself and can be treated by common antibiotics and local wound dressing. The second type is caused by atypical mycobacteria and has an incubation period of 3 to 4 weeks and do not respond to common antibiotics.

It has been shown that endospores of atypical mycobacteria, particularly *M. chelonae* and *M. fortuitum,* both of which belong to the group of rapidly growing mycobacteria, widely colonize soil, and water. This mycobacterial complex primarily presents itself as localized cutaneous infection 3–4 weeks after surgery. These bacteria have an affinity for the dermis and the subcutaneous area and protective factors within the peritoneum destroy the mycobacteria and prevent infection within. After laparoscopic procedures, the infection starts at the 10 mm port sites such as the epigastric or umbilical ports after which it spreads sequentially to the other ports. It is very important to make clinical diagnosis based on the signs, since culture of the pus collected from the port sites is negative for mycobacterial culture and AFB staining. The only method to obtain microbiological evidence is through

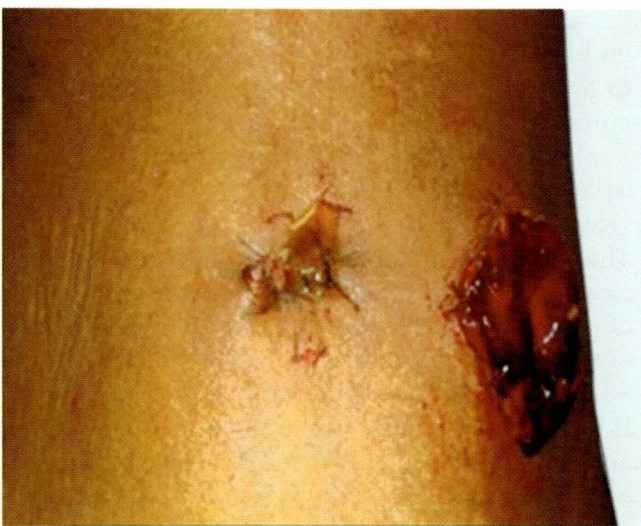

Fig. 23.31: Port site infection

tissue culture from the wall of the cavity, which is very difficult to obtain and takes 3 weeks to isolate from culture leading to delayed treatment, which makes clinical diagnosis the best option.

The presentation can be described in five stages. The first stage is characterized by **tender nodules** which appears 4 weeks after the laparoscopic surgery and projects out in the vicinity of the port site. During the second stage, the nodules get bigger in size, become more tender and inflamed and eventually form **a sinus discharging white pus**. In the third stage of infection, there is a reduction of pain following discharge of pus with **necroses of overlying skin**. In the fourth stage, the area develops into a chronic sinus discharging white fluid followed by the fifth stage where the area **darkens with necrosed skin.** If left untreated, the infection can continue for months and multiple nodules appear in different areas.

Infections with atypical mycobacteria have been primarily reported after laparoscopic procedures. This is because, unlike open surgery, the instruments used here have a layer of insulation that restricts the use of the autoclave in the sterilization process. Also, proper mechanical cleaning of the instruments is not done, which leaves the deposit of blood and charred tissue that collects in the joints of the instruments during surgery. Contaminated instruments deposit the endospores on to the subcutaneous tissue during the surgical process, which then germinate following which clinical symptoms appear after an incubation period of 3 to 4 weeks. The current practice in India is to immerse instruments in 2–2.5% glutaraldehyde solution for 20 minutes which achieves disinfection but does not kill the mycobacterial spores. Furthermore, the source of infection is often the boiled tap water used for cleansing of the instruments after immersion in glutaraldehyde.

In light of the **current evidence and guidelines** on hospital infection control, it is recommended that several steps be utilized to ensure proper sterilization of laparoscopic instruments and other invasive surgical devices.

1. The instruments should be thoroughly mechanically cleansed after each use, with complete dismantling of parts to ensure removal of all organic soil. This is best achieved by using an ultrasonic technology which is available in some hospitals. ,

2. It is necessary to limit glutaraldehyde disinfectants and replace it with ethylene oxide gas sterilization, as this is highly effective in reducing atypical mycobacterial infections following laparoscopy. When liquid chemical sterilants are used, higher concentrations (3.4%) must be used and the exposure time should be increased to 8–12 hours to activate sporicidal activity. Furthermore, the water used to rinse the instruments should be autoclaved to prevent recontamination with spores post-sterilization. Conventional autoclave can be used for sterilization of the metallic cannula of the ports.

3. The use of advanced sterilization systems such as STERRAD, which uses gas plasma technology to kill spores at low temperatures, or the use of ethylene oxide gas is strongly recommended for sterilization of insulated laparoscopic instruments. Another option is to keep instruments for 24 hours in a formalin gas chamber. However, the instruments must be thoroughly cleansed and dried for this process to be effective, as the presence of dirt and moisture prevents the penetration of formalin gas, thus giving the same disastrous results.

4. The use of disposable laparoscopic instruments is strongly advocated.

Treatment

- Oral treatment with clarithromycin and ciprofloxacin (500 mg each, twice daily) for 28 days to 3 months.
- For persistent local nodules, direct injection of amikacin into the nodules for five days (500 mg, twice daily).

Once clinical diagnosis of atypical mycobacterial infection of laparoscopic port sites is made, treatment with a combination of second line antituberculosis drugs is started. Of the different antimicrobial drugs used, aminoglycosides have been highly effective in the treatment of atypical mycobacterial infections of laparoscopic wounds. The course of antibiotic treatment for these organisms is often prolonged, for up to 6 months. In some cases, surgical excision of the wound may be necessary followed by prolonged antimicrobial therapy. However, this process of surgical wound debridement is generally not desired as it leaves a nasty wound and poses the risk of bacteria spreading into non-invaded zones. This method should only be reserved for critical cases, where there is gross tissue destruction with necrosis of skin.

Port Site Metastasis

The rate of port site metastases in patients with gynecological malignancies is 1.1 to 2.3%. This rate is similar to the rate of wound metastasis seen in laparotomic gynecologic malignancy operations. Risk factors proposed for port site metastasis are:

1. Aggressive disease
2. CO_2 compared with other insufflating agents is associated with significantly increased tumor growth.
3. Pneumoperitoneum increases risk compared with gasless laparoscopy.
4. High efflux of gas from the abdominal cavity through the space around the trocars.
5. Decreased influence of the local immune system during laparoscopy.

The risk of port site metastases is highest in patients with recurrence of ovarian or primary peritoneal malignancies with ascites. The lavage of port sites with cytotoxic agents (heparin, taurolidine, 5-fluorouracil, doxorubicin and methotrexate) can act as a preventive measure.

RCOG Guidelines

1. *How should women be counselled prior to laparoscopic surgery?*

Women must be informed of the risks and potential complications associated with laparoscopy. This should include discussion of the risks of the entry technique used: specifically, injury to the bowel, urinary tract and major blood vessels, and later complications associated with the entry ports: specifically, hernia formation.

Surgeons must be aware of the increased risks in women who are obese or significantly underweight and in those with previous midline abdominal incisions, peritonitis or inflammatory bowel disease.

These factors should be included in patient counseling where appropriate.

2. *How should the closed laparoscopic entry technique be performed?*

In most circumstances, the primary incision for laparoscopy should be vertical from the base of the umbilicus (not in the skin below the umbilicus). Care should be taken not to incise so deeply as to enter the peritoneal cavity.

The Veress needle should be sharp, with a good and tested spring action. A disposable needle is recommended, as it will fulfil these criteria.

The operating table should be horizontal (not in the Trendelenburg tilt) at the start of the procedure. The abdomen should be palpated to check for any masses and for the position of the aorta before insertion of the Veress needle.

The lower abdominal wall should be stabilized in such a way that the Veress needle can be inserted at right angles to the skin and should be pushed in just sufficiently to penetrate the fascia and the peritoneum. Two audible clicks are usually heard as these layers are penetrated.

Excessive lateral movement of the needle should be avoided, as this may convert a small needlepoint injury in the wall of the bowel or vessel into a more complex tear.

3. *What intra-abdominal pressure should be achieved to safely insert the primary trocar?*

An intra-abdominal pressure of 20–25 mm Hg should be used for gas insufflation before inserting the primary trocar.

The distension pressure should be reduced to 12–15 mm Hg once the insertion of the trocars is complete.

This gives adequate distension for operative laparoscopy and allows the anesthetist to ventilate the patient safely and effectively.

4. *Where should the primary trocar be inserted?*

The primary trocar should be inserted in a controlled manner at 90° to the skin, through the incision at the thinnest part of the abdominal wall, in the base of the umbilicus. Insertion should be stopped immediately the trocar is inside the abdominal cavity.

Once the laparoscope has been introduced through the primary cannula, it should be rotated through 360° to check visually for any adherent bowel. If this is present, it should be closely inspected for any evidence of hemorrhage, damage or retroperitoneal hematoma.

If there is concern that the bowel may be adherent under the umbilicus, the primary trocar site should be visualized from a secondary port site, preferably with a 5 mm laparoscope.

On completion of the procedure, the laparoscope should be used to check that there has not been a through-and-through injury of bowel adherent under the umbilicus by visual control during removal.

5. *Hasson (open) entry technique: How should the open entry technique be performed?*

When the Hasson open laparoscopic entry is employed, confirmation that the peritoneum has been opened should be made by visualising bowel or omentum before inserting the blunt tipped cannula.

The Hasson technique of open laparoscopic entry is an alternative to closed laparoscopy that avoids the use of sharp instruments after the initial skin incision. It allows the insertion of a blunt-ended trocar under direct vision.

Once the fascial edges are incised, they should be held by a lateral stay suture on either side of the incision. Once the peritoneum is opened, the fascial sutures are then pulled firmly into the suture holders on the cannula to produce an airtight seal with the cone of the cannula. Gas is insufflated directly through the cannula to produce the pneumoperitoneum. The blunt trocar is withdrawn only after the abdomen is partially distended. At the end of the procedure, the fascial defect should be closed using the stay sutures (and possibly additional sutures) to minimize the risk of herniation.

6. *What alternative entry techniques are available?*

Direct trocar insertion is an acceptable alternative trocar insertion method.

This technique was developed to overcome the difficulty associated with grasping the abdominal wall already distended by the pneumoperitoneum. Although in experienced hands it is the most rapid method of entry and can be safely used, if the cases are carefully selected.

7. *What alternative sites can be safely used for primary trocar or Veress needle insertion?*

Palmer's point is the preferred alternative trocar insertion site, except in cases of previous surgery in this area or splenomegaly. The rate of adhesion formation at the umbilicus may be up to 50% following midline laparotomy and 23% following low transverse incision. The umbilicus may not, therefore, be the most appropriate site for primary trocar insertion following previous abdominal surgery. The point of entry is 3 cm below the left costal margin in the mid-clavicular line. A small incision is made and a sharp Veress needle inserted vertically. Testing for correct placement using the pressure/flow test is performed. CO_2 is then instilled to 25 mm Hg pressure and a 2–5 mm endoscope is used to inspect the undersurface of the anterior abdominal wall in the area beneath the umbilicus. If this is free of adhesions, the trocar and cannulae can be inserted under direct laparoscopic vision. If there are many adhesions present, it is possible to dissect these

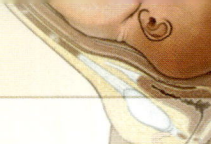

free via secondary ports in the lower left abdomen or an alternative entry site can be selected visually.

8. *How should secondary ports be inserted?*
Secondary ports must be inserted under direct vision perpendicular to the skin, while maintaining the pneumoperitoneum at 20–25 mm Hg. During insertion of secondary ports, the inferior epigastric vessels should be visualized laparoscopically to ensure the entry point is away from the vessels.

During insertion of secondary ports, once the tip of the trocar has pierced the peritoneum it should be angled towards the anterior pelvis under careful visual control until the sharp tip has been removed.

Secondary ports must be removed under direct vision to ensure that any hemorrhage can be observed and treated, if present.

9. *What specific measures are required for laparoscopic surgery in the obese woman?*

The open (Hasson) technique or entry at Palmer's point are recommended for the primary entry in women with morbid obesity. If the Veress needle approach is used, particular care must be taken to ensure that the incision is made right at the base of the umbilicus and the needle is inserted vertically into the peritoneum.

10. *What specific measures are required for laparoscopic surgery in the woman who is very thin?*

The Hasson technique or insertion at Palmer's point is recommended for the primary entry in women who are very thin.

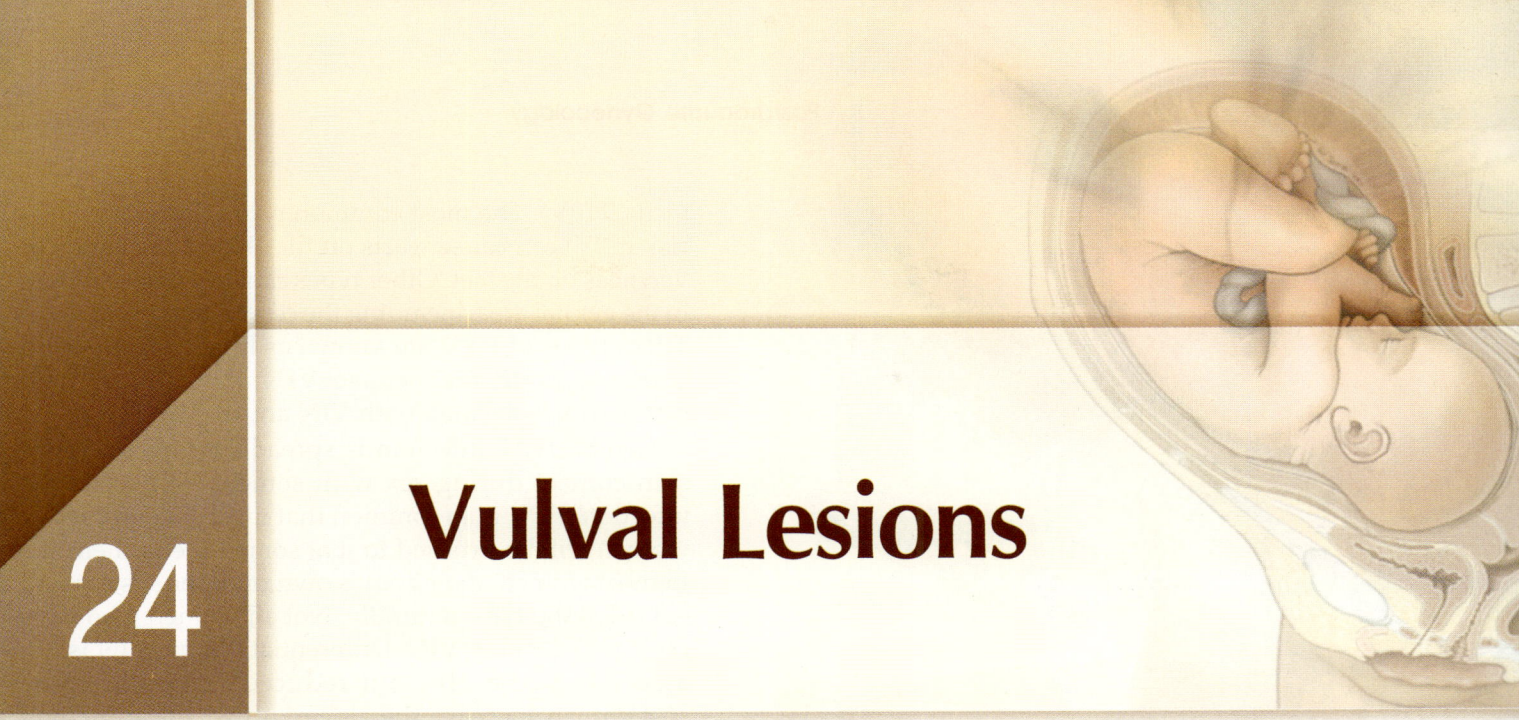

24 Vulval Lesions

Vulval intraepithelial neoplasia (VIN) is a skin condition that can affect the vulva and, in some women, may develop into cancer after many years.

ISSVD Classification

Medically speaking, the term denotes a squamous intraepithelial lesion of the vulva that shows dysplasia with varying degrees of atypia. The epithelial basement membrane is intact and the lesion is thus not invasive but has invasive potential.

The terminology of VIN evolved over several decades. In 1989, **International Society for the Study of Vulvar Disease** (ISSVD) replaced older terminology such as vulvar dystrophy, Bowen's disease, and Kraurosis vulvae by a new classification system for *epithelial vulvar disease*:

- Non-neoplastic epithelial disorders of vulva and mucosa:
  - Lichen sclerosus
  - Squamous hyperplasia
  - Other dermatoses
- Mixed neoplastic and non-neoplastic disorders
- Intraepithelial neoplasia
  - Squamous vulvar intraepithelial neoplasia (VIN)
    - VIN 1, mildest form
    - VIN 2, intermediate
    - VIN 3, most severe form including carcinoma in situ of the vulva.
  - Non-squamous intraepithelial neoplasia
    - Extramammary Paget's disease
    - Tumors of melanocytes, non-invasive

- Invasive disease (vulvar carcinoma)

The ISSVD further revised this classification in 2004, replacing the three-grade system with a single-grade system in which only the high-grade disease is classified as VIN.

I. VIN, usual type
  a. VIN warty type
  b. VIN basaloid type
  c. VIN, mixed (warty/basaloid type)
II. VIN, differentiated type
  1. The term VIN 1 will no longer be used. Histologic changes previously encompassed within the term VIN 1 is described as *flat condyloma acuminatum*.
  2. The term VIN should apply only to histologically high grade squamous lesions (former terms, VIN 2, VIN 3 and differentiated VIN3).
  3. Two categories of VIN should be used to describe squamous VIN:
    a. The more common type of VIN will be termed *VIN usual type.* This encompasses the previous VIN 2, VIN 3, Bowen's disease, hisgtologically older terms like dysplasia, carcinoma in situ etc. These lesions are generally associated with high-risk HPV types, especially HPV 16. VIN, usual type can be subcategorized histologically as warty (condylomatous), basaloid or mixed (present within the same lesion of warty and basaloid VIN).
    b. The less common type of VIN lesion will be termed *VIN, differentiated type*. These lesions are not associated with HPV (Fig. 24.1).

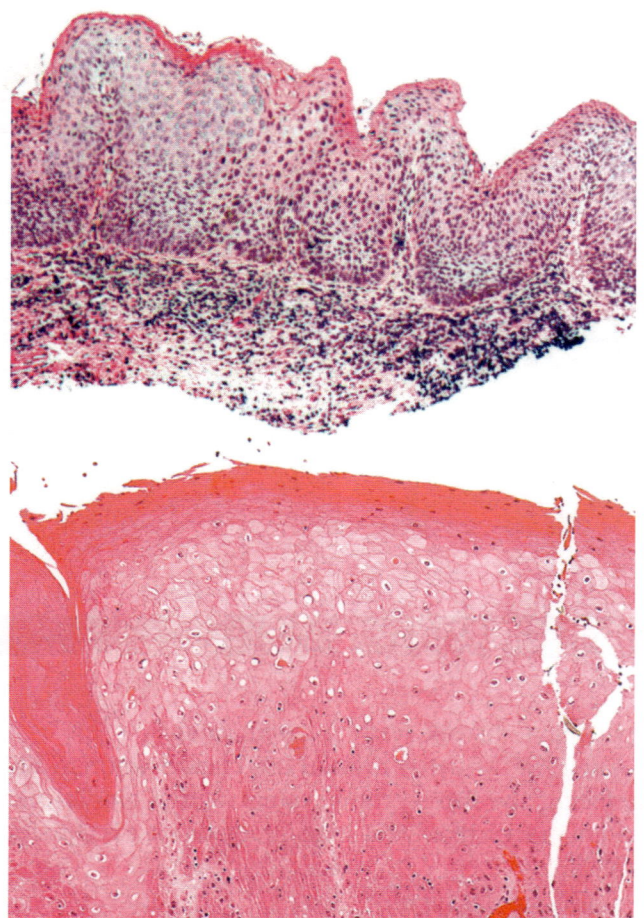

Fig. 24.1: Vulvar intraepithelial neoplasia 3 differentiated vulvar intraepithelial neoplasia

4. The occasional example of VIN that cannot be classified into either of the above VIN categories (usual and differentiated types) may be classified as VIN unclassified type or VIN, NOS. The rare variety VIN of pagetoid type may be placed in this category.
5. Classification is performed on the basis of morphologic criteria only and not on HPV type or clinical appearance.

Causes of VIN

The exact cause of VIN is unknown. The following factors have been associated with VIN:
- HPV (human papillomavirus).
- HSV-2 (herpes simplex virus—type 2).
- Smoking.
- Immunosuppression.
- Chronic vulvar irritation.
- Conditions such as lichen sclerosus

Usual type VIN is associated with an infection in the skin of the vulva by a virus known as human papilloma-

virus (HPV). The most common types (known as low-risk HPV) can cause warts on the skin of the hands or verrucas on the feet. Other types can cause cell changes in the genital area, including the cervix, vulva and anus. These types of HPV are known as high-risk HPV and some of them may cause VIN. The types most commonly associated with VIN are 16, 18 and 31.

Genital HPV infection is spread by direct skin-to-skin contact during sex with someone who has the infection. HPV is so common that most sexually active women will be exposed to it at some time in their life. In most women, their body's own immune system will get rid of the HPV naturally. Not all women who have HPV will develop VIN. Differentiated type VIN is not associated with HIV but reduced body's immune system can increase the risk of VIN. These include smoking, immunosuppressive drugs, inherited immunity problems and some rare bone marrow and blood disorders.

Signs and Symptoms of VIN

The signs and symptoms vary, and may include some, or all, of the following:
- The patient may have no symptoms.
- Itching and soreness in the vulva.
- Burning, or a severe tingling sensation, that can become worse when passing urine.
- One or more areas of reddened, white or discolored skin in the vulva.
- Raised areas of skin that can vary in size.
- The skin with warty appearance.
- Pain during sex.

The diagnosis is always based on a careful inspection and a targeted biopsy. If the changes become more severe, there is a chance that cancer might develop after many years, and so VIN is referred to as a pre-cancerous condition.

Diagnosis

By clinical examination of the affected area. The vaginal area can be assessed by colposcopy. This will be followed by excisional biopsy from the junction of healthy and unhealthy areas.

Indications

Indications for vulvar biopsy include the following:
- Visible lesion for which definitive diagnosis cannot be made on clinical grounds.
- Possible malignancy.
- Visible lesion with presumed clinical diagnosis that is not responding to usual therapy.

- Lesions with atypical vascular patterns.
- Benign appearing lesions requiring definitive diagnosis (e.g. acrochordon).
- White lesions failing empiric therapy.

Contraindications

No absolute contraindications exist for vulvar biopsy. Relative contraindications include the following:
- Infected site
- Coagulopathy
- Allergy to local anesthetic

Technique

Choice of Biopsy Site

Suspected inflammatory diseases, neoplasia, ulcers, and pigmented lesions should be sampled using punch biopsy that includes the edge of the lesions. Sometimes, multiple biopsies may be necessary. If possible, one should avoid taking the biopsy from the clitoris, labia minora, urethra and near rectum because these areas are particularly sensitive.

The biopsy is performed using a Keyes punch biopsy or scalpel or scissors. Punch biopsy is used for flat or slightly raised lesions, and scalpel or scissors for raised or pedunculated lesions.

The Keyes punch biopsy is particularly useful when the depth of the lesion is of importance. The Keyes punch is a pen-sized instrument with a sharp, circular cutting edge that is used to cut tissue in a twisting motion.

Punch Biopsy

Punch biopsy is useful, if the lesion is small enough for complete excision by the biopsy tip. Punch biopsies are available in sizes from 2 to 10 mm. Punch biopsies may heal without suturing; however, if hemostasis cannot be achieved within a few minutes, sutures may be considered for hemostasis. Post-procedural discomfort secondary to the location of sutures and keloid formation is possible complication.

In general, the smallest punch biopsy that will adequately sample the lesion should be used. Typically, 4- or 5 mm punch biopsies are used to achieve an adequate sample for tissue diagnosis. A larger lesion can be excised using a punch biopsy of larger size that completely circumscribes the lesion.

Keyes Punch Biopsy (Fig. 24.2)

After adequate local anesthesia, the punch biopsy placed firmly against the skin is rotated with a constant firm pressure for penetration through the skin.

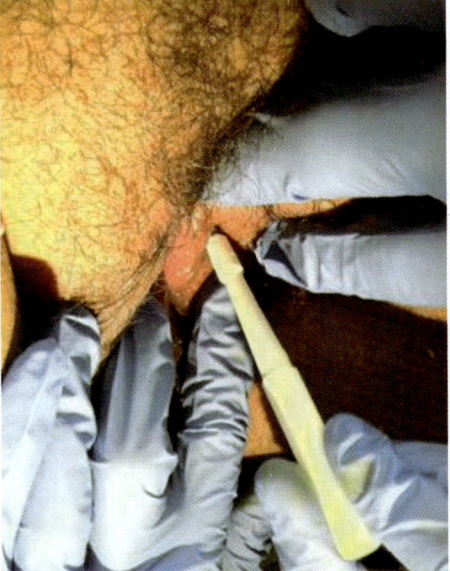

Fig. 24.2: Keyes punch biopsy

Generally, there is a change in resistance of the Keyes punch on the skin once the biopsy has reached the subcutaneous fat. At this time, the Keyes punch is removed and forceps is used to elevate the core of skin and subcutaneous tissue and the base of the biopsied tissue is cut with curved iris scissors.

Shave Biopsy (Fig. 24.3)

A shave biopsy is performed using a scalpel or scissors. Injecting the anesthetic underneath the lesion also helps to elevate the lesion. With scalpel, the lesion is excised.

Curved scissors are beneficial for lesions that may need more depth removal of tissue.

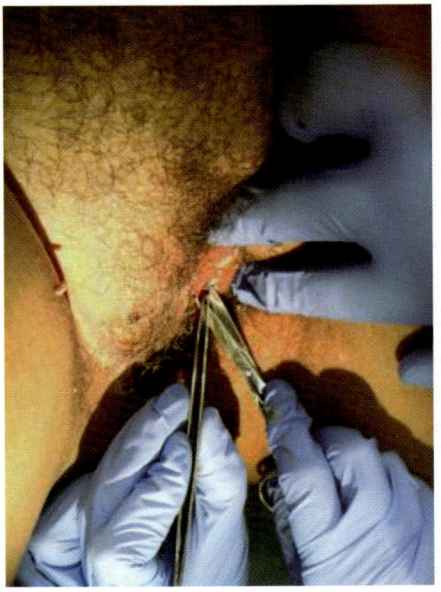

Fig. 24.3: Grasping the biopsy site with toothed forceps and excising it with scissors

Fixation

Once an adequate sample has been excised, the specimen is placed carefully in a fixative solution, such as 10% formalin.

Hemostasis

Bleeding can be stopped in a number of ways. Shave biopsies may not bleed much and pressure alone may provide hemostasis. Silver nitrate sticks are applied. Monsel solution can also be used, but it may be more irritating to surrounding skin. It is important to know that silver nitrate and Monsel solution may also potentially cause increased skin pigmentation. When using these hemostatic agents, it is important to dry the area with sterile gauze and then apply the hemostatic agent only to the bleeding area. A suture can be placed if necessary with suture, such as 2-0 monofilament or polygalactin, for reapproximation and hemostasis.

Treatment for VIN

Treatment depends on the symptoms and the type of lesions. The type of treatment will depend on:
- The size of the affected area.
- The estimated risk of the area developing into cancer.

Surgery

In women who need treatment, most of the affected areas are removed by local surgical excision. Rarely, if the affected area is large or there are several areas, the whole vulva is removed by vulvectomy with or without grafting.

Ablation Treatment

Ablation means destroying the affected area. It may be used for areas where it is difficult to surgically remove the VIN, such as around the clitoris. Ablation can be done using a high-energy beam (laser) or diathermy.

The laser beam or diathermy is focused on the affected areas to destroy the abnormal cells.

New Treatments that are Being Researched

The following treatments (imiquimod, cidofovir and photodynamic therapy) are experimental and are being investigated in research trials to see how useful they might be for VIN.

Imiquimod

Imiquimod is an antiviral drug. It stimulates the immune system to get rid of the HPV infection, which in turn will allow the vulva cells to return to normal.

Cidofovir

Research is also looking into another antiviral drug treatment for VIN called cidofovir, but this is at an early stage.

Photodynamic Therapy (PDT)

PDT uses laser light to activate a light-sensitive drug. The drug is given either as a cream that is applied to the vulva or intravenously. A laser light is then shone on to the affected area which activates the drug to destroy the abnormal cells.

Creams to relieve symptoms: Steroid cream can be applied to the affected areas. It reduces inflammation and can control symptoms, but does not cure the condition. Sometimes a local anesthetic cream/gel can be used to ease any soreness or discomfort.

Prognosis of VIN

If left untreated, VIN may go away by itself or it may turn into an invasive cancer in later years. Careful follow-up after treatment is essential long term, as VIN may recur in about half of women treated during their lifetime. It grows slowly so most women are reviewed every 6 to 12 months. Up to 50% of women with VIN develop cervical intraepithelial neoplasia (CIN), anal intraepithelial neoplasia (AIN), vaginal intraepithelial neoplasia (VAIN) or invasive cancer of the genital tract. It is particularly important to have regular cervical smears.

Vulval Lichen Sclerosus (Fig. 24.4)

Etiology

This is an inflammatory condition of unknown etiology. It is thought to be an autoimmune condition and recent evidence has shown autoantibodies to extracellular matrix protein 13. There is an increased frequency of other autoimmune disorders in females with lichen sclerosus.

The etiology and pathogenesis of lichen sclerosus is unknown but may include genetic, infectious, environmental, and hormonal factors. Local irritation or trauma seems to play a role in some cases of lichen sclerosus, especially in genetically predisposed individuals. However, the sequence of events that leads to the altered fibroblast function, microvascular changes, and hyaluronic acid accumulation in the upper dermis is still not known. Oral contraceptives in premenopausal women have been shown to give a relative risk of 2.5, which suggests an altered hormonal axis as a possible contributory factor.

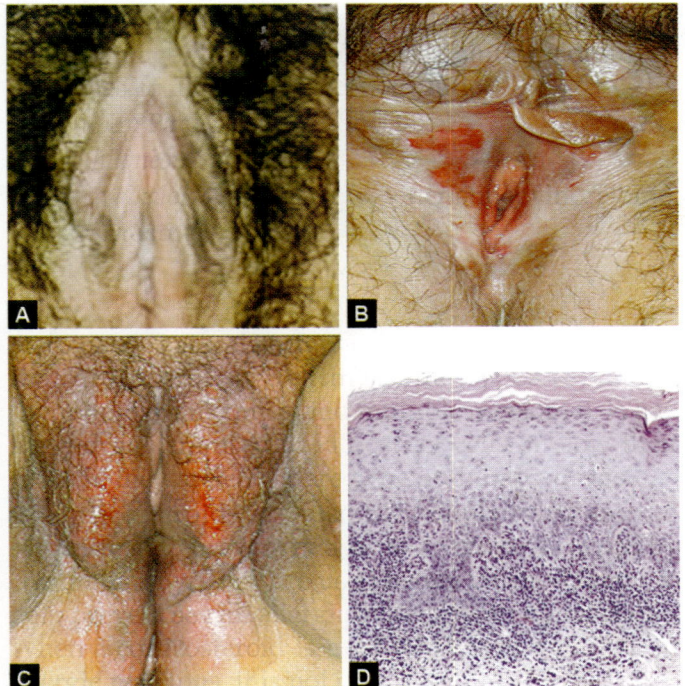

Fig. 24.4: Lichen sclerosus

Pathophysiology

Inflammation and altered fibroblast function in the papillary dermis leads to fibrosis of the upper dermis. Genital skin and mucosa are affected most frequently, but extragenital lichen sclerosus does occur. Several studies have recently identified the presence of autoantibodies to the glycoprotein extracellular matrix protein 1 (ECM 1). The role that hypoxia and ischemia have in the initial cellular and vascular damage is supported by the finding of increased glut-1 and decreased vascular endothelial growth factor (VEGF) expression in affected skin.

Most cases are in postmenopausal women, although it can occur in prepubescent girls and young women. It can be familial and may affect the male prepuce too. 21% of patients have autoimmune disease, like thyroid disorder. 22% have a family history and 44% have various autoantibodies.

Lichen sclerosus and squamous cell hyperplasia present with pruritus vulvae, vulvodynia, superficial dyspareunia, or visible lesions. It has an appearance called "cigarette paper" skin as it is thin, white, and brittle. The introitus may shrink with fusion of the labia minora. Biopsy under local anesthetic may need to be repeated from time to time, to exclude malignant change.

Clinical Features

Three clinical variants: Erosive (most common), papulosquamous, hypertrophic. Vulvar lichen sclerosus may progress to gradual obliteration of the labia minora and stenosis of the introitus. The most common variation occurs when the inflammation is intense enough to cause separation of a large area of epidermis, creating blisters or large, occasionally hemorrhagic, bullae. Because this occurs more often in genital cases, it may be confused with the trauma of sexual abuse or other genital ulcerative disease.

I. **Symptoms**
- Itching
- Soreness
- Dyspareunia
- Urinary symptoms
- Other symptoms, e.g. constipation, can occur as a result of disruption of the normal architecture
- Can be asymptomatic

II. **Signs**
- Patchy pale, atrophic appearance
- Erosions, blistering and purpura in some cases
- Fissuring
- Hyperkeratosis can occur
- Changes may be localized or in a 'figure of eight' distribution including the perianal area

Diagnosis

- Characteristic clinical appearance.
- **Skin biopsy** is the primary study to perform for diagnosis of lichen sclerosus. Punch biopsy in the most mature area of the lesion usually is diagnostic. Ulcerative or vegetative genital lesions may need to be biopsied more than once to screen for squamous cell carcinoma. Epidermal hyperplasia and/or dysplasia associated with lichen sclerosus on vulvar biopsy specimens is associated with an increased risk of malignant transformation.
- Despite the presence of autoantibodies described in several studies, an autoimmune workup (e.g. antinuclear antibody, vitamin B_{12} levels, thyroid function tests) is still not generally recommended because the frequency of multiple autoimmune diseases associated with lichen sclerosus is not high enough to justify the expense of screening all patients.
- Imaging studies are not needed unless urinary obstruction secondary to severe, stenosing genital lichen sclerosus is present. Intravenous pyelogram might be appropriate in this situation.

Histologic Features

- Epidermal atrophy with loss of rete pegs, homogenized collagen of papillary dermis and underlying band of lymphocytes.

- Lymphocytic infiltrate (without plasma cells) with lichenoid pattern involving superficial dermis and extending into basilar and parabasilar epithelium.
- Epithelium may have prominent acanthosis with prominent granular layer and hyperkeratosis.
- In older lesions, acanthosis may be absent and epithelium is thinned with loss of rete ridges.
- Ulceration and bullae may occur in severe lesions.

Complications

- Loss of architecture may be manifested as loss of the labia or midline fusion.
- Development of squamous cell carcinoma (actual risk uncertain but small, 1–4%).

Treatment

General Advice

Patients should be informed about the condition and made aware of the small risk of neoplastic change.

Recommended Regimen

- *Topical steroid:* Clobetasol proprionate with daily use for one month is very useful. Maintenance treatment may be required with weaker steroid preparations.
- The calcineurin inhibitors (i.e. tacrolimus, pimecrolimus) have been found to help some patients, but they do not work as fast or as effectively as potent topical corticosteroids.
- *Surgery:* A variety of destructive procedures have been reported to be of benefit. Nonablative lasers, such as Er:YAG lasers, have been reported to benefit persons with lichen sclerosus. Cryotherapy of affected genital lesions is also reported to reduce the area involved after one or series of treatment.

Mortality/Morbidity

Lichen sclerosus has no associated increased mortality unless the patient develops malignancy in the area. Many pediatric cases will improve with puberty, although other expressions of vulvodynia may persist. The rate of spontaneous resolution may be lower than 25%. Extragenital cases and many genital cases are asymptomatic except for the cosmetic aspect or pruritus. Resistant cases especially those associated with erosion or progressive scarring, may result in severe sexual dysfunction.

Squamous Cell Hyperplasia (SCH) (Fig. 24.5)

Squamous cell hyperplasia (formerly called hyperplastic dystrophy or leukoplakia) represents

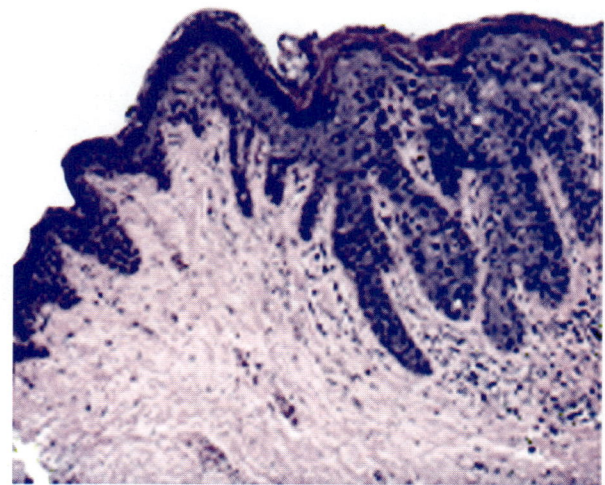

Fig. 24.5: Squamous cell hyperplasia

about 40 to 45% of patients with non-neoplastic epithelial disorders. Approximately two-thirds of the patients are premenopausal. It is related to chronic irritation.

The skin of the vulvar area is permeable to water in respect to the skin of other body sites. In this way, the vulvar region is moist and prone to absorb many compounds which occasionally come in the area. Almost any irritative condition may lead to hyperplastic changes. Among the factors implicated in the pathogenesis of hyperplasia, intrinsic (physiologic sweat, psychogenic sweat, psychogenic pruritus, pruritus as the result of systemic disease) and extrinsic factors (physical, mechanical and chemical factors) are recognized.

Presentation

Squamous cell hyperplasia is characterized by a pink-red vulva with overlying gray-white keratin. Areas most frequently involved on the vulva are the prepuce, labia majora, interlabial sulci, outer aspect of the labia minora, and the posterior commissure. Lesions may be present to the adjacent thighs. Pruritis is generally present. Itching, scrubbing and scratching are consequence of the initial event and contribute to sustain and promote the circle leading to squamous cell hyperplasia.

Histopathology

Microscopic findings consist of elongation, widening of the rete ridges and irregular thickening of the Malpighian layer of rete ridges (acanthosis), hyperkeratosis, and chronic inflammation in dermis. Parakeratosis may also be present. Inflammatory reactions within the dermis consist of lymphocytes and a small number of plasma cells.

Treatment

The relief of itching seems, therefore, the first aim of any therapy. If symptoms of anxiety and irritability are present, oral tranquillizers may be used, especially at bedtime. Topical corticosteroids are the mainstay of therapy for squamous cell hyperplasia. The fluorinated compounds in ointment base applied twice daily generally cure the lesion. If the vulva is extremely thickened and a large area is involved with squamous cell hyperplasia, a Class 1 topical steroid may be required. If an antihistamine is added, the antipruritic effect will be improved. Rarely it is necessary to inject triamcinolone acetonide. Once the relief of itching has been achieved, the identification and removal of any irritant cause should be undertaken.

Malignant Potential

Squamous cell hyperplasia is sometimes observed as precancerous stage of invasive squamous cell cancer although the risk of development of invasive cancer for women treated for squamous cell hyperplasia without intraepithelial neoplasia is minimal. It has been found that women with squamous cell hyperplasia occurring in a background of lichen sclerosus constitute a distinct group at higher risk of developing invasive cancer and require histologic assessment.

Prognosis

- Lichen sclerosus usually responds to steroid therapy in a month or less. Long-term follow-up care is necessary.
- Squamous hyperplasia usually responds to adequate therapy within 2 to 3 weeks.
- Any chronic vulvar irritation may increase the risk of cancer and must, therefore, be carefully monitored by multiple biopsies to be examined at regular intervals. Sometimes associated with carcinoma, however, it is not considered a premalignant lesion unless there is atypia.

Squamous Papilloma (Fig. 24.6)

Condylomata acuminata are commonly transmitted through sexual intercourse or where there is labioscrotal contact. They are hyperplastic, pedunculated or sessile growth which appear red or pink, forming soft exuberant masses strangulated at their bases.

Condyloma acuminatum refers to an epidermal manifestation attributed to the epidermotropic human papillomavirus (HPV). Approximately 90% of condyloma acuminata are related to HPV types 6 and 11. These two types are the least likely to have a

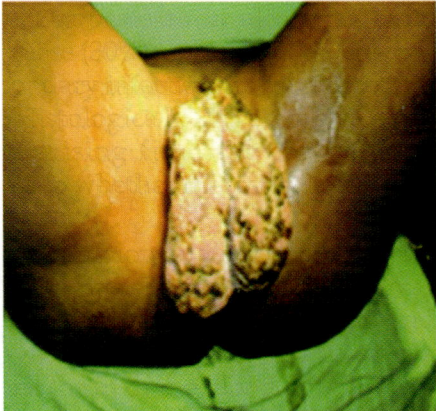
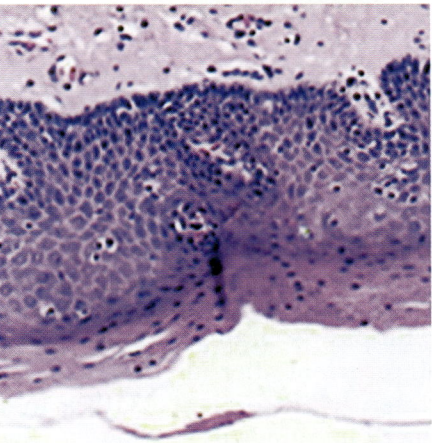

Fig. 24.6: Squamous papilloma

neoplastic potential. Risk for neoplastic conversion has been determined to be moderate (types 33, 35, 39, 40, 43, 45, 51–56, 58) or high (types 16, 18).

Annual incidence of condyloma acuminatum is 1%. It is considered the most common sexually transmitted disease (STD).

Prevalence is greatest in persons aged 17–33 years, with incidence peaking in persons aged 20–24 years.

History

- Smoking, oral contraceptives, multiple sexual partners, and early coital age are risk factors for acquiring condylomata acuminata.
- Generally, two-thirds of individuals who have sexual contact with a partner with condyloma acuminatum develop lesions within 3 months.
- The chief complaint usually is one of painless bumps, pruritus, or discharge. Involvement of more than 1 area is common. History of multiple lesions, rather than 1 isolated wart, is common.
- Coital bleeding may occur. Vaginal bleeding during pregnancy may be due to condyloma eruptions.
- Latent illness may become active, particularly with pregnancy and immunosuppression.

- Lesions may regress spontaneously, remain the same, or progress.
- Pruritus and discharge may be present.

Signs

Single or multiple papular eruptions may be observed. Eruptions may appear pearly, filiform, fungating, cauliflower-, or plaque-like around vulvovaginal and cervical areas in women. More than 50% of female patients with external lesions have been found to have negative Papanicolaou (Pap) tests but tested positive for HPV infection.

Laboratory Studies

- Test for other STDs, such as HIV, gonorrhea, chlamydia, and syphilis.
- Pap smear from the lesions for koilocytic and nuclear abnormality.
- Filter or in situ hybridization, and polymerase chain reaction (PCR) for diagnosis and HPV typing.
- Colposcopy to identify cervical and vaginal lesions.
- *Biopsy:* Biopsy is indicated for lesions that are atypical, recurrent after initial success, or resistant to treatment or in patients with a high risk for neoplasia or immunosuppression.
- Anoscopy

Treatment

Cryotherapy

Cryotherapy may be performed using an open spray or cotton-tipped applicator for 10–15 seconds and repeated as needed. Lift away mobile skin from underlying normal tissue before freezing.

Response rates are high with few adverse sequelae.

Adverse reactions include pain at time of treatment, erosion, ulceration, and post-inflammatory hypo-pigmentation of skin.

Cryotherapy is safe during pregnancy.

Surgical Excision

Excision has highest success rate and lowest recurrence rate with initial cure rates of 63–91%.

Carbon dioxide laser is used in treatment for extensive or recurrent condylomata acuminata. Potentially infectious HPV-6 DNA has been detected in the carbon dioxide laser plume.

Cytotoxic Agents

1. **Podophyllum resin:** Purified podophyllotoxin is antimitotic, and cytotoxic. While exact mechanism of action on condyloma is unknown, podofilox results in necrosis of genital condyloma acuminatum.
2. **Trichloroacetic acid topical:** Up to 80% of these agents rapidly penetrate and cauterize skin, keratin, and other tissues. It causes less local irritation and systemic toxicity. Response is often incomplete, and recurrence is frequent.
3. **5-Fluorouracil:** It is no longer recommended for routine use. It has antimetabolic , antineoplastic and immunostimulative activity. It is useful in prevention of recurrence after condyloma ablation, if started within 4 wk, especially in immunocompromised patients.
4. **Bleomycin:** It inhibits DNA synthesis with some evidence of RNA and protein synthesis inhibition to a lesser degree; may cause a variety of adverse effects.
5. **Imiquimod:** It induces interferon production and is a cell-mediated immune response modifier. It has minimal systemic absorption but causes erythema, irritation, ulceration, and pain.
6. **Interferon alfa:** Alpha interferon has been approved by FDA for injectional use in refractory condylomata acuminata with some possible benefit. Recurrence rate of 20–40% exists with intralesional interferon. Numerous adverse reactions may occur which include myalgias, fever, chills, GI symptoms, transient leukopenia, thrombocytopenia, LFT abnormalities, serum lipid abnormalities with intramuscular interferon.
7. **Vaccines:** *Papillomavirus vaccine (HPV):* This is quadrivalent human papillomavirus (HPV) recombinant vaccine indicated to prevent cervical cancer, genital warts (condyloma acuminata), and precancerous genital lesions (e.g. cervical adenocarcinoma in situ; cervical intraepithelial neoplasia grades 1, 2, and 3; vulvar intraepithelial neoplasia grades 2 and 3; vaginal intraepithelial neoplasia grades 2 and 3) due to HPV types 6, 11, 16, and 18. Vaccine efficacy is mediated by humoral immune responses for prevention of condylomata acuminata caused by HPV types 6 and 11 in boys, men, girls, and women aged 9–26 years.

Conclusions and Recommendations by ACOG

The American College of Obstetricians and Gynecologists and the American Society for Colposcopy and Cervical Pathology make the following conclusions and recommendations:

- Immunization with the quadrivalent HPV vaccine has been shown to decrease the risk of VIN and should be recommended for women in target populations.

- No screening strategies have been developed for the prevention of vulvar cancer through early detection of VIN.
- Diagnosis is limited to visual assessment. Biopsy is indicated for most pigmented vulvar lesions.
- Presumed genital warts should be biopsied in postmenopausal women and in women in whom topical treatments have failed.
- Treatment is indicated for all cases of VIN. Wide local excision is recommended when cancer is suspected, despite a biopsy diagnosis of only VIN, to identify occult invasion.
- When occult invasion is not a concern, VIN can be treated with excision, laser ablation, or topical imiquimod (off-label use).
- Women with VIN should be considered at risk of recurrent VIN and vulvar cancer throughout their lifetime. After resolution, women should be monitored at 6 and 12 months and annually thereafter.

Bartholin Gland Lesions

Bartholin glands were first described by Caspar Bartholin, a Dutch anatomist, in 1677. These paired glands are approximately 0.5 cm in diameter and are found in the labia minora in the 4 and 8 o'clock positions. Typically, they are nonpalpable. Each gland secretes mucus into a 2.5 cm duct. These two ducts emerge into the vestibule at either side of the vaginal orifice, inferior to the hymen. Their function is to maintain the moisture of the vaginal mucosa's vestibular surface.

Pathophysiology

Bartholin glands are known to form cysts and abscesses in women of reproductive age. Cysts and abscesses are often clinically distinguishable. Bartholin cysts form when the ostium of the duct becomes obstructed, leading to distention of the gland or duct with fluid. Obstruction is usually secondary to nonspecific inflammation or trauma. The cyst is usually 1–3 cm in diameter and often asymptomatic, although larger cysts may be associated with pain and dyspareunia.

Bartholin abscesses result from either primary gland infection or infected cyst. Patients with abscesses complain of acute, rapidly progressive vulvar pain. These abscesses are usually polymicrobial and rarely attributable to sexually transmitted pathogens.

Adenocarcinoma of the Bartholin glands is rare, accounting for 1–2% of all vulvar malignancies. Typically, this lesion presents as a gradually enlarging gland in an asymptomatic, postmenopausal woman.

Epidemiology

Frequency

Approximately 2% of women of reproductive age will experience swelling of one or both Bartholin glands.

Mortality/Morbidity

Bartholin gland diseases are rarely complicated by systemic infection, sepsis, and bleeding secondary to surgical treatment. Missed diagnosis of malignancy may result in poorer outcome for those patients.

Age

These diseases typically occur in women between the ages of 20 and 30 years. Bartholin gland enlargement in patients older than 40 years is rare and should be referred to a gynecologist for possible biopsy.

History

Patients with cysts may present with painless labial swelling. Abscesses may present spontaneously or after a painless cyst with the following symptoms:
- Acute, painful unilateral labial swelling
- Dyspareunia
- Pain with walking and sitting
- Sudden relief of pain followed by spontaneous rupture.

Physical Examination

The following physical examination findings are seen in Bartholin abscess (Fig. 24.7):
- Patients typically have an exquisitely tender, fluctuant labial mass with surrounding erythema and edema.

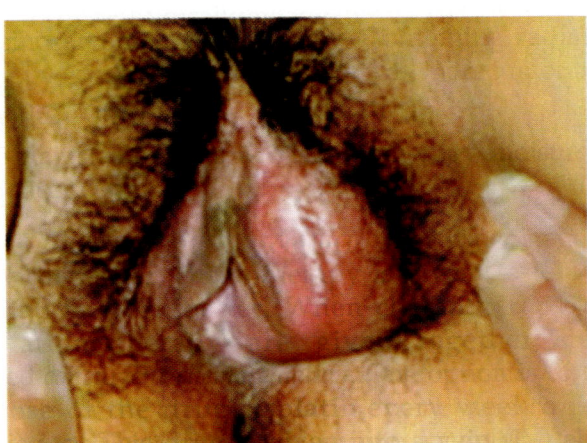

Fig. 24.7: Bartholin abscess

- In some cases, areas of cellulitis surrounding the abscess may be present.
- Fever, though not typical in healthy patients, may occur.
- If the abscess has spontaneously ruptured, purulent discharge may be noted. If completely drained, no obvious mass may be observed.

The following physical examination findings are seen in Bartholin cysts:

- Patients may have a painless, unilateral labial mass without signs of surrounding cellulitis.
- If large, the cyst may be tender.
- Discharge from ruptured cyst is nonpurulent.

Causes

The most common bacterial pathogens responsible for Bartholin abscess was previously named *Neisseria gonorrhoeae* and *Chlamydia trachomatis.* More recent studies report the predominance of opportunistic bacteria such as *Staphylococcus* species, *Streptococcus* species, and most commonly, *Escherichia coli* as conservative organism.

Differential diagnosis

Bartholin gland malignancy	Sebaceous cysts
Chancroid	Skene duct cyst
Endometriosis	Syphilis
Gartner duct cyst	Vestibular mucous cysts
Hematoma	Vulvar malignancy
Hidradenoma	Genital warts
Lipoma	

Laboratory Studies

In otherwise healthy, afebrile adults, blood tests are not necessary to evaluate an uncomplicated abscess or cyst. Sexually transmitted disease (STD) testing should be available at the request of the patient; however, Bartholin abscesses are very rarely caused by sexually transmitted pathogens.

Cultures are rarely useful in treatment of abscess; furthermore, routine culturing of drained fluid is not recommended.

Features suggestive of Bartholin gland malignancy:

- Age older than 40 years
- Chronic or gradually progressive, painless mass
- Solid, nonfluctuant, painless mass
- Prior history of labial malignancy

Treatment

Those with an uncomplicated, asymptomatic cyst may be discharged with sitz bath instructions. Sitz baths (3 times daily) for several days may promote improvement with resolution or spontaneous rupture with resolution of the cyst.

A Bartholin abscess is generally painful, and, thus, usually requires incision and drainage. The goal of abscess treatment is to allow drainage and to prevent rapid reaccumulation of fluid.

Incision and Drainage

This technique consists of traditional incision, drainage, irrigation, and packing. Packing should be removed 2 days after the procedure. This technique requires multiple, painful packing changes and has a higher rate of abscess recurrence.

Word Catheter (Fig. 24.8)

The word catheter is a small catheter with a saline inflatable balloon at the distal end (Fig. 24.9). This procedure should be performed using sterile technique.

Using an #11 blade a 0.5 cm incision is made into the abscess cavity on the mucosal surface of the labia minora. Contents of the cavity are expressed manually or by hemostat. The tip of the catheter is inserted into the cavity, and the balloon is inflated with 4 mL normal saline.

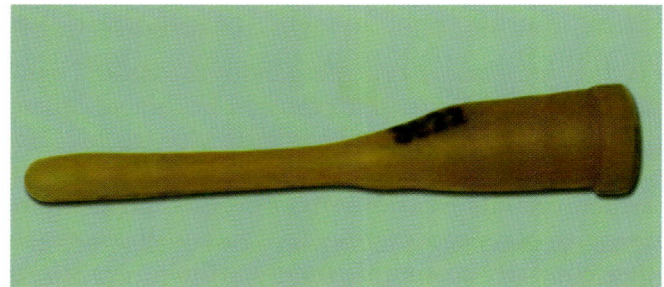

Fig. 24.8: Word catheter

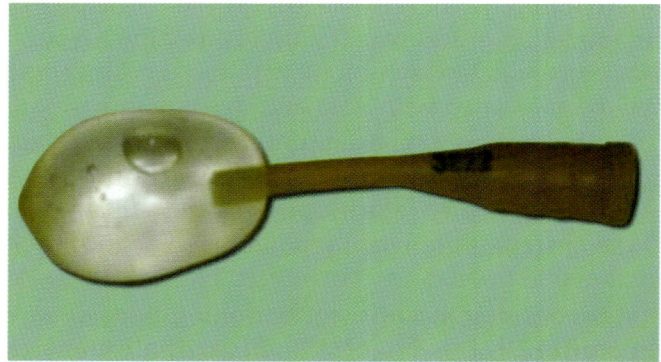

Fig. 24.9: Word catheter with inflated balloon

The free end of the catheter may be inserted into the vagina for patient comfort. The catheter allows for abscess drainage acutely and is left in place for several weeks to promote fistula formation.

Patients should be advised to take sitz baths 2–3 times a day for 2 days following the procedure and to abstain from sexual intercourse until the catheter is removed.

Marsupialization

This procedure is reserved for recurrent abscesses. The acute abscess is drained prior to marsupialization. This procedure consists of a wide incision of the mass followed by suturing the inner edge of the incision to external mucosa.

Excision

This procedure requires excision of the Bartholin gland and surrounding tissue. It is disfiguring, painful, and seldom indicated in the treatment of abscess, although it may be used to treat malignancy.

Recent Techniques

1. Carbon dioxide laser therapy as well as alcohol sclerotherapy to treat Bartholin abscesses show promising results with a cure rate of nearly 96%.
2. Silver nitrate gland ablation is safe and effective treatment for both simple cysts and abscesses.

Antibiotics

Most Bartholin abscesses are caused by opportunistic pathogens. Uncomplicated abscesses in otherwise healthy women may not require antibiotic therapy after successful drainage. Treatment of *N. gonorrhoeae* and *C. trachomatis* should be initiated only in patients with confirmed disease.

Ceftriaxone: An effective monotherapy against *N. gonorrhoeae*, ceftriaxone is a third-generation cephalosporin with broad-spectrum efficiency against gram-negative organisms, lower efficacy against gram-positive organisms, and higher efficacy against resistant organisms.

Ciprofloxacin: It is a bactericidal antibiotic that inhibits bacterial DNA synthesis and, consequently, growth by inhibiting DNA-gyrase in susceptible organisms.

Doxycycline: This inhibits protein synthesis and bacterial replication by binding with 30S and, possibly, 50S ribosomal subunits of susceptible bacteria. It is indicated for treatment of *C. trachomatis*.

Azithromycin: This is used to treat mild-to-moderate infections caused by susceptible strains of microorganisms specifically for *C. trachomatis*.

Complications

- The most common complication of treatment of Bartholin abscess is recurrence.
- Rare reports of necrotizing fasciitis after abscess drainage are found.
- Development of toxic shock syndrome with packing.
- Nonhealing of wounds.
- Bleeding, especially in patients with a coagulopathy, may be a complication.
- Cosmetic scarring may result.

Prognosis

If abscesses are properly drained and reclosure is prevented, most abscesses have a good outcome.

Recurrence rates are generally reported to be less than 20%.

24B. VULVAL CANCER

Vulvar carcinoma encompasses any malignancy that arises in the skin; glands; or underlying stroma of the perineum, including the mons, labia minora, labia majora, Bartholin glands, or clitoris. Tumors can also arise in ectopic breast tissue that can be located in the vulva along the milk line. Metastatic tumors have also been described but occur relatively infrequently.

Frequency

Cancer of the vulva is the fourth most common malignancy of the female genital tract. The incidence of preinvasive disease of the vulva has almost doubled over the past decade, and this may translate into a marked increase in the incidence of invasive vulvar carcinoma in the future. Since vulvar cancer is rare and is not monitored by the World Health Organization, the global incidence of this disease is not precisely known.

Incidence

The incidence of vulvar carcinoma has a bimodal peak. Currently, development of vulvar carcinoma in situ in young women is suggested to correlate to human papillomavirus (HPV) infection. In older women, the etiology of the carcinoma is attributed to chronic irritation or other poorly understood cofactors. Estimates indicate that women who smoke cigarettes have a 4- to 5-fold increase in the incidence of carcinoma in situ of the vulva and a 20% increase in vulvar carcinoma. The incidence of vulvar carcinoma in situ and vulvar carcinoma is higher in women with multiple sexual partners and in women with a history of HPV infection. For women who report a history of genital warts or HPV-related disease, the relative risk for carcinoma in situ is 18.5 and for invasive cancer is 14.5.

Vulval cancer (Fig. 24.10) is uncommon and accounts for approximately 1–4% of all gynecological cancers.

Its incidence is 1.8 /100.000. It is predominantly seen in postmenopausal and old women (mean age 65 years) and only 2% in less than 30 years.

Pathophysiology

The development of vulvar dysplasia and cancer in most patients is related to HPV infection. Certain strains of HPV are known to be more oncogenic than others. HPV types 16, 18, 31, 33, 35, 45, and 54 are more likely to be associated with cervical neoplasia and are

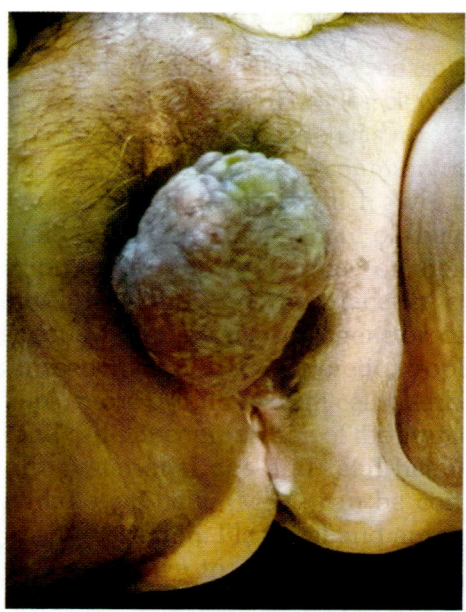

Fig. 24.10: Vulval growth

suspected to be responsible for vulvar cancers. The DNA from HPV 16 and 18 has been detected in up to 60% of patients with vulvar cancer.

The mechanism of HPV transformation into dysplasia and cancer is not well understood. Two gene products from HPV are known to immortalize cells in culture and are probably responsible for malignant transformation. The HPV E6 protein does have the ability to bind the host p53 protein. The HPV E7 protein binds the Rb gene product. The oncogenic viral types are thought to have a greater affinity for these cellular proteins, which would explain the increased risk of malignant transformation. Some infections may lead to integration of the viral DNA into the host, with disruption of the normal regulation of the E6 and E7 oncoproteins. This increased production of the E6 and E7 gene products then results in oncogenic transformation.

Clinical Presentation

Diagnosis of vulvar carcinoma is often delayed. Women neglect to seek treatment for an average of 6 months from the onset of symptoms. In addition, a delay in diagnosis often occurs after the patient presents to physician. In many cases, a biopsy of the lesion is not performed until the problem fails to respond to numerous topical therapies. A biopsy should be performed when any discrete lesion of the vulva is discovered.

The most common presentation is pruritic lesion of the vulva or a mass detected by the patient herself. However, early vulvar cancer may be asymptomatic and recognized only with careful inspection of the vulva. A biopsy should be performed on all visible lesions on the vulva. More advanced vulvar carcinomas present with bleeding, pain, or discharge. Most patients with invasive disease complain of:

- Irritation or pruritis in 70% of cases
- Vulvar mass or ulcer in 55% of cases
- Bleeding in 28% of cases
- Discharge in 2–3% of cases

Laboratory Studies

Routine preoperative laboratory studies for vulvar cancer include serum electrolyte evaluations and a complete blood cell count.

No special testing is needed, except as indicated by the patient's medical condition.

Imaging Studies

- Imaging studies other than routine chest radiographs have not been helpful in the evaluation of women with vulvar carcinoma, except to evaluate specific symptoms or nodal enlargement.
- A CT scan may be useful to help evaluate nodal spread in the pelvis in women with evidence of groin node metastasis, but the sensitivity of a CT scan to help detect pelvic lymphadenopathy is approximately 30%. Because of the low sensitivity of imaging in detecting pelvic node metastasis, some authors have suggested laparoscopic assessment of the pelvic lymph nodes as an alternative.
- MRI can be used to evaluate lymphatic spread but is of limited use because of the expense and the difficulty of evaluating the pelvic nodal group.
- Positron emission tomography (PET) scanning holds some promise in improving the sensitivity of detecting small nodal metastasis. PET is used in patients with vulvar cancer, but the clinical impact has not been established.

Other Tests

- ECG prior to surgery, if indicated.
- Pulmonary function tests may be appropriate in women who smoke and are older than 50 years to help in perioperative management. Evaluation should also include an arterial blood gas analysis.

Diagnostic Procedures

Colposcopy can be performed on the vulva but is more difficult than colposcopy of the cervix because of the large surface area of the vulva and the variability in premalignant lesions. Because of the keratinized skin, acetic acid should be placed for at least 5 minutes prior to colposcopy. A punch biopsy tool can be used to take a representative sample of the vulva. A biopsy should be performed on all lesions to ensure that a cancer is not missed when multiple dysplastic lesions are present.

Histologic Findings (Table 24.1)

Squamous carcinoma is the most common pathologic type of vulvar carcinoma. Various grading systems are described and may be prognostic. Other prognostic features include confluent growth patterns and lymph vascular involvement.

Melanoma accounts for approximately 10% of vulvar cancers. The staging and treatment is similar to other melanomas.

Sarcoma is relatively uncommon. Subtypes include leiomyosarcoma, malignant fibrous histiocytoma, and epithelioid sarcoma. In addition, a sarcoma can arise from any structure in the vulva; including blood vessels, skeletal muscle, and fat.

Basal cell carcinoma of the vulva is uncommon, but it can occur in elderly women. As with other basal cell carcinomas, local excision is usually curative.

Verrucous carcinoma resembles condylomata acuminata and is also called a Buschke-Lowenstein giant condyloma. This type of carcinoma is locally aggressive but does not have a propensity to spread via lymphatics. These tumors are thought to be associated with HPV type 6.

Table 24.1: Types of vulval cancer	
Type	*Percent*
Squamous	92
Melanoma	2–4
Basal cell	2–3
Bartholin gland (adenocarcinoma, squamous cell, transitional cell, adenoid cystic)	1
Metastatic	1
Verrucous	<1
Sarcoma	<1
Appendage (e.g. hidradenocarcinoma)	Rare

Adenocarcinoma may arise in the Bartholin gland, and it represents approximately 40% of tumor types from this location. This type of tumor may attain considerable size before detection. Removal of the Bartholin gland to exclude an underlying carcinoma is indicated for recurrent Bartholin gland abscesses or cysts or if asymptomatic enlargement occurs in persons older than 50 years.

Paget's disease usually manifests as a red, raised, pruritic lesion. Histologically, the lesion is noted to contain cells with prominent nuclei and an increased amount of cytoplasm. Paget's disease has been associated with underlying adenocarcinoma of the colon or sweat glands in 15% of cases. Although Paget's disease does not metastasize, because the histologic changes often extend past the gross extent on the skin, it is known to have a high rate of local recurrence. For this reason, a clinical margin of 2 cm is recommended at the time of excision.

Other carcinomas of the vulva are rare. Tumors can occur in the apocrine sweat glands, and breast carcinoma can also develop from ectopic breast tissue contained within the milk line that extends down into the vulva.

The New FIGO Staging for Carcinoma of the Vulva

Stage I: Tumor confined to vulva.
IA Tumor confined to the vulva or perineum, ≤2 cm in size with stromal invasion ≤ 1mm^3, negative nodes
IB Tumor confined to the vulva or perineum, >2 cm in size or with stromal invasion >1 mm^3, negative nodes

Stage II: Tumor of any size with adjacent spread (1/3 lower urethra, 1/3 lower vagina, anus), negative nodes

Stage III: Tumor of any size with or without any extension to adjacent perineal structures (lower third of urethra, lower third of vagina, anus) with positive inguinofemoral nodes.

IIIA Tumor of any size with positive inguinofemoral lymph nodes
    i. 1 lymph node metastasis greater than or equal to 5 mm
    ii. 1–2 lymph node metastases of less than 5 mm

IIIB
    i. 2 or more lymph node metastases greater than or equal to 5 mm
    ii. 3 or more lymph node metastases less than 5 mm

IIIC Positive node(s) with extracapsular spread

Stage IV: Tumor invades other regional (upper 2/3rd urethra, upper 2/3rd vagina), or distant structures.

IVA
    i. Tumor invades other regional structures (2/3rd upper urethra, 2/3rd upper vagina), bladder mucosa, rectal mucosa, or fixed to pelvic bone
    ii. Fixed or ulcerated inguinofemoral lymph nodes.

IVB Any distant metastasis including pelvic lymph nodes

The 2 systems used for staging most types of vulvar cancer—the *FIGO* (International Federation of Gynecology and Obstetrics) system and the American Joint Committee on Cancer TNM staging system—are very similar. They both classify vulvar cancer on the basis of 3 factors: The extent of the tumor (T), whether the cancer has spread to lymph nodes (N) and whether it has spread to distant sites (M). The system described below is the most recent AJCC system, which went into effect January 2010. Any differences between the AJCC system and the FIGO system are explained in the text.

Tumor Extent (T)

Tis: The cancer is not growing into the underlying tissues. This stage, also known as *carcinoma in situ*, is not included in the FIGO system.

T1: The cancer is growing only in the vulva or perineum
- *T1a:* The cancer has grown no more than 1 mm into underlying tissue (stroma) and is 2 cm or smaller in size (about 0.8 inches).
- *T1b:* The cancer is either more than 2 cm or it has grown more than 1 mm into underlying tissue (stroma).

T2: The tumor can be any size. The cancer is growing into the anus or the lower third of the vagina or urethra. (stage 2/3 in the FIGO system).

T3: The tumor can be of any size. The cancer is growing into the upper urethra, bladder or rectum or into the pubic bone (stage 4 in the FIGO system).

Lymph Node Spread of Cancer (N)

N0: No lymph node spread
N1: The cancer has spread to 1 or 2 lymph nodes in the groin with the following features:
- **N1a:** The cancer has spread to 1 or 2 lymph nodes and the areas of cancer spread are both less than 5 mm (about 1/5th of an inch) in size.
- **N1b:** The cancer has spread to one lymph node and the area of cancer spread is 5 mm or greater.

N2: The cancer has spread to groin lymph nodes with the following features:

- **N2a:** The cancer has spread to 3 or more lymph nodes, but each area of spread is less than 5 mm.
- **N2b:** The cancer has spread to 2 or more lymph nodes with each area of spread 5 mm or greater.
- **N2c:** The cancer has spread to lymph nodes and has started growing through the outer covering of at least one of the lymph nodes (extracapsular spread).

N3: The cancer has spread to the lymph nodes causing open sores (*ulceration*) or causing the lymph node to be stuck (*fixed*) to the tissue below it.

Distant Spread of Cancer (M)

M0: No distant spread.
M1: The cancer has spread to distant sites (includes spread to pelvic lymph nodes).

Stage Grouping

The grouping of T, N, and M determines the stage:

Stage 0 (Tis, N0, M0): This is a very early cancer found on the surface of the skin of the vulva only. It is also known as *carcinoma in situ* and as *Bowen disease*. This stage is not included in the FIGO system.

Stage I (T1, N0, M0): The cancer is in the vulva or the perineum (the space between the rectum and the vagina) or both. The tumor has not spread to lymph nodes or distant sites.

Stage IA (T1a, N0, M0): These are stage I cancers with tumors that are 2 cm or less that have grown into the underlying tissue no deeper than 1 mm (about 1/25 inch).

Stage IB (T1b, N0, M0): These are stage I cancers that have invaded deeper than 1 mm and/or are larger than 2 cm.

Stage II (T2, N0, M0): The cancer has grown outside the vulva or perineum to the anus or lower third of the vagina or urethra (T2). It has not spread to lymph nodes (N0) or distant sites (M0). In FIGO, this grouping is T2/T3, N0, M0, but it is still stage II.

Stage IIIA (T1 or T2, N1a or N1b, M0): Cancer is found in the vulva or perineum or both (T1) and may be growing into the anus, lower vagina, or lower urethra (T2). Either it has spread to a single nearby lymph node with the area of cancer spread 5 mm or greater in size (N1a); OR it has spread to 1 or 2 nearby lymph nodes with both areas of cancer spread less than 5 mm in size (N1b). It has not spread to distant sites (M0). In FIGO, this stage is also called IIIA.

Stage IIIB (T1 or T2, N2a or N2b, M0): Cancer is found in the vulva or perineum or both (T1) and may be growing into the anus, vagina, or lower urethra (T2). Either, the cancer has spread to 3 or more nearby lymph nodes, with all areas of cancer spread less than 5 mm in size (N2a); OR the cancer has spread to 2 or more lymph nodes with each area of spread 5 mm or greater in size (N2b). The cancer has not spread to distant sites (M0). In FIGO, this stage is IIIB.

Stage IIIC (T1 or T2, N2c, M0): Cancer is found in the vulva or perineum or both (T1) and may be growing into the anus, lower vagina, or lower urethra (T2). The cancer has spread to nearby lymph nodes and has started growing through the outer covering of at least one of the lymph nodes (extracapsular spread; N2c). The cancer has not spread to distant sites (M0). In FIGO, this stage is IIIC.

Stage IVA: Either of the following:

T1 or T2, N3, M0: Cancer is found in the vulva or perineum or both (T1) and may be growing into the anus, vagina, or lower urethra (T2). Cancer spread to nearby lymph nodes has caused them to be fixed to the underlying tissue or caused open sores (ulceration) (N3). It has not spread to distant sites. In FIGO, this stage is also called IVA. OR

T3, any N, M0: The cancer has spread beyond nearby tissues to the bladder, rectum, pelvic bone, or upper part of the urethra (T3). It may or may not have spread to nearby lymph nodes (any N). It has not spread to distant sites (M0). In FIGO, this stage is also called IVA.

Stage IVB (any T, any N, M1): Cancer has spread to distant organs or lymph nodes (M1). This is the most advanced stage of cancer. In FIGO, this stage is also called IVB.

Treatment

History of the Procedure

In the early part of the 20th century, patients with vulvar cancer diagnosed usually died of disease. The overall survival rate for vulvar cancer after simple surgical excision was less than 25%. Attempts to improve outcomes for patients with vulvar cancer by performing more radical surgery were first described by Basset in 1912.

Stanley Way described an improved survival rate using an en bloc dissection of radical vulvectomy with an inguinal and pelvic lymphadenectomy. The Bassett-Way operation resulted in a 5-year survival rate of 74%.

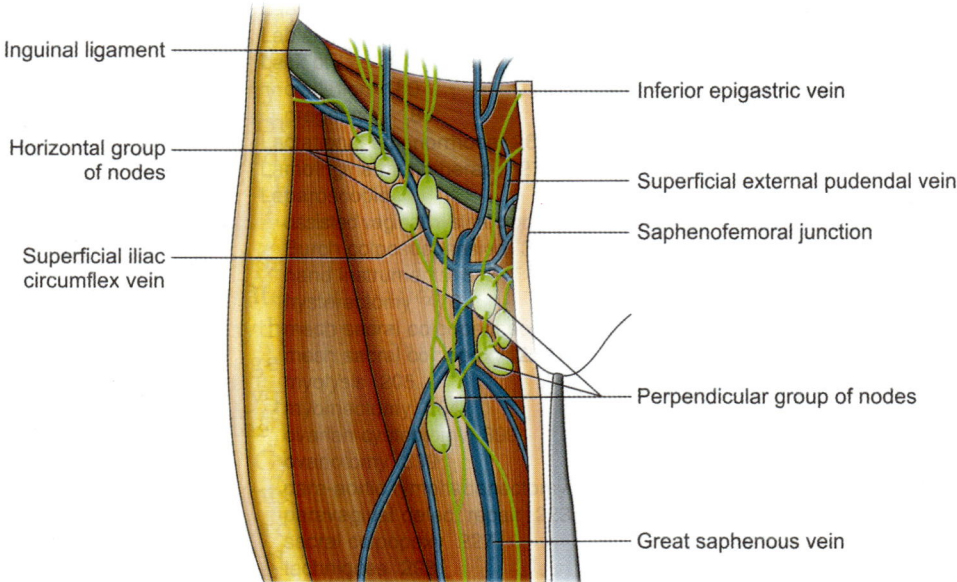

Fig. 24.11: Groin nodal groups. Direct spread to the deep nodalgroups without metastasis to the superfcial group has been documented using lymphatic mapping. This type of direct spread is uncommon and represents fewer than 5% of cases

Major morbidity from this procedure included poor wound healing and long-term lymphedema.

Fred Taussig used separate incisions for the groin dissection and the vulvar excision. He reported using three separate incisions for patients with clinical stage I disease. The 5-year survival rate was 97%.

Relevant Anatomy (Fig. 24.11)

The vulva includes all external genital structures, including the mons pubis, labia majora, labia minora, clitoris, vaginal vestibule, perineum, and supporting structures exterior to the urogenital diaphragm.

The femoral triangle is bounded by the inguinal ligament superiorly, the adductor longus medially, and the sartorius laterally. The superficial groin nodes lie above the cribriform fascia in the femoral triangle. Careful dissection generally reveals 5 vessels in the femoral triangle above the cribriform fascia, the largest of which is the saphenous vein. Often, a lateral accessory saphenous vein can be identified. The other vessels include the superficial circumflex, the superficial epigastric, and the external pudendal. Below the cribriform fascia are the deep inguinal nodes. Three to four nodes can be found medial to the femoral vein. The most superior of these is the sentinel node to the pelvic lymphatics and is known as the node of Cloquet.

The lymphatics of the vulva and distal third of the vagina drain into the superficial inguinal node group and travel through the deep femoral lymphatics and the node of Cloquet to the pelvis.

Most lymphatics flow through the superficial inguinal nodes, deep inguinal nodes, and the node of Cloquet to the pelvic lymph node chains. Deep inguinal node findings are positive approximately 3% of the time when superficial inguinal node findings are negative. Lymphatic mapping studies indicate that 13% of cases demonstrate findings consistent with flow to the pelvis that does not involve the node of Cloquet (Fig. 24.12).

Lymphatic mapping studies have also demonstrated that 10–20% of lymphatic flow from the superficial node group travels directly to the pelvis without passage through the deep inguinal nodes. A direct pathway from the clitoris or vulva to the pelvic nodes has not been identified. Therefore:

- Left-sided lesion will spread to the left groin lymph node.
- Right-sided lesion will spread to the right groin lymph node.

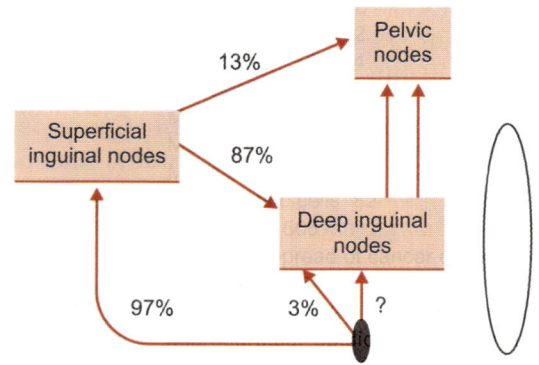

Fig. 24.12: Diagram of lymphatic drainage of a lateral lesion

- Bilateral nodes involvement is seen in 14% of cases.
- Contralateral node involvement without ipsilateral disease is seen in 5% of cases.
- Pelvic nodes are not involved in the absence of inguinal nodes metastases.

Surgical Approach

Principles

1. Three basic types of surgery include *wide local excision* or simple partial vulvectomy, *radical partial vulvectomy*, *radical complete vulvectomy* (Fig. 24.13).
2. In wide local excision 1–2 cm tumor free margins are excised around the lesion. The depth of surgery usually confines up to 1 cm into the superficial perineal fascia.
3. With radical partial vulvectomy, tumor-containing portion of vulva is completely removed with tumour free skin margins of 1–2 cm and the excision deep to the perineal membrane. In unilateral well-lateralized lesion, unilateral hemivulvectomy and anterior or posterior hemivulvectomy is adequate in case of anterior and posterior lesion, respectively (Fig. 24.14).
4. With radical complete vulvectomy, dissection is done around 1–2 cm free margin and depth 1 cm up to superficial perineal fascia. It is appropriate in bilateral or midline lesions.
5. Currently three separate incisions—two separate groin and one vulval incision are given to avoid postoperative morbidity and skin disruption (Fig. 24.15).

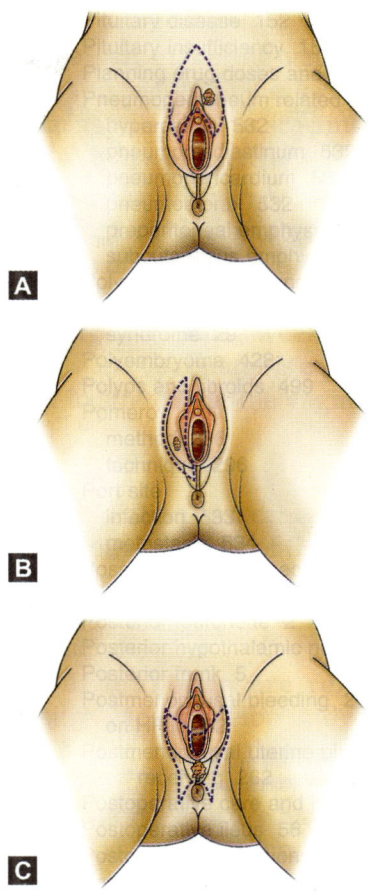

Fig. 24.14: Modified radical vulvectomy. (A) Anterior hemivulvectomy. (B) Right hemivulvectomy with clitoral sparing. (C) Posterior hemivulvectomy

6. *Inguinofemoral lymphadenectomy* can be unilateral. In unilateral well-lateralized lesions or bilateral in midline incisions. Rarely cribriform fascia is penetrated to avoid skeletonisation of major femoral

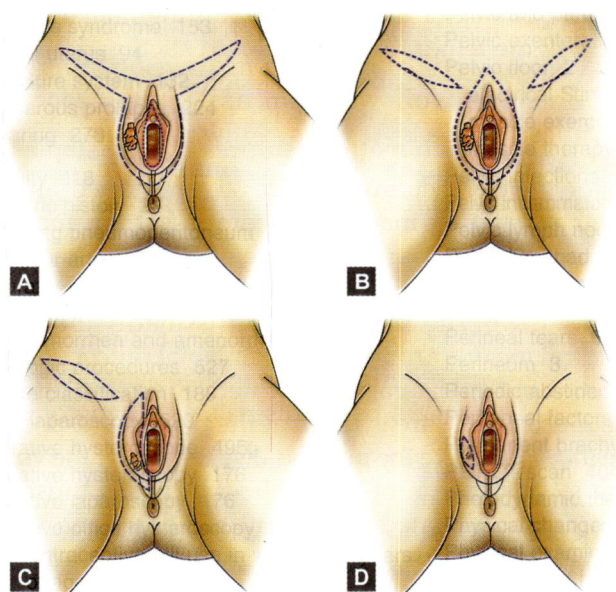

Fig. 24.13: Different incisions

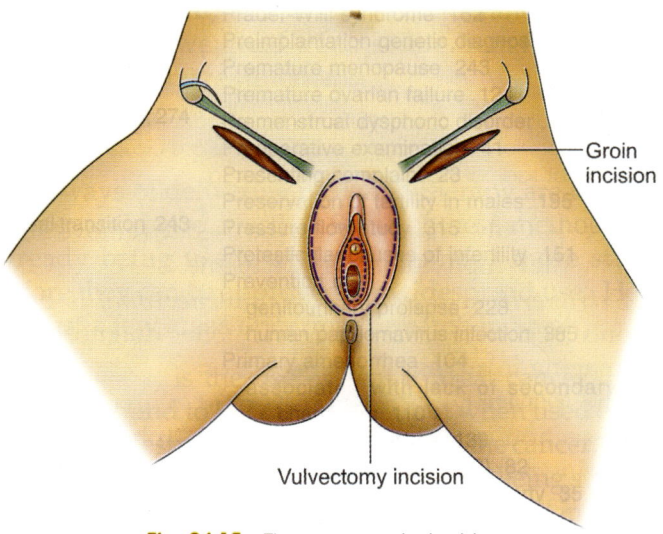

Fig. 24.15: Three separate incisions

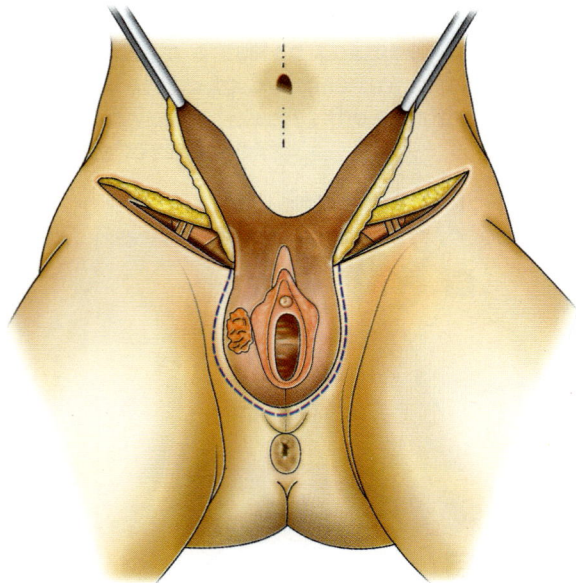

Fig. 24.16: Bilateral inguinofemoral lymphadenectomy is complete. Planned incisions for the en bloc radical vulvectomy are shown

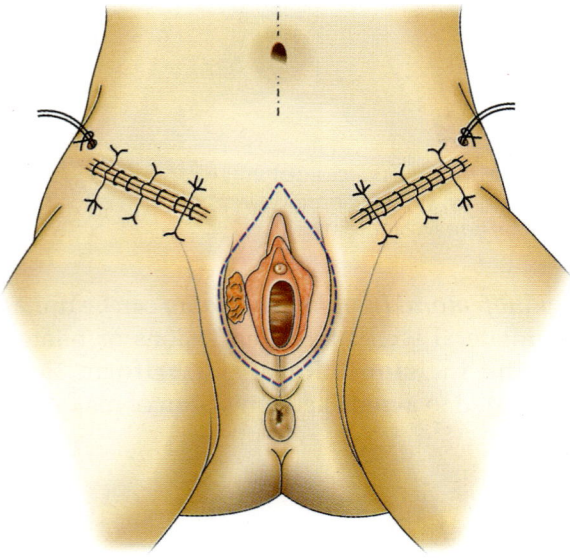

Fig. 24.17: Bilateral inguinofemoral lymphadenectomy through separate incisions is completed and wounds are closed. Separate incisions for radical vulvectomy are marked

vessels. Only fossa ovalis can be used to remove deep femoral lymph node (Figs 24.16 and 24.17).

7. ***Extraperitoneal pelvic lymphadenectomy*** is done only in case of enlarged pelvic nodes diagnosed on imaging in advanced stage.

8. The traditional description of a groin node dissection includes ligation of the saphenous vein during removal of the superficial groin lymphatics. But it is currently observed that if saphenous vein is preserved, the incidence of wound cellulitis and

acute and chronic lymphedema is significantly lower.

9. Many physicians now omit deep groin node dissection. Opening the femoral sheath and removing the deep nodes is not without morbidity. Deep lymph node dissection may increase the incidence of lymphedema. In addition, infection of the groin over the femoral vessels after deep groin dissection can result in catastrophic bleeding. The sartorius muscle historically was transferred to the inguinal ligament to cover the exposed femoral vessels.

Intraoperative Details

Surgery for vulvar carcinoma is often performed with the woman's legs in adjustable stirrups to facilitate both the groin node dissection and the perineal phase of the operation. A surgical team can greatly reduce operative time. After the patient is prepared and draped, an incision is made approximately 2 cm below the inguinal ligament. The tissue is undermined below the Scarpa fascia and the dissection is carried down upto the tensor fasciae latae. Then, the superficial inguinal nodal group—lateral and medial group is dissected off the cribriform fascia, taking care not to injure the great saphenous vein. The fatty tissue with all lymphatic channels are removed en bloc.

If the deep nodes are to be dissected, open the cribriform fascia laterally and take it as part of the specimen. Then, dissect the femoral vein free and remove the nodes from the medial portion of the femoral vein. After a deep groin node dissection, the sartorius muscle can be divided at its insertion on the anterior iliac spine and sutured to the inguinal ligament to cover the femoral vessels. Closed suction drains are placed through a separate incision and suture to the skin. Scarpa fascia is closed with 3-0 absorbable sutures and the skin with mattress sutures or with staples.

For the vulvectomy, the lesion is outlined and an outer incision is made to encompass 1 cm margins around the tumor. In contrast to a simple vulvectomy, the dissection is carried deep to the perineal membrane (Fig. 24.18). The inner incision is made above the urethral meatus around the inner labial mucocutanous junction at 1 cm lateral to the growth all around through the fourchette. Care is taken at the posterior aspects of the incision where the pudendal vessels enter the vulva. The lower portion of the bulbocavernosus muscle is clamped and ligated to prevent bleeding. The whole vulval skin along with the growth is removed (Fig. 24.19). The vagina and vulvar skin can be mobilized to reduce the tension on the incision. It is

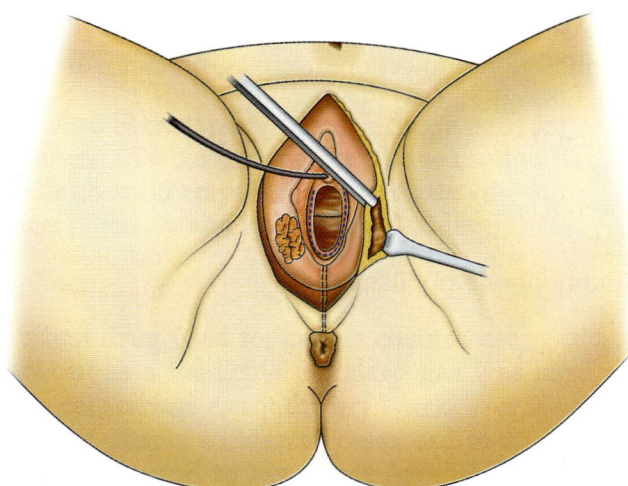

Fig. 24.18: Labiocrural incisions extended to the deep fascia of the urogenital diaphragm

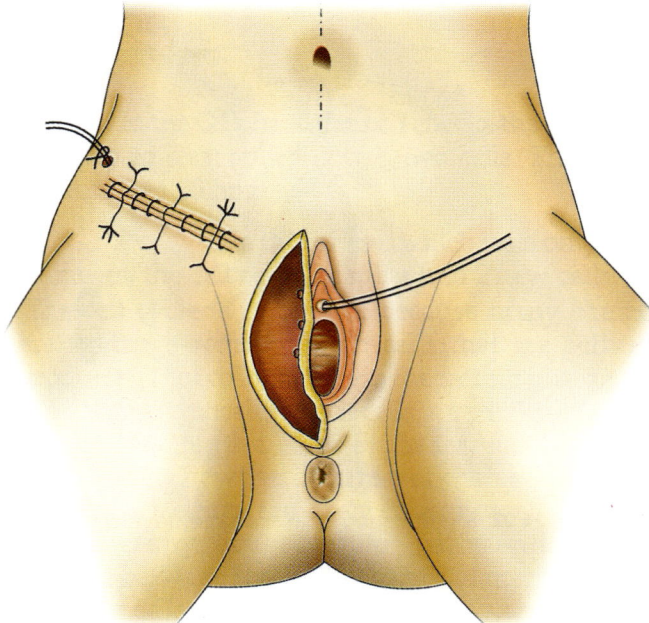

Fig. 24.20: Unilateral groin and hemivulvectomy

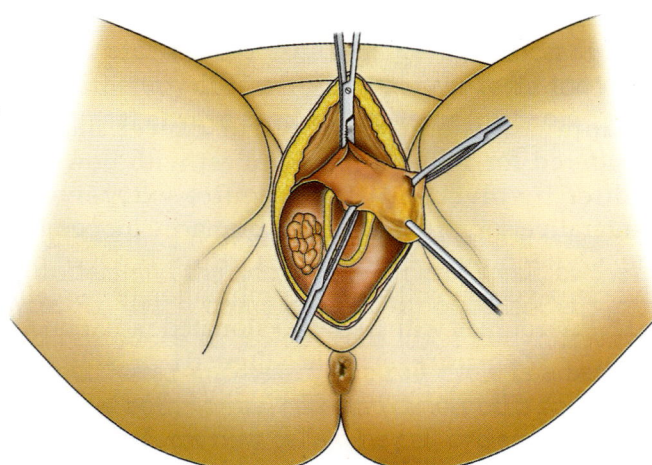

Fig. 24.19: Disection proceeds dorsally off of the pubic bone. The vascular base of the clitoris clamped, followed by transaction and ligation

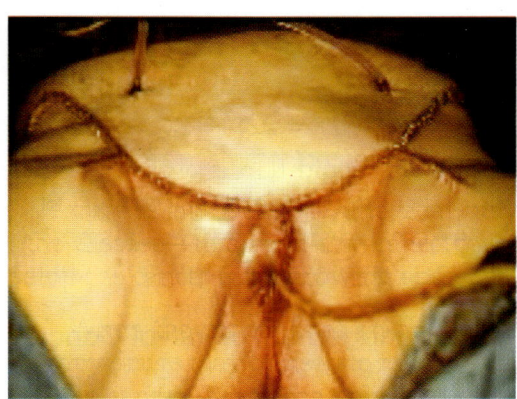

Fig. 24.21: Postoperative incision scar

closed in layers with absorbable suture, and the skin is closed with horizontal or vertical absorbable 3-0 mattress sutures. Figure 24.20 shows incisions of unilateral groin and hemivulvectomy in unilateral lesion. Figure 24.21 shows postoperative incision scar after bilateral inguinofemoral lymphadenectomy.

Split-thickness Skin Grafting

When wide local excision of vulvar lesions create large defects, a segmental skin graft can be applied so that skin approximation without tension will ensure a better cosmetic result.

The technique of removing just the vulvar skin (i.e. skinning vulvectomy) and preserving the subcutaneous tissue and vulva blood supply is preferred. Although operative time and hospital stay are lengthened when skinning vulvectomy and grafting are performed, better cosmetic results with few residual sequelae are obtained. Among these sequelae are graft-take failure in the range of 5 to 15% and an impairment of sensation in both the grafted area and the graft site. The mons pubis is a potential graft selection site.

Use of the Labia Minora (Full-thickness Graft)

Patients with vulvar surgery may experience complications such as dyspareunia, introital stenosis, hoods over the urethral orifice, vulvar scarring, and vulvar breakdown with infection. In these patients, vulvar reconstruction can be performed by using full-thickness grafts. Full-thickness grafts use both the

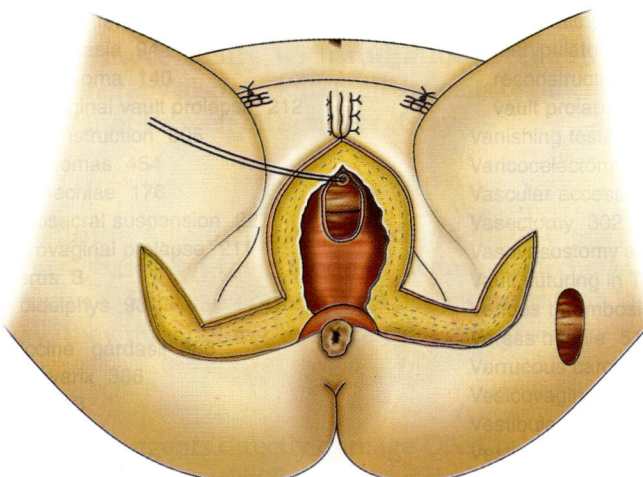

Fig. 24.22: Bilateral rhomboid flaps are developed

epidermis and the dermis. The possible donor sites include the labia minora, upper medial thigh, and groin. The size of the graft should be larger than the area to be covered secondary to the high primary contracture rate. The use of skin grafting at the time of initial vulvar surgery can circumvent many of the aforementioned complications.

Rhomboid Flap (Fig. 24.22)

Creation of a rhomboid flap is a useful approach for repairing defects occurring after partial vulvectomy. The flaps are created such that a graft is not necessary and adequate closure without tension is obtained.

Stage-wise Management of Vulval Cancer

See Table 24.2.

Early Postoperative Complications

- Groin wound infection, necrosis, breakdown
- En bloc operation: 53–85%
- Separate-incision approach – 44%
- UTI
- Seromas
- DVT
- Pulmonary embolism
- MI
- Hemorrhage

Late Complications

- Chronic lymphedema (30%)
- Recurrent lymphagitis or cellulitis (10%)
  - Usually responds to oral antibiotics
- SUI (10%)
- Femoral hernia (uncommon)
- Depression, altered body image and sexual dysfunction

Adjuvant Therapy

Neoadjuvant therapy for vulvar cancer may be considered for tumors that manifest with bowel or bladder involvement that require extensive or exenterative surgery or tumor is primarily inoperable. The Gynecologic Oncology Group (GOG) has advocated good result with a combination of cisplatin and 5-fluorouracil with hyperfractionated radiation for patients with unresectable stage III or stage IV squamous cell carcinoma of the vulva. Except in the neoadjuvant setting, chemotherapy for vulvar

Table 24.2: Stage-wise management of vulval cancer	
Features of carcinoma	*Management*
1. ≤ 2 cm lesion size ≤ 1 mm depth invasion No lymph-vascular space involvement. Well or mod.diff.	Radical local excision only (excision with 2 cm margins, down to super, aponeurosis of the original diaph +/-pubic periosteum)
2. >2 cm lesion size Or > 1 mm depth invasion Or lymph-vascular space involvement Or poorly diff	Radical local excision and inguinofemoral node dissection. Unilateral, if lesion unilateral not involving midline; bilateral, if lesion midline
3. Involves clitoral	Anterior redical vulvectomy (including removal of clitoris but preserving post.vulva). Bilat inguinal–femoral nerve dissection
4. Post. vulva/perineum	Posterior radical vulvectomy (preserving clitoris and anterior vulva). Bilat inguinal-femoral nerve dissection
5. Locally advanced	Pelvic exenteration (ant, post, total as indicated by structures involved) Anovalvetomy (for lesion involving anus/and vulva). Chemoradiation followed by limited surgery
6. Bone involvement fixed groin nodes	Chemoradiation followed by limited surgery, if locally resectable

carcinoma is palliative and often ineffective. Only bleomycin has been reported to produce a complete clinical response. The only other agent that has been reported to be effective in recurrent vulvar cancer is doxorubicin.

In women with locally advanced vulvar cancer, no significant differences in survival or adverse events were found when primary chemoradiation or neoadjuvant chemoradiation were compared with primary surgery. However, these findings were based on small numbers and few studies in this Cochrane review. Good, quality studies that compare primary treatments in locally advanced vulvar cancer are needed.

Cisplatin and 5-fluorouracil (5-FU) is also used in recurrent vulvar cancer though adequate reports are yet to establish this.

Follow-up

Studies indicate these women after surgery are at high risk for sexual dysfunction, even in the absence of a functional problem after surgery. Sexual dysfunction seems to be related to a disturbance in body image, leading to hypoactive sexual disorder and aversion disorder. Depression and increasing age are risk factors for sexually active women to discontinue intercourse after surgery. Interestingly, sexual dysfunction with extent of surgery s reduced if the clitoris is preserved.

Women who have positive findings from more than one node are likely to benefit from adjuvant radiation therapy to the inguinal and pelvic nodes. The GOG studied the use of pelvic node resection compared with radiation of the groin and pelvis. The cancer-related death rate at 6 years for women having a pelvic lymph node resection is 51% compared with 29% in women who have underwent radiation. Therefore, radiation after vulvectomy and inguinal lymphadenectomy significantly reduces local relapses and decreases cancer-related deaths for patients with node-positive vulvar cancer. A clear benefit for radiation has not been proven in women with positive microscopic findings from one node, but, because groin recurrence is almost universally fatal, adjuvant radiation is often recommended.

Follow-up of patients with physical examinations every 3 months for the first 2 years is often recommended because more than two thirds of recurrences occur in this time period. Detection of local recurrence of vulvar carcinoma is important because it can be treated by radical surgical excision.

The long-term survival rate after radical excision of a vulvar recurrence has been reported as 50–60%. Survival is better in women who originally presented with early-stage disease. Other factors that diminish the cure rate after local recurrence include disease at sites other than the vulva and a short interval from initial treatment to recurrence. For a large recurrence, an exenterative procedure can be attempted. A long-term survival rate of 38% has been reported after exenterative surgery for vulvar carcinoma.

Resection of a groin recurrence is not usually recommended. Often, this area heals slowly if radiation has already been used. Generally, the procedure should not be considered curative. The only situation in which resection of a groin node recurrence should be attempted is when the groin node is an isolated recurrence and the patient has not been previously irradiated.

Positive groin nodes at the time of initial surgery increase the risk of recurrence in the groin in the first 2 years. After the first 2 years, the risk of groin recurrence is low, regardless of the status of the nodes at the time of the initial surgery. It has been noted that up to 10% of patients treated for vulvar cancer had a local recurrence more than 5 years after the original diagnosis.

Complications

Lymphocyst formation is noted in 7–19% of patients after groin lymphadenectomy. Although cellulitis after vulvectomy is associated with an increase in the incidence of lymphedema, it has not been associated with an increase in lymphocyst formation. Therefore, drains are not removed after inguinal node dissection until the daily output of the drain is less than 25 mL.

Lymphocysts usually manifest as an asymptomatic mass in the groin. To exclude a groin recurrence, fluid is aspirated from the cyst and sent for cytologic evaluation. Multiple aspirations are often required and may not be curative. If the mass is symptomatic, the lymphocyst can be removed surgically. Sometimes, lymphocysts are successfully treated by placing a drain in the groin until the output is less than 25 mL/day. A pressure dressing is placed to prevent reaccumulation of the fluid.

Cellulitis and lymphangitis can occur after groin node dissection. The incidence rate of cellulitis requiring antibiotics ranges from 20–40%. Often, patients who develop lymphocysts are at increased risk of lymphangitis. The etiologic agent is most often a streptococcal species, and treatment with penicillin is adequate. If drains are still in place, first-generation cephalosporins may be more appropriate to treat *Staphylococcus aureus*.

Chronic lymphedema has been reported in 10–20% of women after groin node dissection. This can be a disabling problem and is more common if radiation is required after groin dissection. Limiting groin node dissection in women with early cancers and preserving the saphenous vein decreases the incidence of this problem. The use of graduated compression stockings after lymphadenectomy can help prevent lymphedema. If edema develops, the use of compression stockings, massage therapy, and limb wraps can help control the accumulation of fluid.

Morbidity Related to Surgery (RCOG)

- Wound breakdown
- Wound infection
- Deep vein thrombosis and pulmonary embolism
- Pressure sores
- Introital stenosis
- Fecal incontinence
- Inguinal lymphocyst
- Lymphedema

- Hernia
- Psychosexual complications

- Urinary incontinence
- Rectocele

Prognosis

Overall survival for patients with vulvar carcinoma is excellent, especially in those with early-stage disease. The overall survival rate for women with vulvar carcinoma is 75%, The 5-year survival rates after surgery for vulvar cancer are as follows:

- Stage I—90%
- Stage II—81%
- Stage III—68%
- Stage IV—20%

It is noteworthy that more than 95% of these patients are treated with vulvar-conserving surgery in stages I and II.

Future Therapy

A prophylactic quadrivalent vaccine is now approved by the Food and Drug Administration (FDA) in 2006 for the prevention of anogenital lesions including genital warts, vulvar and vaginal intraepithelial neoplasia, and cervical lesions associated with HPV 6, 11, 16 and 18.

A sentinel lymph node (SLN) can be identified and can be predictive of patients who will have other involved nodes. The technique of SLN dissection is attractive in vulvar carcinoma since most women will have negative lymph nodes. If the sentinel node dissection proves to be sufficiently sensitive, full groin node dissection could be limited only to women with positive lymph nodes. A sentinel node can be identified in approximately 85% of women with isosulfan blue dye and 100% with the injection of Tc-99 labeled albumin. Intraoperative lymphatic mapping is accomplished by injecting radionucleolide intradermally at the border of the primary tumour which is closest to the groin. For midline tumour both sides of the tumour are injected. Then Isosulfan blue is injected at the same primary tumour location followed by groin skin incision approximately 5 minutes later. The tracer and dye are taken up by specific node that drains the tumour site. The handheld gamma counter assist in localizing the sentinel node or it can be identified by the blue colour and can be made separated from the other nodes within the regional group. The GOG lymphatic mapping and SLNB study supports the use of SLNB for women with primary tumors smaller than 4 cm performed by well-trained gynecologic oncologists.

Melanoma

This is a rare condition in vulva. Incidence is: 0.1–0.19/100,000 women though this is the second most common of vulvar malignancy. Mostly seen in postmenopausal white women. The patients are mostly asymptomatic. The other features are Itching, bleeding, groin mass. It involves mainly labia minora, and clitoris.

Histopathology

- Mucosal lentiginous melanoma: These are flat freckle, quite extensive, superficial lesions.
- Superficial spreading melanoma: Most common variety.
- Nodular melanoma: Most aggressive, raised lesion which penetrate deeply and metastasize widely.

The one-fourth of cases of melanomas are macroscopically amelanotic and spread early.

Staging

The FIGO staging used for squamous lesions is not applicable to melanomas because the lesions are usually much smaller and the prognosis is related to the depth of tumor invasion rather than to the diameter of the lesion.

Treatment

- It has more conservative surgical management. In case of <1 mm invasion: Radical local excision of the primary tumor and regional groin node dissection is recommended with 2 cm surgical margin (1–4 mm).

- 10-year survival rate with lateral lesion has 61% and medial lesion has 37% survival rate.
- Superfical lesion (Breslow tumor thickness <0.76 mm) Lymphadenectomy is not indicated
- Intermediate-thickness (1–4 mm)—lymph node dissection is recommended.
- Deeply invasive cutaneous melanoma (>4 mm) Benefit from regional lymphadenectomy and chemotherapy with interferon-α.

Bartholin Gland Carcinoma (Fig. 24.23)

- It is rare; found in both postmenopausal and premenopausal women
  – Honan's criteria
  – The tumor is in the correct anatomic position
  – The tumor is located deep in the labium majus
  – The overlying skin is intact
  – There is some recognizable normal gland present

Signs and Symptoms

- Vulvar mass or perineal pain
- 10% of patients may be mistaken for benign cysts or abscesses

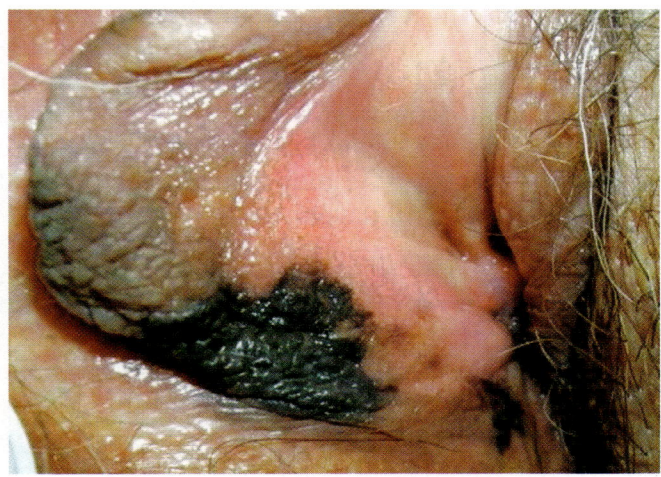

Fig. 24.23: Bartholin gland cancer growth

Treatment

- Radical vulvectomy with bilateral groin and pelvic LN dissection.
- If the lesion is fixed, involves adjacent structures, postoperative radiation and chemotherapy is preferable.

RCOG Guidelines

In women who present with vulval bleeding, pruritus, pain and ulceration, it is reasonable to use a period of 'treat, watch and wait' as a method of management. This should include the offer of active follow-up until these symptoms resolve or a diagnosis is confirmed. If symptoms persist, referral should be routine, preferably without recourse to biopsy, which may influence subsequent assessment and introduce delay. [C]

- Vulval cancer should be managed in gynecological cancer centres/networks by multidisciplinary teams. [B/C]
- The woman should be seen and managed according to current national directives on waiting times and time from diagnosis to treatment.
- Radical treatment should not be undertaken without prior biopsy confirmation of malignancy. [C]

Biopsy

All diagnoses should be based upon a representative biopsy of the tumour that should include the area of epithelium where there is a transition of normal to malignant tissue. Diagnostic biopsies should be of a sufficient size (greater than 1 mm depth to allow differentiation between superficially invasive and frankly invasive tumours) and orientated to allow quality pathological interpretation.

Biopsies should be referred to a pathologist with a specialist interest in gynaecological pathology.

The following investigations are suggested for the majority of patients, although one must accept that, in a predominantly elderly population, this cannot be considered either complete or proscriptive, as each case must be fully assessed according to individual need:

- Full blood count (pretreatment assessment)
- Biochemical profile (pretreatment assessment, abnormal liver function might suggest metastatic disease)
- Chest X-ray (preoperative assessment, exclude metastases)
- Electrocardiogram (preoperative assessment)
- Cervical smear
- Locally available imaging to assess for concurrent pelvic pathology and retroperitoneal nodes
- Fine-needle aspiration of any clinically suspicious nodes or other metastases where the result will alter management (i.e. may elect for radiation therapy).
- Wide radical local excision of the primary tumour with a minimum margin of 15 mm of disease-free tissue is often sufficient. [C]

Surgery to the primary tumour should be radical enough to remove the tumour with adequate margins. The incidence of vulval recurrence has been shown to be related to the measured disease-free surgical margin, as measured in the fixed histopathological specimen.

Given the reduction and contraction of tissues following excision and fixation, this equates to at least a 15 mm margin on the fresh surgical specimen. The risk of recurrence increases as the disease-free margins decrease (> 8.0 mm: 0%; 8.0–4.8 mm: 8%; <4.8 mm: 54%).

Therefore, wide radical local excision with a minimum margin of 1 cm of disease free tissue should be sufficient.

Depth of Invasion

Lesions less than 2 cm in diameter and confined to the vulva or perineum, with stromal invasion less than or equal to 1.0 mm (FIGO Stage Ia) can be managed by wide local excision only, without groin node dissection. This is because the risk of lymph node metastases is negligible.

Dissection of the groin nodes should be performed when the depth of invasion is greater than 1 mm (FIGO Stage 1b or worse) or the maximum diameter of

This surgery can often be undertaken through separate incisions (triple incision technique) to reduce morbidity

- Groin node dissection should be omitted in stage 1a squamous cancer, verrucous tumour, basal cell carcinoma and melanoma. [B]
- Surgery is the cornerstone of therapy for the groin nodes in women with vulval cancer. Individual women who are not fit enough to withstand surgery can be treated with primary radiotherapy. [A/B]
- Groin node surgery can often be undertaken through separate incisions (triple incision technique) to reduce morbidity. The incidence of skin bridge recurrence in early-stage disease is low. [B]
- Superficial groin node dissection alone should not be performed, as it is associated with a higher risk of groin node recurrence. [B]
- In lateral tumours, only an ipsilateral groin node dissection need initially be performed. Contralateral lymphadenectomy may be required if ipsilateral nodes are positive. [B]
- Preservation of the long saphenous vein may reduce both groin wound and subsequent lower limb problems. [C]

Advanced vulval cancer

- Surgery to the primary lesion
- Resection of advanced disease involves careful preoperative planning and, if reconstruction is required, this should be planned jointly with a plastic surgeon.

The size and location of the tumour will influence the surgical approach. Wide, radical, local excision with a minimum of 1 cm disease-free margin may be used but some tumours will require a radical vulvectomy. If these surgical approaches risk sphincter damage leading to urinary or faecal incontinence, treatment by radiotherapy should be considered, either with curative intent or to reduce tumour volume to permit less destructive surgery.

Management of the groin nodes

Groin node dissection should be undertaken when there are clinically suspicious groin nodes present. In cases with large primary lesions and clinically suspicious nodes, a radical vulvectomy with 'en bloc' groin node dissection should be considered. In cases with fixed or ulcerated groin nodes, surgery and or radiotherapy should be considered. Surgical management of nonsquamous vulval cancer

Carcinoma of the Bartholin Gland

This is a rare vulval cancer. Histologically, it is usually a squamous carcinoma or adenocarcinoma. The current evidence base is insufficient to suggest different management from squamous tumours. The lesions are often deep-seated or likely to be associated with metastatic disease. The close proximity to the anal sphincter may necessitate partial resection with reconstruction and this may necessitate a defunctioning temporary colostomy. Any perimenopausal or postmenopausal woman with a persisting Bartholin abscess or cyst should be suspected of having a possible carcinoma. Appropriate biopsies and histological review should be undertaken.

Basal cell carcinoma and verrucous carcinoma

These squamous variants are rarely associated with lymph node metastases and can be managed by wide local excision. Basal cell carcinomas are also amenable to treatment by radiotherapy, which should be the preferred treatment if resection would compromise function (i.e. would cause sphincter damage).

Malignant melanoma

This group of tumours has not been shown to benefit from block dissection of the groin. Wide local excision is preferred. Relapse in this subgroup is high and closely correlates with the depth of invasion. On the vulva (which includes mucosal surfaces) Breslow's classification is more appropriate than Clarke's levels. As yet, there are no new strategies to minimise the risk of relapse in melanoma.

Radiotherapy

Adjuvant radiotherapy should be considered when either groin has two or more lymph nodes involved with microscopic metastatic disease or there is complete replacement and or extra capsular spread in any node. There is no evidence to show whether adjuvant radiotherapy should be given to both sides or to the involved side only. Treatment should be to the groins and the pelvic nodes.

Primary Treatment

Radiotherapy, with or without chemotherapy, is increasingly used in themanagement of advanced vulval cancer. Preoperative radiotherapy may allowfor sphincter-preserving surgery. Radiotherapy may also be of use in place of surgery for histologically proven involved groin lymph nodes. It is unknown whether post-radiation groin node removal is advantageous in terms of outcome.

Radical treatment will usually require a prophylactic dose (45–50 Gy) to be delivered to the primary and nodal sites and that the tumour is then boosted by a second phase of treatment by electrons, conformal radiotherapy or brachytherapy, to a total dose of 65 Gy. A Cochrane review has suggested that there is no evidence that prophylactic groin irradiation should be used in preference to surgery.

Chemotherapy

The role of chemotherapy in vulval cancer is still debatable but it is increasingly being used in the primary setting. Chemotherapy can be used as an adjuvant postoperatively, concomitant with radiotherapy for node positive disease. Most recent studies have looked at platinum and 5-fluorouracil-containing regimens or PMB (cisplatin, methotrexate and bleomycin) but mitomycin-C and 5-fluorouracil have also been used.

The following scenarios probably best summarise the likely uses of chemotherapy in vulval cancer:

- As a neo-adjuvant to shrink tumour initially considered unresectable
- As a concomitant to radiation for primary management of unresectable tumours
- As a postoperative adjuvant treatment either alone or concomitant to radiation for the management of relapsed disease.
- Those women with primarily unresectable disease, who are of good performance status and with good renal function, should be considered for platinum- and 5-fluorouracil-based regimens or PMB. The use of cisplatin at a dose of 60–80 mg/m^2 every 3 weeks, together with 5-fluorouracil (often given as a protracted infusion over 96 hours) can be recommended, using 750 mg/m^2 per day

Concomitant chemotherapy and radiotherapy

Chemotherapy used concomitantly with radiation should be considered analogous to use in cervical cancer and either cisplatin alone or cisplatin plus 5-fluorouracil should be considered. If used alone, cisplatin at 40 mg/m^2 weekly, concomitantly with radiotherapy, would be advised. Alternative regimens may include cisplatin and 5-fluorouracil using the regimen above, or PMB given on week-1 and week-4 of a prolonged course of radiation

Postoperative chemotherapy

The use of chemotherapy as a postoperative adjuvant is unproven.

Recurrence rates and survival

Recurrence rates for invasive squamous cell carcinoma range from 15% to 33%. The vulva is the most common site of recurrence (69.5%) with the groin nodes affected in 24.3%, the pelvis in 15.6% and distant metastases in 18.5%.

Groin recurrence

Groin recurrence has a much poorer prognosis and is difficult to manage. In women who have not been treated previously with groin irradiation, radiotherapy (with or without additional surgery) would be the preferred option. The options are much more limited in those who have already been irradiated and palliative surgery may be considered.

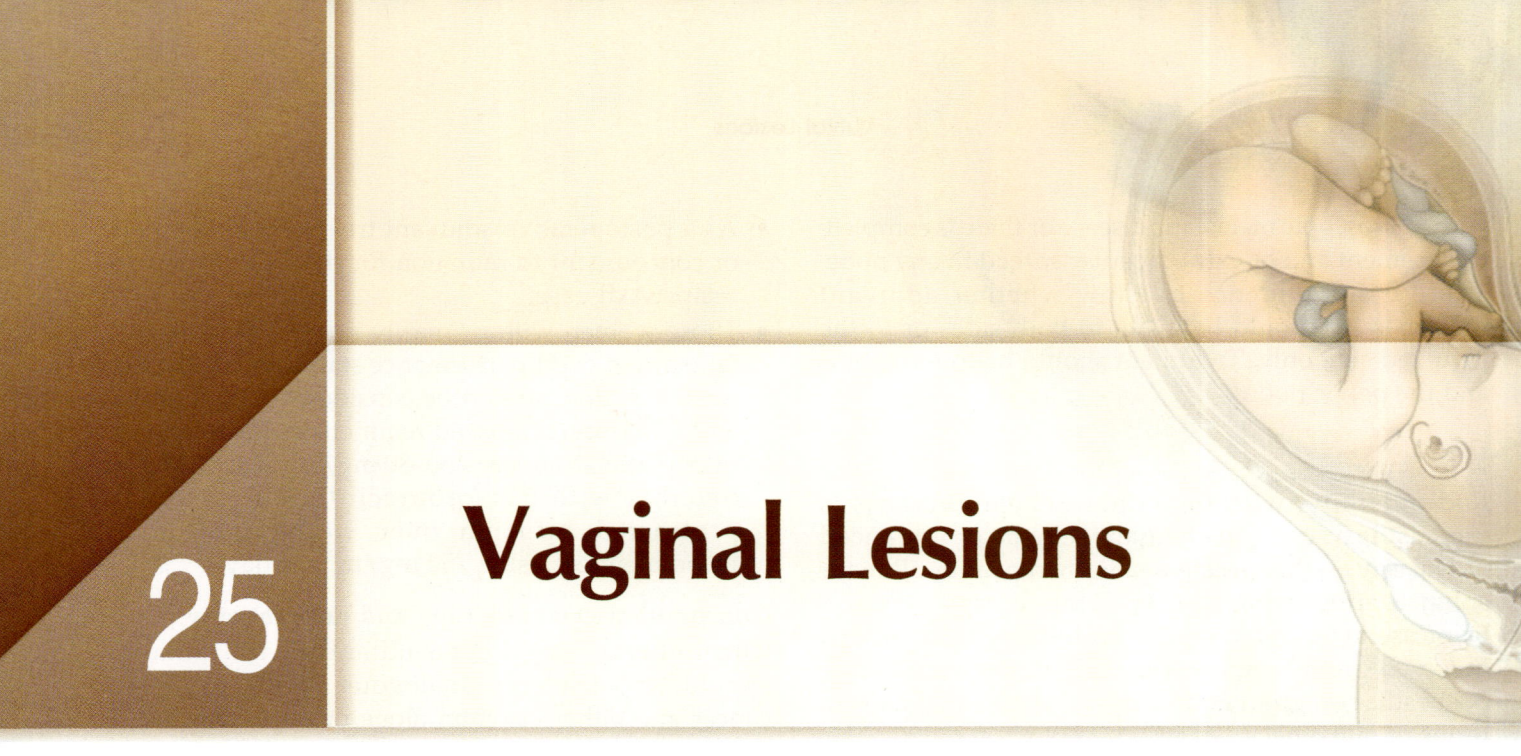

25 Vaginal Lesions

25A. VAGINAL INTRAEPITHELIAL NEOPLASIA (VAIN)

The term VAIN refers to changes that can occur in the skin of the vagina. VAIN is not cancer and in some women it disappears without treatment. However, if the changes become more severe, there is a chance that cancer may develop after many years, and so it is referred to as a precancerous condition.

VAIN can occur in just one area of the vagina, but it more often affects several different areas at once (multifocal). If only one area is affected, it is most often the upper third of the vagina.

Although cases of VAIN is rare, it is now recognised and diagnosed more often. It can affect women of any age, but is more common in women over 50. Occasionally, women may have abnormal changes that affect other areas in addition to the vagina, such as the cervix, vulva and anus.

Causes of VAIN

HPV

It is not fully understood what causes VAIN, but infection in the skin of the vagina caused by certain types of human papilloma virus (HPV), may be a factor. Types 16 and 18 are most commonly associated with VAIN.

HPV infection alone is unlikely to cause VAIN. Other factors that depress the body's immune system also need to be present for VAIN to occur. These include smoking, inherited immunity problems after transplant surgery, and some rare bone marrow and blood disorders.

Other Factors

- VAIN is more common in women following a hysterectomy for cervical cancer or severe precancerous changes (CIN).
- Women who have had previous precancerous or cancerous conditions in the vagina or cervix, or who have been treated with radiotherapy to the pelvis may have a slightly increased risk of developing VAIN.

Symptoms of VAIN

VAIN doesn't cause any symptoms. VAIN may be first detected by a cervical smear test or by a smear taken from the top of the vagina (vaginal vault smear test) following a hysterectomy or diagnosed following investigations for vaginal discharge.

Diagnosis of VAIN

VAIN cannot be detected by the naked eye. It is mainly diagnosed on colposcopy.

Colposcopy

The walls of the vagina are visualized through colposcope and inspected with acetic acid and Lugol's iodine stain. The cervix, vulva and skin around anus are also examined.

During the colposcopy, biopsy is taken from suspicious sites for examination under a microscope under local anesthesia. A cervical smear test, or liquid-based cytology test, may be done at the same time to check for any changes in the cells of the cervix.

The Grades of VAIN

VAIN is divided into grades. They describe how deeply the abnormal cells are embedded in the surface layer of the vagina:

- **VAIN 1 (low-grade VAIN):** One-third of the thickness of the surface layer of the vagina is affected.
- **VAIN 2 (high-grade VAIN):** Two-thirds of the thickness of the surface layer of the vagina is affected.
- **VAIN 3 (high-grade VAIN):** The full thickness of the surface layer of the vagina is affected.

Although VAIN 3 (Fig. 25.1) is also known as **carcinoma in situ**, it is not cancer of the vagina. With all three grades of VAIN, only a small area of the vagina may be affected by abnormal changes or there may be several areas of the vagina affected by a mixture of grades of VAIN.

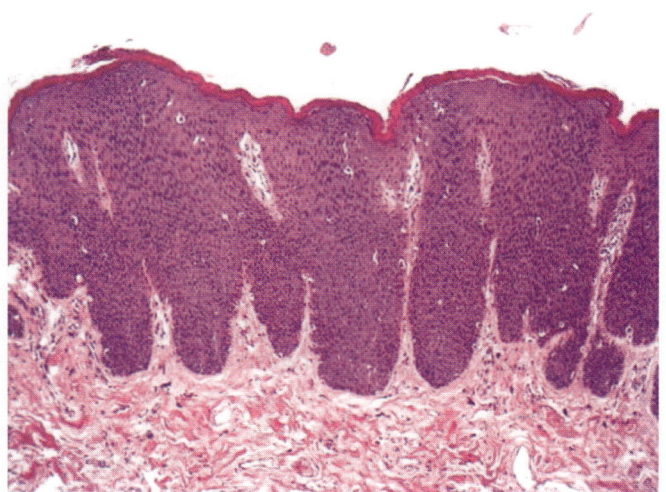

Fig. 25.1: VAIN 3

Treatment of VAIN

VAIN is not cancer, but it can be considered premalignant. If the cell changes are mild (VAIN 1), treatment may not be needed as this will often return to normal. If changes are more severe (VAIN 2 or VAIN 3), treatment is essential.

The type of treatment that is most appropriate will depend on a number of factors, including:

- The cellular abnormality
- The size of the affected area
- The location of the abnormal cells in the vagina
- Any previous treatment

Types of Treatment

Local Ablation (Conservative Treatment)

Local ablation treats VAIN by removing or destroying the abnormal cells in the vagina. This can be done in two ways:

a. *Carbon dioxide (CO_2) laser treatment.* This is the most common method of local ablation. A very fine beam of laser is directed at the abnormal cells through colposcope to destroy the lesion under general anesthesia.

b. *Diathermy treatment.* This is used to remove the abnormal cells under local anesthesia. A thin wire uses an electric current to destroy the affected area.

After laser or diathermy treatment, it is usual to have slight bleeding or discharge for a few days as the vaginal tissue take some time to heal after treatment.

Surgery

Surgery may be recommended when the lesion is suspicious of malignancy or has recurrence after previous treatment.

Wide local excision is appropriate when lesion is small but if it is more widespread, surgery should be partial or total vaginectomy. A new vagina may be created by grafting, using tissue from other parts of the body.

Radiotherapy

Radiotherapy can be effective in treating recurrence of VAIN or the lesion is widespread.

VAIN may be treated with internal radiotherapy (brachytherapy) when an applicator containing a radioactive substance is placed in the vagina for several hours or a few days.

Chemotherapy Cream

Sometimes chemotherapy cream called 5-fluorouracil is used. It can cause irritation to the vaginal skin so it is not used often.

25B. CANCER VAGINA

Malignant diseases of the vagina are either primary vaginal cancers or metastatic cancers from adjacent or distant organs. Primary vaginal cancers are defined as arising solely from the vagina, with no involvement of the external cervical os proximally or the vulva distally.

According to the International Federation of Gynecology and Obstetrics (FIGO), a vaginal lesion involving the external os of the cervix should be considered cervical cancer and treated as such; a tumor involving both the vulva and the vagina should be considered vulvar cancer.

About 80% of vaginal cancers are metastatic, primarily from the cervix or endometrium. Metastatic cancer from the vulva, ovaries, choriocarcinoma, rectosigmoid, and bladder are less common. These cancers usually invade the vagina directly. Cancers from distant sites that metastasize to the vagina through the blood or lymphatic system also occur, including colon cancer, renal cell carcinoma, melanoma, and breast cancer.

Incidence

Primary vaginal carcinoma is rare, constituting only 1–2% of all malignant gynecologic tumors. It ranks fifth in frequency behind cancer of the uterus, cervix, ovary, and vulva. The age-adjusted incidence in the United States is 0.6 per 100,000 population. The strict criteria used in defining vaginal carcinoma contribute to this low incidence.

Vaginal Structure

The vagina itself is a muscular tube lined by squamous epithelium that extends from the cervix to the hymenal ring, penetrating the levator ani and the urogenital diaphragm. These latter structures provide vaginal support inferiorly. From the outermost to the innermost layers, the vagina is composed of an endopelvic fascia—which contains an abundant plexus of vessels, lymphatics, and nerves—as well as outer longitudinal and inner circular smooth muscle layers, submucosa, and mucosa.

Levator ani

The levator ani forms the major support of the pelvic structures and is the major component of the pelvic diaphragm. It is penetrated anteriorly by the rectum, vagina, and urethra. It forms the floor of all the planes.

Vaginal Blood Supply

The upper part of the vagina receives its blood supply from the uterine and the internal pudendal arteries, from which the vaginal artery arises. The inferior rectal artery and other branches arising from the internal pudendal artery supply the lower vagina. The vaginal venous plexus mainly drains into the pelvic wall through the parametrial veins, and to a lesser degree to the vesical and rectal plexuses.

Vaginal Lymphatic System

Crossover of the vaginal lymphatic system is extensive. The middle to upper vagina communicates superiorly with the cervical lymphatics and drains into the pelvic obturator node, the internal and external iliac chains, and then the para-aortic nodes. The distal third of the vagina drains to the inguinal and then the pelvic nodes. The posterior wall lymphatics communicate with the rectal lymphatics and drain to the inferior gluteal, sacral, and rectal nodes.

Types of Vaginal Cancer

The etiology of vaginal cancer has not been identified. Note that vaginal cancer is not histologically homogeneous; several types of lesions exist, each with its own characteristics, age predilection, aggressiveness, and prognosis (Table 25.1). This suggests that a single etiologic factor is unlikely. Although some histologic types of vaginal cancer have been associated with exposure to certain agents, so far no clear cause-and-effect relationship has been found between any of those agents and vaginal carcinoma.

Risk Factors

HPV and other Infectious Agents

The identification of HPV deoxyribonucleic acid (DNA) in squamous cell cancer cells by in situ hybridization (21%) and southern blot hybridization (56%) strongly suggests a possible role for developing cancerous change in vagina.

HPV subtypes 16 and 18 have the highest oncogenic potential and are most commonly linked to dysplastic changes in the female genital tract. Because HPV is sexually transmitted, this association raises the question as to whether women who engage in high-risk sexual behaviors, such as sex with multiple partners, are at risk for developing vaginal cancer.

Table 25.1: Common forms of primary carcinoma of the vagina

	Cases of vaginal carcinoma	Peak age	Spread	Characteristics
Squamous cell carcinoma	85–87%	60 yrs	Local, blood, lymphatic	Most common in upper third of vagina
Verrucous carcinoma	Rare	60 yrs	Local	Variant of squamous cell, cauliflower-like, aggressive, radiotherapy contraindicated
Clear cell adenocarcinoma	9%	19 yrs	Local, blood, lymphatic	Associated with in utero exposure to diethylstilbestrol (DES), tubulocystic pattern most favorable prognosis, late recurrence common
Melanoma	0.5–2%	60 yrs	Local, blood, lymphatic	White women, lower anterior vaginal wall, size more prognostically significant than invasion, poor prognosis
Sarcoma botryoides (embryonal rhabdomyosarcoma)	Rare	3 yrs	Local, blood, lymphatic	Most common vaginal cancer among children, grape-like mass, strap cells
Endodermal sinus	Very rare	10 months	Local	Aggressive, alpha-fetoprotein (AFP) as marker tumor (yolk sac tumor)
Leiomyosarcoma	<2%	Wide	Local, blood, lymphatic	Grade is most important prognostic factor, can be secondary to pelvic irradiation range

Another association that strengthens the link between HPV infection and vaginal cancer is the presence of a premalignant lesion in the vagina, known as vaginal intraepithelial neoplasia (VAIN). VAIN may be a precursor to vaginal cancer even though the incidence of VAIN is 0.2–0.3 per 100,000 women, which is less than the incidence of diagnosed vaginal cancer. This is because of the fact that women with VAIN are usually asymptomatic and that screening for VAIN is not recommended for the general population. Still, the true malignant potential of VAIN needs to be clarified.

Other infectious agents that appear to be associated with vaginal cancer are herpes simplex virus (HSV) and *Trichomonas vaginalis*. Young women infected with both HIV and HPV are at increased risk for a more aggressive and less responsive vaginal cancer.

Epidemiology

A history of cervical intraepithelial neoplasia (CIN), invasive cervical carcinoma, or invasive vulvar carcinoma has also been associated with vaginal carcinoma. Several studies indicate that up to 30% of patients with primary vaginal carcinoma have a history of in situ or invasive carcinoma at other sites that was treated at least 5 years before diagnosis.

Diethylstilbestrol

Diethylstilbestrol (DES), a drug previously used in the first trimester to prevent pregnancy loss, has a strong association with clear cell adenocarcinoma of the vagina.

Age

In younger women, the disease occurred in the upper part of the vagina and seem to be related to cervical dysplasia and HPV infection, while in older patients, the tumors are exophytic. There is significant correlation with late menarche, suggesting hormonal factors and trauma to the vagina as probable etiologies.

Additional Factors

Long-term pessary use and chronic irritation of vaginal mucosa in women with procidentia have been associated with vaginal cancer. Other predisposing factors include cigarette smoking, immunosuppressive therapy, chemotherapy, and radiation therapy. Approximately 10% of women diagnosed with primary vaginal carcinoma have a previous history of irradiation to the pelvis.

The presence of different stages of histologic differentiation in vaginal cancer—VAIN, carcinoma in situ, possible microinvasive carcinoma, and invasive cancer—suggests a continuum of transformation from less malignant to more invasive one.

HPV and History of Carcinoma

The significant association of vaginal cancer with a history of cervical or vulvar cancer suggests that the entire genital tract is at risk for squamous cell carcinoma once malignancy has occurred anywhere along the tract; this is a phenomenon known as the "field effect."

HPV infection, which is associated with the pathogenesis of squamous cell vaginal carcinoma, can explain this phenomenon, because HPV is associated with cervical, vaginal, and vulvar disease.

Metastasis

The proximity of the bladder anteriorly and the rectum posteriorly to the vagina predisposes these organs to direct invasion by the tumor. Lymphatic dissemination follows the lymphatic drainage of the vagina. The middle-to-upper vagina communicates superiorly with the lymphatics of the cervix and drains into the pelvic obturator node, the internal and external iliac chains, and then to the para-aortic nodes.

The distal third of vagina drains to the inguinal node and then the pelvic node. Posterior wall lymphatics communicate with rectal lymphatics and drain to the inferior gluteal, sacral, and rectal nodes. Hematogenous dissemination to distant sites includes the lungs, liver, bone, and skin. A submucosal lesion suggests that the malignancy is metastatic via the vaginal lymphatics.

Routine Screening

Routine screening for vaginal carcinoma is not justified for all patients, because it is not cost-effective. Women at risk, however, particularly those with a history of cervical neoplasia and risky sexual behavior, should receive a Papanicolaou test on a regular basis.

Screening after Hysterectomy

Screening women with previous hysterectomy is controversial.

The American College of Obstetricians and Gynecologists recommends discontinuing screening in women who have undergone hysterectomy for benign diseases who have no prior history of high-grade cervical dysplasia. Women with a history of CIN 2 or CIN 3 are at increased risk of developing recurrent dysplasia or carcinoma of the vaginal cuff; therefore, in these women and in those in whom a negative history of high-grade dysplasia could not be verified, screening after hysterectomy should continue

Screening in Women Exposed to DES

Young girls who were exposed to DES in utero should be routinely examined starting at puberty or at the age of 14 years. Examination includes cytologic screening of the cervix and vagina, followed by careful inspection

and palpation of the genital tract. Staining with half-strength Lugol iodine helps to mark areas of adenosis. As long as cytologic findings are negative, colposcopy is unnecessary.

History

The duration of symptoms in vaginal cancer averages 6–12 months before diagnosis, with a range of 0–11 years. Delay in the diagnosis of vaginal carcinoma is not uncommon; this is partially due to the rarity of the disease, as well as with delays in relating patient symptoms to a vaginal origin. As expected, the longer the delay, the more advanced the cancer once the diagnosis is made, resulting in a poorer outcome.

Painless vaginal bleeding is the most common symptom, accounting for 65–80% of all presentations. Bleeding is postmenopausal in about 70% of patients, which is consistent with the peak age of 60 years for squamous cell carcinoma, the most common type. Menorrhagia, intermenstrual bleeding, and postcoital bleeding have also been reported.

Vaginal discharge occurs in 30% of patients, while 20% of patients report urinary symptoms, which are caused by an anterior lesion compressing or invading the bladder, the urethra, or both. This causes bladder pain, dysuria, urgency, and hematuria.

About 15–30% of patients present with pelvic pain. Posterior lesions compress or invade the rectosigmoid, which causes tenesmus or constipation.

About 10–27% of patients are asymptomatic; diagnosis is made during routine pelvic examination. These patients tend to be caught at a much earlier stage than those presenting with symptoms, and their prognosis is much better.

Local Examination

During routine vaginal examination, the speculum blades should be rotated laterally in order to visualize the anterior and posterior vaginal walls. Inspect all vaginal mucosa while withdrawing the speculum. Vaginal cancer is multifocal and, although it is typically located in the vaginal apex, the disease may involve any part of the vagina. Visual inspection alone is not enough, and careful circumferential palpation of the entire vagina is required in order to feel any raised or hardened areas.

Vaginal lesions, particularly when small and located in the lower third of the vagina, are often missed during the first vaginal inspection because the blades of the speculum normally cover the anterior and posterior vaginal walls. This can lead to diagnostic delays.

Other reasons for delay are the rarity of vaginal carcinoma (1–2%) and the similarity of patient symptoms to more common diseases, such as postmenopausal bleeding and endometrial cancer.

Patients with carcinoma in situ or very early invasive carcinoma are usually asymptomatic. Diagnosis is made when a routine Papanicolaou smear identifies abnormal cells. If the cervix is present, then the physician must rule out cervical neoplasia, because cervical cancer is much more common than vaginal cancer.

After a cervical origin has been ruled out through colposcopy, then the physician should perform a vaginal colposcopy. Because this is a time-consuming and difficult procedure, especially in elderly patients, it should be done under general anesthesia. Lugol iodine solution can help to identify regions to obtain biopsies from; malignant cells lack glycogen and so, unlike healthy vaginal mucosa, they do not stain dark brown.

Because healthy vaginal epithelium needs to be estrogenized in order to have sufficient glycogen, use of local estrogen cream for 1–2 weeks before examination may be helpful for postmenopausal patients. Estrogen cream should be discontinued 2 days prior to colposcopy.

Patients with previous hysterectomy and abnormal cytologic findings should also undergo vaginal colposcopy. If no lesion is observed and the abnormal cytology persists, then resecting the vaginal cuff may be considered because the lesion may be buried in the closed vaginal cuff at the time of hysterectomy.

Vaginal Biopsy

All visible lesions should be biopsied using Kevorkian punch biopsy forceps or similar instruments. In elderly patients, particularly those with some degree of vaginal stenosis, the procedure should be performed under general anesthesia to allow adequate biopsy.

Primary vaginal carcinoma is not homogeneous. It is classified into several histologic types, each with its own characteristics.

The following are brief descriptions of the most common types:

Squamous Cell Carcinoma

Squamous cell carcinoma is by far the most common type, accounting for 85–87% of all cases of primary vaginal carcinoma. It generally occurs in women older than 50 years and peak incidence is in people aged 60 years; however, several cases have been reported in women as young as 18 years.

Grossly, it appears as an ulcerating lesion (50%), a fungating mass (30%), or an annular, constricting mass (20%). Secondary infections in an ulcerating tumor are common. Histologically, it resembles squamous cell carcinoma arising from the cervix, confusing the physician as to whether the lesion is cervical or vaginal in origin.

The most common site of occurrence is the upper third of the vagina. Because of the thin vaginal wall, squamous cell carcinoma tends to spread early by directly invading the bladder and rectal walls. It also metastasizes through the blood or lymphatics.

Verrucous Carcinoma

Verrucous carcinoma is rare in the vagina and is more commonly observed in the vulva. It is observed in women older than 50 years and is considered a variant of squamous cell carcinoma. Its clinical and pathologic characteristics are similar to their vulvar counterparts.

On visual examination, verrucous carcinoma has a large, warty, cauliflower-like appearance similar to that of condylomata acuminata, but the papillary fronds lack a central core of connective tissue.

Verrucous carcinoma is slow growing, locally aggressive, and rarely metastatic. Radiation is contraindicated because it has been implicated in potentiating this tumor to a more malignant phenotype.

Clear Cell Adenocarcinoma

This is the second most common type of primary vaginal carcinoma, accounting for about 9% of all cases. Unlike squamous cell carcinoma, clear cell adenocarcinoma manifests in patients at a very early age, usually after age of 14 years, with peak incidence in people aged 19 years. An association with intrauterine exposure to DES has been established. The estimated risk in the exposed population is about 1 in 1000.

Clear cell adenocarcinoma arises mainly from areas of vaginal adenosis but may also arise in wolffian rest elements, periurethral glands, and foci of endometriosis. In patients who have not been exposed to DES, ectopic cervical glands are a possible origin.

Grossly, vaginal adenosis appears as multiple cysts 0.5–4 cm in diameter or as a diffuse, erythematous, granular mucosal lesion. The cancerous lesion appears polypoid, papillary, flat, or ulcerated.

Microscopically, three histologic patterns are predominant—tubulocystic, solid, and papillary. The tubulocystic pattern has the most favorable outcome.

The tumor can spread by local invasion or by hematogenous or lymphatic dissemination. Upon presentation, 70% of cases are stage I disease, but recurrence is frequent and can occur as late as 20 years after initial therapy. Secondary tumors from the colon, endometrium, cervix, breast, or ovary should be considered.

Melanoma

Vaginal melanoma is rare, accounting for 0.5–2% of all primary vaginal cancers. Vaginal melanoma tends to occur in white women; it usually manifests in women older than 50 years, with peak incidence in women aged 60 years.

Melanoma is most commonly found in the lower anterior vaginal wall. Grossly, it appears as blue or black, soft, mucosal or submucosal nodules, but it may also be nonpigmented and is frequently ulcerated, mimicking squamous cell carcinoma. Histologically, it is similar to cutaneous melanoma, except that it is more invasive.

Melanoma is thought to arise from melanocytes, which are present in 3% of healthy vaginas. The source probably is an aberrant melanocyte migration or melanocyte metaplasia.

The Breslow and Clark systems are used as part of staging; however, because deep invasion is invariably present upon presentation, tumor size, rather than depth, is a more significant prognostic factor. Tumors tend to recur locally, and metastasis to the lungs is common.

Sarcoma Botryoides (Embryonal Rhabdomyosarcoma)

Although this tumor is rare, it is the most common vaginal cancer in children. It manifests in girls younger than 8 years, with peak incidence in girls aged 3 years. Sarcoma botryoides is highly malignant and very aggressive. Initially, it tends to invade locally; it then metastasizes to the inguinal, pelvic, retroperitoneal, and mediastinal lymph nodes, as well as to the lungs, pericardium, liver, kidney, and bones.

Grossly, sarcoma botryoides occurs in two structural forms—solid and multicystic grape-like (the term botryoides comes from the Greek word *botrys,* which means grapes.) It originates in the subepithelial layers and expands outward to fill the vaginal cavity. Histologically, it is characterized by a loose, myxomatous stroma with malignant pleomorphic cells and characteristic cross-striated rhabdomyoblasts (strap cells), staining positively for muscle markers. Patients most commonly present with abnormal vaginal bleeding; they occasionally present with a polypoid mass protruding from the introitus.

Endodermal Sinus Tumor (Yolk Sac Tumor)

This type of adenocarcinoma is very rare. It is classified as a germ cell tumor and most commonly occurs in the ovary. It manifests in patients at a very young age, usually girls younger than 2 years, and peak incidence is in babies aged 10 months. Characteristically, it secretes alpha-fetoprotein (AFP), which is frequently used as a marker of recurrence.

Vaginal Leiomyosarcoma

This tumor of smooth muscle origin is rare and accounts for fewer than 2% of all primary vaginal cancers. It occurs over a wide patient age range, from 25 to 86 years, and may follow radiation therapy to the genital tract.

Grossly, vaginal leiomyosarcoma manifests as a bulky submucosal lesion, mainly in the upper vagina. Histologically, it is similar to leiomyosarcoma of the uterus. The microscopic criteria to diagnose leiomyosarcoma of the vagina is moderate to marked atypia with 5 or more mitotic figures per 10 high-power fields (HPF). Histologic grade is the most important predictor of outcome

Staging

Once the diagnosis of cancer is established, staging should proceed to determine the best treatment.

For vaginal cancer, staging is clinical and based on findings during general examination, pelvic examination, cystoscopy (for anterior wall tumors), proctoscopy (for posterior wall tumors), and chest radiography. If the patient reports bone pain, then skeletal radiography should be performed to rule out bone involvement.

Imaging

Computed tomography (CT) scanning or magnetic resonance imaging (MRI) of the upper abdomen and pelvis are not FIGO recommendations, although they are frequently performed because they help in establishing the presence of enlarged lymph nodes, ureteral compression, hydronephrosis, and liver metastasis.

Antigen Testing

Baseline levels of carcinoembryonic antigen (CEA), cancer antigen-125 (CA-125), and squamous cell carcinoma antigen are recommended because they are elevated in patients with some carcinoma types.

Evaluation for Origin and Metastasis of Adenocarcinoma

Patients in whom adenocarcinoma is diagnosed should undergo thorough exploration for possible metastasis, mainly in the uterus, cervix, ovary, and colon. In these patients, a fractional dilatation and curettage is indicated to rule out endometrial origin. A barium enema with either sigmoidoscopy or colonoscopy is also indicated to rule out colonic origin. In addition, mammography, chest radiography, and CT scanning of the abdomen or pelvis should follow. CA-125 should be taken as baseline for post-treatment follow-up.

Surgical Staging

Surgical staging is not usually required, but it is performed in selected premenopausal patients prior to radiotherapy. In these patients, pretreatment laparotomy allows the transposition of at least 1 ovary away from the field of radiation. It also allows for better assessment of the extent of the disease through dissection of the pelvic lymph nodes. In addition, for patients scheduled for exenterative surgery, an exploratory laparotomy is required to rule out metastasis or lateral spread to the pelvic sidewall before proceeding with exenteration.

FIGO Classification

FIGO staging classification of vaginal carcinoma is as follows:

- Stage 0—Carcinoma is carcinoma in situ (VAIN)
- Stage I—Carcinoma is limited to the vaginal wall
- Stage II—Carcinoma involves subvaginal tissue but has not extended to the pelvic wall.
- Stage III—Carcinoma extends to the pelvic wall
- Stage IV—Carcinoma extends beyond the true pelvis or involves mucosa of bladder or rectum; bullous edema as such precludes inclusion in the stage IV classification
- Stage IVA—Carcinoma invades bladder or rectal mucosa or directly extends beyond the true pelvis.
- Stage IVB—Carcinoma spreads to distant organs
  Three types of standard treatment are used:

Surgery

Surgery is the most common treatment of vaginal cancer. The following surgical procedures may be used:

- *Laser surgery:* A surgical procedure that uses a laser beam (a narrow beam of intense light) as a knife to make bloodless cuts in tissue or to remove a surface lesion such as a tumor.

- *Wide local excision:* A surgical procedure that takes out the cancer and some of the healthy tissue around it.
- *Vaginectomy:* Surgery to remove all or part of the vagina.
- *Total hysterectomy:* Vaginal of abdominal hysterectomy can be often undertaken along with vaginectomy.
- *Lymphadenectomy:* If the cancer is in the upper vagina, the pelvic lymph nodes may be removed. If the cancer is in the lower vagina, lymph nodes in the groin may be removed.
- *Pelvic exenteration:* Extensive surgery to remove the lower colon, rectum, and bladder. Along with uterus, cervix, vagina, ovaries, and nearby lymph nodes are also removed. Skin grafting may follow surgery, to repair or reconstruct the vagina.

Radiation Therapy

As most of the vaginal cancers are squamous cell type, they are very radiosensitive. External radiation therapy uses a machine outside the body to send radiation toward the cancer. Internal radiation therapy uses a radioactive substance sealed in needles, seeds, wires, or catheters that are placed directly into or near the cancer. The way the radiation therapy is given depends on the type and stage of the cancer being treated.

Chemotherapy

Both systemic and local chemotherapy is used in vaginal cancers as adjunctive therapy either following primary surgery or during concurrent radiotherapy.

Radiosensitizers

Radiosensitizers are drugs that make tumor cells more sensitive to radiation therapy. Combining radiation therapy with radiosensitizers may kill more tumor cells.

Treatment Options by Stage

Stage 0 vaginal cancer (carcinoma in situ): Treatment of vaginal squamous cell carcinoma in situ may include the following:

- Wide local excision, with or without a skin graft.
- Partial or total vaginectomy, with or without a skin graft.
- Topical chemotherapy.
- Laser surgery.
- Internal radiation therapy.

Stage I vaginal cancer: Treatment of stage I squamous cell vaginal cancer may include the following:

- Internal radiation therapy, with or without external radiation therapy to lymph nodes or large tumors.
- Wide local excision or vaginectomy with vaginal reconstruction. Radiation therapy may be given after the surgery.
- Vaginectomy and lymphadenectomy, with or without vaginal reconstruction. Radiation therapy may be given after the surgery.

Treatment of stage I vaginal adenocarcinoma may include the following:

- Vaginectomy, hysterectomy, and lymphadenectomy. This may be followed by vaginal reconstruction and/or radiation therapy.
- Internal radiation therapy, with or without external radiation therapy to lymph nodes.
- A combination of therapies that may include wide local excision with or without lymphadenectomy and internal radiation therapy.

Stage II vaginal cancer: Treatment of stage II vaginal cancer is the same for squamous cell cancer and adenocarcinoma. Treatment may include the following:

- Both internal and external radiation therapy to the vagina, with or without external radiation therapy to lymph nodes.
- Vaginectomy or pelvic exenteration, with or without radiation therapy.

Stage III vaginal cancer: Treatment of stage III vaginal cancer is the same for squamous cell cancer and adenocarcinoma. Treatment may include both internal and external radiation therapy, with or without surgery.

Stage IVA vaginal cancer: Treatment of stage IVA vaginal cancer is the same for squamous cell cancer and adenocarcinoma. Treatment may include both internal and external radiation therapy, with or without exenteration surgery.

Stage IVB vaginal cancer: Treatment of stage IVB vaginal cancer is the same for squamous cell cancer and adenocarcinoma. Treatment may include the following:

- Radiation therapy as palliative therapy, to relieve symptoms and improve the quality of life. Chemotherapy may also be given.

Indications of Surgery

Consensus as to the proper treatment for vaginal carcinoma is lacking, mainly because of the rarity of the disease. The most commonly used treatment modality is radiotherapy. Surgery, with or without concomitant radiation therapy, is indicated in the following conditions:

- Squamous cell carcinoma—stage I disease in the upper posterior vagina; stage IVA disease, particularly in the presence of a rectovaginal or vesicovaginal fistula; central recurrence after radiotherapy; ovary transposition in young patients prior to radiotherapy.
- Clear cell adenocarcinoma—although the etiology is different, the presentation may be similar to that of squamous cell carcinoma.
- Verrucous carcinoma—radiation therapy is contraindicated because it has been implicated in potentiating this tumor to a more malignant phenotype; therefore, surgery is the only treatment.
- Other cases—melanoma, sarcoma, embryonal rhabdomyosarcoma, endodermal sinus tumor.

Contraindications

Metastasis and extension to pelvic sidewalls are contraindications for exenteration. Microscopic pelvic node involvement is more of a controversy than a contraindication, and patients with positive pelvic nodes and no other poor prognostic factors can be considered candidates for exenteration. Involvement of both the pelvic and para-aortic nodes should warrant aborting the surgery.

Squamous Cell Cancer

Stage I Disease

Stage I disease involving the upper posterior vagina is treated by radical hysterectomy, partial vaginectomy, and bilateral pelvic lymphadenectomy. Lymphadenectomy is required to ensure that metastatic disease is not present.

If the patient had a previous hysterectomy, then a radical upper vaginectomy with pelvic lymphadenectomy is performed after the paravesicular and pararectal spaces are developed to avoid injury to the bladder and rectum, respectively. Each ureter is also dissected out to its point of entry into the bladder.

If the lesion is multifocal or if it extends to the lower third of the vagina, inguinal lymphadenectomy should also be performed, and a total vaginectomy is required. If the depth of the invasion is questioned during the operation, then a frozen section from the margins should be taken to ensure that tumor resection was adequate.

In general, tumors of the upper posterior wall are more operable because the sigmoid reflects away from the posterior vaginal wall while the entire length of the anterior vaginal wall stays in close proximity to the bladder. A lower vaginal lesion can be treated with radical hemivulvectomy and lower vaginectomy with bilateral inguinal node dissection. Radiation therapy is commonly used as an alternative to surgery.

Stages II, III, and IV Disease

Stages II and III are treated with radiation therapy. In premenopausal patients, a pretreatment laparotomy is performed in order to transpose the ovaries away from the field of radiation and to resect any enlarged lymph nodes. If the patient has a central recurrence with no signs of metastasis after radiotherapy, then pelvic exenteration is the only option.

Patients with stage IVA disease have the option of radiation therapy or pelvic exenteration. The latter is highly recommended, if a rectovaginal or vesicovaginal fistula is present. Stage IVB is a contraindication for surgery.

Clear Cell Adenocarcinoma

Therapeutic considerations are very similar to those for patients with squamous cell carcinoma, although most patients are young, and every effort should be made to preserve functional ovaries and a functional vagina. Surgery is the primary treatment modality.

In stage I and early stage II disease, radical hysterectomy, pelvic lymphadenectomy, and vaginectomy with split-thickness skin graft have been successful.

If radiation is used as the sole treatment, then transposition of at least 1 ovary up into the paracolic gutter beyond the radiation field should be done with pelvic lymph node dissection. Local excision without radiation is not recommended, since 16% of patients with stage I disease have positive pelvic nodes. Pelvic exenteration is done for central recurrences after primary irradiation.

Melanoma

The best treatment for vaginal melanoma remains controversial. Radical surgery has been the main treatment modality, although a more conservative approach has been advocated.

Detection of Lymph Node Involvement

Recently, detection of nodal involvement prior to radical procedures has been suggested because positive lymph nodes indicate poor prognosis and radical surgery might be unjustified.

Technetium-99m (^{99m} Tc)-sulfur colloid is injected around the lesion to detect the sentinel lymph node with hot spot by lymphoscintigraphy. Otherwise, 1mL of methylene blue is injected into the subcutaneous layer at the boundary between the lesion and the vaginal mucosa, followed by incision in the ipsilateral groin to detect the stained lymph node.

Radical Surgery

Radical surgery varies depending on tumor size and location. Small lesions in the upper vagina are treated by radical hysterectomy, subtotal vaginectomy, and pelvic lymphadenectomy. Lesions in the lower vagina are managed by partial vaginectomy, total or partial vulvectomy, and bilateral inguinal lymphadenectomy. Larger and more invasive lesions (>3 mm) are treated with exenterative surgery.

Conservative Therapy

Conservative management includes wide local excision and simple hysterectomy combined with radiotherapy and/or chemotherapy. Radiation therapy with high-dose fractions (>400cGy/fx) has been effective in selected patients.

Treatment of other Nonsquamous Cancers

Verrucous Carcinoma

Radiation therapy is contraindicated in verrucous carcinoma because it tends to induce aggressive cancer types. The only treatment option is surgical resection. If the lesion is small, a wide surgical excision is performed. With larger lesions, vaginectomy or exenteration is recommended. Because this tumor rarely metastasizes, dissecting the lymph nodes is unnecessary unless they appear enlarged.

Sarcoma Botryoides

Because the typical patient is prepubertal, ovarian function and reproductive organs are preserved. Currently, a conservative approach is used instead of exenterative surgery. Preoperative and/or postoperative chemotherapy and radiotherapy improve the outcome.

For small, easily resectable tumors, the lesion is excised. Chemotherapy VAC (vincristine, actinomycin D, and cyclophosphamide) and radiotherapy follow. If the tumor is bulky, preoperative chemotherapy or radiotherapy is administered before the lesion is excised.

Endodermal Sinus Tumor

This very rare tumor is treated with chemotherapy VAC to reduce the tumor size. Chemotherapy is followed by partial colpectomy, radiotherapy, or both.

Vaginal Leiomyosarcoma

These tumors vary in their malignancy depending on how well they are differentiated. Well-differentiated tumors are less likely to metastasize and are managed by surgical excision. Frozen sections are taken to ensure that the tumor is well contained within the surgical margins. Poorly differentiated tumors should receive adjuvant radiotherapy.

Simple Vaginectomy

Simple vaginectomy is indicated when invasion is suspected in a patient with VAIN. The approach usually is vaginal. In postmenopausal women with poorly estrogenized vaginal mucosa, estrogen cream can be used 2–4 weeks prior to the operation. Lugol solution is used to delineate the abnormal mucosa. Injecting saline solution into the submucosa elevates the lesion from the underlying tissue layer and helps in the excision. Usually, a 3–5 mm margin of healthy mucosa is adequate. For lesions located in the upper vagina, sutures are placed in the apex to place traction and the upper vagina is excised. The bladder and rectal pillars (lymph vascular pillars) are transected from their vaginal attachments. Blunt dissection is used to further remove the specimen. The surgeon must keep in mind the proximity of the ureters to the corners of the apex. The vagina is closed with interrupted biodegradable sutures.

Radical Vaginectomy

When the uterus is in situ, radical vaginectomy can be approached vaginally or abdominally. If two thirds of the vagina needs to be removed, however, a combined approach is required to mobilize the distant vagina. In patients with previous hysterectomy, the abdominal approach or a combined approach is required because of a higher risk of injury to the ureters during resection of the cardinal ligaments and the proximal bladder pillars.

The vesicovaginal (anterior), rectovaginal (posterior), and 2 lateral paravaginal spaces are developed, and the bladder and rectal pillars are transected at their attachments to the bladder and rectum, respectively (as opposed to their vaginal attachments in simple vaginectomy). The ureters should be dissected away before resection of the vagina with the cardinal and vesicouterine ligaments. The specimen is resected in a manner similar to that used in simple vaginectomy.

Pelvic Exenteration

Pelvic exenteration is classified as follows:
- Total exenteration for apical lesions involving the bladder and rectum.
- Anterior exenteration for anterior lesions involving the bladder.
- Posterior exenteration for posterior lesions involving the rectum.

Vaginal Reconstruction

A neovagina can be constructed in several ways. The procedure depends on how much vaginal tissue is preserved after the exenteration as well as the size of the pelvic or perineal defect.

Split-thickness Graft

A split-thickness graft is usually used when an anterior or a supralevator exenteration has been performed, because these procedures leave a smaller defect. The mobilized omentum is used to create a pocket to receive the neovagina. A split-thickness skin graft is obtained from either the buttock or the anterior or medial thigh. The skin graft is sewn over a vaginal stent. The stent is inserted through the introitus into the omental pocket, which provides a blood supply to the graft.

Myocutaneous Flaps

Myocutaneous flaps are preferred whenever the defect is larger, such as after a total exenteration. The two most common flaps are the TRAM flap and the gracilis myocutaneous flap.

Postoperative Complications

- Hemorrhage should be dealt with promptly with percutaneous embolization because reexploration carries high mortality and morbidity rates. Intravascular fluid loss from wound oozing and third spacing is expected.
- Pelvic sepsis (10%) and wound sepsis and dehiscence (12%) are minimized by bowel preparation, but the risk is still present because of the radical nature of the surgery, the length of the operation, and the age of the patient.
- Pulmonary embolus occurs in 1.5% of patients despite prophylaxis. This is also due to the length of •the operation and prolonged bedrest after surgery.

Lower Rectal Anastomosis Complications

- Anastomotic leakage depends on the distance of the anastomosis from the anus, as well as on the vascularity and tension on the anastomotic site. Along with fistulae, it carries a very high mortality rate of approximately 50%.
- Rectovaginal fistulae and strictures are more common in patients with previous irradiation.
- Small bowel obstruction occurs in 4–9% of patients.
- Fistulae (12–32%) are more common with ileoileal anastomosis and previous irradiation. With the use of a transverse colon conduit for urinary diversion, this complication now is uncommon.
- Complications from vaginal reconstruction include necrosis of the graft and stenosis of the neovagina.

In general, the operative mortality rate in exenteration is less than 5%, and the 5-year survival rate is about 40%. Improved hemodynamic monitoring, nutritional support, and advances in surgical techniques and instruments have contributed to the decrease in intraoperative mortality and morbidity. Anterior exenteration has a better survival rate than total exenteration (30–60% versus 20–46%, respectively).

Clinical Factors that Affect Survival

These include the following:
- Length of time from initial radiation therapy to exenteration—less than 1 year is a poor prognostic sign.
- Size of the central mass (>3 cm).

Pathologic factors that Affect Survival

- Tumor extension—most important risk factor for reduced survival is the extension of the tumor laterally into the surgical margins.
- Positive nodes—5-year survival rate of 70% for negative nodes versus 0% for positive nodes.
- Spread of tumor to adjacent organs.

Special Topics

Hirsutism is one of the most common endocrine disorders, affecting approximately 7% of women. Hirsutism is defined as excess terminal hair that commonly appears in a male pattern in women. It is generally associated with hyperandrogenemia. Hirsutism should be distinguished from hypertrichosis, which is generalized excessive hair growth not caused by androgen excess. Hypertrichosis may be congenital or caused by metabolic disorders such as thyroid dysfunction, anorexia nervosa and porphyria.

Physiology of Hair Growth (Fig. 26.1)

- *The cuticle:* Outermost layer consisting of scale-like overlapping cells, 5 to 12 layers deep. It is formed from dead cells and gives the hair shaft strength and provides protection for the softer inner structures.

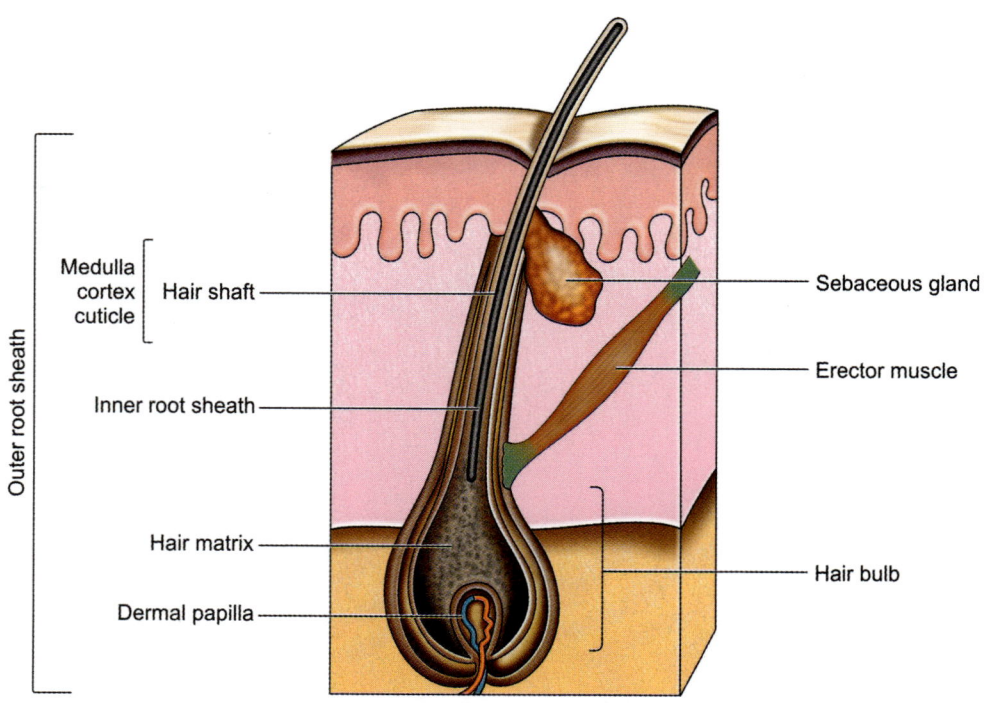

Fig. 26.1: Hair growth cycles

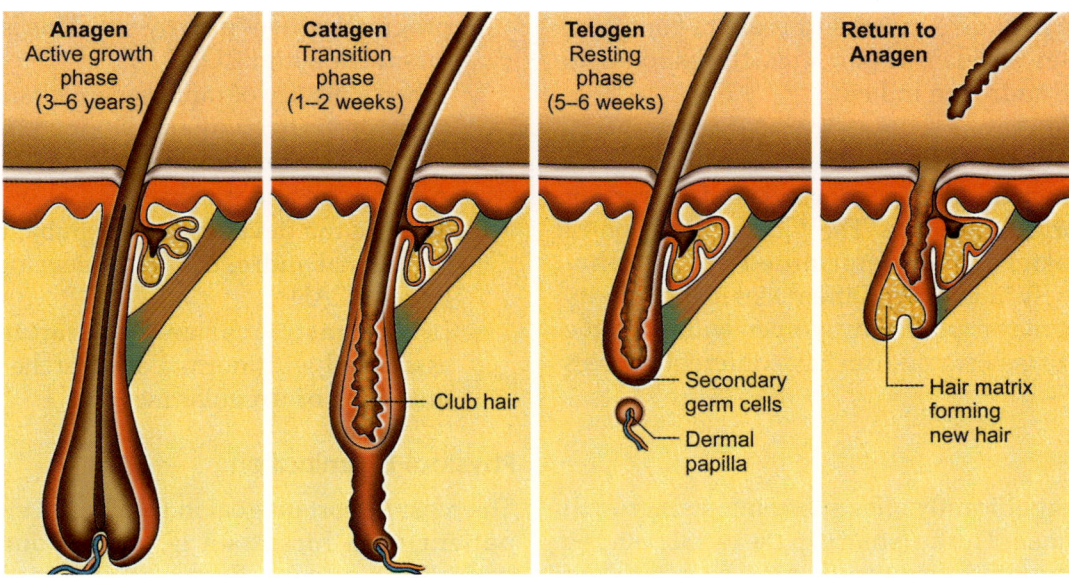

Fig. 26.2: Growth cycle of hair

- *The cortex:* The fibrous middle layer of hair, consisting of keratin-filled, elongated cells that are cemented together with lipid rich, flexible keratin. This gives the cortex the properties of elasticity and a high tensile strength. The cortex contains the pigment melanin that gives hair its color.
- *The medulla:* The inner most layer of the hair structure, consisting of sparse cells and air bubbles. Its role in humans is unknown, however, in animals it helps to control body temperature.

There are three stages to the growth cycle of hair. The entire cycle can be as short as 1 year to as long as 7 years, with the average growth cycle being 4 years. Many factors can interrupt the cycle and induce hair into the telogen stage (hair shedding). It is understood that the protein FGF-5 triggers the hair to change from anagen to catagen and then to shed (Fig. 26.2).

The anagen phase: Lasts 1–7 years. The active growing phase.
- 80–90% of hair is in the anagen phase.
- Hair growth is approximtely 1.25 cm a month.
- The hair bulb produces the hair colour pigment, melanin in the growth cycle.
- The blood supply provides nutrients and minerals to the hair.

The catagen phase: Lasts 1–3 weeks. The transition phase.
- The hair detaches from the blood supply.
- The detached follicle will slowly shrink to about 1/6th of its size.
- The hair bulb stops producing the color pigment.

- The bulb will be pushed upwards towards the surface when the new hair is formed.
- Approximately 2–3% of the hair is in this phase.

The telogen phase: Lasts up to 3 months. The resting phase.
- 10–15% of hair is in telogen phase.
- Up to 100 hairs a day can be shed in a normal telogen phase.

Pathophysiology of Hirsutism

Hormones and the intrinsic characteristics of the hair follicle determine the quality of hair growth. **Vellus** hairs are fine, lightly pigmented hairs that cover most of the body before puberty. Pubertal androgens promote the conversion of these vellus hairs to coarser, pigmented **terminal** hairs. The level and duration of exposure to androgens, the local 5-alpha-reductase activity, and the intrinsic sensitivity of the hair follicle to androgen action determine the extent of conversion from vellus to terminal hair. However, some terminal hair growth is androgen-independent (e.g. scalp, eyebrows, eyelashes).

The development of terminal hair or reversion back to a vellus pattern may not be immediately evident because of the characteristics of the hair cycle. This cycle has 2 phases that include active hair growth (anagen phase) and a resting period (telogen phase), which follows the anagen phase. During the resting period, the hair shaft separates from the dermal papillae at the follicle base, and no further growth takes place. Eventually, growth restarts and the new hair shaft formed by the reactivated papillae pushes the old hair out. The cycle may take months to years to complete, and this causes a delay in hair growth response to changes in the androgen milieu.

Dihydrotestosterone is the androgen that acts on the hair follicle to produce terminal hair. This hormone is derived from both the bloodstream and local conversion of a precursor, testosterone. The local production of dihydrotestosterone is determined by 5-alpha-reductase activity in the skin. Differences in the activity of this enzyme may explain why women with the same plasma levels of testosterone can have different degrees of hirsutism.

Race

Ethnic origin significantly affects terminal hair growth in healthy women. The difference in the racial patterns of normal terminal hair growth may be related to genetic differences of 5-alpha-reductase activity in the skin.

Age

The age of onset of hirsutism depends on the etiology. Most forms of non-neoplastic hirsutism become evident around puberty. This includes polycystic ovary syndrome (PCOS), CAH, and idiopathic hirsutism.

Hirsutism may also develop after weight gain and cessation of the use of oral contraceptives in young women. Normally, terminal hair growth becomes apparent after adrenarche and accelerates after puberty. Terminal hair continues to develop gradually in healthy women until after menopause, when loss of ovarian androgen leads to a loss of hair. Rapidly worsening hirsutism, especially in older women, should raise the suspicion of an androgen-secreting tumor.

History

An accurate history of the patient's onset of hirsutism and developmental milestones can be helpful in the etiologic diagnosis.

- Age of onset
- Idiopathic hirsutism usually begin at puberty.
- Conversely, hirsutism that occurs in middle-aged or older women should suggest an adrenal or ovarian tumor.
- Family history: A patient with a family history of hirsutism is consistent with congenital adrenal hyperplasia (CAH); however, idiopathic hirsutism and polycystic ovary syndrome can also be familial.
  - Hirsutism severity and rate of progression:
  - The history of a benign form of hirsutism is usually characterized by pubertal onset with slow

progression over many years. This is often true of hirsutism with PCOS.
- When a history of rapid severe hirsutism or other signs of virilization are obtained, an androgen-secreting tumor is a possibility.
- Adrenarche and puberty
- Because the development of pubic hair depends on adrenal androgens, early development points toward CAH.
- In contrast, ovarian hyperandrogenism is associated with normal adrenarche and delayed menarche or irregular menses.

Physical Examination

The most important goal in the clinical evaluation of a patient with hirsutism is to rule out significant underlying disease. Excess androgens can be from either an exogenous or an endogenous source.

- An exogenous source of androgens can usually be elicited by history findings as sometimes reported in female athletes.
- Endogenous androgens originate from either the adrenal cortex or the ovary. Therefore, the evaluation of androgen excess can focus on disorders of these 2 glands. The principal possibilities are tumors of the ovary or the adrenal cortex, Cushing syndrome, CAH, and PCOS. Idiopathic hirsutism is the most common etiology, but it is a diagnosis of exclusion.
- The initial task in the evaluation of hirsutism via the physical examination is to quantitate the disorder. This task requires that terminal hair, which depends on androgen, be differentiated from vellus hair, which is androgen-independent.
  - Vellus hair is fine, soft, and lightly pigmented. An excess of vellus hair (hypertrichosis) is usually idiopathic, but may be associated with metabolic disorders (e.g. hyperthyroidism, anorexia nervosa, porphyria) and with some medications (e.g. phenytoin, diazoxide, minoxidil, glucocorticoids, cyclosporine, hexachlorobenzene).
  - By contrast, terminal hair is coarse, curly, and pigmented. Because small amounts of terminal hair are normal in women, quantification is important.
- The most widely accepted method of quantification uses the Ferriman and Gallwey scale (Fig. 26.3). In this approach, hair growth is judged in each of 11 androgen-sensitive areas.
  - The grade for each area ranges from 0 (no terminal hair) to 4 (frankly virile).
  - The body areas used to grade hirsutism are: (1) the upper lip, (2) chin, (3) chest, (4) leg, (5) thigh,

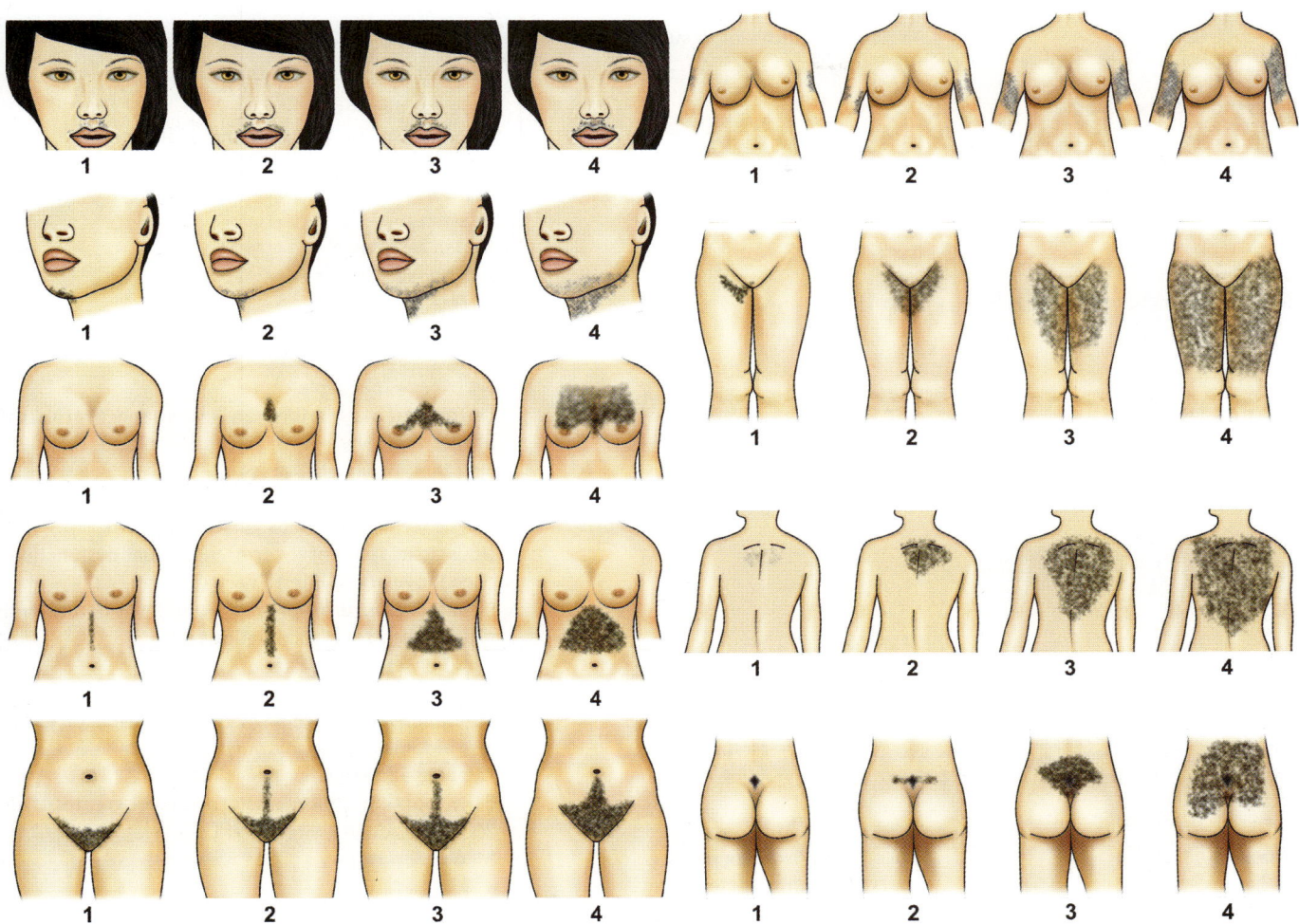

Fig. 26.3: The Ferriman-Gallwey scale for hirsutism. A score of 1 to 4 is given for nine areas of the body. A total score less than 8 is considered normal, a score of 8 to 15 indicates mild hirsutism, and a score greater than 15 indicates moderate or severe hirsutism. A score of 0 indicates absence of terminal hair

(6) upper arm, (7) forearm, (8) upper back, (9) lower back, (10), upper abdomen, and (11) lower abdomen.

– Areas such as the axilla and pubis are not included because terminal hair grows in these places at normal androgen levels in women.

- The total score correlates roughly with the elevation of androgen levels. A woman with a score of 8 or higher is considered to have hirsutism. Most women who seek medical attention for the disorder have scores of 15 or higher.

- In women with moderate-to-severe hirsutism (score >15), additional signs of hyperandrogenism, are looked for which includes (1) temporal hair recession, (2) oily skin, (3) masculine voice, (4) well-developed musculature, (5) enlargement of the clitoris (>35 m^2 in surface area), (6) irregular menses, and (7) psychological changes (e.g. heightened libido, aggressiveness).

- A thorough abdominal and pelvic examination is important in patients with hirsutism because more than half of androgen-secreting adrenal and ovarian tumors are palpable.

- Women with hirsutism are usually obese, with increased waist-hip ratios, and are thought to be at an increased risk for atherosclerosis and coronary heart disease. The presence of acanthosis nigricans shows evidence of insulin resistance.

Causes (Table 26.1)

Multiple diseases can cause hyperandrogenism and hirsutism. The etiologic forms of hirsutism include endocrine-related, idiopathic, medication-related, and miscellaneous. Endocrine-related causes include adrenocortical disorders and ovarian disorders.

Adrenal tumors, Cushing syndrome, and CAH are the adrenocortical causes. Ovarian tumors (malignant or benign) and PCOS are the ovarian causes of hirsutism.

Table 26.1: Causes of hirsutism and their diagnostic clues

Diagnosis	Percentage of hirsutism cases	Distinguishing historical and clinical clues
Polycystic ovary syndrome	72 to 82	Irregular menses Normal to mildly elevated androgen levels Polycystic ovaries on ultrasonography Central obesity Infertility Insulin resistance Acanthosis nigricans
Idiopathic hyperandrogenemia	6 to 15	Normal menses Normal ovaries on ultrasonography Elevated androgen levels No other explainable cause
Idiopathic hirsutism	4 to 7	Normal menses, androgen levels, and ovaries on ultrasonography No other explainable cause
Adrenal hyperplasia	2 to 4	Family history of congenital adrenal hyperplasia Classic form: ambiguous genitalia at birth Nonclassic, late-onset form: menstrual dysfunction, oligoanovulation, infertility Elevated 17-hydroxyprogesterone level before and after corticotropin stimulation test
Androgen-secreting tumors	0.2	Rapid onset of hirsutism Progression of hirsutism despite treatment Virilization (e.g. clitoromegaly, increased muscle mass, loss of female body contour) Palpable abdominal or pelvic mass Early morning total testosterone level greater than 200 ng per dL (6.94 nmol per L)
Iatrogenic hirsutism	Uncommon (exact percentage not well-defined in the literature)	Medication history
Acromegaly	Rare to present with isolated hirsutism	Frontal bossing, increased hand and foot size, mandibular enlargement, coarse facial features, hyperhidrosis, deepened voice
Cushing syndrome	Rare to present with isolated hirsutism	Central obesity, moon facies, purple skin striae, proximal muscle weakness, acne Hypertension, impaired glucose tolerance Elevated 24-hour urine free cortisol level
Hyperprolactinemia	Rare to present with isolated hirsutism	Galactorrhea, amenorrhea, infertility Elevated prolactin level
Thyroid dysfunction	Rare to present with isolated hirsutism	Hypothyroidism: Fatigue, cold intolerance, dry skin, hair loss, myxedema, weight gain, difficulty concentrating, irregular menses Hyperthyroidism: Hyperactivity, heat intolerance, moist skin, palpitations, oligomenorrhea, goiter, exophthalmos Abnormal thyroid function tests

Adrenal Tumors

Adrenocortical tumors are almost always malignant in patients who present with hirsutism. These tumors are usually large and are associated with a very poor prognosis.

Cushing Syndrome

In most instances, Cushing syndrome is caused by glucocorticoid therapy. Because pure glucocorticoids have no androgenic activity, the treatment rarely produces hirsutism. Instead, glucocorticoid therapy is one of the causes of hypertrichosis, resulting in vellus hair growth, especially on the face. Thus, excess growth of terminal hair in a patient with the clinical stigmata of Cushing syndrome suggests that the syndrome has an endogenous origin, i.e. a pituitary tumor that secretes adrenocorticotropin hormone (ACTH), an

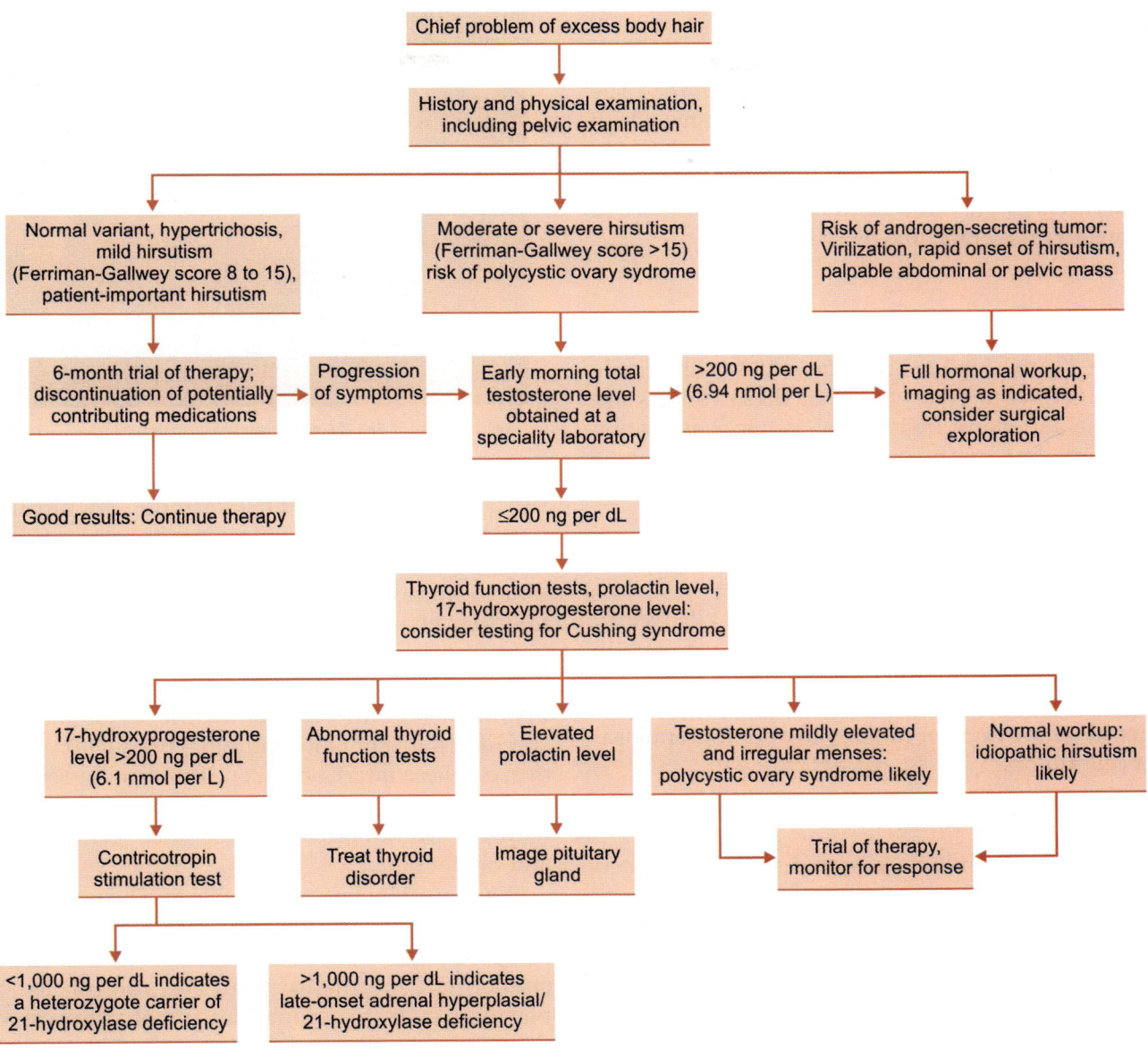

Fig. 26.4: Algorithm of management plan for hirsutism

adrenal tumor that secretes both cortisol and androgens, or an ectopic tumor that secretes ACTH. The pituitary tumor is the most likely possibility. Cushing syndrome, as a cause of hirsutism, is diagnosed based on the presence of dexamethasone suppression test that fails to suppress both androgens and cortisol.

CAH

CAH is actually a family of defects in 1 of 5 enzymes that are responsible for the biosynthesis of cortisol. The resulting cortisol deficiency heightens the secretion of ACTH and thereby leads to adrenal cell proliferation. However, only 3 of these defects can produce hirsutism—21-hydroxylase (most frequent), 3β-hydroxysteroid dehydrogenase (less frequent), and 11-β-hydroxylase deficiency (least frequent).

If CAH is considered, an ACTH-stimulation test is indicated, which search for causes of exaggerated quantities of the precursors of cortisol. The stimulation test is required because baseline elevation of these steroids may be in the reference range.

Hyperandrogenism in CAH can cause infertility, but dexamethasone therapy in this setting may induce ovulation. Two important reasons for the diagnosis of CAH are that specific therapy is available and genetic counseling may be necessary.

Ovarian Tumors

Ovarian tumors may be malignant though androgen-secreting ovarian tumors are a less serious threat. The most common among them is arrhenoblastoma, which accounts for less than 1% of all ovarian tumors. In patients with this neoplasm, the serum testosterone level is always elevated, and most patients have amenorrhea and a palpable ovarian mass.

Gonadoblastomas

Gonadoblastomas usually develop in younger persons (aged 10–30 yrs) who are genetic males with female external genitalia. Nearly half of these tumors are malignant, and many are bilateral. Pelvic examination findings are abnormal because internal female genitalia are absent.

Lipoid Cell Tumors

Lipoid cell tumors are of 2 histologic types—adrenal-like cells (in younger patients) and hilar or Leydig-like cells (in older patients). These tumors are usually palpable but are seldom malignant. Ovarian tumors, which are even less frequently encountered, include dysgerminomas, Brenner tumors, and cystic granulosa-theca cell tumors.

PCOS (Figs 26.5 and 26.6)

PCOS is the most common ovarian disorder associated with hirsutism. Although the cause of PCOS is not known, the etiology is speculated to be multifactorial. By definition, polycystic ovaries have 20 or more subcapsular follicles, which range from approximately 1–15 mm in diameter. The follicles are at various states of atresia, and hyperplasia of the theca interna, the anatomic source of ovarian androgens, is present.

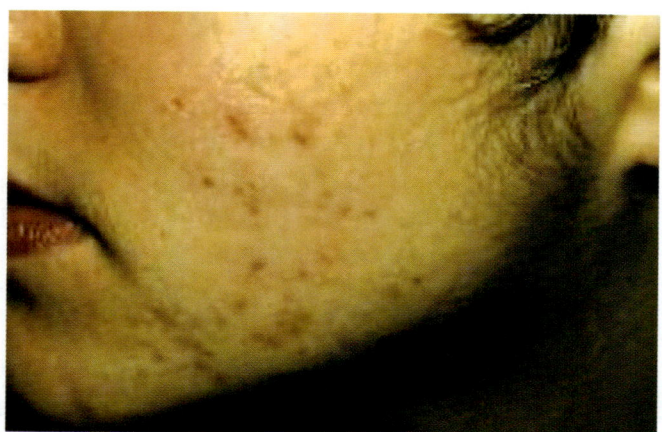

Fig. 26.5: The photograph depicts hirsutism in a young woman with polycystic ovary syndrome. Note the acne lesions and excessive hair on her face and neck

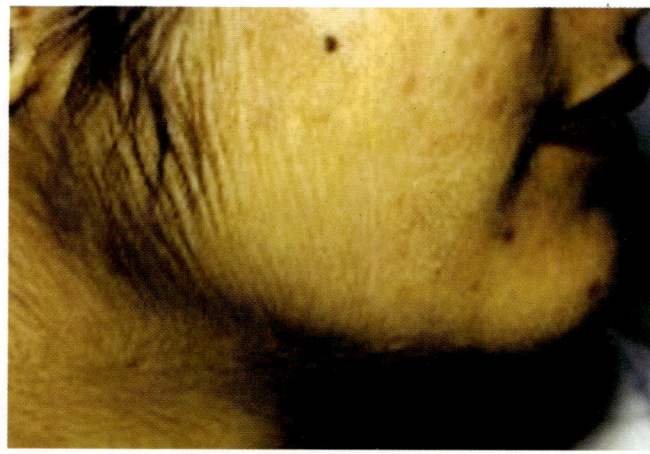

Fig. 26.6: Excessive facial hair

However, the basic abnormalities in PCOS are functional, rather than anatomic, in nature. In particular, levels of luteinizing hormone (LH) are tonically elevated (with LH levels higher than those of follicle-stimulating hormone FSH 3:1 from the early follicular phase).

Many women with PCOS have insulin resistance, manifested by acanthosis nigricans and elevated plasma insulin levels. Increased insulin levels have been speculated to stimulate androgen production from the ovarian theca interna cells. For this, insulin-sensitizing medications (e.g. metformin, thiazolidinediones) are used to restore normal ovarian androgen production and ovulation.

PCOS usually begins at puberty. The incidence has been estimated to be approximately 5% among adolescent girls and adult women. The characteristic endocrine abnormality is an elevation in levels of plasma free testosterone that is not suppressed by dexamethasone; however, as many as 50% of patients also show abnormal adrenal androgen secretion.

Idiopathic Hirsutism

Idiopathic hirsutism is a diagnosis of exclusion. The patient's hirsutism is not caused by well-defined abnormalities such as an androgen-secreting tumor or CAH.

The spectrum of clinical presentations ranges from normal menses and mild hirsutism to amenorrhea and signs of virilization, and testosterone levels range from normal to frankly elevated. The hirsutism usually begins at puberty. The disorder is often familial and may be associated with obesity and insulin resistance. There are some patients with elevated adrenal androgen levels (dehydroepiandrosterone sulfate [DHEAS]); in these cases, the disorder is called idiopathic adrenal hyperandrogenism.

Some patients with idiopathic hirsutism have normal plasma androgen levels. The underlying mechanism in these patients may be an increase in androgen sensitivity or in 5-alpha-reductase activity in the skin. This enzyme is located in the skin near the hair follicle, and it converts plasma testosterone to the androgen metabolite dihydrotestosterone.

Laboratory Studies

Approximately 50% of women with even minimal hirsutism have excessive androgen. Laboratory studies in hirsutism serve both to confirm the clinical impression of hyperandrogenism and to identify the source of excess androgens, either adrenal or ovarian.

- *Testosterone:* The most important assay is the level of serum testosterone, the major circulating androgen. If the total serum testosterone level is normal, the free serum level is measured because hyperandrogenism (and insulin resistance, if present) decreases sex steroid-binding globulin, such that the unbound, biologically active testosterone moiety may be elevated even if the total level is unremarkable. A total testosterone level greater than 200 ng per dL (6.94 nmol per L) should prompt evaluation for an androgen-secreting tumor of the adrenal or ovary, whereas idiopathic and benign etiologies result in very mild elevations. Indeed, in idiopathic hirsutism, the androgen levels are often normal.

- *Dehydroepiandrosterone sulfate (DHEAS):* Because testosterone can originate in either the adrenal cortex or the ovary, an elevated testosterone level does not indicate the gland of origin. Accordingly, measurement of elevated plasma levels of DHEAS, an androgen synthesized almost exclusively by the adrenal cortex, can indicate excess adrenal function. Elevations in both testosterone and DHEAS suggest an adrenal origin, whereas an isolated testosterone elevation indicates an ovarian source.

- *Dexamethasone suppression:* Laboratory testing of testosterone (free or total) and DHEAS can be performed on the initial visit. At the same time, a diagnostic trial of dexamethasone therapy for 7–14 days can be initiated to help exclude adrenocorticotropin hormone (ACTH)-dependent hirsutism. When the patient returns, free testosterone, DHEAS, and plasma cortisol levels are measured. Dexamethasone-mediated suppression of androgens is observed in healthy women who do not have hirsutism and in those with congenital adrenal hyperplasia (CAH) and idiopathic hirsutism.

- *Adrenocorticotropin stimulation:* An ACTH-stimulation test (250 µg for 30 min) can help differentiate between CAH and idiopathic hirsutism because CAH produces abnormal findings (elevations in metabolic precursors of cortisol).
  - Hirsutism caused by CAH is due to 1 of 3 cortisol biosynthetic defects, i.e. 21-hydroxylase deficiency, 3β-hydroxysteroid dehydrogenase, or 11-β-hydroxylase deficiency.
  - Because 21-hydroxylase deficiency accounts for the vast majority of cases of CAH (approximately 90%), the presence of possible 21-hydroxylase deficiency is determined by measuring plasma 17-hydroxyprogesterone levels obtained between 0700 and 0900 hours. Values of less than 7 nmol/L exclude the diagnosis, and values of greater than 45 nmol/L in nonpregnant women confirm 21-hydroxylase deficiency. When basal values of 17-hydroxyprogesterone are between 7 and 45 nmol/L, an ACTH-stimulated concentration of greater than 45 nmol/L is also diagnostic.

- *Cortisol suppression:* Investigation of subnormal dexamethasone suppression of androgens can be guided by the patient's cortisol level, without the need for an ACTH-stimulation test. PCOS and adrenal and ovarian tumors are associated with normal suppression of cortisol by dexamethasone, whereas cortisol levels in patients with Cushing syndrome are not suppressed.

Other laboratory tests include the following:

- *Serum prolactin and FSH:* Women with hirsutism and amenorrhea of unknown cause should have a serum prolactin and FSH test to evaluate for prolactinoma and ovarian failure respectively.

- *Diabetes screening:* Women with hirsutism, PCOS, obesity, or acanthosis nigricans may have insulin resistance, and screening for diabetes and hyperlipidemia is warranted. Approximately 50% of these women have increased insulin levels and 5% have undiagnosed diabetes mellitus.

- *Prostate-specific antigen (PSA):* Ultrasensitive assays can detect PSA in women and is a potential marker for androgen excess.

Imaging Studies

If indicated based on the findings from the clinical evaluation and laboratory testing, ovarian ultrasonography and adrenal computed tomography scanning or magnetic resonance imaging is done to evaluate for either ovarian or adrenal sources of androgen production.

Medical Care (Table 26.2)

The treatment of hirsutism begins with a careful explanation about the cause of the problem and reassurance that the patient is not losing her femininity. Then, direct intervention, if possible, is instituted for the underlying disorder. If hirsutism persists (or the patient has idiopathic hirsutism), other cosmetic or systemic treatment may be necessary. In some cases, cosmetic measures may be sufficient. In others, the slow progress of systemic therapy may necessitate more immediate cosmetic treatment. The most effective strategy is to combine systemic therapy, which has a slow onset of effectiveness, with mechanical depilation (shaving, plucking, waxing, depilatory creams) or light-based (laser or pulsed-light) hair removal.

Hirsutism requires a careful and systematic clinical evaluation coupled with a rational approach to treatment. For the patient who desires treatment, a wide variety of pharmacologic strategies are available.

- Systemic therapies directed at hirsutism can be divided into those that decrease ovarian or adrenal androgen production and those that inhibit androgen action in the skin. The systemic therapies include glucocorticoids, oral contraceptives (OCs), spironolactone, flutamide, finasteride, cyproterone acetate and insulin sensitizers (metformin and rosiglitazone).
  - *Glucocorticoids:* Glucocorticoids (dexamethasone or prednisone), which suppress adrenocortico-tropin hormone (ACTH)-dependent adrenal androgen synthesis, have been used with variable success in women with adrenal hirsutism, as in congenital adrenal hyperplasia (CAH) or idiopathic adrenal hyperandrogenism. Usually, 0.5–1 mg of dexamethasone at bedtime is sufficient to suppress ACTH and adrenal androgen production. Unfortunately, some patients gain weight and develop cushingoid features, even with this small dose. Further investigations may establish that lower doses (perhaps 0.25 mg) can be effective without adverse effects.
  - *Oral contraceptives:* These drugs are widely used to suppress ovarian androgen production. They are probably the first choice for young women with hirsutism who do not want to become pregnant.
- OCs are inexpensive and promote regular uterine bleeding. In addition, OCs can be used in combination with one of the antiandrogens. But OC are not used in women with a history of migraines, known or possible thrombotic disease, or breast or uterine cancer.
- Moreover, for several reasons, OCs have a significant failure rate in patients with hirsutism. Low-dose OCs and progestin-only minipills fail to suppress ovulation in as many as 50% of women. This is because ovarian function continues at a variable rate, and ovarian androgens continue to be produced. Secondly, the progestins in OCs are attenuated derivatives of testosterone and have variable degrees of androgenic activity in women.

Tabel 26.2: Medications commonly used for treatment of hirsutism				
Medication	*Dosage*	*Adverse effects*	*Comments*	*FDA pregnancy category*
Oral contraceptives (various)	One tablet daily	Gastrointestinal upset, headache	Recommended first-line agents; formulations containing norgestimate, desogestrel, or drospirenone are preferred	X
Metformin (glucophage)	500 to 1,000 mg twice daily	Gastrointestinal upset	Useful for treating polycystic ovary syndrome, but no data to support primary use for hirsutism	B
Spironolactone (aldactone)	100 to 200 mg daily	Hyperkalemia, irregular menses	Risk of pseudohermaphroditism in male fetuses if used during pregnancy	D
Finasteride (propecia)	2.5 mg daily	Hepatotoxicity		X
Glucocorticoids (prednisone)	5 to 10 mg daily	Weight gain, bone density loss, adrenal suppression	Indicated in congenital adrenal hyperplasia	C
Leuprolide (lupron)	3.75 to 7.5 mg intramuscularly monthly	Hot flashes, atrophic vaginitis, bone density loss	Consider adding back hormone therapy; expensive	X
Ketoconazole	400 mg daily	Dry skin, headache, hepatotoxicity	Typically used only after failure of other therapies	C
Eflornithine (vaniqa)	Apply topically twice daily	Acne, erythema, burning	FDA approval is only for use for unwanted facial hair	C

- *Spironolactone:* Spironolactone, in daily doses of 50–200 mg, blocks androgen receptors. Spironolactone also decreases testosterone production, making it additionally effective for hirsutism. Spironolactone is especially useful in a patient with hypertension or edema because the drug is a mild diuretic.

  With current systemic therapies for hirsutism, 6 months to a year of therapy is usually required before results are noticeable. Even then, only approximately one-half to three-quarters of patients show improvement. The problem may lie partially in the nature of the hair follicle, which persists for 6 months to a year even after androgen levels have been normalized. Ineffectiveness may also be due to the inability of treatment to completely normalize elevated tissue dihydrotestosterone levels. Newer therapies directed at inhibition of 5-alpha-reductase or blockade of the androgen receptor may improve the ability to treat patients.

  - *Finasteride:* Finasteride is a 5-alpha-reductase inhibitor approved for the treatment of benign prostatic hyperplasia. No adverse effects have been reported in women, and the efficacy is similar to that of spironolactone. The main concern with finasteride, however, is the risk of ambiguous genitalia in male fetuses exposed to the enzyme inhibitor during the first trimester. Therefore, use this drug only in women who are postmenopausal with no chance of becoming pregnant.

  - *Flutamide:* Flutamide, is a potent nonsteroidal selective antiandrogen without progestational, estrogenic, corticoid, or antigonadotropin activity. Preliminary data indicate that it is effective as therapy for hirsutism and acne; however, flutamide is expensive and has caused fatal hepatitis.

  - *Cyproterone acetate* has been effective in the treatment of hirsutism. When added to ethinyl estradiol, it is as effective as flutamide in the treatment of hirsutism.

  - *Insulin sensitizers:* Both metformin and rosiglitazone improve insulin resistance and have been shown to be effective in lowering androgen levels and in treating hirsutism.

  - *Eflornithine* is a topical agent that reduces hair growth through inhibition of ornithine decarboxylase. When used for excess facial hair, results are noticed in about eight weeks. Eflornithine can be used alone or in conjunction with other therapies. Hair growth resumes after discontinuation

Cosmetic measures for hirsutism and their disadvantages are as follows:

- Hydrogen peroxide bleaching is not suitable for severe hirsutism.
- Plucking can cause skin irritation, folliculitis, and scarring.
- Waxing can cause skin irritation, folliculitis, and scarring. The wax used has a low melting point.
- Shaving may be psychologically unacceptable.
- Chemical depilatories can cause skin irritation.
- Electrolysis can be painful, and short-wave diathermy can cause scarring.
- Laser therapy has been shown not only to reduce unwanted hair but also to improve depression and anxiety in women with hirsutism. In many patients, hirsutism can be controlled just with laser, without using any drugs.

Prognosis

Prognosis depends on the etiology of the hirsutism and whether it is benign or malignant. Hirsutism requires a careful and systematic clinical evaluation coupled with a rational approach to treatment. Although diagnostic testing can be time consuming and even inconclusive, it is sometimes essential for the determination of an effective intervention. In other cases, counseling and education may be all that is needed.

For the patient who desires treatment, a wide variety of pharmacologic strategies are available. Informing the patient that current systemic therapy is imperfect is important. Furthermore, none of the drugs used to treat hirsutism has FDA approval for such use. Therapy is initiated only in patients who give informed consent after a complete explanation of the potential benefits and risks of a particular treatment and alternative approaches.

SOGC Recommendations

1. Referral to endocrinologist is indicated in the presence of (a) virilism, (b) when testosterone and DHEA-S levels are more than upper limit of normal, or (c) signs or symptoms o Cushing's disease. (IIIB)

2. In addition to medical treatment, all patients suffering from hirsutism should be offered oral contraceptive therapy. (IIIB)

3. Antiandrogens should be added for moderate to severe hirsutism or to ensure an optimal response for milder hirsutism. (IA)

4. Any treatment protocol using CPA should be stopped for at least two cycles prior to attempting

pregnancy in order to avoid the risk of feminizing a male fetus. (IIIB)

5. Antiandrogens are best used in combination with OCs which is particularly effective in women with moderate to severe hirsutism. (IA)

6. Antiandrogen therapy should be stopped prior to patients discontinuing contraceptive measures to prevent feminization of the male fetus. (IIIB)

7. All physicians counseling women with hirsutism should explore the long-term health sequelae of hyperandrogenism including abnormal uterine bleeding/endometrial hyperplasia, infertility, pre-eclampsia, heart disease. Physicians should also discuss lifestyle modifications including exercise, healthy eating habits and smoking cessation. (IIIB)

26B. RADIATION THERAPY IN GYNECOLOGY

Introduction

Radiation therapy is an essential component in gynecology in the primary nonsurgical management and the adjuvant postoperative treatment of selected malignancies arising in the female reproductive tract.

Mode of Action

Radiation is energy that is carried by waves or a stream of particles. Radiation works by damaging the genes (DNA) in cells. Genes control how cells grow and divide. When radiation damages the genes of a cancer cell, it cannot grow and divide any more and over a period of time, the cells die. This means radiation can be used to kill cancer cells and shrink tumors.

To understand how radiation works as a treatment, it is essential to know the normal life cycle of a cell. The cell cycle goes through 5 phases, one of which is the actual splitting of the cell. When a cell splits, or divides, into 2 cells, it is called *mitosis*. This 5-phase process is controlled by proteins known as *cyclin-dependent kinases* (CDKs). Because CDKs are so important to normal cell division, they too have a number of control mechanisms.

The cell life cycle (Fig. 26.7):

G0 = Cell rests from dividing and does its normal work in the body
G1 = RNA and proteins are made for dividing
S = Synthesis (DNA is made for new cells)
G2 = Apparatus for mitosis is built
M = Mitosis (the cell divides into 2 cells)

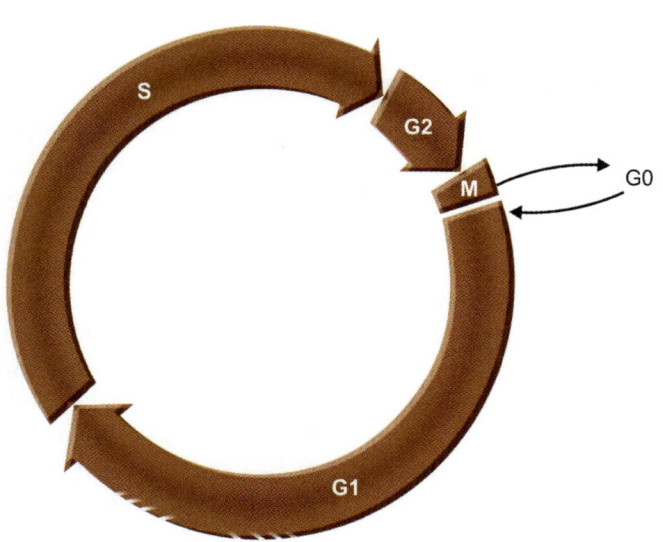

Fig. 26.7: Life cycle of cell

G0 phase (resting stage): The cell has not yet started to divide. Cells spend much of their lives in this phase, carrying out their day-to-day body functions, not dividing or preparing to divide. Depending on the type of cell, this stage can last for a few hours to many years. When the cell gets the signal to reproduce (divide), it moves into the G1 phase.

G1 phase: The cell gets information that determines when it will go into the next phase. It starts making more proteins to get ready to divide. The RNA needed to copy DNA is also made in this phase. This phase lasts about 18 to 30 hours.

S phase: In the S phase, the chromosomes (which contain the genetic code or DNA) are copied so that both of the new cells to be made will have the same DNA. This phase lasts about 18 to 20 hours.

G2 phase: It is provided with more information about when to proceed with cell division. The G2 phase happens just before the cell starts splitting into 2 cells. It lasts from 2 to 10 hours.

M phase (mitosis): In this phase, which lasts only 30 to 60 minutes, the cell actually splits into 2 new cells that are exactly the same.

Cells and Radiation

The cell cycle phase is important in cancer treatment because usually radiation first kills the cells that are actively dividing. It does not work very quickly on cells that are in the resting stage (G0) or are dividing less often. The amount and type of radiation that reaches the cell and the speed of cell growth affect whether and how quickly the cell will die or be damaged. The term *radiosensitivity* describes how likely the cell is to be damaged by radiation.

Cancer cells tend to divide quickly and grow out of control. Radiation therapy kills cancer cells that are dividing but it also affects dividing cells of normal tissues. The damage to normal cells causes unwanted side effects. Radiation therapy is always a balance between destroying the cancer cells and minimizing damage to the normal cells.

Radiation does not always kill cancer cells or normal cells right away. It might take days or even weeks of treatment for cells to start dying, and they may keep dying off for months after treatment ends. Tissues that grow quickly, such as skin, bone marrow, and the lining of the intestines are often affected fast. In contrast, nerve, breast, brain, and bone tissue show later effects. For this reason, radiation treatment can have side effects that might not be seen until long after treatment is over.

Types of Radiation used to Treat Cancer

Radiation used for cancer treatment is called *ionizing radiation* because it forms ions (electrically charged particles) in the cells of the tissues it passes through. It creates ions by removing electrons from atoms and molecules. This can kill cells or change genes so the cells stop growing.

Other forms of radiation such as radio waves, microwaves, and light waves are called *non-ionizing*. They do not have much energy and are not able to form ions. Ionizing radiation can be sorted into two major types:

- *Photons* (X-rays and gamma rays), which are most widely used in cancer treatment.
- *Particle radiation* (such as electrons, protons, neutrons, carbon ions, alpha particles, and beta particles)

Some types of ionizing radiation have more energy than others. The higher the energy, the more deeply the radiation can penetrate the tissues. The way a certain type of radiation behaves is important in planning radiation treatments.

Photon Radiation

By far the most common form of radiation used for cancer treatment is a high-energy photon beam. This comes from radioactive sources such as cobalt, cesium, or a machine called a *linear accelerator*. Photon beams of energy affect the cells along their path as they go through the body to get to the cancer, pass through the cancer, and exit the body.

Particle Radiation

Electron beams *or* particle beams are also produced by a linear accelerator. Electrons are negatively charged parts of atoms. They have a low energy level and do not penetrate deeply into the body, so this type of radiation is used most often to treat the skin, tumors, and lymph nodes that are close to the surface of the body.

Proton beams are a form of particle beam radiation. Protons are positively charged parts of atoms. They cause less damage to tissues they pass through but are very good at killing cells at the end of their path. Because of this, proton beams are thought to be able to deliver more radiation to the cancer while causing fewer side effects to normal tissues. Protons are used routinely for certain types of cancer.

Some of the techniques used in proton treatment can also expose the patient to neutrons. Proton beam radiation therapy requires highly specialized equipment and is not widely available.

Neutron beams are used for some cancers of the head, neck, and prostate and for certain inoperable tumors. A neutron is a particle in many atoms that has no charge. Neutron beam radiation can sometimes help when other forms of radiation therapy do not work. But its use has declined partly because of problems of getting the beams on target. Because neutrons can damage DNA more than photons, effects on normal tissue can be more severe. Still, neutron beams show great promise with salivary gland cancers that cannot be cured with surgery.

Carbon ion radiation is also called *heavy ion radiation* because it uses a particle that is heavier than a proton or neutron. The particle is part of the carbon atom, which itself contains protons, neutrons, and electrons. Because it is so heavy, it can do more damage to the target cell than other types of radiation. As with protons, the beam of carbon ions can be adjusted to do the most damage to the cancer cells at the end of its path. But the effects on nearby normal tissue can be more severe. This type of radiation is only available in a few centers in the world. It can be helpful in treating cancers that do not usually respond well to radiation (called *radioresistant*).

Alpha and beta particles are mainly produced by special radioactive substances that may be injected, swallowed, or put into the body of a person with cancer. They are most often used in imaging tests, but can be helpful in treating cancer.

Goals of Radiation Therapy

Most types of radiation are considered *local* treatments because the radiation is aimed at a specific area of the body where there is a tumor. Only cells in that area are affected. Most forms of radiation therapy cannot reach all parts of the body and so may not be helpful in treating cancer that has spread to many distant areas. Radiation is used to treat cancer in several ways:

1. *To cure or shrink early stage cancer:* Some cancers are very sensitive to radiation. Radiation may be used by itself in these cases to make the cancer shrink or disappear completely. It may be used before surgery (as *preoperative* or *neoadjuvant therapy*) to shrink the tumor, or after surgery to prevent the cancer recurrence (this is called *adjuvant therapy*).

For certain cancers that can be cured either by radiation or by surgery, radiation may be preferred because it can sometimes preserve the organ's function (such as that of the larynx or the anus). In treating some types of cancer, radiation may also be used along with chemotherapy. This is because the drug acts as a radiosensitizer to make the cancer cells more sensitive to radiation. These drugs like 5-FU, cisplatin make the radiation work better and are known to be radiosensitizers. The drawback of giving chemo and radiation together is that side effects tend to be worse. In some other types of cancer, it is better to use radiation before or after chemotherapy.

2. *To stop cancer from recurrence:* If a type of cancer is known to spread to a certain area, even though imaging scans (such as CT or MRI) show no tumors, that area may be treated to keep these cells from growing into tumors. Sometimes, radiation to prevent future cancer can be given at the same time that radiation is given to treat existing cancer, especially if the prevention area is close to the tumor itself.

3. *To treat symptoms caused by advanced cancer:* Sometimes cancer spreads too far to be cured. But even some of these tumors can still be treated to make them smaller so that the person can feel better. Radiation might help relieve symptoms such as pain, troublesome swallowing or breathing, or bowel blockages that can be caused by advanced cancer. This is often called *palliative radiation*.

Who Gives Radiation Treatments?

During radiation therapy, a team comprising of the following speciality are needed:

- A *radiation oncologist* is a doctor specially trained to treat cancer with radiation.
- The *radiation physicist* makes sure that the radiation equipment is working the way it should and it delivers the correct dose of radiation.
- The *dosimetrist* helps plan and calculate the needed number of treatments. The dosimetrist is supervised by the radiation physicist.
- The *radiation therapist* or *radiation therapy technologist* operates the radiation equipment and positions for treatment.
- A *radiation therapy nurse* is a registered nurse with special training in cancer treatment.

External Beam Radiation

External beam radiation is the most widely used type of radiation therapy, and it most often uses photon beams.

The radiation comes from a machine outside the body and is focused on the cancer. This type of radiation is most often given by machines called *linear accelerators*.

External beam radiation can be used to treat large areas of the body. It also can treat more than one area, such as the main tumor and nearby lymph nodes. External radiation is usually given daily over several weeks. It is given in an outpatient clinic. The radiation is aimed at the cancer, but it affects the normal tissue as it passes through on its way into and out of the body.

Special ways to Deliver External Beam Radiation

Three-dimensional conformal radiation therapy (3D-CRT): This technique uses imaging scan pictures and special computers to map the location of a tumor very precisely in three dimensions. The patient is fitted with a plastic mold or cast to keep the body part still during treatment. The radiation photon beams are matched to the shape of the tumor and delivered to the tumor from several directions. Careful aiming of the radiation beam reduces radiation damage to normal tissues. A drawback of 3D-CRT is that it can be hard to see the full extent of some tumors on imaging tests, and any part not seen will not get treated with this therapy.

Intensity modulated radiation therapy (IMRT): This is an advanced form of external radiation therapy. As with 3D-CRT, computer programs are used to precisely map the tumor in three dimensions. But along with aiming photon beams from several directions, the intensity of the beams can be adjusted. This gives even more control over the dose, decreasing the radiation reaching sensitive normal tissues while delivering higher doses to the tumor.

A variation of IMRT is called *volumetric modulated arc therapy*. It uses a machine called *Rapid Arc* that delivers the radiation quickly as it rotates once around the body. This allows each treatment to be given over just a few minutes. Although this can be more convenient for the patient, it is not yet clear, if it is more effective than regular IMRT.

Because IMRT uses a higher total dose of radiation, it may slightly increase the risk of secondary cancers later on.

Image-guided radiation therapy (IGRT) is an option on some newer radiation machines that have imaging scanners built into them. This advance lets the doctor take pictures of the tumor and make minor aiming adjustments just before giving the radiation. This may help deliver the radiation even more precisely. This might result in fewer side effects.

Intensity modulated proton therapy (IMPT) is IMRT using proton beams instead of photon beams. Protons are parts of atoms that in theory can deliver radiation to the area that they are aimed at while doing less damage to nearby normal tissues. Though, there have been no studies showing that proton beam radiation is better than the more common photon beam in terms of cancer outcomes or side effects. Meanwhile, IMPT is often used for tumors near critical body structures such as the eye, the brain, and the spine.

Protons can only be sent out by a special machine called a *cyclotron* or *synchrotron*. This machine is very costly and requires expert staff to use and maintain it. Because of this, proton beam therapy is expensive, and very few treatment centers offer it.

Stereotactic radiosurgery (SRS) and fractionated stereotactic radiotherapy: These advanced image-guided techniques are used to deliver a large, precise dose of radiation to a small, well-defined tumor. This technique is used to treat tumors that start in or spread to the brain or head and neck region. If the radiation is given as a single dose, it is called *stereotactic radiosurgery*. If the radiation is spread out over several doses, it is called *fractionated stereotactic radiotherapy*.

Once the exact location of the tumor is mapped, narrow radiation beams from a machine called a *gamma knife* are focused at the tumor from hundreds of different angles for a short time. The process may be repeated, if needed. Another approach uses a movable linear accelerator controlled by a computer. The linear accelerator moves around to deliver radiation to the tumor from different angles.

Intraoperative radiation therapy (IORT): With this technique, radiation is given to the cancer during surgery. The radiation may be given using a linear accelerator for external beam radiation. Another option is to place a radioactive substance into the area that needs treatment for a short time. It is often used along with a course of external radiation given before or after the operation.

IORT is useful for cancers that are deep inside the body, because normal tissues can be moved aside during surgery, exposing the cancer. After as much tumor is removed as possible, one large dose of radiation is directed straight at the cancer without going through normal tissues. Shielding can also be used to protect the nearby normal tissues further. IORT is given in a special operating room lined with radiation-shielding walls.

IORT is most often used for abdominal or pelvic cancers that cannot be completely removed and for cancers that tend to grow back after treatment. This technique is not widely available.

Electromagnetic-guided radiation therapy (IMRT): This is another way of aiming the radiation beam that can be used with 3D and IMRT. It uses tiny electromagnetic implants (called *transponders*) that are placed into the area being treated. These implants send out radio waves to direct the radiation therapy machines where to aim. It helps to refocus radiation beams as organs shift or cancer shrinks over time. It is sometimes known as *4-D therapy*, because it includes time in the radiation planning formula.

Treatment Planning for External Beam Radiation

The process of planning external beam radiation therapy has many steps and may take several days to complete. The treatment will give the strongest dose of radiation to the cancer while sparing normal tissue as much as possible.

The first part of treatment planning is called *simulation*. It is sometimes referred to as a "marking session." The health care team works out the best treatment position and will then mark the *radiation field*, which is the exact place on the body where the radiation will be aimed. The marks may be done with permanent markers or with tattoos to outline normal tissues in the treatment area, to take measurements, and plan treatment. Computer programs are also used through a complex process called *dosimetry* to find out how much radiation the nearby normal structures would be exposed to if the prescribed dose is delivered to the cancer.

Dosing and Treatment with External Beam Radiation

The total amount of radiation is measured in units called *Gray* (Gy). Often the dose is expressed in *centigray* (cGy), which is one-hundredth of a Gray.

For external radiation, the total dose is often divided into smaller doses (called *fractions*) that are most often given over a number of weeks. This allows the best dose to be given with the least damage to normal tissues. Treatments are usually given 5 days a week for about 5 to 8 weeks.

Some cancers may be treated more often than once a day.

- *Hyperfractionated radiation* divides the daily dose into 2 treatment sessions without changing the length of the treatment. In this case, one would be treated twice a day for several weeks.

- *Accelerated radiation* gives the total dose of radiation over a shorter period of time. In other words, giving more frequent doses (more than once a day) to get the same total dose of radiation; it may shorten the course of treatment by a week or two.

- *Hypofractionated radiation* breaks radiation into fewer doses, so that each dose is larger. Sometimes, it is given less often than once a day.

Internal Radiation Therapy (Brachytherapy)

Internal radiation therapy is also known as *brachytherapy*, means short-distance therapy. With this method, sources of radiation are put in or near the area that needs treatment. The radiation only travels a short distance, so there is less risk of damaging nearby normal tissues. Brachytherapy can be used to deliver a high dose of radiation to a small area in a fairly short period of time. It is useful for tumors that need a high dose of radiation or are near normal tissues that are easily hurt by radiation.

The main types of internal radiation are:

- *Interstitial radiation:* The radiation source is placed directly into or next to the tumor using small pellets, seeds, wires, tubes, or containers.
- *Intracavitary radiation:* A container of radioactive material is placed in a cavity of the body such as the chest, rectum, uterus, or vagina.

Ultrasound, X-rays, or CT scans are used to put the radioactive source in the right place. The placement can be permanent or temporary.

Permanent brachytherapy uses small containers, often called *pellets* or *seeds*, which are about the size of a grain of rice. They are put right into the tumors using thin, hollow needles. Once in place, the pellets give off radiation for several weeks or months. Because they are very small and cause little discomfort, they are simply left in place after their radioactive material is used up.

Temporary brachytherapy can be *high-dose rate* (HDR) or *low-dose rate* (LDR). Either type places cylinders, hollow needles, tubes (catheters), or fluid-filled balloons into the area to be treated that are removed after treatment. Radioactive material can be put in these containers for a short time and then removed. This may be done by hospital staff or the radioactive material can be put into the device remotely by machine.

For HDR brachytherapy, the radiation source is put into place for a few minutes at a time, and then removed. This process may be repeated twice a day for up to a week, or once a week for a few weeks.

For LDR brachytherapy, the radiation source stays in place for up to 7 days. To keep the implant from moving, one will need to stay in hospital bed and lie fairly still during LDR therapy.

Treatment with Internal Radiation

Anesthesia usually is not needed to take out temporary brachytherapy implants in a hospital room specially shielded to contain the radioactivity and the staff use shields to protect themselves while handling radioactive materials. Once implants are removed, there is no radioactivity in the body. The area that has been treated with an implant may be sore or sensitive for some time after treatment.

Radioembolization: This is a special type of internal radiation that is now used only for cancer in the liver that cannot be surgically removed. Small radioactive beads (called *microspheres*) are injected into the artery that feeds the tumor. Once infused, the beads lodge in blood vessels near the tumor, where they give off small amounts of radiation to the tumor site for several days. The radiation travels a very short distance, so its effects are limited mainly to the tumor. In some cases, it can cause ulcers in the intestine, low white blood cell counts, lung damage, or serious damage to the normal liver cells.

Radiopharmaceuticals: Radiopharmaceuticals are drugs that contain radioactive materials called *radioisotopes*. They may be put into a vein, taken by mouth, or placed in a body cavity. Depending on the drug and how it is given, these materials travel to various parts of the body to treat cancer or relieve its symptoms. They put out radiation, mostly in the form of alpha and beta particles that target the affected areas. They are most often used in small amounts for imaging tests, but larger doses can be used to deliver radiation.

Phosphorus 32: This form of phosphorus (also known as *chromic phosphate P 32*) is put inside brain tumors that are cystic to kill the tumor without hurting the healthy parts of the brain.

In the past, P-32 was given intravenous as a common treatment for a blood disease called *polycythemia vera*. P-32 was also placed inside the abdomen as a treatment for ovarian cancer. It is rarely used in these ways today, because there are better drugs with fewer side effects.

Radiolabeled antibodies: *Monoclonal antibodies* are man-made versions of immune system proteins that attack only a specific molecular target on certain cancer cells. Scientists have learned how to pair these antibodies with radioactive atoms. When put into the bloodstream, the antibodies act as *homing* devices. They attach only to their target, bringing tiny packets of radiation directly to the cancer.

Cancer Cervix

Treatment Combining Chemotherapy with Radiotherapy

Patients who have undergone radical hysterectomy with histopathologic evidence of tumoral spread to regional lymph nodes, tumor at the surgical margin, and/or with microscopic involvement of the parametrium are considered to be at high risk for recurrence, and postoperative adjuvant therapy is generally indicated. GOG has demonstrated a survival advantage for patients who received chemoradiation as compared with radiation therapy alone.

Similarly, postoperative pelvic chemoradiation is recommended for patients with cancers of stage IB1 or higher that are incidentally found after simple hysterectomy for presumed benign disease. Alternatively, such patients may be offered completion surgery consisting of radical upper vaginectomy, parametrectomy, and pelvic lymphadenectomy.

The addition of concurrent chemotherapy to radiation in the treatment of cervical cancer, both in the postoperative adjuvant setting for early stage disease and as definitive primary therapy for advanced disease, has emerged as one of the major breakthroughs in the treatment of gynecologic cancer in the last decade.

FIGO stage*	Treatment
IB2	Radiotherapy plus weekly cisplatin followed by extrafascial hysterectomy
IIB-IVA	Radiotherapy plus weekly cisplatin or radiotherapy plus cisplatin, 5-fluorouracil, and hydroxyurea
IB2-IVA	Pelvic radiotherapy plus cisplatin and 5-fluorouracil
IIB-IVA	Radiotherapy plus cisplatin and 5-fluorouracil
IB (postoperative) or IIA (postoperative)	Radiotherapy plus cisplatin and 5-fluorouracil

The treatment of bulky stage I (stage IB2, clinical tumor diameter >4 cm) cervical cancer remains controversial.

a. Common treatment strategies consist of primary radical hysterectomy, with postoperative adjuvant chemoradiation administration tailored to histopathologic findings,

b. Definitive primary chemoradiotherapy. Proponents of definitive primary chemoradiation are of the view that most patients undergoing radical surgery demonstrate surgical-pathologic risk factors that may ultimately require them to receive adjunctive postoperative chemoradiation with an attendant increase in morbidity.

c. Neoadjuvant chemotherapy administration (to reduce tumor volume preoperatively) followed by radical hysterectomy and chemoradiotherapy followed by type I extrafascial hysterectomy are additional treatment strategies that are less-commonly used.

Because direct extension of tumor into adjacent structures limits the ability of surgery to gain clear surgical margins and the presence of the uterus is critical for the anatomy of brachytherapy insertion in this setting, primary chemoradiotherapy is generally indicated for the management of stage IIB-IVA locally advanced cervical cancer. Tumoral resection with anterior and/or posterior pelvic exenteration is technically possible in some cases. However, this procedure entails diversion of the urinary tract and/or bowel, and it is usually reserved for patients with isolated central pelvic disease that persists or recurs after definitive chemoradiotherapy.

Brachytherapy (Fig. 26.8)

Brachytherapy involves the temporary placement of intrauterine tandem and intravaginal ovoid that are loaded with radioactive material. The devices are placed with the patient under general anesthesia or heavy sedation. Radiopaque vaginal gauze is applied to secure the devices in place and fix their position relative to the bladder and rectum. Intraoperative radiographs or digital fluoroscopic images document appropriate device positioning. Contrast material in a Foley catheter and a rectal tube can be used to identify

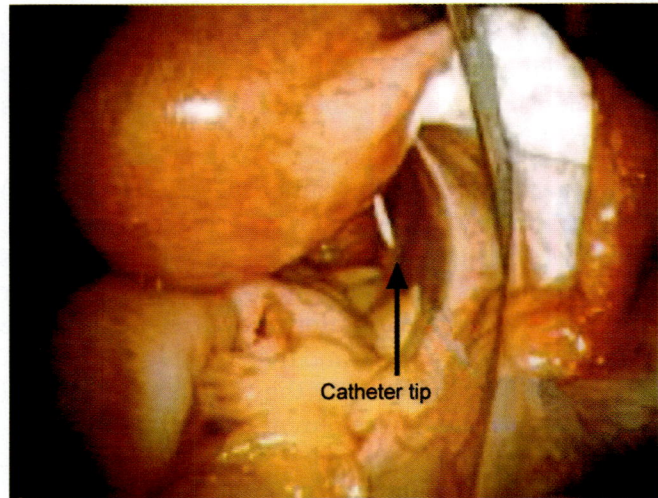

Fig. 26.8: Laparoscopic view of the pelvis during application of the device for interstitial brachytherapy. When the right parametrial tissues are retracted, penetration of the catheter into the peritoneal cavity can be observed. The catheter is then repositioned to avoid exposing its sharp end to the mobile bowel in the low pelvis

the International Commission of Radiological Units (ICRU) reference points of interest.

ICRU reference points for gynecologic brachytherapy doses are as follows:

- Point A = 2 cm cephalic to the external os along the tandem and 2 cm perpendicular to the plane of the tandem
- Point B = 2 cm cephalic to the os and 5 cm lateral to the patient's midline
- Bladder point = Most posterior point in the bulb of the Foley catheter along a direct AP line through the center of the bulb
- Rectal point = 0.5 cm posterior to the vaginal mucosa in the patient's midline at the level of the posterior aspect of the ovoid

Doses are prescribed to ICRU points A and B. The reference point of origin for points A and B is the cervical os, which is identified by using a radiopaque flange adjusted and fixed at the time of tandem placement.

Brachytherapy may be performed with low dose rate (LDR) or high dose rate (HDR) applications. LDR is defined as a dose of 0.4–2 Gy per hour and HDR is defined as a dose of greater than 12Gy per hour. HDR brachytherapy typically involves 5–7 weekly outpatient procedures in which the radioactive source is iridium-192 of high activity. Point A is given a dose of 5–7 Gy during each treatment, which is typically accomplished in less than an hour. LDR brachytherapy usually involves 1 or 2 placement procedures in which the radioactive source is cesium-137. Each time, the sources are left in place for approximately 2 days, during which a dose of 20–40 Gy is administered to point A.

Intracavitary brachytherapy devices are sometimes difficult to position because of anatomic distortion due to tumoral infiltration into surrounding structures. In high-stage disease, the vaginal fornices are commonly effaced because tumor erodes the cervix. The lateral distribution of the radiation dose to the parametrium is compromised when ovoids cannot be placed to a level near the cervical os. The net result can be that the devices cannot be appropriately arranged to avoid excessive doses to the bladder and rectal reference points while giving an adequate dose to point A.

One solution is to administer pelvic external RT and brachytherapy in moderately high doses and then perform extrafascial hysterectomy to resect the residual cervical tumor. However, this option is generally not feasible for disease of stage IIB or higher. An alternative is to use interstitial brachytherapy, wherein blind-ended catheters are placed through the perineum into areas of tumor infiltration in the lower pelvis lateral to the cervix.

Treatment Combining XRT and Brachytherapy

Comprehensive radiotherapy for stage IB–IVA cervical cancer involves both XRT and brachytherapy. Initial external-beam fields encompass a clinical target volume including the primary tumor and the adjacent areas at risk for direct occult invasion or regional lymph node metastases. The superior border of the field is typically placed at the L4–L5 interspace.

A typical regimen includes an initial external-beam dose of 40–45 Gy to the pelvis in fractions of 1.8–2 Gy. Cisplatin is usually given weekly at a dose of 40 mg/m^2 of body surface area, with a maximum weekly dose of 70 mg.

Carcinoma of the Body Uterus

When hysterectomy is medically contraindicated, primary radiotherapy can offer 5-year disease-specific survival rates of 80–90%, approaching those achieved with surgery.

Indications for adjuvant radiation after surgery for endometrial cancer are somewhat controversial. Whole-pelvis external-beam radiotherapy (XRT, or EBRT) and intravaginal brachytherapy are potential adjuvant postoperative therapies for patients with advance stages.

XRT Protocol

Whole-pelvis XRT is administered by using a 4-field setup involving parallel opposed anteroposterior (AP), posteroanterior (PA), right lateral, and left lateral fields. Patients are positioned prone on a partially depressed surface that allows for anterior displacement of the small intestines away from the lateral fields. A radiopaque marker is placed in the vagina. During simulation, this marker facilitates identification of the vaginal cuff. Typical field borders are the following:

- Superior (all fields)— L4–L5 or L5–S1 interspace.
- Inferior (all fields)— middle or inferior aspect of the obturator foramen or at least 5 cm below the vaginal cuff.
- Lateral (AP and PA fields)—1.5–2 cm lateral to bony pelvis.
- Anterior (lateral fields)—anterior pubic symphysis, with portions of small bowel anterosuperior to the external iliac nodal chain blocked out.
- Posterior (lateral fields)—posterior aspect of S3, covering the region of insertion of the uterosacral ligament, with a 2 cm or greater margin posterior to the vagina inferiorly.

Brachytherapy

- Since the vaginal cuff is well recognized to be a common site of recurrence in many patients with early stage disease. Intravaginal brachytherapy may be administered with an afterloading device to deliver a low dose rate (LDR) or a high dose rate (HDR).
- The HDR technique has become popular because of its convenience as a well-tolerated outpatient regimen. When intravaginal brachytherapy is given after pelvic XRT, a typical dosage schedule for intravaginal brachytherapy is 15 Gy prescribed to a depth of 0.5 cm over 3–4 cm of the upper vagina, given in 3 weekly fractions of 5 Gy each. When intravaginal brachytherapy is administered without pelvic XRT, a dose of 21 Gy to a depth of 0.5 cm given in 3 fractions is commonly prescribed.

Additional Observation

- For stage II endometrial carcinoma, preoperative or postoperative radiotherapy may be administered. The goals of preoperative treatment are to facilitate hysterectomy by reducing tumoral bulk, by clearing microscopic infiltration from the upper vaginal mucosa, or by rendering cells incapable of local implantation. Pelvic XRT may be combined with brachytherapy in this setting.
- For stage III–IV disease, patients are treated with combinations of pelvic XRT, whole-abdomen radiotherapy (WAR), intravaginal brachytherapy, and chemotherapy.
- Histologic variants of endometrial carcinoma require special consideration. Uterine papillary serous cancer (UPSC) is characterized by a propensity for local and distant recurrence.
- Carcinosarcoma, formerly called malignant mixed müllerian tumor (MMMT), is associated with a particularly high rate of treatment failure after hysterectomy. Patients may benefit from postoperative pelvic XRT in all stages of disease. The rate of distant recurrence is higher with carcinosarcomas than with endometrial adenocarcinomas.

Vulvar and Vaginal Cancer

- Although primary nonsurgical treatment is usually preferable for stage I or II vaginal lesions, partial or total vaginectomy followed by postoperative radiotherapy is the treatment of choice. Postoperative radiotherapy for stage I or II is indicated when pathologic evidence suggests inguinal node metastasis or close (<8 mm) resection margins around the primary site. A dose of 45–50 Gy is given in fractions of 1.8–2 Gy to regions at risk for residual microscopic disease.
- For stage III–IVA disease, the management strategy is tailored to the individual. A common policy is to surgically remove all resectable regional and iliac nodes larger than 1cm in diameter. Since the resection of the primary tumor entails permanent diversion of the lower urinary or gastrointestinal tract, combined-modality therapy is now offered. A chemoradiotherapy schedule involving 5-fluorouracil and mitomycin-C is used. This regimen is highly effective.

Ovarian Cancer

The current regimen for adjuvant therapy after surgery is intravenous combination chemotherapy with carboplatin and paclitaxel or, in optimally debulked patients, intraperitoneal cisplatin and paclitaxel. Whole-abdomen radiation (WAR) has been used, but its popularity has waned because of the favorable toxicity profiles of current chemotherapeutic regimens. Techniques for WAR include AP-PA field treatment to the entire peritoneal cavity at doses of 25–30 Gy given in fractions of 1–1.5 Gy. Renal doses of less than 20 Gy and whole-liver doses of less than 30 Gy is recommended using shielding techniques.

Palliative Radiotherapy

Palliative radiotherapy is frequently offered to patients who have focally symptomatic recurrences of ovarian cancer. The field arrangements and dose schedules are based on the site of recurrence and the patient's overall status. For patients with painful or hemorrhagic pelvic masses refractory to chemotherapy, a hypofractionated schedule of 14.8 Gy given in 4 fractions within 2 days may be administered by using AP-PA fields and then repeated once or twice at 2- to 4-week intervals. This regimen has been found to reduce symptoms for most patients.

Radiotherapy in Hormonal Ablation

Radiotherapy can also be applied when ovarian hormonal ablation is indicated, most commonly in the treatment of estrogen receptor-positive breast cancer in premenopausal women. Tamoxifen is widely given to premenopausal women with estrogen receptor–positive breast cancer. However, low-dose radiotherapy is sometimes administered. Radiotherapy can be highly effective and cost-effective. A dose of 10–20 Gy in 5–10 fractions is usually sufficient to eliminate ovarian hormone production.

Possible Side Effects of Radiation Therapy

Normal body tissues vary in their response to radiation. As with tumors, normal tissues in which cells are quickly dividing may be affected. Since radiation is a local treatment, side effects depend on the area of the body being treated. The early effects of radiation may be seen a few days or weeks after treatments have started and may go on for several weeks after treatments have ended. The most common side effects are briefly discussed below.

Fatigue

Fatigue is a common effect of radiation, but the exact cause is unknown. Sometimes tumors cause the immune system breakdown or it may be caused by anemia and poor nutrition.

Skin Changes

Current mode of radiation therapy causes less skin damage. Dryness and peeling may occur in 3 to 4 weeks. The skin over the treatment area may become darker. This is because of the effect of radiation on the cells in the skin that produce pigment. The skin in the treatment area may also become dry and itchy. Moisturizing the skin with aloe vera, lanolin, or vitamin E may help.

Later effects of radiation may include thinning of the skin. The skin may feel hard, especially if surgery has also been done in the same area.

Mouth and Throat Problems

Mucositis of gum and throat is a short-term side effect that can happen when radiation is given to the head and neck area. It can make swallowing painful. It usually gets better within a few weeks after treatments end. Dry mouth and loss of taste can be caused by radiation damage to the salivary glands and taste buds.

Reproductive/Sex Organs

Fertility in men: Radiation to the testicles can cause permanent loss of sperm production. Unless the cancer is in the testicles, they can usually be protected from radiation by using a shield called a *clam shell*.

Fertility in women: It is harder to protect the ovaries when women are getting radiation to the abdomen. If both ovaries are exposed to radiation, early menopause and permanent infertility can result. Sparing one ovary can prevent these side effects. If the uterus is exposed, radiation can cause scarring and fibrosis.

Sexual effects of radiation therapy on women: Radiation to the pelvic area can make the vagina tender and inflamed during and for a few weeks after treatment. The area may scar as it heals. This scarring can interfere with the vagina's ability to stretch.

The scarring can also shorten or narrow the vagina to produce dysparunia. This can often be prevented by stretching the walls of the vagina a few times a week. One way to do this is to have sex that includes vaginal penetration at least 3 to 4 times a week. Another option is to use a *vaginal dilator*. A dilator is a plastic or rubber rod or tube used to stretch out the vagina.

Secondary Cancers

The link between radiation and cancer was confirmed many years ago through studies of the survivors of the atomic bombs in Japan, the exposures of workers in certain jobs, and patients treated with radiation therapy for cancer and other diseases.

Some cases of leukemia are related to past radiation exposure. Most develop within a few years of exposure, with the risk peaking at 5 to 9 years, and then slowly declining. Other types of cancer that develop after radiation exposure have been found to take much longer to show up. These are solid tumor cancers, like cancer of the breast or lung. Most are not seen for at least 10 years after radiation exposure, and some are diagnosed even more than 15 years later.

Radiation therapy techniques have steadily improved over the last few decades. Treatments now target the cancers more precisely, and more is known about setting radiation doses. These advances are expected to reduce the number of secondary cancers that result from radiation therapy. Overall, the risk of second cancers is low and must be weighed against the benefits gained with radiation treatments.

What is new in radiation therapy?

New ways of delivering radiation therapy are making it safer and more effective. Some of these methods are already being used, while others need more study before they can be approved for widespread use. Here are just a few areas of current research interest:

Hyperthermia is the use of heat to treat cancer. Heat has been found to kill cancer cells, but when used alone it does not destroy enough cells to cure the cancer. Heat created by microwaves and ultrasound is being studied in combination with radiation and appears to improve the effect of the radiation.

Hyperbaric oxygen therapy consists of breathing pure oxygen while in a sealed chamber that has been pressurized at 1½ to 3 times normal atmospheric pressure. It helps to increase the sensitivity of certain cancer types to radiation.

Radiosensitizers are a growing field in cancer treatment. Researchers are continuing to look for new substances that will make tumors more sensitive to radiation without affecting normal tissues.

Radioprotectors are substances that protect normal cells from radiation. These types of drugs are useful in areas where it is hard not to expose vital normal tissues to radiation when treating a tumor, such as the head and neck area.

26C. CHEMOTHERAPY IN GYNECOLOGIC CANCER

The word *chemotherapy* refers to drugs used for cancer treatment. Two other medical terms used to describe cancer chemotherapy are *antineoplastic* (meaning anti-cancer) therapy and *cytotoxic* (cell-killing) therapy.

History of Chemotherapy

The first drug used for cancer chemotherapy did not start out as a medicine. Mustard gas was used as a chemical warfare agent during World War II where a group of people accidentally exposed to mustard gas were later found to have very low white blood cell counts. In the 1940s, several patients with advanced lymphomas were given the drug by vein, rather than by breathing the irritating gas. Their improvement, although temporary, was remarkable. Treatments like radiation and surgery are considered *local treatments*. They act only in one area of the body such as the breast, lung, or prostate and usually target the cancer directly. Chemotherapy differs from surgery or radiation in that it is almost always used as a *systemic treatment*.

Mode of Action

To understand how chemotherapy works, it is essential to understand the normal life cycle of a cell, or the *cell cycle*. All living tissue is made up of cells. Cells grow and reproduce to replace cells lost through injury or normal "wear and tear." The cell cycle is a series of steps that both normal cells and cancer cells go through in order to form new cells. The cell cycle has 5 phases and the resting phase (G0) is the starting point.

After a cell reproduces, the two new cells are identical. Each of the two cells made from the first cell can go through this cell cycle again when new cells are needed (*see* Fig. 26.7).

G0 phase (resting stage): The cell has not yet started to divide. Cells spend much of their lives in this phase. Depending on the type of cell, G0 can last from a few hours to a few years. When the cell gets a signal to reproduce, it moves into the G1 phase.

G1 phase: During this phase, the cell starts making more proteins and growing larger, so the new cells will be of normal size. This phase lasts about 18 to 30 hours.

S phase: In the S phase, the chromosomes containing the genetic code (DNA) are copied so that both of the new cells formed will have matching strands of DNA. The S phase lasts about 18 to 20 hours.

G2 phase: In the G2 phase, the cell checks the DNA and gets ready to start splitting into two cells. This phase lasts from 2 to 10 hours.

M phase (mitosis): In this phase, which lasts only 30 to 60 minutes, the cell actually splits into 2 new cells.

The cell cycle is important because many chemotherapy drugs work only on cells that are actively reproducing (not cells that are in the resting phase, G0). Some drugs specifically attack cells in a particular phase of the cell cycle (the M or S phases, for example). Understanding how these drugs work helps oncologists predict which drugs are likely to work well together. Chemotherapy drugs cannot differentiate the difference between reproducing cells of normal tissues and cancer cells. This means normal cells are damaged and this results in side effects. Therefore, during selection of chemotherapy drugs, it is necessary to find a balance between destroying the cancer cells and sparing the normal cells.

Goals of Chemotherapy

There are 3 possible goals for chemotherapy treatment:
Cure: Chemotherapy is used to cure the cancer.

Control: If cure is not possible, the goal may be to control the disease—to shrink any cancerous tumors and/or stop the cancer from growing and spreading.

Palliation: When the cancer is at an advanced stage, chemotherapy drugs may be used to relieve symptoms caused by the cancer. When the only goal of a certain treatment is to improve the quality of life but not treat the disease itself, it is called *palliative treatment* or palliation.

Chemotherapy Given with Other Treatments

Sometime, chemotherapy may be given along with other treatments. It may be used as *adjuvant therapy* or *neoadjuvant therapy*.

Adjuvant chemotherapy: After surgery to remove the cancer, there may still be some cancer cells left behind that cannot be seen. When drugs are used to kill those unseen cancer cells, it is called adjuvant chemotherapy. Adjuvant treatment can also be given after radiation

Neoadjuvant chemotherapy: Chemotherapy can be given before the main cancer treatment (such as surgery or radiation). Giving chemotherapy first can shrink a large cancerous tumor, making it easier to remove with surgery. Shrinking the tumor may also allow it to be treated more easily with radiation. Neoadjuvant chemotherapy also can kill small deposits of cancer cells that cannot be seen on scans or X-rays.

Different Types of Chemotherapy Drugs

Chemotherapy drugs can be divided into several groups based on their mode of action and chemical structure. Because some drugs act in more than one way, they may belong to more than one group.

Alkylating Agents

Alkylating agents directly damage DNA to prevent the cancer cell from reproducing. As a class of drugs, these agents are not phase-specific; in other words, they work in all phases of the cell cycle. Alkylating agents are used to treat many different cancers, including leukemia, lymphoma, Hodgkin disease, multiple myeloma, and sarcoma, as well as cancers of the lung, breast, and ovary.

Because these drugs damage DNA, they can cause long-term damage to the bone marrow. The risk of leukemia from alkylating agents is "dose-dependent," meaning that the risk is small with lower doses, but goes up as the total amount of the drug used gets higher. The risk of leukemia after getting alkylating agents is highest about 5 to 10 years after treatment.

There are different classes of alkylating agents, including:
- *Nitrogen mustards:* Such as mechlorethamine (nitrogen mustard), chlorambucil, cyclophospha-mide, ifosfamide, and melphalan
- *Nitrosoureas:* Which include streptozocin, carmustine, lomustine
- *Alkyl sulfonates:* Busulfan
- *Triazines:* Dacarbazine and temozolomide
- *Ethylenimines:* Thiotepa and altretamine (hexame-thylmelamine)

The **platinum** drugs (cisplatin, carboplatin, and oxalaplatin) are sometimes grouped with alkylating agents because they kill cells in a similar way. These drugs are less likely than the alkylating agents to cause leukemia later on.

Antimetabolites

Antimetabolites are a class of drugs that interfere with DNA and RNA growth by substituting for the normal building blocks of RNA and DNA. These agents damage cells during the S phase. They are commonly used to treat leukemias, cancers of the breast, ovary, and the intestinal tract, as well as other types of cancer. Examples of antimetabolites include:

- 5-fluorouracil (5-FU)
- 6-mercaptopurine (6-MP)
- Capecitabine
- Cladribine
- Clofarabine
- Cytarabine
- Floxuridine
- Fludarabine
- Gemcitabine
- Hydroxyurea
- Methotrexate
- Pemetrexed
- Pentostatin
- Thioguanine

Anthracyclines

Anthracyclines are anti-tumor antibiotics that interfere with enzymes involved in DNA replication. These drugs work in all phases of the cell cycle. They are widely used for a variety of cancers though they are mostly cardiotoxic. Examples of anthracyclines include:
- Daunorubicin
- Doxorubicin
- Epirubicin
- Idarubicin

Other Antitumor Antibiotics

Antitumor antibiotics that are not anthracyclines include:
- Actinomycin-D
- Bleomycin
- Mitomycin-C

Topoisomerase Inhibitors

These drugs interfere with enzymes called topoisomerases, which separate the strands of DNA so they can be copied. They are used to treat certain leukemias, as well as lung, ovarian, gastrointestinal, and other cancers.

Examples of topoisomerase I inhibitors include topotecan and irinotecan (CPT-11).

Examples of topoisomerase II inhibitors include etoposide (VP-16) and teniposide. Mitoxantrone also inhibits topoisomerase II.

Treatment with topoisomerase II inhibitors increases the risk of a second cancer—acute myelogenous leukemia (AML). With this type of drug, secondary leukemia can be seen as early as 2 to 3 years after the drug is given.

Mitotic Inhibitors

Mitotic inhibitors are often plant alkaloids and other compounds derived from natural products. They can stop mitosis or inhibit enzymes from making proteins needed for cell reproduction.

These drugs work during the M phase of the cell cycle but can damage cells in all phases. They are used to treat many different types of cancer including breast, lung, myelomas, lymphomas, and leukemias. These drugs are known for their potential to cause peripheral nerve damage, which can be a dose-limiting side effect. Examples of mitotic inhibitors include:

- *Taxanes:* Paclitaxel and docetaxel
- *Epothilones:* Ixabepilone
- *Vinca alkaloids:* Vinblastine, vincristine, vinorelbine
- Estramustine

Corticosteroids

Steroids are natural hormones and hormone-like drugs that are useful in treating some types of cancer (lymphoma, leukemias, and multiple myeloma). When these drugs are used to kill cancer cells or slow their growth, they are considered chemotherapy drugs.

Corticosteroids are also commonly used as *antiemetics* to help prevent nausea and vomiting caused by chemotherapy. They are used before chemotherapy to help prevent severe allergic hypersensitivity reactions. When a corticosteroid is used to prevent vomiting or allergic reactions, it is not considered chemotherapy.

Examples include prednisone, methylprednisolone (solumedrol), and dexamethasone (decadron).

Miscellaneous Chemotherapy Drugs

Some chemotherapy drugs act in slightly different ways and do not fit well into any of the other categories.

Examples include drugs like L-asparaginase, which is an enzyme, and the proteosome inhibitor bortezomib.

Enzyme Inhibitors

Some targeted therapies block (inhibit) enzymes that are signals for cancer cells to grow. These drugs are called *enzyme inhibitors*. Blocking these cell signals can keep the cancer from getting bigger and spreading. So even if the tumor is not getting smaller, its out-of-control growth has been interrupted. This may help *regular chemotherapy* drugs a better chance to work. Slowing or stopping out-of-control growth may also help people live longer, even without adding other drugs.

Enzyme inhibitors may be called different names based on the enzymes they block:

- Tyrosine kinase inhibitors
- mTOR inhibitors
- Proteosome inhibitors
- Growth factor inhibitors
- Signal-transduction inhibitors
- Multi-targeted kinase

A multi-targeted kinase drug blocks many different enzymes. It may also be called a *multikinase inhibitor*.

Apoptosis-inducing Drugs

Some targeted therapies change proteins within the cancer cells and cause the cells to die. These are called *apoptosis-inducing drugs*. Apoptosis is the medical word for cell death. These drugs cause or induce cell death by producing cell changes that lead to apoptosis.

Angiogenesis Inhibitors

Angiogenesis is the process of making new blood vessels. In most cases, this is a normal, healthy process. But in a person with cancer, this same process creates new blood vessels that give a tumor its own blood supply. This blood brings nutrients that allow the cancer to grow and spread. Angiogenesis inhibitors target and inhibit this process. This helps cut off the tumors' blood supply, and without blood, tumors cannot grow.

Many of these drugs work by blocking *vascular endothelial growth factor* (VEGF). VEGF is a family of protein growth factors made by some tumors. The VEGF proteins can attach to the VEGF receptors of blood vessel cells. This causes new blood vessels to form around the tumors. Blocking this process prevents angiogenesis.

Other Types of Cancer Drugs

Other drugs and biological treatments are used to treat cancer but are not usually considered chemotherapy. While chemotherapy drugs take advantage of the fact that cancer cells divide rapidly, these other drugs target different properties that set cancer cells apart from normal cells. They often have less serious side effects than those commonly caused by chemotherapy drugs because they are targeted to work mainly on cancer cells, not normal, healthy cells. Many are used along with chemotherapy. Most of these drugs attack cells with mutant versions of certain genes, or cells that express too many copies of a particular gene. These drugs can be used as part of the main treatment, or they may be used after treatment to maintain remission or decrease the chance of recurrence.

Examples of targeted therapies include imatinib, gefitinib, sunitinib and bortezomib.

How does Targeted Therapy Work?

Targeted therapy is used to keep cancer from growing and spreading. The drugs target certain parts of the cell and the signals that are needed for a cancer to develop and keep growing. These drugs are often grouped by how they work or what part of the cell they target.

There are two main types of targeted therapy drugs:
- **Antibody drugs** that have been designed to attack certain targets on cancer cells.
- **Small-molecule drugs** are not antibodies which are large molecules.

Targeted Therapy Drugs

There are many different targeted therapy drugs. Here are a few examples:

Imatinib mesylate: This is one of the first targeted therapy drugs ever used to treat cancer. It is used to treat gastrointestinal stromal tumor and certain kinds of leukemia. Imatinib is a tyrosine kinase inhibitor that targets abnormal proteins, or enzymes, in cancer cells and promote uncontrolled growth. Blocking these enzymes inhibits cancer cell growth.

Gefitinib: Gefitinib is used to treat advanced non-small cell lung cancer. This drug targets the epidermal growth factor receptor (EGFR). These receptors are found on the surface of many normal cells as well as on cancer cells. When gefitinib blocks this signal, it can slow or stop cell growth.

Sunitinib: This drug is used to treat advanced *kidney cancer* and some *gastrointestinal stromal tumors.* It is considered a multi-targeted kinase inhibitor because it is a type of vascular endothelial growth factor (VEGF) receptor inhibitor, an angiogenesis inhibitor, and it blocks an enzyme called tyrosine kinase. By doing all of this it slows cancer growth and keeps tumors from making their own blood vessels to help them grow and spread.

Bortezomib: This enzyme inhibitor may be used to treat *multiple myeloma* that does not respond to other treatments. Bortezomib is a proteasome inhibitor. A proteasome is a complex of enzymes that helps destroy proteins that the cell no longer needs. Some of these proteins help to regulate cell function and growth. Bortezomib stops the proteasome from breaking down these proteins, which in turn causes the cancer cells to die.

Other drugs that may be called targeted therapies: There are other cancer treatments that can be included in the group of drugs called targeted therapies. Some examples of these are:

Monoclonal antibodies, such as:
- Alemtuzumab
- Cetuximab
- Rituximab
- Trastuzumab
- Bevacizumab

Immunomodulating drugs, such as:
- Thalidomide
- Lenalidomide

Cytokines, such as:
- Interleukins
- Interferons
- Granulocyte-macrophage colony-stimulating factor

Common Side Effects

Skin problems: Many of the targeted therapy drugs can cause a rash or other skin changes. These problems usually develop slowly over days to weeks. Allergic reactions to drugs tend to start suddenly, usually within minutes to hours after taking the drug. They may include hives (raised skin erythema that often go away within a day or so), and intense itching. Besides, other serious symptoms such as breathing problems, dizziness, tightness in the throat or chest, or swelling of the lips or tongue also can occur.

Why do targeted therapies cause skin changes? Some targeted therapy drugs target the epidermal growth factor receptor (EGFR) protein, which is also present in normal skin cells. Drugs that target or block EGFR often affect skin cells, too.

Hand-foot syndrome: Hand-foot syndrome (HFS) has been linked to many cancer treatment drugs, including some targeted therapies. It is due to damage to the tiny blood vessels in the hands and feet, or with the drugs themselves leaking out of the blood vessels and causing tissue damage.

Hormone Therapy

Drugs in this category are sex hormones, or hormone-like drugs, that change the action or production of female or male hormones. They are used to slow the growth of breast, prostate, and endometrial cancers, which normally grow in response to natural hormones in the body. Examples include:

- *The anti-estrogens:* Fulvestrant, tamoxifen, and toremifene
- *Aromatase inhibitors:* Anastrozole, exemestane, and letrozole
- *Progestins:* Megestrol acetate
- Estrogens
- *Antiandrogens:* Bicalutamide, flutamide, and nilutamide
- *Gonadotropin-releasing hormone (GnRH), GnRH agonists or analogs:* Leuprolide and goserelin.

Immunotherapy

Some drugs are given to people with cancer to stimulate their natural immune systems to recognize and attack cancer cells. These drugs are often considered to be separate from chemotherapy.

There are different types of immunotherapy. *Active immunotherapies* stimulate the body's own immune system to fight the disease. *Passive immunotherapies* do not rely on the body to attack the disease; instead, they use immune system components (such as antibodies) created outside the body. Types of immunotherapies include:

- Monoclonal antibody therapy (passive immunotherapies), such as rituximab and alemtuzumab .
- Non-specific immunotherapies and adjuvants that boost the immune response such as BCG, interleukin-2 (IL-2), and interferon-alfa.
- Immunomodulating drugs, for instance, thalidomide and lenalidomide.
- Cancer vaccines (active specific immunotherapies). In 2010, the FDA approved the first vaccine to treat cancer (the Provenge vaccine for advanced prostate cancer);

Types of Monoclonal Antibodies

Two types of monoclonal antibodies are used in cancer treatments:

- *Naked mAbs* are antibodies that work by themselves. There is no drug or radioactive material attached to them. They work mainly by attaching to and blocking specific antigens that are important signals for cancer cells. For example, trastuzumab is an antibody against the HER2/neu protein. A large amount of this portein is present on the cells in some types of cancer. When HER2/neu is activated, it helps these cells grow. Trastuzumab stops these proteins from becoming active. It is used to treat breast and stomach cancers that have large amounts of this protein.
- *Conjugated mAbs* are those joined to a chemotherapy drug, radioactive particle, or a toxin. These mAbs work, at least in part, by acting as homing devices to take these substances directly to the cancer cells. They can be divided into groups depending on what they are linked to.
- mAbs with radioactive particles attached are referred to as *radiolabeled*, and treatment with this type of antibody is known as *radioimmunotherapy* (RIT).
- mAbs with chemotherapy drugs attached are referred to as *chemolabeled*.
- mAbs attached to cell toxins are called *immunotoxins*.

Planning Drug Doses and Schedules

Most chemotherapy drugs are strong medicines that have a fairly narrow range of safe and effective doses. Taking too little of a drug will not effectively treat the cancer and taking too much may cause life-threatening side effects. For this reason, dose calculation of chemotherapy drugs is done very precisely.

Doses

Depending on the drug(s) to be given, there are different ways to determine chemotherapy doses. Most chemotherapy drugs are measured in milligrams (mg). The overall dose may be based on a person's body weight in kilograms or body surface area (BSA) expressed in meters squared (m^2).

Dosages for children and adults differ, even after BSA is taken into account. This is because children's bodies process drugs differently. They may have different levels of sensitivity to the drugs, too. For the same reasons, dosages of some drugs may also be adjusted for people who:

- Are elderly?
- Have poor nutritional status?
- Are obese?
- Have already taken or are currently taking other medicines?
- Have already had or are currently receiving radiation therapy?
- Have low blood cell counts?
- Have liver or kidney diseases?

Schedule (Cycles)

Chemotherapy is generally given at regular intervals called *cycles*. A chemotherapy cycle may involve a dose of one or more drugs followed by several days or weeks without treatment. This gives normal cells time to recover from the drug's side effects.

How is Chemotherapy Given?

Systemic Chemotherapy

Drugs used for systemic (total body) chemotherapy can be given in these ways:

- Oral (PO) — taken by mouth
- Intravenous (IV) — infused through a vein
- Intramuscular (IM) — injected into a muscle
- Subcutaneous (SQ) — injected under the skin

Central venous catheters (CVCs) or vascular access devices (VADs) may be needed: Central venous catheters are also known as *vascular access devices*. They are used for these reasons:

- To give several drugs at one time
- For long-term therapy
- For continuous infusion chemotherapy
- To give drugs that can cause serious damage to skin and muscle tissue, if they leak outside of a vein (these drugs are known as *vesicants*). Delivering these through a CVC provides more reliable access to a vein than a short-term IV.

Regional Chemotherapy

Regional chemotherapy directs the anticancer drugs into the part of the body where the cancer is. The purpose is to get more of the drug to the cancer, while trying to minimize side effects on the whole body. Side effects will often still happen because the drugs can be partly absorbed into the bloodstream and travel throughout the body. Examples of regional chemotherapy include drugs given into these parts of the body:

- Intra-arterial—injected into an artery that goes to a certain area of the body
- Intravesical—infused into the bladder
- Intrapleural—infused into the chest cavity between the lung and chest wall
- Intraperitoneal—infused into the abdomen around the intestines and other organs
- Intrathecal—infused into the central nervous system via spinal fluid
- Intralesional/intratumoral—injected directly into the tumor
- Topical—applied to the skin as a cream or lotion

Chemotherapy Side Effects

Although chemotherapy is given to kill cancer cells, it also damages normal cells. The normal cells most likely to be damaged are those that divide rapidly, for instance:

- Bone marrow/blood cells
- Cells of hair follicles
- Cells lining the digestive tract
- Cells lining the reproductive tract

What is new in chemotherapy research?

- New classes of chemotherapy medicines and combinations of medicines are being developed.
- Some newer medicines, called *targeted therapies,* are designed to attack a particular target on cancer cells.
- Other approaches to targeting drugs more specifically at the cancer cells—such as attaching drugs to *monoclonal antibodies*—may make them work

better and cause fewer side effects. Monoclonal antibodies, which are special types of proteins made in the lab, can be designed to guide chemotherapy drugs directly to the cancer cells.

- Monoclonal antibodies (without attached chemotherapy) can also be used as immunotherapy drugs, to strengthen the body's immune response against cancer cells.
- *Liposomal therapy* uses chemotherapy drugs that have been packaged inside liposomes (synthetic fat globules). The liposome helps the drug penetrate the cancer cells more selectively and decreases possible side effects (such as hair loss and nausea and vomiting). Examples of liposomal medicines already being used are the encapsulated form of doxorubicin and daunorubicin.
- Chemoprotective agents are being developed to protect against specific side effects of certain chemotherapy drugs. For example, dexrazoxane helps prevent heart damage, amifostine helps protect the kidneys, and mesna protects the bladder.
- Some new agents may be given along with chemotherapy to help overcome drug resistance. Cancer cells often become resistant to chemotherapy by developing the ability to pump the drugs out of the cells. These new agents inactivate the pumps, which allows the chemotherapy to remain in the cancer cells longer, which might make it more effective.

Chemotherapy for Ovarian Cancer

Chemotherapy for Epithelial Ovarian Cancer

Chemotherapy for ovarian cancer most often is a combination of 2 or more drugs, given IV every 3 to 4 weeks.

The standard approach is the combination of a platinum compound, such as cisplatin or carboplatin, and a taxane, such as paclitaxel or docetaxel used for 3 to 6 cycles.

Epithelial ovarian cancer often shrinks or regresses after 3–6 cycles of combination chemotherapy. Some of the chemo drugs that are helpful in treating ovarian cancer include (in alphabetical order):

- Albumin bound paclitaxel
- Altretamine
- Capecitabine
- Cyclophosphamide
- Etoposide (VP-16)
- Gemcitabine
- Ifosfamide
- Irinotecan liposomal doxorubicin

- Melphalan
- Pemetrexed
- Topotecan
- Vinorelbine

Common temporary side effects include:

- Nausea and vomiting
- Loss of appetite
- Loss of hair
- Hand and foot rashes
- Mouth sores
- Increased chance of infection due to leucopenia.
- Bleeding or bruising after minor cuts or injuries due to thrombocytopenia
- Fatigue due to low RBC

Most side effects disappear once treatment is stopped. Hair will grow back after treatment ends, although it may look different. Some drugs may have long-term or even permanent side effects. For example, cisplatin can cause kidney damage. Both cisplatin and the taxanes can cause nerve damage (*neuropathy*). This can lead to problems with numbness, tingling, or even pain in the hands and feet. Cisplatin can also damage the nerves to the ear, which can lead to hearing loss (od*ototoxicity*). Rarely, some drugs can permanently damage bone marrow. This can later cause a bone marrow problem like myelodysplastic syndrome or even acute myeloid leukemia. This is called a *secondary malignancy.*

Intraperitoneal Chemotherapy

In intraperitoneal (IP) chemotherapy for ovarian cancer, in addition to giving the drugs systemic route cisplatin and paclitaxel are injected into the abdominal cavity through a catheter . The tube can be placed during the staging/debulking surgery, but sometimes it is placed later by laparoscopy or by an interventional radiologist. This drug also gets absorbed into the bloodstream and can reach cancer cells outside the abdominal cavity. IP chemotherapy works well, but the side effects are often more severe than with regular chemotherapy like abdominal pain, nausea, vomiting.

Germ Cell Tumors

Patients with germ cell cancer often need to be treated with combination chemotherapy. The combination used most often is called PEB and includes the chemotherapy drugs cisplatin, etoposide, and *bleomycin*. Dysgerminomas are usually very sensitive to chemotherapy, and can sometimes be treated with the less toxic combination of carboplatin and etoposide.

These include:

- *TIP:* Paclitaxel, ifosfamide, and cisplatin
- *VeIP*: Vinblastine, ifosfamide, and cisplatin
- *VIP:* Etoposide (VP-16), ifosfamide, and cisplatin

The side effects of these drugs include nausea/vomiting, hair loss, and low blood counts. Neuropathy, infertility, and premature menopause can also occur. Rarely, bleomycin can lead to lung damage, ifosfamide can cause hemorrhagic cystitis. This can usually be prevented by giving the drug mesna with ifosfamide.

Stromal Tumors

Ovarian stromal tumors are not often treated with chemotherapy, but when they are, the combination of carboplatin plus paclitaxel or PEB is most often used.

Chemotherapy for Endometrial Cancer

Chemotherapy in endometrial cancer is usually adjunctive therapy following staging laparotomy. Drugs used in treating endometrial cancer may include:

- Paclitaxel
- Carboplatin
- Doxorubicin (adriamycin) or liposomal doxorubicin
- Cisplatin

Most often, two or more drugs are combined for treatment. The most common combinations include carboplatin with paclitaxel and cisplatin with doxorubicin.

For carcinosarcoma, the drug ifosfamide, either alone or in combination with either carboplatin, cisplatin or paclitaxel, is often used. However, the combination of carboplatin and paclitaxel is also often being used for carcinosarcoma.

Sometimes chemotherapy is given for a few cycles, followed by radiation. Again chemotherapy is given. This is called *sandwich therapy* and is sometimes used for endometrial papillary serous cancer and uterine carcinosarcoma.

Chemotherapy for Cervical Cancer

The mainstay of treatment is radiotherapy and surgery in cancer cervix.

As a part of the main treatment: For some stages of cervical cancer, chemotherapy is given to help the radiation work better. When chemotherapy and radiation therapy are given together, it is called *concurrent chemoradiation*. One option is to give a dose of the drug cisplatin every week during radiation. This drug is given into a vein (IV) about 4 hours before the radiation appointment. Another choice is to give cisplatin along with 5-fluorouracil (5-FU) every 4 weeks during radiation.

To treat cervical cancer recurrence as palliative measure: Drugs most often used to treat cervical cancer include:

- Cisplatin
- Carboplatin
- Paclitaxel
- Topotecan
- Gemcitabine

Some other drugs can be used as well, such as docetaxel, ifosfamide, 5-fluorouracil (5-FU), irinotecan, and mitomycin.

Chemotherapy for Gestational Trophoblastic Disease

Gestational trophoblastic disease (GTD) is one of the few cancers that can almost always be cured by chemotherapy drug no matter how advanced it is. The best indicator of which drug to use is the prognostic score. The drugs that can be used to treat GTD include:

- Methotrexate (with or without leucovorin)
- Chlorambucil
- Cisplatin
- Fluorouracil

Actinomycin-D

Vincristine
Ifosfamide
Paclitaxel

Cyclophospha mide

Etoposide
Bleomycin

Single Drug Treatment

Methotrexate: Chemotherapy with methotrexate alone can be used in most women with low-risk disease. The methotrexate can be given as IV or IM every day for 5 days. This can be repeated again after a rest period based on the hCG level. Another way to give methotrexate is to give a larger dose once a week.

Another option is to give methotrexate along with folinic acid (*leucovorin*). Leucovorin is not a chemo drug, but instead is a type of vitamin related to folic acid that reduces the toxic effects of methotrexate. In this course of treatment, methotrexate is given on days 1, 3, 5, and 7, and leucovorin is given on days 2, 4, 6, and 8. Each cycle has 8 days of drug treatment, followed usually by a 7 day rest period and then the cycle is repeated. In all cases, methotrexate is given in cycles that are repeated until blood levels of hCG remain normal for a few weeks. Vitamins such as folic acid can make methotrexate less effective and so should not be taken with this drug.

Actinomycin-D: Another option is to give actinomycin-D instead of methotrexate. This drug may be especially

useful in patients with liver problems, because it is less toxic to the liver than is methotrexate. Actinomycin-D is given IV every day for 5 days, followed by several days without treatment. It is also given as a larger single dose once every 2 weeks. The cycles are repeated until hCG levels have stayed in the normal range for several weeks.

Etoposide: It is given IV, every day for 3 to 5 days, followed by several days of treatment. This is used much less often by itself than either actinomycin or methotrexate.

Combinations of Drugs

Women with higher-risk disease will receive combinations of drugs such as methotrexate, actinomycin-D, and cyclophosphamide. Other drugs such as etoposide, vincristine and cisplatin may also be used.

Some of the more commonly used combinations include:

- MAC: Methotrexate/leucovorin, actinomycin-D, and cyclophosphamide or chlorambucil
- EMA-CO: Etoposide, methotrexate/leucovorin, and actinomycin-D, followed a week later by cyclophosphamide and vincristine)
- EMA-EP: Etoposide, methotrexate/leucovorin, and actinomycin-D, followed a week later by etoposide and cisplatin
- VBP: Vinblastine, bleomycin, and cisplatin
- BEP: Bleomycin, etoposide, cisplatin
- Common side effects of methotrexate are diarrhea and sores in the mouth. This drug can also cause mild liver dysfunction, conjunctivitis, pain in the chest or abdomen or skin rash. Hair loss and blood side effects do not usually occur with single-drug methotrexate therapy.
- Actinomycin-D can cause severe nausea, vomiting and hair loss.
- Bleomycin can cause pulmonary fibrosis
- Cyclophosphamide and ifosfamide can cause nausea and hair loss. They can also cause bladder irritation and rarely cause severe lung problems.
- In rare cases, etoposide treatment has been linked with the development of leukemia several years later. Cisplatin has also been linked to this, although it occurs less often than with etoposide.
- Vincristine and cisplatin can damage nerves (called *neuropathy*).

Chemotherapy for Vulvar Cancer

Drugs most often used in treating vulvar cancer include cisplatin with or without fluorouracil (5-FU). Mitomycin-C may rarely be used.

The role of chemotherapy in treating vulvar cancer remains to be determined. In more advanced disease, it might be given with radiation therapy before surgery. This combined treatment may shrink the tumor, making it easier to remove it with surgery.

Chemotherapy for Vaginal Cancer

Systemic chemotherapeutic drugs has not been shown to work well in treating vaginal cancer. It may be helpful as a way to shrink tumors before surgery. The treatment is similar to that used for cervical cancer. Drugs that have been used include cisplatin, fluorouracil (5-FU), paclitaxel, and docetaxel.

Chemotherapy for Cancer of Fallopian Tube

The National Comprehensive Cancer Network (NCCN) guidelines suggest administering 3–6 cycles of chemotherapy for stage IA–IC disease and 6–8 cycles for stage II–IV disease. As in ovarian cancer, the use of intraperitoneal (IP) chemotherapy must be considered the current standard treatment option in patients with stage II–IV disease.

In the treatment recommendations, carboplatin is dosed to achieve a targeted area under the curve (AUC), which is defined as the area under the concentration-versus-time curve and expressed in mg/mL/min.

Treatment Recommendations for Stage I Disease

Treatment recommendations for stage I fallopian tube cancer include the following:

- Paclitaxel 135–175 mg/m^2 IV infused over 3 hr plus carboplatin AUC 5–7.5 IV infused over 30–60 min every 21 days for 3–6 cycles or
- Docetaxel 60–75 mg/m^2 IV infused over 1 hr plus carboplatin AUC 5–6 IV infused over 1 hr every 21 days for 3–6 cycles.

Treatment Recommendations for Stages II–III Disease

Patients who have undergone optimal tumor debulking should be offered IP chemotherapy. The following dosing regimen is recommended:

- Paclitaxel 135 mg/m^2 IV infused over 24 hr on day 1 (may be given over 3 hr if tolerated) plus cisplatin 100 mg/m^2 IP on day 2 (may be reduced to 75 mg/m^2 and given on day 1 or day 2 to allow an outpatient regimen) plus paclitaxel 60 mg/m^2 IP on day 8 every 21 days for 6 cycles.

Treatment Recommendations for Stage IV Disease

If the patient is unable to tolerate IP chemotherapy, debulking has been suboptimal (i.e. disease >1 cm), disease has spread to the liver parenchyma, or the patient has malignant plural effusions, one of the following IV regimens should be considered:

- Paclitaxel 135–175 mg/m^2 IV infused over 3 hr plus carboplatin AUC 5–7.5 IV infused over 30–60 min every 21 days for 6 cycles, or
- Docetaxel 60–75 mg/m^2 infused over 1 hr plus carboplatin AUC 5–6 IV infused over 1 hr every 21 days for 3–6 cycles.

26D. STEM CELL THERAPY

Introduction

Reproductive tissues are now recognised as sources of stem/progenitor cells and as targets for regenerative medicine. Stem cells sourced from reproductive tissues have been used or investigated for their potential use in other areas such as hematological disease, traditionally treated with hematopoietic stem cells (HSC) from adult sources but for which toxic adjuvant treatments, or bone tissue engineering, are concurrently needed. Briefly, stem cells have two properties. The first is the ability to self-renew or undertake numerous cell divisions, while maintaining an undifferentiated state. The second is that of multipotency; the capacity to differentiate into a mature cell type. **Totipotent stem cells**, from the morula, can differentiate into embryonic and extraembryonic cell types, and can produce a complete and viable organism. **Pluripotent stem cells** descend from totipotent cells and differentiate into tissues derived from any of the three germ layers, including fetal tissues (amniotic fluid cells, the amnion, umbilical cord and placenta). **Embryonic stem cells** are pluripotent, having been derived from the inner cell mass of a blastocyst. **Multipotent stem cells** differentiate into various tissues originating from a single germ layer, for example, mesenchymal or hemopoietic stem cells. **Unipotent cells** such as muscle satellite cells on the other hand, produce only their own cell type but show greater self-renewal than fully mature cells. Theoretically, the more primitive or "potent" a stem cell is, the more predisposed it is to uncontrolled cell division, and the greater its potential for oncogenesis. Although there is some concern regarding the oncogenic potential of pluripotent stem cells such as embryonic stem cells and induced pluripotent stem cells, nonpluripotent cell sources are not inherently oncogenic.

Embryonic stem (ES) cells offer the prospect of novel treatments in regenerative medicine although progress has been impeded by controversies surrounding the source. However, multipotent cells are now being isolated from several fetal tissues, readily obtained as products of diagnostic tests, at disruption of pregnancy and at birth. In the field of gynecology, regenerative medicine approaches to repair or replace damaged or diseased urogenital tract organs, such as the urinary sphincter, pelvic floor, uterus, ovaries and vagina, are currently in the preclinical and clinical phases of study. In obstetrics, the area of stem cell transplantation has been largely focused on fetal therapy.

Stem Cells from Reproductive Tissues

Over the past decade, stem cells have been isolated from embryonic, fetal and extra-fetal tissues, as well as adult gonads. Extra-fetal tissues such as the amniotic membranes and placenta share a common origin; the inner cell mass of the blastocyst, which gives rise to the embryo, yolk sac, mesenchymal core of the chorionic villi, chorion and amnion. Because of their shared origin, amniotic fluid and the placenta contain a heterogeneous population of progenitor cells. This includes mesenchymal, hematopoietic, trophoblastic and, perhaps, more primitive stem cells. Although the chemical and cellular composition of the amniotic fluid varies with gestational age and fetal health status, mesenchymal stem cells (MSC) can be consistently isolated at any gestation. Placental and amniotic fluid MSC have been shown to differentiate into most cell types of mesodermal lineage, as well as into a few cells of ectodermal and endodermal lineages.

Fetal stem cells have been isolated from various parts of the fetus. Early gestation HSC from the bone marrow and liver are well characterized, with placental HSC being described more recently.

Primitive human fetal MSC (hfMSC) have been isolated from virtually every part of the developing fetus, have higher proliferative capacity, express significant higher amounts of telomerase. They differentiate efficiently into neuronal and muscle lineages and have shown more robust differentiation down the osteogenic lineage than the later perinatal and adult sources of MSC, suggesting their utility for postnatal applications for bone tissue engineering.

Sample Collection and Stem Cell Banking

The use of fetal and perinatal stem cells in regenerative medicine should be regulated through appropriate institutional and regulatory boards. Protocols for optimal collection of such tissues should maximize the quantity and quality of stem cells derived prior to their banking within **good manufacturing practice (GMP)** facilities. The banking of umbilical cord blood (UCB) is an established process in many centers worldwide. It is a source of HSC12 and MSC13 and has established utility for allogeneic postnatal treatment of hematological diseases such as leukemia and bone marrow failure. Although there is a trend towards nondirected autologous banking of umbilical cord blood (UCB) in low-risk families promulgated largely by private cord blood banks, this practice has not been supported by several academic institutions. However, there may be an advantage to private banking for directed use in a family with a sibling affected by a medical condition that can potentially benefit from UCB.

Harvesting of stem cells from fetal tissue following medically indicated pregnancy termination should be guided by the specific cell targeted, if the harvested cells are intended for a particular application. hfMSC have been collected from the liver for intrauterine transplantation targeting osteogenesis imperfecta and for the treatment of hemoglobinopathies, both of which should be processed in GMP conditions. However, as a source for donor cells, the majority of the parts of a fetus can be harvested; from the central nervous system for neural stem cells, to the skin for epidermal progenitors.

Approaches for Regeneration of Urogenital Tract

Several studies have focused on the use of regenerative medicine to correct insufficiencies in the urogenital tract.

Stem/Progenitor Cell Treatment of Stress Urinary Incontinence (SUI)

Biomaterials aim to resolve SUI by providing structural/mechanical bladder neck support. This is executed via the injection of autologous stem or urethral tract progenitor cells, which has been culture-expanded before retransplantation, into the urethral sphincter. This aims to restore and regenerate rhabdomyo-sphincter muscle content and function. Continuing clinical and animal studies suggest that injected autologous cells may integrate into the sphincteric complex and differentiate, leading to "sphincter regeneration". However, it is unclear as to the precise fate of injected cells, such as the extent to which injected cells integrate and adopt a functional myogenic phenotype, or perform a growth factor secreting function to stimulate regeneration. Nevertheless, the concept of stem cell injection for sphincteric muscle regeneration is the subject of research in a number of centres and the development of improved forms of treatment for SUI might yet prove to be one of the major clinical benefits of regenerative medicine.

Bladder Reconstruction

A tissue-engineered and urothelial-lined bladder provides a functional barrier against urine exposure and could help to overcome most of the serious complications associated with conventional entero-cystoplasty. The requirements of such "engineered" tissue are more complex than just structural support and need to fulfil the functions of the normal healthy bladder wall by combining compliance (normally conferred by the detrusor smooth muscle) with a urinary barrier (normally provided by the specialized urothelial lining).

Three fundamentally different strategies have been investigated to augment or reconstruct the urinary bladder:

- *Use of acellular natural or synthetic biomaterials:* With this approach, an acellular biomaterial graft is used as a tissue implant which becomes incorporated through the ingrowth of cells from the surrounding native host bladder. As biomaterials can be produced, stored and used as "off-the-shelf" materials, this approach circumvents technically demanding and expensive cell-based and patient-specific procedures. The best studied of these biomaterials are small intestinal submucosa and bladder-derived acellular matrix. Success varies with these materials and seems to be dependent on the graft size and biomaterial processing.

- *Implantation of scaffolds preincubated with autologous cells in vitro:* Tissue is engineered by seeding cultured cells (usually autologous urothelial and smooth muscle cells) onto a biodegradable scaffold in vitro prior to implantation. Autologous urothelial cells from bladder biopsies are cultured in vitro for 7–8 weeks prior to seeding on collagen or collagen coated polyglycolic acid (PGA) scaffolds. Functional urodynamic data reveal best outcomes in patients receiving cell-seeded collagen coated PGA scaffolds wrapped in omentum as a vascular bed at the time of reconstruction.

- *Combining tissue-engineered urothelium with a host of vascularized smooth muscle segment ("composite cystoplasty"):* Composite cystoplasty describes an approach to combine autologous urothelial cell sheets grown and expanded in vitro with a de-epithelialized pedicled smooth muscle segment from the host. There are advantages of this strategy over a completely tissue-engineered organ. The first is that the in vitro component of the procedure is confined to the propagation of urothelium and the second is that a single, highly regenerative cell type is combined with a preformed, vascularised smooth muscle tissue. The rationale stems from long term complications of conventional enterocystoplasty which arise almost entirely from the unsuitable properties of the intestinal epithelium rather than the smooth muscle component of the bowel wall.

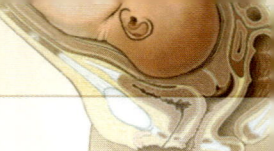

Biomaterials for Pelvic Floor Prolapse (POP) and Urinary Incontinence (UI)

There are two distinct requirements of bioengineered materials in this area. The first requirement is to provide mechanical support to the pelvic organs. The second is to generate new muscle which can perform in an integrated manner with the existing organs, such as with new sphincters. The main disadvantages of synthetic meshes for POP and pelvic floor related UI are the complications of erosion and extrusion. Biomaterial developed to replace meshes need to contain the strength of meshes and also be bioabsorbable. Hybrid biomaterials may be fabricated using a combination of synthetic and naturally derived polymers and can possess many desired characteristics of replacement tissues, including good biocompatibility and appropriate biomechanical and biochemical properties. Fiber diameter can be altered by changing the relative concentration of the two polymers, which in turn can be used in producing the most appropriate biomaterial for use.

Uterine Reconstruction

Factors that affect the integrity of the uterus, such as congenital/acquired malformations or disease, often compromise a woman's reproductive potential. The uterus is a source of progenitor cells that enhance the ability of self-repair. Studies have demonstrated that bone marrow stem cells can engraft and produce endometrium from the beginning. This finding suggests that cell therapy may be used to regenerate uterine tissues for women with uterine factor infertility.

Vaginal Reconstruction

The first-line treatment for vaginal agenesis is vaginal dilatation therapy. However, vaginal reconstruction is often performed as a treatment for vaginal agenesis using nonvaginal tissue substitutes, such as segments of large intestine or skin. These materials are not functionally or anatomically ideal. It has been reported that construction of a functional vagina using autologous cells expanded from a small vaginal biopsy is possible with the neovagina demonstrating wide, patent vaginal calibers without strictures and histological analysis revealing well-organized epithelial and muscle cell layers.

Opportunities for Intrauterine Stem Cell Transplantation (IUSCT) for Monogenic Diseases

Rationale for IUSCT

The objective of IUSCT is to correct a genetic disorder early in the evolution of disease through the engraftment of normal functional stem cells. There are several aims of IUSCT; replacing the missing or aberrant protein before permanent organ damage occurs, rescuing an affected fetus from a perinatally lethal condition or improving postnatal survival and preserving vital functions. The fetal milieu offers the best chance of cure for diseases that cause end organ damage in utero, because of the opportunity to correct pathology at the early stages of cellular damage. Tolerance toward the transplanted cells may be induced in the preimmune fetus before antigen recognition develops at the end of the first trimester, in order to facilitate engraftment in an immature bone marrow compartment where there is little competition from host cells. Because of the physical limitation on the quantity of donor stem cells that can be harvested and transplanted, fetal size offers a distinct advantage over the several fold larger neonate, because it allows a greater concentration of stem cells to be achieved within the target organ compared to a larger postnatal recipient. Potential target organs in early development such as the central nervous system have a greater susceptibility to transduction by vectors or engraftment by stem cells. Restrictive barriers, such as the blood–brain barrier, are also more permissive in early development which may contribute to more efficient stem cell engraftment in the fetus.

Applications of IUSCT

The most important challenge for IUSCT would be to treat diseases which can result in perinatal lethality, such as α-thalassemia and those which cause irreversible end organ damage such as some mucopolysaccharidoses (MPS). Besides because of lack of immune response it allows for the use of normal allogeneic cells to treat diseases of early postnatal onset, such as β-thalassemia and sickle cell anemia, muscular dystrophies and other lysosomal enzyme disorders. However, human experience with in utero hematopoietic stem cell transplantation (IUHSCT), performed for a spectrum of genetic diseases, reveals that successful treatment has only been achieved in a few fetuses with inherited immunodeficiencies. But IUSCT has been performed unsuccessfully in fetuses with hemoglobinopathies or enzyme deficiency disorders at a time in gestation when immune-competency has been attained. Important barriers include a normal host hemopoietic microenvironment that competitively inhibits donor stem cell proliferation in bone marrow. It is likely that the use of paternal HSC and the avoidance of breastfeeding may be required to negate these immune barriers. Successful IUSCT will potentially negate the need to find a haplo-identical allogeneic donor and avoid the myeloablative side effects associated with postnatal bone marrow transplantation.

The use of hfMSC has been explored for diseases involving a mesenchymal origin, where they undergo site-specific differentiation and contribute to the repair of the tissues after IUSCT with hfMSC in both muscular dystrophy and osteogenesis imperfecta (OI). While there was no cure in the case of muscular dystrophy, hfMSC-IUSCT may lead to normalization of bone indices, and two-thirds reduction in fracture frequencies.

Allogeneic versus Autologous Approaches

The fetus can be a recipient for autologous or allogeneic transplantation of HSC to treat monogenic disorders which have been shown to benefit from bone marrow transplantation in the postnatal patient, such as β-thalassemia major, severe combined immunodeficiency (SCID) or selected lysosomal storage disease (LSD). Allogeneic donor stem cells that are transplanted before the onset of fetal immune maturity can achieve central tolerance and avoid rejection. An ex vivo gene transfer approach via the harvest of autologous stem cells through fetal blood sampling or fetal liver biopsy in early gestation is another approach. Here, defective autologous stem cells are corrected through gene transfer technologies before reintroduction into the fetus, reducing the risk of immune rejection. Whilst this approach may appear attractive, it may also present significant technical obstacles for clinical translation. This is because it require confirmation of pregnancy, molecular diagnosis, fetal stem cell harvesting, gene correction and reintroduction into the fetus towards the end of the first/early second trimester window. Though the harvest of these fetal liver cells through a 20G needle can result in a loss of 47% fetuses, ultrasound or fetoscopy guided human fetal liver biopsies result in a far lower procedure-related pregnancy loss rate. Highly proliferative first trimester fetal HSC circulate in significant numbers, have favourable engraftment kinetics, and are thus a possible source of autologous HSC. Amniotic fluid may be a feasible and safer alternative source, if significant HSC numbers can be derived.

Tissue Engineering using Fetal Stem Cells for Specific Intrauterine Applications

Fetal stem cells, as a source of material for tissue bioengineering, have the potential for far-reaching application. These applications include the utility of fetal mesenchymal stem cells for bone therapies and the potential application of amniotic membrane and fluid-derived stem cells for diseases of the skin, liver and heart. Stem cells derived from fetal sources may have specific intrauterine application for sealing amniotic membranes following preterm rupture or amniocentesis. They may also be a valuable source for developing autologous implants to be used in reconstructive surgery for congenital heart disease, craniofacial and neural tube defects.

Conclusion

Stem cells from reproductive tissues have now been isolated and well characterized, with significant advances made in directing their differentiation, genetic manipulation and integration into scaffolds and bioreactors. The opportunity to widen such applications within reproductive medicine is becoming apparent. Progenitor cells are likely to play an important role in normal uterine and ovarian physiology and are probably involved in the response of these tissues to injury and disease. These cells may also be used as a platform for in place organ regeneration. In addition, stem cells are likely to play a role in reproductive tract pathology in some cancers, endometriosis and other diseases. Greater understanding of stem cell biology and the processes that result in uncontrolled reproductive cell proliferation may prove helpful in the treatment of these conditions and yield novel alternatives to standard treatments for urinary incontinence, infertility and structural repair. In the field of obstetrics, particularly fetal medicine, the twin advances made in prenatal molecular diagnosis and the advent of stem cell transplantation and ex vivo gene transfer may impact greatly in the treatment of a wide range of inherited genetic disorders.

Given the burden of β-globinopathies and the progress made in the preclinical field, it is likely that the haemoglobinopathies will be one of the first diseases to reach broad clinical translation. Women with a prenatal diagnosis of severe lethal genetic disease are currently faced with the choice of having an affected baby with only palliative postnatal therapy available or pregnancy termination and possibly future pre-implantation genetic diagnosis and embryo selection. The unrealised potential of IUSCT may be the only therapeutic option. Thus, IUSCT may alter the outcome from perinatal demise to survival of a severely disabled child who may still require postnatal therapy. Bystander maternal effects will also be an important consideration which may mitigate the desire to treat the fetus. Potential adverse effects may be related to the procedure by which the material is injected, including transplacental cell trafficking.

It is recommended that clinicians are aware of the various ethical issues at play when IUSCT is contemplated. A multidisciplinary approach is adopted with a transparent discussion about the known limitations, putative benefits and unknown or unquantifiable risks. Therefore, each clinical case should be considered on its individual merits until there is a greater body of evidence on the efficacy of fetal therapy from which to draft guidelines. Centers of excellence in fetal medicine and the rapeutics research should take the lead in developing the scientific expertise in this field and the clinical guidelines for future trials, in discussion with the regulatory and ethical authorities.

26E. MEDICAL ETHICS

The practice of medicine has changed in ways that highlight the relevance of ethical issues. Medical science can intervene in ways (such as genetics, stem cells) that were not previously possible; patients are better informed; litigation is more common; physicians have to be aware of the cost implications of their treatment for society; they have to juggle obligations to the hospital, the health region and the government.

Ethics deals with right and wrong conduct, with what we ought to do and what we should refrain from doing. Medical ethics concerns how to handle moral problems arising out of the care of patients; often clinical decisions must consider more than just the patient's medical condition.

"Ethical issues arise when not all values can be respected. The values in conflict must then be prioritized and the essence of 'doing ethics' is to justify breaching the values that are not respected."

The Four Traditional Pillars of Medical Ethics

Traditional approaches to medical ethics quote the four fundamental principles described below.

1. Respect for *autonomy* of the patient. Autonomy refers to the capacity to think, decide and act on one's own free initiative. Physicians and family members, therefore, should help the patient come to their own decision by providing full information; they should also uphold a competent, adult patient's decision, even if it appears medically wrong.

2. *Beneficence:* Promoting what is best for the patient. The definition of 'what is best' may derive from the health professional's judgment or the patient's wishes; these are generally in agreement, but may diverge. Beneficence implies consideration of the patient's pain; their physical and mental suffering; the risk of disability and death; and their quality of life. At times, beneficence can imply not intervening, if the benefit of therapy would be minimal.

3. *Non-maleficence:* Do no harm. In most cases of treating sick patients, this adds little to the beneficence principle. But most treatments involve some degree of risk or have side effects, so this principle reminds us to ponder the possibility of doing harm, especially when you cannot cure.

4. *Justice:* Resources are limited; one cannot cure everybody and so priorities must be set (hence the notion of triage). In allocating care, the Justice principle holds that patients in similar situations should have access to the same care, and that in allocating resources to one group we should assess the impact of this choice on others. While our primary duty is to our patient, others will be affected by our decisions and there may be a tension between beneficence, autonomy and justice.

Related Principles

Confidentiality forms a cornerstone of the doctor–patient relationship; it implies respecting the patient's privacy, encouraging them to seek care and preventing discrimination on the basis of their medical condition. In order to protect the trust between doctor and patient, the physician should not release personal medical information without the patient's consent. It can be necessary to override privacy in the interests of public health, as in contact tracing for partners of a patient with a sexually transmitted disease. Note that we are legally obligated to report a possibly HIV-infected patient to the public health authorities. However, this should always be done in a way that minimizes harm to the patient.

Discussion topic: A patient's relative gives us information on the patient but asks not to reveal where the information came from. Do we have to keep this secret?

Disclosure: For the patient to be well informed and to make informed choices (i.e. autonomy), the doctor must disclose information that is materially relevant to the patient's understanding of their condition, their treatment options and likely outcomes.

Discussion topic: A teenage patient requests an abortion but asks not to tell her parents. How do we balance protection of the patient's confidentiality against the rights of her parents?

Informed consent follows from the principle of patient autonomy, and consent is required before providing care. "No medical intervention done for any purpose—whether diagnostic, investigational, cosmetic, palliative, or therapeutic—should take place unless the patient has consented to it". Informed consent also serves as a significant protection against possible litigation.

In the shorter Oxford dictionary, *consent is defined as "the voluntary agreement to or acquiescence in what another person proposes or desires; agreement as to a course of action."*

In the medical context and as the law on consent to medical treatment has evolved, it has become a basic accepted principle that "every human being of adult years and of sound mind has the right to determine what shall be done with his or her own body." Clearly physicians may do nothing to or for a patient without valid consent. This principle is applicable not only to surgical operations but also to all forms of medical treatment and to diagnostic procedures that involve intentional interference with the person.

Disclosure of Information

For consent to treatment to be considered valid, it must be an "informed" consent. The patient must have been given an adequate explanation about the nature of the proposed investigation or treatment and its anticipated outcome as well as the significant risks involved and alternatives available. The information must be such as will allow the patient to reach an informed decision. In situations where the patient is not mentally capable, the discussion must take place with the substitute decision maker.

The obligation to obtain informed consent must always rest with the physician who is to carry out the treatment or investigative procedure. This obligation may be delegated in appropriate circumstances to junior worker but before assigning this duty to another, the treating physician should be confident the delegate has the knowledge and experience to provide adequate explanations to the patient.

Types of Consent

I. Implied consent

Much of a physician's work is done on the basis of consent which is implied either by the words or the behavior of the patient or by the circumstances under which treatment is given. For example, it is common for a patient to arrange an appointment with a physician, to keep the appointment, to volunteer a history, to answer questions relating to the history and to submit without objection to physical examination. In these circumstances, consent for the examination is clearly implied. To avoid misunderstanding, however, it may be prudent to state to the patient an intention to examine the breasts, genitals or rectum. The foregoing notwithstanding, in many situations the extent to which consent was implied may later become a matter of disagreement. Physicians should be reasonably confident the actions of the patient imply permission for the examinations, investigations and treatments proposed. When there is doubt, it is preferable the consent be expressed, either orally or in writing.

II. Expressed consent

Expressed consent may be in oral or written form. It should be obtained when the treatment is likely to be more than mildly painful, when it carries appreciable risk, or when it will result in ablation of a bodily function. Although orally expressed consent may be acceptable in many circumstances, frequently there is need for written confirmation. As physicians have often observed, patients can change their minds or may not recall what they authorized after the procedure or treatment has been carried out. Consent may be confirmed and validated adequately by means of a suitable notation by the treating physician in the patient's record.

Expressed consent in written form should be obtained for surgical operations and invasive investigative procedures. It is prudent to obtain written consent also whenever analgesic, narcotic or anesthetic agents will significantly affect the patient's level of consciousness during the treatment. For consent to serve as a defence to allegations of negligence , it must meet certain requirements. The consent must have been **voluntary**, the patient must have had the **capacity** to consent and the patient must have been **properly informed.**

Patients must always be free to consent to or refuse treatment, and be free of any suggestion of duress or coercion. Consent obtained under any suggestion of compulsion either by the actions or words of the physician or others may be no consent at all and, therefore, may be successfully repudiated. In this context, physicians must keep clearly in mind there may be circumstances when the initiative to consult a physician was not the patient's, but was rather that of a third party, a friend, an employer, or even a police officer. Under such circumstances the physician may be well aware that the patient is only very reluctantly following the course of action suggested or insisted upon by a third person. Then, physicians should be more than usually careful to assure themselves patients are in full agreement with what has been suggested, that there has been no coercion and that the will of other persons has not been imposed on the patient.

Consent obtained under any suggestion of compulsion either by the actions or words of the doctor or others may be no consent at all and therefore may be successfully repudiated.

Capacity to Consent

An individual who is able to understand the nature and anticipated effect of proposed medical treatment and alternatives, and appreciate the consequences of refusing treatment, is considered to have the necessary capacity to give valid consent. However, there are special circumstances to which particular attention must be mgiven.

Age of Consent

The legal age of majority has become progressively irrelevant in determining when a young person may consent to his or her medical treatment. As a result of consideration and recommendations by law reform groups as well as the evolution of the law on consent, the concept of maturity has replaced chronological age.

The determinant of capacity in a minor has become the extent to which the young person's physical, mental, and emotional development will allow for a full appreciation of the nature and consequences of the proposed treatment, including the refusal of such treatments. Generally, where the minor patient lacks the necessary capacity, the parents or guardian are authorized to consent to treatment on the minor's behalf. In doing so, the parents or guardian must be guided by what is in the best interests of the minor.

Mental Incapacity and Substitute Decision-making

Many individuals who may be mentally infirm or who have been committed to a psychiatric facility continue to be capable of controlling and directing their own medical care, including the right to consent to treatment or to refuse treatment; legal requirements vary with jurisdiction, so physicians should be generally familiar with the applicable mental health legislation in their jurisdiction. In circumstances where there are questions or doubts about what is in the patient's best interests or whether a proposed treatment is "therapeutic" or not, physicians are encouraged to consult with other physicians and, when warranted, legal counsel.

Patient Comprehension

Physicians have a duty to take reasonable steps so as to be relatively satisfied that the patient does understand the information being provided, particularly where there may be language difficulties or emotional issues involved.

Consent Disclosure in Research and Experimentation

The issue of consent merits careful consideration by those physicians who may become involved in any research work in which patients or human volunteers are asked to participate. In such circumstances, a standard of full disclosure may be applicable when obtaining consent. A fair explanation must always be given about what is proposed, its risks and discomforts, what, if any, benefits might accrue and, if applicable, what appropriate alternative treatments or procedures might be offered. If a blind study is involved, patients must be aware they could stand to derive no benefit at all. Researchers should emphasize to patients or subjects they are free to withdraw consent and discontinue participation in the project at any time without prejudice.

Informed Refusal

Our courts have reaffirmed repeatedly a patient's right to refuse treatment even when it is clear treatment is necessary to preserve the life or health of the patient. However, difficulty may arise, if it should later be claimed the refusal had been based on inadequate information about the potential consequences of declining what had been recommended. In the same way as valid consent to treatment must be "informed," so it may be argued a refusal must be similarly "informed." Physicians thus may be seen to have the same obligations of disclosure as when obtaining consent, that is, disclosure of the risk to be accepted. When patients decide against recommended treatment, particularly urgent or medically necessary treatment, discussions about their decision must be conducted with some sensitivity. While recognizing an individual's right to refuse, physicians must at the same time explain the consequences of the refusal without creating a perception of coercion in seeking consent. Refusal of the recommended treatment does not necessarily constitute refusal for all treatments. Reasonable alternatives should be explained and offered to the patient. As when documenting the consent discussion, notes should be made about a patient's refusal to accept recommended treatment.

A Consent Form itself is not Consent

The consent form itself is not the "consent." It is simply evidentiary, written confirmation that the explanations were given and that the patient agreed to what was proposed.

Basic Elements of a Consent Form

Consent to investigation, treatment or operative procedure
1. I,_____ , hereby consent to undergo the investigation, treatment or operative procedure, _____, ordered by or to be performed by Dr._____.

2. The nature and anticipated effect of what is proposed including the significant risks and alternatives available have been explained to me. I am satisfied with these explanations and I have understood them.

3. I also consent to such additional or alternative investigations, treatments or operative procedures as in the opinion of Dr._____ are immediately necessary.

4. I further agree that in his or her discretion, Dr._____ may make use of the assistance of other surgeons, physicians, and hospital medical staff (including trainees) and may permit them to order or perform all or part of the investigation, treatment, or operative procedure, and I agree that they shall have the same discretion in my investigation and treatment as

Dr. _____

Dated_____(Day/month/year)

Witness_____

Patient_____

26F. MANAGEMENT OF PERINEAL TEAR

Fecal incontinence is one of the most psychologically and socially debilitating conditions in an otherwise healthy individual. It can lead to social isolation, loss of self-esteem and self-confidence, and depression.

Fecal incontinence is a syndrome that involves the unintentional loss of solid or liquid stool. Many definitions of fecal incontinence exist, some of which include flatus (passing gas), while others are confined to stool. True anal incontinence is the loss of anal sphincter control leading to the unwanted or untimely release of feces or gas. This must be distinguished from other conditions that lead to stool passing through the anus. Stool seepage that produces soilage of undergarments may result from hemorrhoids, enlarged skin tags, poor hygiene, fistula-in-ano, and rectal mucosal prolapse.

Other conditions that result in poor bowel control are inflammatory bowel disease, laxative abuse, parasitic infection, and toxins. Fecal urgency also must be differentiated from fecal incontinence because urgency may be related to medical problems other than anal sphincter disruption.

Epidemiology

Frequency

The reported prevalence of fecal incontinence in the general population is approximately 2–3%. At 3–6 months after vaginal or cesarean delivery, as many as 13–25% of women report fecal incontinence.

Etiology

Fecal incontinence has many etiologies. One or a combination of several factors can lead to the inability to control passage of stool or flatus. Congenital abnormalities such as spina bifida and myelo-meningocele with resultant spinal cord damage can result in fecal incontinence. Inflammatory bowel disease may lead to decreased compliance of the rectum and may manifest as fecal urgency, frequency, soilage, or incontinence. Anal surgery, such as hemorrhoidectomy and sphincterotomy, has been associated with internal sphincter injury and subsequent urgency and incontinence.

Medical conditions that may result in fecal incontinence include diabetes mellitus, stroke, spinal cord trauma, and degenerative disorders of the nervous system. These conditions may alter normal sensation, feedback, or function of the complex mechanism of anal continence.

Vaginal delivery is widely accepted as the most common predisposing factor to fecal incontinence in an otherwise young and healthy woman. Vaginal delivery may result in internal or external anal sphincter disruption, or may cause more subtle damage to the pudendal nerve through overstretching and/or prolonged compression and ischemia (Fig. 26.9). This mechanical sphincter disruption result in fecal incontinence to the extent of 16.7% after vaginal delivery (14% with external, 1.7% internal, and 1% both). In addition, inadequate repairs of obstetric sphincter injuries may contribute to delayed symptoms of fecal incontinence.

Factors that are significantly associated with an increased risk of third-degree obstetric sphincter tears are primiparity, occiput posterior presentation, use of forceps, fetal weight greater than 4000 g, perineal tears, episiotomy, and prolonged second stage of labor.

Pudendal nerve injury may also be a mechanism in fecal incontinence. The pudendal nerve innervates the external anal sphincter muscle, anal canal skin, and coordinates reflex pathways.

Successive vaginal deliveries increase the risk of developing fecal incontinence. 13% of primiparous patients and 23% of multiparous patients undergoing

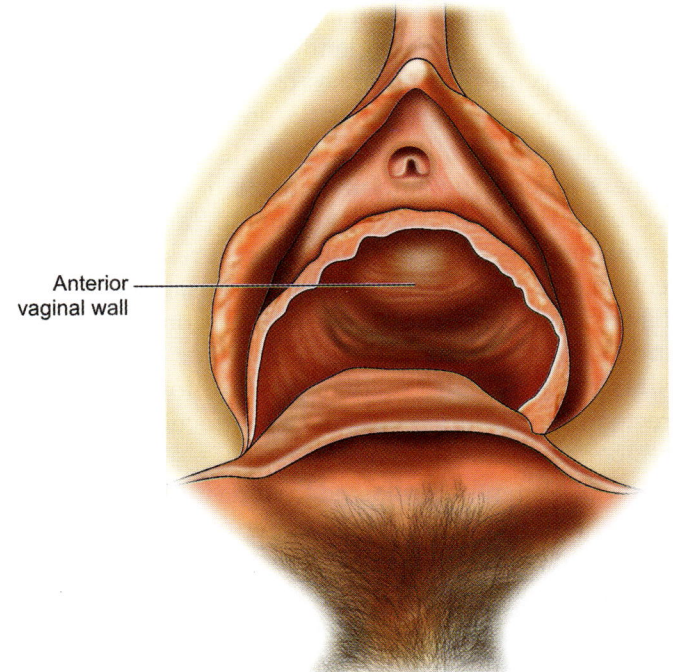

Anterior vaginal wall

Fig. 26.9: An attenuated perineal body results from trauma to the perineum and damage to the structures that normally compose the perineal body

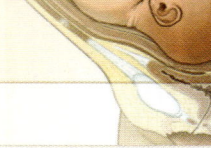

vaginal delivery often complain of fecal incontinence or fecal urgency at 6 weeks postpartum.

Pathophysiology

Bowel function is controlled by multiple factors including anal sphincter pressure, anorectal sensation, rectal compliance, colonic transit time, and stool volume and consistency. If any of these factors are compromised, incontinence can occur.

Fecal continence is maintained by the structural and functional integrity of the anorectal unit. Normal anal sphincter function is a critical part of continence. The anal sphincter is comprised of 2 components: the internal anal sphincter (IAS), which is a 0.3–0.5 cm expansion of the circular smooth muscle layer of the rectum and the external anal sphincter (EAS), a 0.6–1.0 cm expansion of the levator ani muscles. The IAS is chiefly responsible for maintaining continence at rest and contributes approximately 70–80% of the resting sphincter tone. This barrier is reinforced during voluntary squeeze by the EAS, the anal mucosal folds, and the anal endovascular cushions.

These barriers are further augmented by the puborectalis muscle, which forms a sling around the rectum and creates a forward pull to reinforce the anorectal angle. The anorectal angle, which is approximately 90° at rest, is created as the rectum perforates the levator complex. During voluntary squeeze, the angle becomes more acute, whereas during defecation, the angle becomes more obtuse. Innervation of the EAS is from the pudendal nerve, a mixed motor and sensory nerve that arises from the second, third, and fourth sacral nerves (S2, S3, and S4).

Continence requires the complex integration of signals among the smooth muscle of the colon and rectum, the puborectalis muscle, and the anal sphincters. As colonic contents are presented to the rectum, the rectum distends. The sensation of rectal distension is most likely transmitted along the S2, S3, and S4 parasympathetic nerves. This results in a parasympathetically mediated relaxation of the IAS (rectoanal inhibitory reflex) and a contraction of the EAS (rectoanal contractile reflex).

Rectal contents are allowed to come into contact with the very sensitive epithelial lining of the upper anal canal. The epithelial lining of the upper anal canal has a rich supply of sensory nerve endings, especially in the region of the anal valves. The contents are then sampled as to their nature (i.e. gas, liquid, or solid). This sampling is described as an equalization of the rectal and upper anal canal pressures. The decreased anorectal sensation and abnormal sampling likely contribute in the pathogenesis of anal incontinence as sampling facilitates the fine tuning of the continence barrier. This process is incompletely understood.

When defecation is desired, the anorectal angle straightens (which is facilitated by squatting or sitting), and abdominal pressure is increased by straining. This results in descent of the pelvic floor, contraction of the rectum, inhibition of the external anal sphincter, and subsequent evacuation of the rectal contents.

If evacuation of the rectum is not socially appropriate, sympathetically mediated inhibition of the smooth muscle of the rectum and voluntary contraction of EAS and puborectalis musculature occur. The anorectal angle becomes more acute and prevents the bolus of stool from descending further. The contents of the rectum are forced back into the compliant rectal reservoir above the levators, which allows the IAS to recover and contract again. A decrease in the compliance of this rectal reservoir has been associated with fecal urgency and anal incontinence. The exact mechanism of this is unclear.

In essence, any process that interferes with these mechanisms, including trauma from vaginal delivery or a neurological insult, can result in fecal incontinence.

Presentation

The history should include a thorough account of the type and duration of fecal incontinence, frequency of incontinent episodes, type of stool lost, impact of the disorder on the patient's life, history of associated trauma or surgery, and associated factors such as protective undergarment use. True incontinence must be differentiated from pseudoincontinence, and patients may perceive drainage of mucous, pus, or blood from the perianal region as incontinence. Medications and dietary habits should be reviewed to determine if an easily remedied cause exists.

An obstetric history should be taken carefully. Information about the number of vaginal deliveries and the presence of any risk factors for fecal incontinence pertaining to those deliveries should be obtained. As previously mentioned, prolonged second stage of labor, forceps delivery, significant tears, and episiotomy, among other causes, are associated with increased risk for anal sphincter disruption and pudendal nerve injury.

Once a complete history has been obtained, a focused physical examination should be performed. The examination should consist of a careful visual inspection of the perineal body and anus. The vagina should be inspected with the aid of a speculum. Examination of the anal region may reveal skin tags, hemorrhoids, anal fissures, scars, or chemical dermatitis. Rectal prolapse or fistulae may also be present.

After obstetric injuries, a discrete sphincter defect will almost always be anterior in location and be associated with loss of the perineal body or attenuation of the rectovaginal septum. Sometimes, however, the connective tissue of the perineal body is intact and only the sphincter has failed to heal. With an intact anal sphincter, the creases in the anal skin are arranged radially around the anal canal. When the sphincter is disrupted and the perineal skin is intact, there is a classic dovetail appearance to the anus, in which the radial distribution of the anal skin creases is absent anteriorly.

After inspection, sensation of the perianal region should be assessed. This is performed by gently stroking the skin surrounding the anus and observing a reflex contraction of the external anal sphincter. The absence of this anocutaneous reflex suggests interruption of the spinal arc.

Digital examination should be performed to detect obvious anal pathology and provide an initial assessment of the anal resting tone. At the beginning the rectal examination, resistance is met at the anal verge. If the examining finger meets little resistance and the anus feels patulous, significant sphincter dysfunction may be present. Deformity may be due to fistulotomy, fissurectomy, or hemorrhoidectomy.

A bimanual digital rectal examination is performed using 1 digit in the rectum and 1 digit in the vagina. This examination is mandatory to palpate the anal sphincters, determine perineal body thickness, evaluate anal sphincter and levator tone, and test for perineal body hypermobility. The external anal sphincter is palpable as a 1.5–2 cm, moderately firm, doughnut-shaped mass within the perineal body. If, upon palpation of the perineal body, the examining fingers are not separated by much tissue or the muscle mass is not palpated, damage to the anal sphincter is likely. Palpation from a midline position to lateral helps to define where normal muscle exists.

The patient is asked to tighten the sphincter around the examining finger. A circumferential increase in the pressure should be felt. Patients who have a disrupted anal sphincter may have adequate innervation to the existing muscle bellies, and equal pressure may be felt on the examining finger. Evaluating the nature and location of increases in muscle tone is important. Pressure may be placed on the finger laterally from existing functional muscle, but no or very little pressure may be felt anteriorly. Disruption of the muscle sphincter allows the muscle bellies to retract laterally and posteriorly, similar to the ends of a rubber band that is cut after being placed on gentle stretch. Scar tissue may develop anteriorly between the two ends of muscle and, with contraction of the lateral muscle bellies, gives the impression of an intact anal sphincter. Palpation of the muscle can assist in this situation.

During rectal examination, the tip of the examining finger is gently flexed and traction is placed on the perineal body. The perineal body is normally supported by the perineal membrane (urogenital diaphragm), which originates from the ischiopubic rami bilaterally. The perineal membrane, along with other fascial supports, inhibits the caudad displacement of the perineal body. Birth trauma sufficient enough to result in detachment or tearing of this support also may have resulted in damage to the anal sphincters.

Although the physical examination is a standard part of any evaluation for fecal incontinence, there is no exact correlation between digital assessment of sphincter tone and contractility. Physical examination results have also been noted to conflict with anal manometry.

Relevant Anatomy

A clear understanding of anatomy is mandatory for any surgical procedure, including surgical procedures of the perineum and anal sphincter. The perineal body is composed of a fusion of several structures. The Denonvilliers fascia is fused, which serves to suspend the perineal body from the sacrum via the endopelvic fascia. The bulbospongiosus and superficial transverse perineum muscles insert onto the perineal body. The bulbospongiosus originates from the pubic rami and inserts into the anterior aspect of the central tendon of the perineum. The superficial transverse perineum muscle originates on the ischial tuberosities and approaches the perineal body from a lateral position. The perineum is innervated by the labial nerve and inferior rectal nerve, which are branches of the pudendal nerve. The external anal sphincter is fused to the perineal body more posteriorly.

The anatomy of the external anal sphincter continues to be debated. Some suggest that it is composed of three parts that are fused, while others maintain that it is composed of two more distinct parts. A subcutaneous portion (just deeper than the perineal skin), a superficial portion, and a deep portion exist. Some combine the subcutaneous and superficial components into a single component. The separation of these components is indistinct in a surgical repair. The deep portion of the external anal sphincter is fused to the puborectalis muscle of the levator complex, and some even suggest that it is a continuation of it. It receives innervation from the pudendal nerve.

The internal anal sphincter is a continuation of the inner circular smooth muscle of the bowel wall. This musculature thickens over the last 2.5–4 cm of the rectum. The internal anal sphincter lies deep to the external anal sphincter, and an identifiable and surgically important plane exists between them. The internal anal sphincter begins at the level of the levator complex, and its distal extent is just proximal to the subcutaneous portion of the external sphincter. The internal anal sphincter is supplied by the autonomic nervous system. It exists in a state of continuous maximal contraction and provides a barrier to the involuntary loss of stool.

The levator complex is composed of the pubococcygeus, the iliococcygeus, and the coccygeus muscles. The most medial fibers of the pubococcygeus make up the puborectalis. These fibers loop around the posterior aspect of the rectum and create an anterior displacement of the rectum known as the anorectal angle. The pelvic surface of the levator complex is innervated by sacral efferents from S2 through S4. The inferior surface is supplied by the perineal and inferior rectal branches of the pudendal nerve. Consequently, pudendal block does not abolish voluntary contraction of the pelvic floor but completely abolishes external anal sphincter function.

Imaging Studies

Ultrasonography

The standard diagnostic imaging study for the anal sphincters is transanal or endoanal ultrasonography. Ultrasonography allows the provider to perform a real-time, 360-degree evaluation of both the internal and external anal sphincters. Sensitivity and specificity of ultrasonography findings are 98–100% for the external anal sphincter and 95.5% for the internal anal sphincter. Endoanal ultrasonography is performed in the left lateral or lithotomy position.

Traditionally, three regions of the rectum are evaluated ultrasonographically. The areas of focus are distal, where only the external anal sphincter is observed (Fig. 26.10); at the level where both the internal and external anal sphincters can be observed in the mid anal canal (Fig. 26.11); and proximal at the level of the levators (pubococcygeus) (Fig. 26.12).

Normal thickness for the external anal sphincter is 6–9 mm and mean internal anal sphincter thickness is 6.5 mm. Inflammatory disorders can increase the thickness of these sphincters.

The external anal sphincter appears as a hyperechoic ring that is circumferential. It is striated muscle, which is echogenic in nature. The internal anal sphincter is

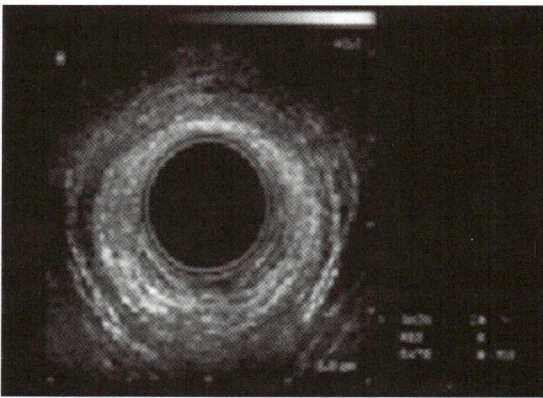

Fig. 26.10: Fecal incontinence. External anal sphincter sho wing normal narrowing anteriorly

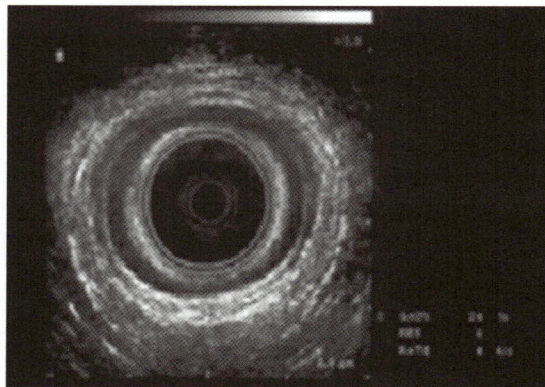

Fig. 26.11: Fecal incontinence. Ultrasound of mid-anal canal taken with the patient in the low lithotomy position showing intact internal and external anal sphincters

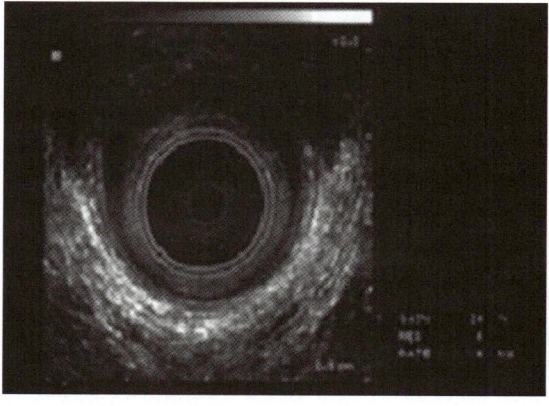

Fig. 26.12: Fecal incontinence. Internal anal sphincter at the level of the levators. The levators are demonstrated by the U-shaped echogenic band posteriorly

composed of smooth muscle and appears as a hypoechoic or sonolucent ring that is medial to the external anal sphincter. It can be viewed from the level of the levators to just inside the anal verge. The puborectalis muscle appears as a hyperechoic U-shaped muscle approximately 4 cm into the anal canal. It has been observed that ultrasonography is preferable to EMG in mapping anal sphincter defects, especially for evaluation of the internal anal sphincter.

Diagnostic Procedures

Anal Manometry

Anal manometry is used to evaluate both the resting and squeeze pressures of the rectum. It can also be used to evaluate the rectoanal inhibitory reflex, rectal capacity, and rectal compliance.

Normal values for manometry vary. Currently, no uniformly accepted standard exists for performing manometry. Normal resting pressures are 40–70 mm Hg. Normal squeeze pressures are 100–180 mm Hg .

Mean resting and mean squeeze pressures are lower in women who have had a vaginal delivery, regardless of sphincter disruption. Low manometric pressures are not predictive of anal sphincter defects. Women with known sphincter defects tend to have lower mean resting pressures; however, mean squeeze pressures may be unaffected. Squeeze pressures are not significantly related to the presence of an external anal sphincter defect.

Pudendal Nerve Terminal Motor Latency

PNTML helps evaluate the length of time required for a fixed electrical stimulus to travel along the pudendal nerve from the ischial spine to the anal verge. Findings reflect the myelin function of the peripheral nerve, and the test allows for the evaluation of pelvic floor neuromuscular integrity. The pudendal nerve is stimulated at the ischial spine transanally. The latency period between stimulation of the nerve and evoked response of the muscle is measured. Any damage to the neuromuscular unit results in the prolongation of the latency. Normal latency has been described as 2 milliseconds.

Several studies have found that persistent prolongation of PNTML occurs in incontinent women after vaginal delivery at three months postpartum. In addition, the only predictor for the development of anal incontinence at 2–4 years postpartum in women with rupture of the anal sphincter is abnormal PNTML.

Electromyelography

EMG helps evaluate the electrical activity generated by muscle fibers during voluntary muscle contraction, rest, and Valsalva-type activities. The motor unit includes the anterior horn cell, its axon with axonal branches, the motor end plates, and the muscle fibers supplied.

Abnormal findings after EMG evaluation are present in more than 90% of patients with fecal incontinence. Although EMG is able to help quantitate denervation, findings do not alter clinical management. EMG as a means to locate the sphincter defect has also lost its place in the preoperative assessment of anal sphincter defects.

Defecography

Evacuation proctography (defecography) involves imaging the rectum with contrast material to observe the rate of progress and completeness of rectal evacuation using fluoroscopic techniques. A variety of contrast materials have been used, including esophageal contrast barium and barium mixed with oatmeal or other viscous materials. Images are obtained by lateral fluoroscopy and taken during attempted defecation. Defecography helps to assess qualitatively the function of the anorectum and the adequacy of rectal emptying; static images measure the length of the anal sphincter, the anorectal angle, and perineal descent. Diagnosis of rectoceles, enteroceles, and internal or occult rectal prolapse is possible. The true benefit in evaluation of patients with fecal incontinence is unclear, because most incontinent patients cannot tolerate the procedure.

Treatment

I. Medical Therapy

The goal of medical therapy is to reduce stool frequency and improve stool consistency.

1. A regular bowel regimen including daily laxatives should be established.

2. If impacted, manual disimpaction and a daily tap-water enema may help prevent reaccumulation.

3. For patients with infrequent, low volume stools, bulking agents are helpful, as formed stools are easier to control than liquid stools.

4. In patients with diarrhea due to noninfectious etiologies or with reduced rectal compliance due to radiation proctitis or inflammatory bowel disease, agents that slow the motility of the gut may be helpful. Loperamide hydrochloride increases gut transit time, allowing for increased absorption of water from the volume of stool. This results in a firmer, more easily controlled stool. The maximum daily dosage is 16 mg. The usual dose regimen is 2–4 mg twice or three times daily to control symptoms. An additional benefit of the opiate derivative loperamide is that it increases internal anal sphincter tone and may improve rectal compliance.

5. Biofeedback is a safe, minimally invasive behavioral technique that uses auditory or visual feedback to reeducate the pelvic floor musculature.

II. *Surgical Therapy*

Usually, sphincter complex defects are secondary to obstetric injury, fistula repair, or lateral internal sphincterotomy. The standard procedure for anal incontinence due to anal sphincter disruption is the anterior overlapping sphincteroplasty.

Aim

- Correct identification and classification of 3rd and 4th degree tears.
- Performing repair under optimal circumstances without delay using correct surgical technique to obtain optimal anatomical repair.
- Reduce the risk of developing a hematoma/ infection/wound breakdown.
- Preserving long term sphincter function.

Woman sustaining 3rd or 4th degree perineal tear as defined below (Fig. 26.13):

- **First degree:** Injury to perineal skin, includes the fourchette, the hymen, labia and vaginal mucosa.

- **Second degree:** Injury to perineum involving perineal muscles but not involving the anal sphincter.
- **Third degree:** Injury to perineum involving the anal sphincter complex:
  - 3a: Less than 50% of external anal sphincter (EAS) thickness torn
  - 3b: More than 50% of EAS thickness torn
  - 3c: Both EAS and internal anal sphincter (IAS) torn
- **Fourth degree** : Injury to perineum involving the anal sphincter complex (EAS and IAS) and anal epithelium.

Can obstetric anal sphincter injury be predicted?

Clinicians need to be aware of the risk factors for obstetric anal sphincter injuries (OASIS). Clinicians should be aware, however, that risk factors do not allow the accurate prediction of OASIS.

Can obstetric anal sphincter injury be prevented?

Clinicians should explain to women that the evidence for the protective effect of episiotomy is conflicting. Mediolateral episiotomy should be considered in instrumental deliveries. Where episiotomy is indicated, the mediolateral technique is recommended, with careful attention to ensure that the angle is 60° away from the midline when the perineum is distended. Perineal protection at crowning can be protective.

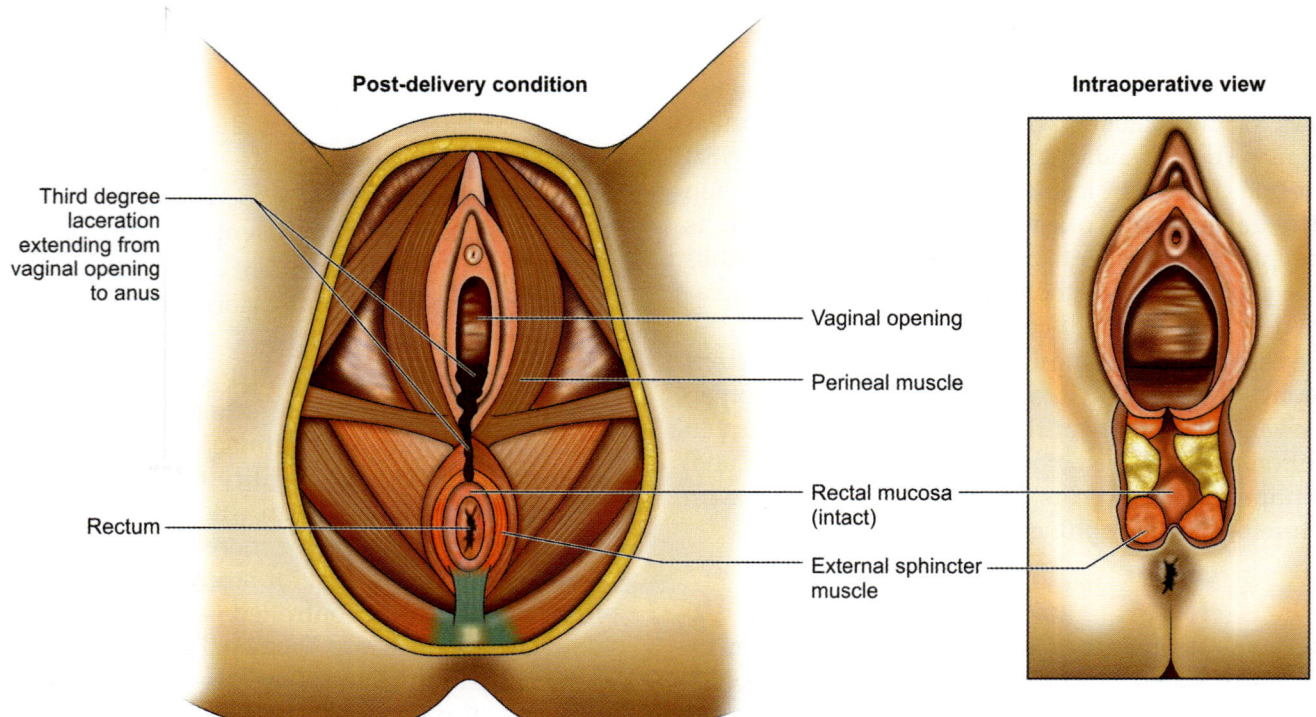

Fig. 26.13: Complete perineal tear

Physical findings of CPT:

1. Absent gynecological perineum
2. Complete blending of red anal mucosa below and pink vaginal mucosa above
3. Absent anal sphincter rugosity anteriorly (round spoke of wheel) and presence of dimple on two sides of the tear indicating retracted anal sphincters
4. Involvement of anal mucosal tear.
5. Fecal incontinence

RCOG Guidelines

Repair of Complete Perineal Tear

General Principles

- Repair of third- and fourth-degree tears should be conducted by an appropriately trained clinician.
- Repair should take place in an operating theatre, under regional or general anesthesia, with good lighting and with appropriate instruments.
- Repair of OASIS in the delivery room may be performed, if the wound is fresh. Old Complete perineal tear should be repaired after 3 months.
- Wide mobilization of the vaginal and anal mucosa is essential.
- Gasproof repair of anal mucosa in two layers continuous with delayed absorbable suture is needed.
- *Figure of eight sutures should be avoided* during the repair of OASIS because they are hemostatic in nature and may cause tissue ischemia.
- A rectal examination should be performed after the repair to ensure that sutures have not been inadvertently inserted through the anorectal mucosa. If a suture is identified, it should be removed.
- Three-step approach in complicated injury, or recurrent failed repair of CPT. Colostomy → primary repair → colostomy closure after 3 months.

Which techniques should be used to accomplish the repair of the anorectal mucosa?

The torn anorectal mucosa should be repaired with sutures using either the continuous or interrupted technique.

Which techniques should be used to accomplish the repair of the internal anal sphincter?

It is advisable to repair this separately with interrupted or mattress sutures without any attempt to overlap the IAS. The surgical approach requires dissection along the intersphincteric plane and identification of the internal anal sphincter. The sphincter is then dissected free from the rectal mucosa and mobilized. The surgical technique varies depending on the bulk of scar tissue. The scar tissue is either divided or left intact as the sphincter is plicated.

Which techniques should be used to repair the external anal sphincter?

For repair of a full thickness external anal sphincter (EAS) tear, either an overlapping or an end-to-end (approximation) method can be used with equivalent outcomes. For partial thickness (all 3a and some 3b) tears, an end-to-end technique should be used. Anterior sphincteroplasty consists of dissecting out the external anal sphincter, dividing the scar tissue in the midline, and then overlapping the scar so that muscle is approximated to muscle as closely as possible.

Which suture materials should be used to accomplish repair of anal sphincter injuries?

3-0 polyglactin should be used to repair the anorectal mucosa as it may cause less irritation and discomfort than polydioxanone (PDS) sutures. When repair of the EAS and/or IAS muscle is being performed, either monofilament sutures such as 3-0 PDS or modern braided sutures such as 2-0 polyglactin can be used with equivalent outcomes. When obstetric anal sphincter repairs are being performed, the burying of surgical knots beneath the superficial perineal muscles is recommended to minimise the risk of knot and suture migration to the skin.

How should women with anal sphincter injury be managed postoperatively?

- The use of broad-spectrum antibiotics is recommended following repair to reduce the risk of postoperative infections and wound dehiscence.
- The use of postoperative laxatives is recommended to reduce the risk of wound dehiscence. Bulking agents should not be given routinely with laxatives.
- Women should be advised that physiotherapy following repair could be beneficial.
- If a woman is experiencing incontinence or pain at follow-up, referral to a colorectal surgeon should be considered.

What advice should women be given following an anal sphincter injury concerning future pregnancies and mode of delivery?

All women who sustained anal sphincter injury in a previous pregnancy should be counseled about the mode of delivery. The role of prophylactic episiotomy in subsequent pregnancies is not known and, therefore, an episiotomy should only be performed, if clinically indicated. All women who have sustained OASIS in a previous pregnancy and who are symptomatic or have abnormal endoanal ultrasonography and/or manometry should be counseled regarding the option of elective cesarean birth.

Other approaches

- **Muscle-wrap techniques** have been developed in which striated muscles from the gracilis or gluteus muscles are transposed and wrapped around the anal canal to increase tone. These techniques create a neosphincter when there is not enough muscle present to repair. The procedure may be indicated in patients who have congenital absence of the anal sphincter or in those who have lost the anal sphincter as a result of disease and in those after several attempts at sphincter repair have failed.
- **The artificial bowel sphincter** is designed to act as a patient's own anal sphincter in cases of severe fecal incontinence.

Complications

- The most common complication is superficial separation of skin and subcutaneous tissues, and the frequency rate is as high as 25%.
- Risk of infection is 3–5%. Opening the wound to allow for drainage and treatment with antibiotics may allow the physician to salvage the surgical repair. Fistula formation occurs in fewer than 1% of cases where infection sets in.
- Bleeding and hematoma formation are also possible complications. Bleeding can usually be controlled with pressure achieved with packing. Hematoma formation into the perirectal space can go unnoticed and result in the sequestration of large amounts of blood. Treatment requires evacuation of the hematoma and surgical hemostasis.
- Other complications include anal stricture, fecal impaction, and pain. Pain may be associated with bowel movements and intercourse. Many of these problems improve with time.

Follow-up

- Postoperative evaluation should be scheduled for 4–6 weeks after the procedure. At this time, most postoperative swelling and tissue distortion is usually resolved.
- A history of the patient's bowel habits should be taken and problems addressed. If modification of the stool softener regimen is required, it can be done at this time.

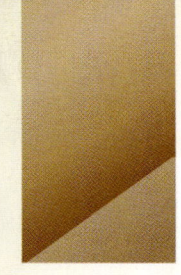
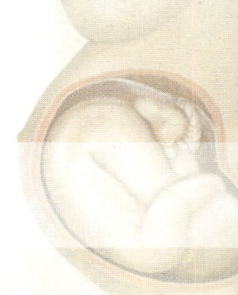

Index

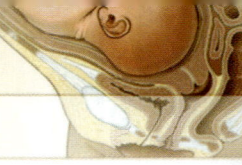

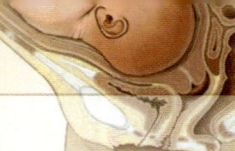